AF767298

Pathology of the Skin

Atlas of Clinical-Pathological Correlation

Pathology of the Skin

Atlas of Clinical-Pathological Correlation

Robert M. Hurwitz, MD
Clinical Associate Professor
Department of Dermatology
Indiana University School of Medicine
Indianapolis, Indiana

Antoinette F. Hood, MD
Professor
Department of Pathology and Laboratory Medicine,
Department of Dermatology
Indiana University School of Medicine
Indianapolis, Indiana

Appleton & Lange
Stamford, Connecticut

Notice: The authors and the publisher of this volume have taken care to make certain that the doses of drugs and schedules of treatment are correct and compatible with the standards generally accepted at the time of publication. Nevertheless, as new information becomes available, changes in treatment and in the use of drugs become necessary. The reader is advised to carefully consult the instruction and information material included in the package insert of each drug or therapeutic agent before administration. This advice is especially important when using, administering, or recommending new or infrequently used drugs. The authors and publisher disclaim all responsibility for any liability, loss, injury, or damage incurred as a consequence, directly or indirectly, of the use and application of any of the contents of this volume.

Copyright © 1998 by Appleton & Lange
A Simon & Schuster Company

All rights reserved. This book, or any parts thereof, may not be used or reproduced in any manner without written permission. For information, address Appleton & Lange, Four Stamford Plaza, PO Box 120041, Stamford, Connecticut 06912-0041

98 99 00 00 01 02 / 10 9 8 7 6 5 4 3 2 1

Prentice Hall International (UK) Limited, *London*
Prentice Hall of Australia Pty. Limited, *Sydney*
Prentice Hall Canada, Inc., *Toronto*
Prentice Hall Hispanoamericana, S.A., *Mexico*
Prentice Hall of India Private Limited, *New Delhi*
Prentice Hall of Japan, Inc., *Tokyo*
Simon & Schuster Asia Pte. Ltd., *Singapore*
Editora Prentice Hall do Brasil Ltda., *Rio de Janeiro*
Prentice Hall, *Upper Saddle River, New Jersey*

Library of Congress Cataloging-in-Publication Data

Hurwitz, Robert M.
Pathology of the skin : atlas of clinical-pathological correlation / Robert M. Hurwitz, Antoinette F. Hood.
p. cm.
Companion v. to: Pathology of the skin / editors, Evan R. Farmer, Antoinette F. Hood. c1990.
ISBN 0-8385-7689-3 (Case : alk. paper)
1. Skin—Diseases—Atlases. I. Hood, Antoinette F. II. Title.
[DNLM: 1. Skin Diseases—pathology—atlases. WR 17 H967p 1998]
RL81.H87 1998
616.5'0022'2—dc21
DNLM/DLC
for Library of Congress 97-37911
CIP

ISBN 0-8385-7689-3

Acquisitions Editor: Michael P. Medina
Production Editor: Sondra Greenfield
Designer: Libby Schmitz

Printed in Hong Kong

In memory of my parents

Samuel Hurwitz, MD
Matilda Hurwitz

Who inspired me to pursue the practice of medicine, impressed upon me the importance of clinical pathological correlation in the field of medicine, and who by their example made me aware of the laws of heaven.

Robert M. Hurwitz, MD

In memory of my parents

Mildred Howe Foote, RN
Capt. John Joseph Foote, USN

Antoinette Foote Hood, MD

CONTENTS

PREFACE

When the time came to plan the second edition of *Pathology of the Skin* we were urged by many of our friends and colleagues to use color photomicrographs. However, to do so would significantly increase the cost of the book, and with a large number of authors contributing to the book, we were concerned that it would be difficult to maintain consistency in image quality. It was then that the concept of a companion color atlas was born—an atlas that was complementary to but also independent of the textbook. Our intent was to create a stand-alone supplement with full color reproductions of both the clinical and histologic features of diseases, with special emphasis on 1) the variability of disease presentation, and 2) the chronology of disease manifestation. It was very important to us to show the evolution of diseases whenever possible because we felt this was an essential aspect in understanding disease, and this concept was too often omitted in other published works. It also was important to build a bridge between the many different concepts and terms applied to similar disease processes by other authors, which heretofore has resulted in confusion.

Because we were working within the outline of the textbook, we were freed from the necessity of providing lengthy descriptions. We feel comfortable referring to the fifty-four authors contributing to *Pathology of the Skin*, 2nd edition, for clinical and histologic details of the diseases covered in the atlas, and for appropriate literature review.

Because we were also working independently of the textbook, we were permitted to be selective in our choice of material. In general we chose to emphasize the common over the esoteric diseases; however, occasionally the collector within us forced the inclusion of a few unusual entities.

A word about the authors. People who know us consider us two unlikely collaborators, the "odd couple" of dermatopathology. We certainly differ in many respects: background, education, training, experience, and sometimes philosophy. But we share a fundamental desire to teach dermatopathology in a clear and unambiguous manner, and we appreciate good images. By learning to bridge our differences and respect our diversities we believe we were able to create a cogent and more balanced book.

Robert M. Hurwitz, MD
Antoinette F. Hood, MD

ACKNOWLEDGMENTS

The publication of an atlas of this size requires the support and assistance of many people. We wish to acknowledge our appreciation and thanks to them at this time.

Dr. A. Bernard Ackerman, Director, Institute for Dermatopathology at Jefferson Medical College, has had a profound influence on our understanding of many cutaneous disorders. He has always emphasized the importance of recognizing the evolutionary process and stages of cutaneous disease, concepts we have attempted to incorporate into this book.

Dr. Evan R. Farmer, Chairman of the Department of Dermatology at the Indiana University School of Medicine, encouraged us to take on the challenge of creating an atlas to accompany the *Pathology of the Skin*. He not only created an environment conducive for the project, but he also contributed generously from his personal collection.

Many faculty members unselfishly contributed material, including Drs. Tsu-Yi Chuang, Holly Faust, Charles Lewis, Patrick Logan, Ginat Mirowski, Arthur Norins, Jeffrey Travers, and Stephen Wolverton, Dale Kephart and Rebecca Bushong. We also wish to thank other dermatologists in the community whose patients attended our weekly Grand Rounds, and whose photographs form the basis of the department teaching collection.

Residents at Indiana University who took many of the clinical photographs include Drs. Alfred Knable, Brian Williams, Scott Fretzin, David Gerstein, Sonya Campbell-Johnson and Christine Kuhn. Drs. Larry Buckel, Howard Gray and William Moores, associated with Dermatopathology, Inc., generously shared their excellently prepared microscopic material. Drs. William B. Ober, Bradley Thurston, John Randall, Jackie Junkins Hopkins and Martha McCullough freely contributed clinical or histologic material. Dr. Diya Mutasim provided many of the immunofluorescent photomicrographs. Dr. Charles Tomich advised us in the preparation of the chapter on mucous membrane disorders and provided material for the chapter.

We are also indebted to Appleton & Lange editors Michael Medina and Sondra Greenfield. For their patience and their attention to detail we are forever grateful.

We recognize and thank the following medical journals for giving permission to reproduce illustrations previously published by them:

Figure 2–12b (p. 27). Hurwitz RM, Tisserand ME. Erythema ab igne. *Arch Dermatol.* 1987;123:21–23. Copyright 1987, American Medical Association.

Figure 2–43b (p. 40). Kephart DC, Hood AF, Provost TT. Neonatal lupus erythematosus: New serologic findings. *J Invest Dermatol.* 1981;77:331–333. Copyright 1981, American Medical Association.

Figure 3–27 (p. 53). Wilkeson RW, Nguyen TH, Guill M. Erythematous, vesicular lesions in a newborn. *Arch Dermatol.* 1992;128:1395–1400. Copyright 1992, American Medical Association.

Figure 4–45 (p. 71). Oursler JR, Goldblum OM. Blistering eruption in a diabetic. *Arch Dermatol.* 1991;127:247–252. Copyright 1991, American Medical Association.

Figure 10–15b (p. 136). Goldman MP. Ascites, gastrointestinal bleeding, and leg nodules. *Arch Dermatol.* 1985;121:673–678. Copyright 1985, American Medical Association.

Figure 11–41 (p. 158). Hurwitz RM, Egan WT, Murphy SH, Pontius EE, Foster ML. Bowenoid papulosis and squamous cell carcinoma of the genitalia: suspected sexual transmission. *Cutis.* 1987;39:193–196. Copyright 1987, American Medical Association.

Figures 11–43, 11–44 & 11–45 (p. 159). Echt AF, Hurwitz RM, Davis TE. Warts: benign or malignant? *Indiana Med.* 1991;84:476–479. Copyright 1991, American Medical Association.

Figure 12–8 (p. 164). Joyce JP, Waldman PC, Hood AF. Persistent genital ulceration. *Arch Dermatol.* 1989;125:551–556. Copyright 1989, American Medical Association.

Figure 12–9 (p. 164). Margolis RJ, Hood, AF. Chancroid: diagnosis and treatment. *J Am Acad Dermatol.* 1982;6:493–499. Copyright 1982, American Medical Association.

Figures 15–9 & 15–10c (p. 191) Triana AF, Matis WL, Peterman AR. Annular plaque on the shoulder. *Arch Dermatol.* 1987;123:1707–1712. Copyright 1987, American Medical Association.

Robert M. Hurwitz, MD
Antoinette F. Hood, MD

Pathology of the Skin

Atlas of Clinical-Pathological Correlation

1

SPONGIOTIC AND PSORIASIFORM DERMATITIS

- Allergic contact dermatitis
- Irritant contact dermatitis
- Atopic dermatitis
- Dyshidrotic dermatitis
- Nummular dermatitis
- Seborrheic dermatitis
- Pityriasis rosea
- Pruritic urticarial papules and plaques of pregnancy (PUPPP)
- Psoriasis
- Guttate parapsoriasis
- Pityriasis rubra pilaris
- Reiter's syndrome

ALLERGIC CONTACT DERMATITIS

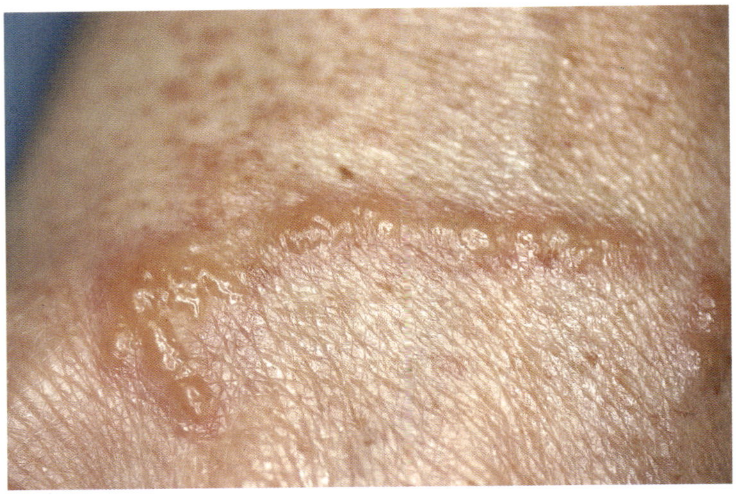

Figure 1–1. Allergic contact dermatitis. Allergic contact dermatitis due to poison ivy. Confluent, linear, eruptive vesicles with surrounding erythema.

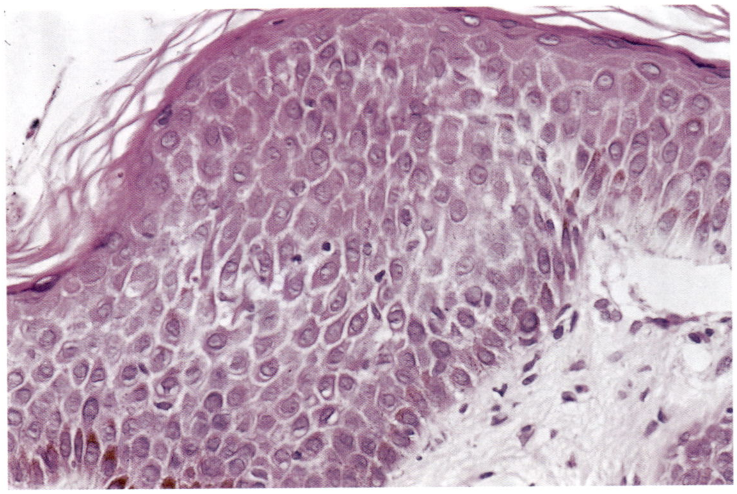

Figure 1–2. Allergic contact dermatitis. Early lesion of allergic contact dermatitis. There is basket-weave orthokeratosis, slight epidermal hyperplasia, and prominent spongiosis.

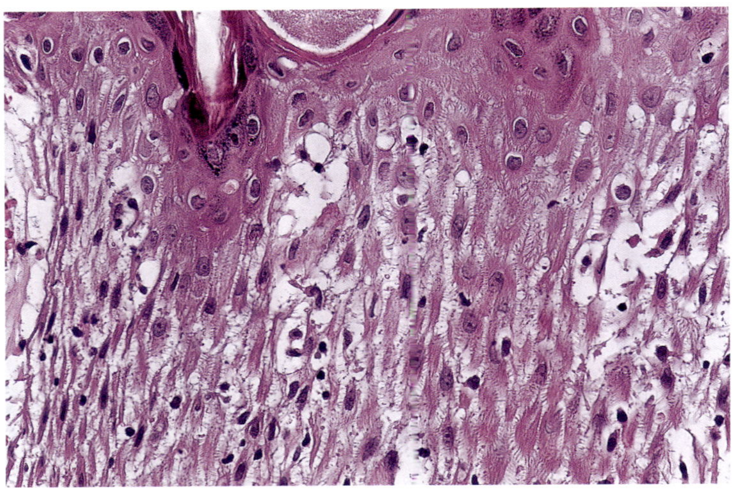

Figure 1–3. Allergic contact dermatitis. Allergic contact dermatitis with severe spongiosis and a scatter of lymphocytes.

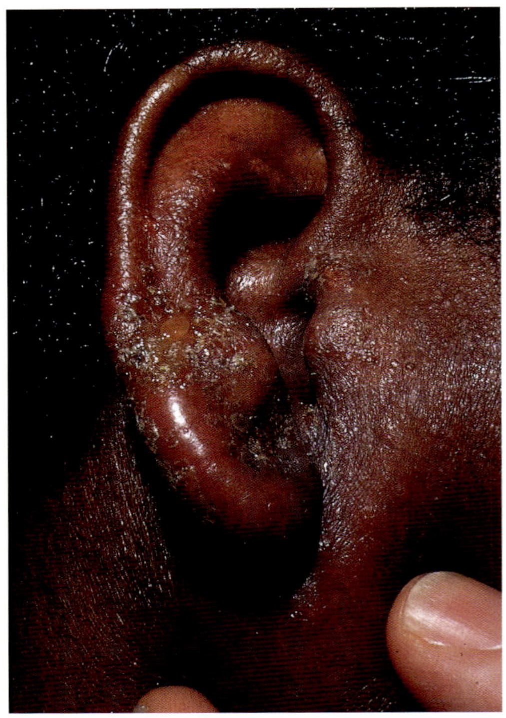

Figure 1–4. Allergic contact dermatitis. Allergic contact dermatitis to an antibacterial ointment. Severe edema, erythema, and vesicles involving the ear and cheek.

ALLERGIC CONTACT DERMATITIS

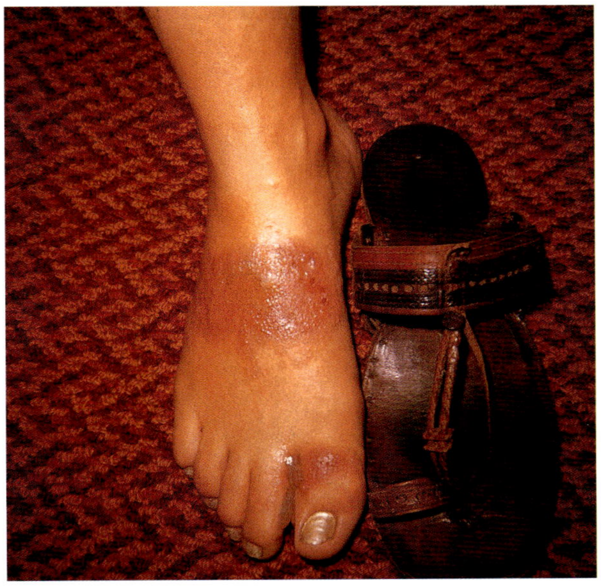

Figure 1–5. Allergic contact dermatitis. Allergic contact dermatitis on the foot secondary to chemicals in leather sandals. Erythema, edema, vesicles, and bullae match the points of contact of the leather straps on the foot.

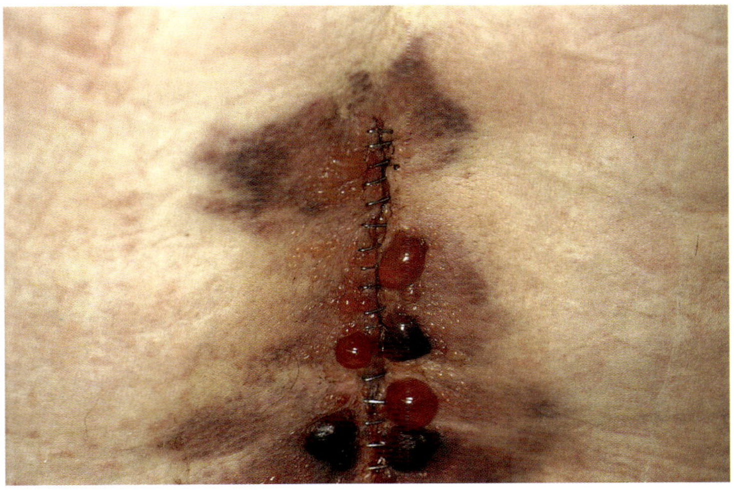

Figure 1–6. Allergic contact dermatitis. Severe allergic contact dermatitis to topical medicament used postoperatively. Erythematous, purpuric vesicles and hemorrhagic bullae along the line of staple closure.

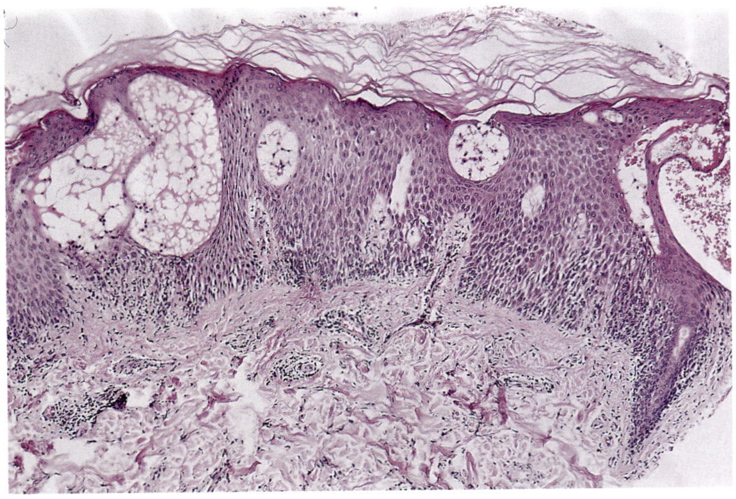

Figure 1–7. Allergic contact dermatitis. Severe spongiosis, microvesiculation, and bullae formation. There is epidermal hyperplasia with a moderately dense mixed dermal infiltrate composed of lymphocytes, eosinophils, and dilated blood vessels.

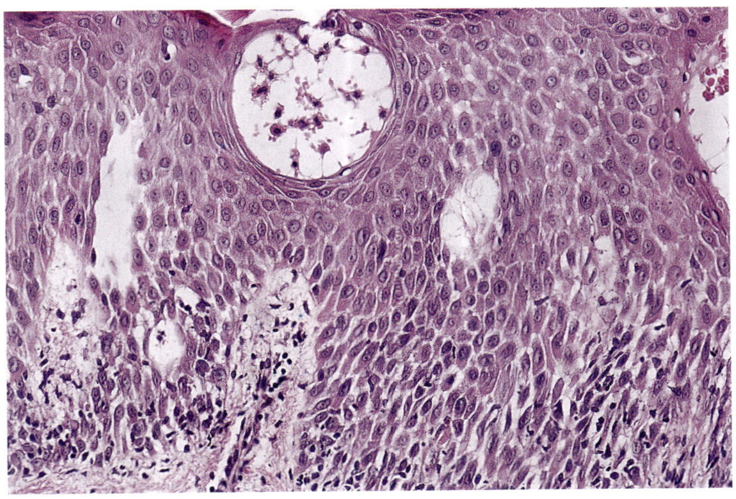

Figure 1–8. Allergic contact dermatitis. Vesiculation and bullae formation with lymphocytic infiltration.

IRRITANT CONTACT DERMATITIS

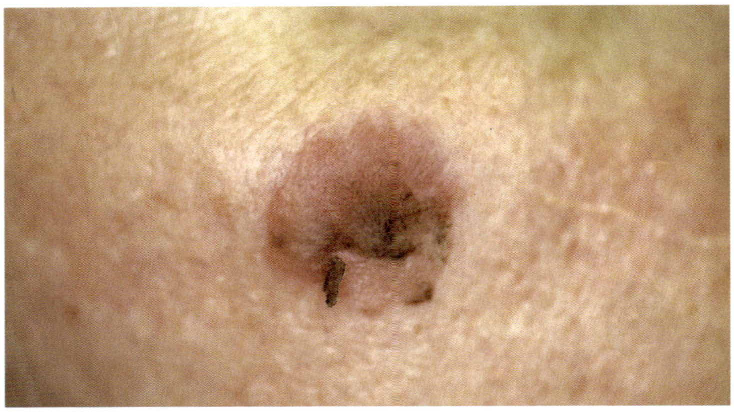

Figure 1–9. Irritant contact dermatitis. Crusting, peeling, and erythema surround a solar lentigo on the cheek treated with a bleaching cream.

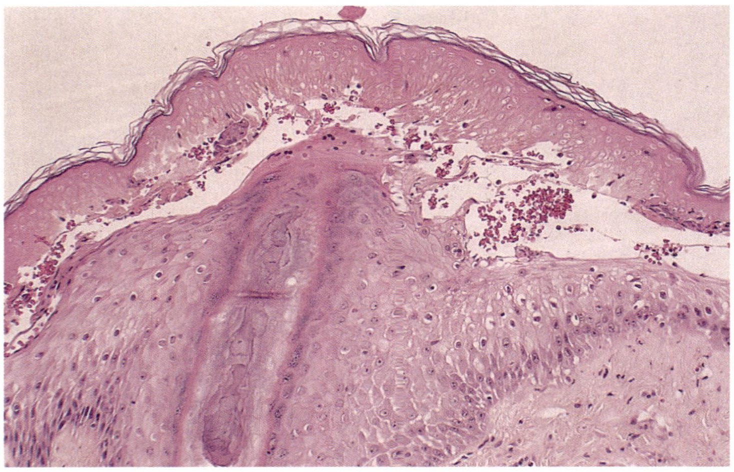

Figure 1–11. Irritant contact dermatitis. There is confluent epidermal necrosis with basket-weave orthokeratosis separated from a viable spongiotic epidermis. Within the cleft is hemorrhage with a mixed-cell infiltrate with neutrophils. The papillary dermis is edematous and contains lymphocytes and neutrophils.

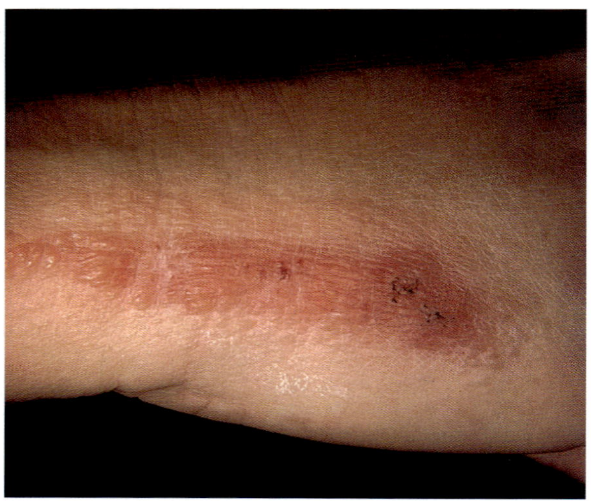

Figure 1–12. Black spot poison ivy dermatitis. At one end of a linear, erythematous, vesicular area of the hand is a group of black spots that correspond to concentrated deposits of the poison ivy oleoresin.

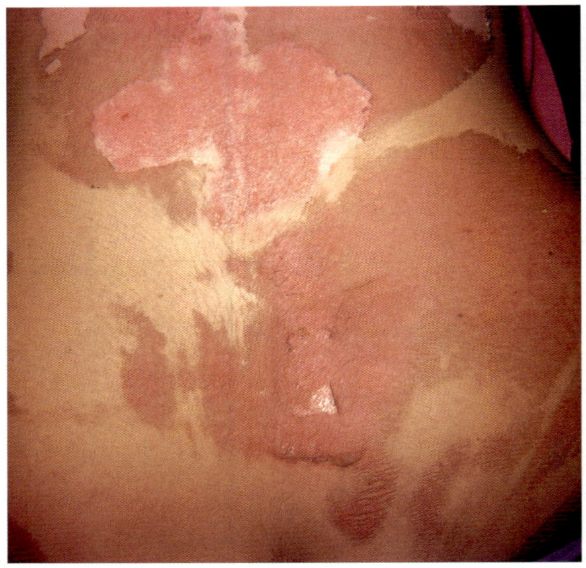

Figure 1–10. Irritant contact dermatitis. Vesiculation and denuded epidermis overlying an erythematous oozing dermis resulting from the application of a toxic chemical to the abdomen.

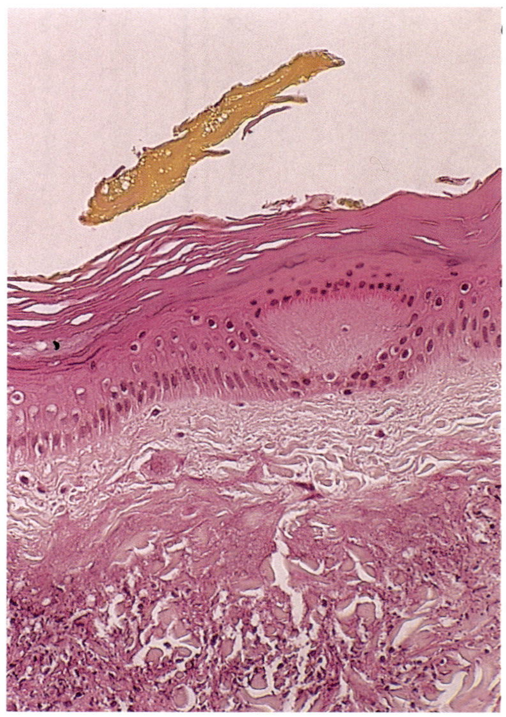

Figure 1–13. Black spot poison ivy dermatitis. Yellow-stained globules, which represent concentrated deposits of poison ivy oleoresin, sit atop the stratum corneum. Subjacent confluent epidermal necrosis lies over the dermis, which is edematous and degenerated in areas. In addition, the dermis contains a dense infiltrate of neutrophils and nuclear fragments, common findings in irritant contact dermatitis.

ATOPIC DERMATITIS

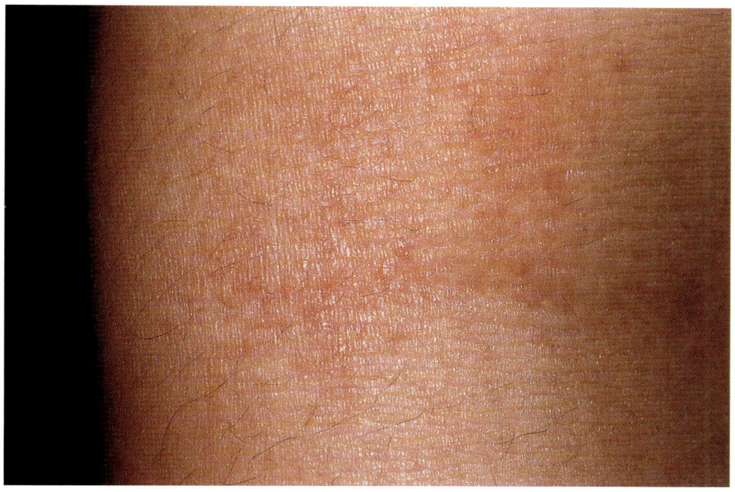

Figure 1–14. Atopic dermatitis, early. Grouped pinpoint erythematous papules involving the antecubital fossa.

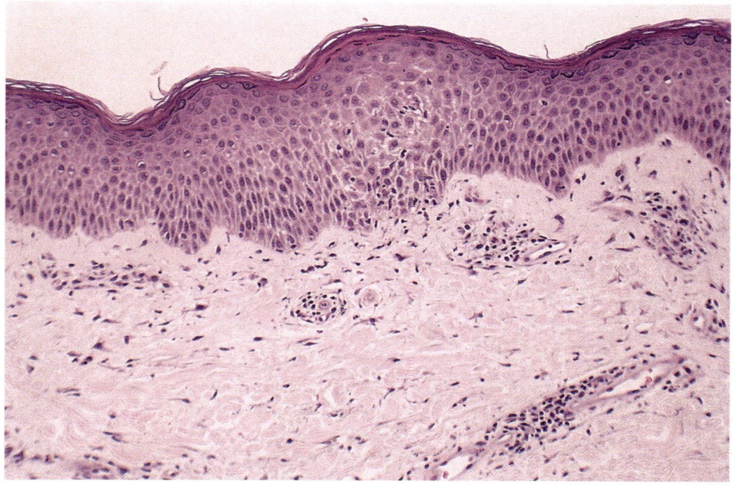

Figure 1–15. Atopic dermatitis, early. There is mild spongiosis with basket-weave orthokeratosis, and a perivascular and interstitial mixed-cell dermal infiltrate comprising lymphocytes, eosinophils, and neutrophils.

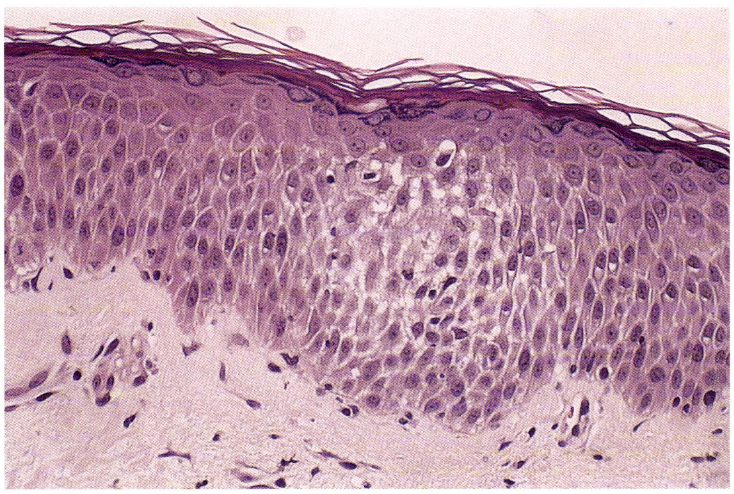

Figure 1–16. Atopic dermatitis. Spongiotic epidermis with overlying basket-weave orthokeratosis.

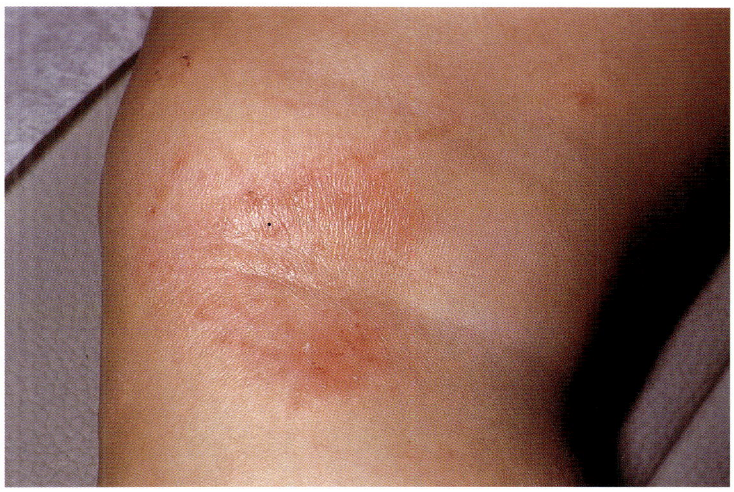

Figure 1–17. Atopic dermatitis. Antecubital fossa with erythematous and crusted papules.

ATOPIC DERMATITIS

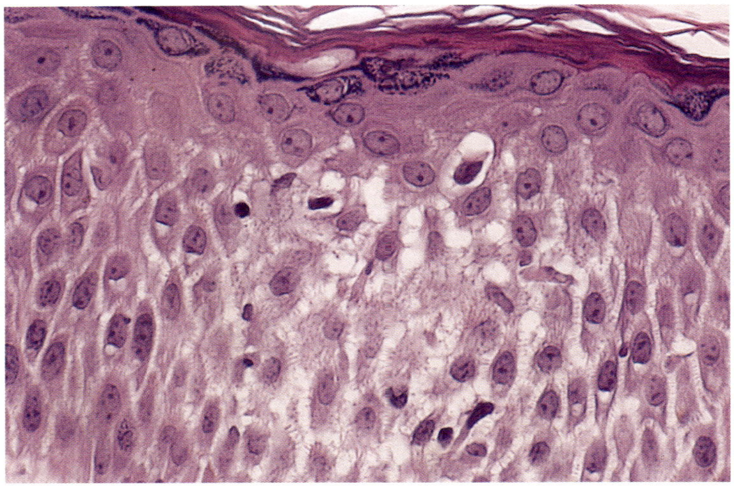

Figure 1–18. Atopic dermatitis. Spongiotic epidermis with orthokeratosis.

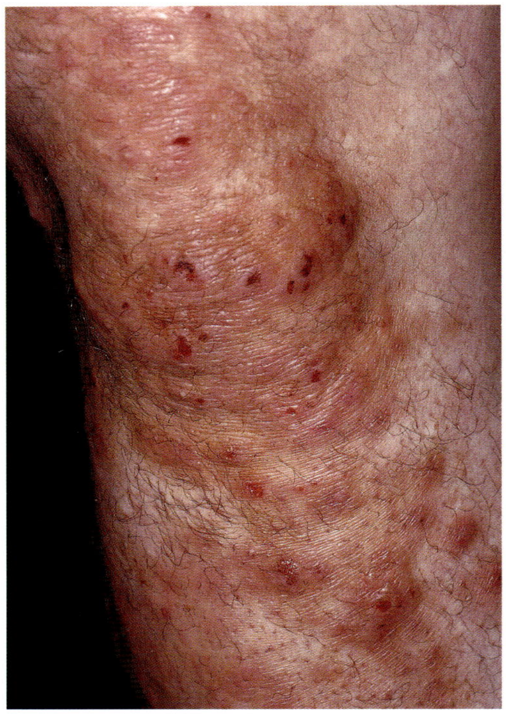

Figure 1–19. Atopic dermatitis, later stage. Some erythematous papules are crusted, while others appear excoriated.

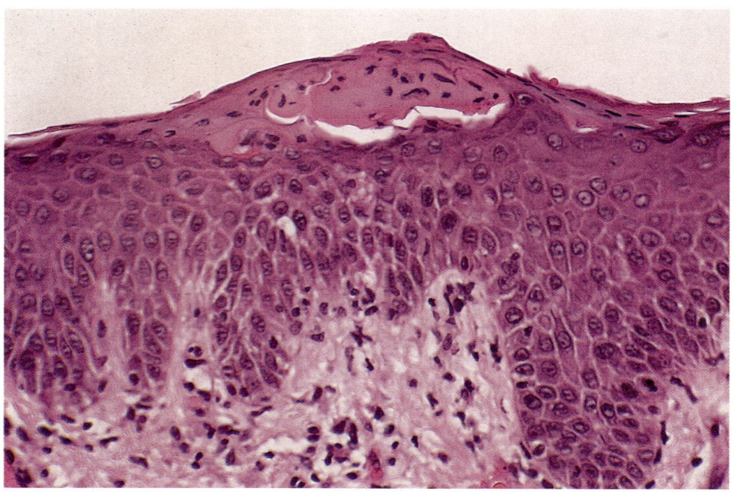

Figure 1–20. Atopic dermatitis, later stage. There is scale-crust atop a spongiotic psoriasiform epidermis.

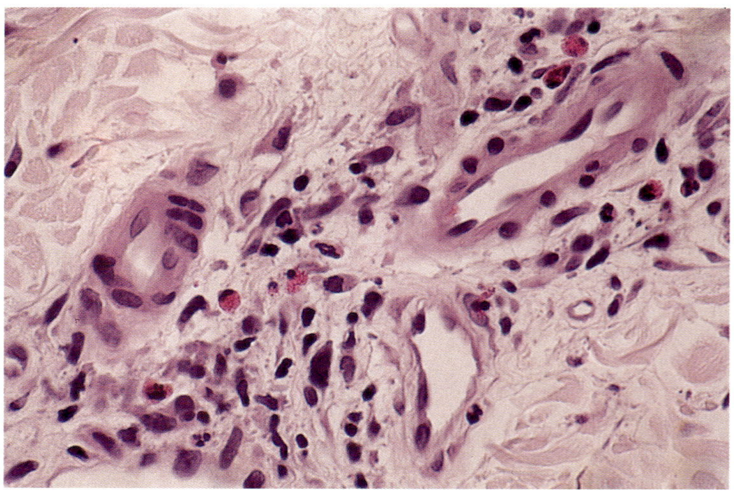

Figure 1–21. Atopic dermatitis. Perivascular and interstitial mixed-cell infiltrate, with lymphocytes, eosinophils, and neutrophils.

ATOPIC DERMATITIS

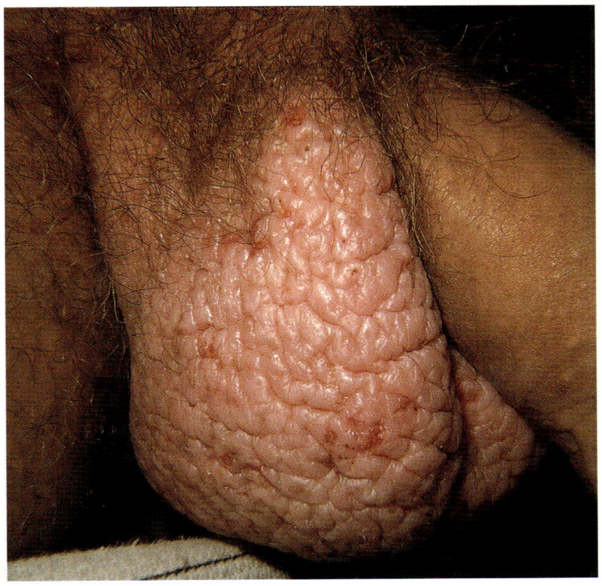

Figure 1–22. Atopic dermatitis, Lichen simplex chronicus. Markedly thickened scrotum of a patient with atopic dermatitis, resulting from chronic rubbing and scratching.

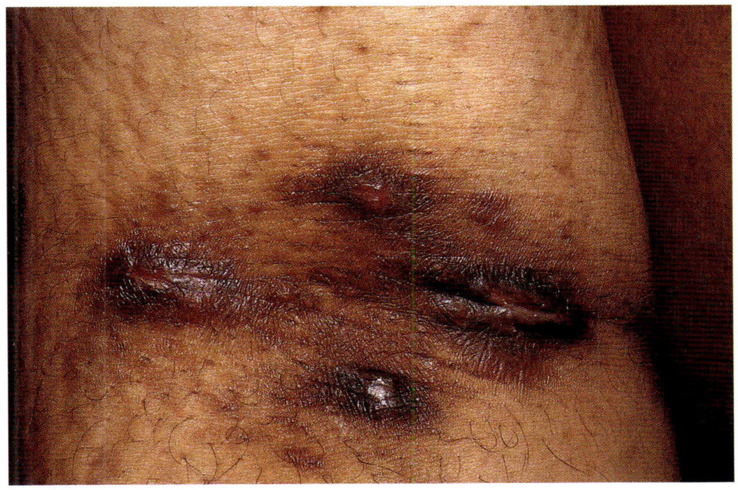

Figure 1–23. Atopic dermatitis. Lichen simplex chronicus and prurigo nodularis within an antecubital fossa of older patient with classic atopic dermatitis. These lesions result from chronic rubbing and scratching, because of the intense pruritus. The lesions are sharply circumscribed, raised, dome-shaped, and hyperpigmented.

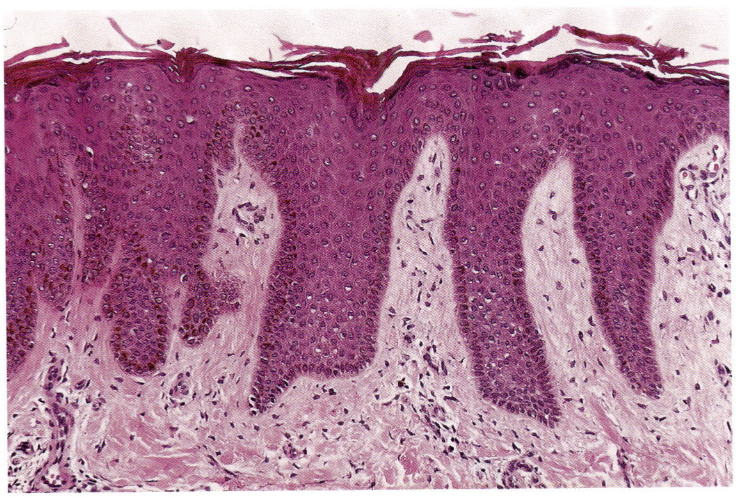

Figure 1–24. Atopic dermatitis, later lesion. Hyperkeratosis, hypergranulosis, adnexal and epidermal hyperplasia, thickened collagen bundles, dilated blood vessels, and lymphohistiocytic infiltrate.

DYSHIDROTIC DERMATITIS

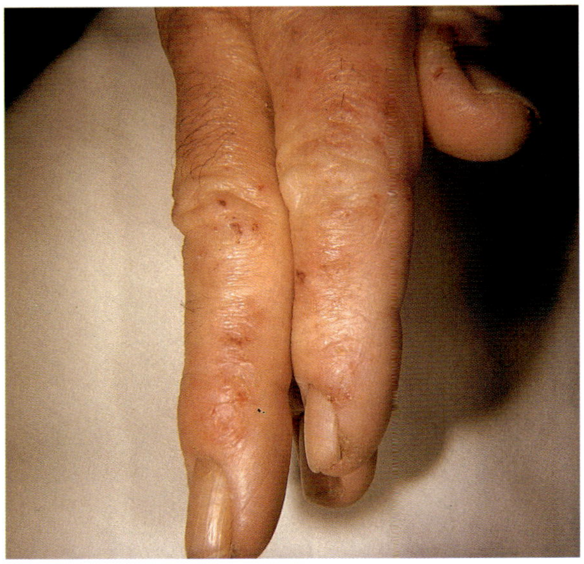

Figure 1–25. Dyshidrotic dermatitis. Grouped, pruritic, erythematous, and flesh-colored papules on the fingers. Some are excoriated and crusted.

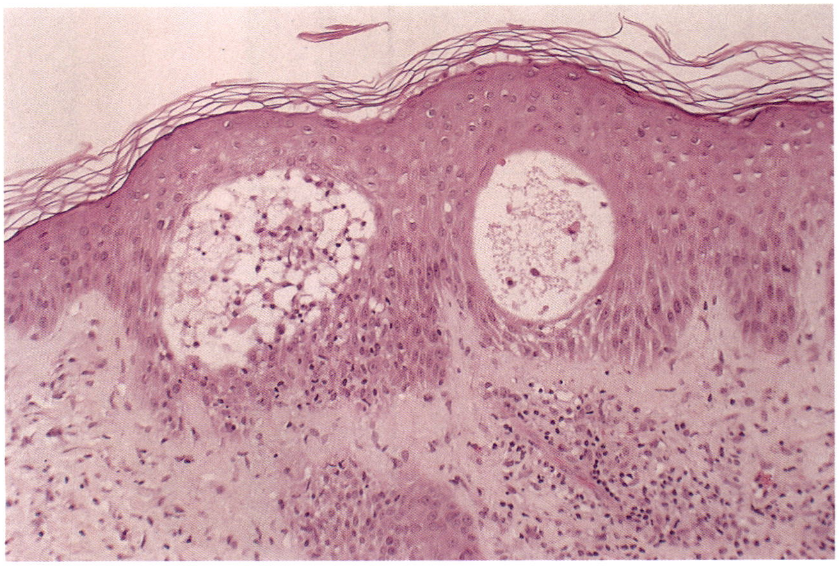

Figure 1–26. Dyshidrotic dermatitis. Intraepidermal spongiosis and vesiculation, acanthosis, and a mixed-cell infiltrate within the thickened papillary dermis.

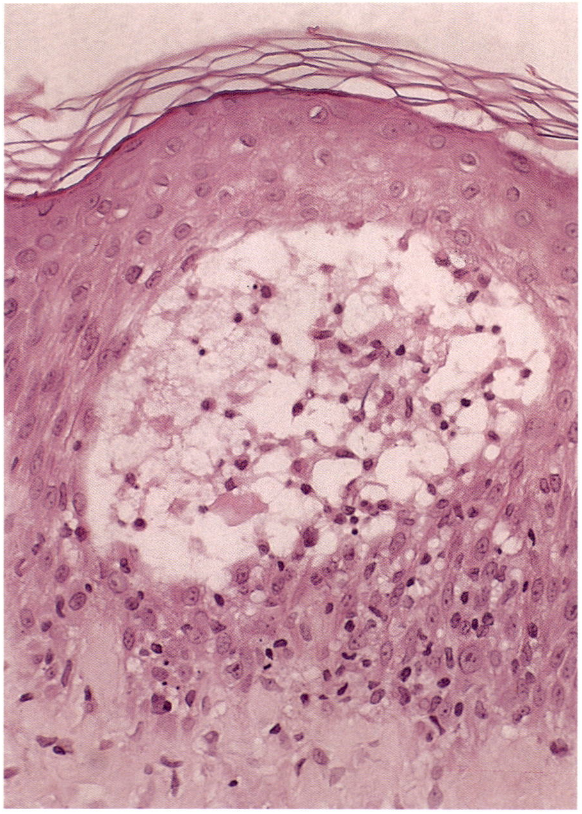

Figure 1–27. Dyshidrotic dermatitis. Intraepidermal spongiosis, vesiculation, and mixed-cell epidermal and dermal infiltrate.

NUMMULAR DERMATITIS

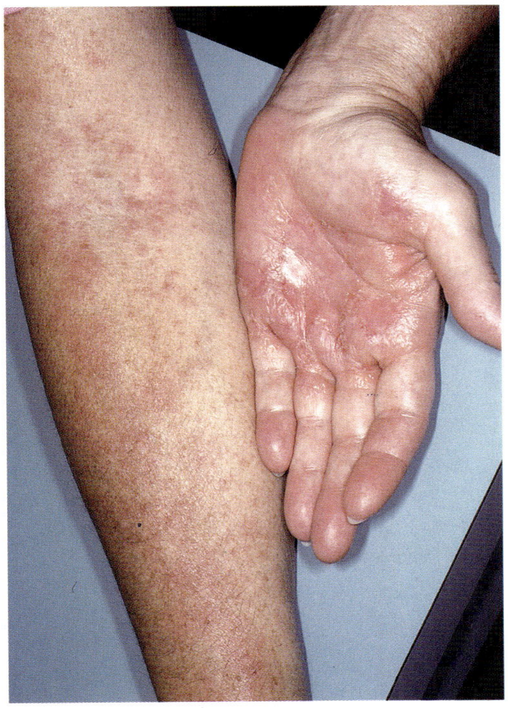

Figure 1–28. **Nummular dermatitis.** Atopic patient with both nummular dermatitis and hand dermatitis. There are erythematous crusted papules on the arm and antecubital fossa as well as palmar erythema, and erythematous papulovesicles on the fingers.

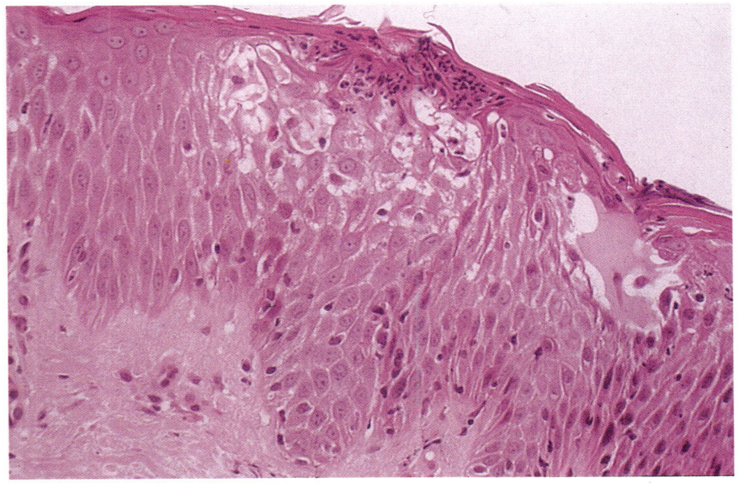

Figure 1–29. **Nummular dermatitis.** Epidermal hyperplasia, spongiosis, microvesiculation, and scale-crust.

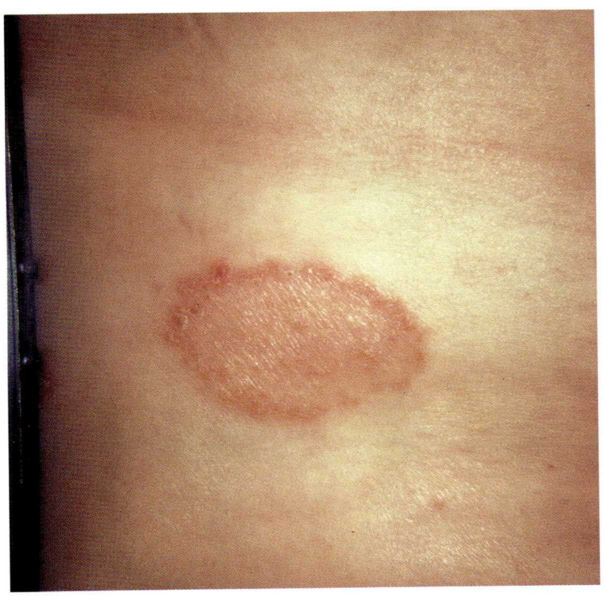

Figure 1–30. **Nummular dermatitis.** Classic "coin shape" lesion on the leg.

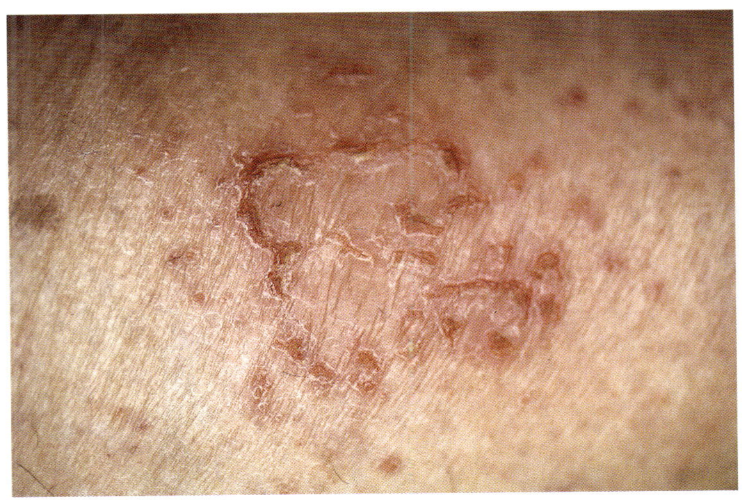

Figure 1–31. **Nummular dermatitis.** Pruritic annular, agminated, crusted papules on the lower leg.

NUMMULAR DERMATITIS

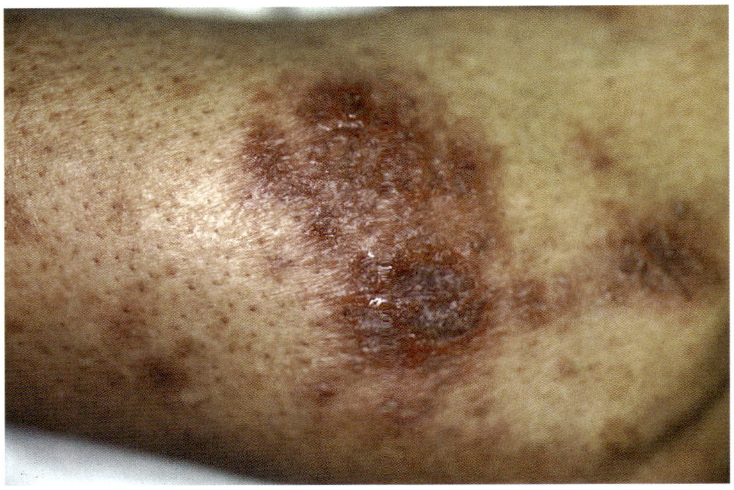

Figure 1–32. Nummular dermatitis, later stage. Grouped, crusted, oozing plaques on lower leg associated with intense pruritus.

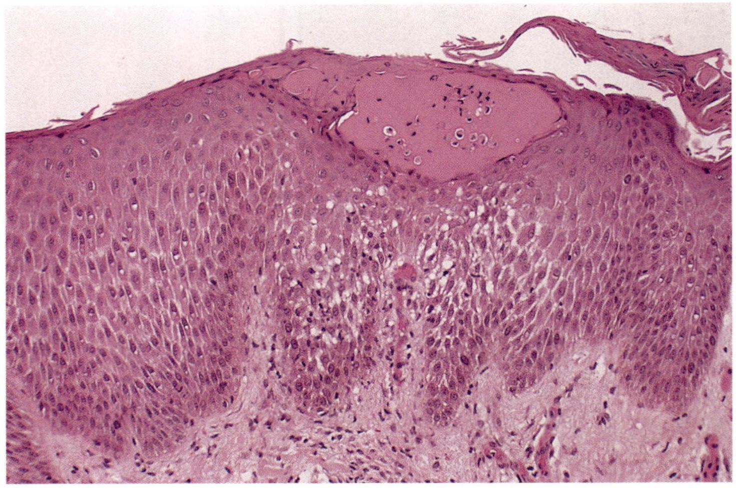

Figure 1–33. Nummular dermatitis, later stage. Psoriasiform epidermal hyperplasia, severe spongiosis, and vesicle formation. The dermis contains a perivascular and interstitial mixed-cell infiltrate of lymphocytes and some eosinophils.

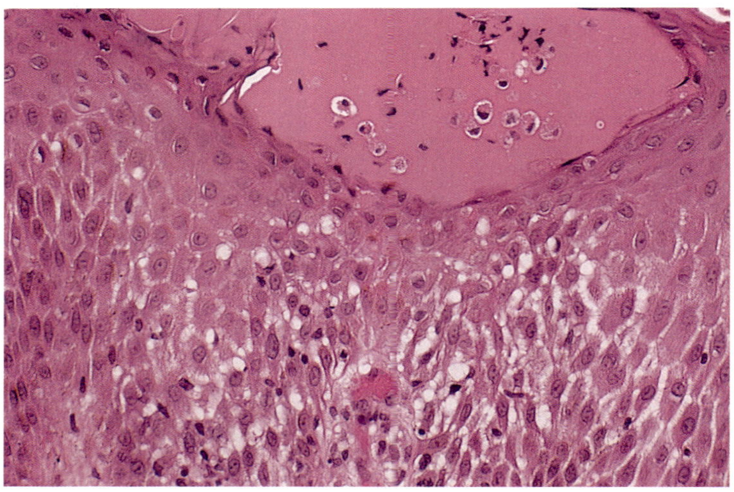

Figure 1–34. Nummular dermatitis. Severe spongiosis and vesiculation.

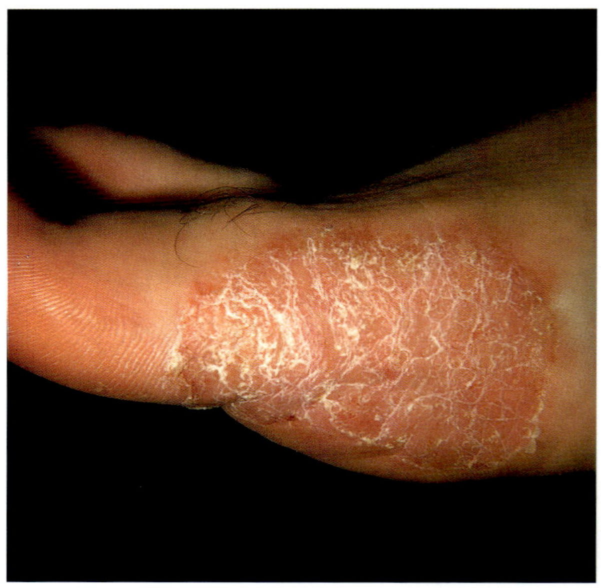

Figure 1–35. Nummular dermatitis evolving into lichen simplex chronicus. The circular plaque is slightly raised, sharply circumscribed, erythematous, thickened, and scaly.

NUMMULAR DERMATITIS

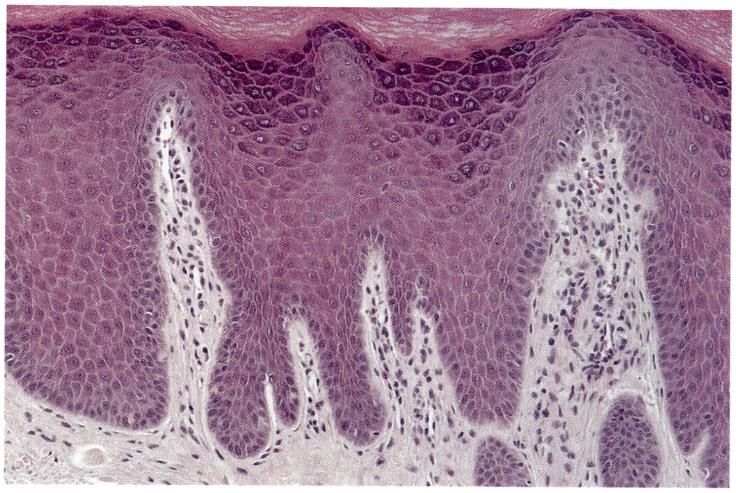

Figure 1–36. Nummular dermatitis, later stage. Hyperkeratosis, hypergranulosis, and hyperplasia of the epidermal and adnexal epithelium. The papillary dermis is thickened with coarse collagen bundles, dilated blood vessels, and a lymphohistiocytic infiltrate.

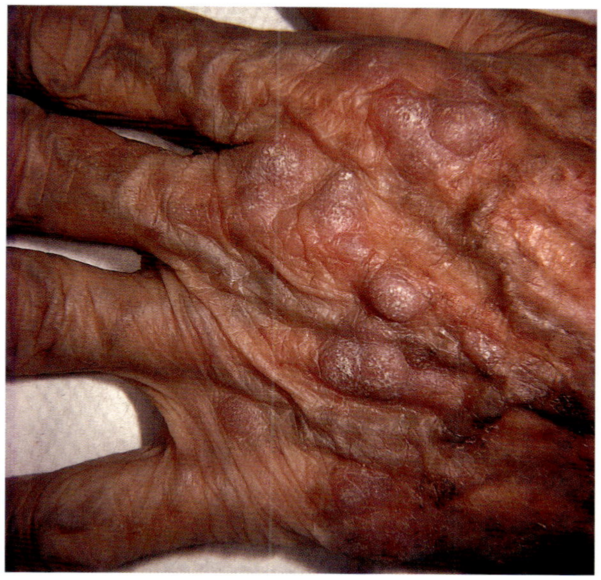

Figure 1–37. Nummular dermatitis, evolving into prurigo nodularis. Thickened, raised, dome-shaped nodule on the dorsum of the hand.

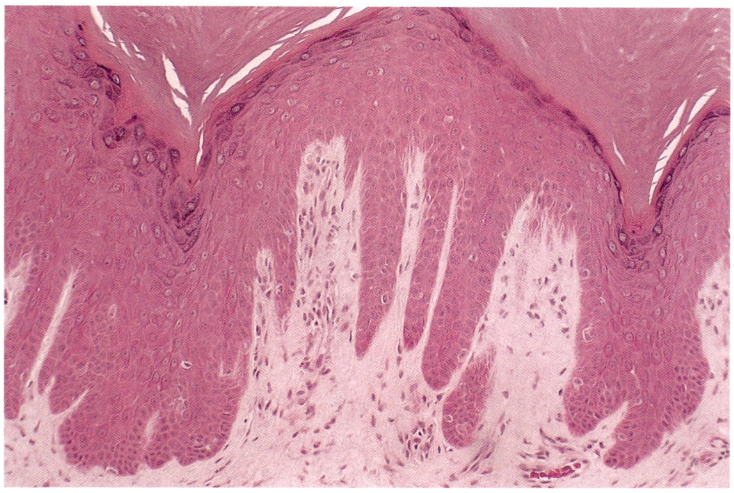

Figure 1–38. Nummular dermatitis, prurigo nodularis. Compact orthohyperkeratosis, focal parakeratosis, and hypergranulosis, with adnexal and epidermal hyperplasia. The papillary dermis is markedly thickened with coarse collagen bundles, dilated blood vessels, and a lymphohistiocytic infiltrate.

SEBORRHEIC DERMATITIS

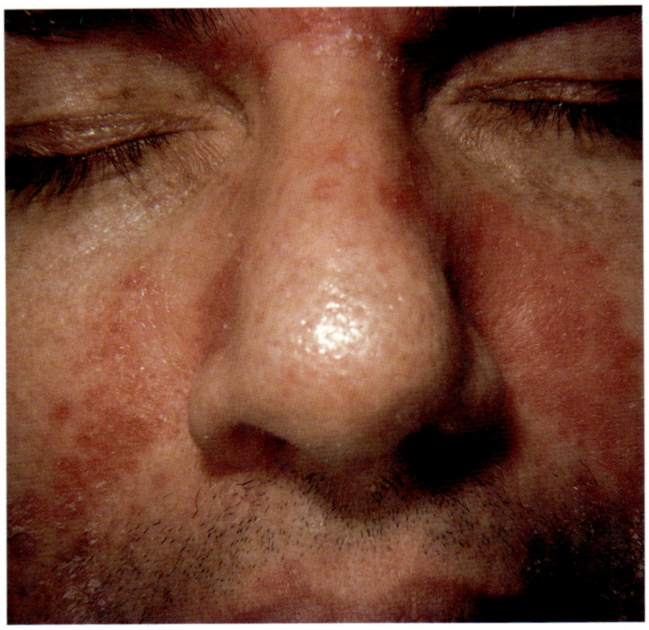

Figure 1–39. Seborrheic dermatitis. Greasy scales atop bright macular erythema involving the central face. This eruption characteristically includes the nose, cheeks, eyebrows, and periorbital regions.

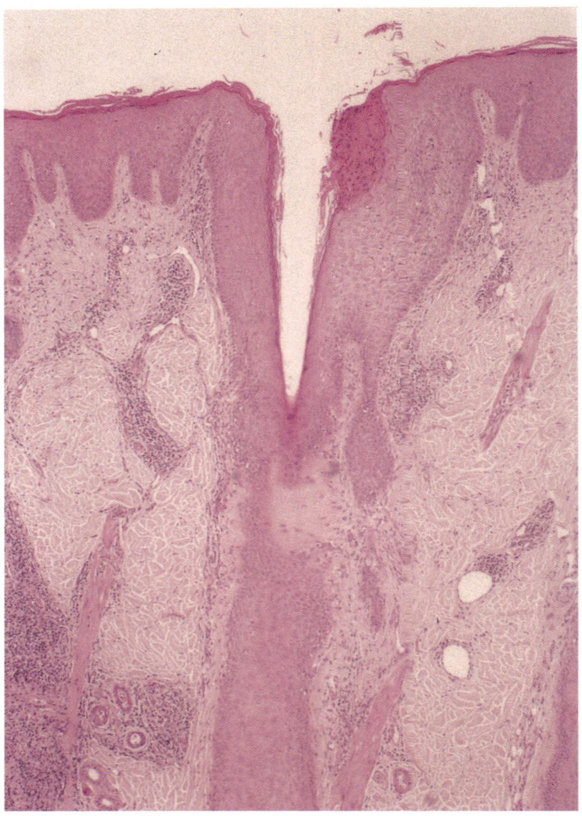

Figure 1–40. Seborrheic dermatitis. Infundibular spongiosis, focal scale-crust at tip of a follicular ostium, and epidermal hyperplasia with compact orthokeratosis. In the dermis there are dilated blood vessels, and a moderately dense perivascular and perifollicular lymphohistiocytic infiltrate.

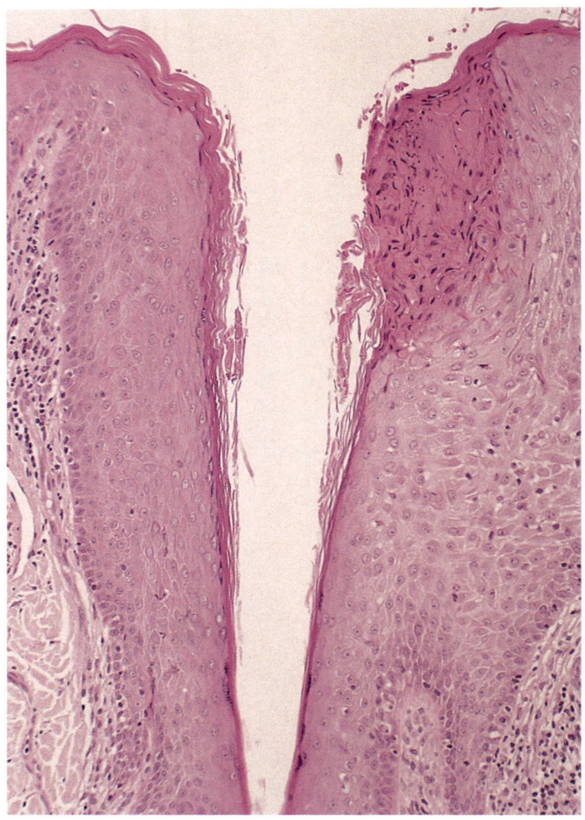

Figure 1–41. Seborrheic dermatitis. Epidermal spongiosis with a mound of scale-crust containing neutrophils.

PITYRIASIS ROSEA

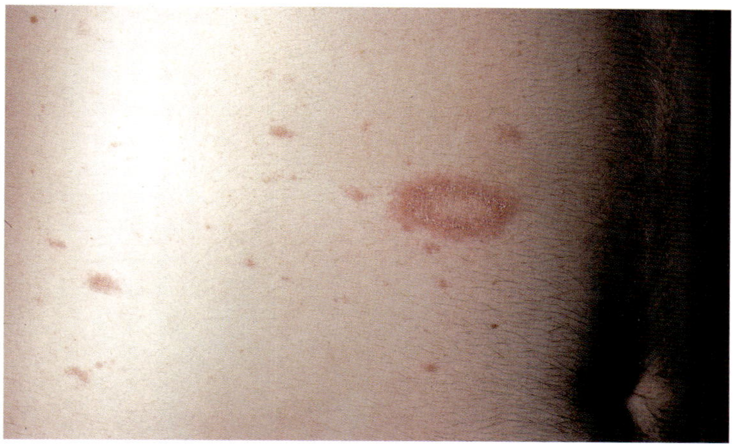

Figure 1–42. Pityriasis rosea. Large, erythematous, oval plaque with peripheral scale, commonly referred to as the "herald" or "mother" patch. This lesion commonly precedes the generalized papulosquamous eruption by several weeks.

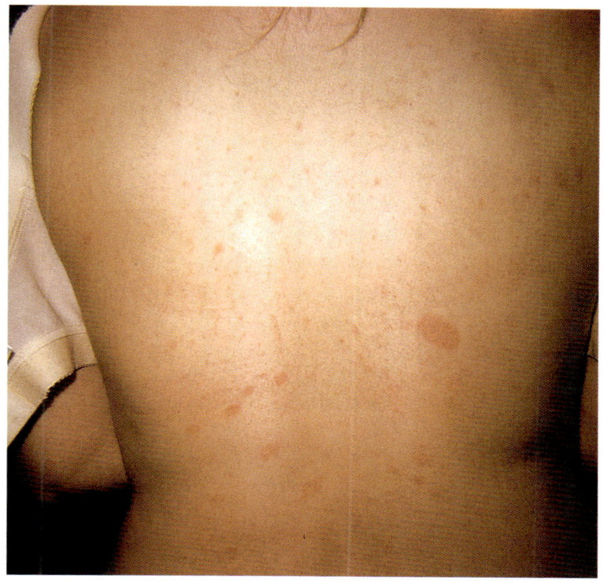

Figure 1–43. Pityriasis rosea. The herald patch and numerous oval-shaped lesions aligned along normal skin cleavage lines. This distribution is often referred to as the "Christmas tree pattern" on the back and "chevron pattern" on the front of the trunk.

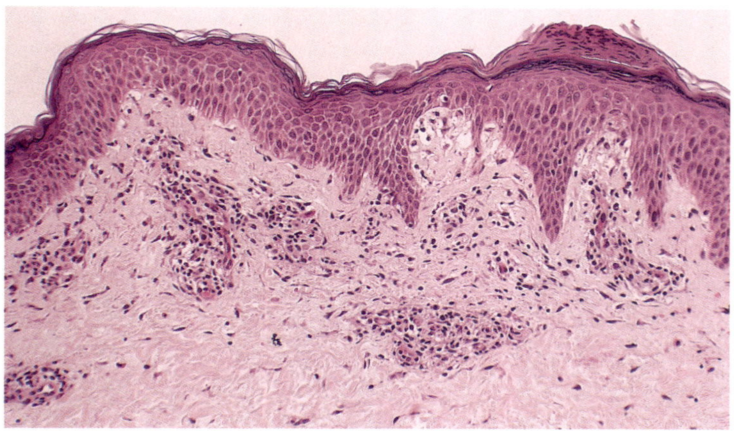

Figure 1–44. Pityriasis rosea. Mild epidermal hyperplasia and spongiosis with a round mound of scale-crust. There is prominent papillary edema, dilated blood vessels, and a perivascular and interstitial lymphohistiocytic infiltrate with occasional eosinophils.

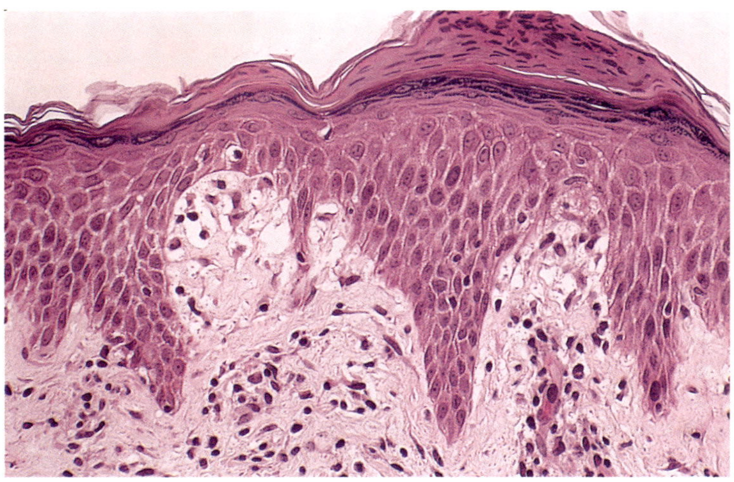

Figure 1–45. Pityriasis rosea. Psoriasiform epidermal hyperplasia, spongiosis, rounded mound of scale-crust with neutrophils, severe papillary edema, and a mixed-cell infiltrate.

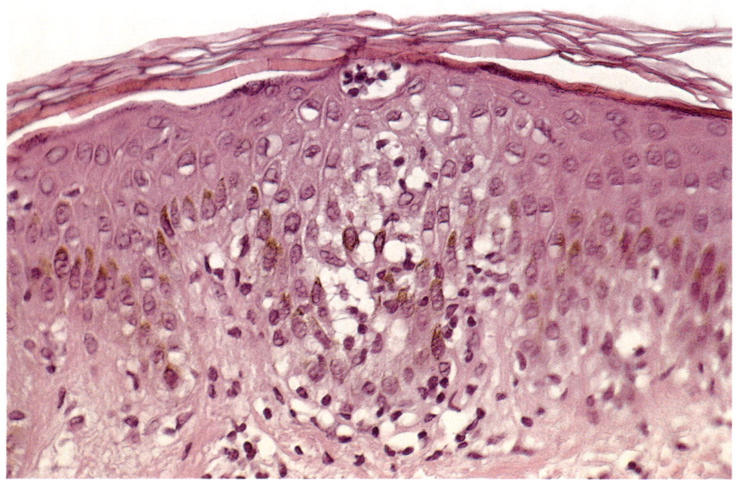

Figure 1–46. Pityriasis rosea. Prominent epidermal spongiosis.

PRURITIC URTICARIAL PAPULES AND PLAQUES OF PREGNANCY (PUPPP)

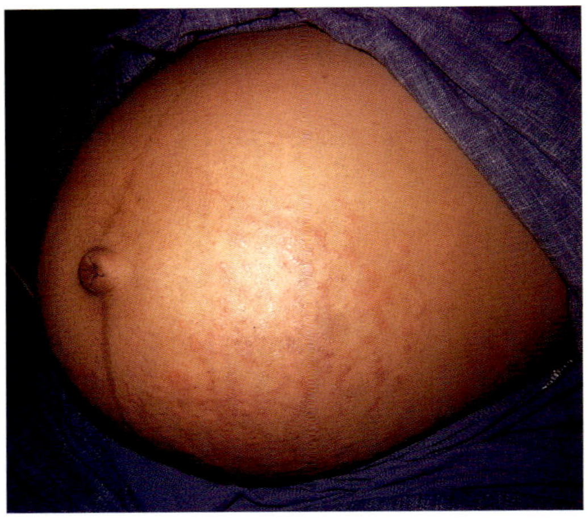

Figure 1–47. Pruritic urticarial papules and plaques of pregnancy (PUPPP). This woman is in her last trimester of pregnancy.

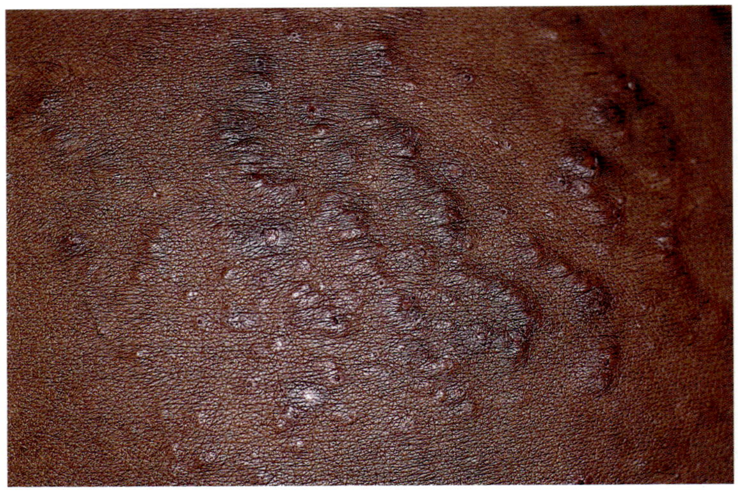

Figure 1–48. PUPPP. Lesions often following striae lines.

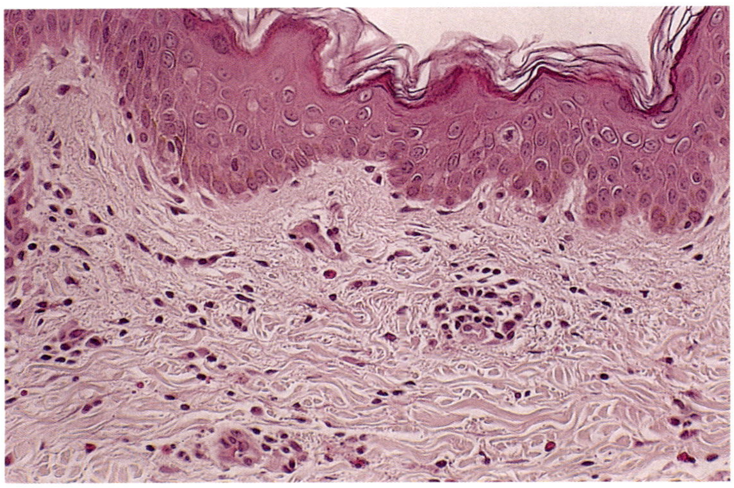

Figure 1–49. PUPPP, early lesions. Mild epidermal hyperplasia, orthokeratosis, and a perivascular and interstitial mixed-cell infiltrate with prominent eosinophils.

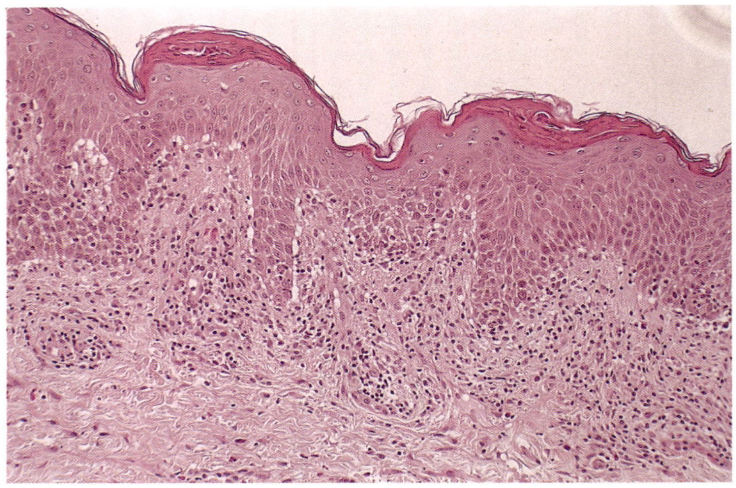

Figure 1–50. PUPPP, later lesion. Psoriasiform epidermal hyperplasia, spongiosis with scale-crust, severe papillary edema, and a perivascular and interstitial mixed-cell infiltrate containing many eosinophils.

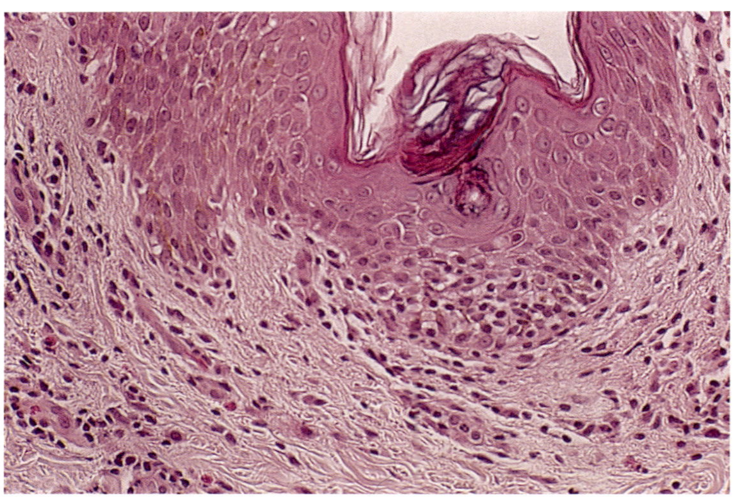

Figure 1–51. PUPPP. Epidermal and infundibular spongiosis.

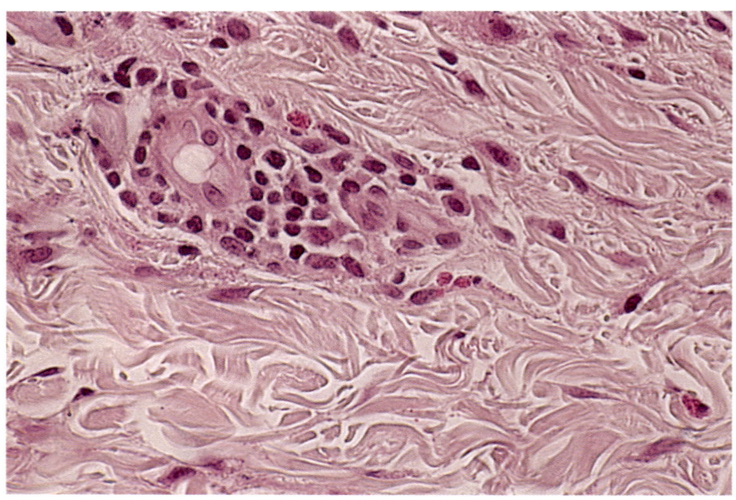

Figure 1–52. PUPPP. Perivascular and interstitial lymphocytes and eosinophils.

PSORIASIS

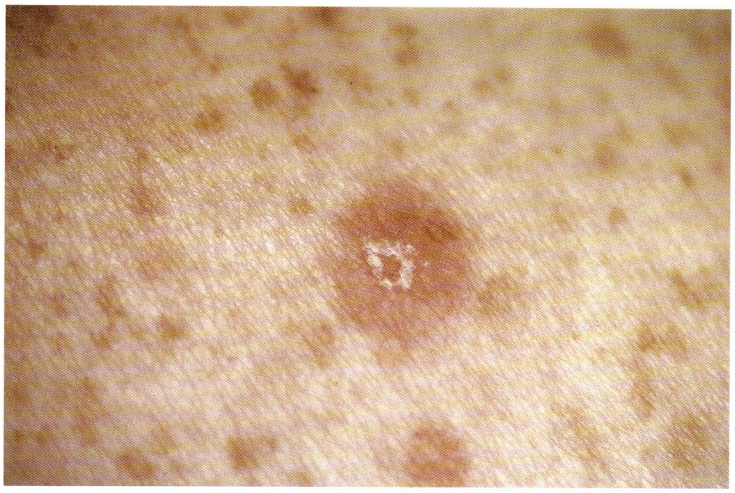

Figure 1–53. Psoriasis, early eruptive stage. Scaly erythematous papule.

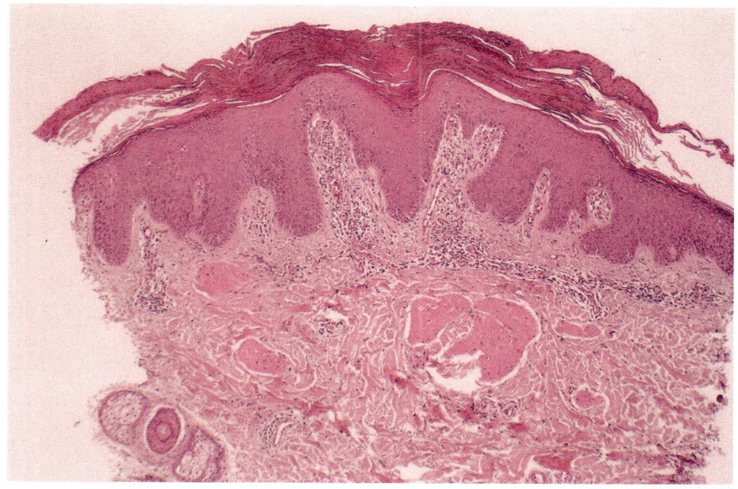

Figure 1–54. Psoriasis, early eruptive stage. Psoriasiform epidermal hyperplasia, hyperkeratosis, parakeratosis with neutrophils, papillary edema, dilated blood vessels, and a perivascular mixed-cell infiltrate with neutrophils.

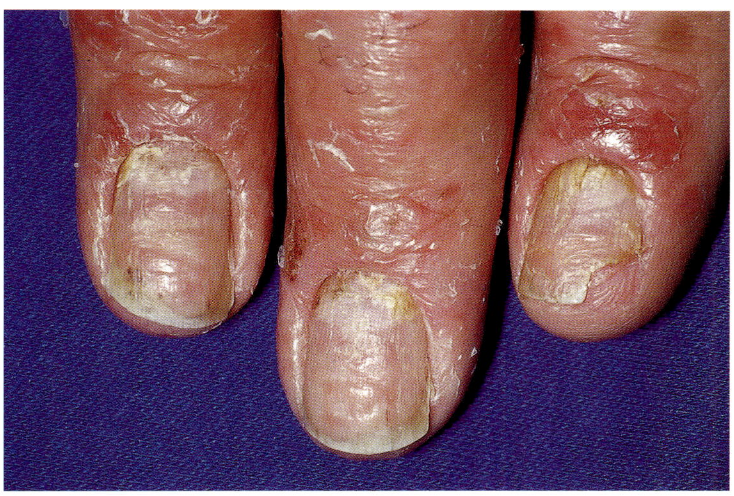

Figure 1–55. Psoriasis. Erythema, scaling, nail dystrophy, and onycholysis.

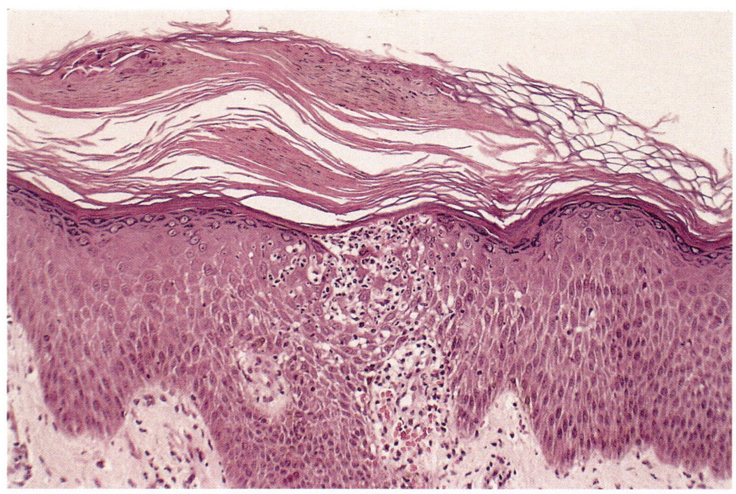

Figure 1–56. Psoriasis, early or eruptive lesion. Collections of neutrophils within the hyperplastic epidermis.

PSORIASIS

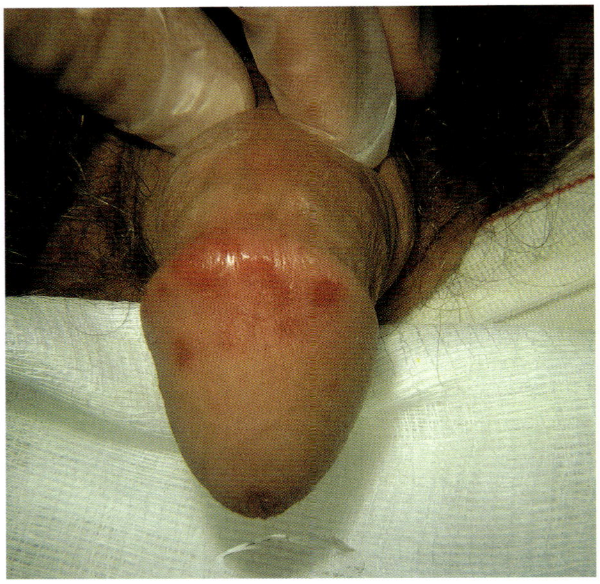

Figure 1–57. Psoriasis, glans penis. Grouped, erythematous, scaly papules.

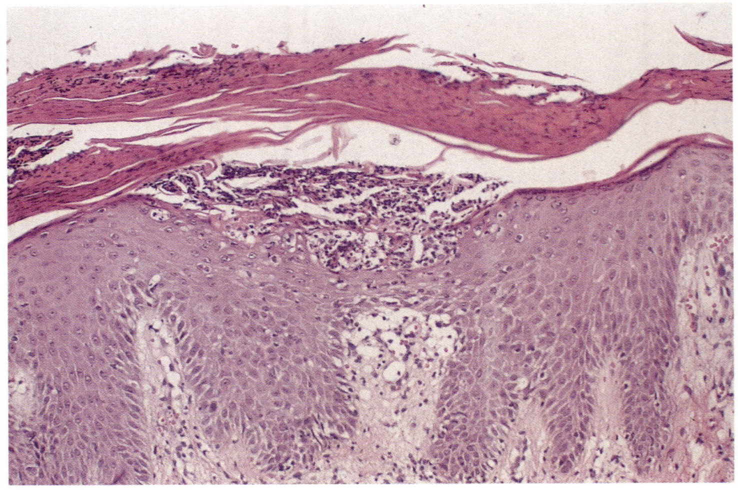

Figure 1–58. Psoriasis, early or eruptive lesion. Subcorneal collection of neutrophils, hyperparakeratosis and psoriasiform epidermal hyperplasia. In the dermis there is severe papillary edema, dilated blood vessels, and a mixed-cell infiltrate with neutrophils.

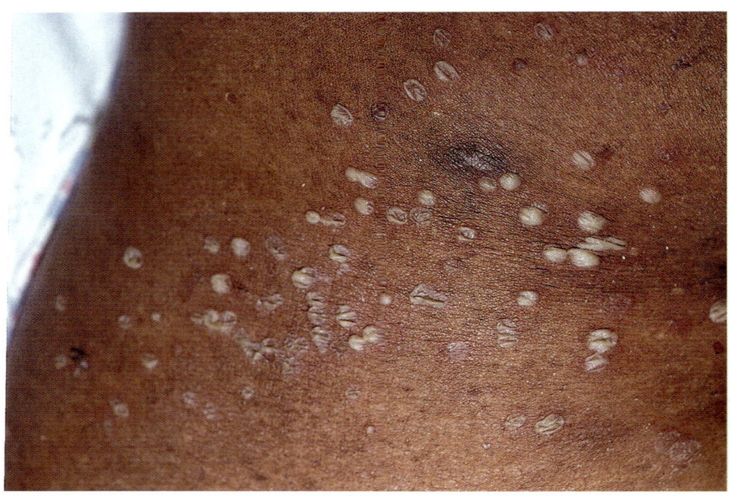

Figure 1–59. Pustular psoriasis. Scattered discrete pustules on the trunk.

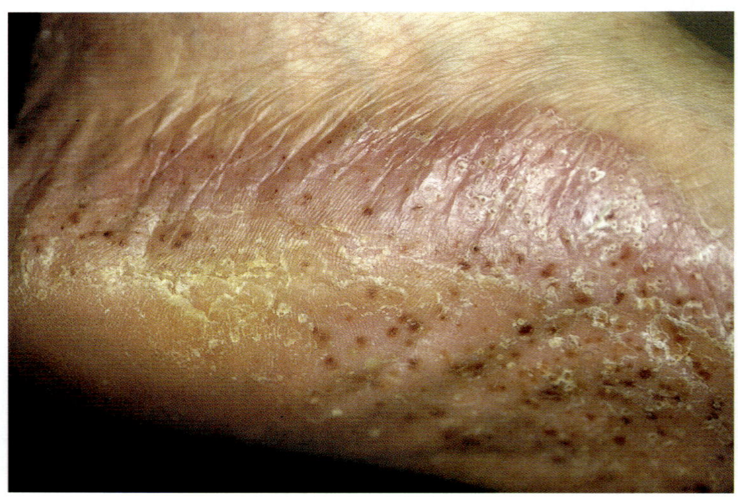

Figure 1–60. Pustular psoriasis. Confluent papulopustules on the sides and sole of the foot.

PSORIASIS

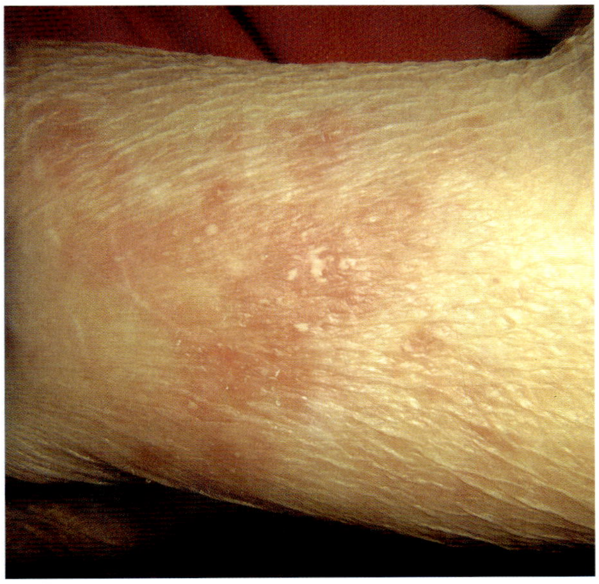

Figure 1–61. Pustular psoriasis. Grouped and confluent pustules overlying macular erythema on the arm.

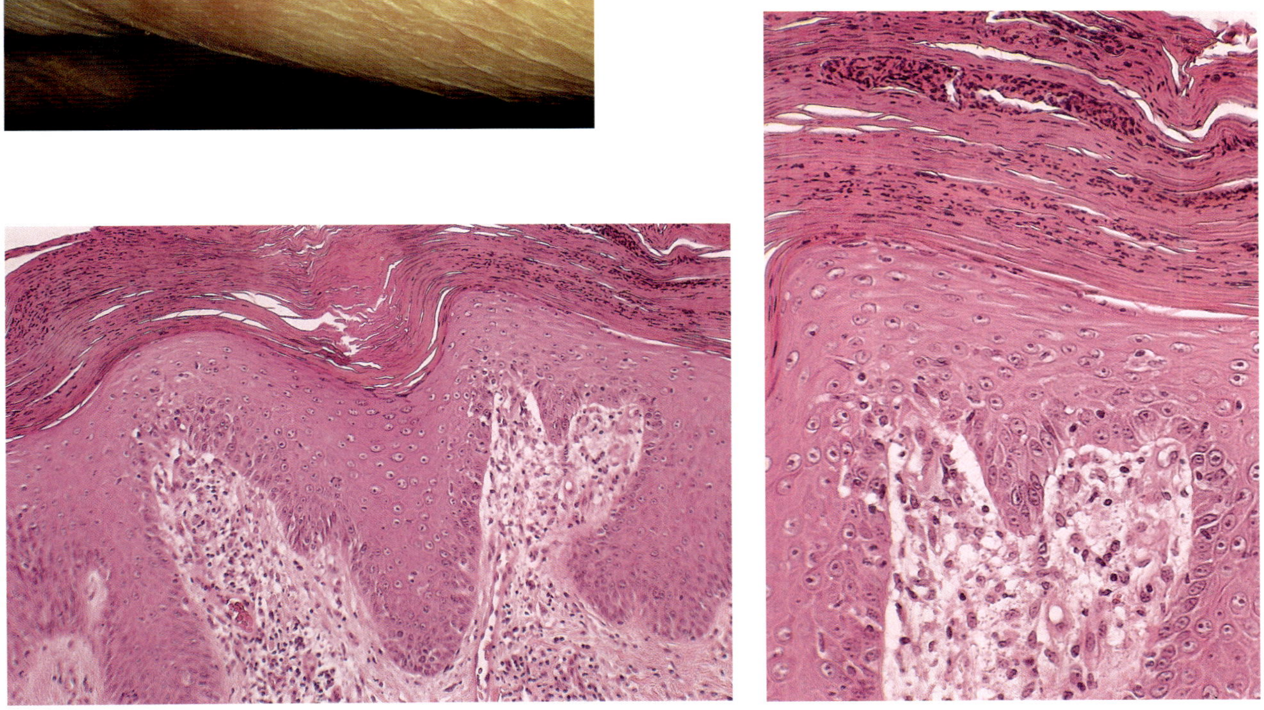

A B

Figures 1–62A, 1–62B. Psoriasis, evolving lesion. Epidermal hyperplasia, with mounds of parakeratosis and neutrophils at all levels of the epidermis. There are dilated blood vessels and a mixed-cell infiltrate within the edematous papillary dermis.

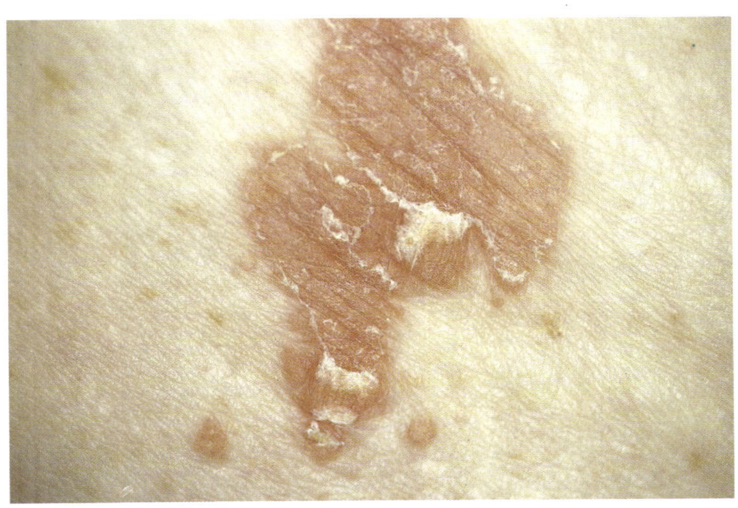

Figure 1–63. Psoriasis, evolving plaque.

PSORIASIS

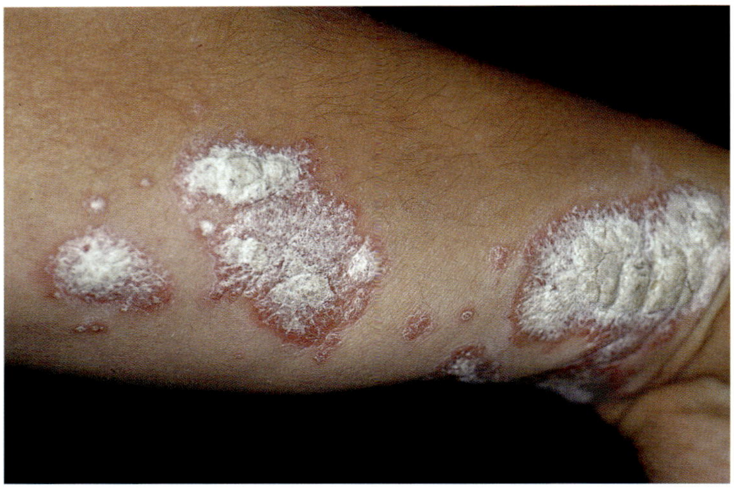

Figure 1–64. Psoriasis, fully developed plaque.

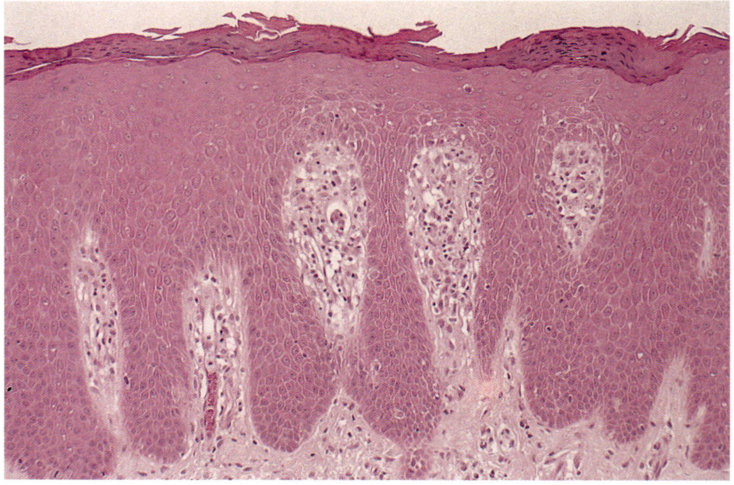

Figure 1–65. Psoriasis, fully developed plaque. Confluent compact orthokeratosis and parakeratosis and occasional neutrophils. There is prominent epidermal hyperplasia with elongated, thin rete ridges of approximate equal length. The papillary dermis is thickened with dilated and congested blood vessels and a mixed-cell infiltrate.

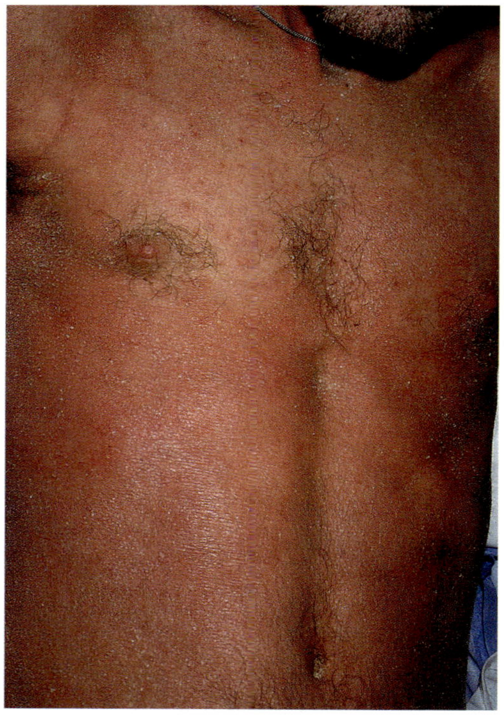

Figure 1–66. Psoriatic erythroderma. There is confluent erythema and scaling.

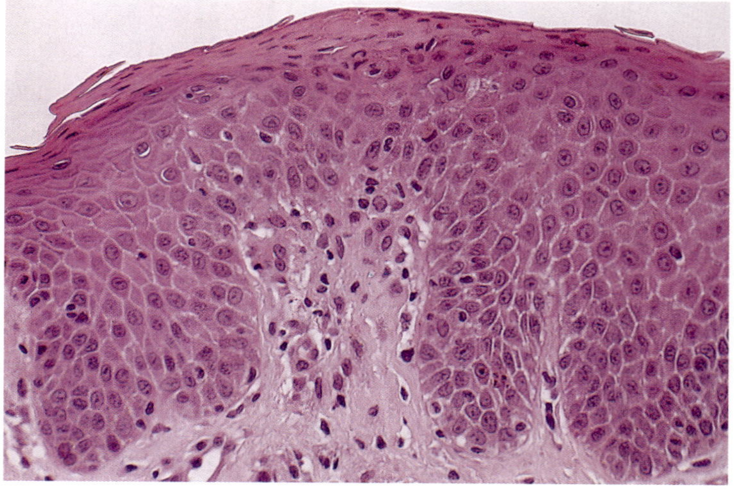

Figure 1–67. Psoriatic erythroderma. Epidermal hyperplasia and diffuse parakeratosis with a scattering of neutrophils in the epidermis and dermis.

GUTTATE PARAPSORIASIS

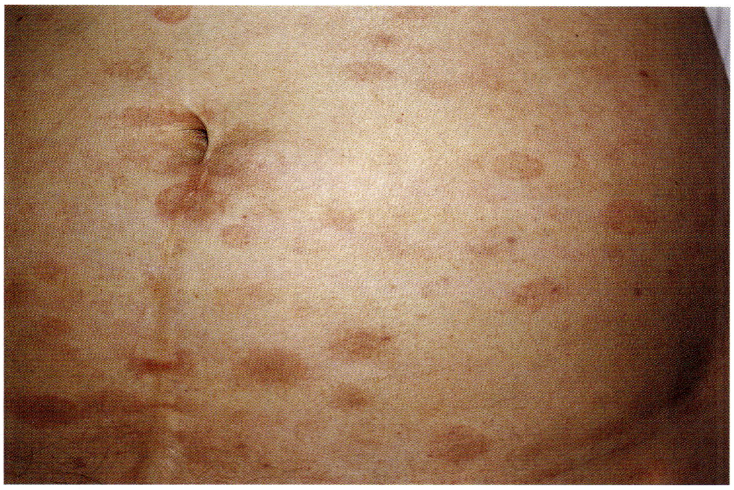

Figure 1–68. Guttate parapsoriasis. Erythematous, scaly macules and patches.

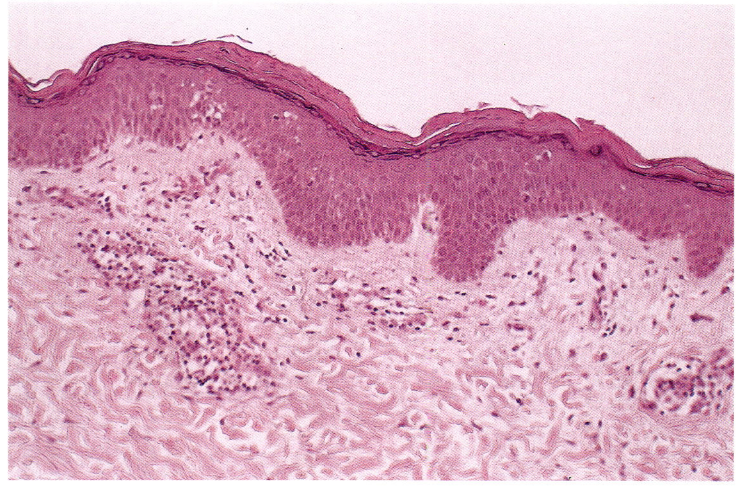

Figure 1–69. Guttate parapsoriasis. Slight epidermal hyperplasia and focal spongiosis, orthokeratosis and parakeratosis with minimal scale-crust. The dermis contains a sparse perivascular lymphohistiocytic infiltrate.

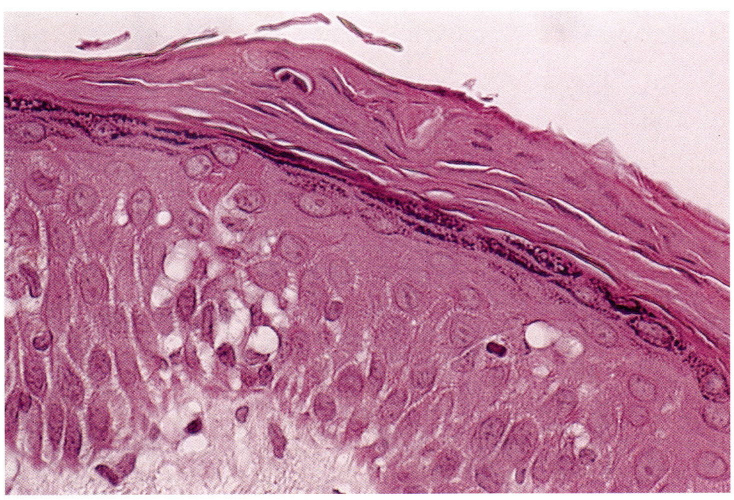

Figure 1–70. Guttate parapsoriasis. Spongiosis, compact orthokeratosis, and parakeratosis.

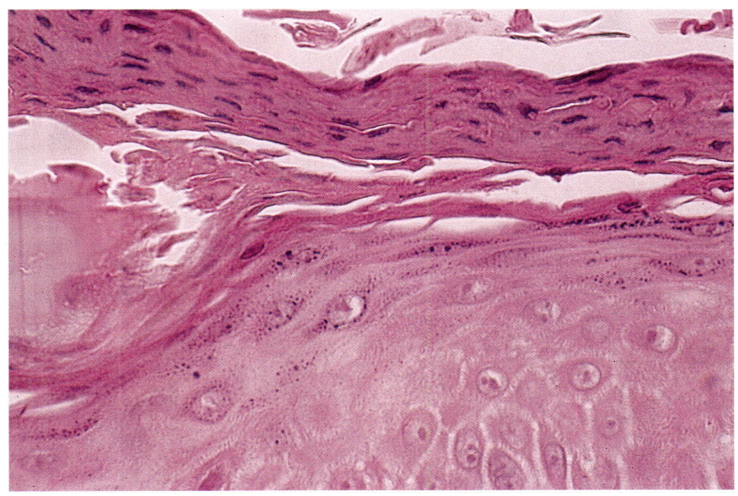

Figure 1–71. Guttate parapsoriasis. Scale-crust.

PITYRIASIS RUBRA PILARIS

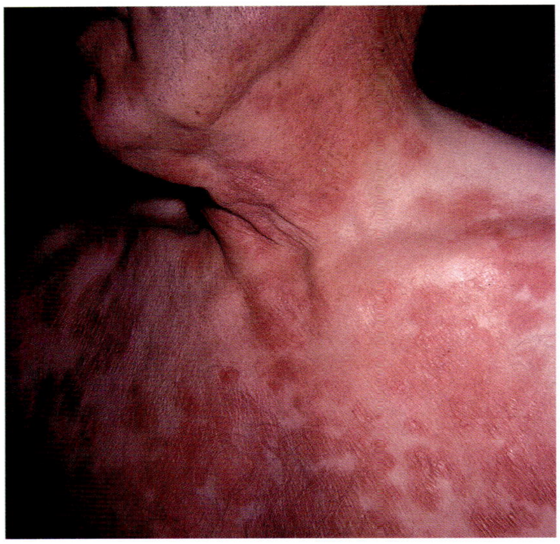

Figure 1–72. **Pityriasis rubra pilaris.** Erythematous scaly patches and plaques on the chest and neck.

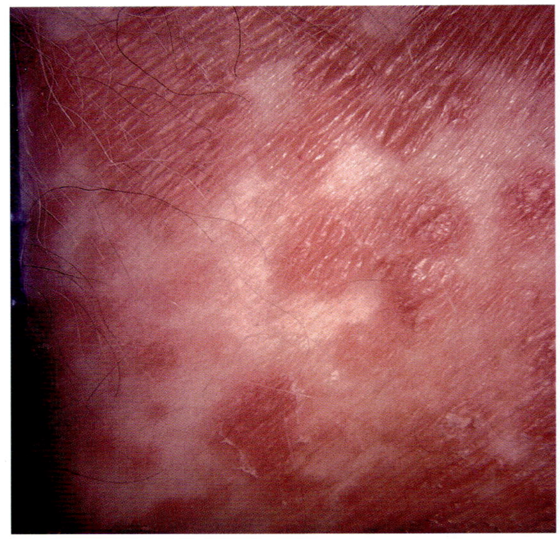

Figure 1–73. **Pityriasis rubra pilaris.** Islands of normal skin within erythematous patches and plaques that are characteristic of this disease.

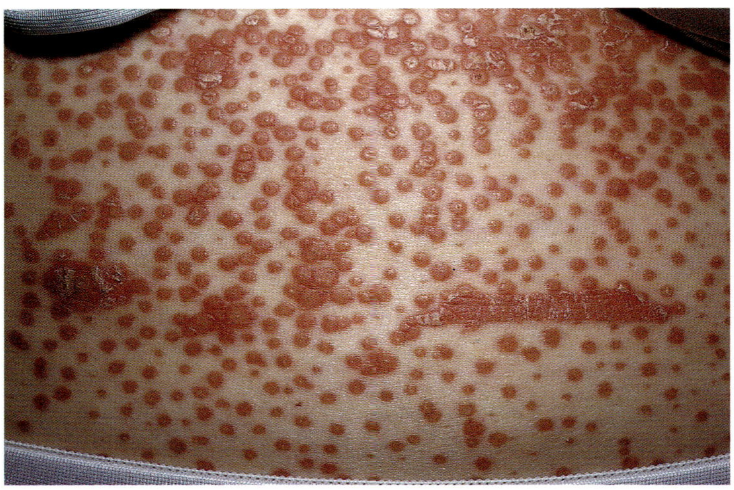

Figure 1–74. **Pityriasis rubra pilaris.** There are both agminated erythematous papules and areas of confluence within areas of normal skin.

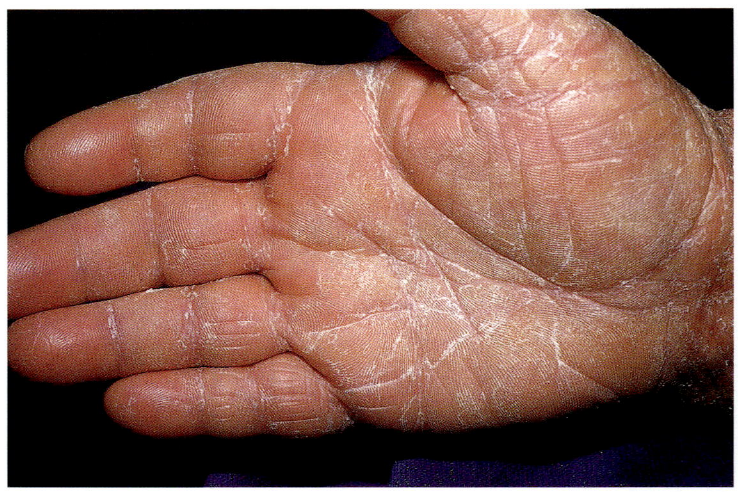

Figure 1–75. **Pityriasis rubra pilaris.** Diffuse thickening and scaling of volar aspect of fingers and palm with accentuation of skin creases.

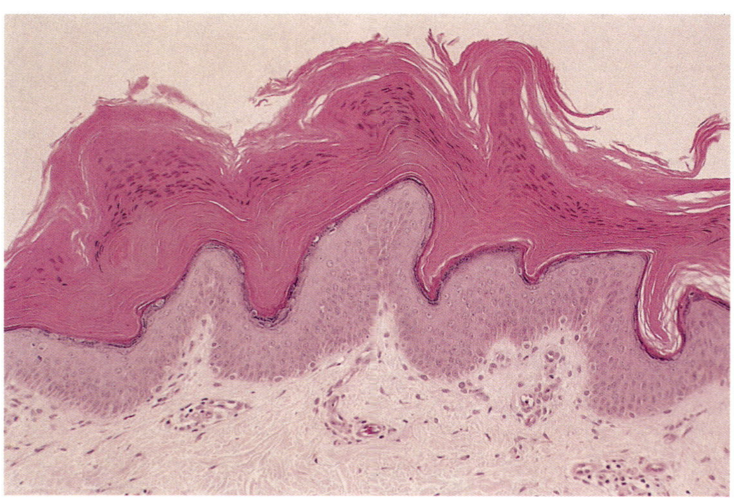

Figure 1–76. **Pityriasis rubra pilaris.** Epidermal hyperplasia with rounded rete ridges, a prominent granular layer, and protuberant hyperkeratosis with alternating orthokeratosis and parakeratosis. In the dermis there is a mild perivascular lymphohistiocytic infiltrate.

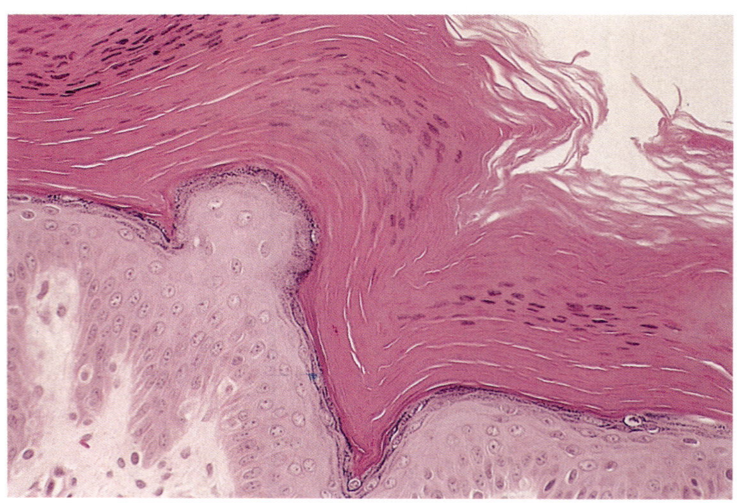

Figure 1–77. **Pityriasis rubra pilaris.** Columns of hyperkeratosis with alternating orthokeratosis and parakeratosis.

REITER'S SYNDROME

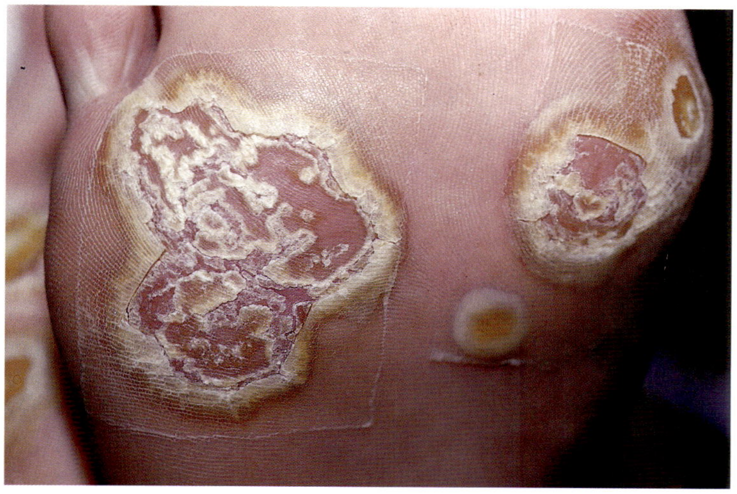

Figure 1–78. Reiter's syndrome, keratoderma blennorrhagica. Multiple, annular, hyperkeratotic plaques with central clearing on the sole of the foot.

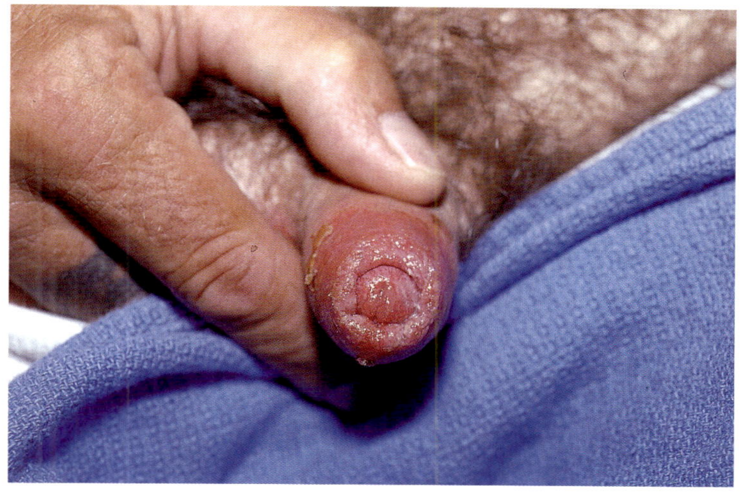

Figure 1–79. Reiter's syndrome, balanitis circinata. Confluent, oozing erythematous papules with crust on the glans penis and foreskin.

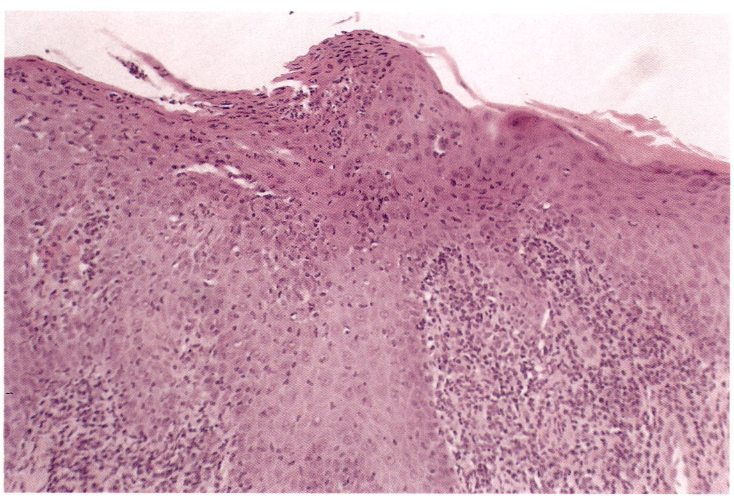

Figure 1–80. Reiter's syndrome. Psoriasiform epidermal hyperplasia with massive parakeratosis. Numerous neutrophils, singly and in collections, are present within the spinous and cornified layers of the epidermis. There is a dense dermal mixed-cell infiltrate with numerous neutrophils.

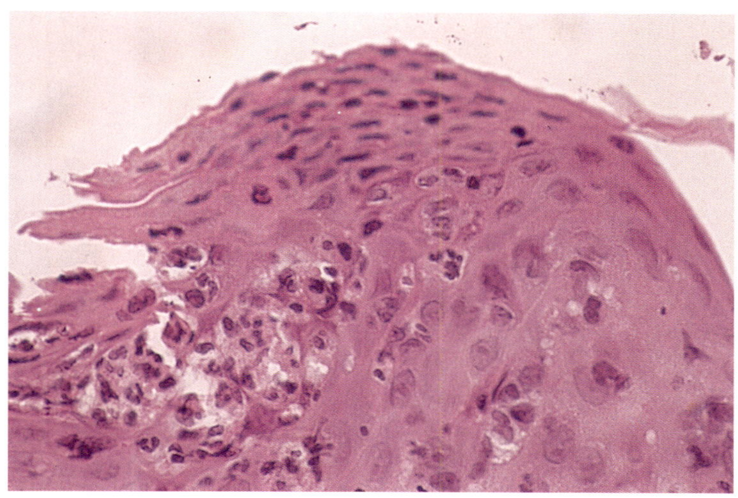

Figure 1–81. Reiter's syndrome. Collections of neutrophils within mounds of parakeratosis.

2

INTERFACE AND LICHENOID DERMATITIS

- Erythema multiforme
- Lichen sclerosus et atrophicus
- Erythema ab igne
- Lichen planus
- Lichenoid purpura (pigmented purpuric dermatosis)
- Pityriasis lichenoides et varioliformis acuta (PLEVA) and chronica (PLC) (Mucha-Habermann disease)
- Discoid lupus erythematosus
- Subacute lupus erythematosus
- Systemic lupus erythematosus
- Neonatal lupus erythematosus
- Dermatomyositis
- Lichen striatus
- Graft-versus-host disease (GVHD)

Acute horn
erythema multiforme
~~lichenoid drug~~
FDE
TEN
GVHD

Vacuolar
SLE
SCLE / DLE
DMM
EM
± GVHD

ERYTHEMA MULTIFORME

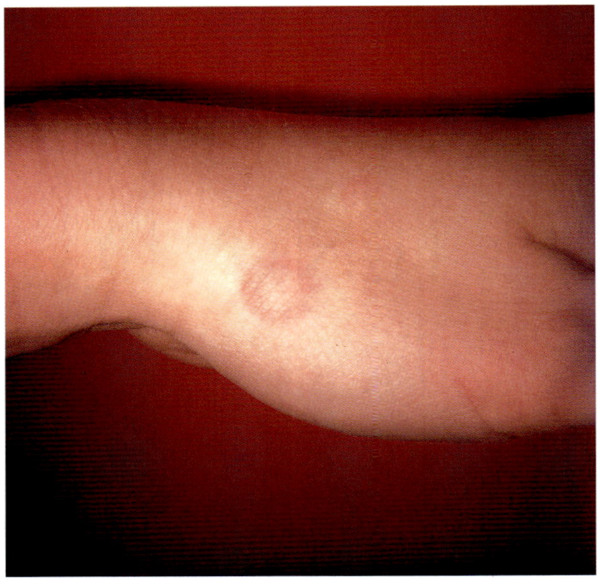

Figure 2–1. Erythema multiforme. Early erythematous papules.

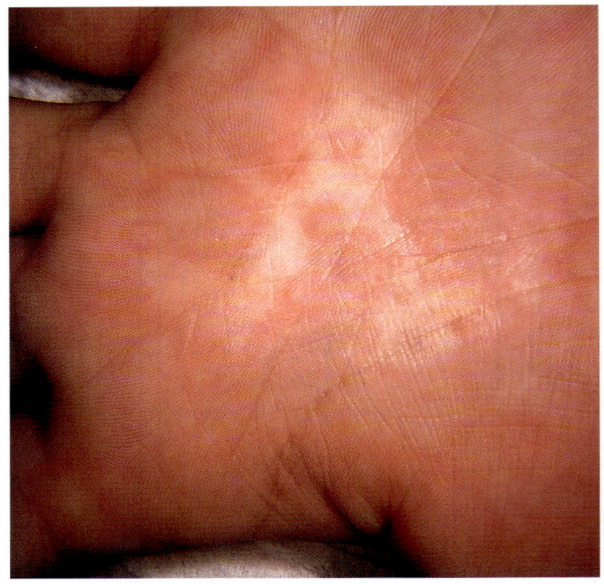

Figure 2–2. Erythema multiforme. Evolving erythematous papules and plaques with targetoid appearance.

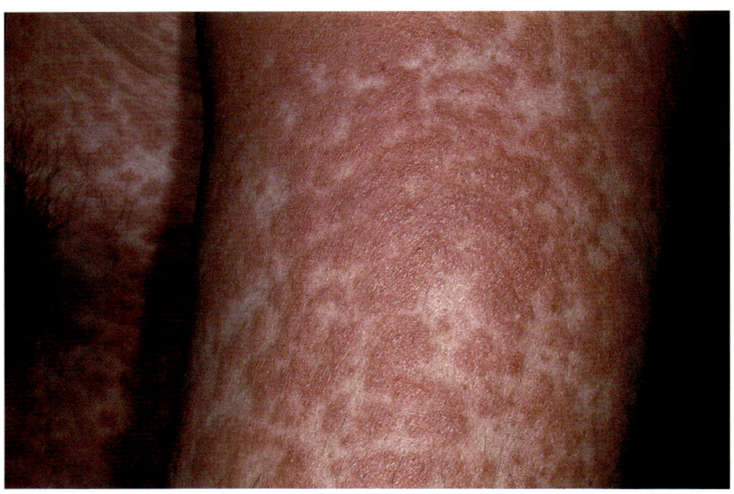

Figure 2–3. Erythema multiforme. Confluent erythematous papules and plaques.

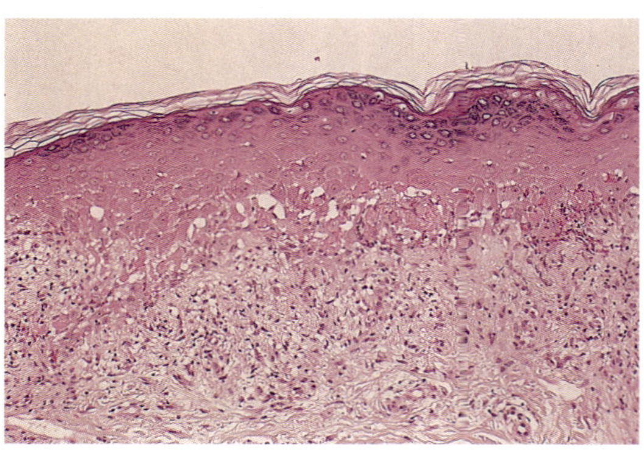

A

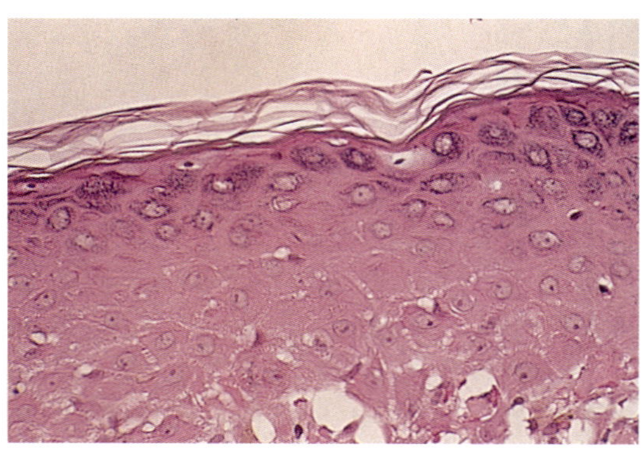

B

Figures 2–4A, 2–4B. Erythema multiforme. An early evolving lesion with basket-weave orthokeratosis, persistent granular layer, spongiosis, ballooned, necrotic keratinocytes and vacuolar alteration. A few neutrophils are associated with necrotic keratinocytes. There is severe papillary edema, dilated blood vessels, and a lymphohistiocytic infiltrate.

ERYTHEMA MULTIFORME

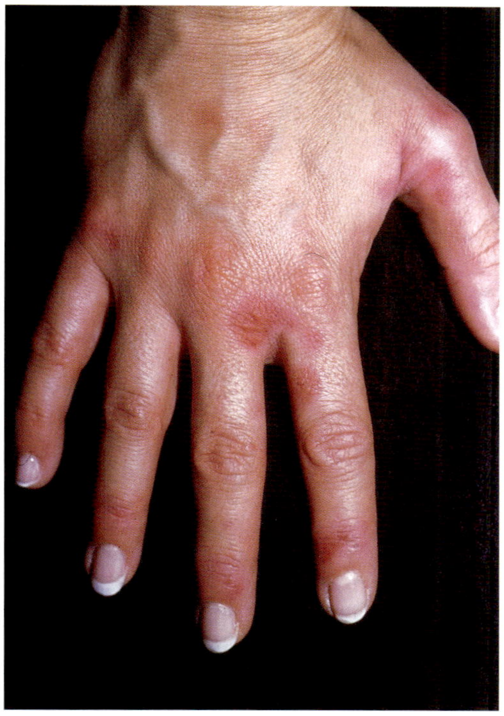

Figure 2–5. Bullous erythema multiforme. Erythematous vesiculo-papules have a targetoid appearance.

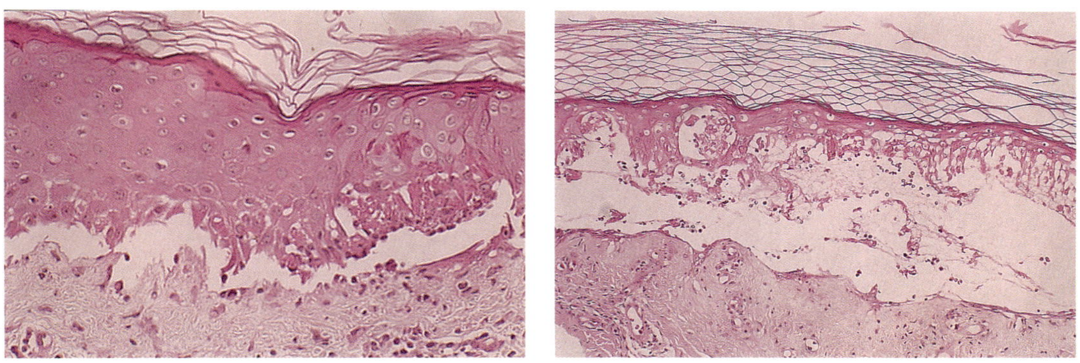

A

B

Figures 2–6A, 2–6B. Bullous erythema multiforme. Fully developed lesions with spongiotic and intraepidermal vesiculation, as well as subepidermal bullae.

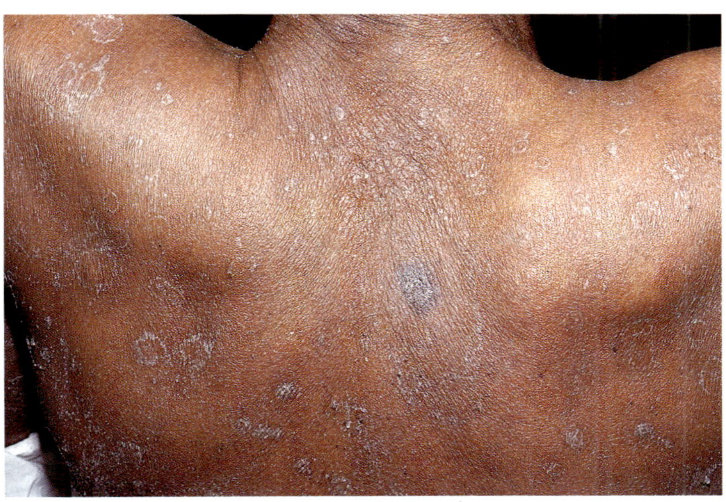

Figure 2–7. Erythema multiforme. Devolution of macular, scaly, and hyperpigmented lesions.

LICHEN SCLEROSUS ET ATROPHICUS

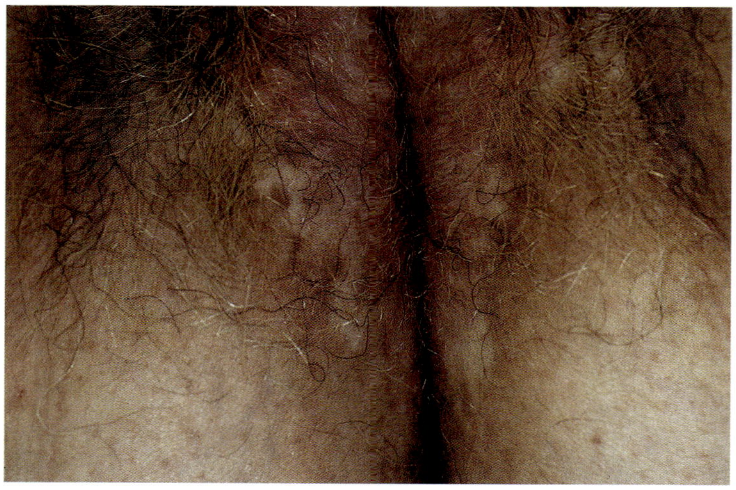

Figure 2–8. Lichen sclerosus et atrophicus. White patches on labia majora.

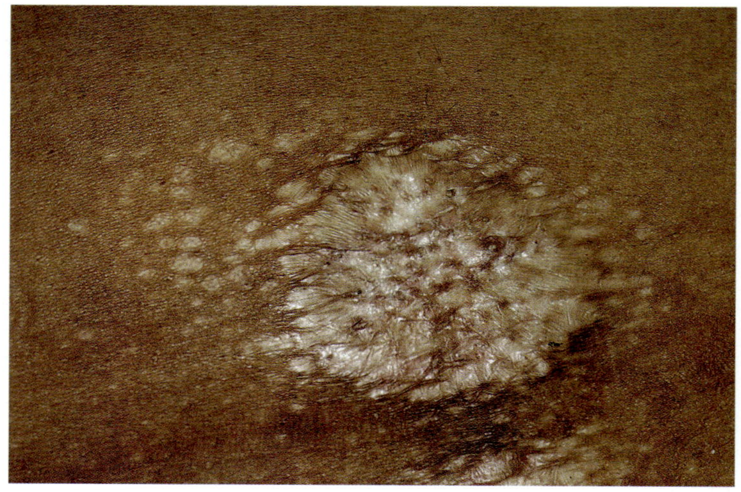

Figure 2–9. Lichen sclerosus et atrophicus. Discrete and confluent white papules with distinctive and characteristic dells, which represent dilated, plugged infundibula.

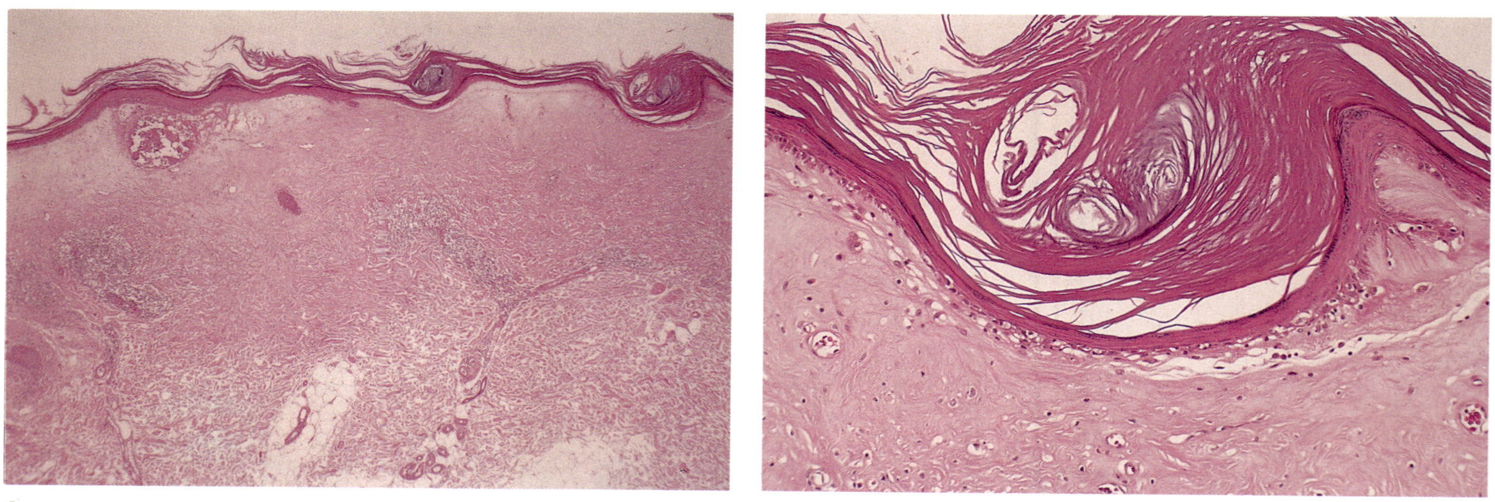

A **B**

Figures 2–10A, 2–10B. Lichen sclerosus et atrophicus. Thinned epidermis, follicular hyperkeratosis, and vacuolar alteration with subepidermal cleft. There is subjacent dermal edema, sclerosis, dilated blood vessels, and a patchy lymphohistiocytic infiltrate.

ERYTHEMA AB IGNE

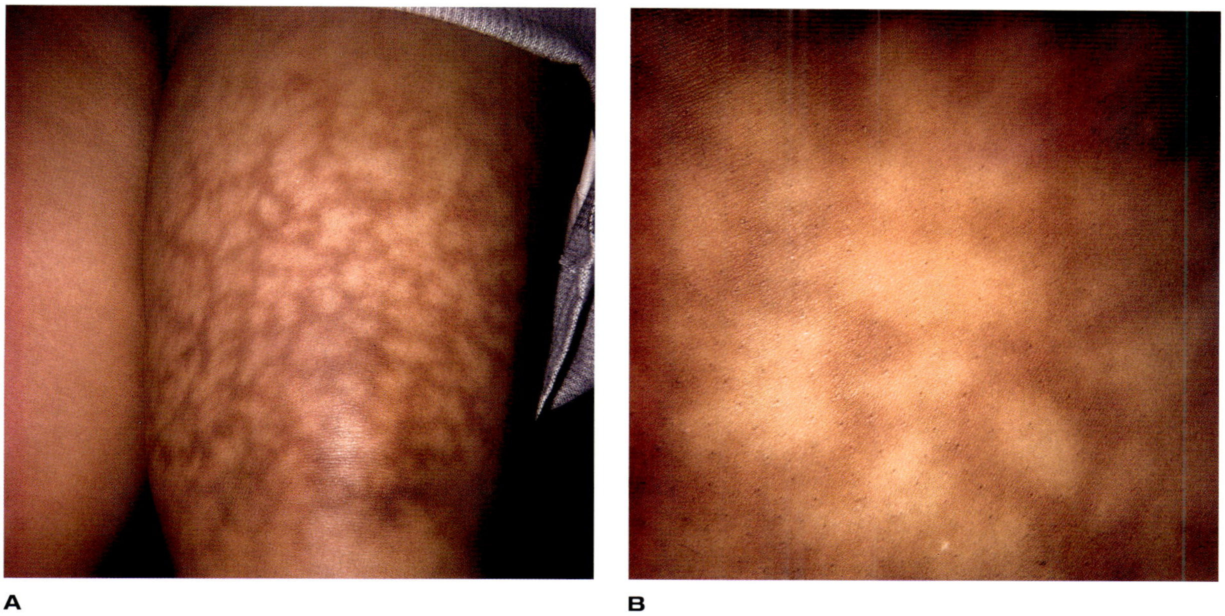

Figures 2–11A, 2–11B. Erythema ab igne. Prolonged application of a heating pad resulting in a localized reticulated area on the thigh.

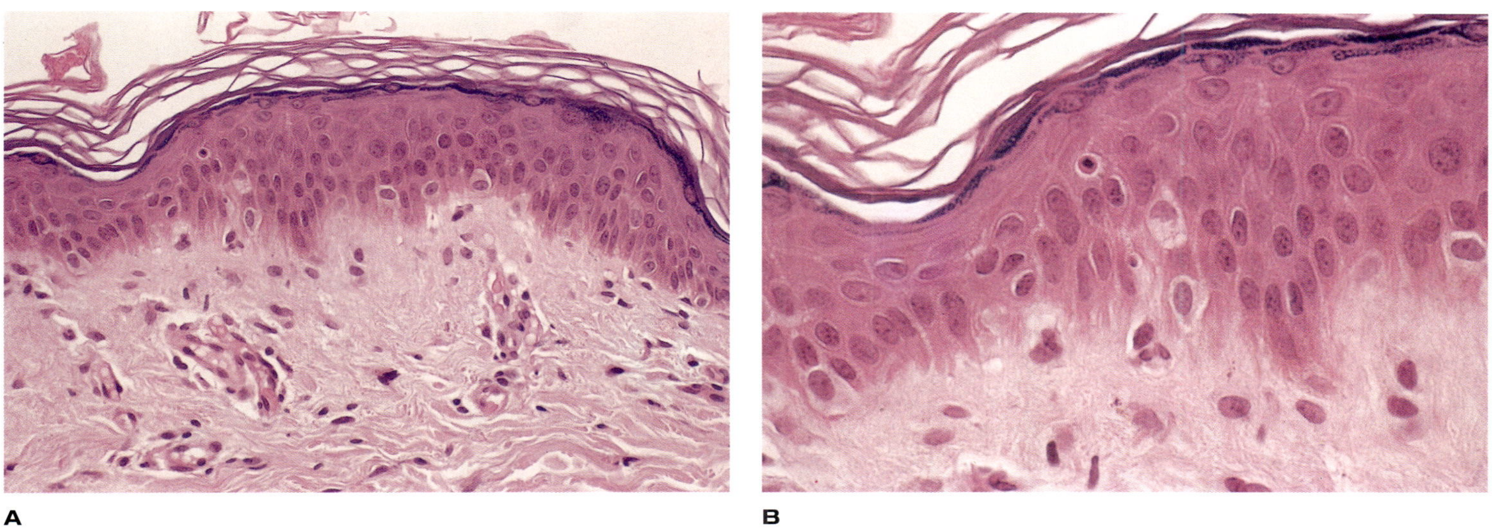

Figures 2–12A, 2–12B. Erythema ab igne. The epidermis has patchy vacuolar alteration and a solitary necrotic keratinocyte. Melanophages and dilated blood vessels with a mild perivascular inflammatory mixed-cell infiltrate fill the dermis.

LICHEN PLANUS

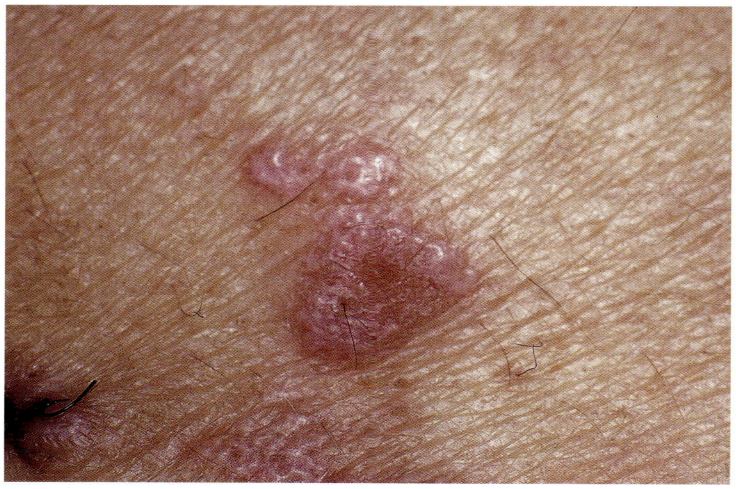

Figure 2–13. Lichen planus. Pink flat-topped papules with reticulate gray lines (Wickham's striae).

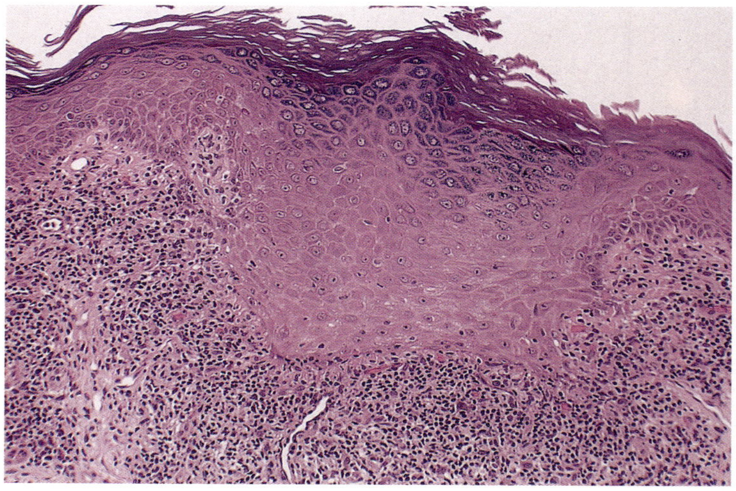

Figure 2–14. Lichen planus. Hyperkeratosis, wedge-shaped hypergranulosis, and irregular epidermal hyperplasia. A dense lichenoid lymphohistiocytic infiltrate obscures the dermoepidermal junction.

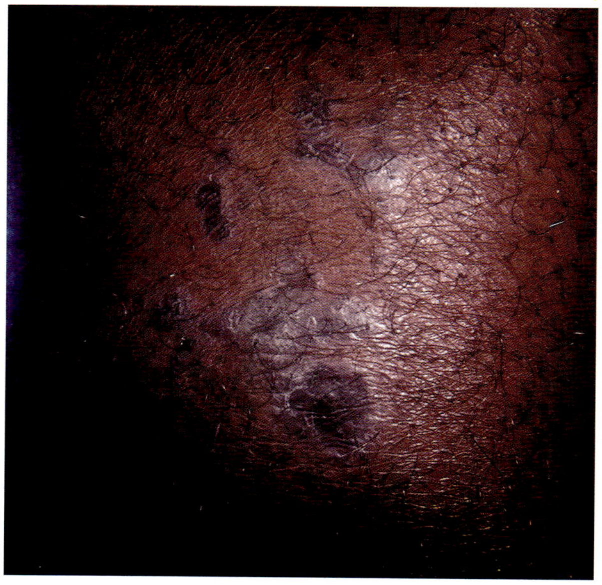

Figure 2–15. Hypertrophic lichen planus. Verrucous, raised hyperpigmented papules and plaques on the lower leg.

LICHEN PLANUS

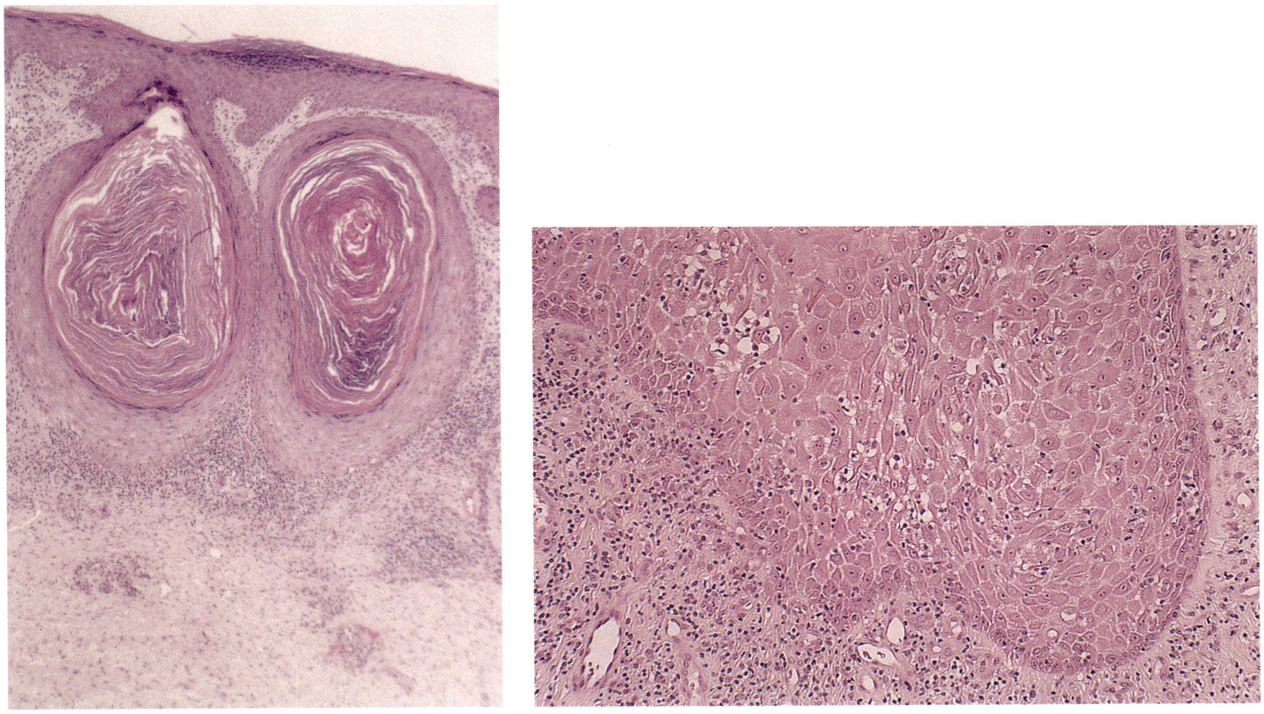

A B

Figures 2–16A, 2–16B. Hypertrophic lichen planus. Dilated, hyperplastic, and bulbous infundibula. At the base of an infundibulum there is a characteristic lichenoid lymphohistiocytic

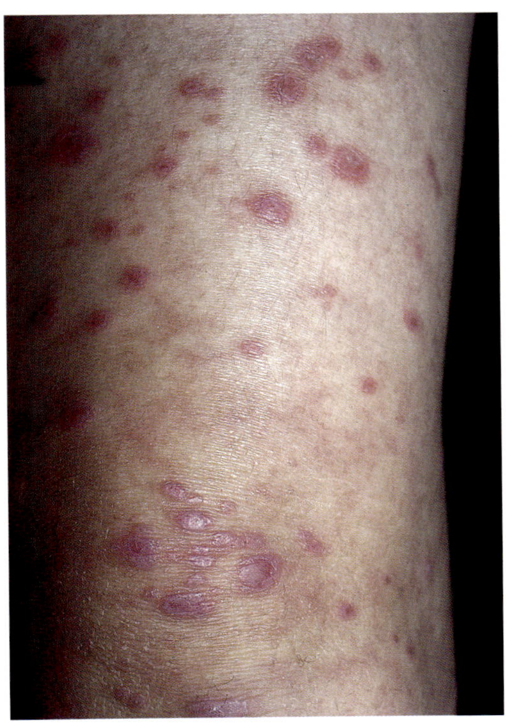

Figure 2–17. Atrophic lichen planus. Flat-topped papules with central depression.

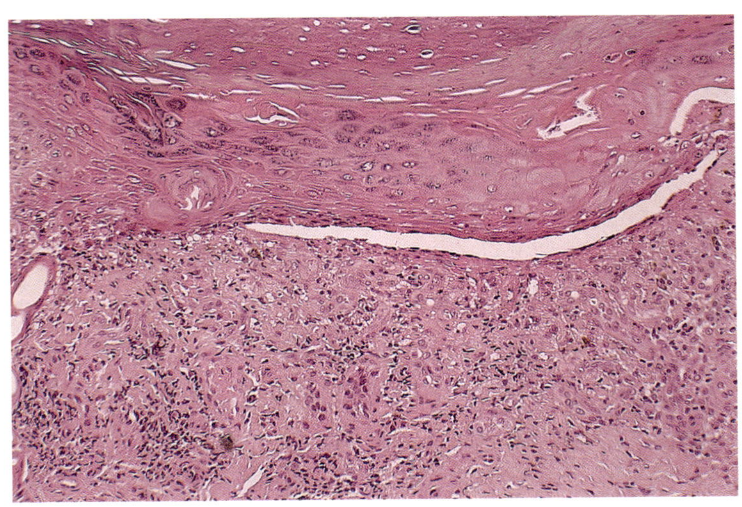

Figure 2–18. Atrophic lichen planus. Epidermal hyperkeratosis, hypergranulosis, subepidermal cleft (Max Joseph space), and a thickened papillary dermis with fibroplasia and a lymphohistiocytic infiltrate.

LICHEN PLANUS

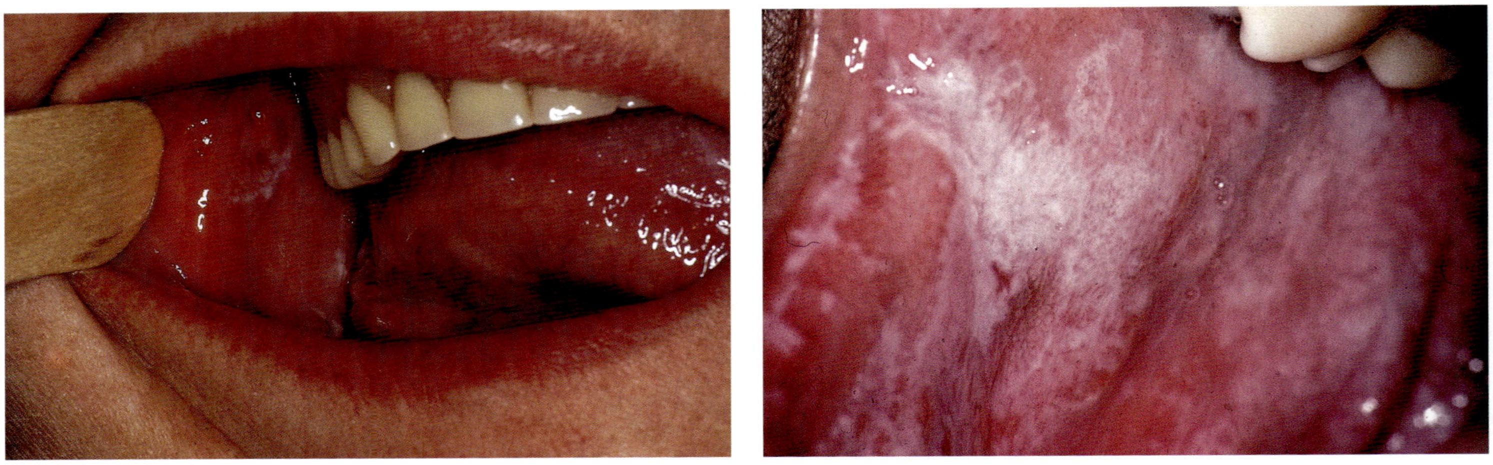

A B

Figures 2–19A, 2–19B. Oral lichen planus. Reticulate gray streaks and patches on the buccal mucosa.

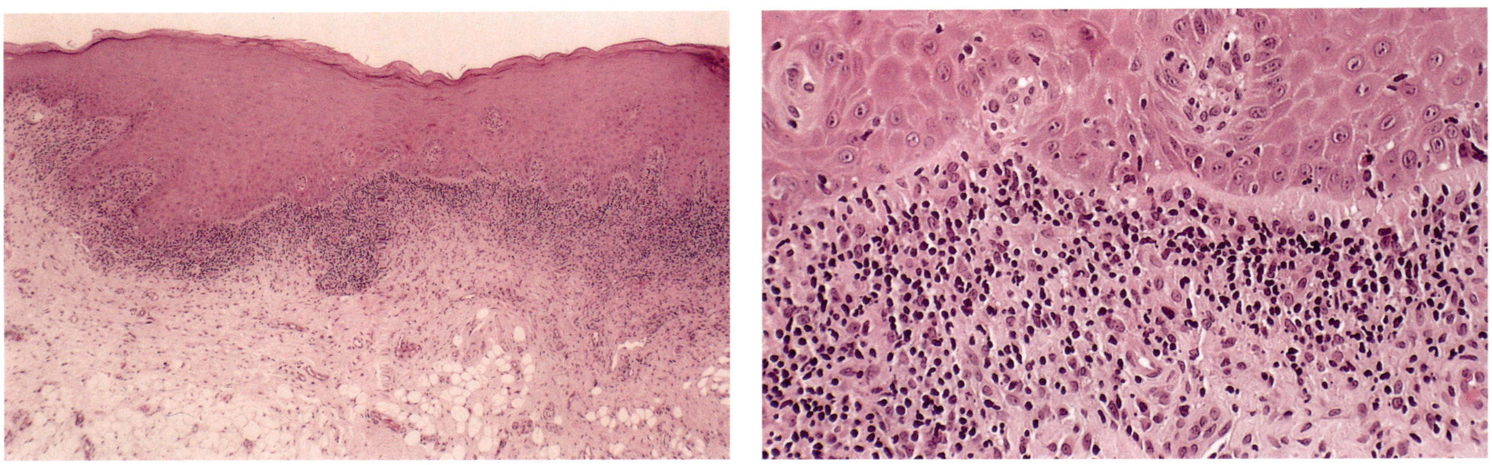

A B

Figures 2–20A, 2–20B. Oral lichen planus. Hyperplastic mucosal epithelium with necrotic epithelial cells. There is a dense lymphohistiocytic infiltrate filling the upper lamina propria.

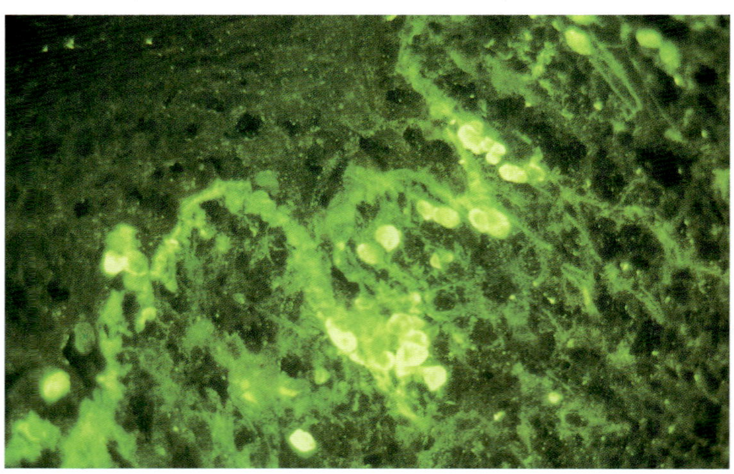

Figure 2–21. Lichen planus. Direct immunofluorescence of lichen planus reveals deposition of fibrinogen in several cytoid bodies and dyskeratotic cells. Note additional fluorescence along the dermo-epidermal junction.

LICHENOID PURPURA (PIGMENTED PURPURIC DERMATOSIS)

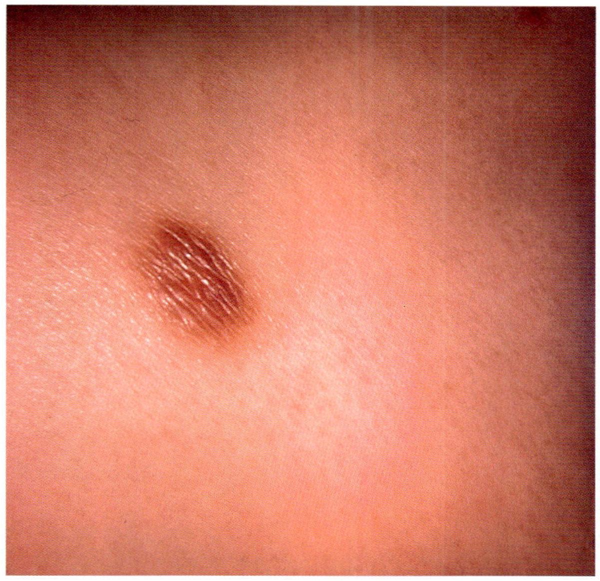

Figure 2–22. Lichenoid purpura. Erythematous dome-shaped nodule on the back.

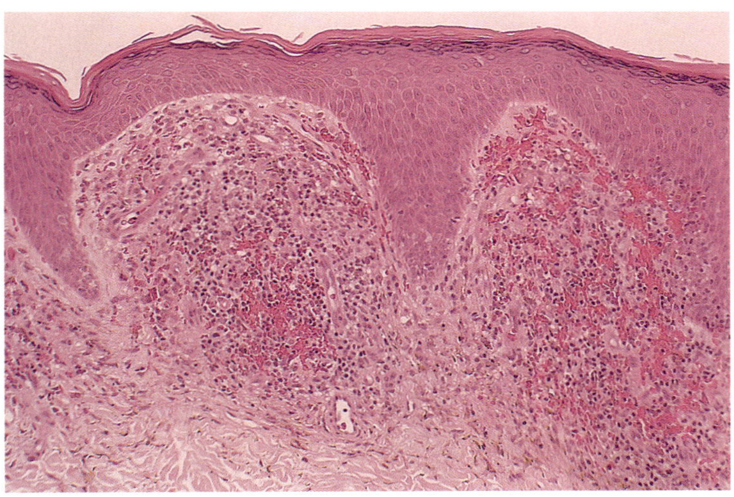

A

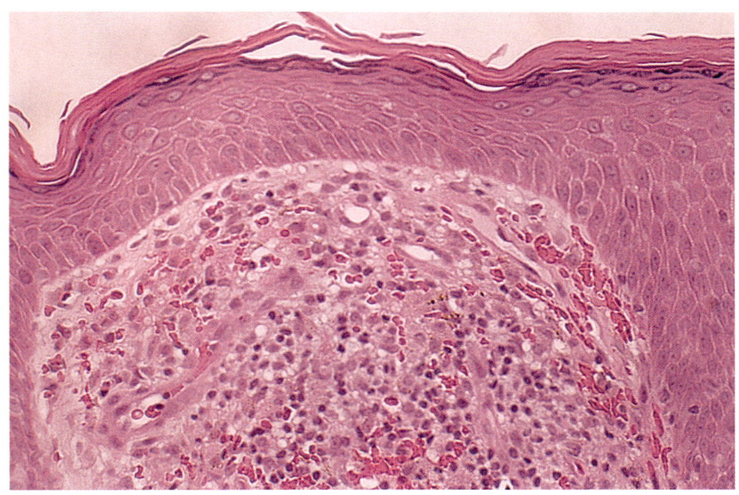

B

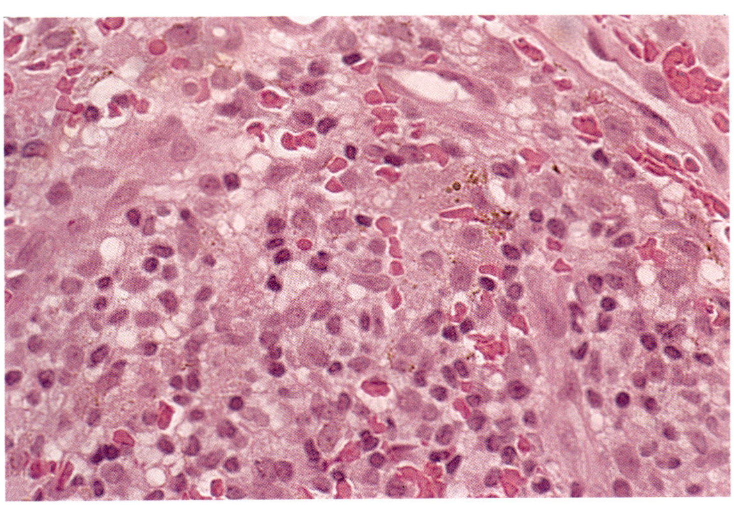

C

Figures 2–23A, 2–23B, 23C. Lichenoid purpura. The dermoepidermal junction is focally obscured by a dense infiltrate composed of lymphocytes and histiocytes, and extravasated erythrocytes. There is a proliferation of dilated and congested venules in the upper dermis.

PITYRIASIS LICHENOIDES ET VARIOLIFORMIS ACUTA (PLEVA) AND CHRONICA (PLC) (MUCHA-HABERMANN DISEASE)

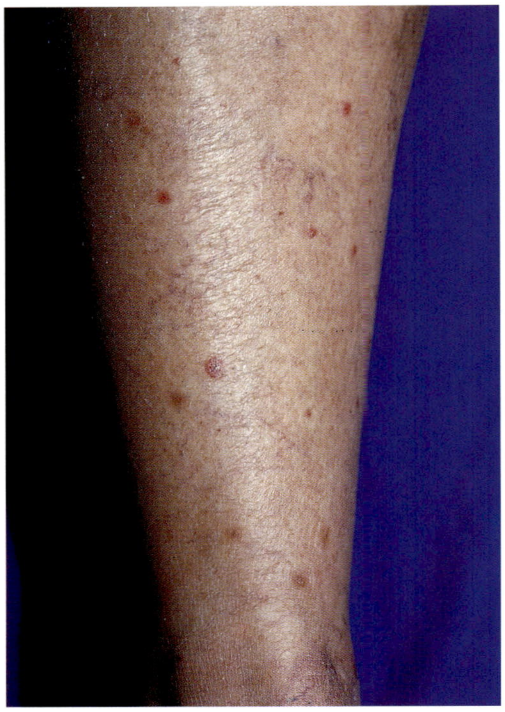

Figure 2–24. PLEVA. Dispersed erythematous papules.

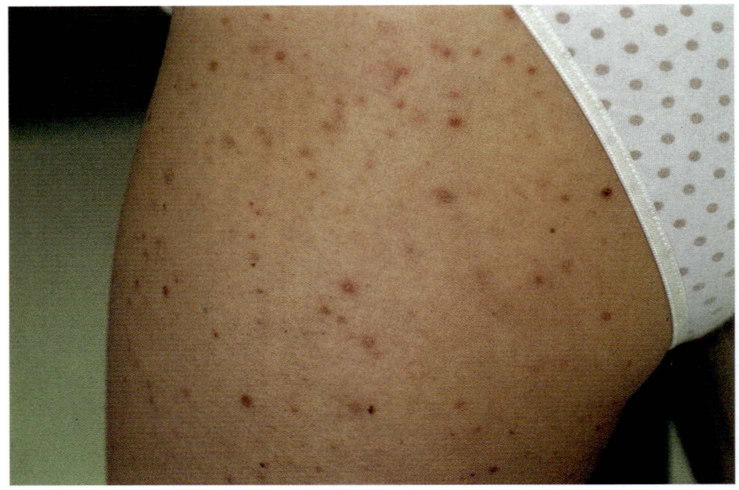

Figure 2–25. PLEVA. There is an assortment of erythematous and crusted papules, pustules, and scaly macules, which are common features of the acute stage of this disease.

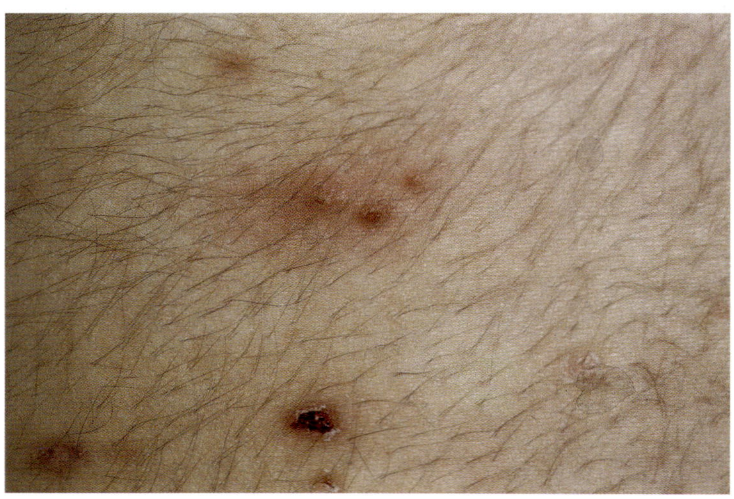

Figure 2–26. PLEVA. Ulcerated and crusted papules.

PITYRIASIS LICHENOIDES ET VARIOLIFORMIS ACUTA (PLEVA) AND CHRONICA (PLC) (MUCHA-HABERMANN DISEASE)

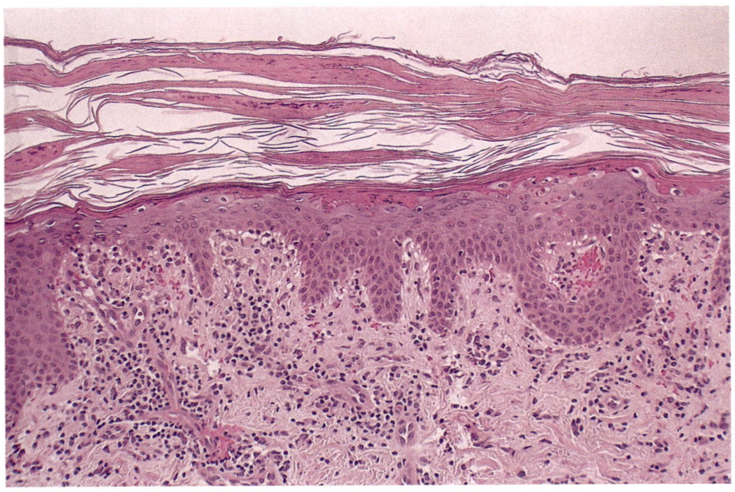

A

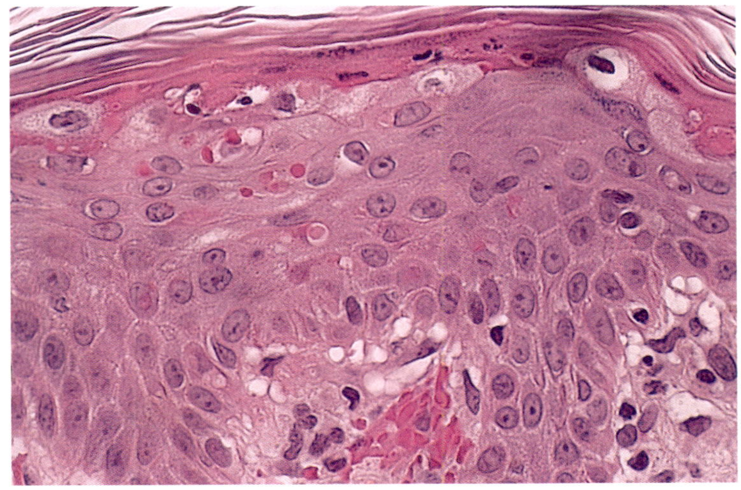

B

Figures 2–27A, 2–27B. PLEVA. Hyperkeratosis, parakeratosis with neutrophils, individual and confluent necrotic keratinocytes, extravasated erythrocytes, and vacuolar alteration. The edematous papillary dermis contains dilated blood vessels, extravasated red blood cells, and a dense lichenoid lymphohistiocytic infiltrate.

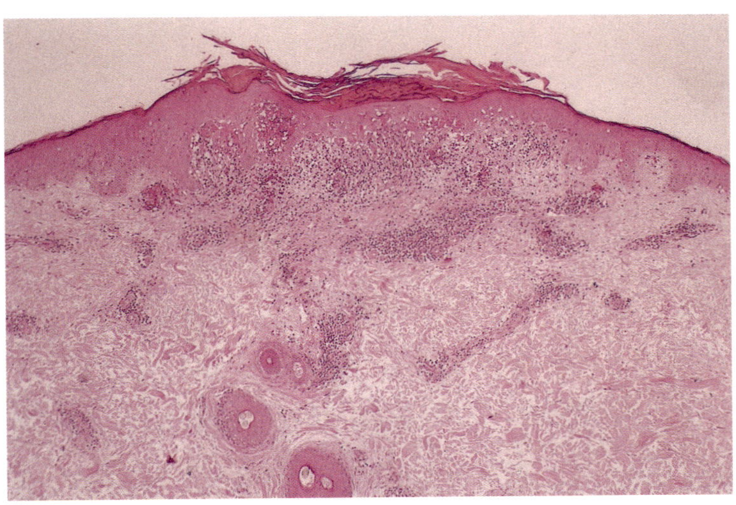

Figure 2–28. PLEVA. Epidermal scale-crust, necrotic keratinocytes, vacuolar alteration, and a dense lichenoid infiltrate, obscuring the dermoepidermal junction. In addition, there is a wedge-shaped perivascular lymphohistiocytic dermal infiltrate.

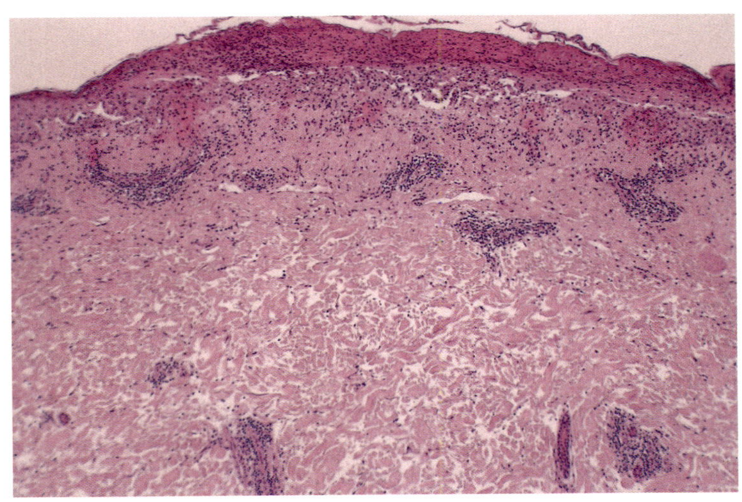

Figure 2–29. PLEVA. Epidermal ulcer, scale-crust, necrotic keratinocytes, vacuolar alteration, and a dermal perivascular lymphohistiocytic infiltrate.

PITYRIASIS LICHENOIDES ET VARIOLIFORMIS ACUTA (PLEVA) AND CHRONICA (PLC) (MUCHA-HABERMANN DISEASE)

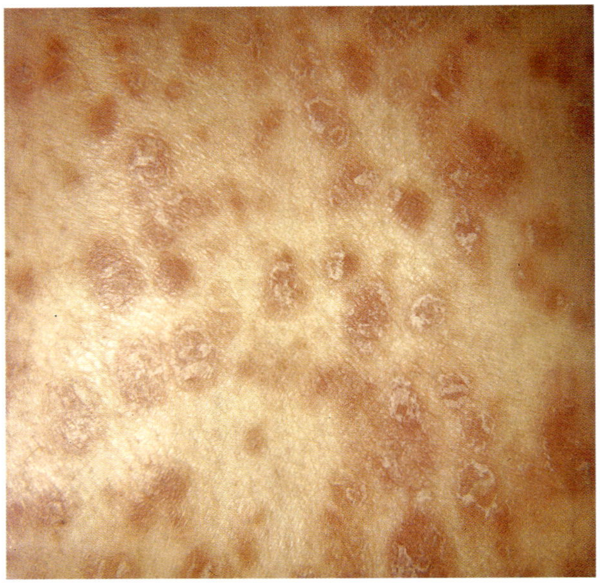

Figure 2–30. PLC. There is an expansive eruption of solitary and coalesced erythematous scaly macules and papules, typical features of the chronic stage.

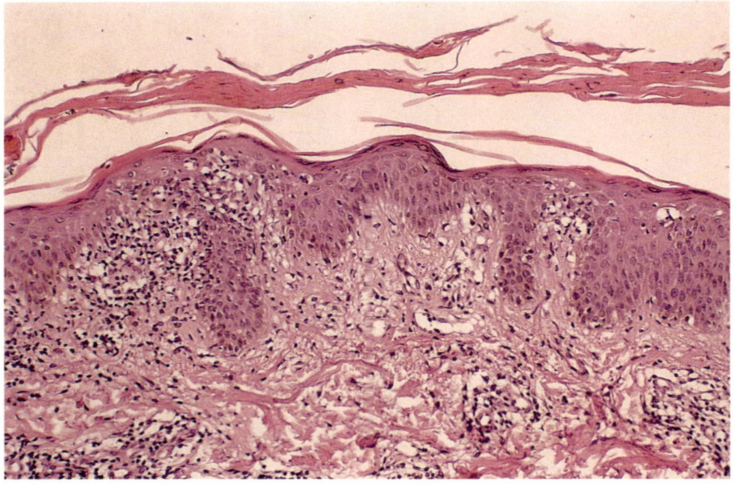

A

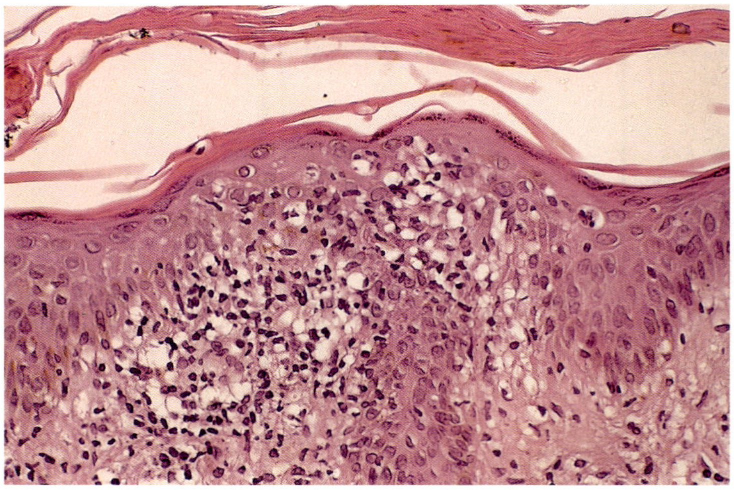

B

Figures 2–31A, 2–31B. PLC. Hyperkeratosis spongiosis, and vacuolar alteration. The dermal lymphohistiocytic infiltrate extends into the epidermis.

DISCOID LUPUS ERYTHEMATOSUS

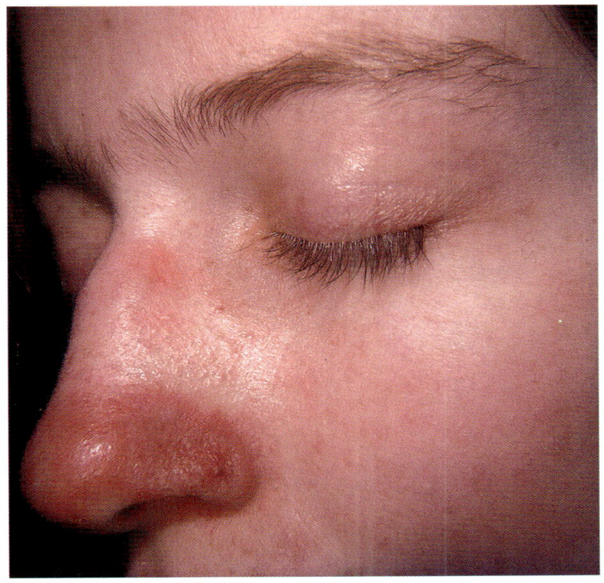

Figure 2–32. Discoid lupus erythematosus. Sharply marginated, erythematous hyperkeratotic plaque involving the tip and ala nasi of the nose.

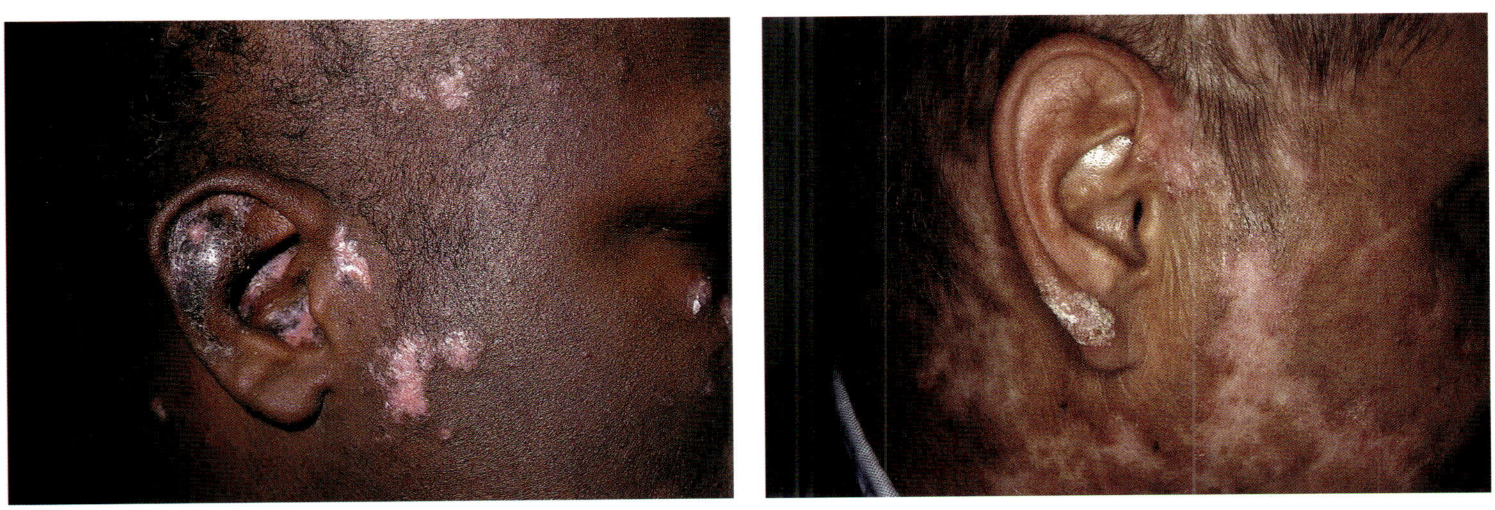

A

B

Figures 2–33A, 2–33B. Discoid lupus erythematosus. Multiple hyperpigmented and hypopigmented raised and atrophic keratotic plaques. The ear is a common site of involvement for discoid lupus erythematosus.

DISCOID LUPUS ERYTHEMATOSUS

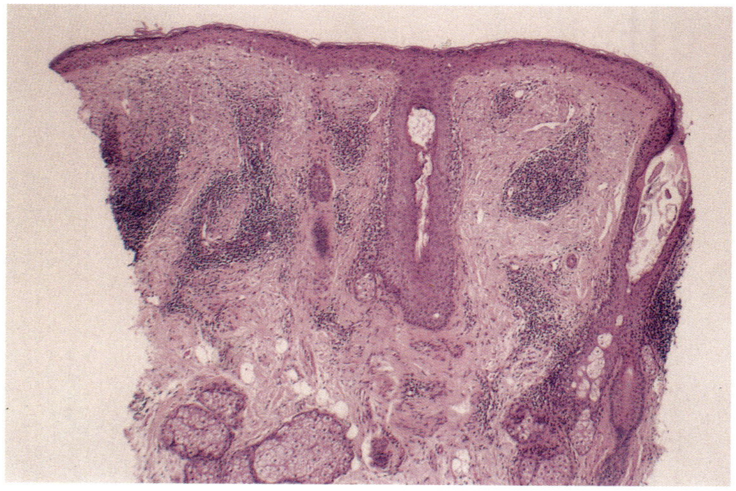

Figure 2–34. Discoid lupus erythematosus. A dense superficial and deep perivascular and periadnexal lymphohistiocytic infiltrate, with vacuolar alteration of the epidermis and infundibular epithelium. The dermis is thickened and sclerotic and there is mucin deposition between collagen bundles.

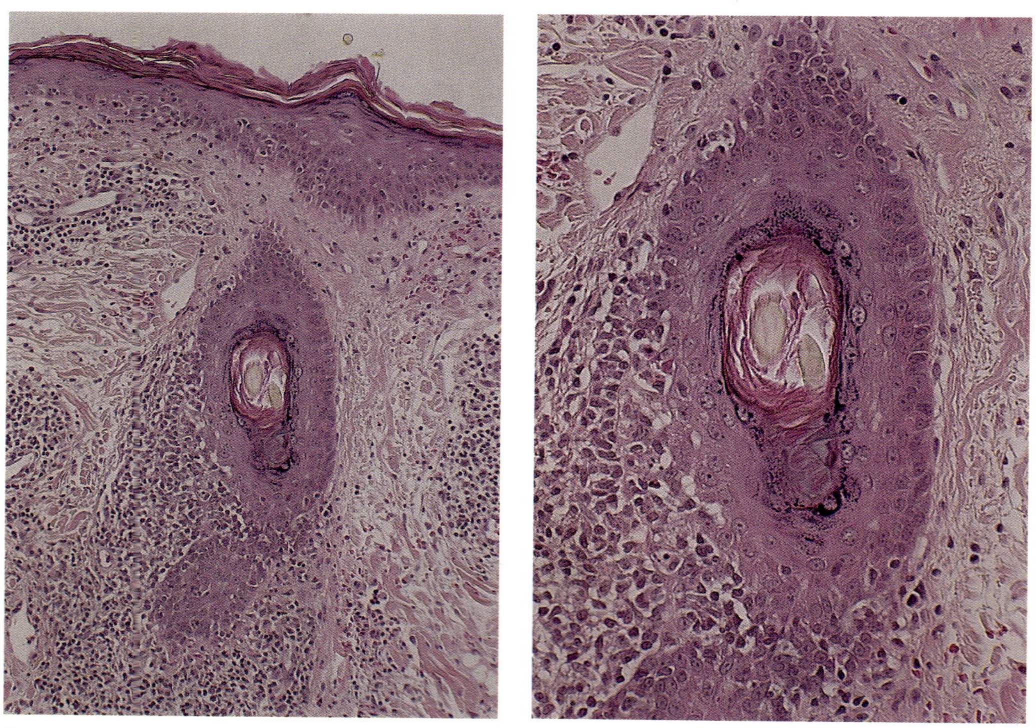

A **B**

Figures 2–35A, 2–35B. Discoid lupus erythematosus. Folliculosebaceous unit involvement with a dense lichenoid lymphohistiocytic infiltrate. Vacuolar alteration and necrotic keratinocytes are prominent.

DISCOID LUPUS ERYTHEMATOSUS

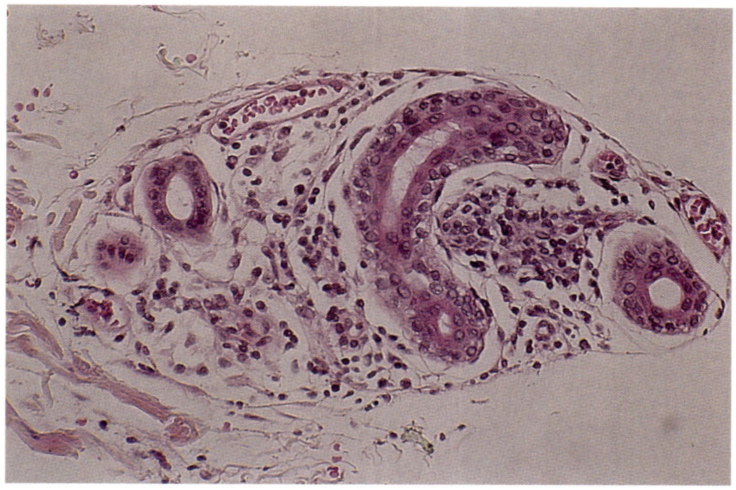

Figure 2–36. Discoid lupus erythematosus. A collection of eccrine glands and ducts surrounded by dilated blood vessels and a lymphohistiocytic infiltrate.

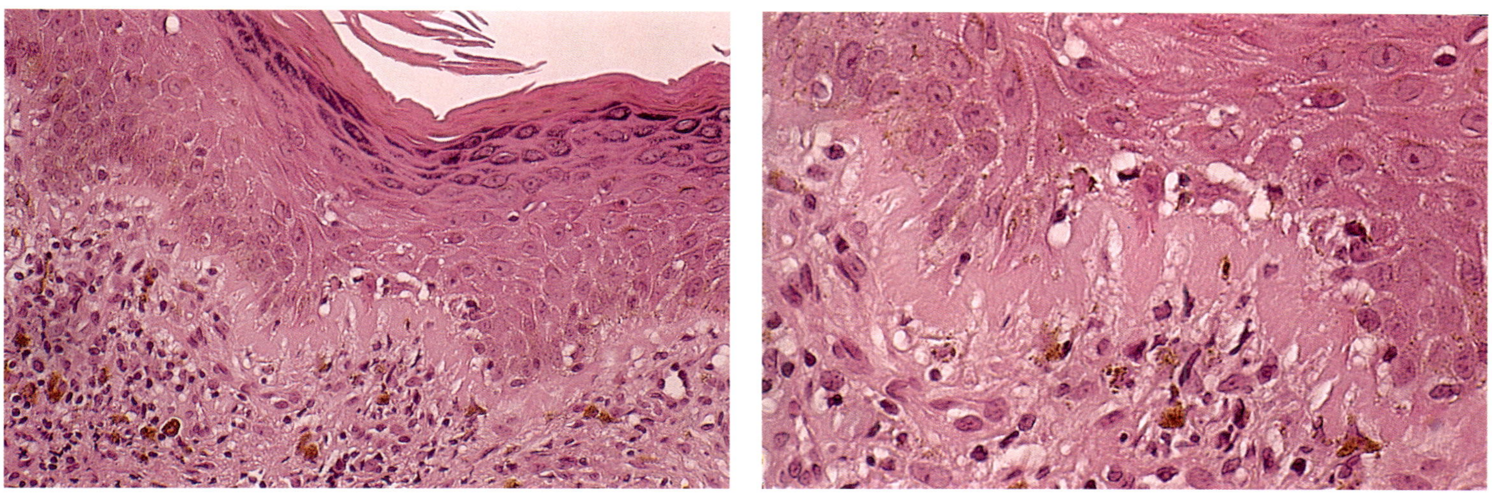

A **B**

Figures 2–37A, 2–37B. Discoid lupus erythematosus. There is a conspicuous thickened, eosinophilic basement membrane, typical of long-standing lesions.

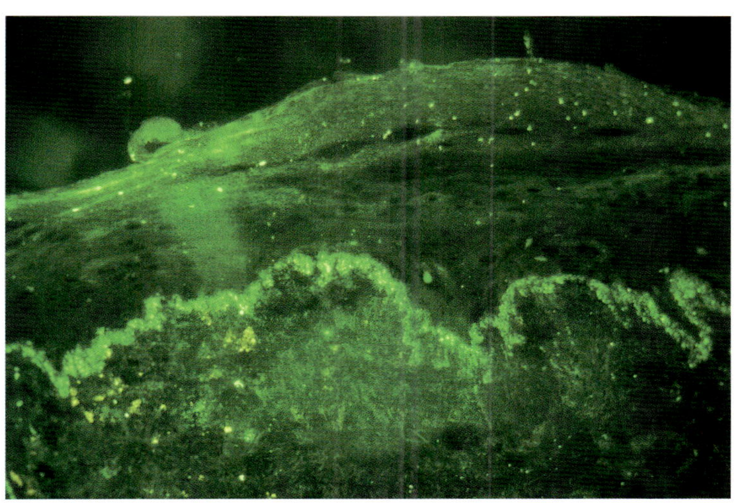

Figure 2–38. Discoid lupus erythematosus. Direct immunofluorescence of discoid lupus erythematosus. Note deposition of IgM along the epidermal basement membrane.

SUBACUTE LUPUS ERYTHEMATOSUS

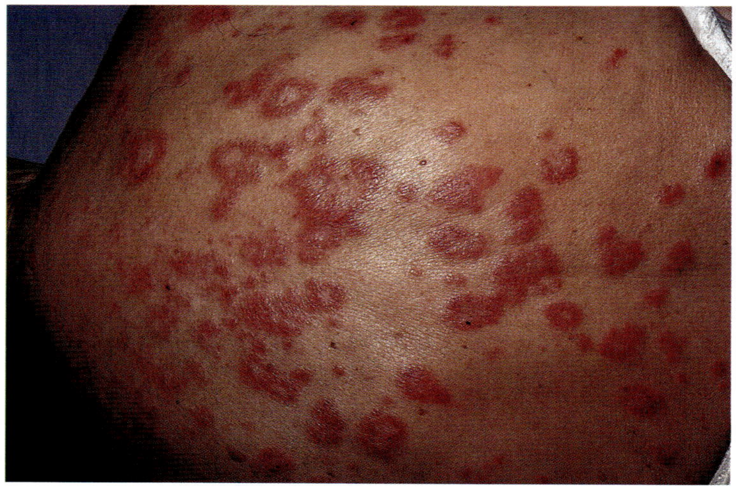

Figure 2–39. Subacute lupus erythematosus. Numerous annular erythematous papules and plaques, many with central clearing.

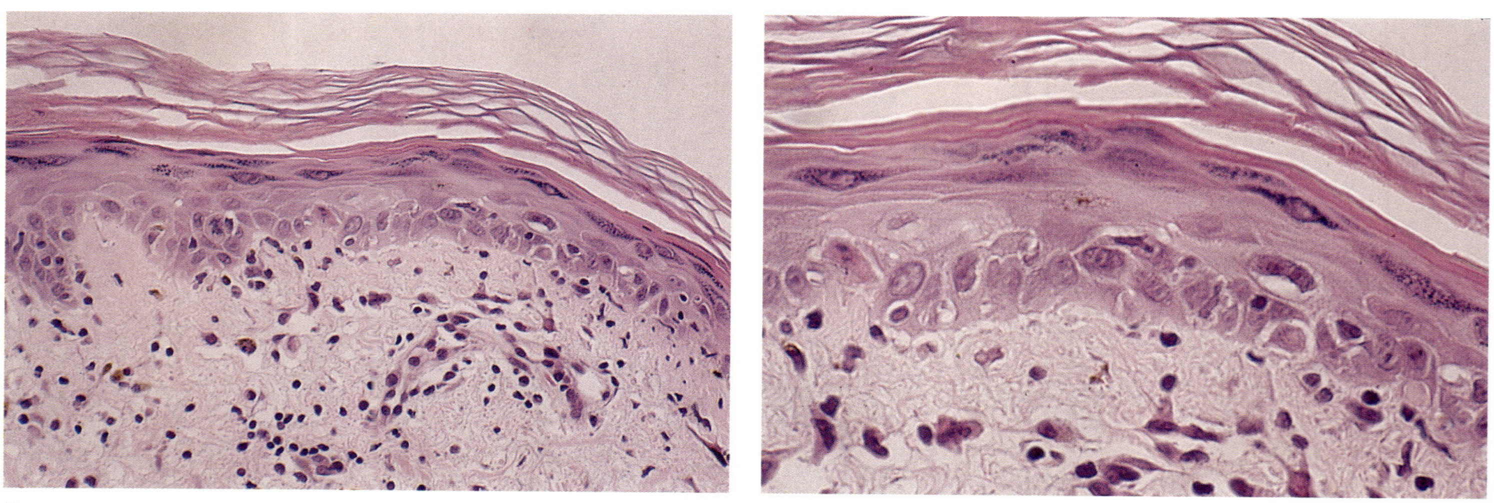

A B

Figures 2–40A, 2–40B. Subacute lupus erythematosus. Hyperkeratosis, vacuolar alteration, and necrotic keratinocytes. There is severe papillary edema, dilated blood vessels, melanophages, and a lymphohistiocytic dermal infiltrate.

SYSTEMIC LUPUS ERYTHEMATOSUS

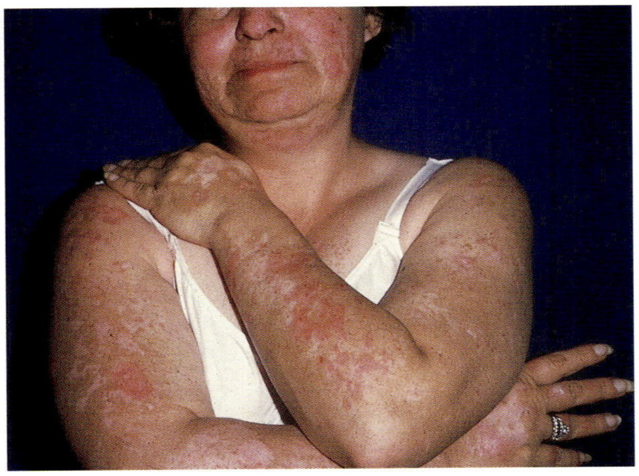

A

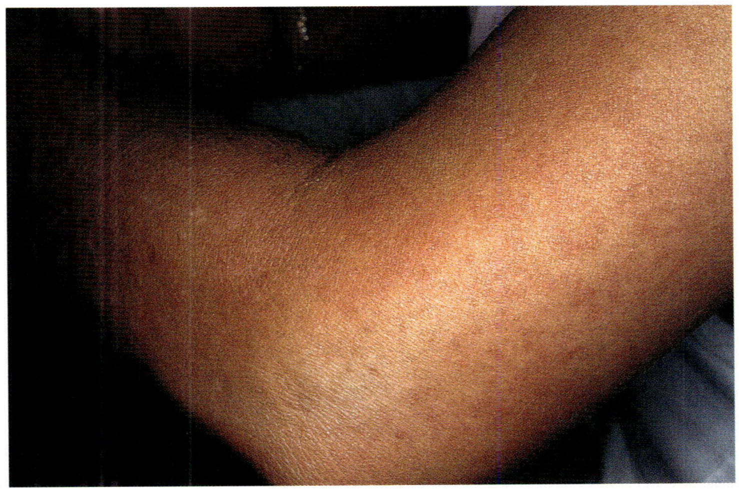

B

Figures 2–41A, 2–41B. Systemic lupus erythematosus. Erythematous patches and plaques, predominantly in sun-exposed areas.

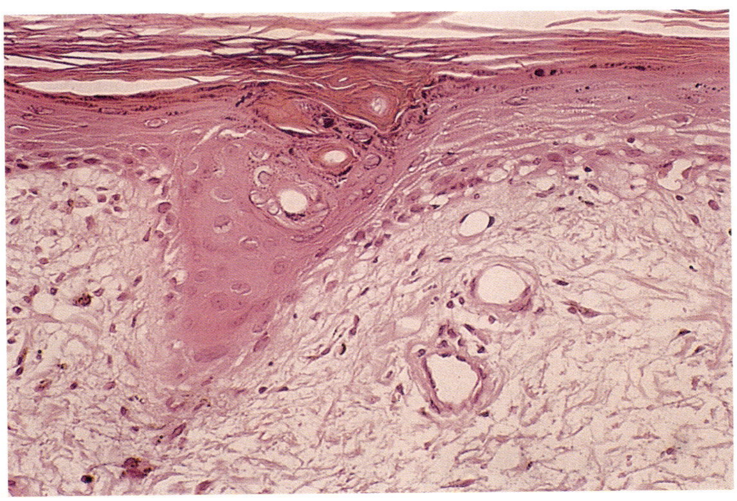

Figure 2–42. Systemic lupus erythematosus. Vacuolar alteration and necrotic keratinocytes involving the epidermis and adnexa. There are dilated venules, solar elastosis, and a sparse dermal mixed-cell infiltrate.

NEONATAL LUPUS ERYTHEMATOSUS

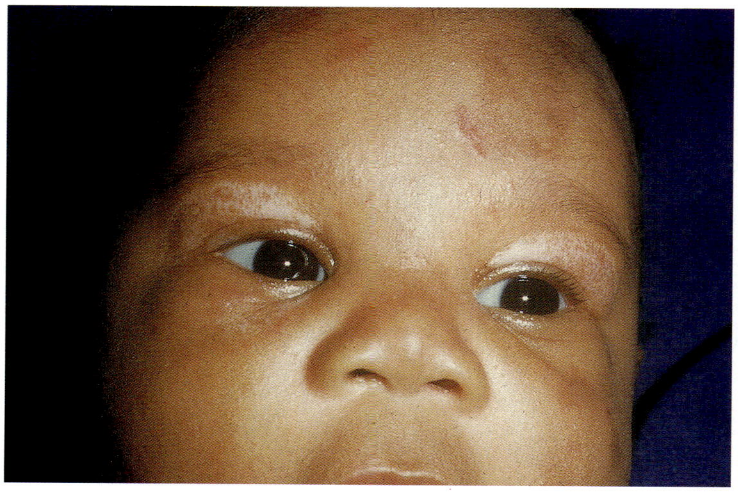

A

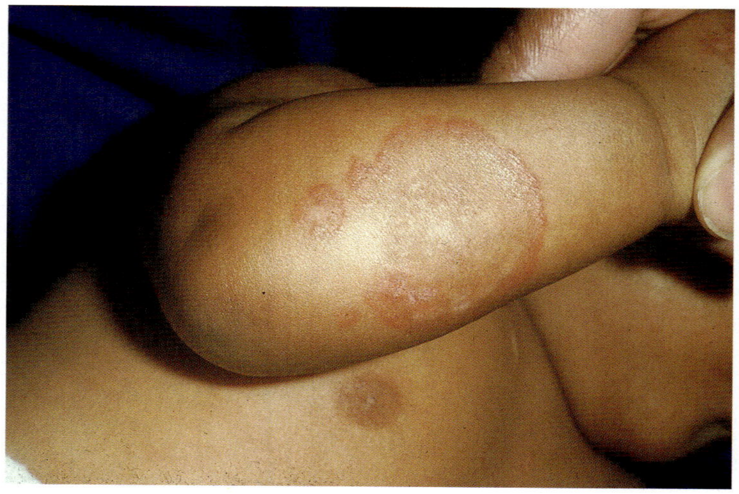

B

Figures 2–43A, 2–43B. Neonatal lupus erythematosus. Annular, scaly, erythematous patches and plaques.

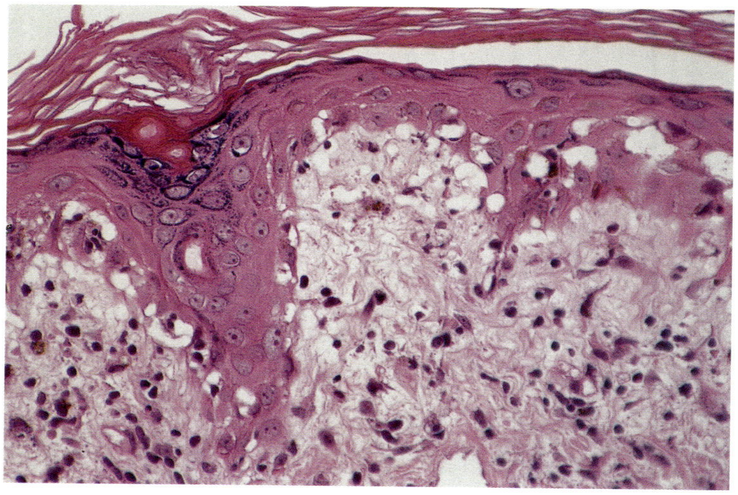

Figure 2–44. Neonatal lupus erythematosus. Hyperkeratosis, focally thinned epidermis, necrotic keratinocytes, extensive vacuolar alteration of the epidermis and adnexa. Severe papillary edema, and a lymphohistiocytic dermal infiltrate are present.

DERMATOMYOSITIS

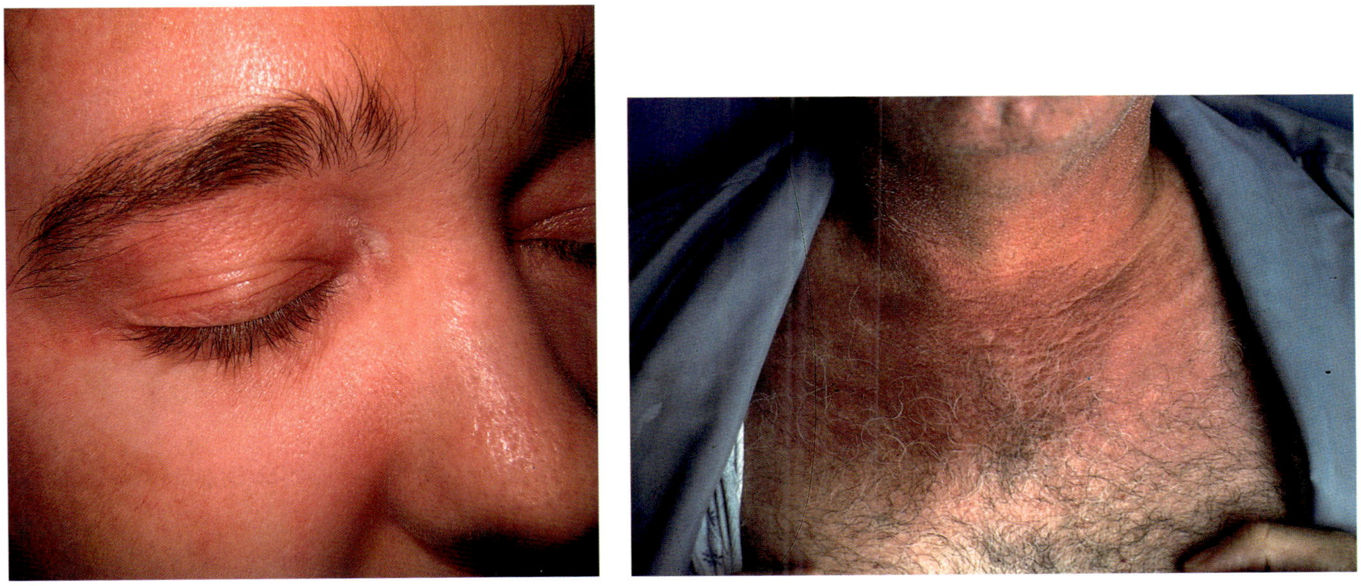

A B

Figures 2–45A, 2–45B. Dermatomyositis. Patchy erythema and scaling. Involvement of the upper eyelid is a classic finding in this disease and is commonly referred to as "heliotrope erythema."

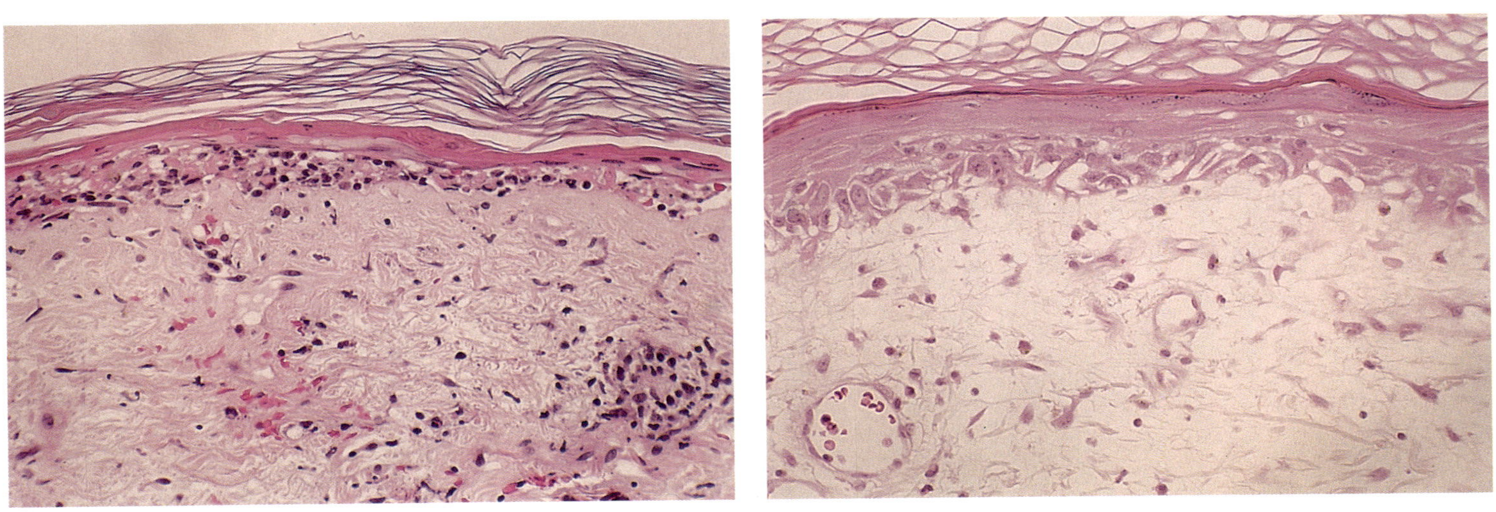

A B

Figures 2–46A, 2–46B. Dermatomyositis. The histopathologic changes are similar to lupus erythematosus. There is hyperkeratosis, focally thinned epidermis, diffuse vacuolar alteration, papillary edema, and dilated blood vessels. However, the lymphohistiocytic infiltrate in the dermis differs from lupus erythematosus in being mostly sparse and superficial.

DERMATOMYOSITIS

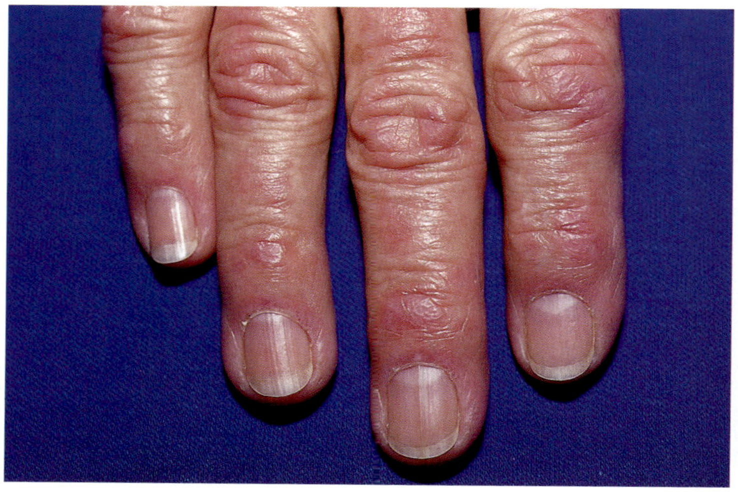

A

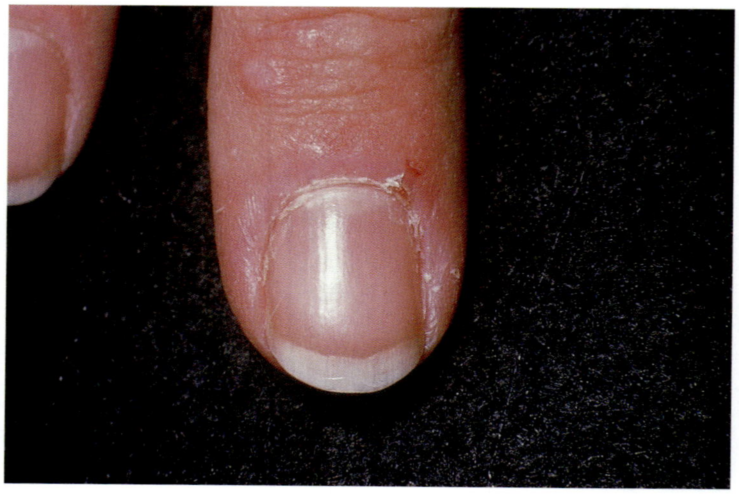

B

Figures 2–47A, 2–47B. Dermatomyositis. Paronychial erythema and scaling. Keratotic papules (Gottron's papules) are present over interphalangeal joints.

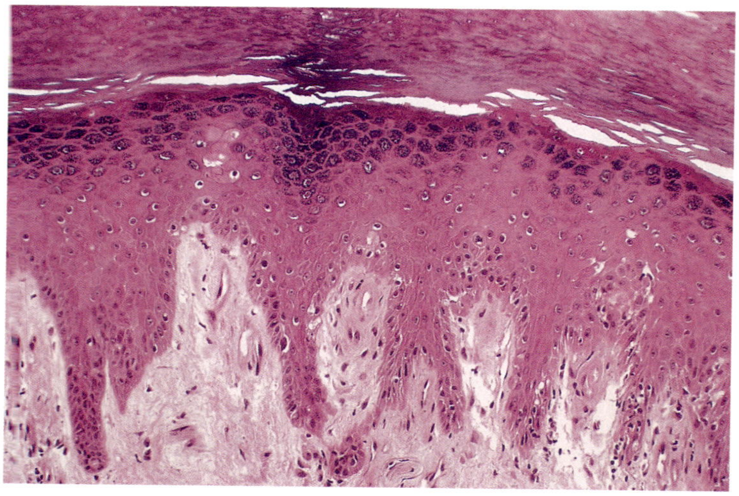

Figure 2–48. Dermatomyositis, Gottron's papule. There is striking psoriasiform epidermal hyperplasia, hyperkeratosis, hypergranulosis, and patchy vacuolar alteration.

LICHEN STRIATUS

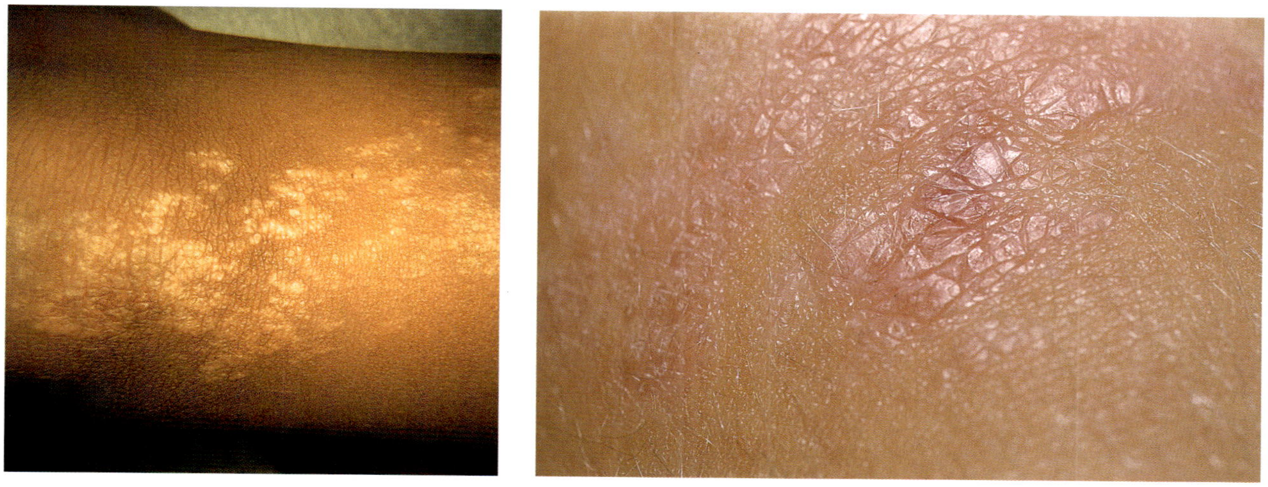

A B

Figures 2–49A, 2–49B. Lichen striatus. Grouped flat-topped papules with characteristic linear configuration.

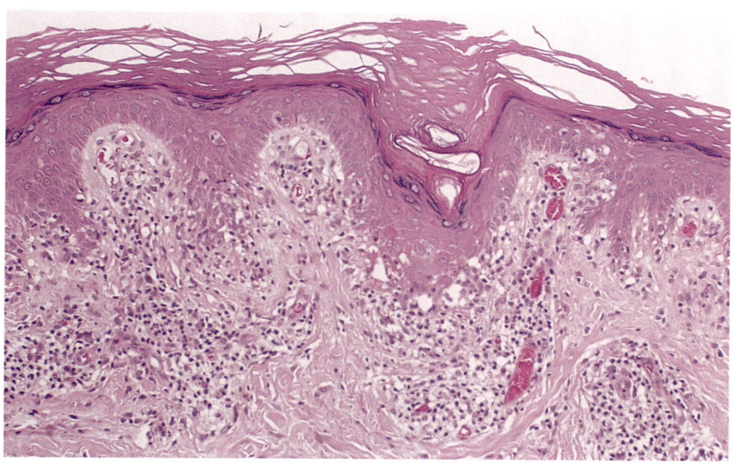

Figure 2–50. Lichen striatus. There is hyperkeratosis, necrotic keratinocytes, and vacuolar alteration involving the epidermis and adnexa. The lymphohistiocytic infiltrate may be lichenoid and follow structures of adnexa far down into the reticular dermis.

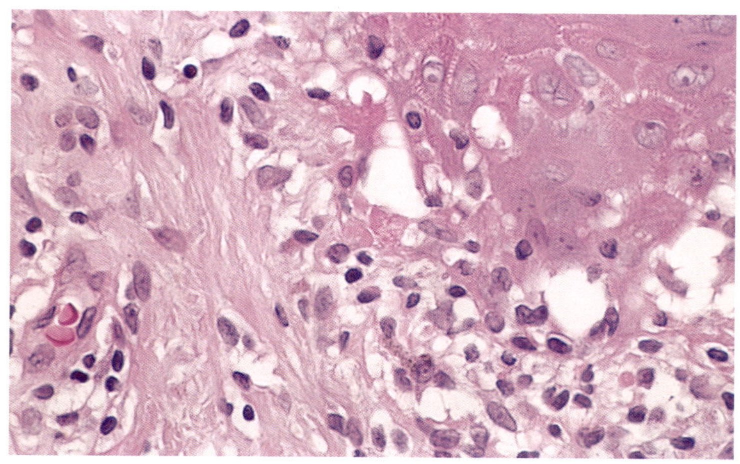

Figure 2–51. Lichen striatus. Prominent vacuolar alteration with necrotic keratinocytes.

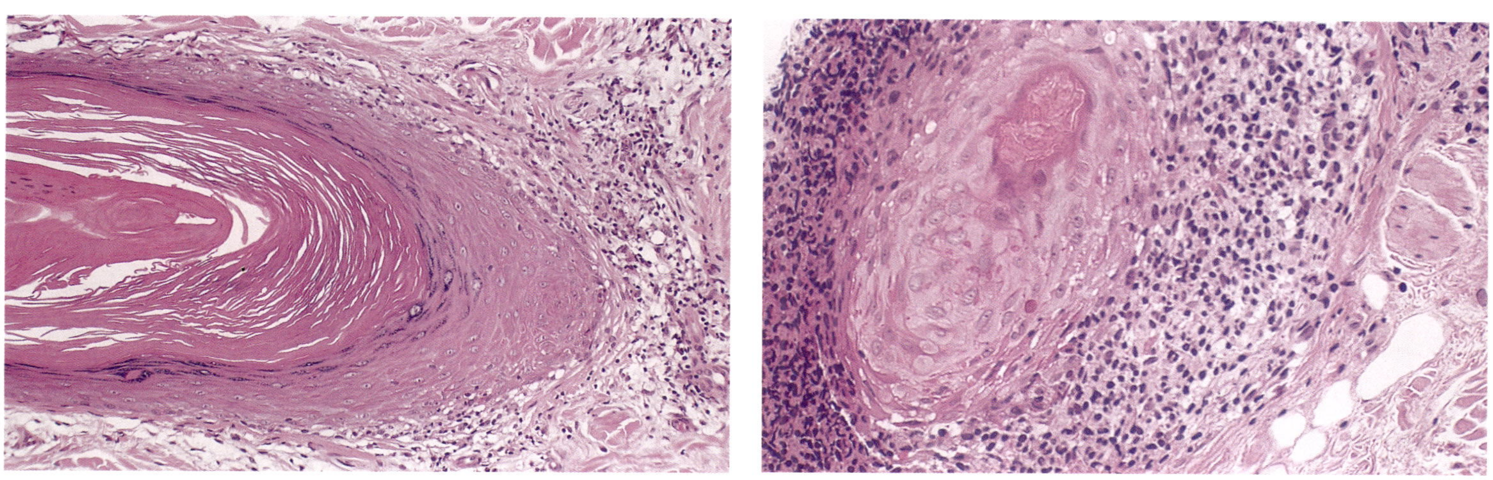

A B

Figures 2–52A, 2–52B. Lichen striatus. Adnexal involvement. Dense mononuclear cell infiltrate obscures interface between epithelium and dermis.

GRAFT-VERSUS-HOST DISEASE (GVHD)

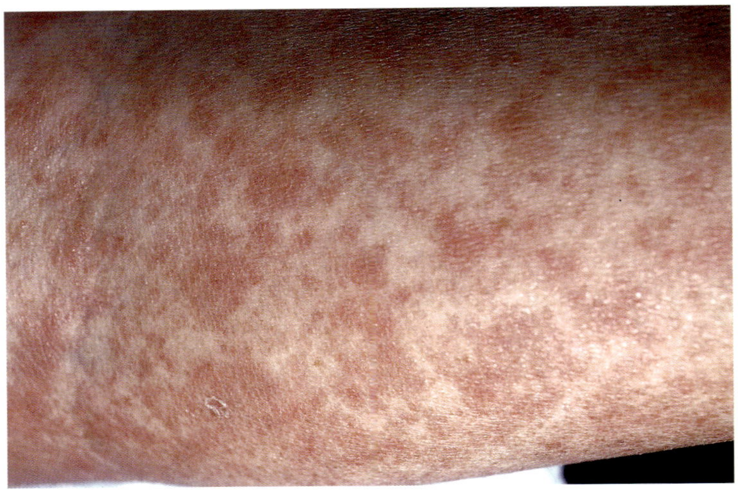

Figure 2–53. Graft-versus-host disease, acute. Patchy erythema on the extremity of a patient who has received an allogeneic bone marrow transplantation.

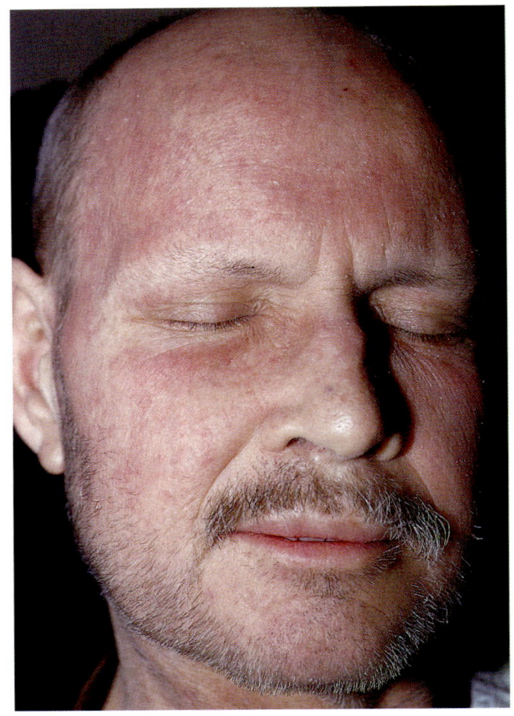

Figure 2–54. Graft-versus-host disease, acute. Progression of GVHD results in confluent erythema, which may be widespread.

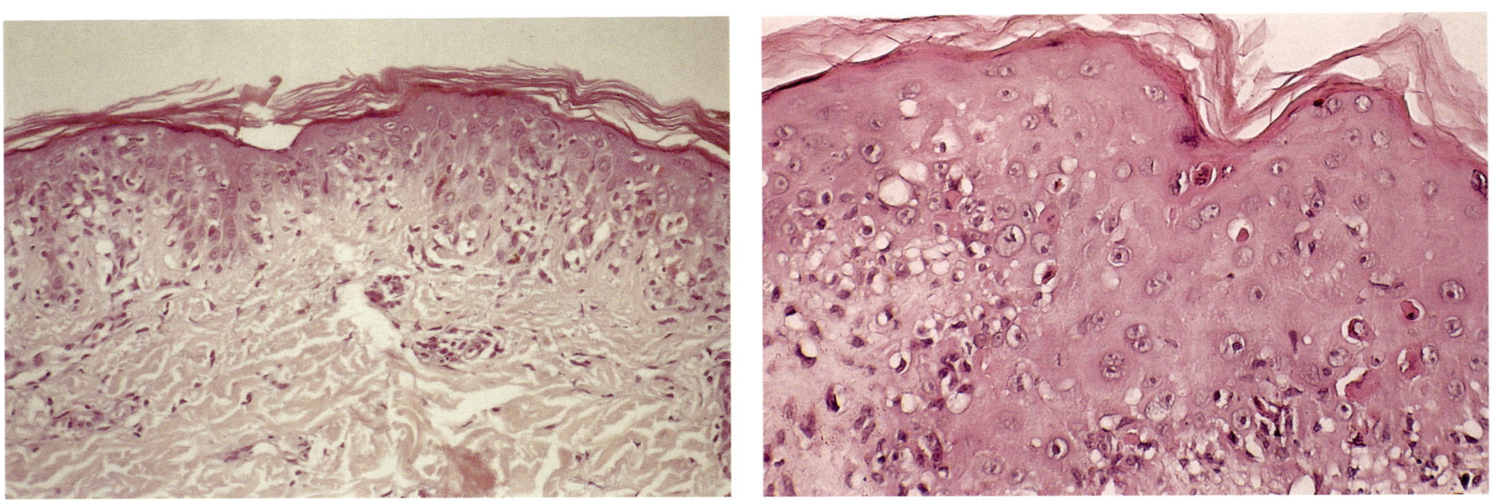

A

B

Figures 2–55A, 2–55B. Graft-versus-host disease, acute. Interface dermatitis with basal vacuolization, dyskeratosis, and exocytosis of lymphocytes into the epidermis. The latter feature distinguishes GVHD from morphologic changes that may be seen in association with the preparatory chemotherapy or radiation regimen.

GRAFT-VERSUS-HOST DISEASE (GVHD)

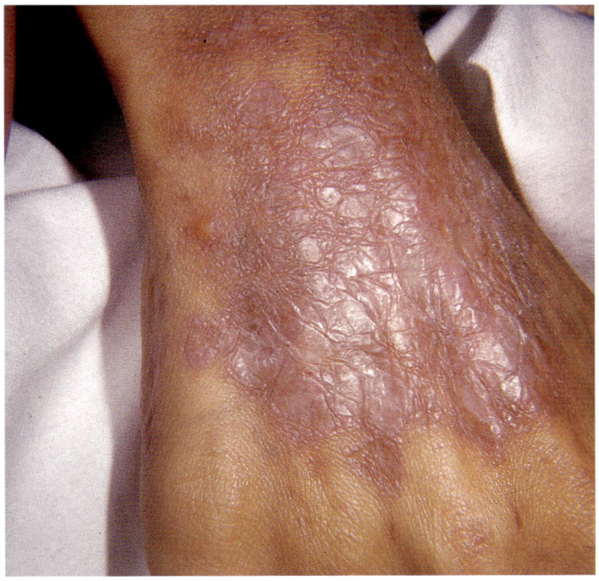

A

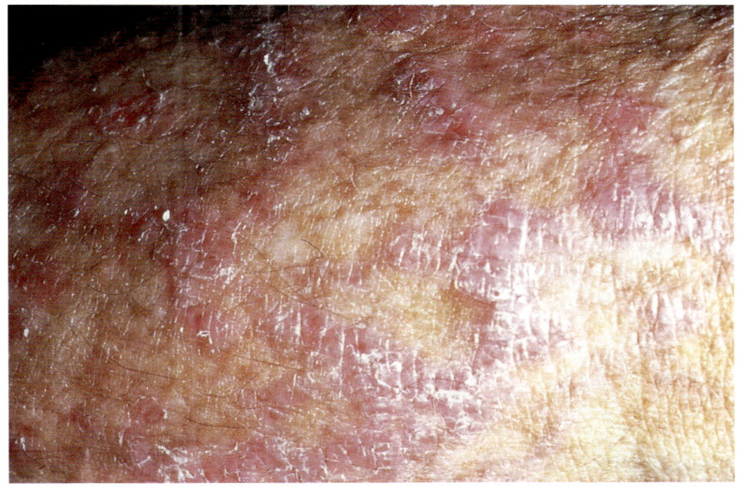

B

Figures 2–56A, 2–56B. Graft-versus-host disease, chronic lichenoid. Violaceous, reticulated, often scaly papular eruption on the extremities of a patient who received an allogeneic bone marrow transplant a few months earlier.

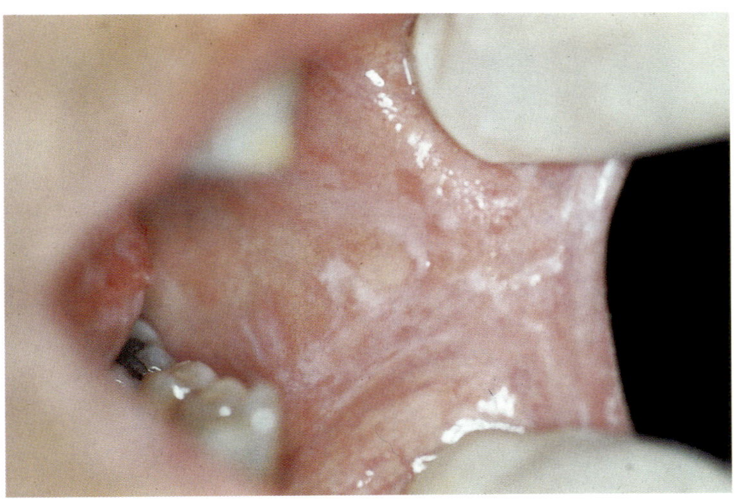

Figure 2–57. Graft-versus-host disease, chronic lichenoid. Oral mucosal changes in lichenoid GVHD may be clinically and histologically indistinguishable from idiopathic lichen planus.

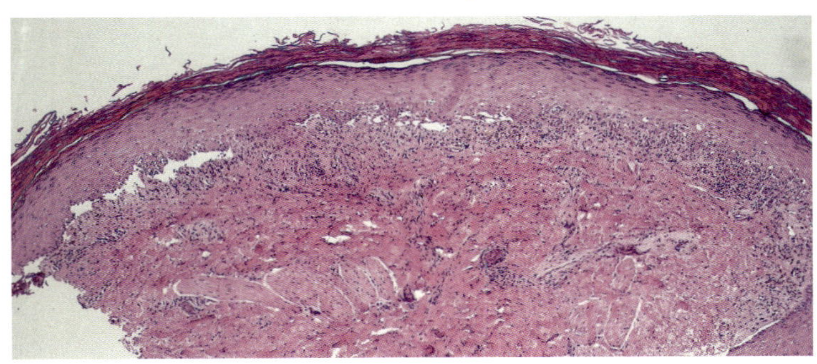

Figure 2–58. Graft-versus-host disease, chronic lichenoid. Hyperkeratosis, irregular acanthosis, basal vacuolization with focal separation of the epidermis from the dermis, and an intense bandlike infiltrate of mononuclear cells in the upper dermis.

GRAFT-VERSUS-HOST DISEASE (GVHD)

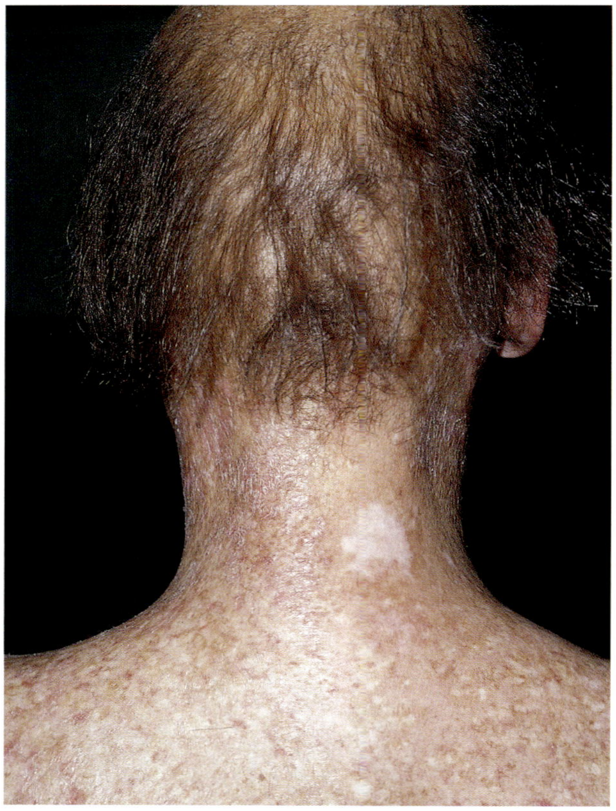

A

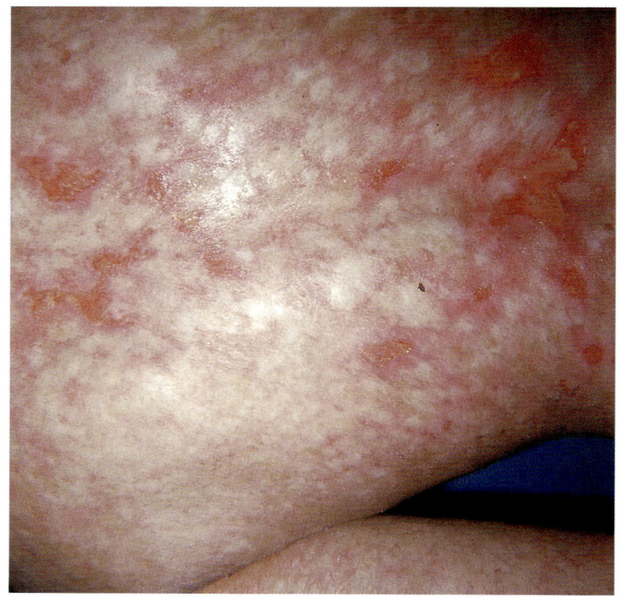

B

Figures 2–59A, 2–59B. Graft-versus-host disease, chronic sclerodermoid. Dermal sclerosis, hyperpigmentation and hypopigmentation, and alopecia (Figure 2–59A), as well as superficial erosions and ulcerations (Figure 2–59B). Both patients received bone marrow transplantations several months earlier.

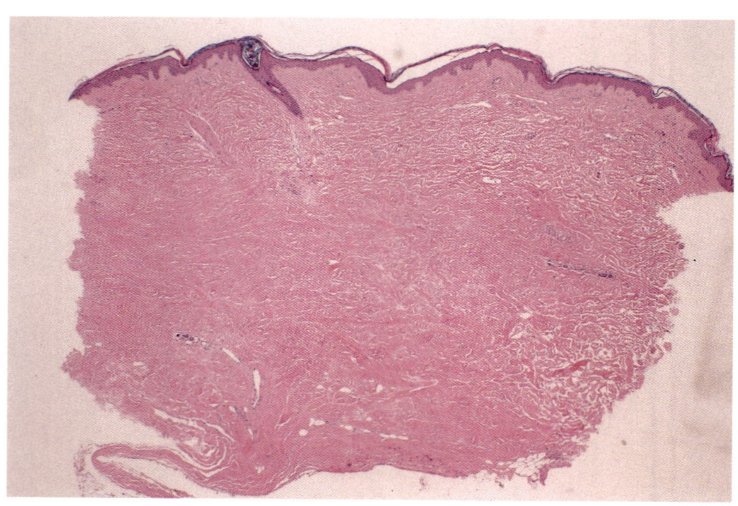

Figure 2–60. Graft-versus-host disease, chronic sclerodermoid. A "square" biopsy specimen with thickened and homogenous collagen replacing normal reticular dermis. Note absence of normal adnexal structures. The epidermis is relatively normal.

3

INTRAEPIDERMAL VESICULAR, BULLOUS, AND PUSTULAR DERMATITIS

- Pemphigus vulgaris
- Pemphigus foliaceous
- Hailey-Hailey disease
- Darier's disease
- Grover's disease (transient acantholytic dyskeratosis)
- Incontinentia pigmenti
- Pustulosis palmaris
- Focal acantholytic dyskeratoma
- Warty dyskeratoma

PEMPHIGUS VULGARIS

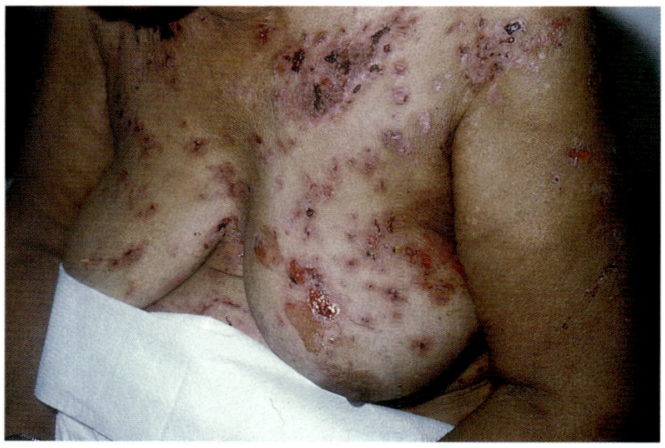

Figure 3–1. Pemphigus vulgaris. Numerous crusted, denuded, and weepy erythematous plaques on the chest, breast, abdomen, and arms.

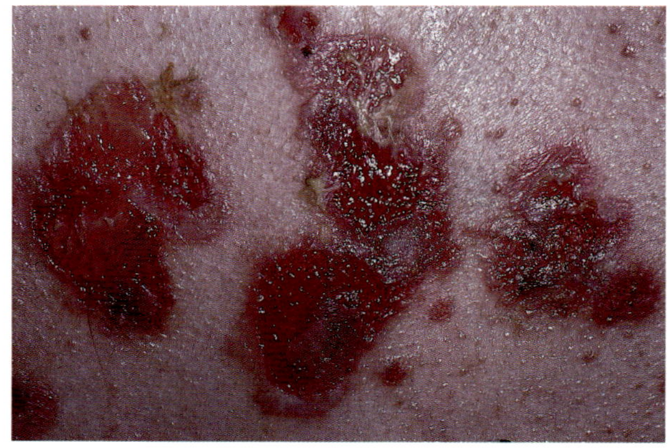

Figure 3–2. Pemphigus vulgaris. Grouped, erythematous, denuded, oozy plaques with vesicular borders and contiguous solitary, erythematous papulovesicles.

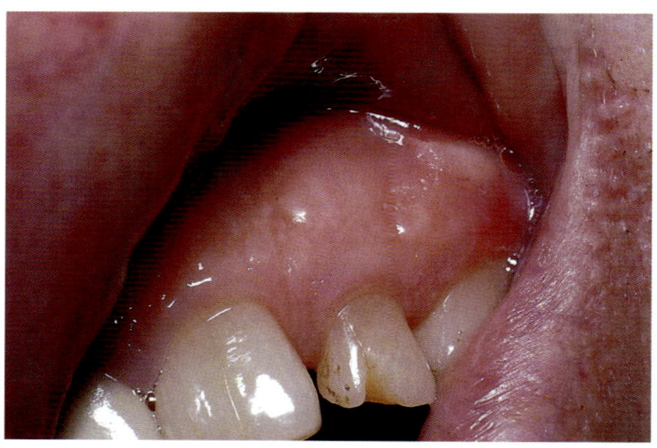

Figure 3–3. Pemphigus vulgaris. Vesicles on the gingiva.

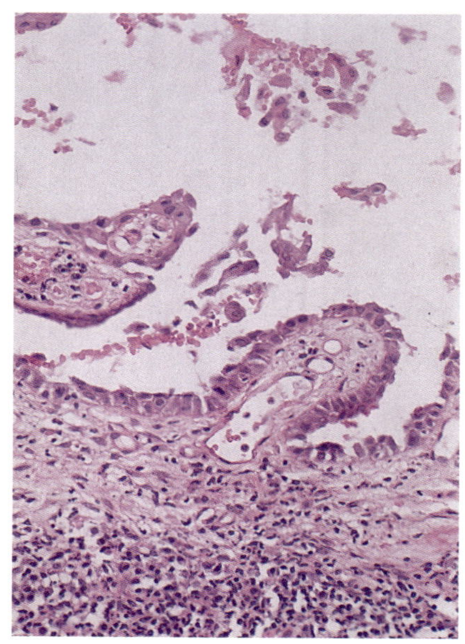

Figure 3–4. Pemphigus vulgaris. Acantholytic keratinocytes singly and in clusters within the vesicular cavity. There are solitary basal keratinocytes lining the dermis, and a dense dermal mixed-cell infiltrate.

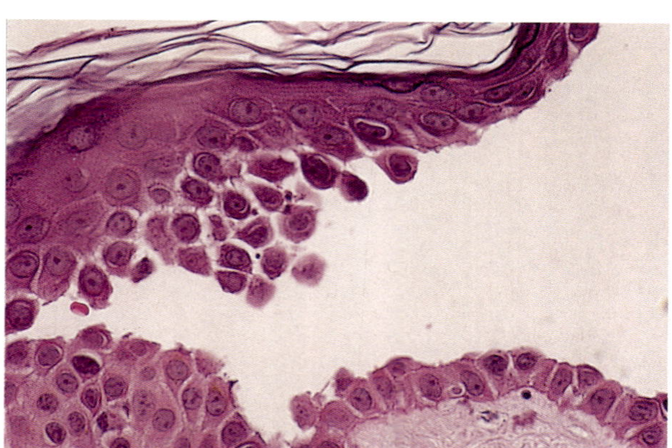

Figure 3–5. Pemphigus vulgaris. Rounded, solitary acantholytic keratinocytes that appear to be floating within the vesicle. The dermis is lined by a single layer of columnar epithelial cells.

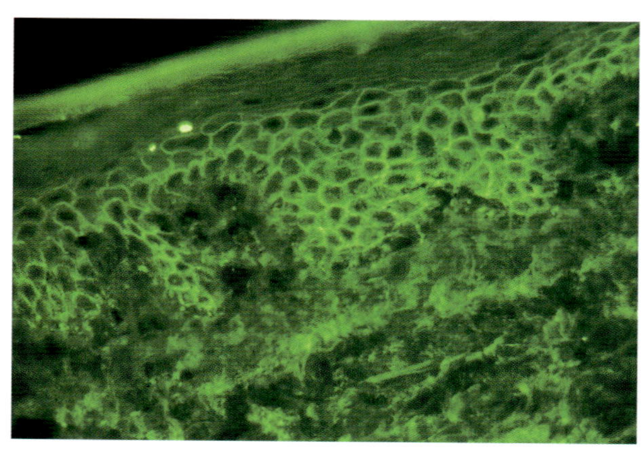

Figure 3–6. Pemphigus vulgaris. Direct immunofluorescence of pemphigus vulgaris. Note deposition of IgG on the surface of epidermal cells. A similar pattern of fluorescence is seen in other forms of pemphigus.

PEMPHIGUS FOLIACEOUS

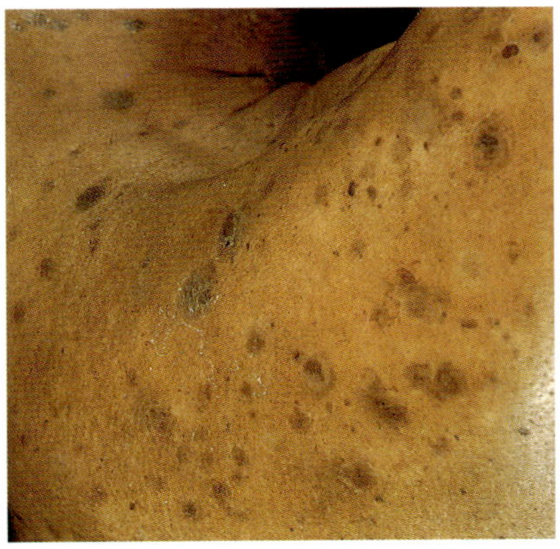

A

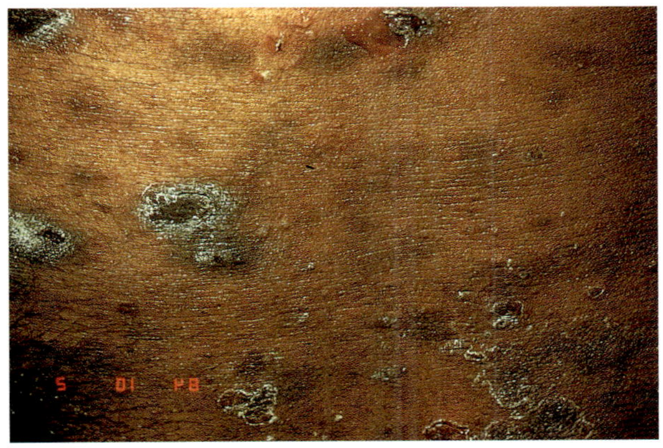

B

Figures 3–7A, 3–7B. Pemphigus foliaceous. Scaly, hyperpigmented macules and patches on the back, arms, and neck.

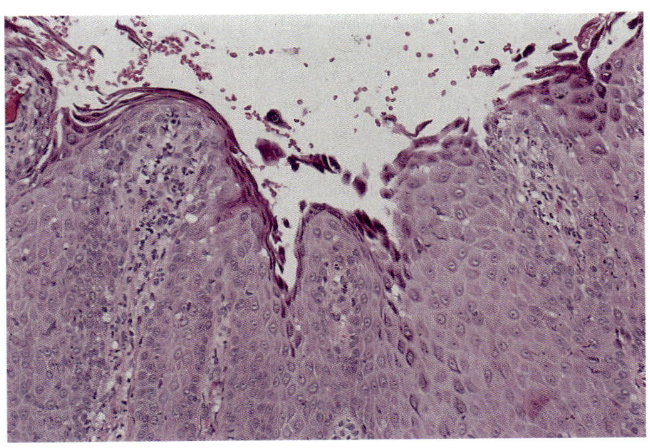

Figure 3–8. Pemphigus foliaceous. Acantholytic keratinocytes within the granular layer of a thickened epidermis. There is a dense dermal mixed-cell infiltrate.

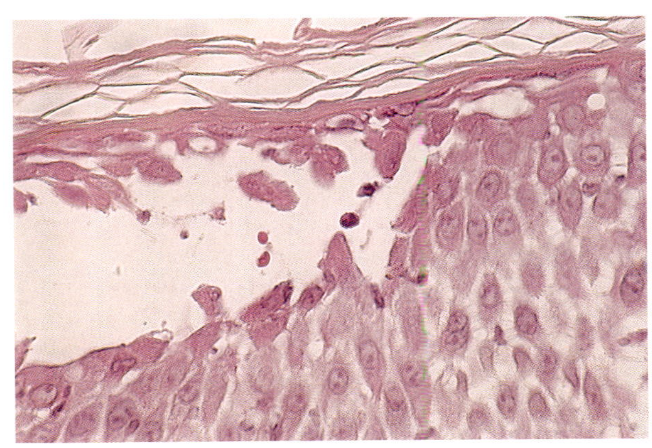

Figure 3–9. Pemphigus foliaceous. Acantholytic keratinocytes within the upper stratum spinosum and stratum granulosum.

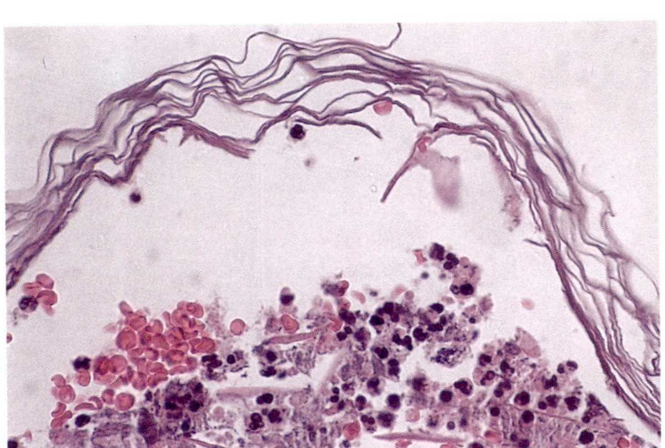

Figure 3–10. Pemphigus foliaceous. Subcorneal collection of acantholytic keratinocytes, neutrophils, and erythrocytes.

HAILEY-HAILEY DISEASE

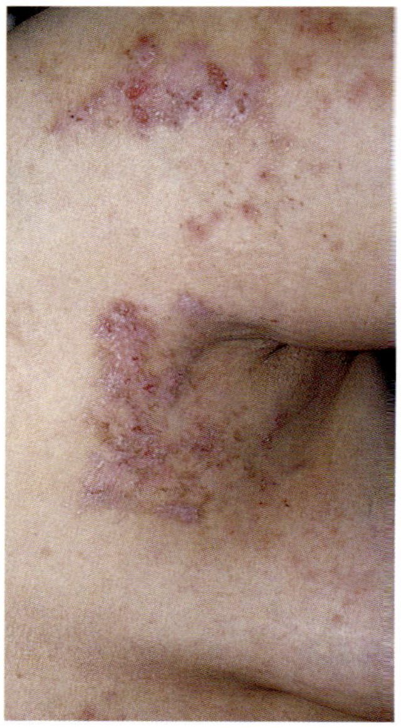

Figure 3–11. Hailey-Hailey disease. Erythematous, crusted papules involving the axilla, breast, and arm.

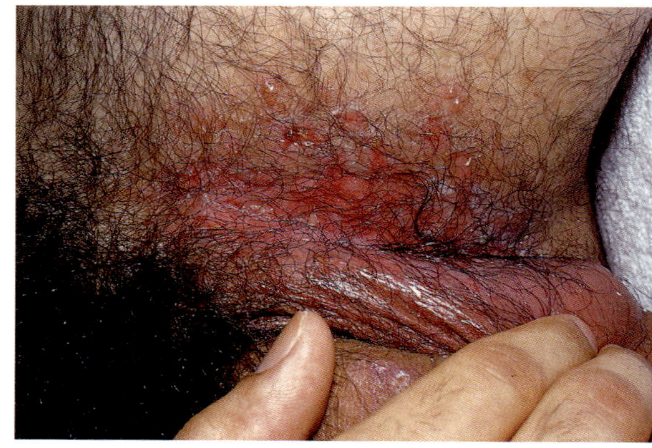

Figure 3–12. Hailey-Hailey disease. Vesicles and erythematous, oozy, denuded papules and plaques on the thigh and groin.

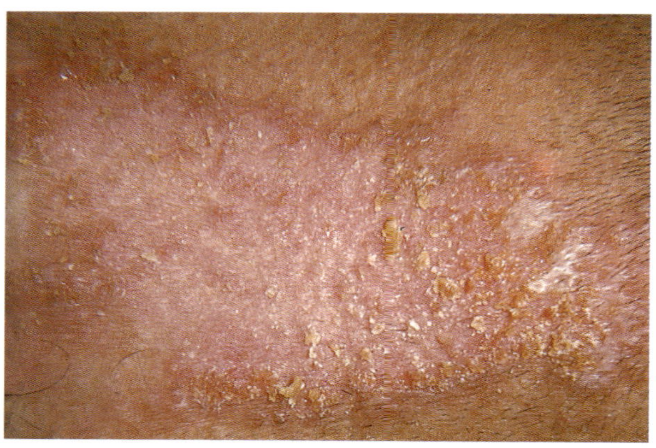

Figure 3–13. Hailey-Hailey disease. Annular thickened plaque with crusted papules and vesicles on the posterior neck.

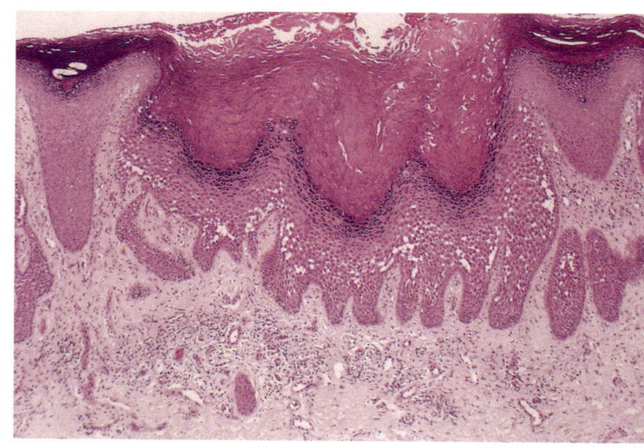

Figure 3–14. Hailey-Hailey disease. Dispersed acantholytic keratinocytes within a hyperplastic epidermis with hypergranulosis and compact hyperkeratosis. There are dilated venules and a mixed-cell dermal infiltrate.

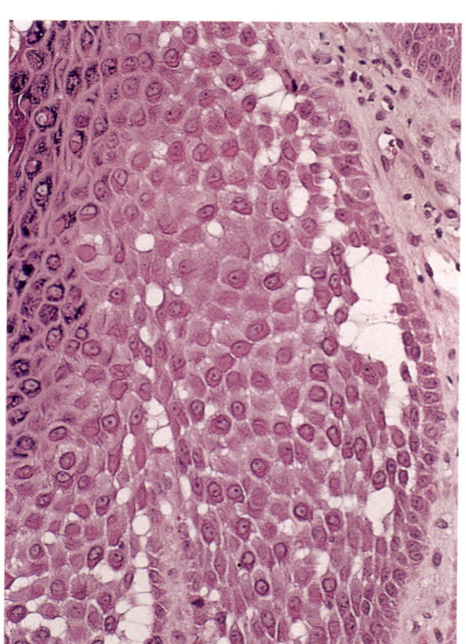

Figure 3–15. Hailey-Hailey disease. Diffusely scattered acantholytic keratinocytes and vesiculation within a bulbous portion of the hyperplastic epidermis.

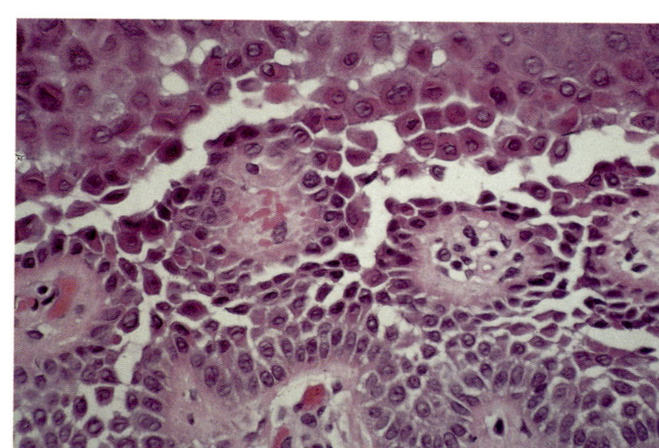

Figure 3–16. Hailey-Hailey disease. Rounded and dyskeratotic, acantholytic keratinocytes are scattered throughout the vesicular epidermis. There are dilated and congested blood vessels, edema, and a mixed-cell infiltrate in the dermis.

DARIER'S DISEASE

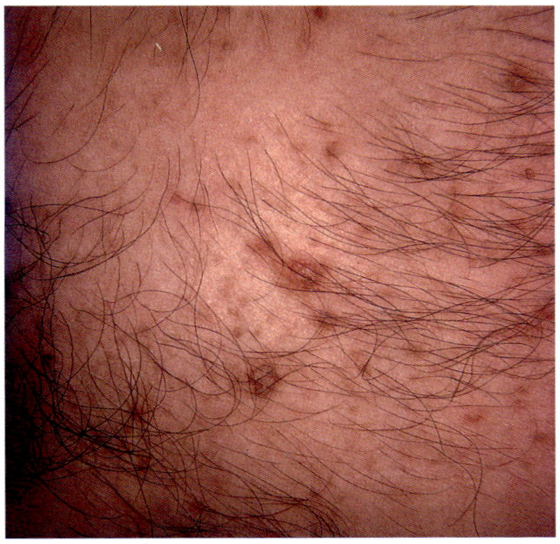

Figure 3–17. Darier's disease. Keratotic, erythematous papules on the chest.

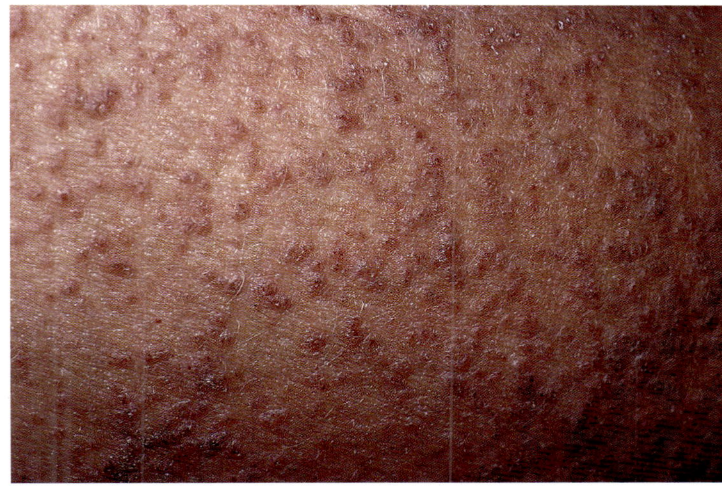

Figure 3–18. Darier's disease. An abundant aggregate of erythematous, keratotic papules on the chest.

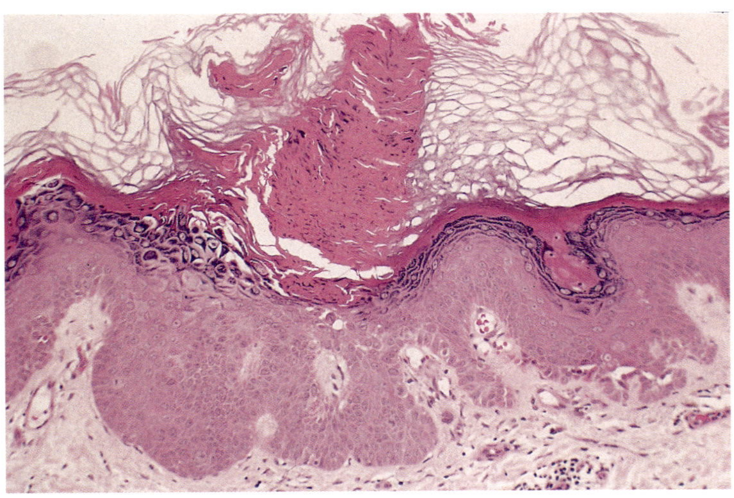

Figure 3–19. Darier's disease. Vertical column of compact parakeratotic cells that overlies a hyperplastic epidermis. There are acantholytic rounded keratinocytes within the spinous and granular layers and acantholytic dyskeratotic keratinocytes within the cornified layer.

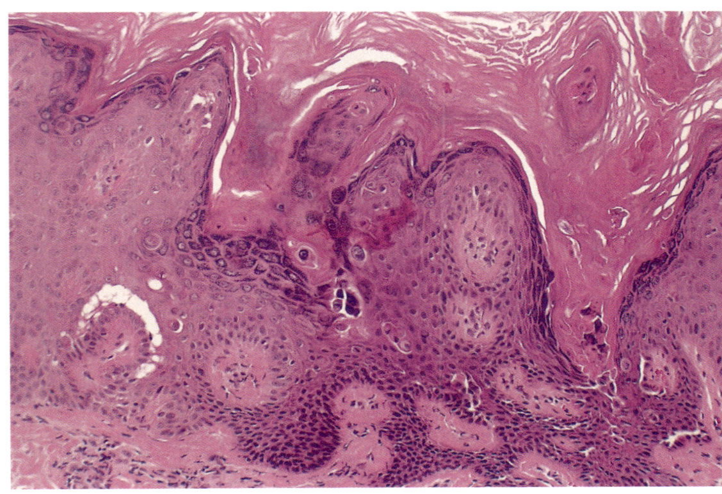

Figure 3–20. Darier's disease. Epidermal vesiculation with dyskeratotic acantholytic keratinocytes within the spinous, granular, and cornified layers (corps ronds and grains). There is dermal fibroplasia and a mixed-cell infiltrate.

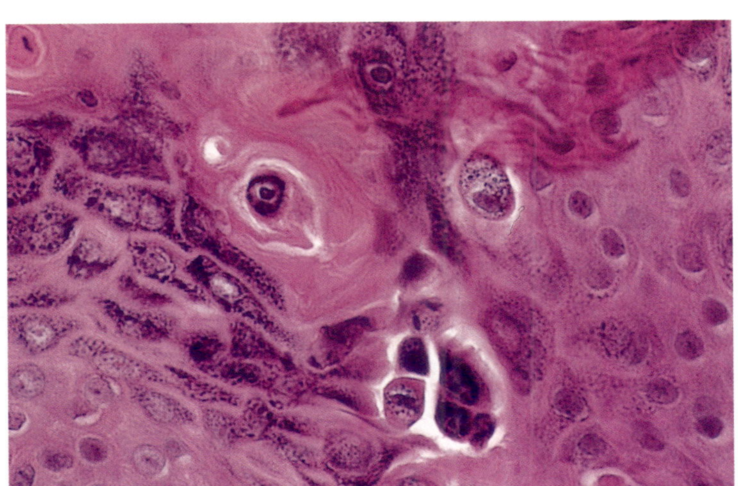

Figure 3–21. Darier's disease. Dyskeratotic acantholytic keratinocytes within the granular and cornified layers.

GROVER'S DISEASE (TRANSIENT ACANTHOLYTIC DYSKERATOSIS)

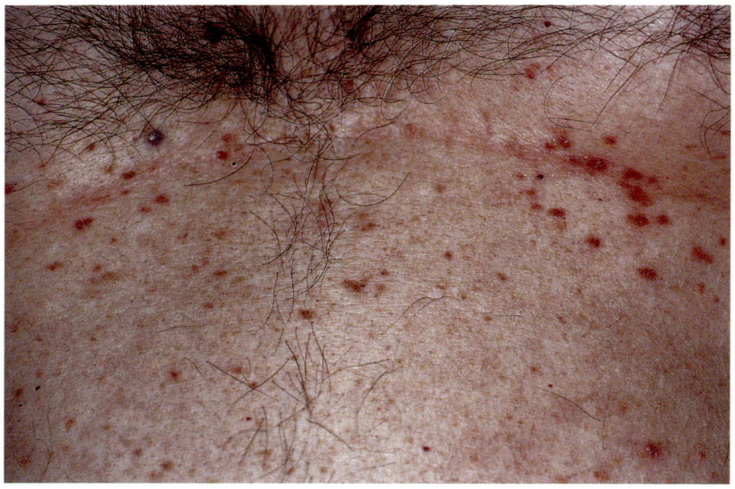

Figure 3–22. Grover's disease. Pru itic erythematous papules on the chest of a middle-aged man.

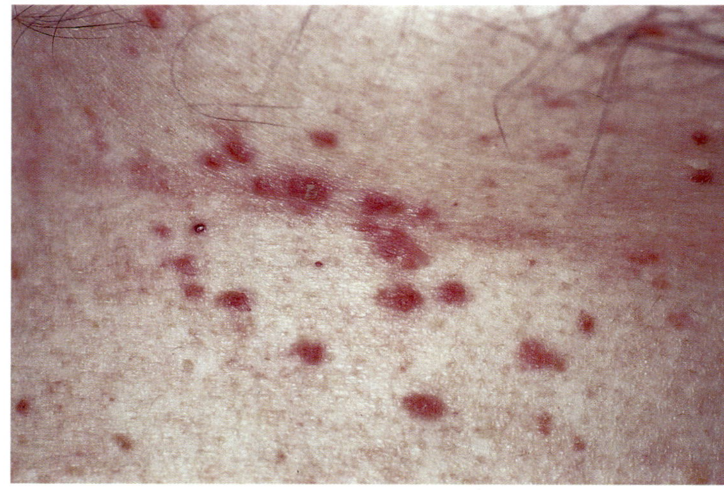

Figure 3–23. Grover's disease. Crusted and scaly erythematous dome-shaped papules.

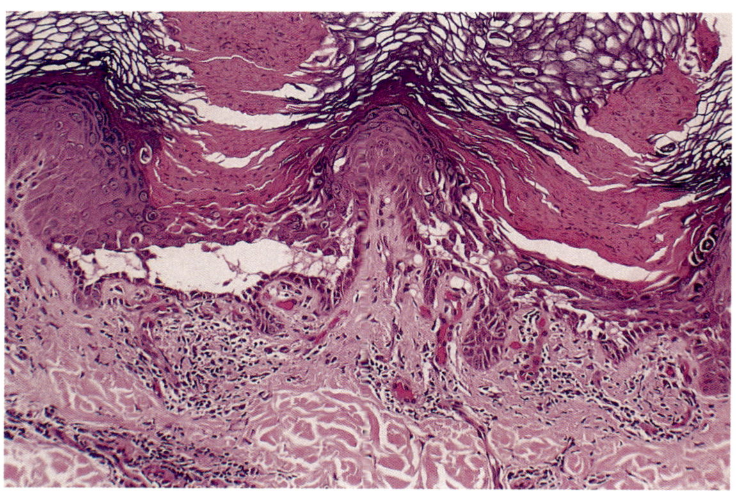

Figure 3–24. Grover's disease. Acantholytic dyskeratotic keratinocytes involve all layers of the epidermis beneath distinct columns of parakeratosis. There are dilated and congested blood vessels and a dermal mixed-cell infiltrate with eosinophils.

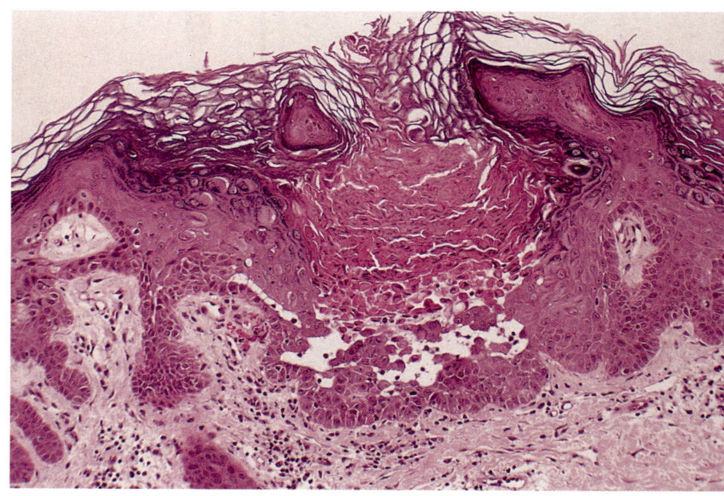

Figure 3–25. Grover's disease. Acantholytic dyskeratotic keratinocytes involving the epidermis in a diffuse pattern.

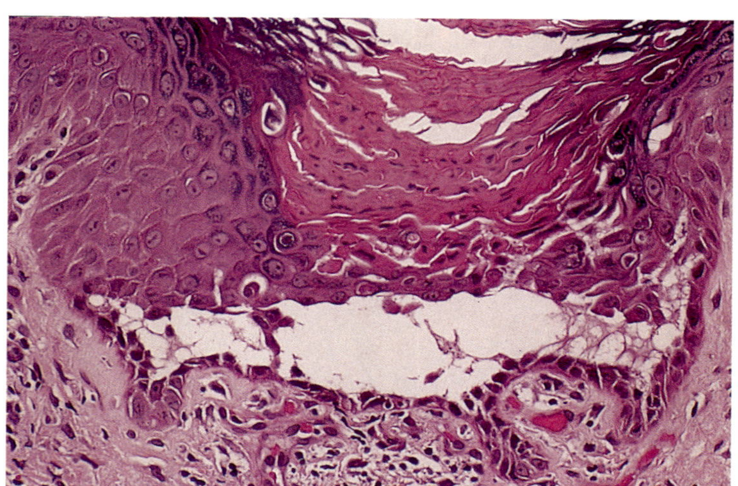

Figure 3–26. Grover's disease. Suprabasilar separation and spongiosis with acantholytic dyskeratotic keratinocytes.

INCONTINENTIA PIGMENTI

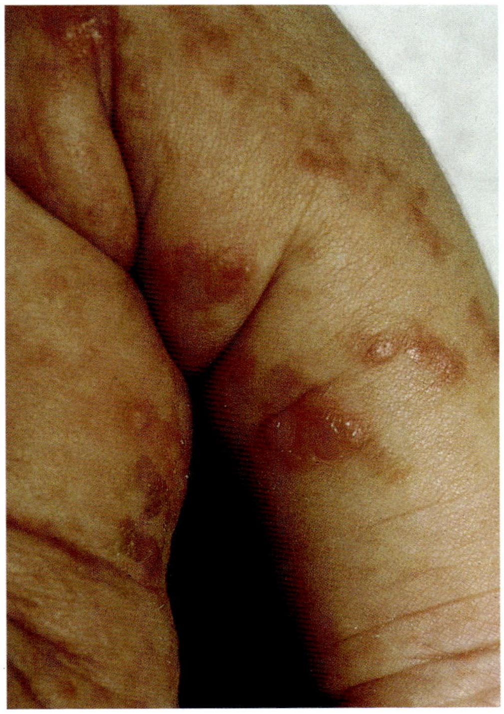

Figure 3–27. Incontinentia pigmenti, early lesions. Erythematous vesiculopapules on the arm and chest of an infant.

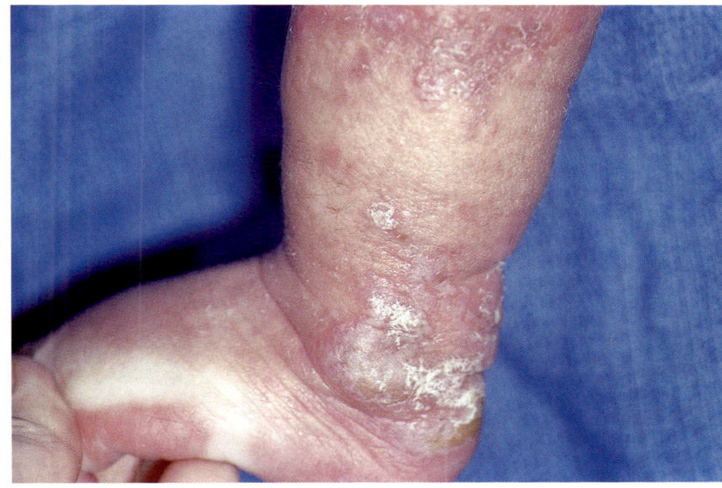

Figure 3–28. Incontinentia pigmenti, later lesions. Verrucous and keratotic papules and plaques on the lower leg of an infant.

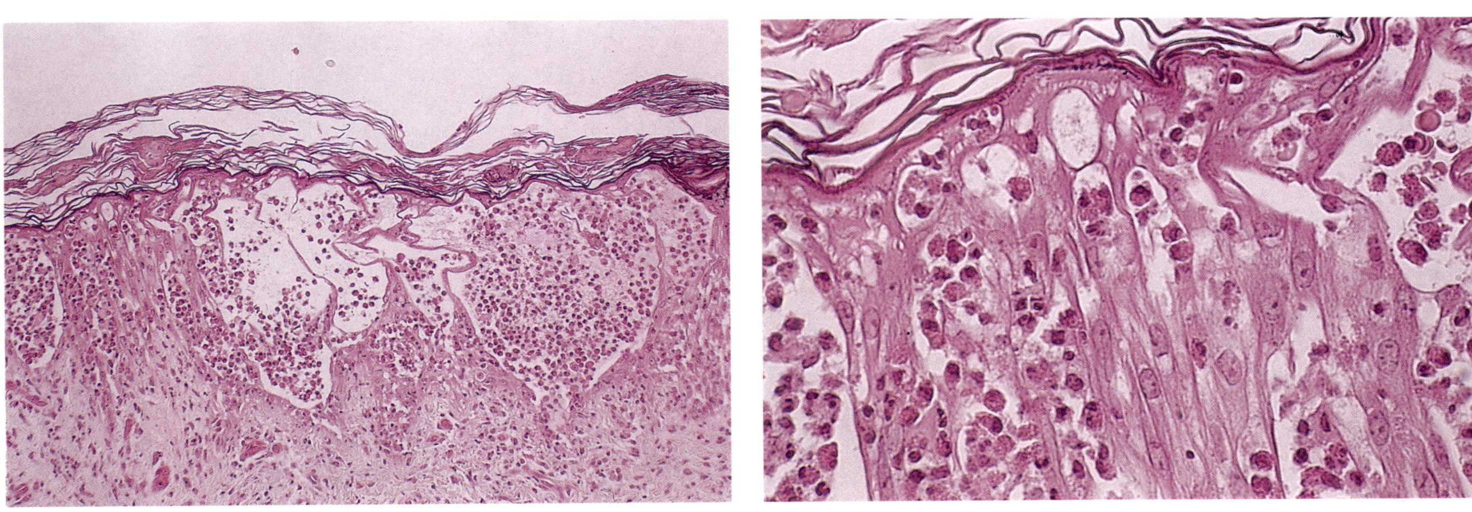

A

B

Figures 3–29A, 3–29B. Incontinentia pigmenti. Intraepidermal vesiculation with eosinophils scattered throughout and in collections. There is dermal edema, dilated blood vessels, and a mixed-cell infiltrate where eosinophils predominate.

PUSTULOSIS PALMARIS

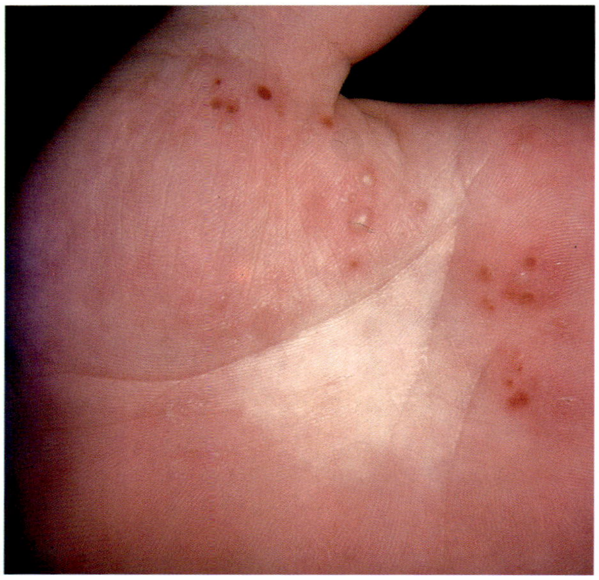

Figure 3–30. **Pustulosis palmaris.** Pustules on the palm.

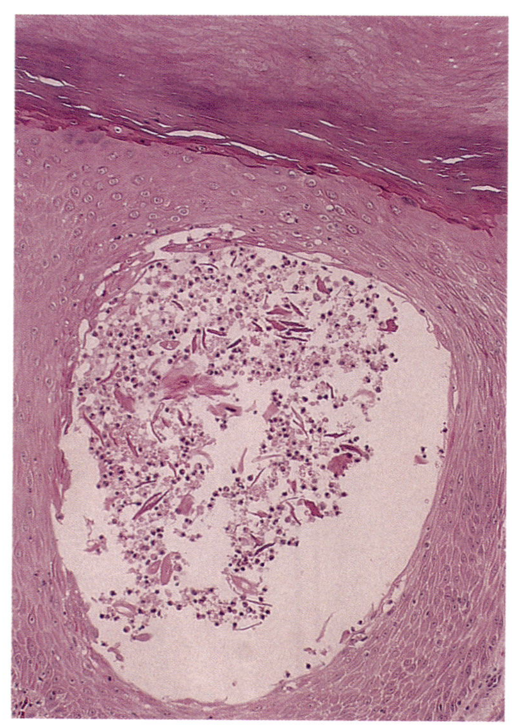

Figure 3–31. **Pustulosis palmaris.** Intraepidermal vesiculopustule with neutrophils.

FOCAL ACANTHOLYTIC DYSKERATOMA

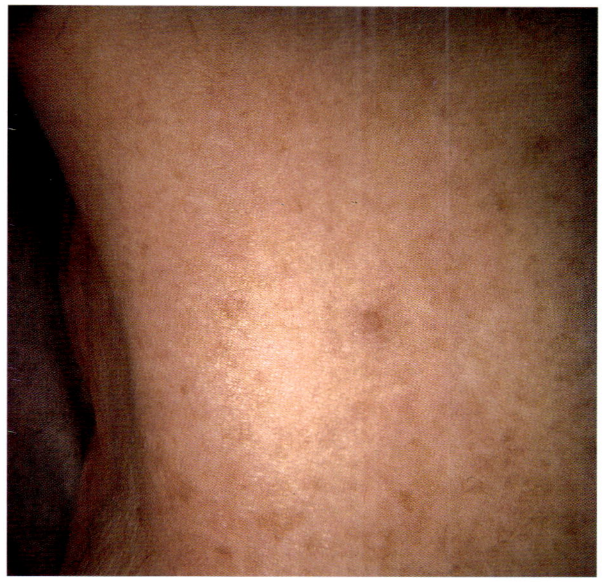

Figure 3–32. Focal acantholytic dyskeratoma. Flat-topped 4-mm keratotic papule on the upper back of a woman.

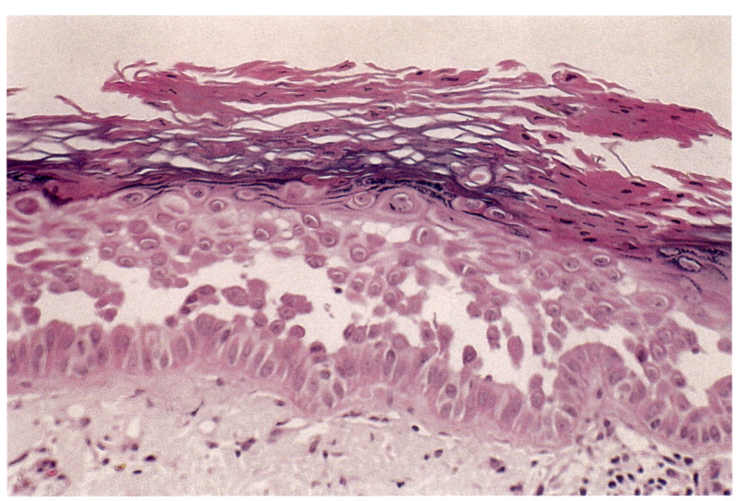

Figure 3–33. Focal acantholytic dyskeratoma. Acantholytic dyskeratotic keratinocytes involve the full thickness of the epidermis, including the hyperkeratotic stratum corneum. There is solar elastosis, dilated blood vessels, and a mixed-cell dermal infiltrate.

WARTY DYSKERATOMA

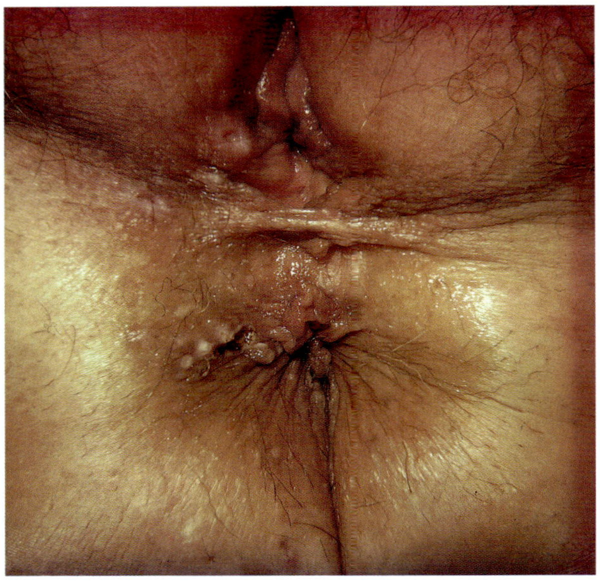

Figure 3–34. Warty dyskeratoma. Perianal keratotic papules.

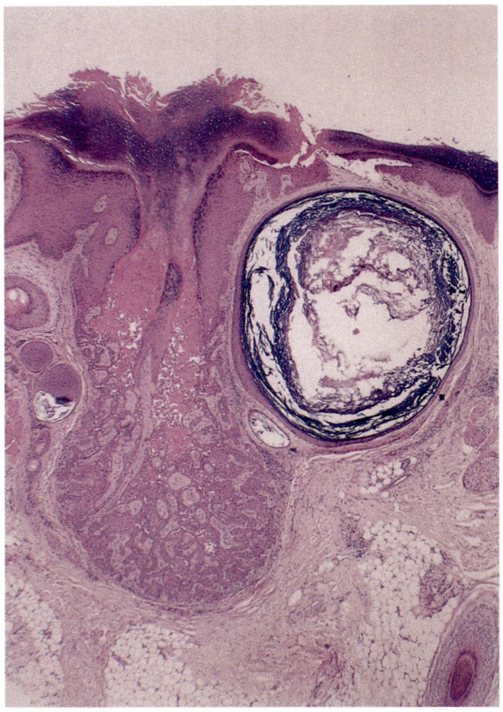

Figure 3–35. Warty dyskeratoma. Dilated and hyperkeratotic infundibulum with acantholytic dyskeratotic keratinocytes. There is fibroplasia, dilated blood vessels, and a mild perivascular lymphohistiocytic infiltrate in the dermis and subcutaneous fat.

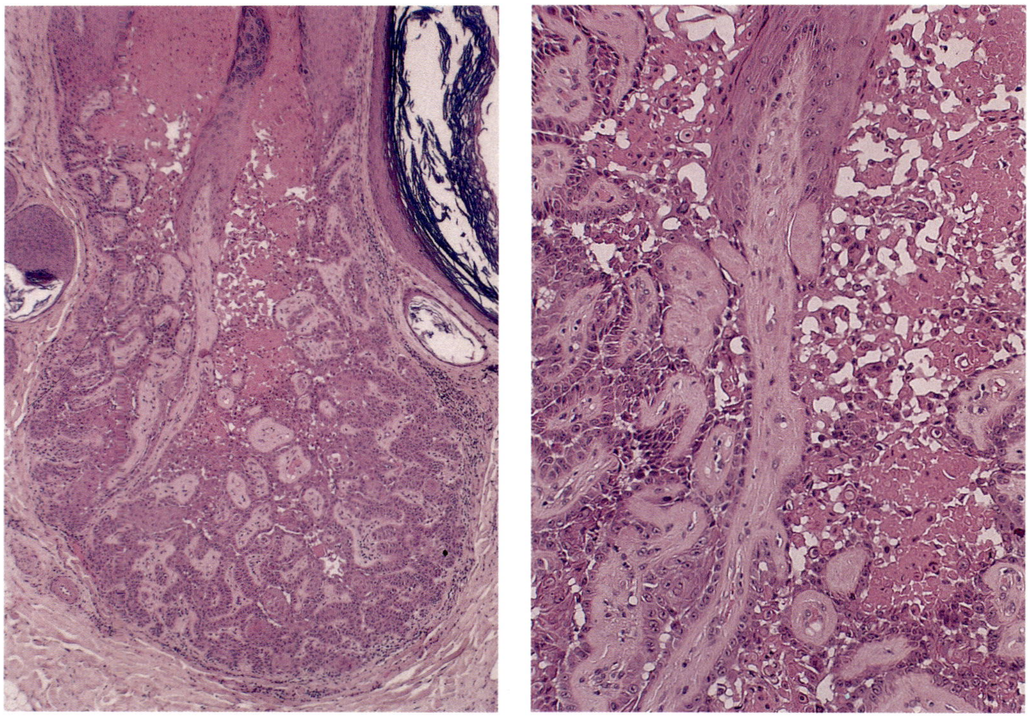

A B

Figures 3–36A, 3–36B. Warty dyskeratoma. Acantholytic dyskeratotic keratinocytes in the dermis.

4

SUBEPIDERMAL BULLOUS DERMATITIS

- Bullous pemphigoid
- Herpes gestationis
- Cicatricial pemphigoid
- Dermatitis herpetiformis
- Bullous systemic lupus erythematosus
- Porphyria cutanea tarda
- Epidermolysis bullosa
- Epidermolysis bullosa aquisita
- Bullous dermatosis of dialysis
- Bullous diabetes mellitus

BULLOUS PEMPHIGOID

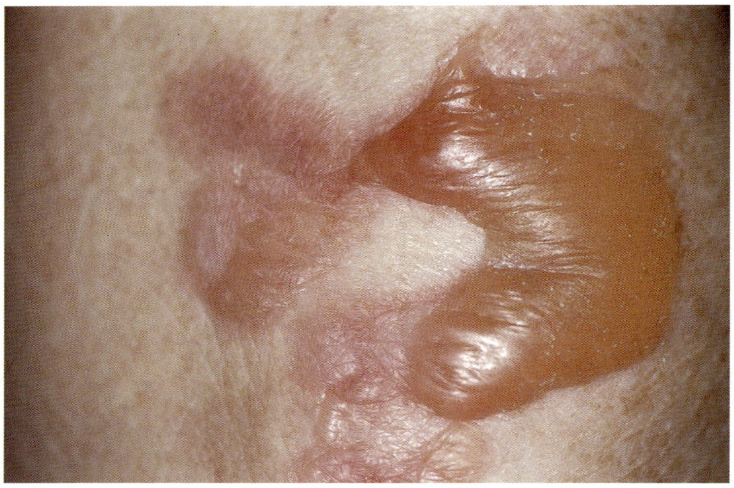

Figure 4–1. Bullous pemphigoid. Erythematous plaques contiguous with small and large bullae.

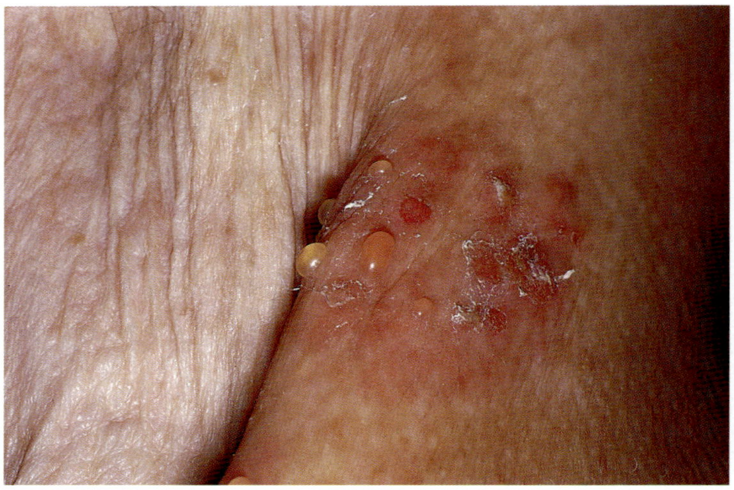

Figure 4–2. Bullous pemphigoid. Vesicles, bullae, erosions, and crusts on an erythematous plaque of the upper arm.

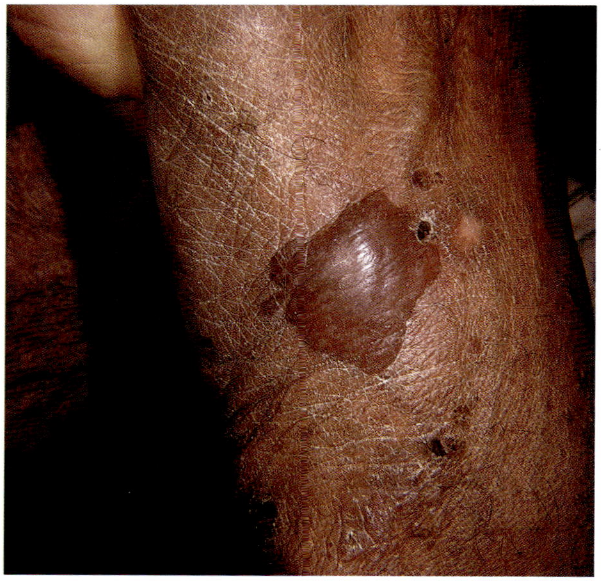

Figure 4–3. Bullous pemphigoid. Bulla on the leg.

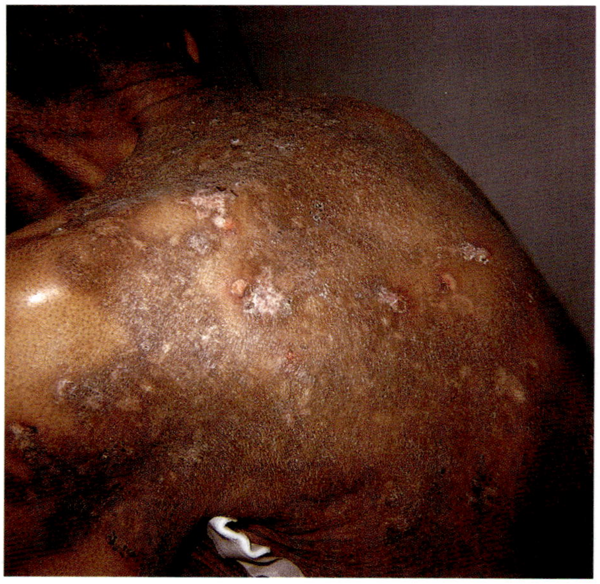

Figure 4–4. Bullous pemphigoid. Hypopigmented, hyperpigmented, and crusted areas from regressed bullous lesions.

BULLOUS PEMPHIGOID

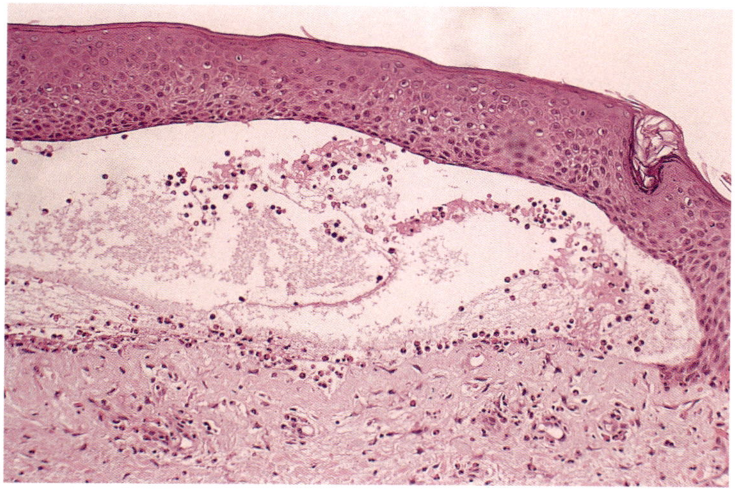

Figure 4–5. Bullous pemphigoid. Subepidermal blister with intact overlying epidermis. There is a mixed-cell infiltrate, where eosinophils predominate within both the bulla and dermis.

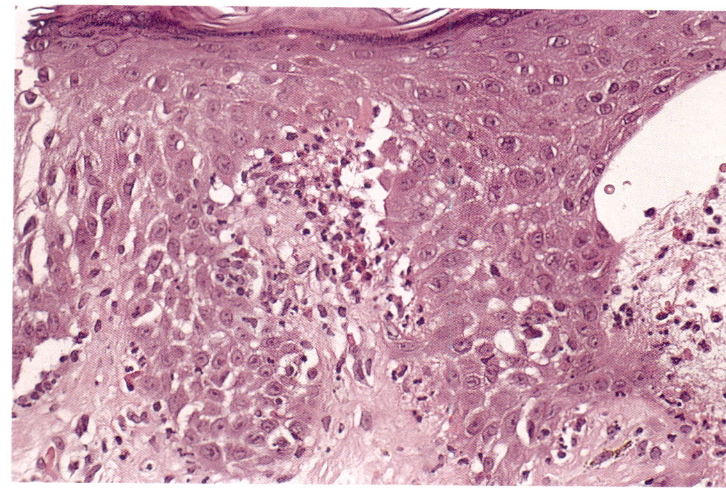

Figure 4–6. Bullous pemphigoid. Edge of subepidermal blister with eosinophils, on the right. The contiguous hyperplastic epidermis on the left contains eosinophils, spongiosis, and vacuolar alteration, which are typical findings in the urticarial stage of pemphigoid. Collections of eosinophils fill a dilated dermal papilla and extend into the epidermis. There are melanophages and a dermal mixed-cell infiltrate with eosinophils.

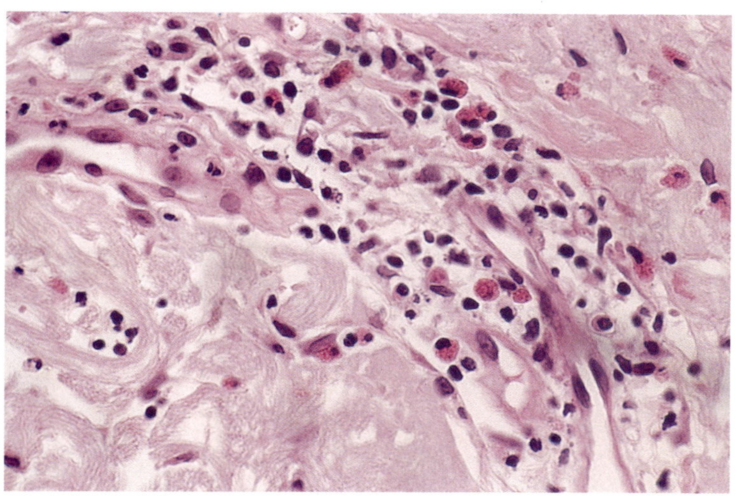

Figure 4–7. Bullous pemphigoid. Dilated dermal venules with perivascular and interstitial eosinophils.

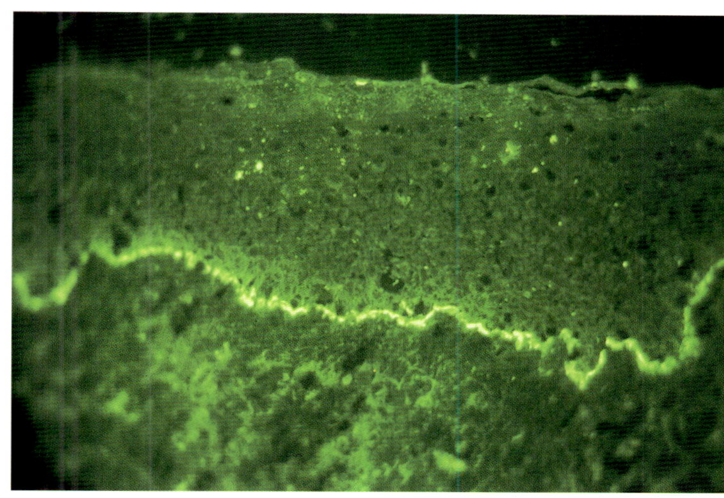

Figure 4–8. Bullous pemphigoid. Direct immunofluorescence of bullous pemphigoid. Note continuous deposition of C3 along the epidermal basement membrane zone.

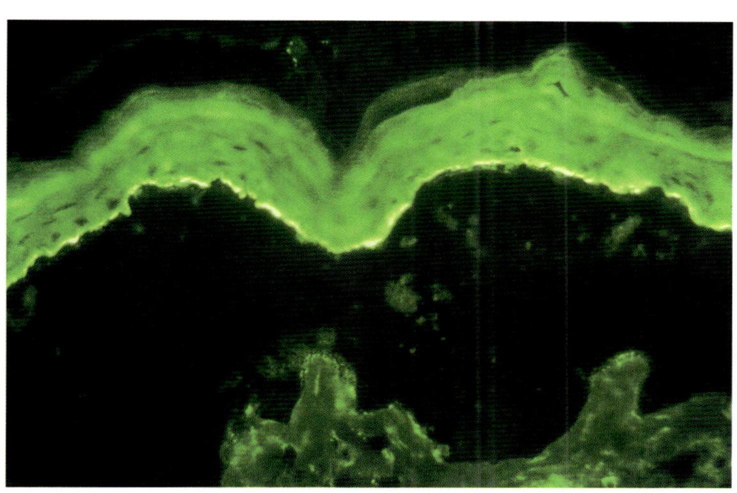

Figure 4–9. Bullous pemphigoid. Indirect immunofluorescence of bullous pemphigoid using salt-split normal human skin as substrate. Note deposition of IgG antibodies limited to the epidermal roof of the split.

HERPES GESTATIONIS

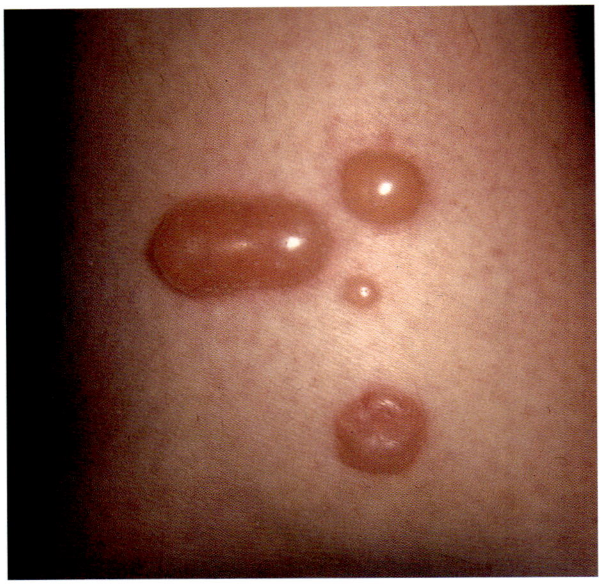

Figure 4–10. Herpes gestationis. Collection of blisters on abdomen of young pregnant woman.

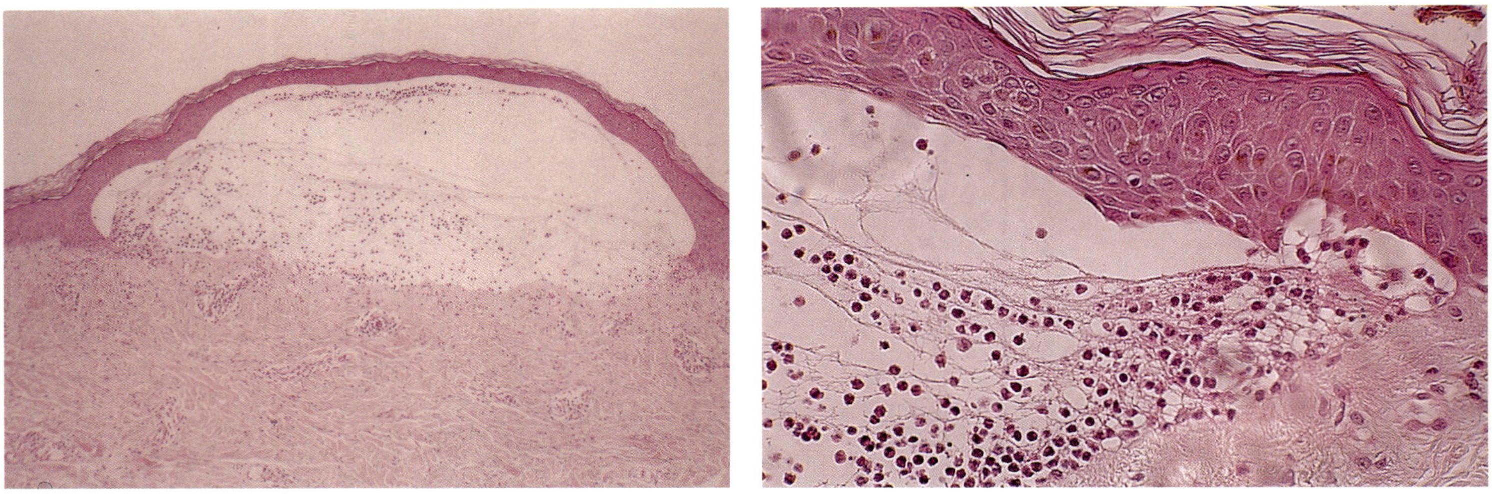

A

B

Figures 4–11A, 4–11B. Herpes gestationis. Subepidermal blister. There are eosinophils and neutrophils in the bulla and dermis.

CICATRICIAL PEMPHIGOID

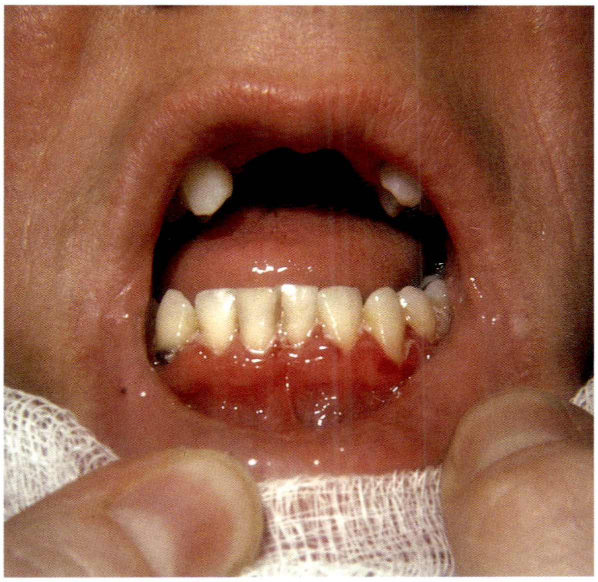

Figure 4–12. Cicatricial pemphigoid. Erythematous gingival erosions.

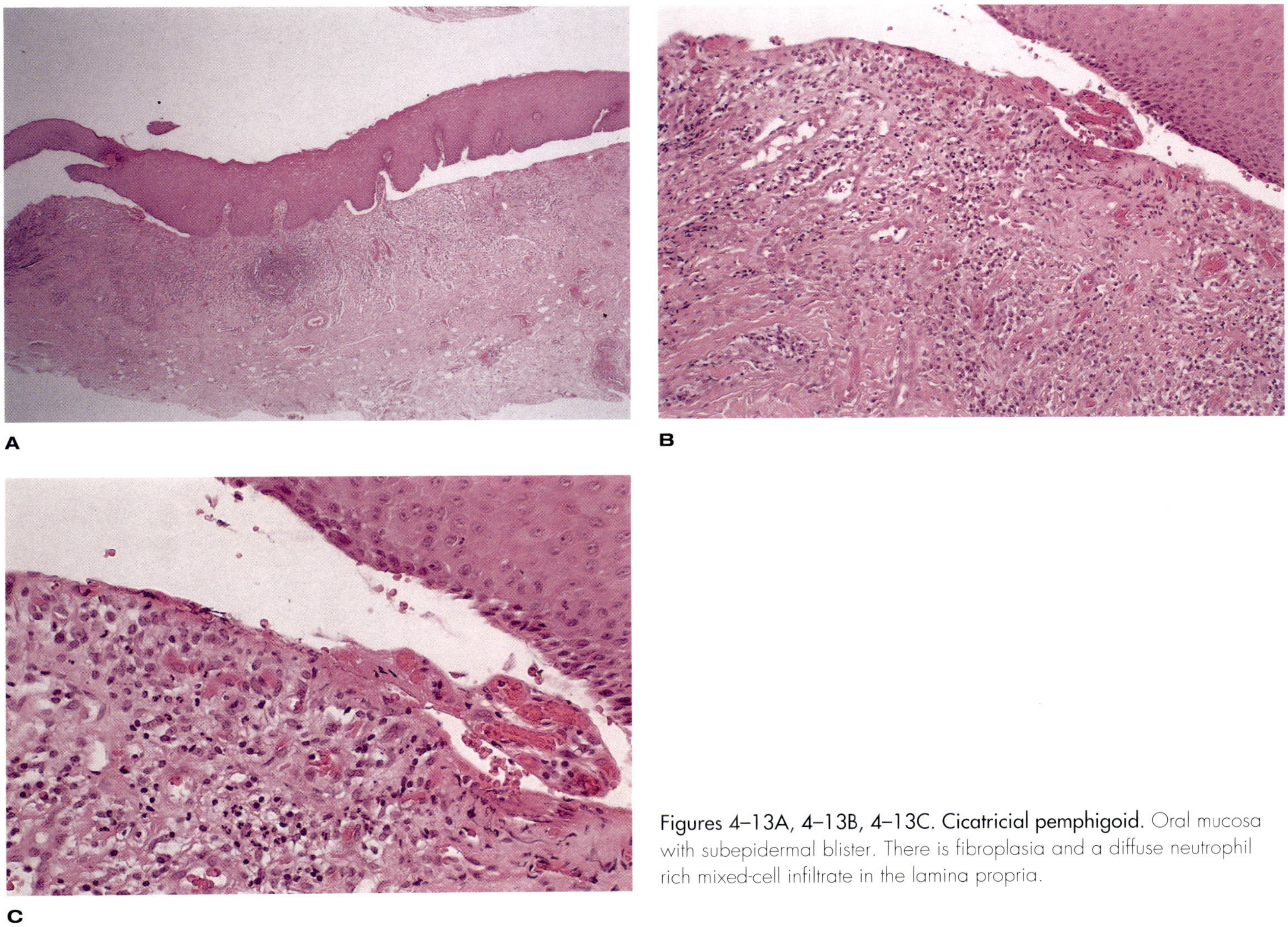

A

B

C

Figures 4–13A, 4–13B, 4–13C. Cicatricial pemphigoid. Oral mucosa with subepidermal blister. There is fibroplasia and a diffuse neutrophil rich mixed-cell infiltrate in the lamina propria.

DERMATITIS HERPETIFORMIS

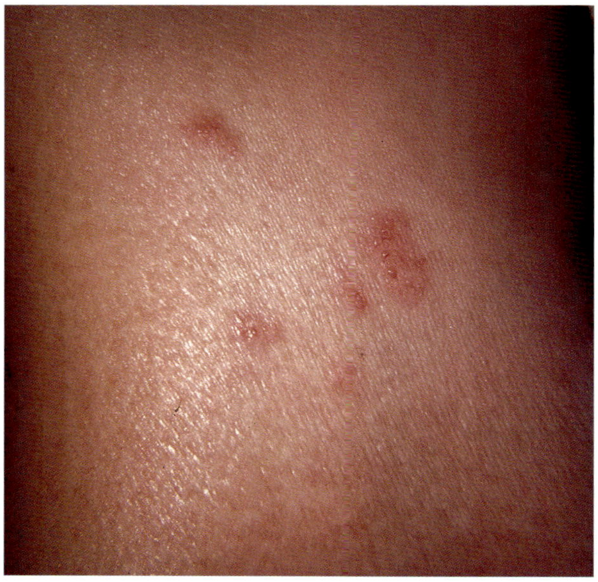

Figure 4–14. Dermatitis herpetiformis. Early erythematous papules with pinpoint vesicles on the arm.

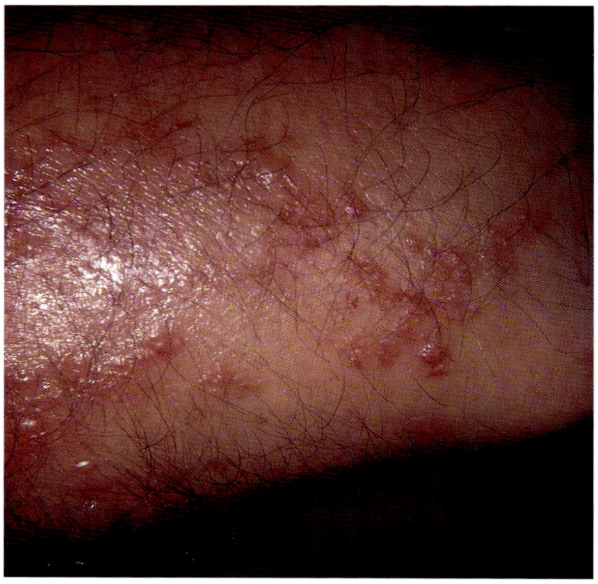

Figure 4–15. Dermatitis herpetiformis. Later erythematous vesiculopapules.

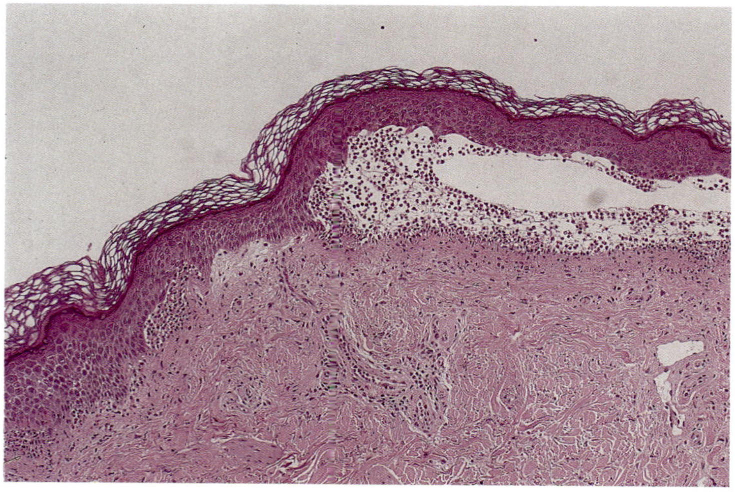

Figure 4–16. Dermatitis herpetiformis. Subepidermal blister where neutrophils predominate. There is dermal edema and a mixed-cell neutrophilic infiltrate. Similar histopathologic changes may be seen in other bullous diseases, such as chronic bullous disease of childhood and linear IgA dermatosis.

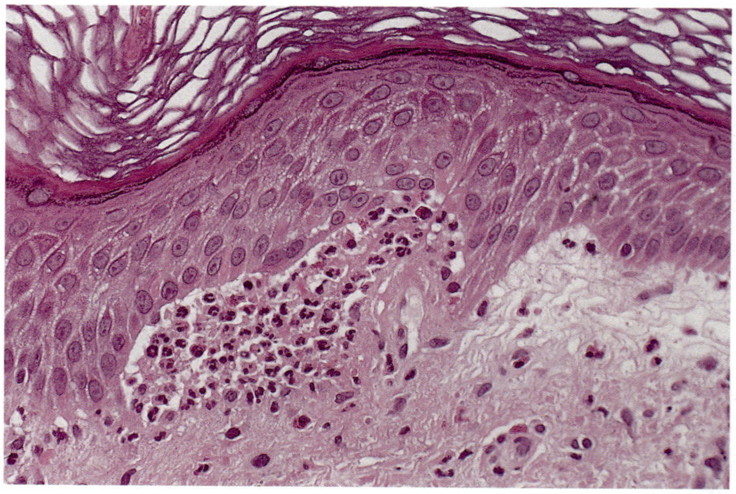

Figure 4–17. Dermatitis herpetiformis. Sharply circumscribed collection of neutrophils fills an edematous dermal papilla.

DERMATITIS HERPETIFORMIS

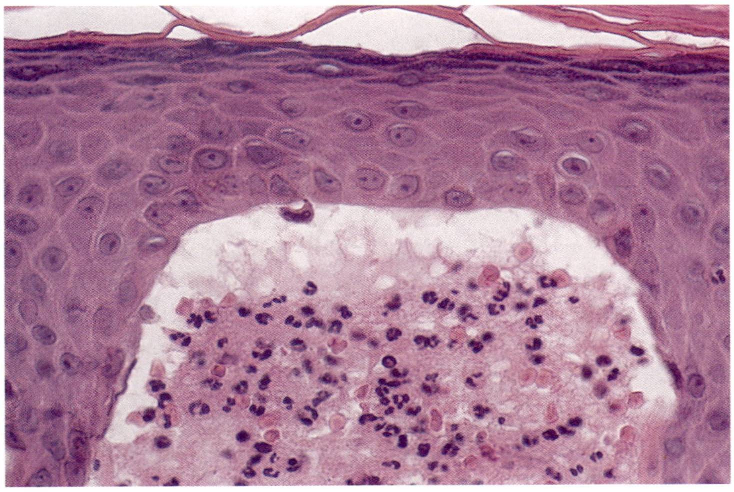

Figure 4–18. Dermatitis herpetiformis. Subepidermal blister with numerous neutrophils. There is an acantholytic keratinocyte at the top of the blister cavity.

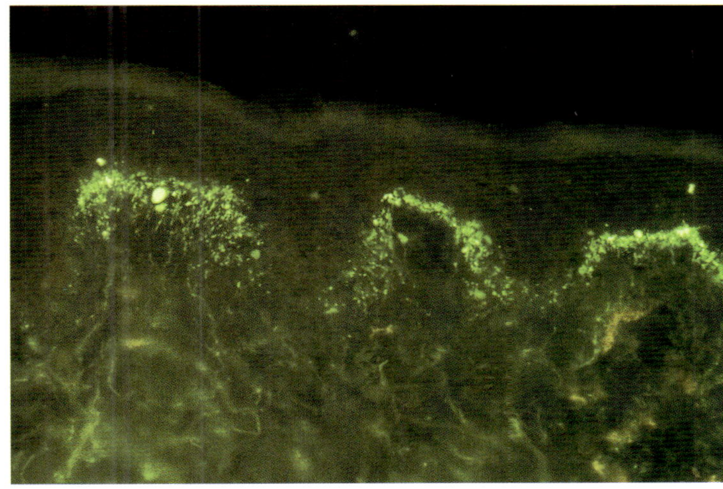

Figure 4–19. Dermatitis herpetiformis. Direct immunofluorescence in dermatitis herpetiformis. Note granular deposition of IgA in dermal/epidermal junction and papillary dermis.

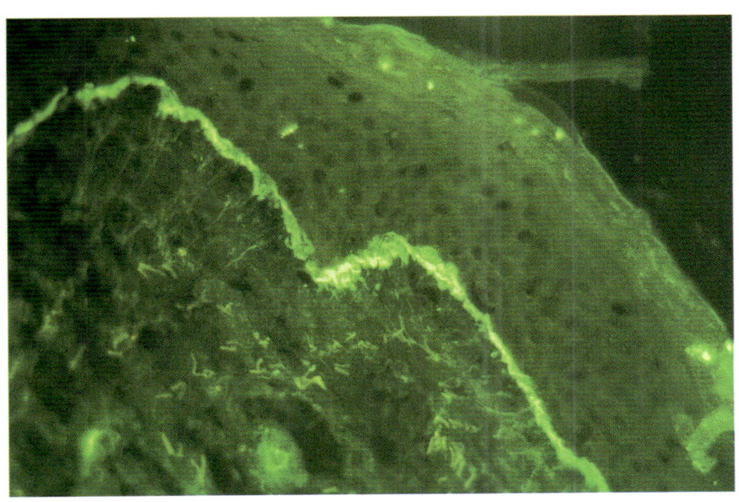

Figure 4–20. Linear IgA disease. Direct immunofluorescence in linear IgA disease. Note deposition of IgA in a continuous pattern along the epidermal basement membrane zone.

BULLOUS SYSTEMIC LUPUS ERYTHEMATOSUS

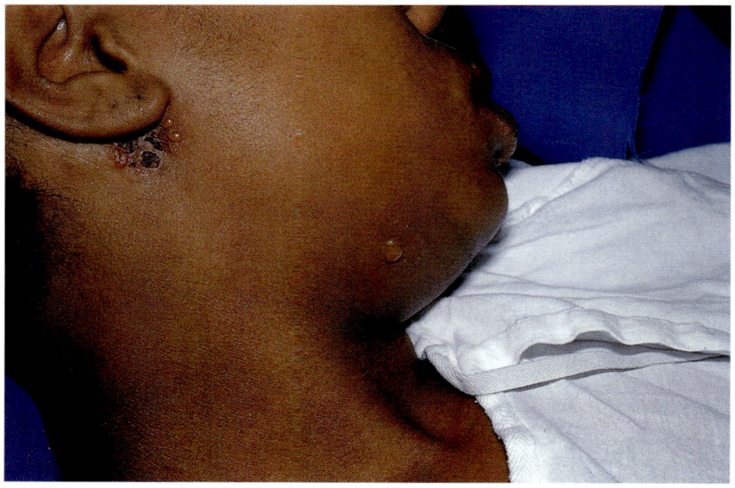

Figure 4–21. Bullous systemic lupus erythematosus. Vesicles on the neck and postauricular area.

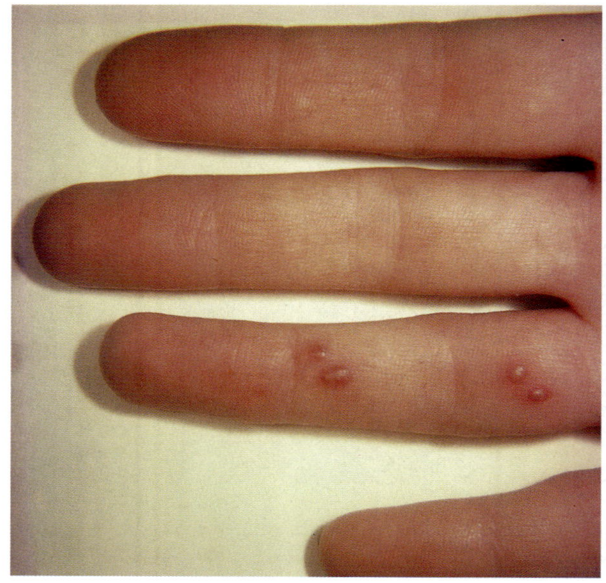

Figure 4–22. Bullous systemic lupus erythematosus. Vesicles on finger of a woman with systemic lupus erythematosus.

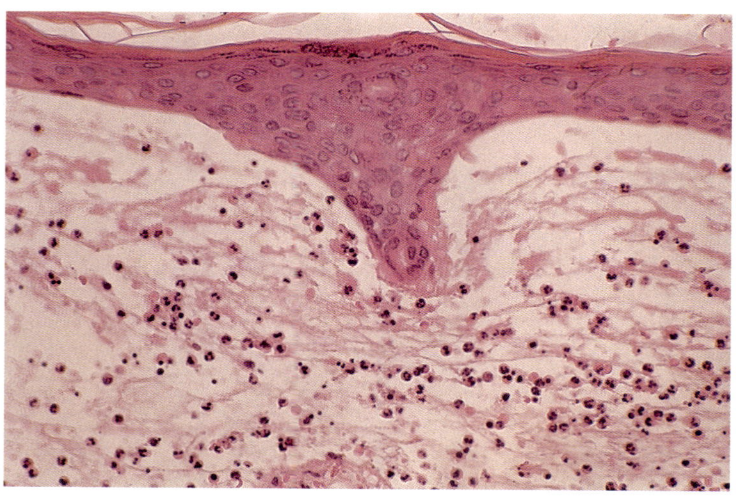

A

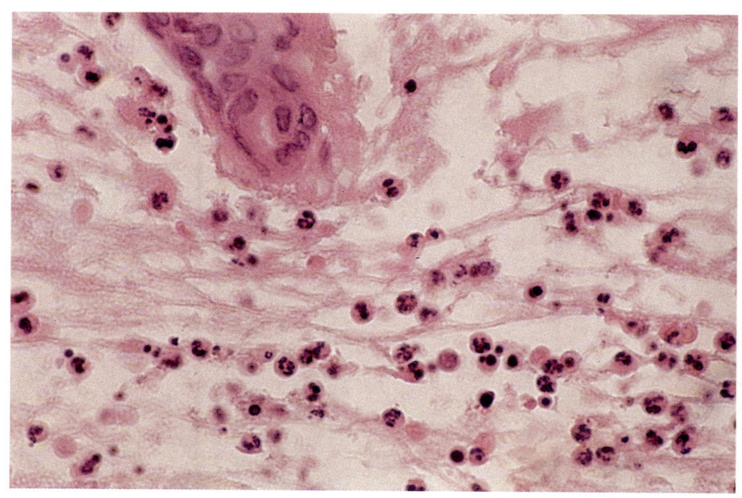

B

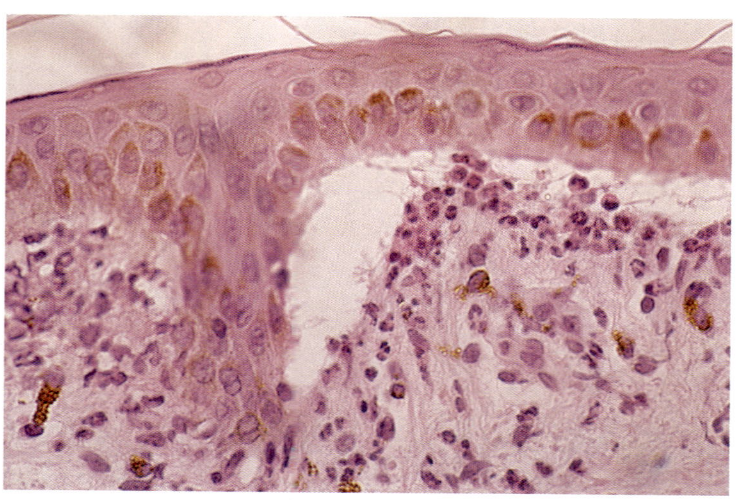

C

Figures 4–23A, 4–23B, 4–23C. Bullous systemic lupus erythematosus. Subepidermal blister with many neutrophils.

PORPHYRIA CUTANEA TARDA

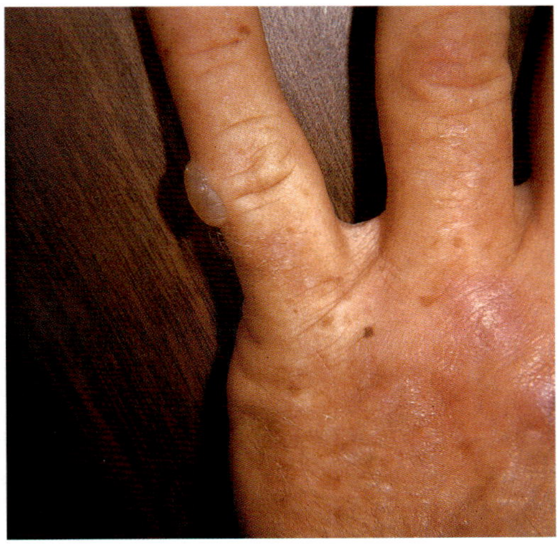

Figure 4–24. Porphyria cutanea tarda. Blister on fifth digit over the proximal interphalangeal joint.

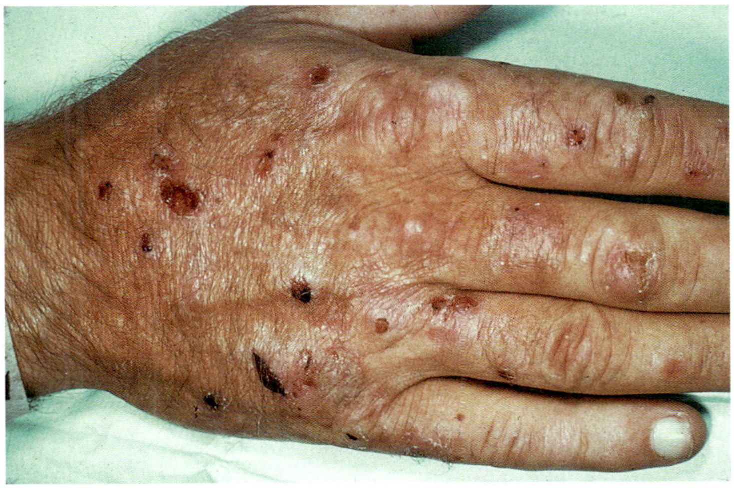

Figure 4–25. Porphyria cutanea tarda. Crusted and erosive lesions on dorsum of hand and fingers.

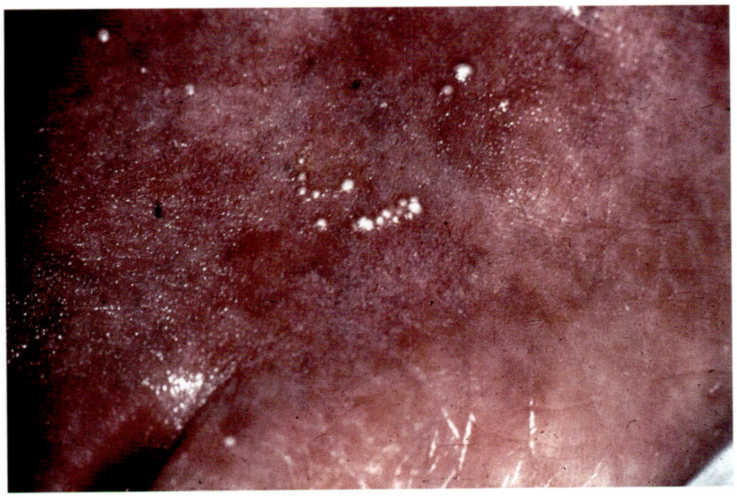

Figure 4–26. Porphyria cutanea tarda. Milia on dorsum of hand.

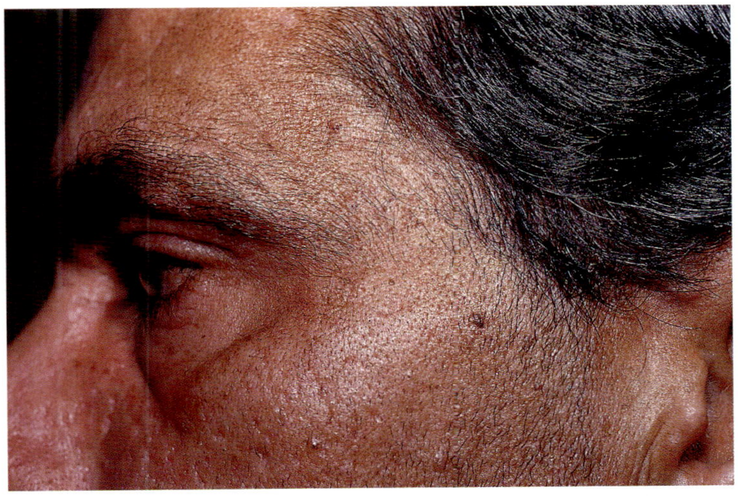

Figure 4–27. Porphyria cutanea tarda. Hypertrichosis.

PORPHYRIA CUTANEA TARDA

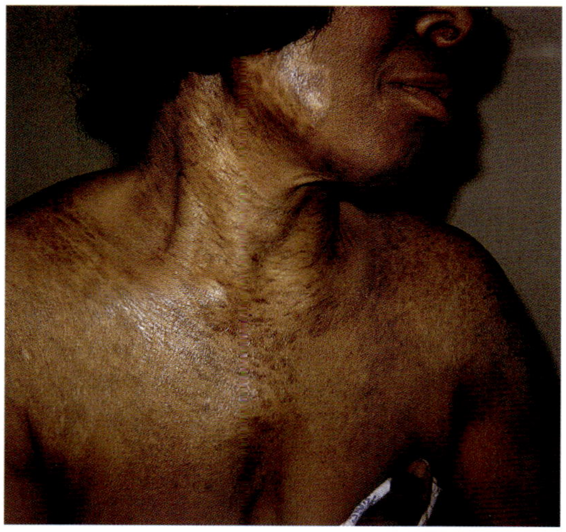

Figure 4–28. Porphyria cutanea tarda. Sclerodermoid changes involving the face, neck, and chest.

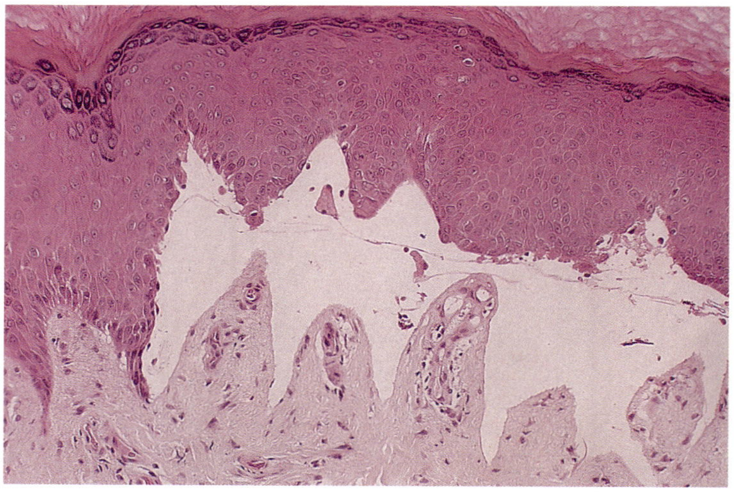

Figure 4–29. Porphyria cutanea tarda. Subepidermal blister on acral skin. Prominent dermal papillae protrude into the subepidermal blister (festooning). There is a paucity of inflammatory cells in the dermis. Blood vessels are dilated and have thickened walls.

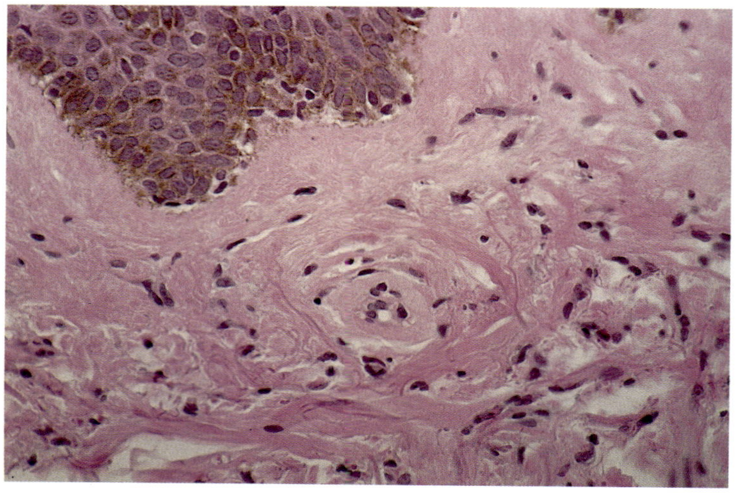

Figure 4–30. Porphyria cutanea tarda. Dermal fibroplasia and thickened blood vessel wall.

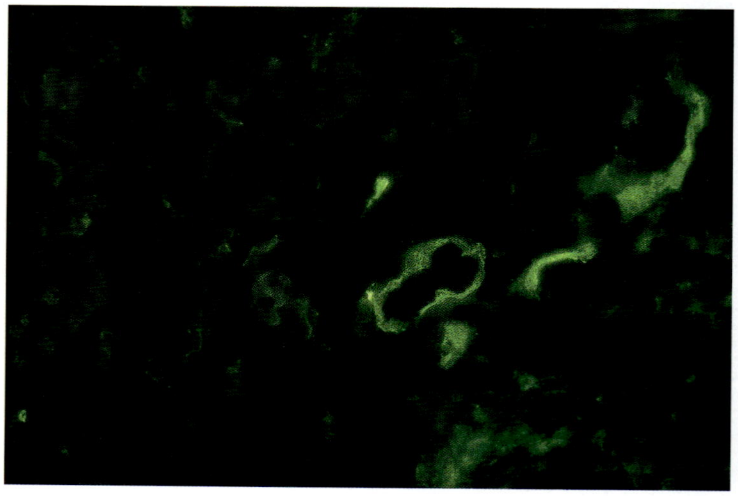

Figure 4–31. Porphyria cutanea tarda. Direct immunofluorescence with positive IgG blood vessel wall deposition.

EPIDERMOLYSIS BULLOSA

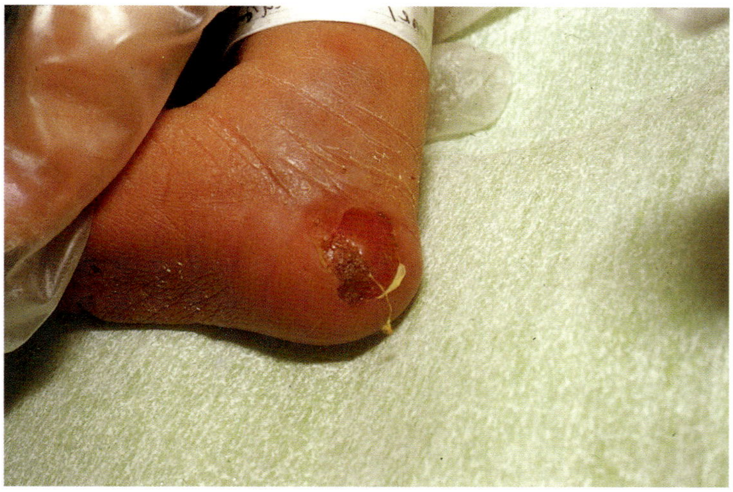

Figure 4–32. Epidermolysis bullosa simplex. Denuded blister on heel of an infant.

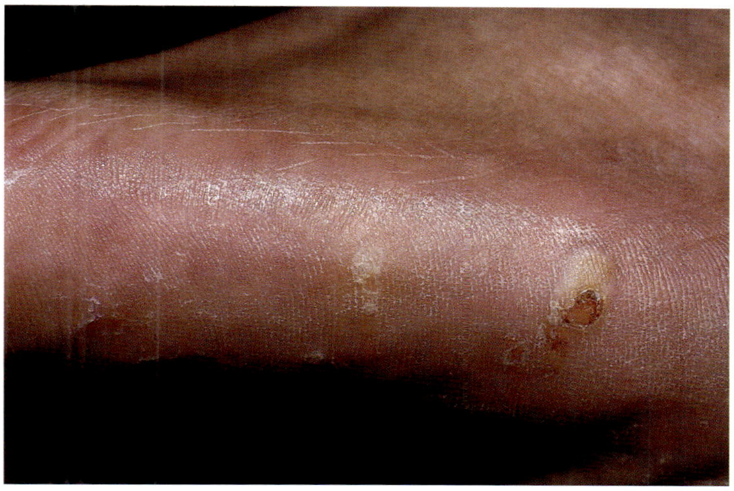

Figure 4–33. Epidermolysis bullosa simplex. Blisters on sole of foot of young man whose father also had blisters on feet.

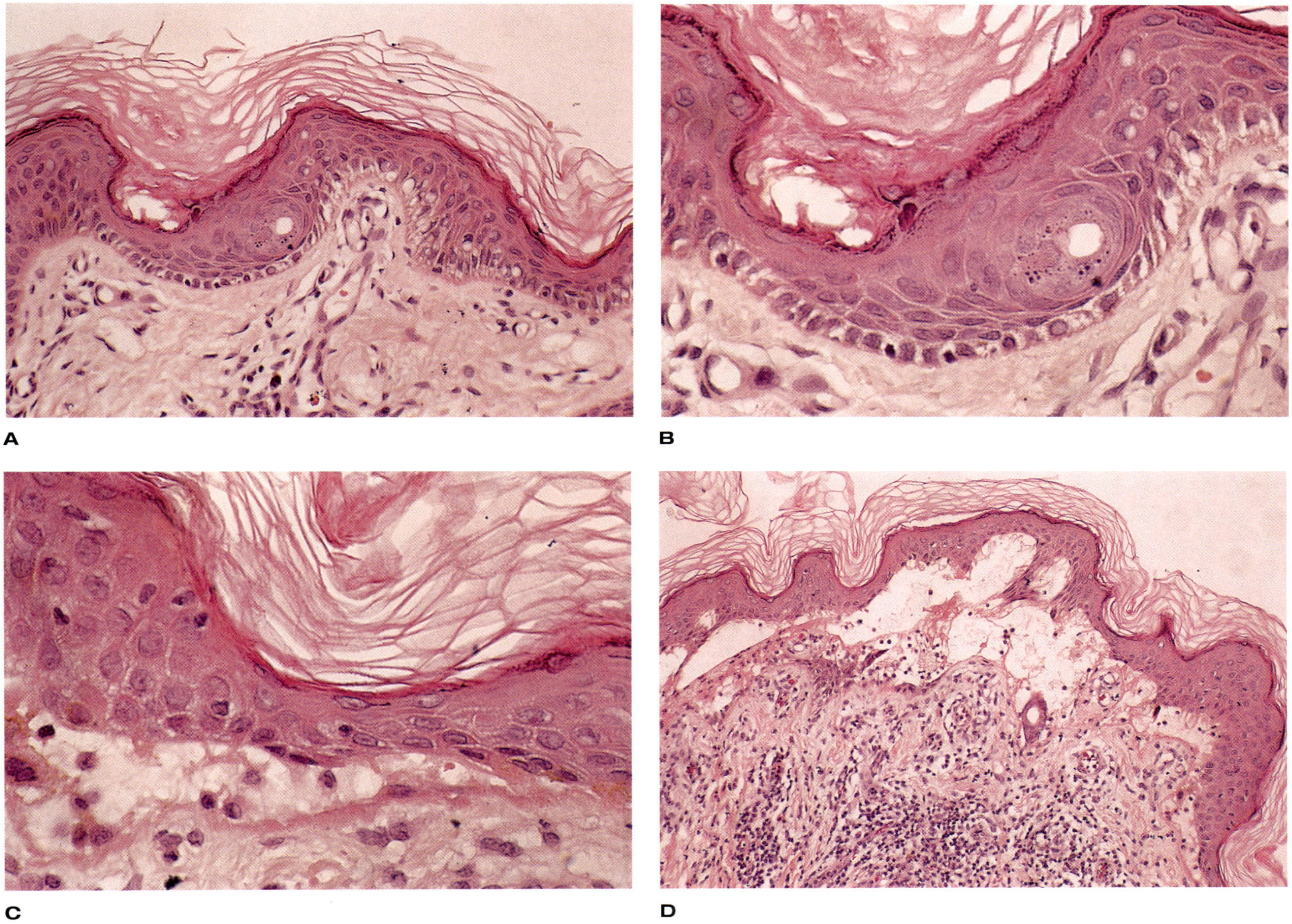

Figures 4–34. Epidermolysis bullosa simplex. Vacuoles initially within the basal cells **(A & B)**. There is subsequent disintegration of the basal cells with subepidermal separation and vesiculation **(C & D)**.

EPIDERMOLYSIS BULLOSA

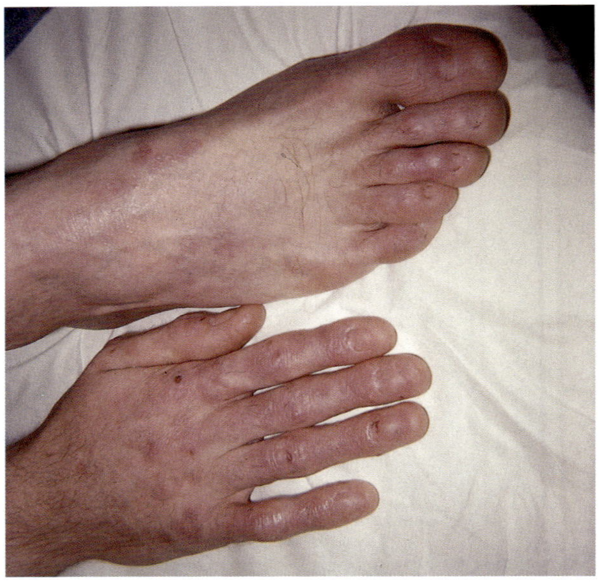

Figure 4–35. Epidermolysis bullosa dystrophica. A few vesicles and erosions on dorsum of foot and hand. Complete absence of all toenails and fingernails with onychial scarring for many years.

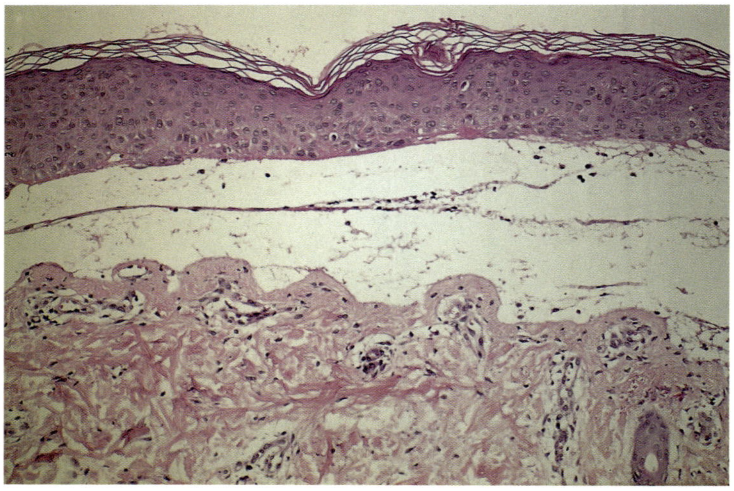

Figure 4–36. Epidermolysis bullosa dystrophica. Subepidermal blister with a sparse inflammatory cell infiltrate.

EPIDERMOLYSIS BULLOSA AQUISITA

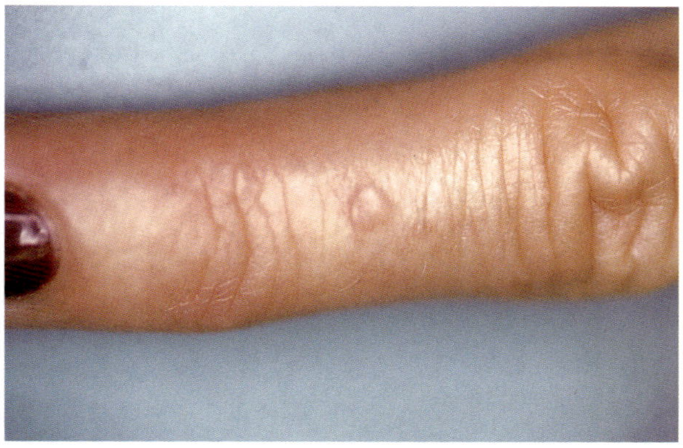

Figure 4–37. Epidermolysis bullosa aquisita. Early blister on finger of a woman with history of recurrent blisters on dorsum of hand for 18 months.

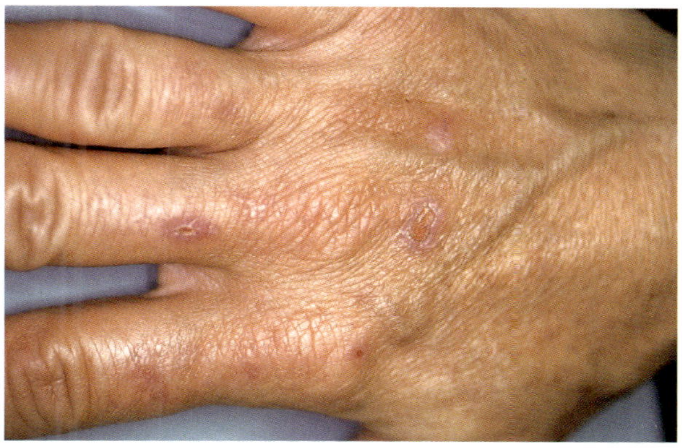

Figure 4–38. Epidermolysis bullosa aquisita Erosions and crusted lesions on dorsum of the hand.

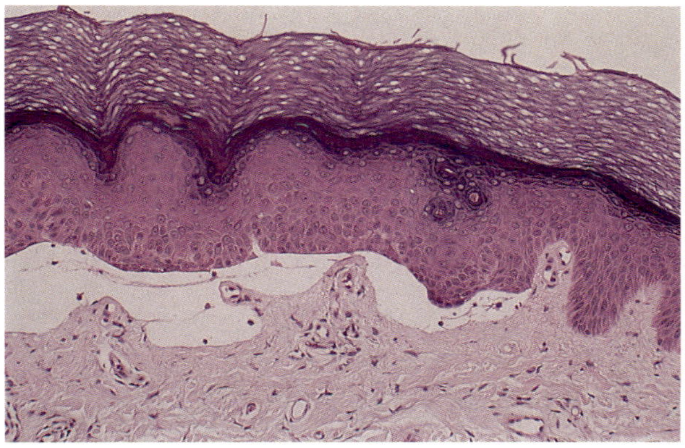

A

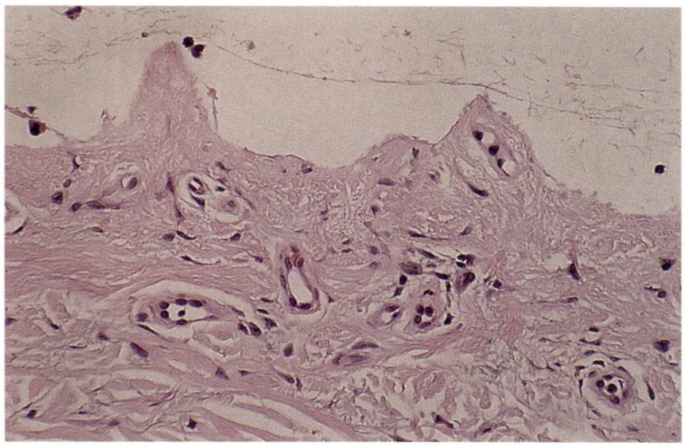

B

Figures 4–39A, 4–39B. Epidermolysis bullosa aquisita. Subepidermal blister. There is a sparse mixed-cell dermal infiltrate and dilated venules.

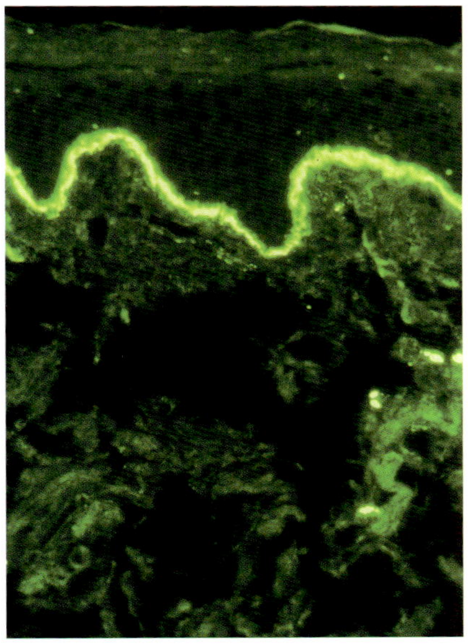

Figure 4–40. Epidermolysis bullosa aquisita. Direct immunofluorescence in epidermolysis bullosa aquisita. Note deposition of IgG in a continuous pattern along the epidermal basement membrane. This pattern is quite similar to that seen in pemphigoid.

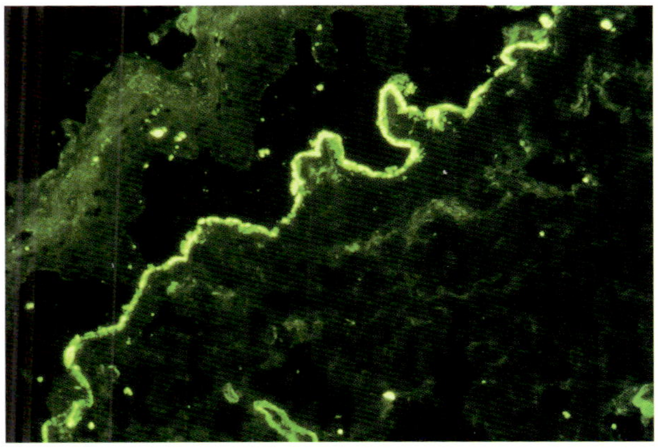

Figure 4–41. Epidermolysis bullosa aqu sita. Direct immunofluorescence in epidermolysis bullosa aquisita after the specimen has been incubated with sodium chloride. Note deposition of IgG limited to the dermal site of the split.

BULLOUS DERMATOSIS OF DIALYSIS

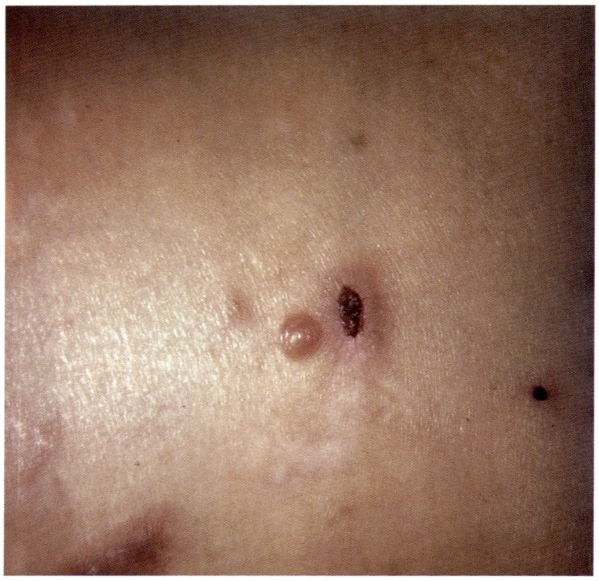

Figure 4–42. Bullous dermatosis of dialysis. Blister and crusted papule.

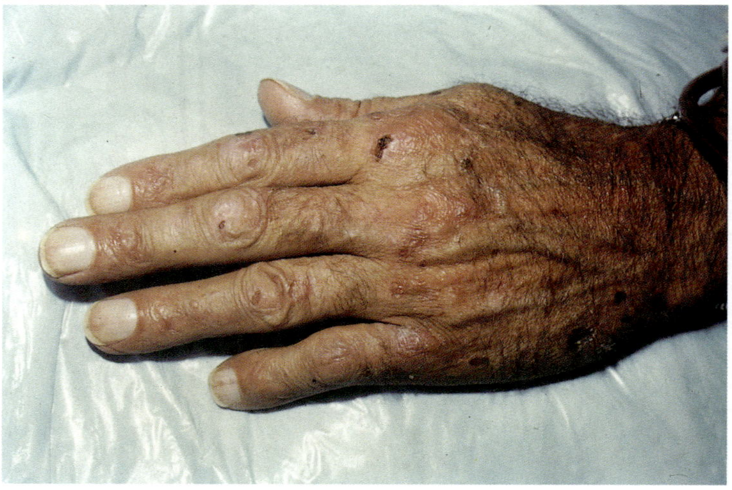

Figure 4–43. Bullous dermatosis of dialysis. Blisters and crusted plaques.

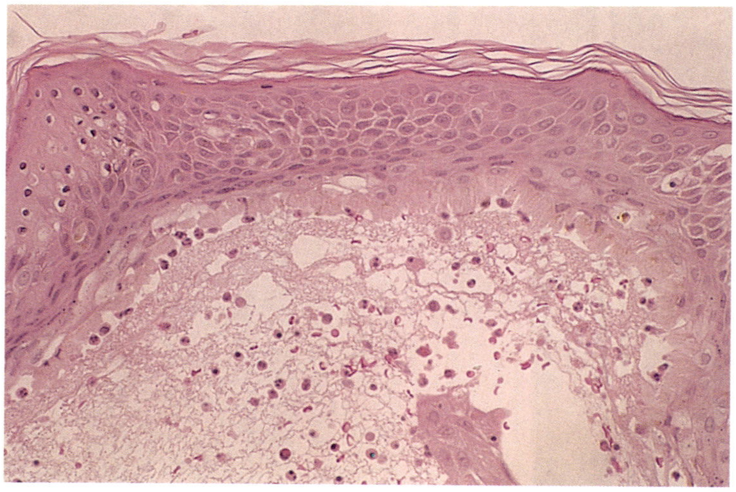

Figure 4–44. Bullous dermatosis of dialysis. Subepidermal blister with a sparse mixed-cell infiltrate with eosinophils and neutrophils.

BULLOUS DIABETES MELLITUS

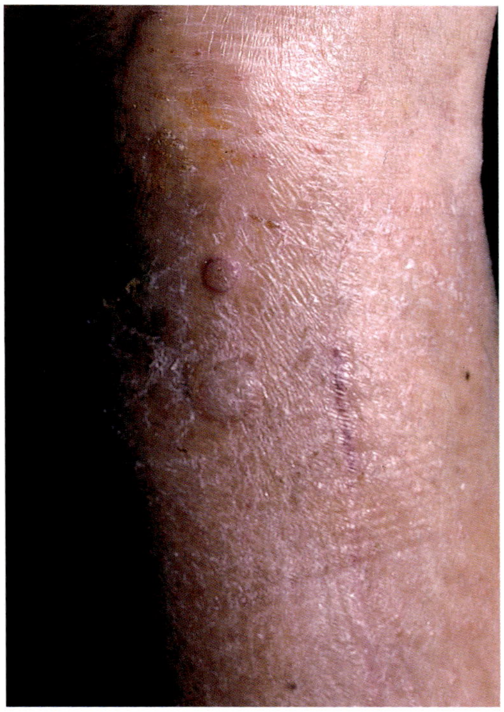

Figure 4–45. Bullous diabetes mellitus. Blisters on the lower leg of a man with diabetes mellitus.

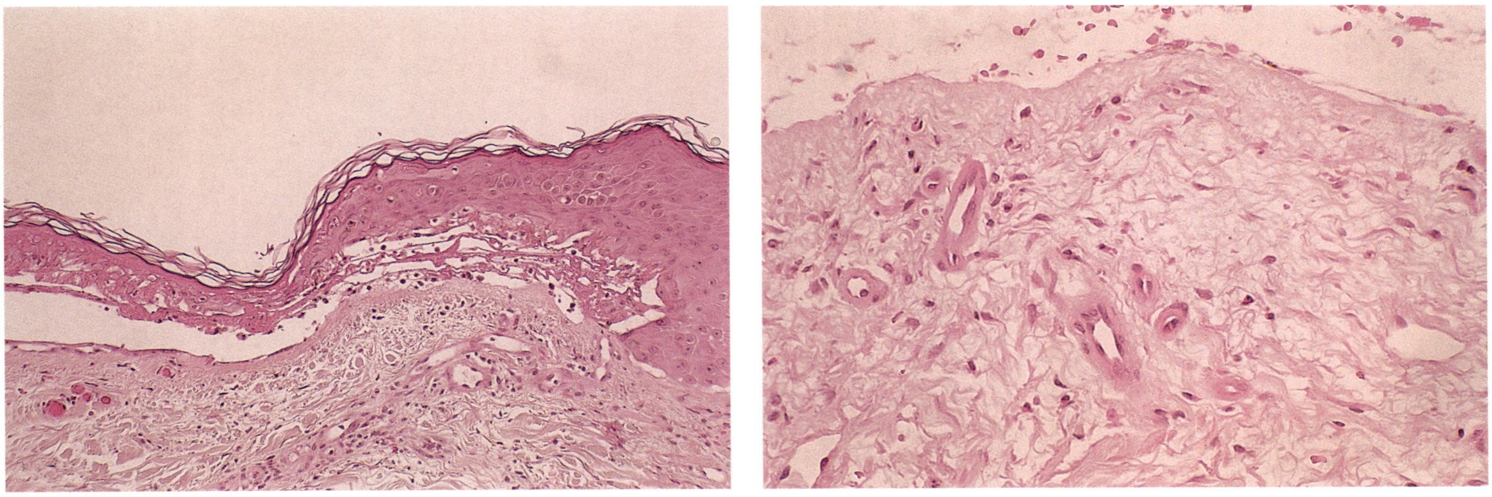

A B

Figures 4–46A, 4–46B. Bullous diabetes mellitus. Subepidermal blister with vacuolar alteration and necrotic keratinocytes. There is a sparse dermal mixed-cell infiltrate and thick-walled venules.

5

Perivascular and interstitial dermatitis

- Urticaria
- Erythema annulare centrificum (EAC)
- Schamberg's disease (pigmented purpuric dermatitis)
- Polymorphous light eruption (PMLE)
- Telangiectasia macularis eruptiva perstans (TMEP)

URTICARIA

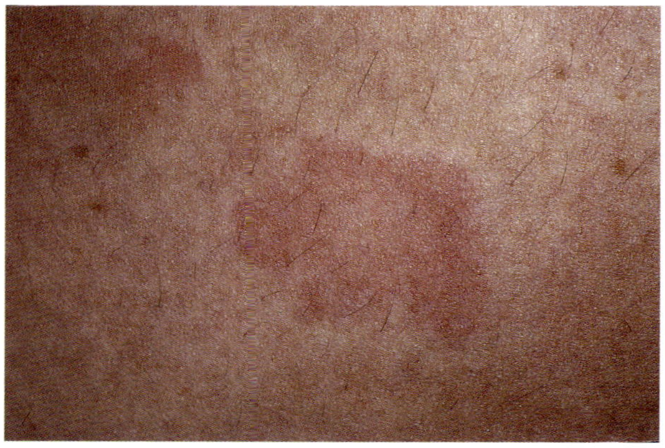

Figure 5–1. Urticaria. Irregular erythematous minimally elevated lesions, which are transient by history.

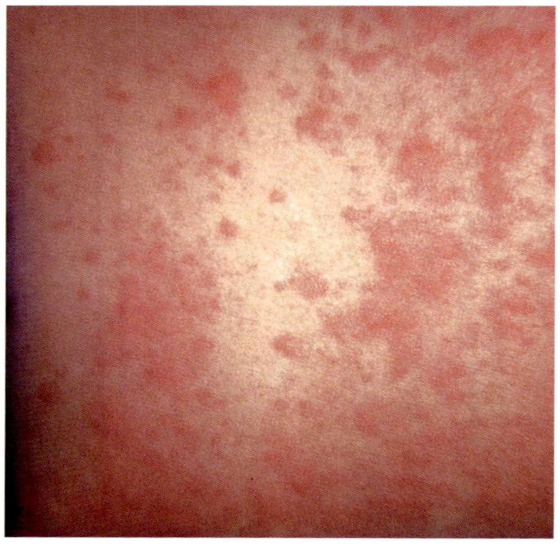

Figure 5–2. Urticaria. Erythematous macules and papules with areas of confluence.

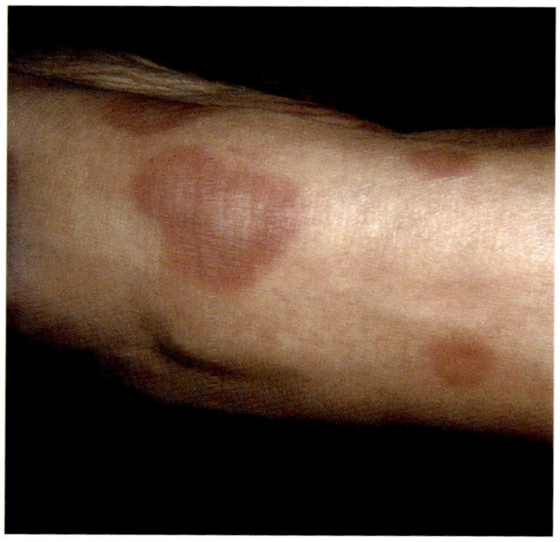

Figure 5–3. Urticaria. Sharply marginated erythematous plaques on the knee and leg.

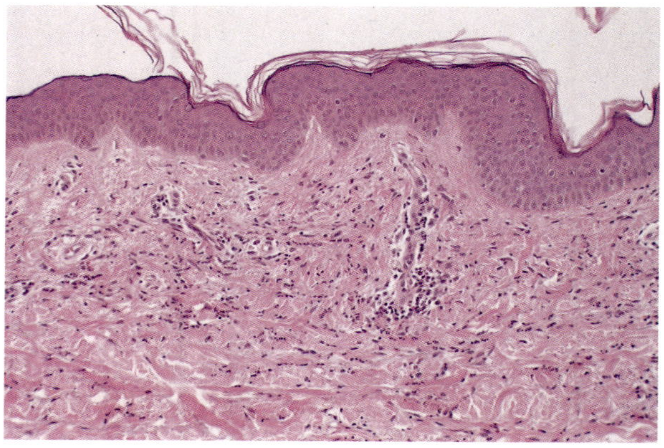

Figure 5–4. Urticaria. Perivascular and interstitial dermal mixed-cell infiltrate with neutrophils and eosinophils. The epidermis is not altered.

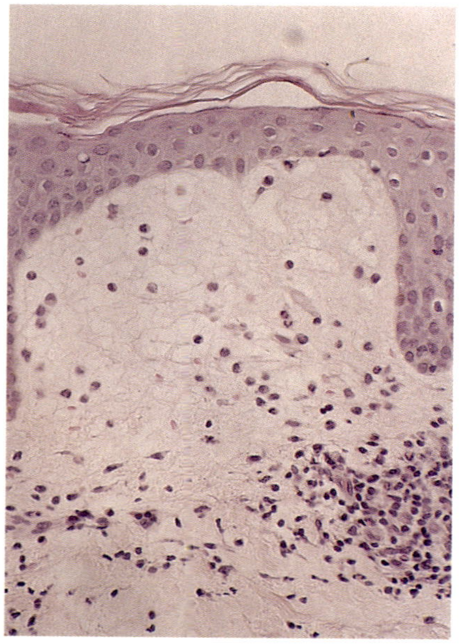

Figure 5–5. Urticaria. Papillary dermal edema with neutrophils and eosinophils.

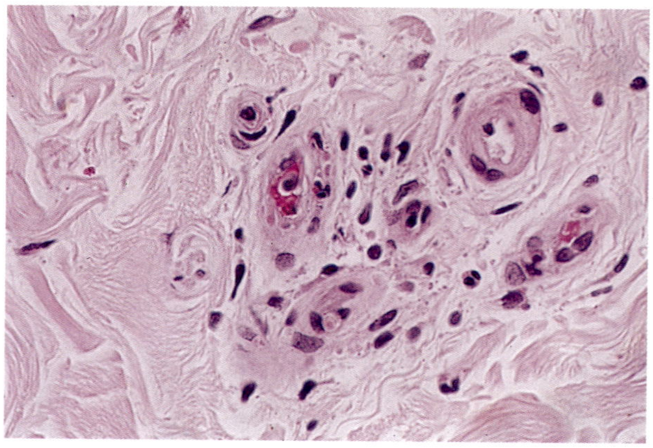

Figure 5–6. Urticaria. Neutrophils perivascularly and interstitially in the reticular dermis.

ERYTHEMA ANNULARE CENTRIFICUM (EAC)

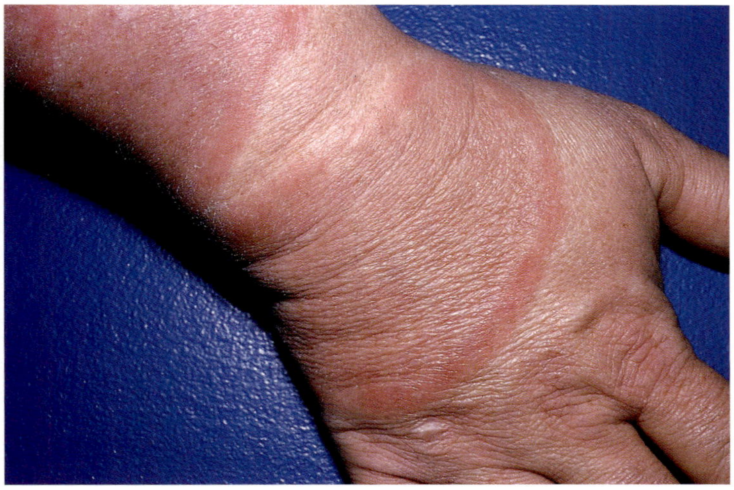

A

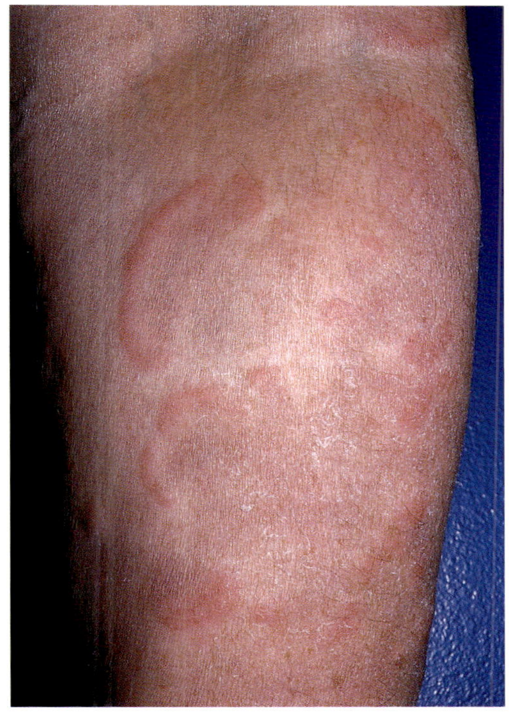

B

Figures 5–7A, 5–7B. Erythema annulare centrificum. Erythematous patches, papules, and plaques with raised margins in annular and arcuate patterns.

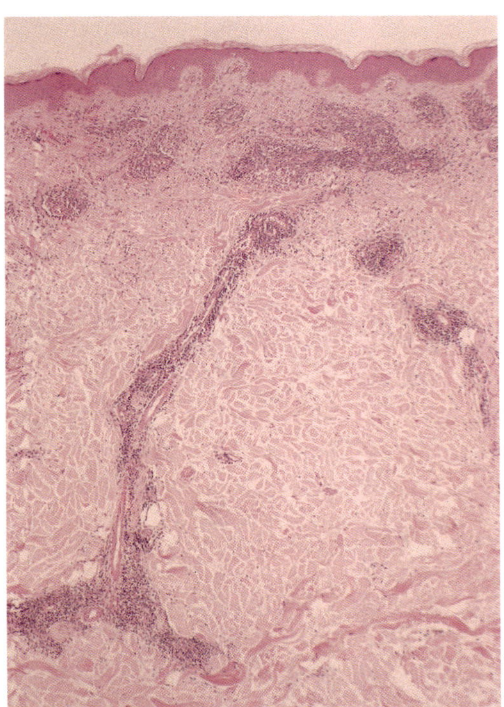

A

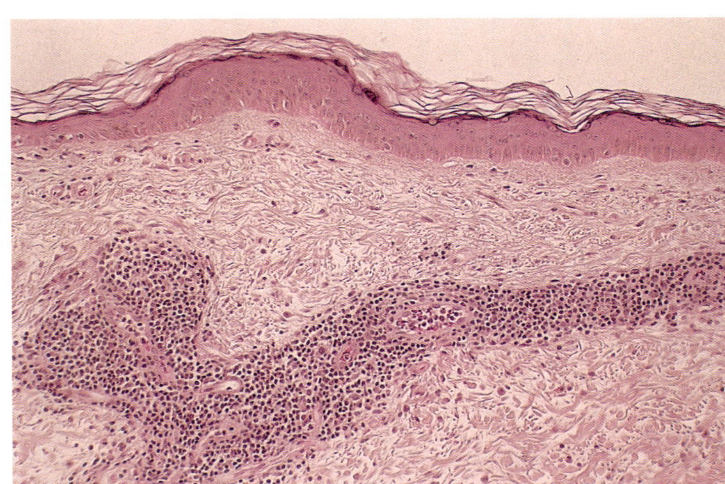

B

Figures 5–8A, 5–8B. Erythema annulare centrificum. Superficial and deep dense perivascular lymphohistiocytic infiltrate.

SCHAMBERG'S DISEASE (PIGMENTED PURPURIC DERMATITIS)

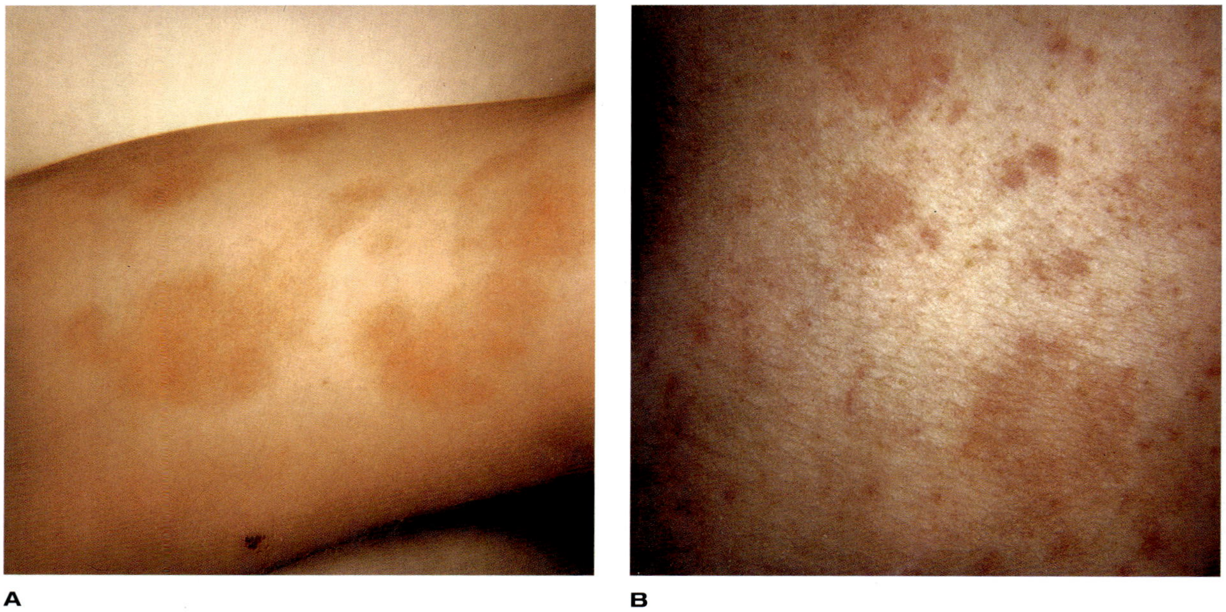

Figures 5–9A, 5–9B. Schamberg's disease. Speckled hyperpigmented macules and patches on the thigh.

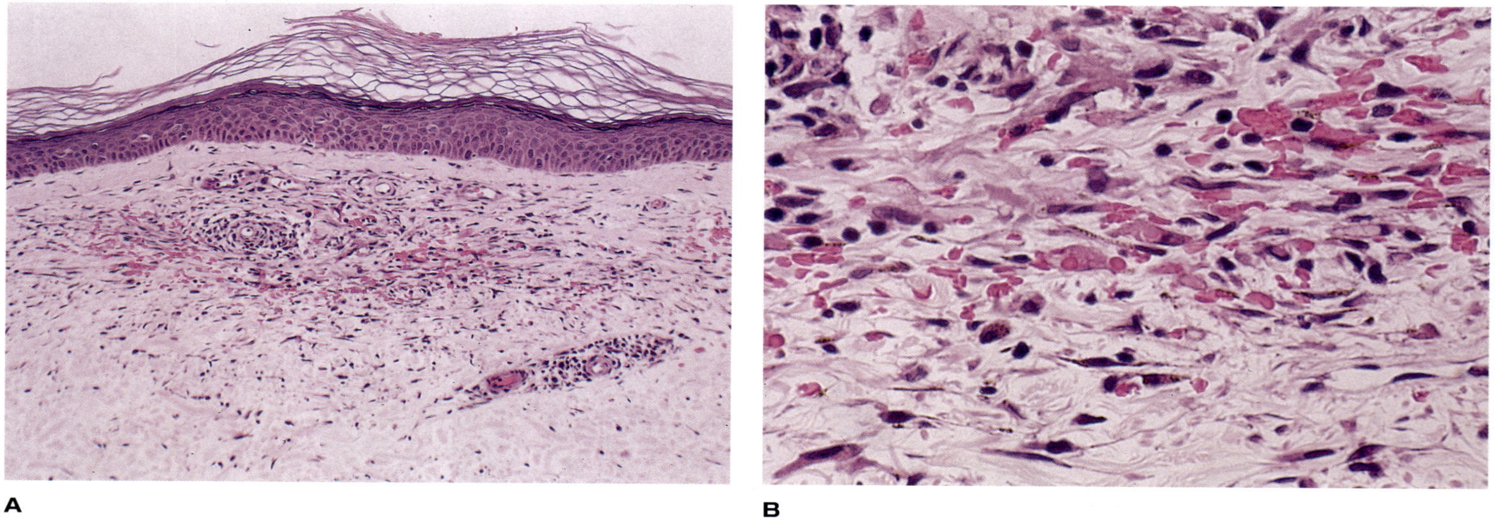

Figures 5–10A, 5–10B. Schamberg's disease. Dilated and congested blood vessels with many extravasated erythrocytes. There are numerous siderophages associated with a mononuclear cell dermal infiltrate.

POLYMORPHOUS LIGHT ERUPTION (PMLE)

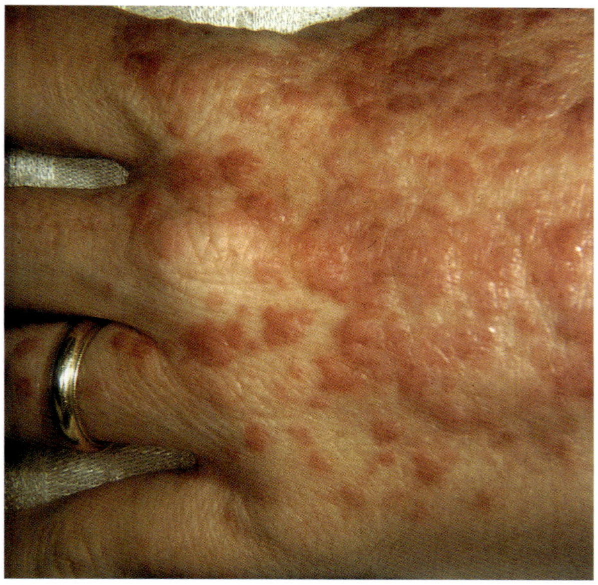

Figure 5–11. **Polymorphous light eruption.** Erythematous papules and plaques on the hand and fingers.

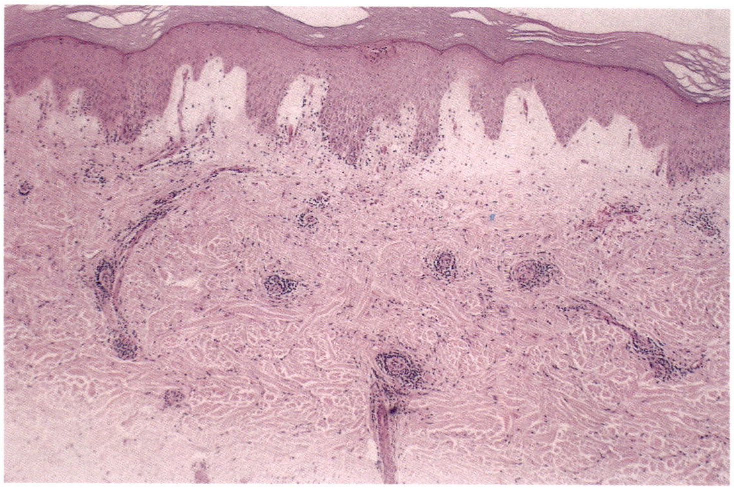

Figure 5–12. **Polymorphous light eruption.** Severe papillary edema and prominent perivascular infiltrate.

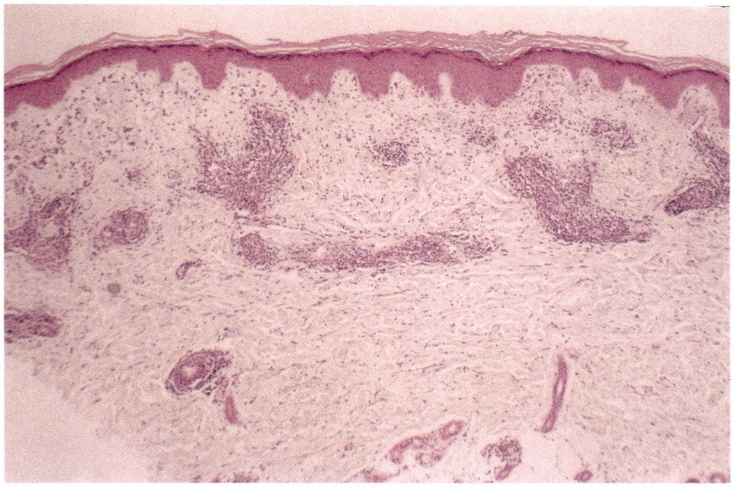

Figure 5–13. **Polymorphous light eruption.** Superficial and deep perivascular infiltrate.

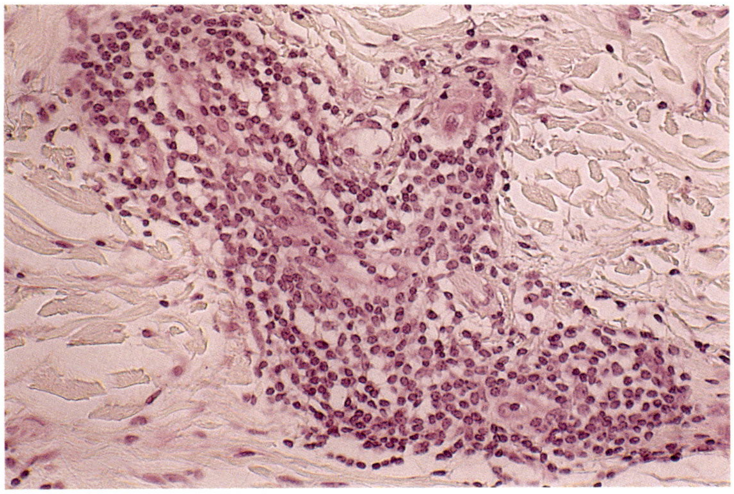

A

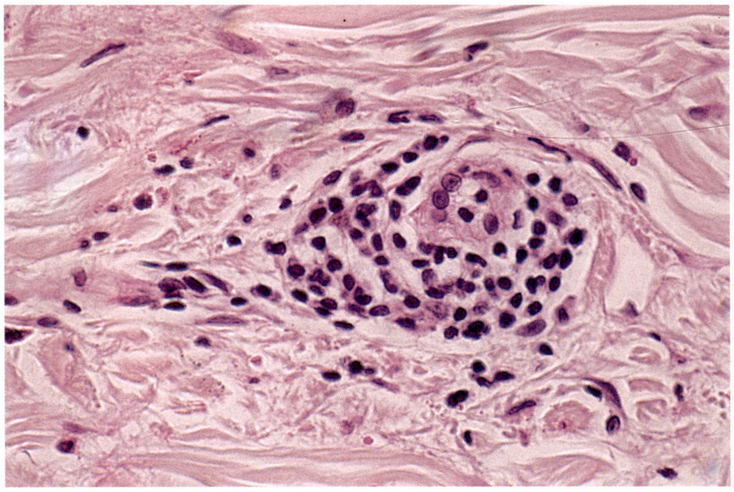

B

Figures 5–14A, 5–14B. **Polymorphous light eruption.** Prominent perivascular lymphohistiocytic infiltrate and sporadic eosinophils.

POLYMORPHOUS LIGHT ERUPTION (PMLE)

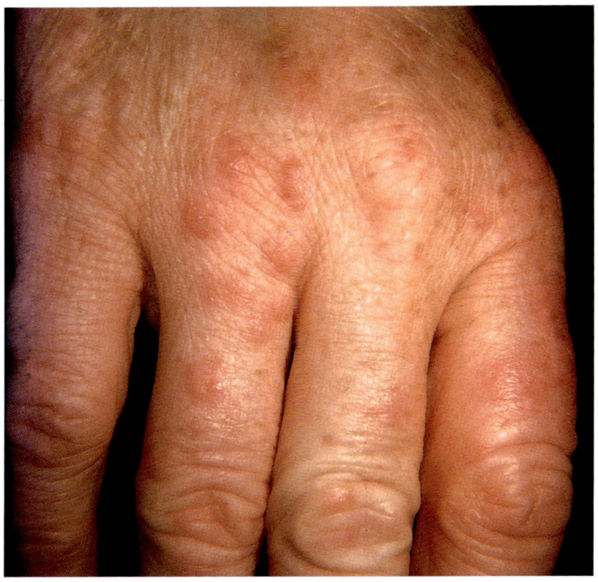

Figure 5–15. Polymorphous light eruption, vesicular type. Erythematous vesiculopapules on the hand and fingers.

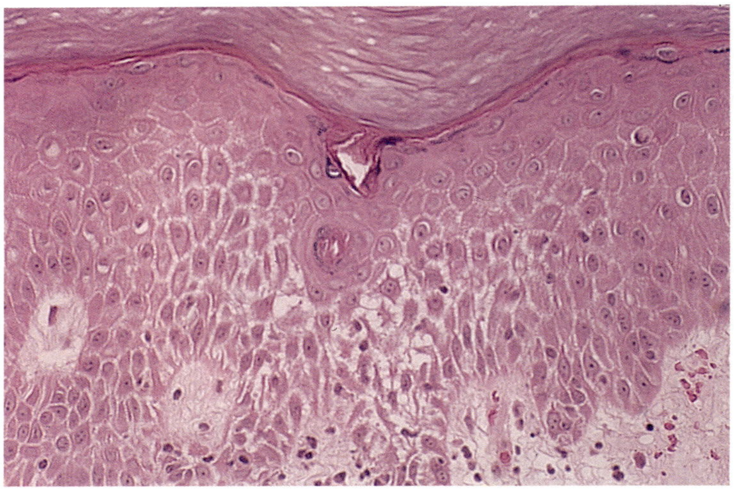

Figure 5–16. Polymorphous light eruption, vesicular type. Spongiosis and severe papillary edema.

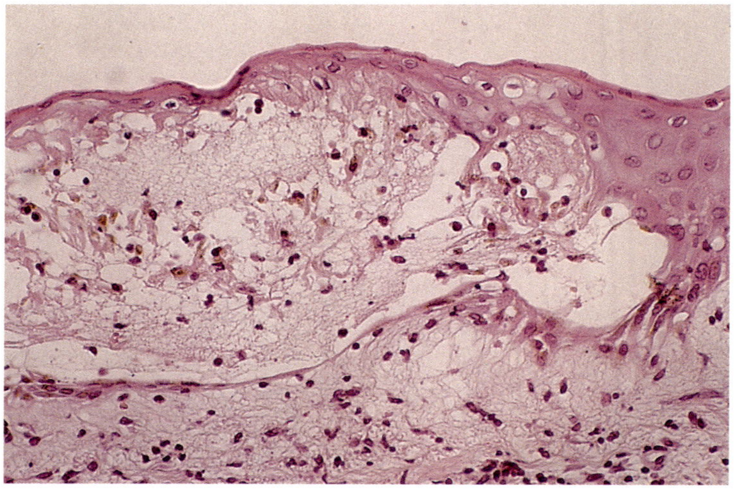

Figure 5–17. Polymorphous light eruption, vesicular type. Intraepidermal vesiculation with spongiosis and ballooned keratinocytes. There is severe papillary edema and a mixed-cell infiltrate with neutrophils and eosinophils.

TELANGIECTASIA MACULARIS ERUPTIVA PERSTANS (TMEP)

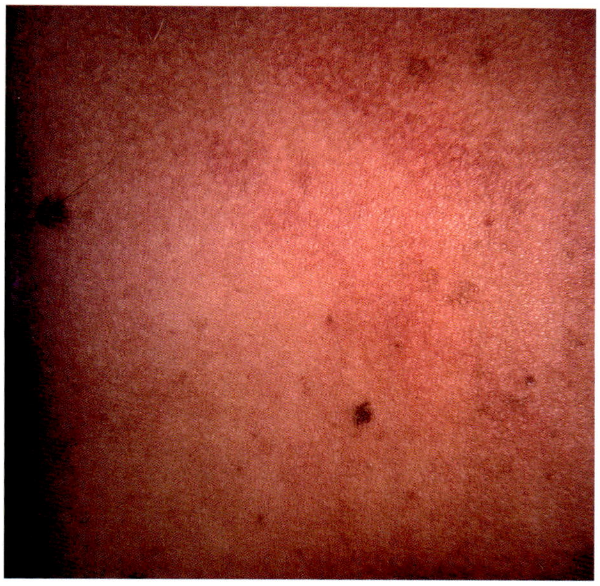

Figure 5–18. Telangiectasia macularis eruptiva perstans. Reticulated erythematous patches.

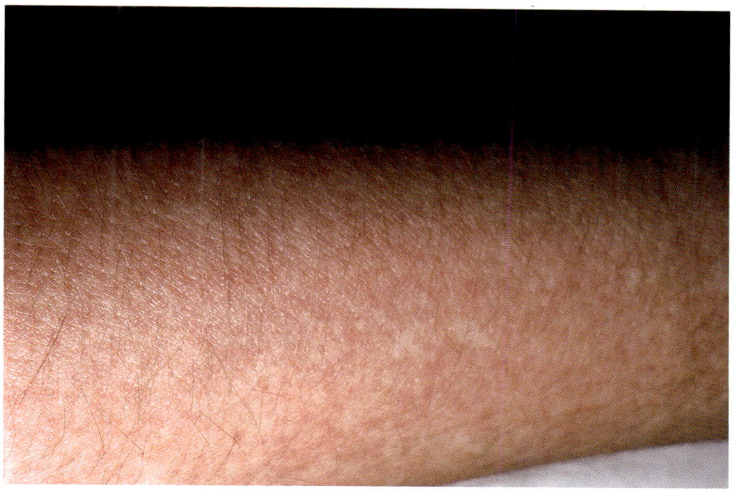

Figure 5–19. Telangiectasia macularis eruptiva perstans. Subtle, spotted, macular erythema on an extremity.

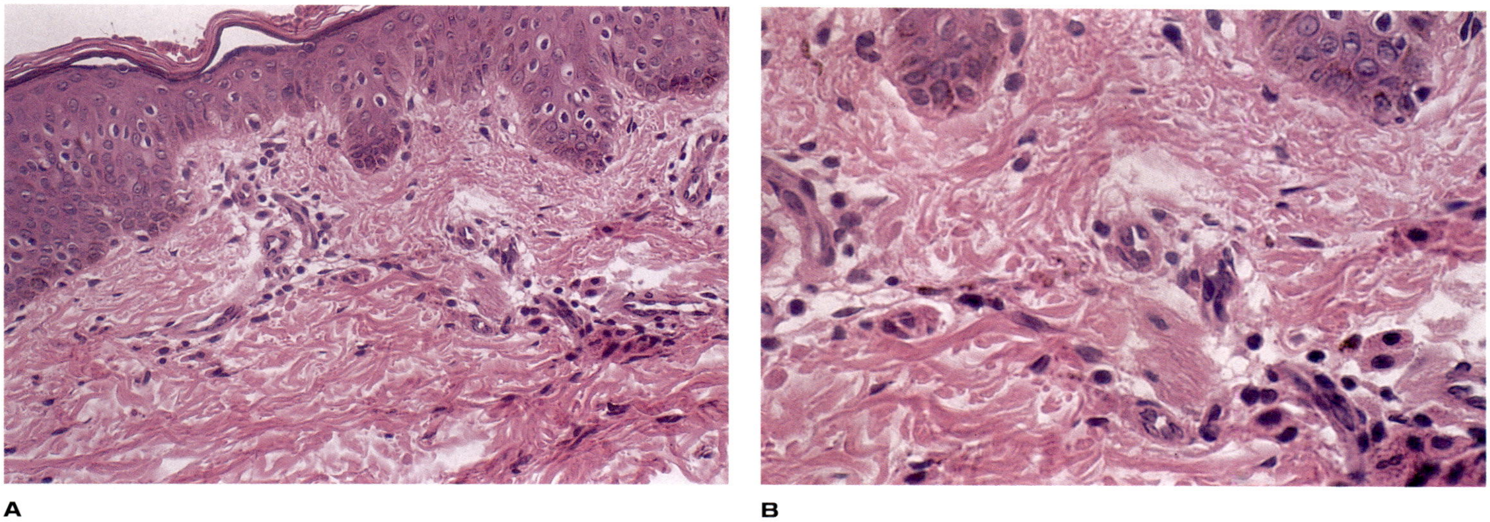

Figures 5–20A, 5–20B. Telangiectasia macularis eruptiva perstans. Prominent mast cells around dilated superficial blood vessels. The mast cells have round or oval nuclei and amphophilic cytoplasmic granules.

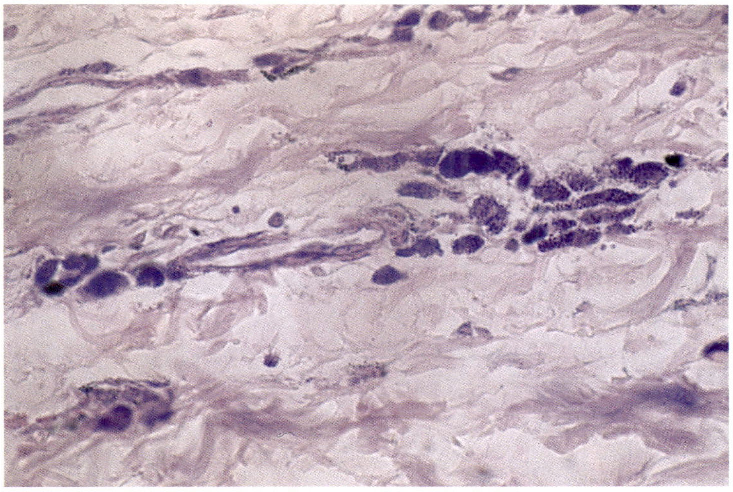

Figure 5–21. Telangiectasia macularis eruptiva perstans. Giemsa stain clearly identifies the mast cells and their cytoplasmic granules.

6

VASCULITIS

- Leukocytoclastic vasculitis
- Disseminated intravascular coagulation (DIC)
- Henoch-Schönlein purpura
- Urticarial vasculitis
- Erythema elevatum diutinum (EED)
- Systemic lupus erythematosus
- Cryoglobulinemia
- Atrophie blanche (livedo vasculitis)
- Polyarteritis nodosa (PAN)
- Nodular vasculitis (erythema induratum)
- Wegener's granulomatosis
- Lymphomatoid granulomatosis
- Rheumatoid vasculitis
- Granuloma faciale
- Degos' disease
- Churg-Strauss syndrome
- Septic vasculitis

LEUKOCYTOCLASTIC VASCULITIS

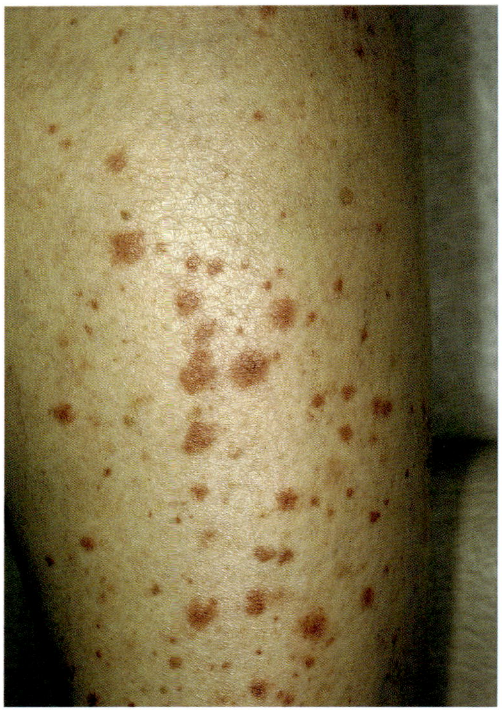

Figure 6–1. Leukocytoclastic vasculitis. Early eruption of erythematous macules and papules.

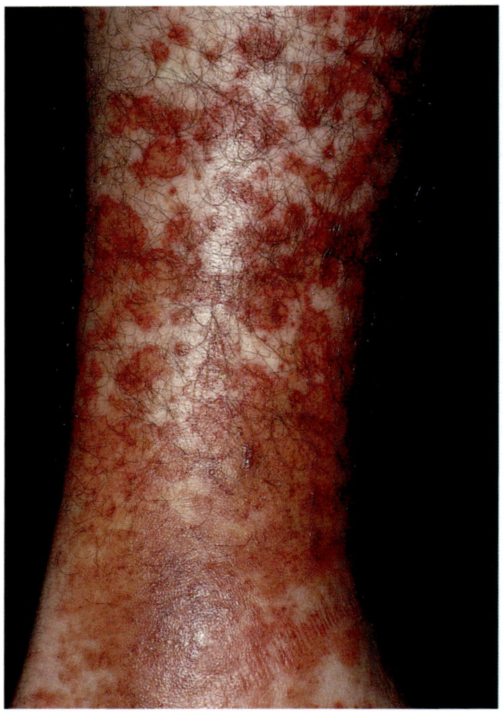

Figure 6–2. Leukocytoclastic vasculitis. Confluent hemorrhagic erythematous papules.

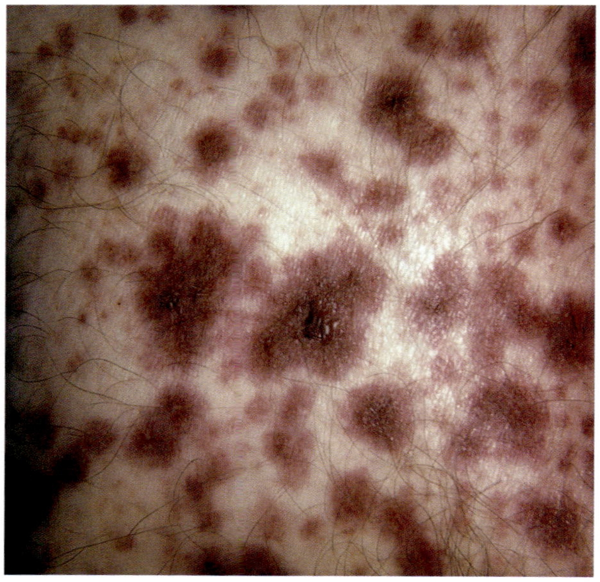

Figure 6–3. Leukocytoclastic vasculitis. Grouped red-brown papules with a few hemorrhagic vesicles.

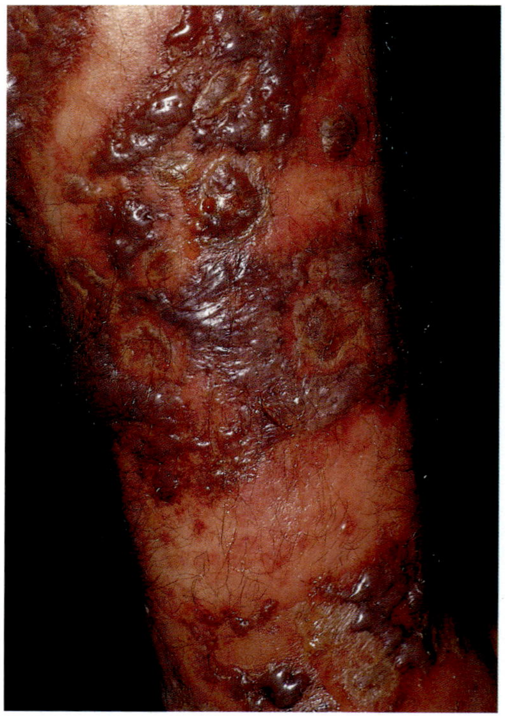

Figure 6–4. Leukocytoclastic vasculitis. Later eruption of confluent violaceous papules, plaques, vesicles, and oozing hemorrhagic blisters.

LEUKOCYTOCLASTIC VASCULITIS

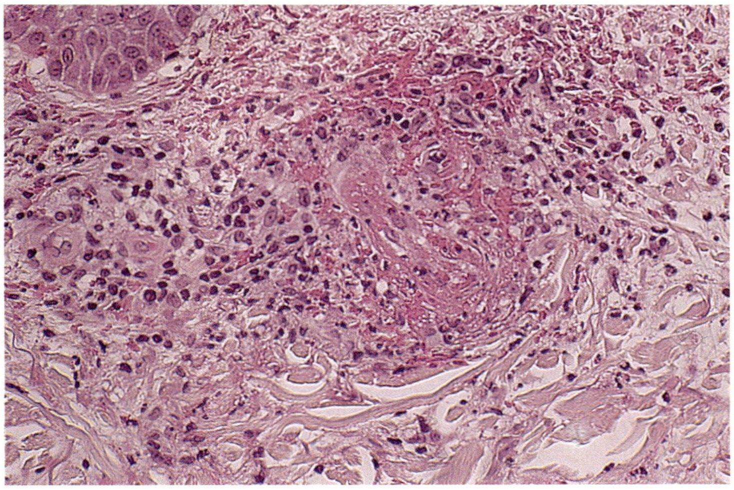
A

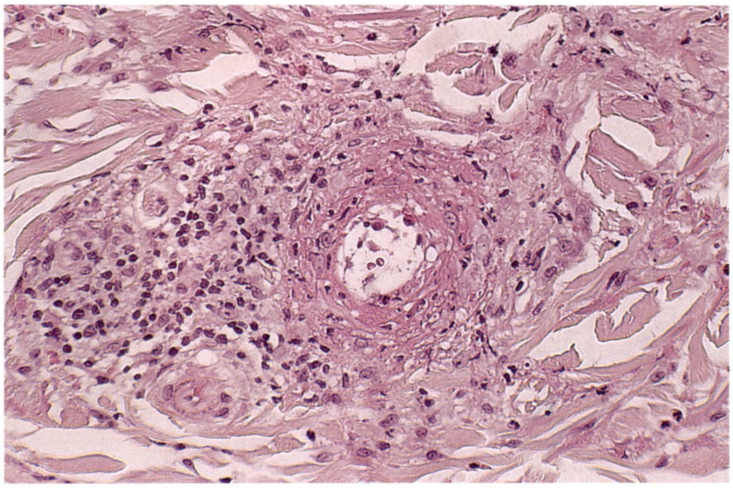
B

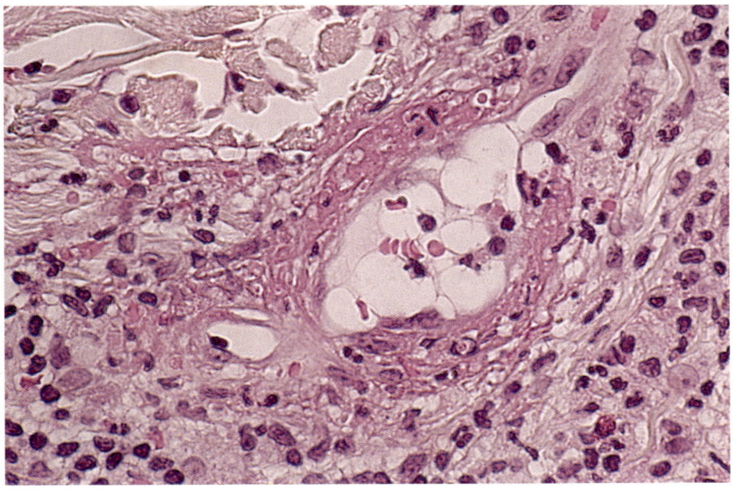
C

Figures 6–5A, 6–5B, 6–5C. Leukocytoclastic vasculitis. Fibrin within wall of a venule. There is a moderately dense dermal mixed-cell infiltrate with neutrophils, nuclear fragments, eosinophils, and extravasated red blood cells.

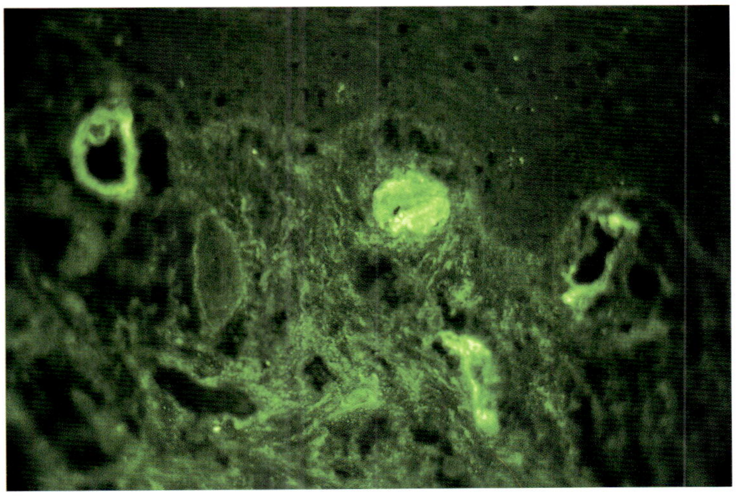

Figure 6–6. Leukocytoclastic vasculitis. Direct immunofluorescence of leukocytoclastic vasculitis. Note granular and fibrillar deposition of C3 within dermal blood vessel walls.

DISSEMINATED INTRAVASCULAR COAGULATION (DIC)

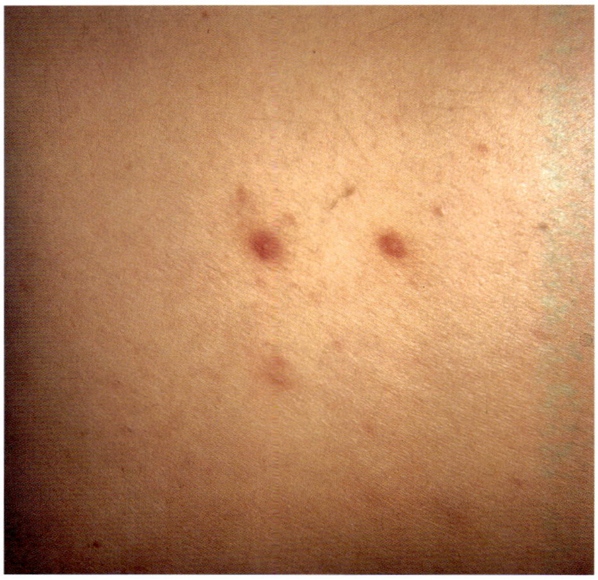

Figure 6–7. Disseminated intravascular coagulation. Early red vesiculopapules.

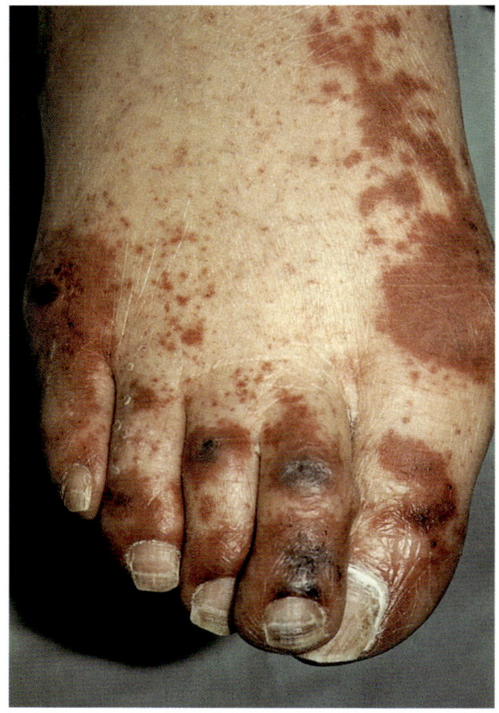

Figure 6–8. Disseminated intravascular coagulation. Later violaceous papules and plaques. There are black hemorrhagic areas involving toe lesions.

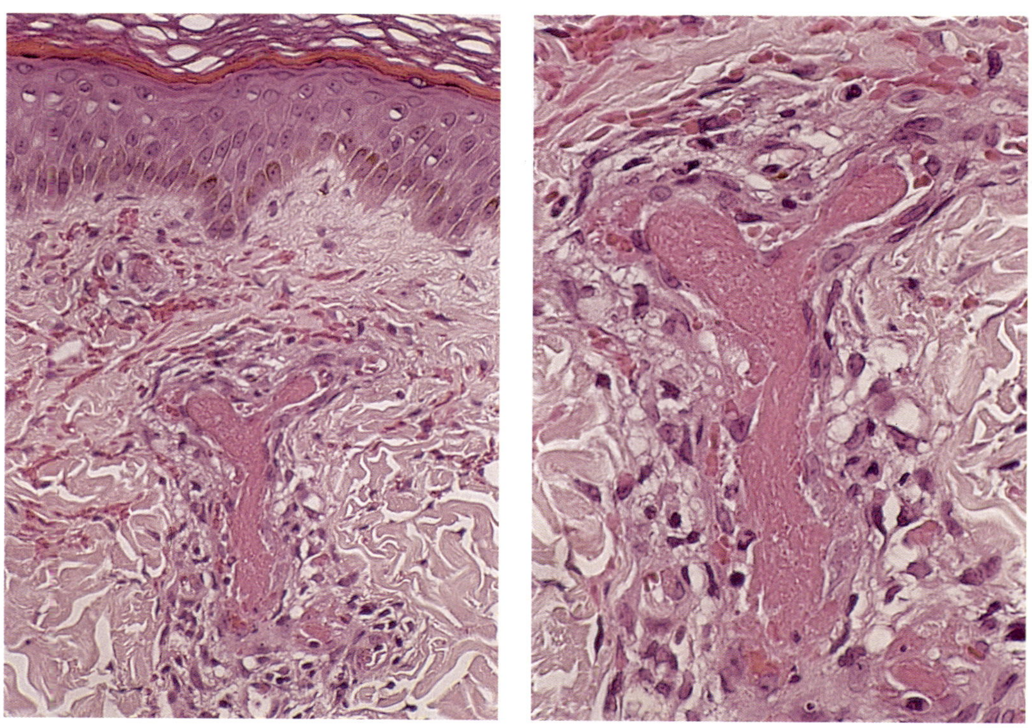

A B

Figures 6–9A, 6–9B. Disseminated intravascular coagulation. Fibrin thombus within a venule. In and around the vessel wall there are neutrophils, eosinophils, nuclear dust, and extravasated erythrocytes.

HENOCH-SCHÖNLEIN PURPURA

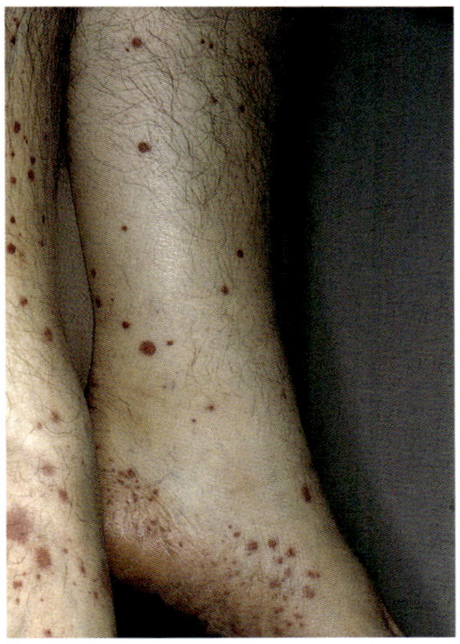

A

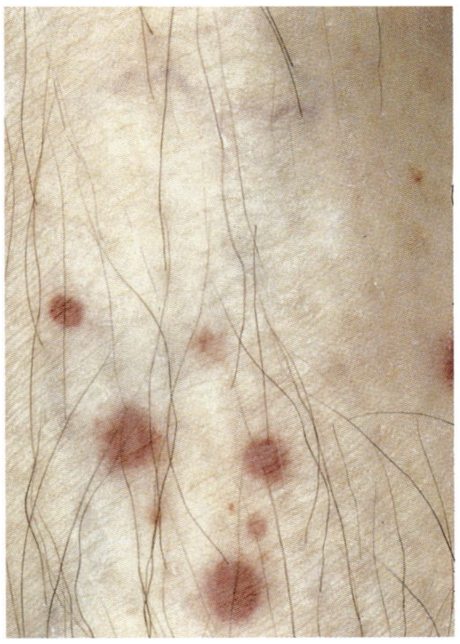

B

Figures 6–10A, 6–10B. Henoch-Schönlein purpura. Early erythematous papules.

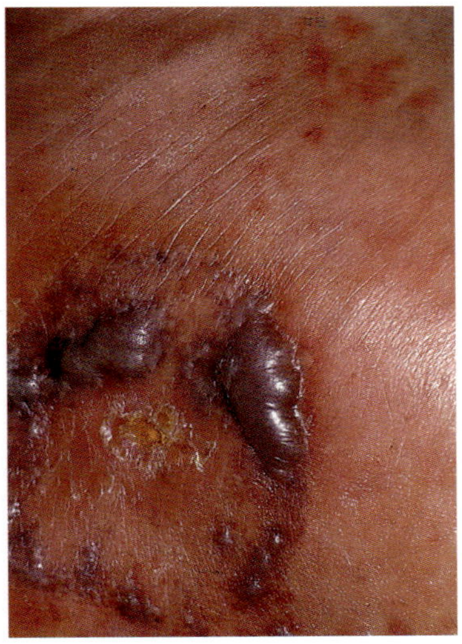

Figure 6–11. Henoch-Schönlein purpura. Later violaceous papules, vesicles, and bullae.

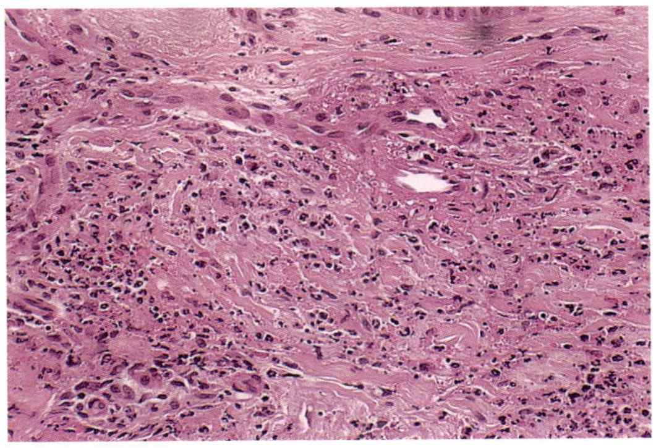

A

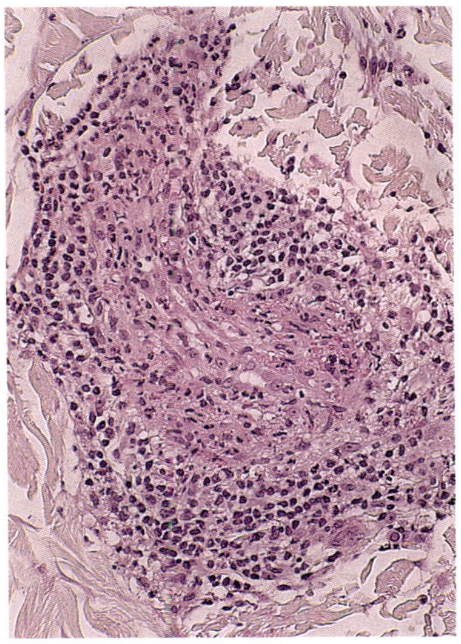

B

Figures 6–12A, 6–12B. Henoch-Schönlein purpura. Destruction of blood vessels with abundant fibrin deposition in and around the vessel wall. A dense mixed-cell dermal infiltrate with neutrophils, nuclear debris, eosinophils, and extravasated erythrocytes accompany the destruction of the venules.

Figure 6–13. Henoch-Schönlein purpura. Direct immunofluorescence staining IgA deposition in blood vessels.

URTICARIAL VASCULITIS

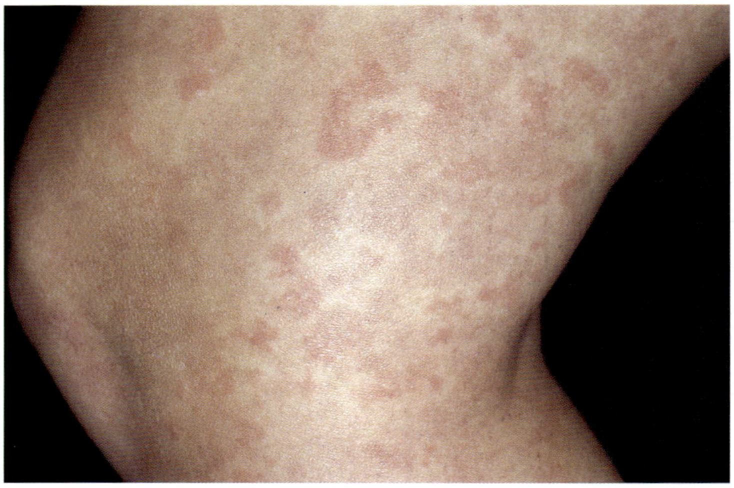

Figure 6–14. Urticarial vasculitis. Recurrent erythematous macules and papules.

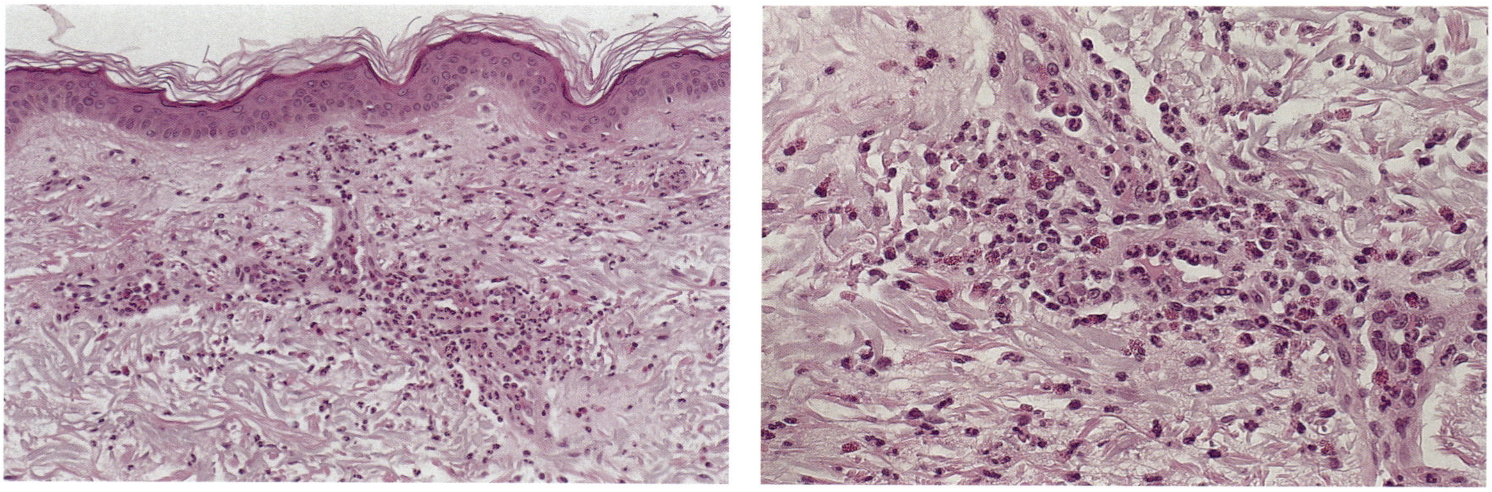

A B

Figures 6–15A, 6–15B. Urticarial vasculitis. The changes of leukocytoclastic vasculitis are present. There is fibrin within blood vessel walls, and a dermal mixed-cell infiltrate with neutrophils, nuclear fragments, eosinophils, and erythrocytes.

ERYTHEMA ELEVATUM DIUTINUM (EED)

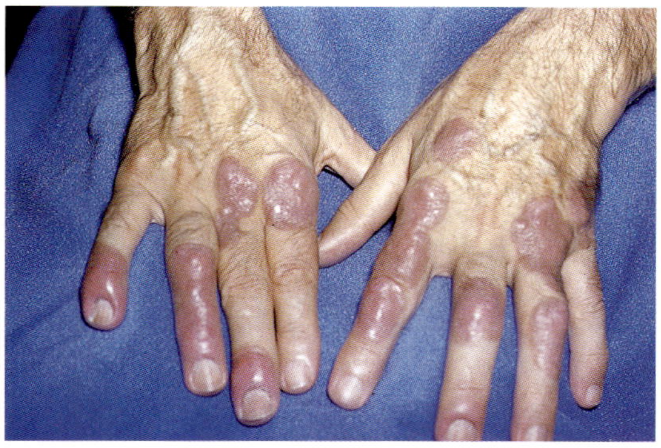
A

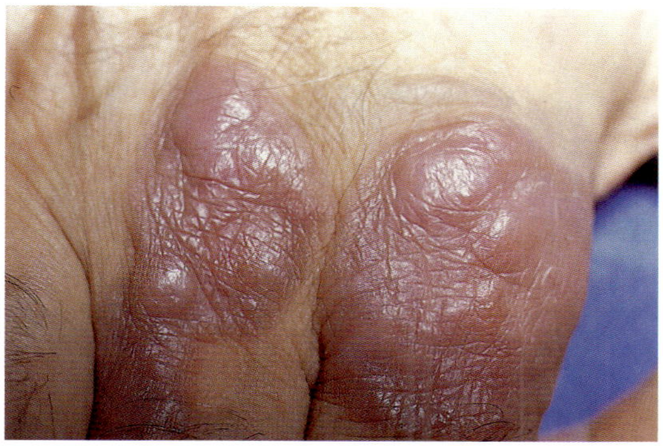
B

Figures 6–16A, 6–16B. Erythema elevatum diutinum. Erythematous nodules on the hands and fingers.

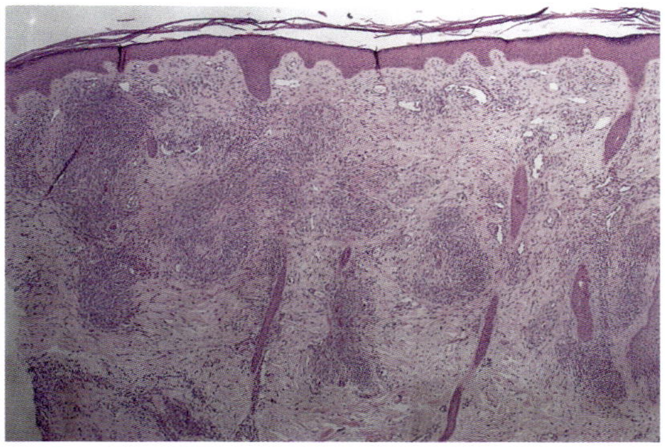

Figure 6–17. Erythema elevatum diutinum. Superficial and deep intravascular, perivascular, and interstitial mixed-cell infiltrate.

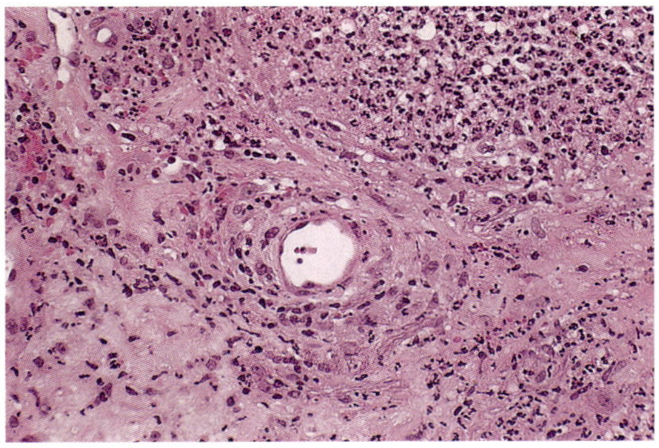
A

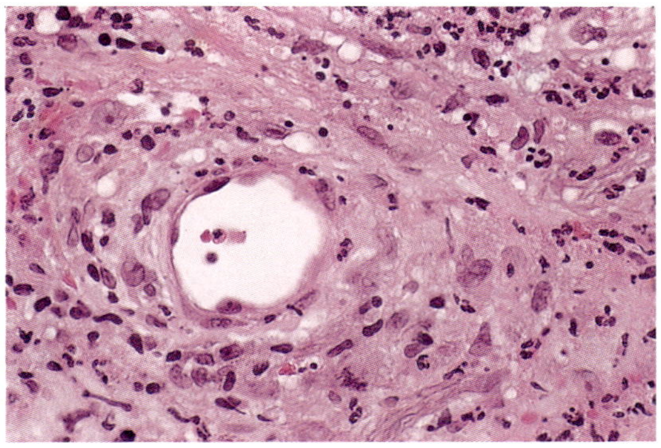
B

Figures 6–18A, 6–18B. Erythema elevatum diutinum, early lesion. There is fibrin within the vessel wall, and a dense mixed-cell infiltrate composed of neutrophils, nuclear fragments, eosinophils, and erythrocytes. These are the characteristic findings of leukocytoclastic vasculitis.

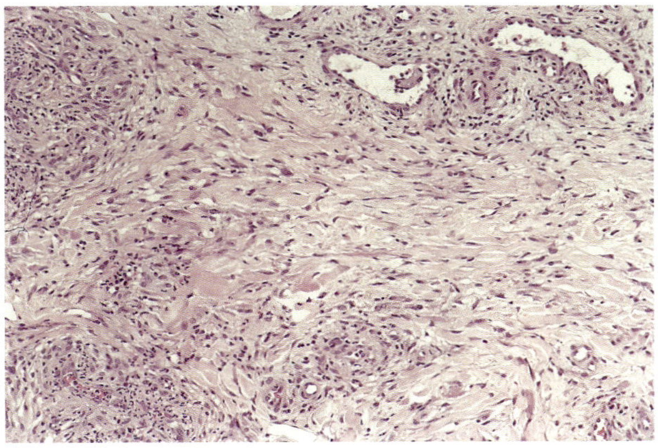

Figure 6–19. Erythema elevatum diutinum, later lesion. Fibroplasia and histiocytes accompany the changes of leukocytoclastic vasculitis.

SYSTEMIC LUPUS ERYTHEMATOSUS

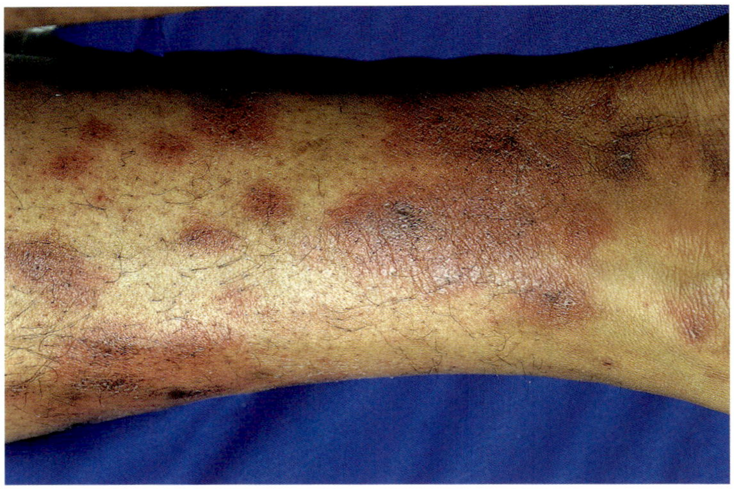

Figure 6–20. Systemic lupus erythematosus. Violaceous and erythematous patches.

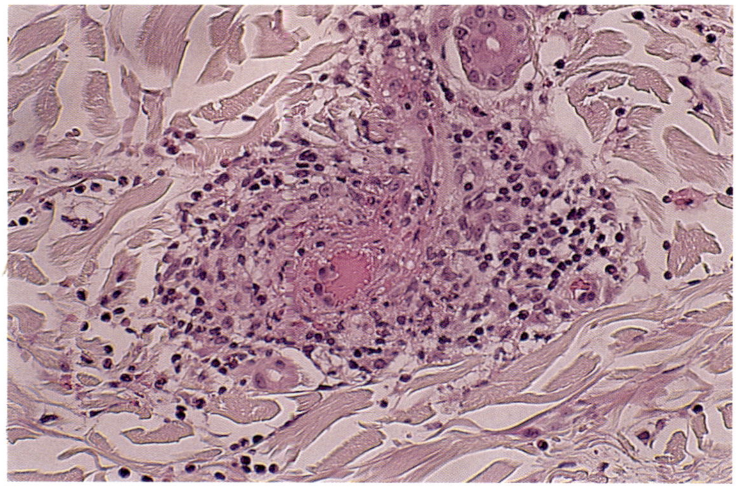

Figure 6–21. Systemic lupus erythematosus with leukocytoclastic vasculitis. Fibrin deposition within the wall of a venule and a mixed-cell infiltrate with neutrophils, nuclear debris, eosinophils, and extravasated red blood cells are present.

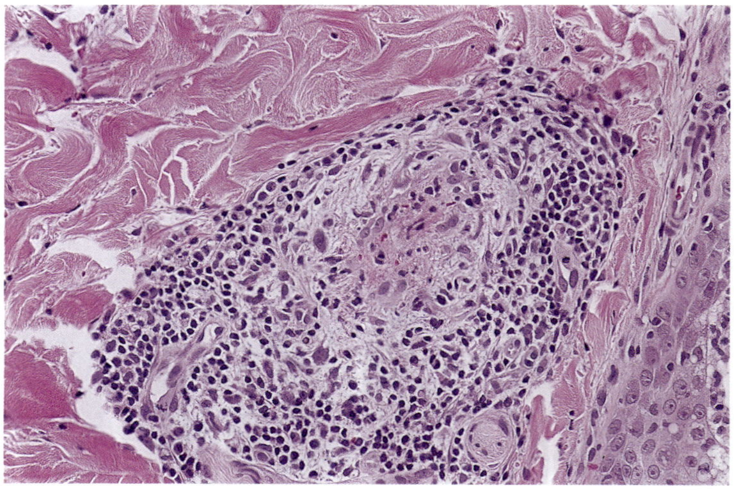

Figure 6–22. Systemic lupus erythematosus with lymphocytic vasculitis. There is a dense mononuclear cell infiltrate around and within a fibrin-laden venule.

CRYOGLOBULINEMIA

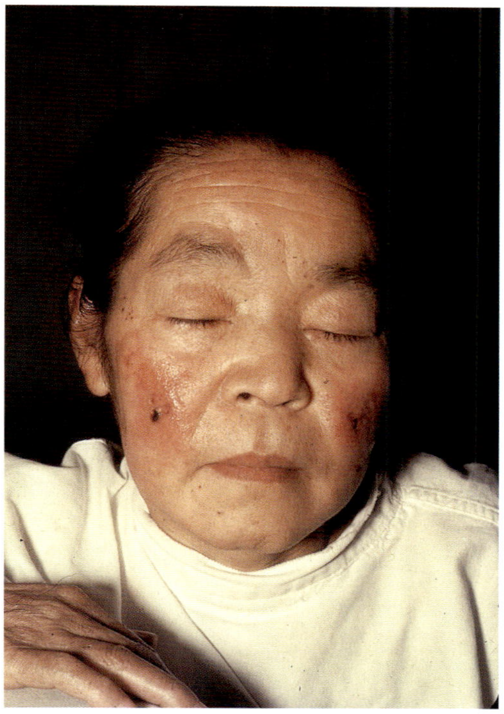

Figure 6–23. Cryoglobulinemia. Erythematous hemorrhagic and crusted plaques on the cheek of a woman with multiple myeloma.

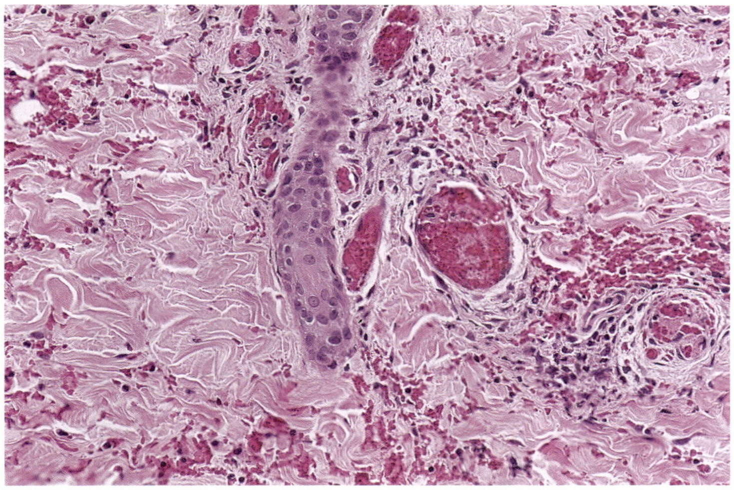

Figure 6–24. Cryoglobulinemia with leukocytoclastic vasculitis. Fibrin thrombi and pink homogenous deposits within dilated and congested blood vessels. There is a sparse infiltrate of neutrophils, nuclear dust, and numerous extravasated erythrocytes.

ATROPHIE BLANCHE (LIVEDO VASCULITIS)

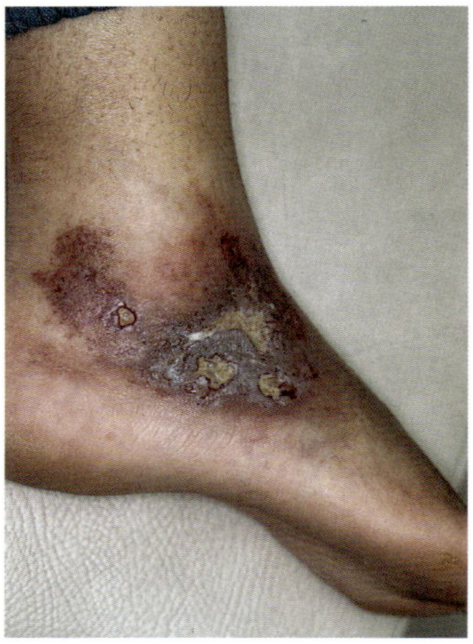

A

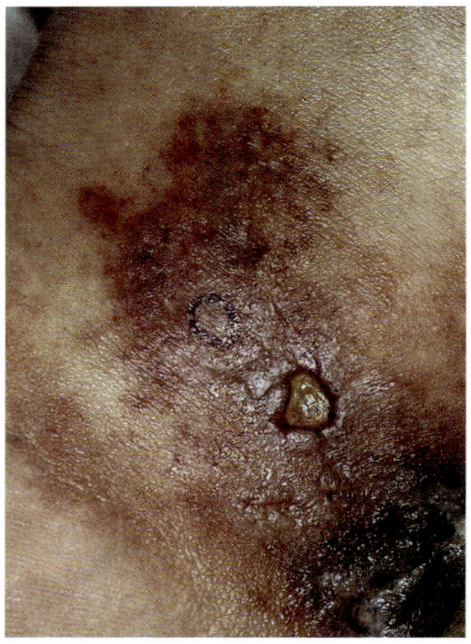

B

Figures 6–25A, 6–25B. Atrophie blanche. Evolving ankle and foot lesions with hemorrhagic plaques and focal ulcerations.

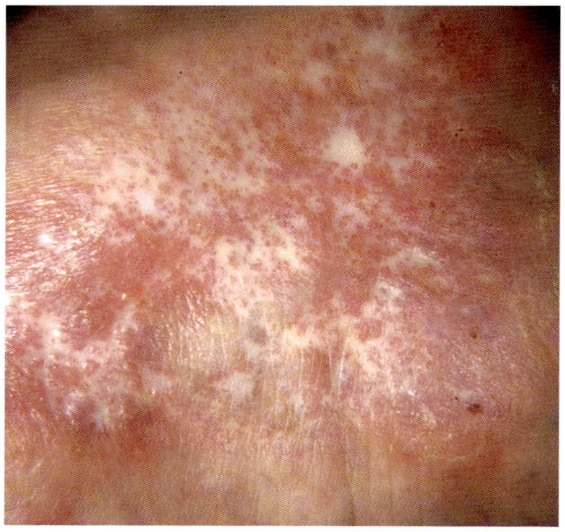

Figure 6–26. Atrophie blanche. Later lesion with reticulated white atrophic scars.

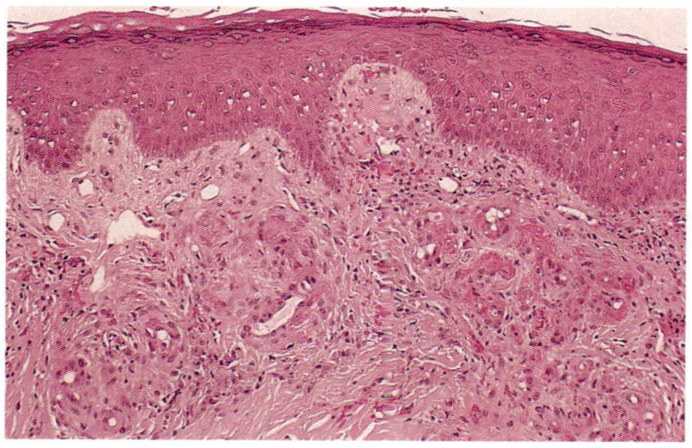

A

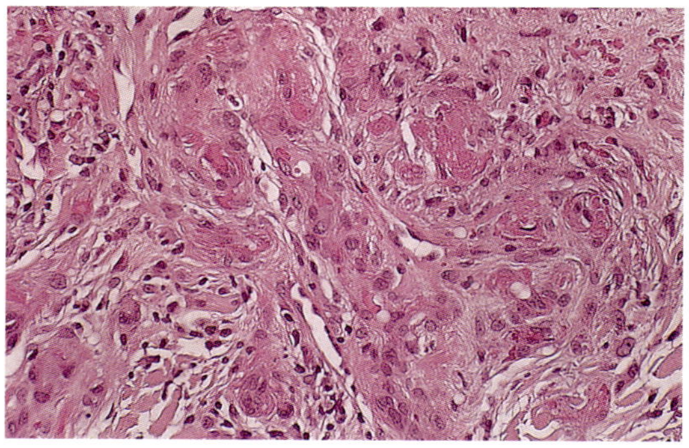

B

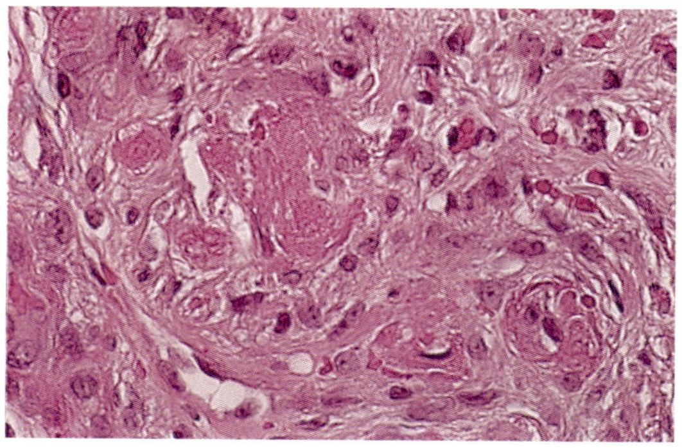

C

Figures 6–27A, 6–27B, 6–27C. Atrophie blanche. Blood vessels containing fibrin thrombi and fibrin within the wall. There is a sparse mixed-cell infiltrate.

POLYARTERITIS NODOSA (PAN)

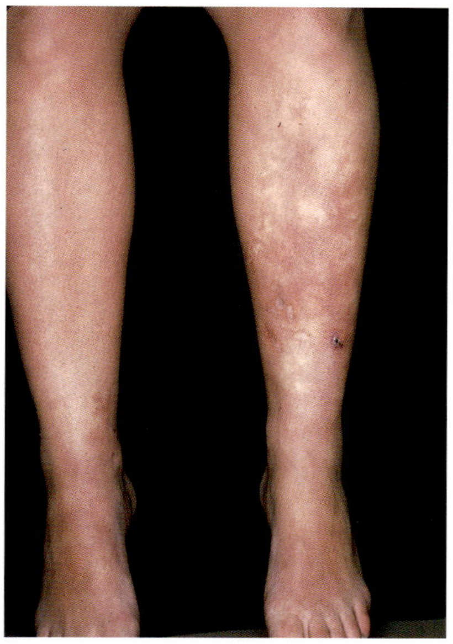

Figure 6–28. Polyarteritis nodosa. Erythematous nodules and plaques on the distal extremities with focal ulcerations and atrophic scars.

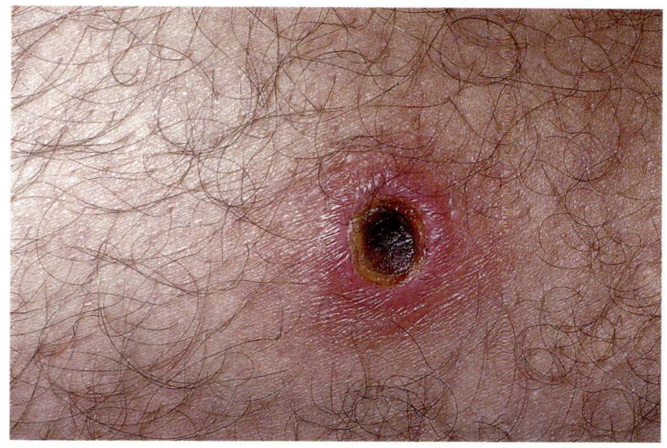

Figure 6–29. Polyarteritis nodosa. Red nodule with central ulceration.

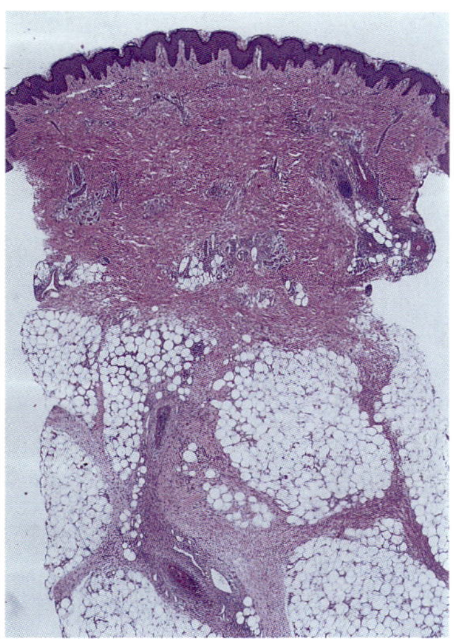

A

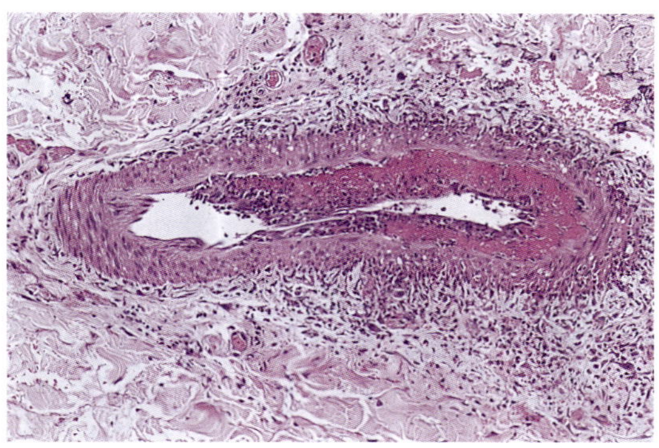

B

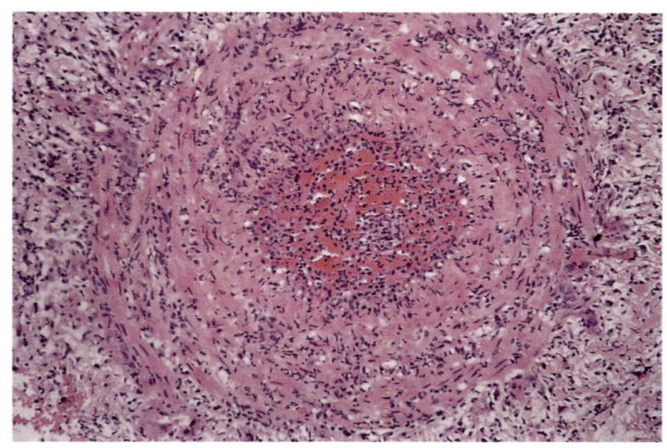

C

Figures 6–30A, 6–30B, 6–30C. Polyarteritis nodosa. Vasculitis involving an artery within the fibrous septa of the subcutaneous fat. Deposits of fibrin and an infiltrate of neutrophils involve all layers of the arterial wall.

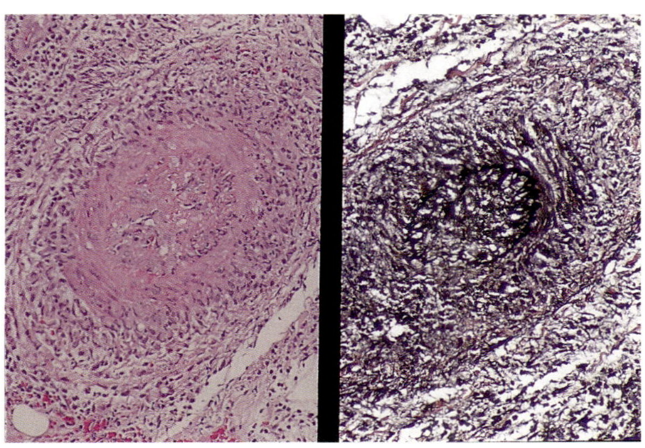

Figure 6–31. Polyarteritis nodosa. Large-vessel vasculitis with hematoxylin and eosin stain on the left and elastic tissue stain on the right. Internal elastic membrane is delineated.

NODULAR VASCULITIS (ERYTHEMA INDURATUM)

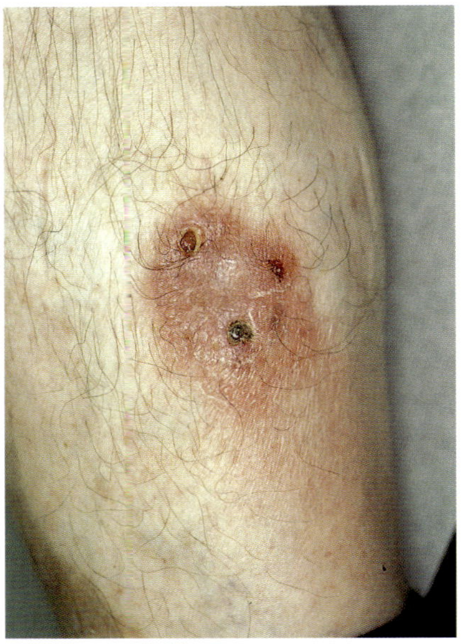

Figure 6–32. Nodular vasculitis, early lesion. Erythematous plaque with focal ulcerations on the calf.

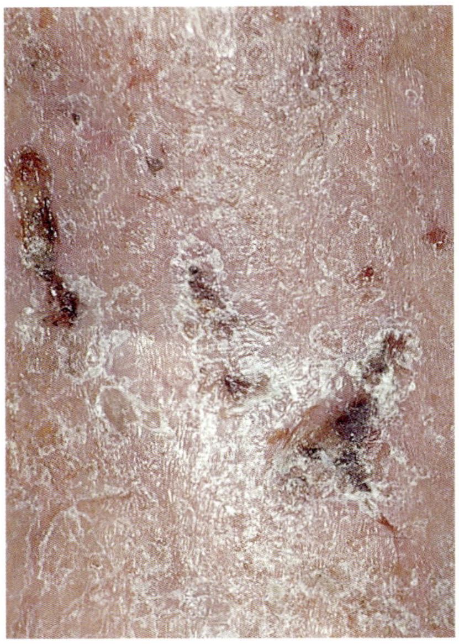

Figure 6–33. Nodular vasculitis, later lesion. Confluent plaques on the lower leg with ulcerations and old hypertrophic scars.

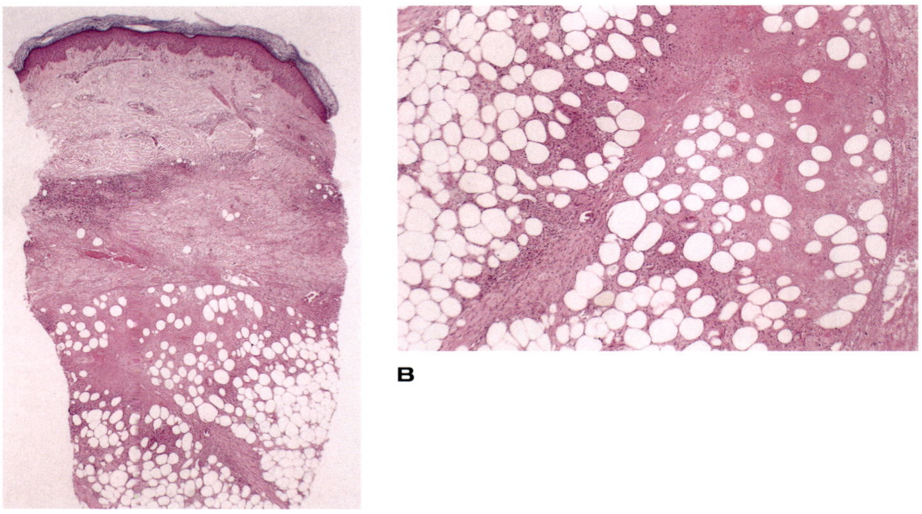

A

B

Figures 6–34A, 6–34B. Nodular vasculitis. Septal and lobular panniculitis with vasculitis. There is extensive fat necrosis.

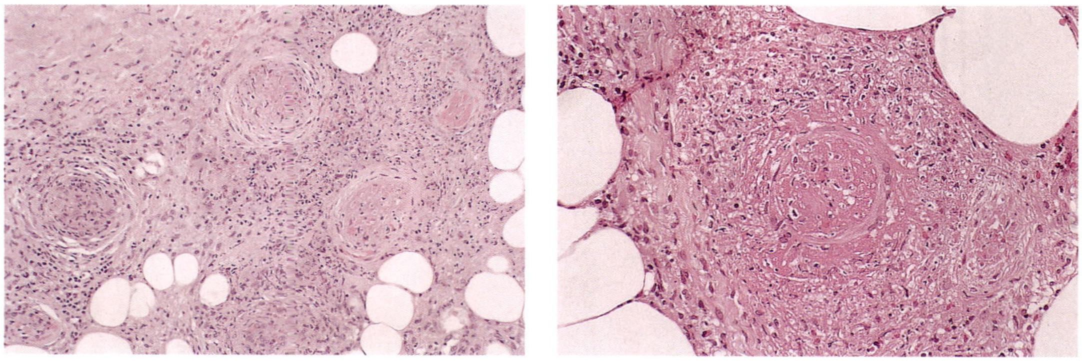

A

B

Figures 6–35A, 6–35B. Nodular vasculitis. Arterial vasculitis with fibrin deposition and a neutrophilic infiltrate occluding the lumen. Around the vessels there is fibroplasia and a dense mixed-cell infiltrate that extends into a thickened fibrous septae and fat lobules.

WEGENER'S GRANULOMATOSIS

Figure 6–36. **Wegener's granulomatosis.** Ulcerated nodule on the tongue.

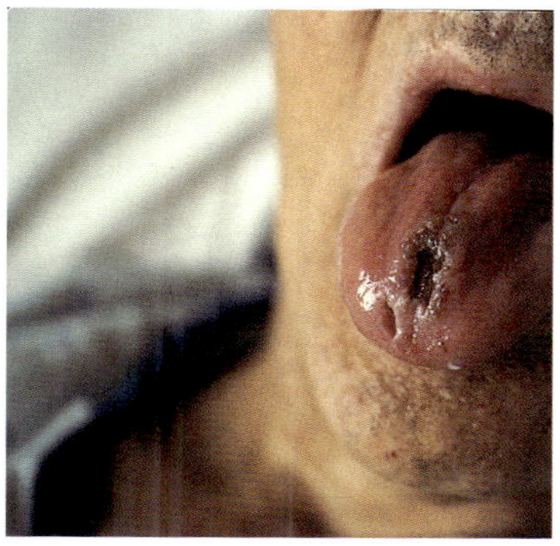

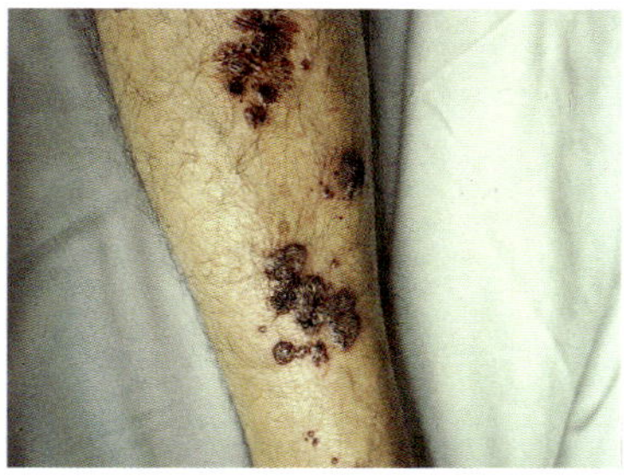

A

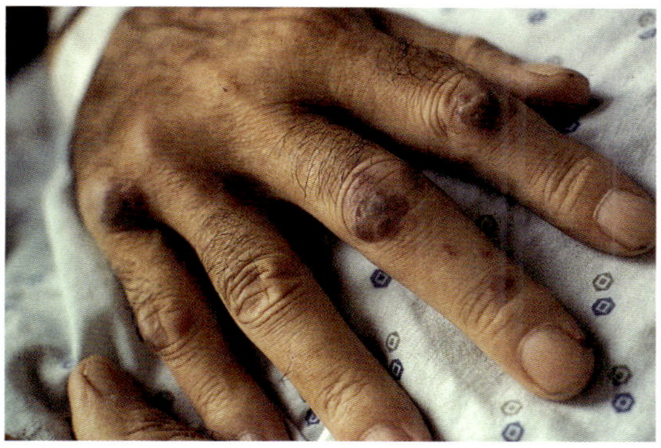

B

Figures 6–37A, 6–37B. **Wegener's granulomatosis.** Hemorrhagic papules and plaques on the lower leg and fingers.

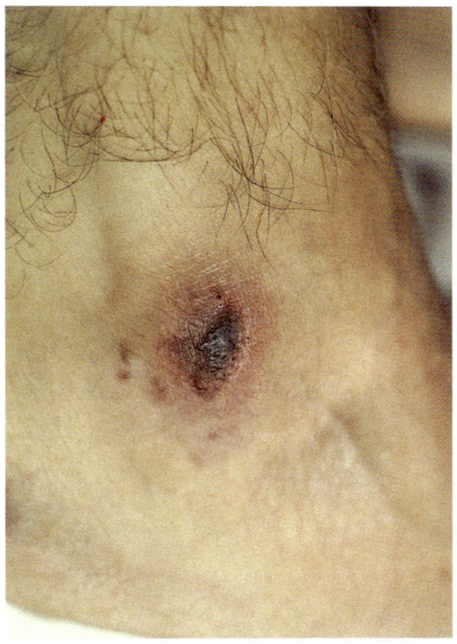

Figure 6–38. **Wegener's granulomatosis.** Solitary ulcerated plaque on the ankle.

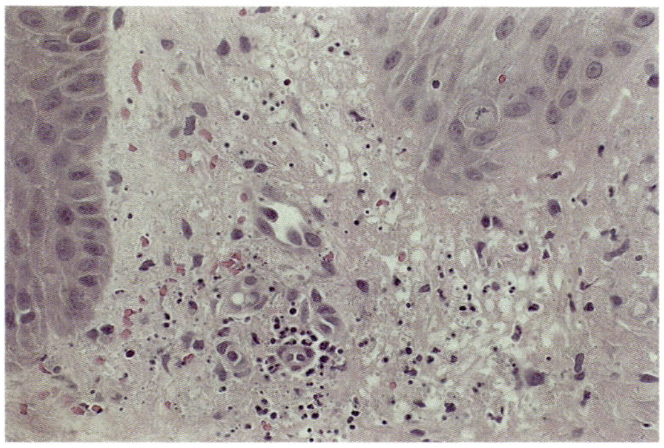

Figure 6–39. **Wegener's granulomatosis.** Leukocytoclastic vasculitis with fibrin deposition, neutrophils, and nuclear fragments surrounding altered blood vessels.

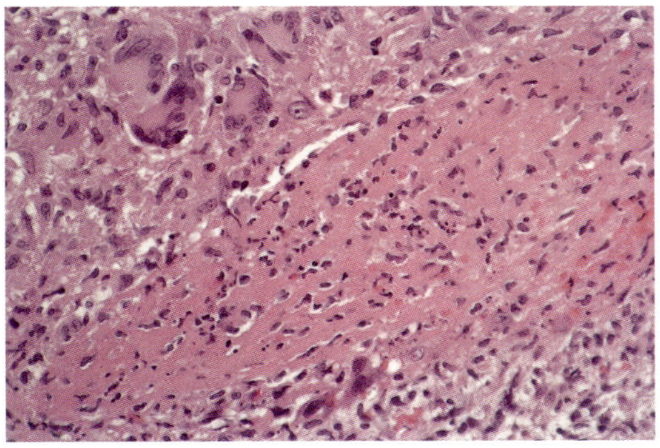

Figure 6–40. **Wegener's granulomatosis.** Granulomatous inflammation with a leukocytoclastic vasculitis. Histiocytes and multinucleated histiocytic giant cells encircle a destroyed blood vessel. The venule contains fibrin, neutrophils, nuclear debris, and erythrocytes.

LYMPHOMATOID GRANULOMATOSIS

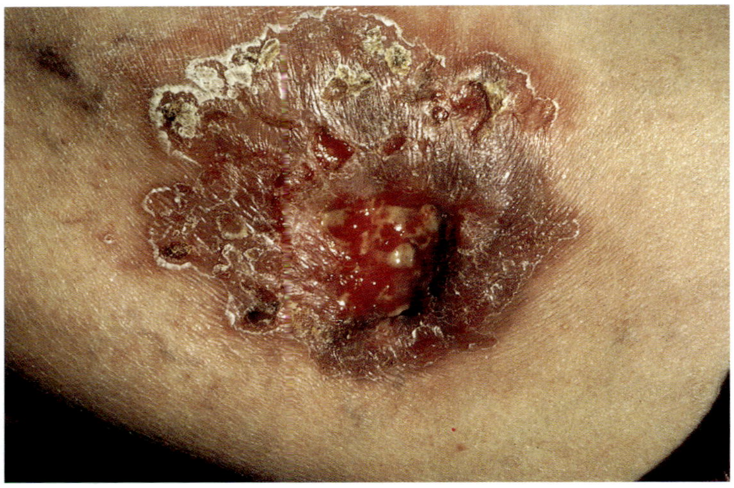

Figure 6–41. Lymphomatoid granulomatosis. Purpuric ulcerative plaque.

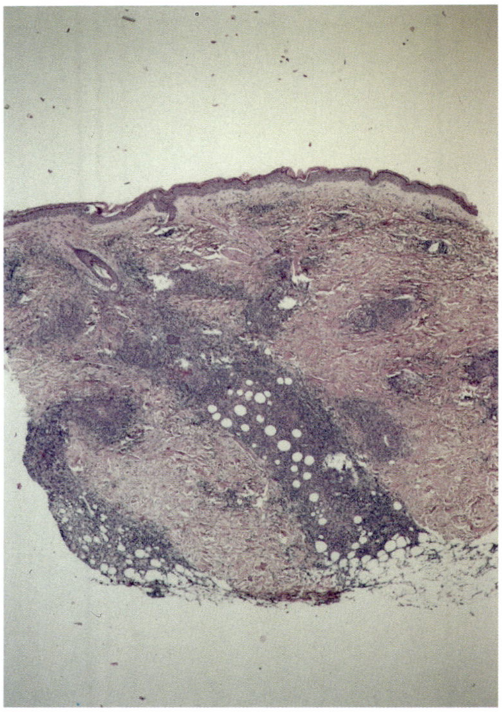

Figure 6–42. Lymphomatoid granulomatosis. Dense superficial and deep vasculitis and panniculitis.

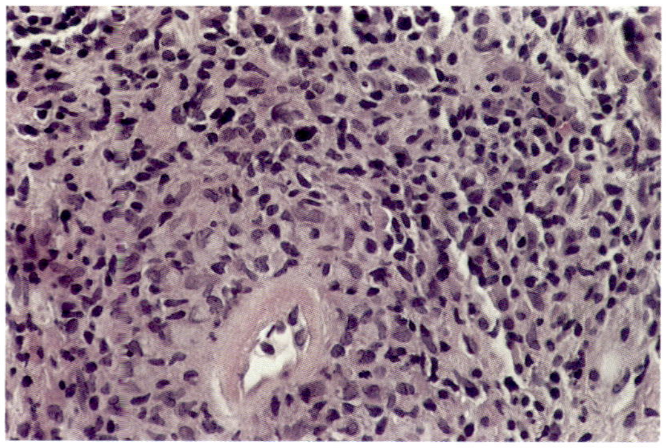

A

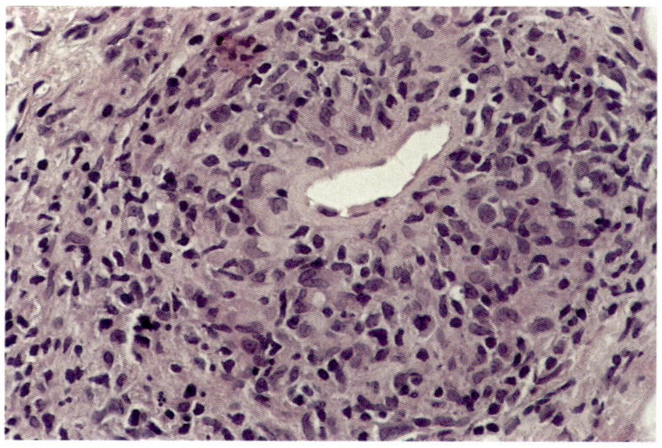

B

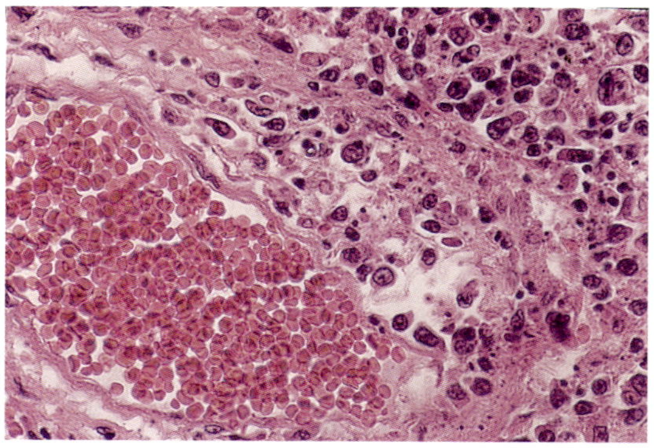

C

Figures 6–43A, 6–43B, 6–43C. Lymphomatoid granulomatosis. Atypical mononuclear cells invade and destroy blood vessels in the dermis and panniculus. The atypical cells have large hyperchromatic and cerebriform nuclei.

RHEUMATOID VASCULITIS

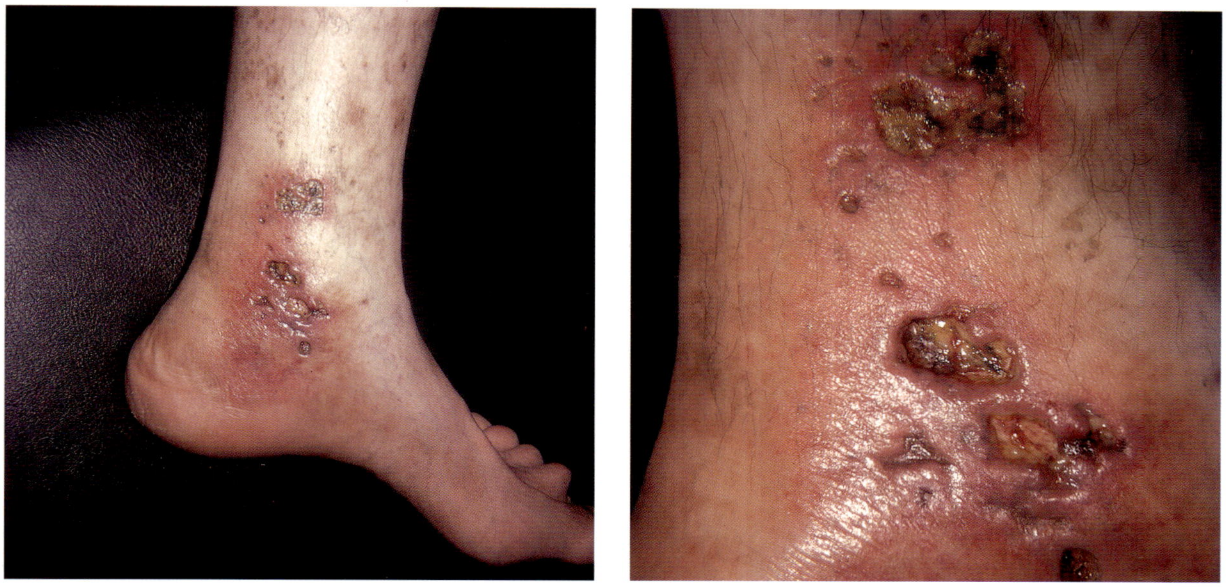

A B

Figures 6–44A, 6–44B. **Rheumatoid vasculitis.** Erythematous ulcerative plaques on the ankle of a man with severe rheumatoid arthritis.

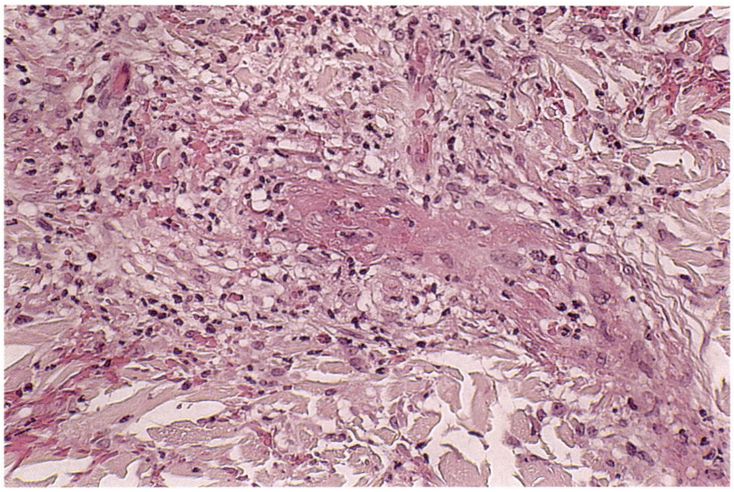

Figure 6–45. **Rheumatoid vasculitis with leukocytoclastic vasculitis.** Blood vessel is destroyed and there is fibrin, neutrophils, nuclear fragments, eosinophils, and erythrocytes.

GRANULOMA FACIALE

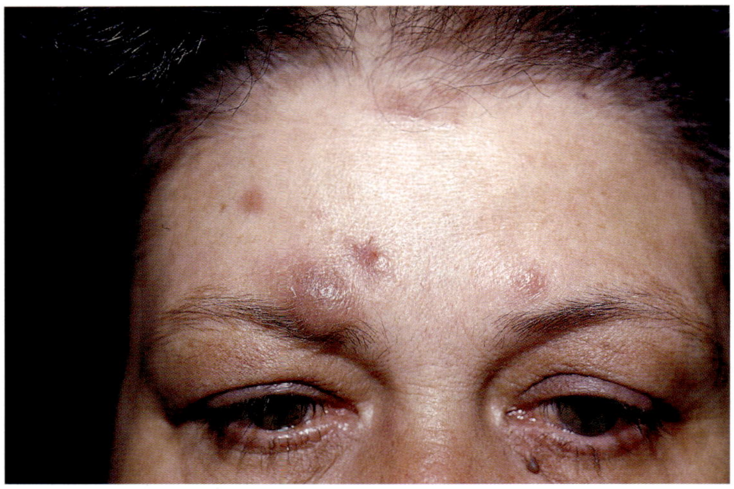

Figure 6–46. Granuloma faciale. Erythematous papules on the forehead and a nodule on the eyebrow.

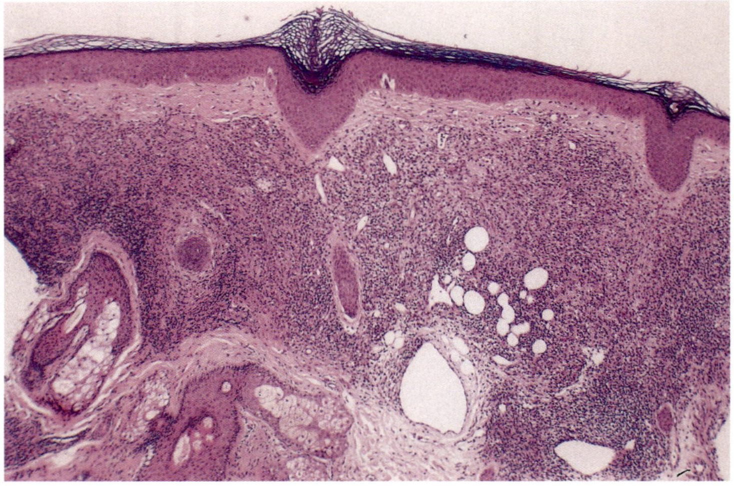

Figure 6–47. Granuloma faciale. Diffuse dermal infiltrate sparing the papillary and adventitial dermis.

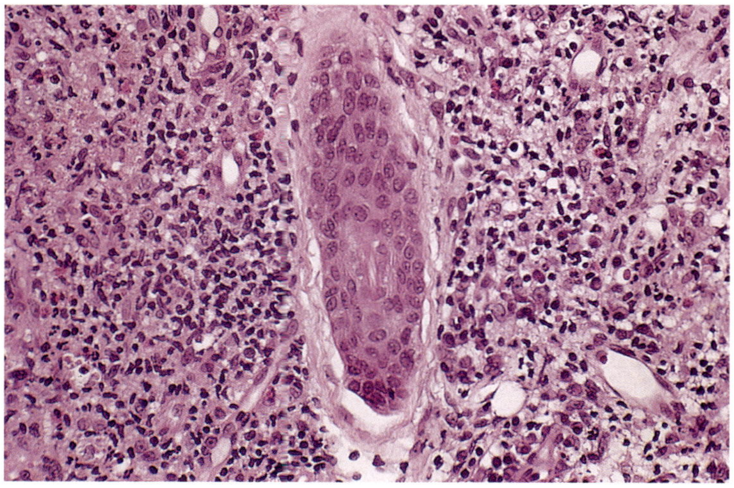

Figure 6–48. Granuloma faciale. Dense mixed-cell dermal infiltrate containing neutrophils, eosinophils, plasma cells, lymphocytes, and histiocytes. There is sparing of the adventitial dermis surrounding the eccrine duct.

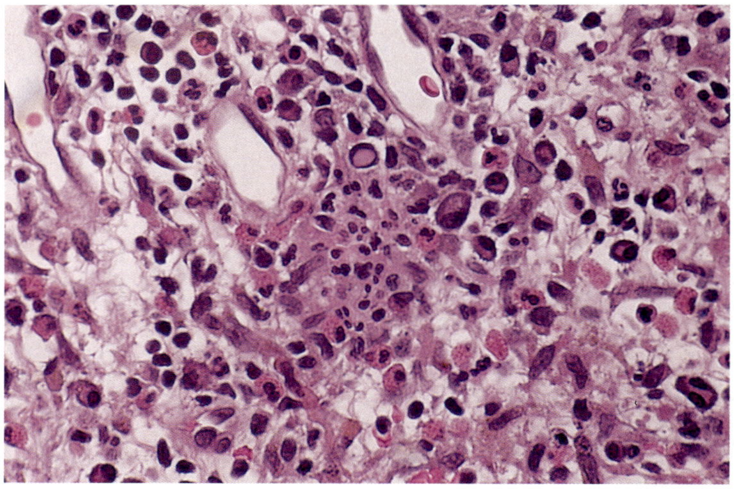

Figure 6–49. Granuloma faciale with leukocytoclastic vasculitis. Destroyed blood vessels with fibrin, neutrophils, and nuclear fragments. The dermal mixed-cell infiltrate includes eosinophils, histiocytes, and plasma cells.

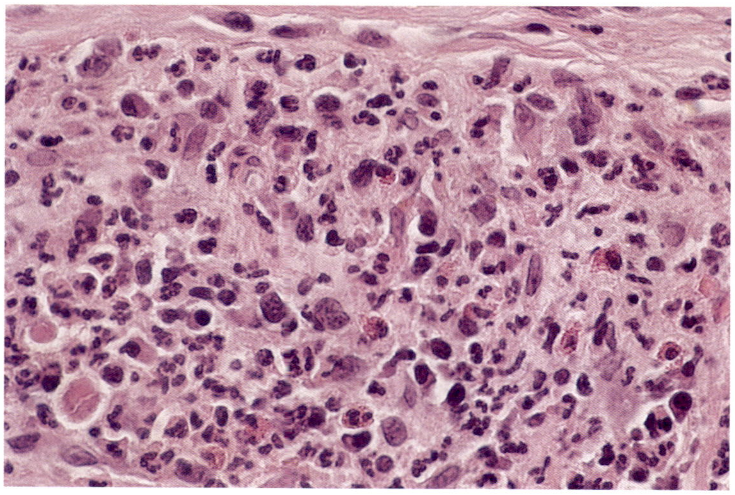

Figure 6–50. Granuloma faciale. Polymorphic dermal infiltrate with neutrophils, eosinophils, lymphocytes, and histiocytic and plasma cells.

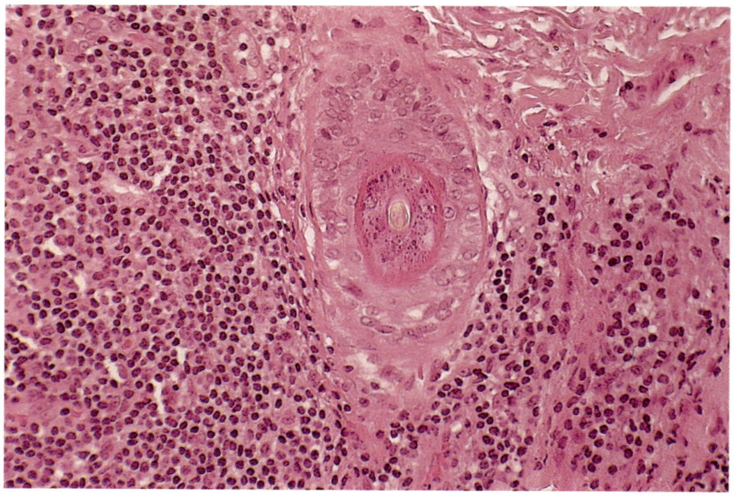

Figure 6–51. Granuloma faciale. Later stage with mononuclear cells only.

DEGOS' DISEASE

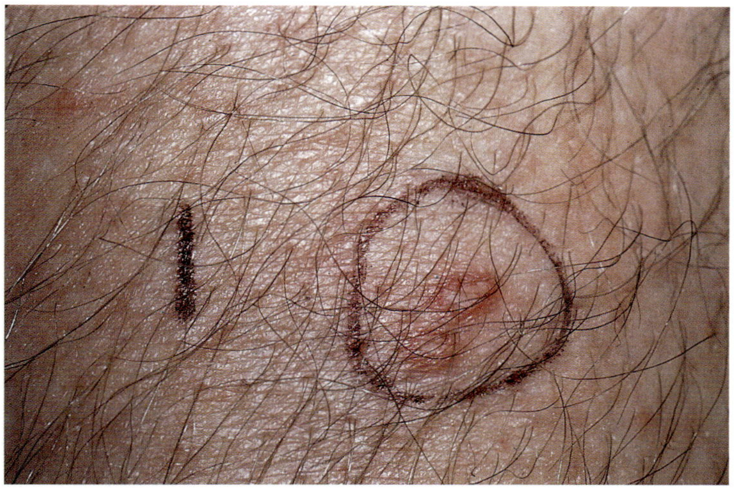

Figure 6–52. Degos' disease. Ink-outlined erythematous papules with atrophic white centers.

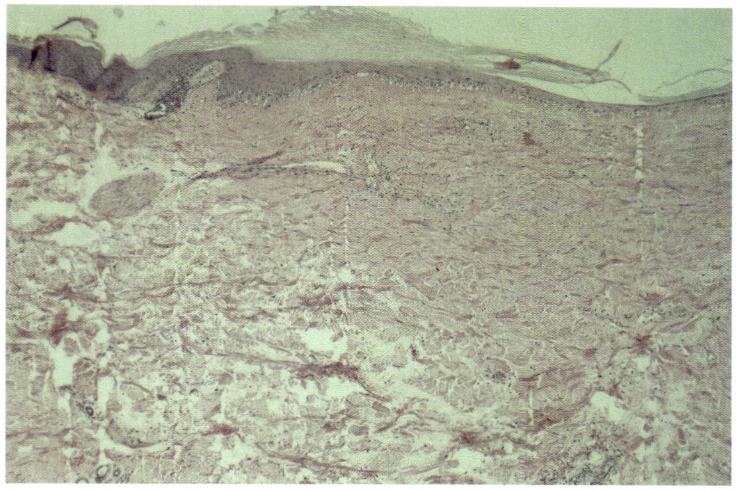

Figure 6–53. Degos' disease. Wedge-shaped area of altered epidermis and dermis.

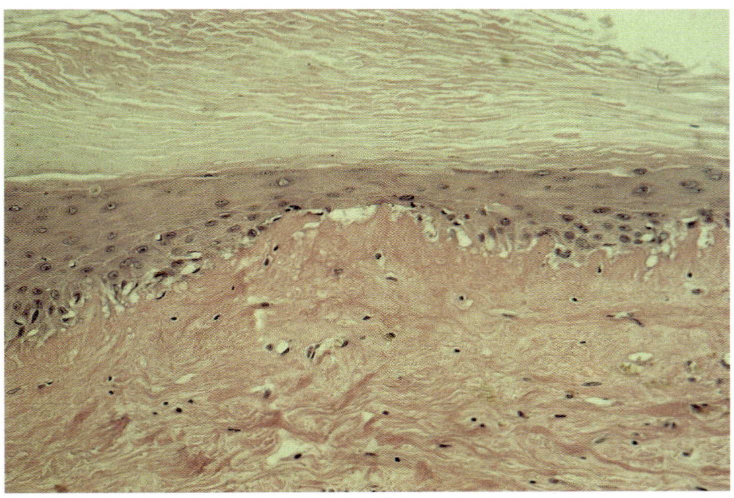

Figure 6–54. Degos' disease. Epidermal hyperkeratosis and necrosis. Necrotic basal cells with vacuolar alteration resulting in focal separation of the epidermis and dermis.

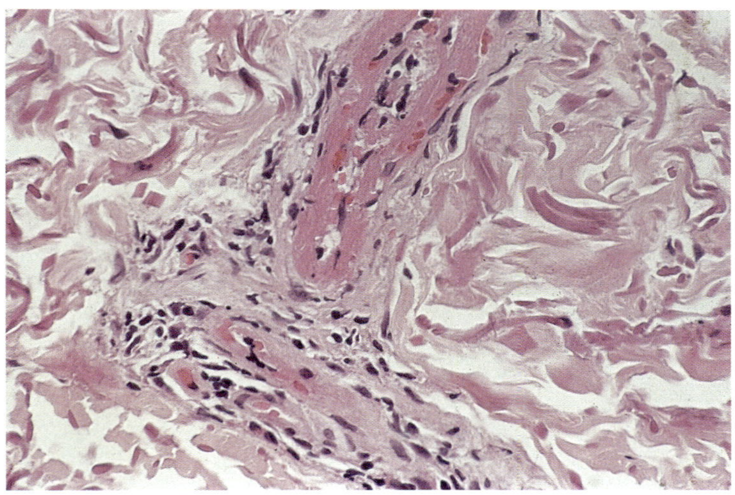

Figure 6–55. Degos' disease. Fibrin thrombus within dermal vessel. There are a few neutrophils, nuclear fragments, and extravasated erythrocytes.

CHURG-STRAUSS SYNDROME

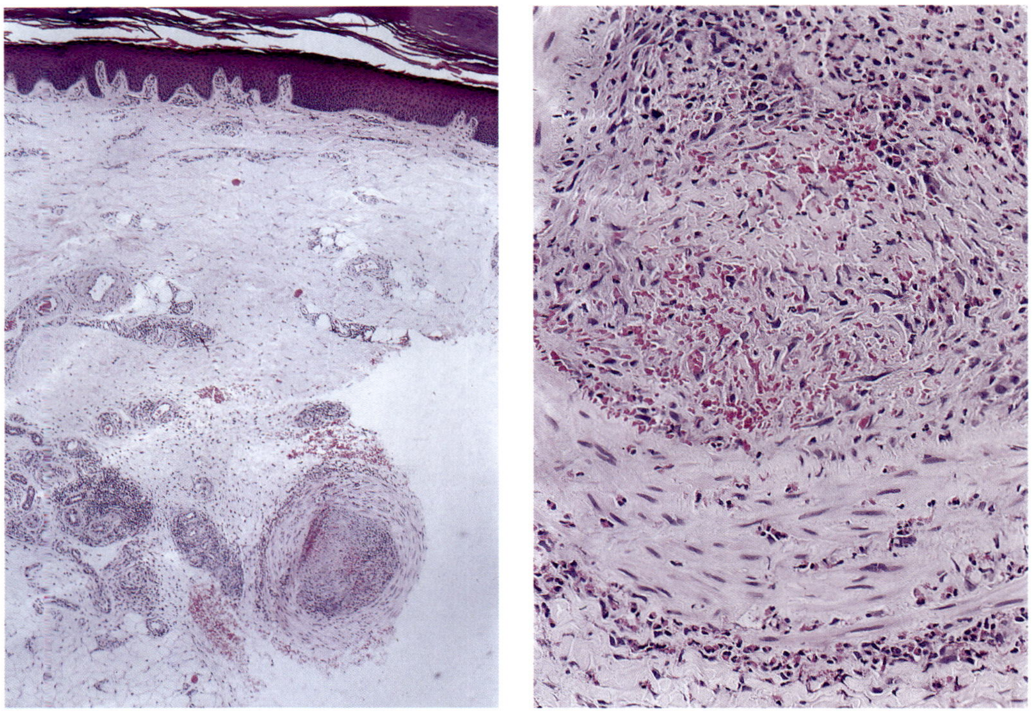

A B

Figures 6–56A, 6–56B. Churg-Strauss syndrome. Occlusion of larger blood vessel in deep dermis and subcutis. In and around the vessel wall there are numerous eosinophils.

SEPTIC VASCULITIS

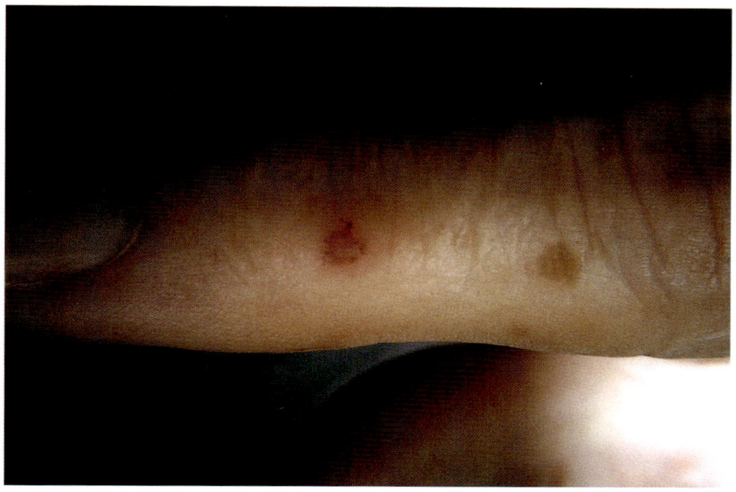

Figure 6–57. Septic vasculitis. Hemorrhagic papule over the distal interphalangeal joint.

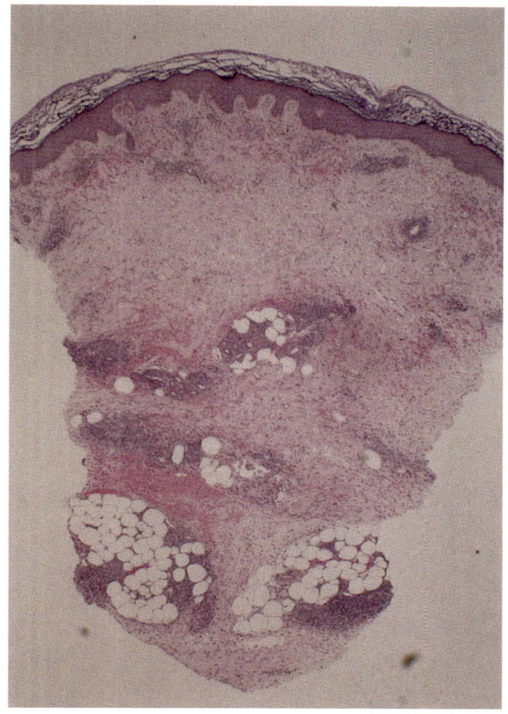

Figure 6–58. Septic vasculitis. Superficial and deep vasculitis and panniculitis.

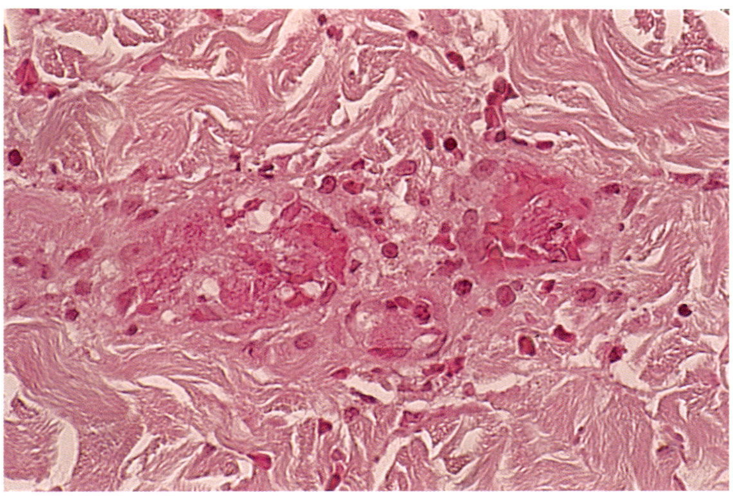

Figure 6–59. Septic vasculitis. Fibrin thrombi within venules. There is disruption of the blood vessel walls, and a mixed-cell infiltrate composed of neutrophils and nuclear debris.

7

Nodular and Diffuse Dermatitis

- Sweet's syndrome (acute febrile neutrophilic dermatosis)
- Pseudolymphoma
- Plasmacytoma
- Mastocytosis (urticaria pigmentosa)

SWEET'S SYNDROME (ACUTE NEUTROPHILIC DERMATOSIS)

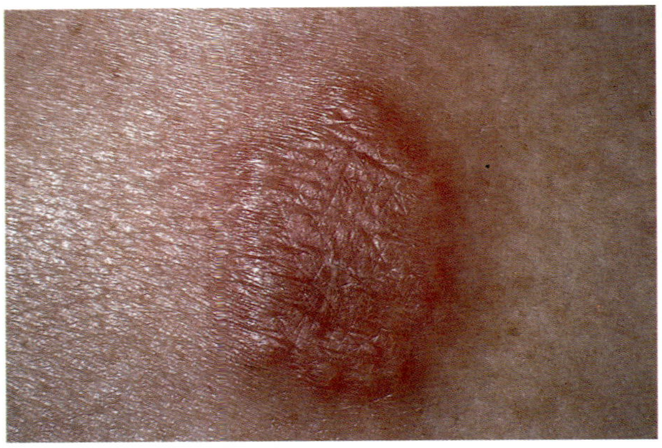

Figure 7–1. Sweet's syndrome. Erythematous and edematous plaque.

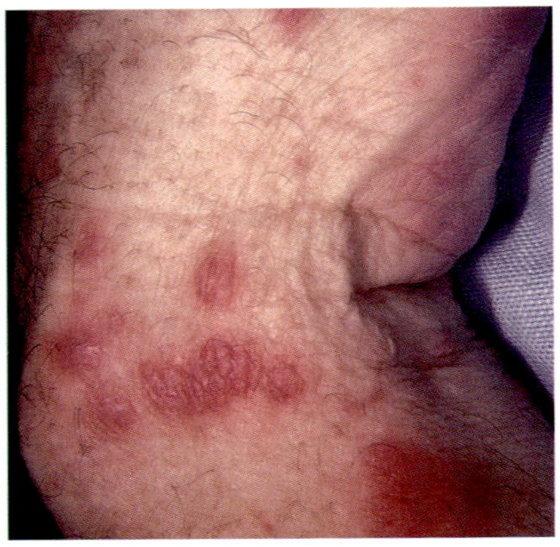

Figure 7–2. Sweet's syndrome. Solitary and confluent erythematous nodules and plaques on the thigh and leg.

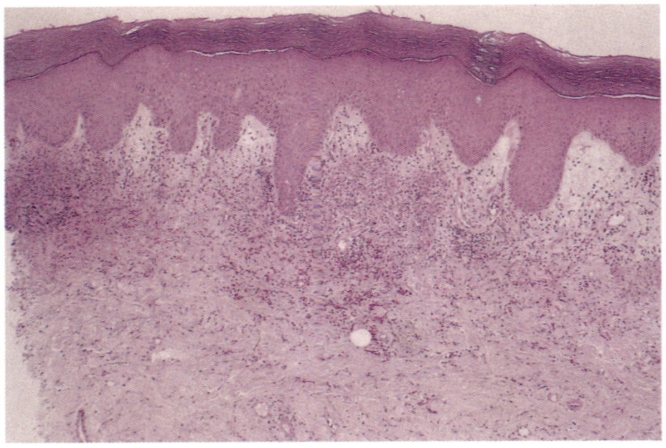

A

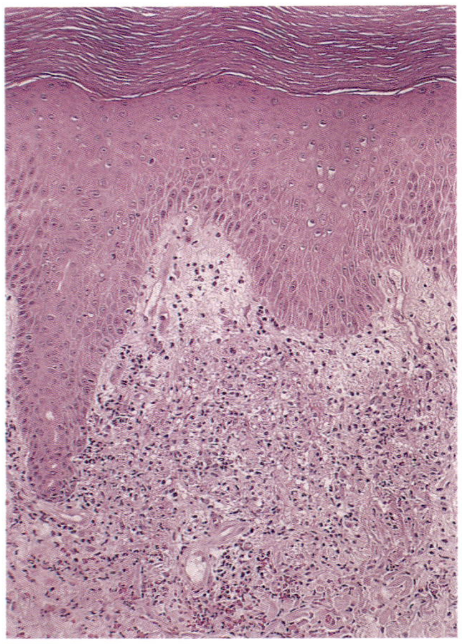

B

Figures 7–3A, 7–3B. Sweet's syndrome. Diffuse dermal infiltrate and prominent papillary edema; neutrophils predominate.

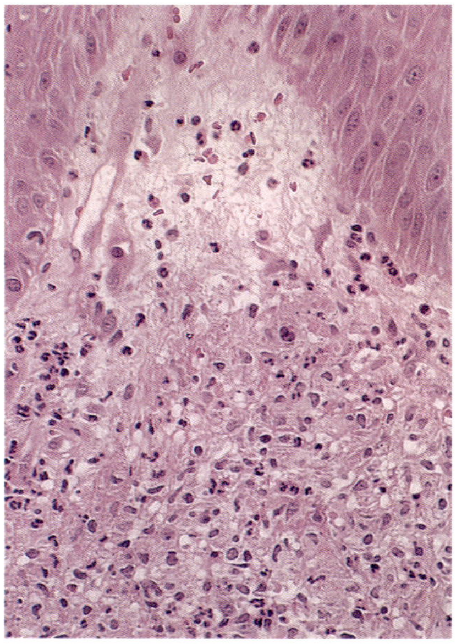

Figure 7–4. Sweet's syndrome. Extensive papillary dermal edema, dilated blood vessels, and a dense infiltrate of neutrophils and nuclear fragments.

PSEUDOLYMPHOMA

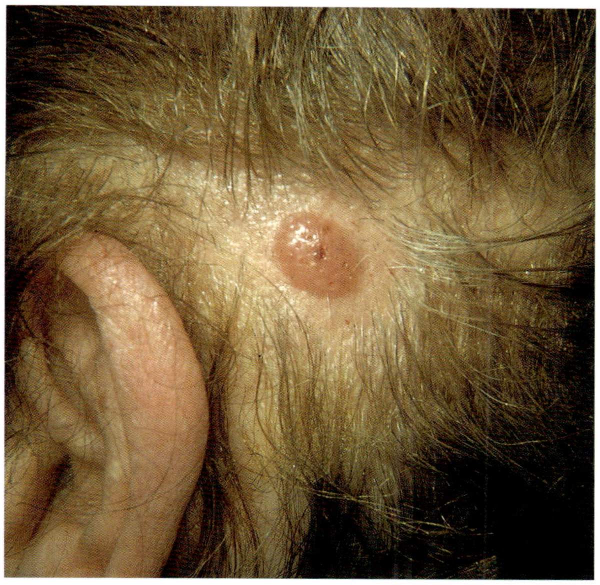

Figure 7–5. Pseudolymphoma. Erythematous nodule on the scalp.

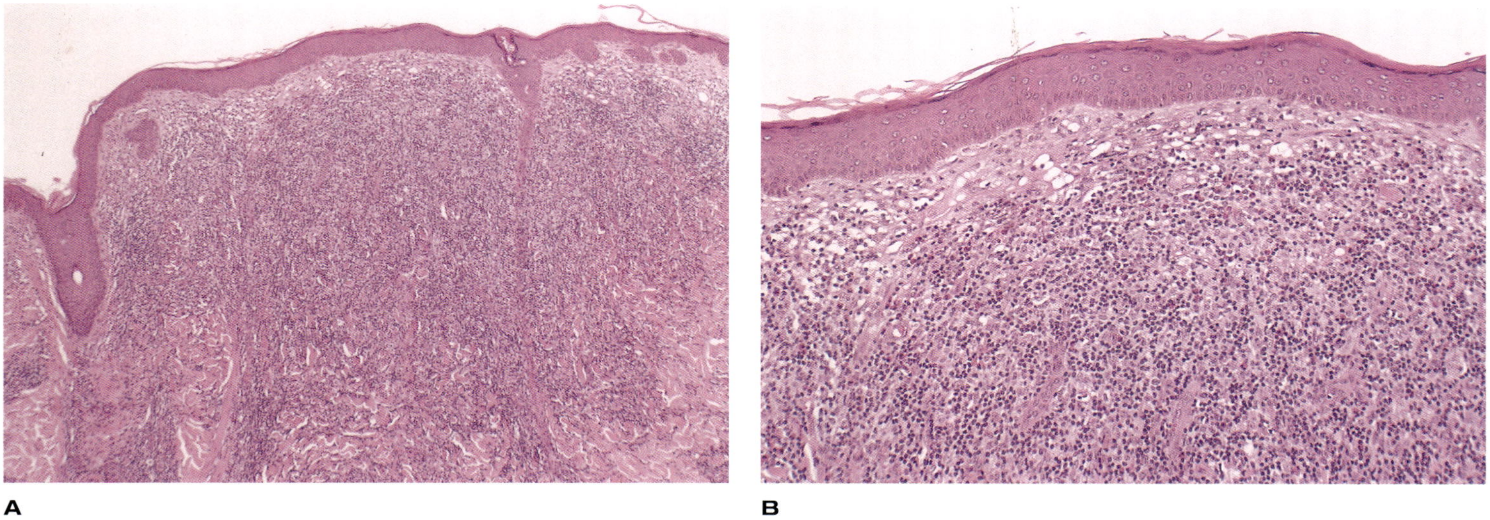

Figures 7–6A, 7–6B. Pseudolymphoma. Diffuse dermal infiltrate sparing adnexal structures and blood vessels.

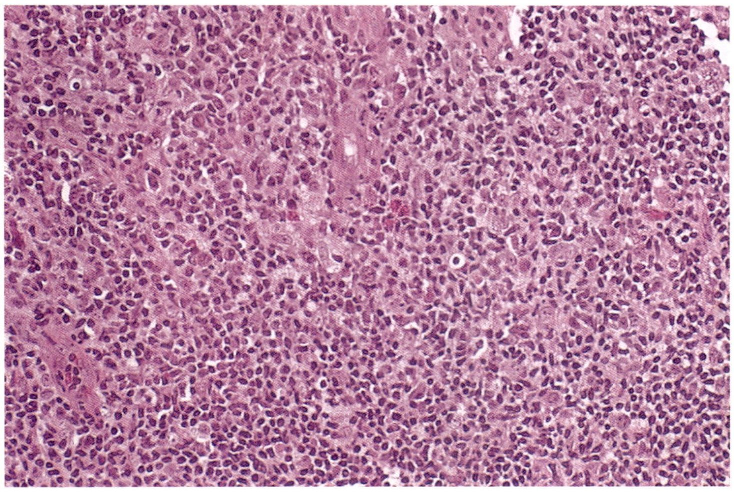

Figure 7–7. Pseudolymphoma. Diffuse infiltrate of lymphocytes, histiocytic cells, plasma cells, and eosinophils around blood vessels with plump endothelial cells.

PLASMACYTOMA

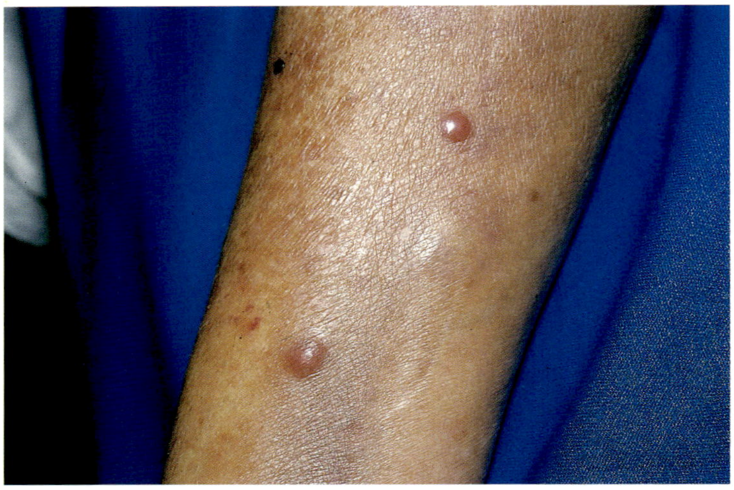

Figure 7–8. Plasmacytoma. Erythematous domed-shaped papules.

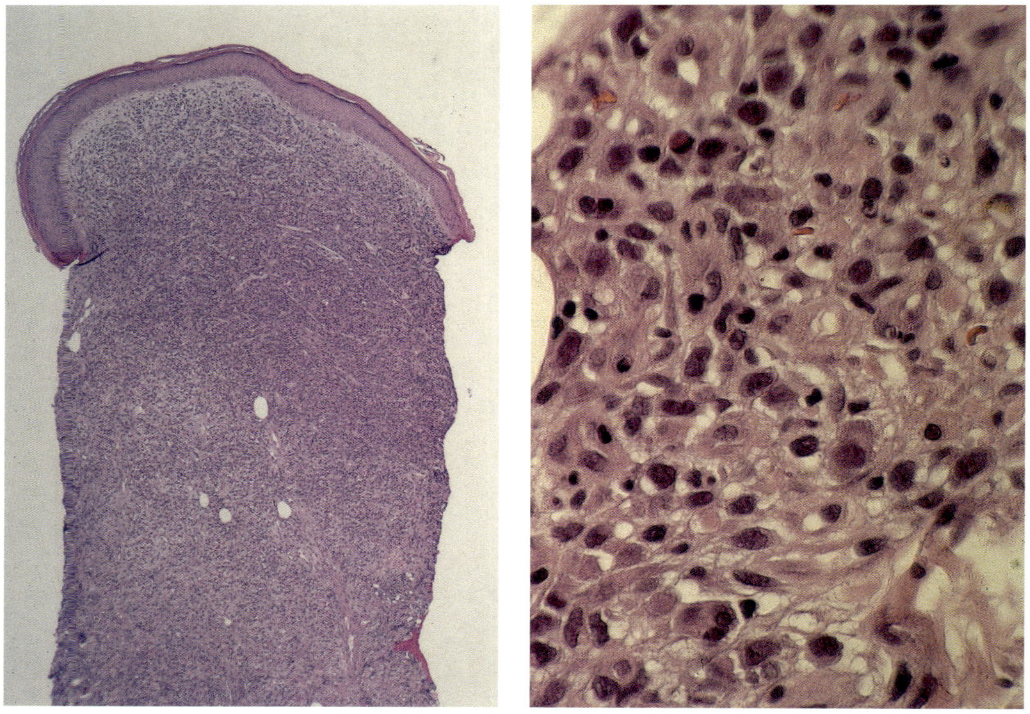

A B

Figures 7–9A, 7–9B. Plasmacytoma. Dense dermal infiltrate involving the entire reticular dermis. There are numerous plasma cells admixed with lymphocytes and histiocytic cells.

MASTOCYTOSIS (URTICARIA PIGMENTOSA)

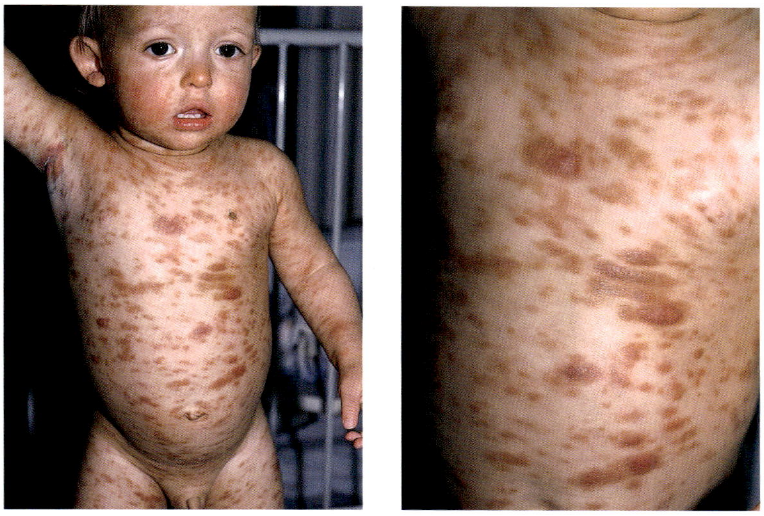

A B

Figures 7–10A, 7–10B. Mastocytosis. Child with numerous hyperpigmented macules and papules involving the trunk and extremities.

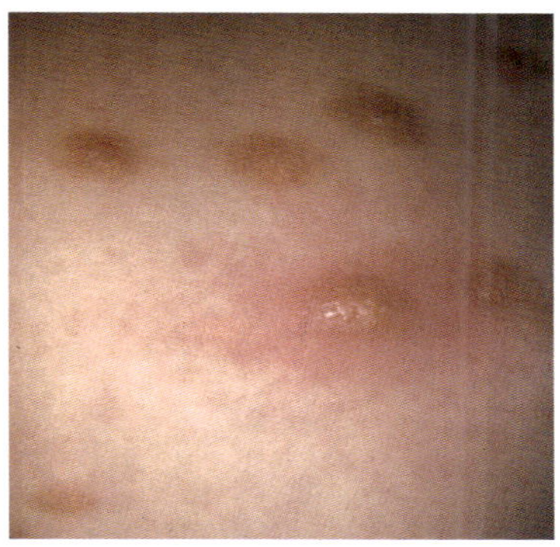

Figure 7–11. Mastocytosis. Enlarged nodule with surrounding erythema induced by rubbing (Darier's sign).

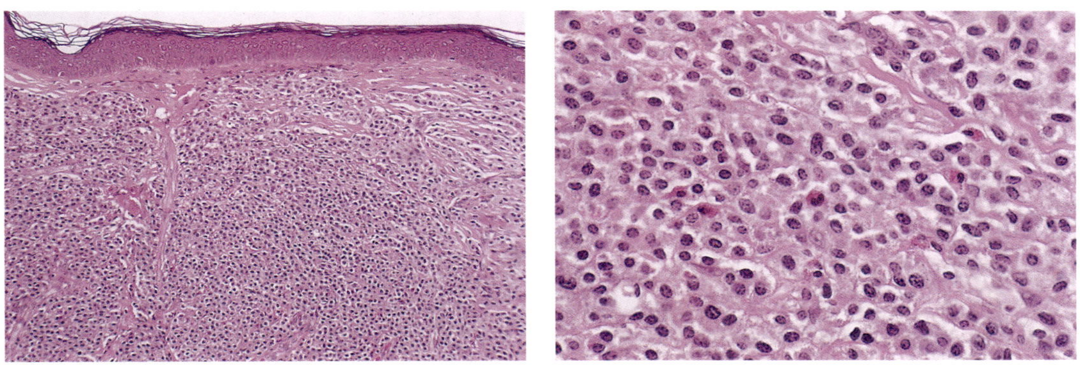

A B

Figures 7–12A, 7–12B. Mastocytosis. Sheets of monomorphous mononuclear cells. There are numerous mast cells with round or oval nuclei and cytoplasmic granules in addition to scattered eosinophils.

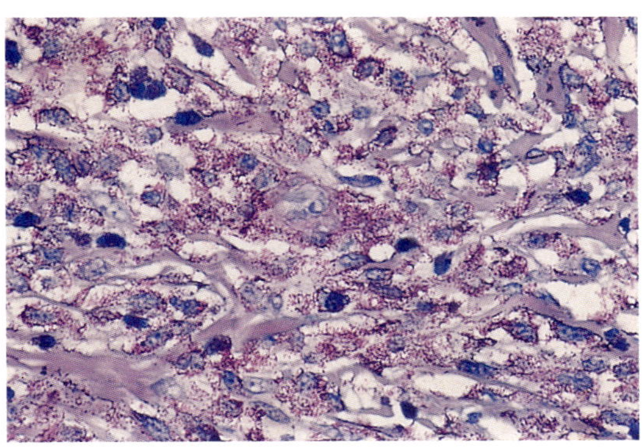

Figures 7–13. Mastocytosis. Giemsa stain shows characteristic amphophilic cytoplasmic granules within mast cells.

8

GRANULOMATOUS DERMATITIS

- Granuloma annulare
- Miescher's granuloma
- Necrobiosis lipoidica
- Necrobiotic xanthogranuloma
- Rheumatoid nodule
- Sarcoidosis
- Cutaneous Crohn's disease
- Lichen nitidus
- Ruptured follicular cyst

GRANULOMA ANNULARE

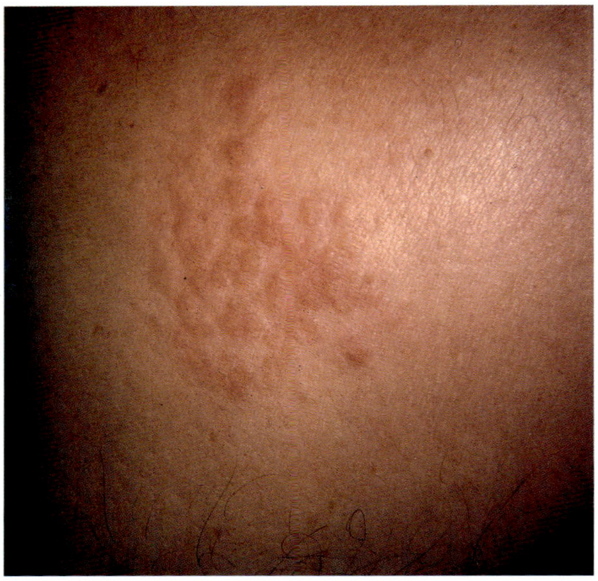

Figure 8–1. Granuloma annulare. Grouped erythematous papules.

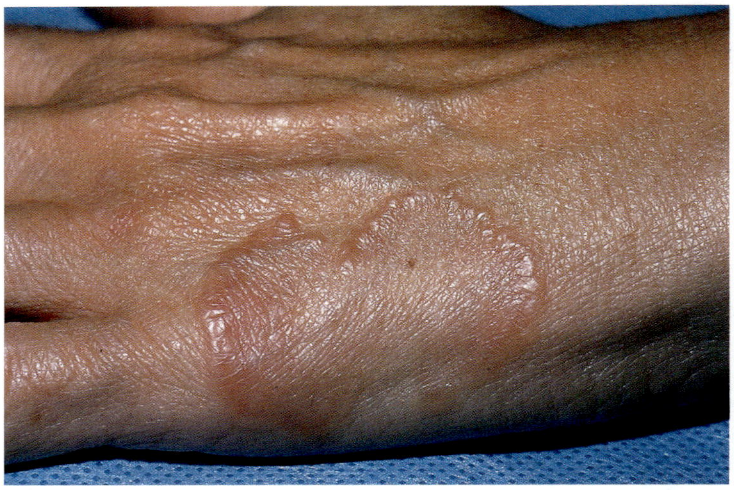

Figure 8–2. Granuloma annulare. Annular erythematous papules on dorsum of hand.

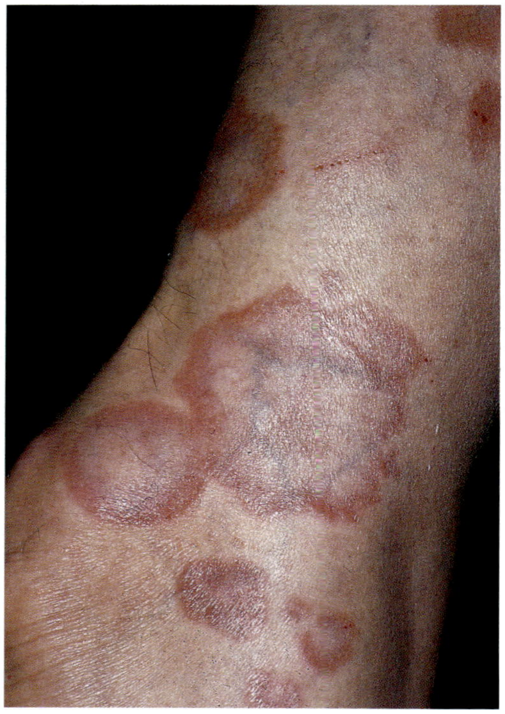

Figure 8–3. Granuloma annulare. Coalescing annular erythematous papules with central clearing on the lower leg and ankle.

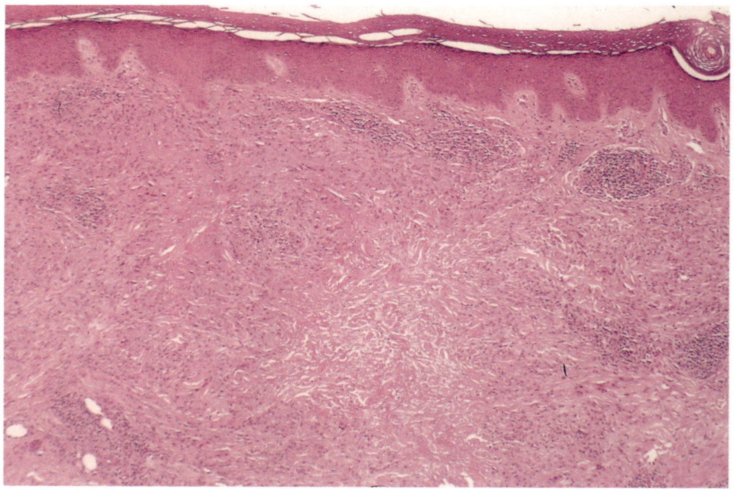

Figure 8–4. Granuloma annulare. Dermal granulomatous infiltrate composed of lymphocytes and histiocytic cells.

GRANULOMA ANNULARE

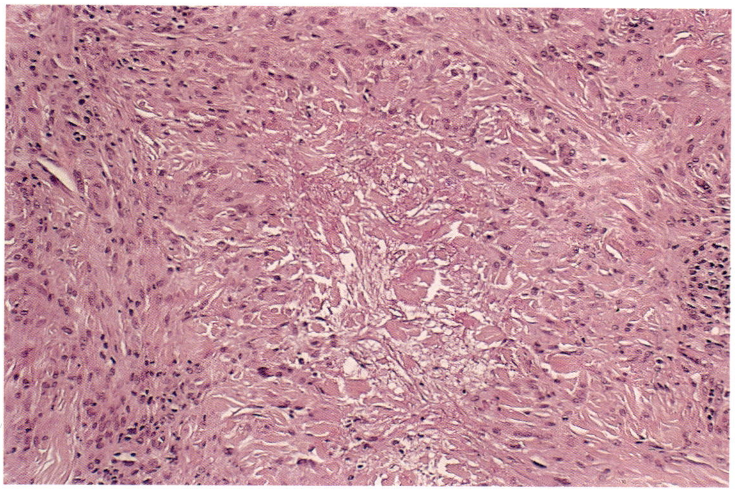
A

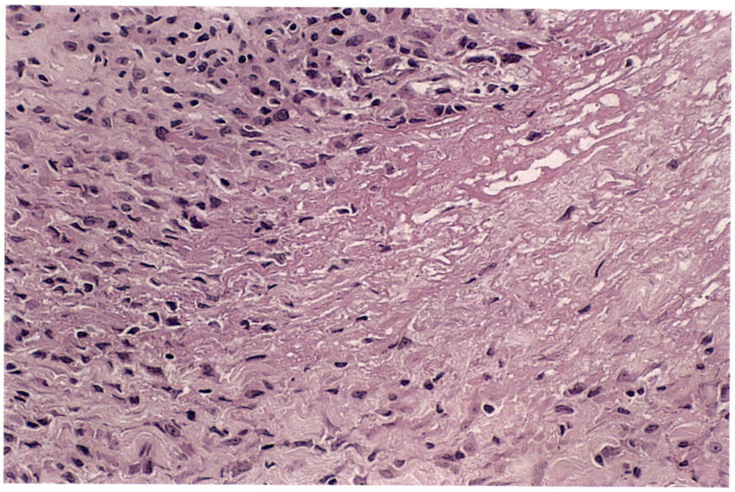
B

Figures 8–5A, 8–5B. Granuloma annulare. Typical palisaded granuloma. There are lymphocytes, histiocytic cells, and multinucleated histiocytic giant cells arranged about collagen bundles that are separated by mucin.

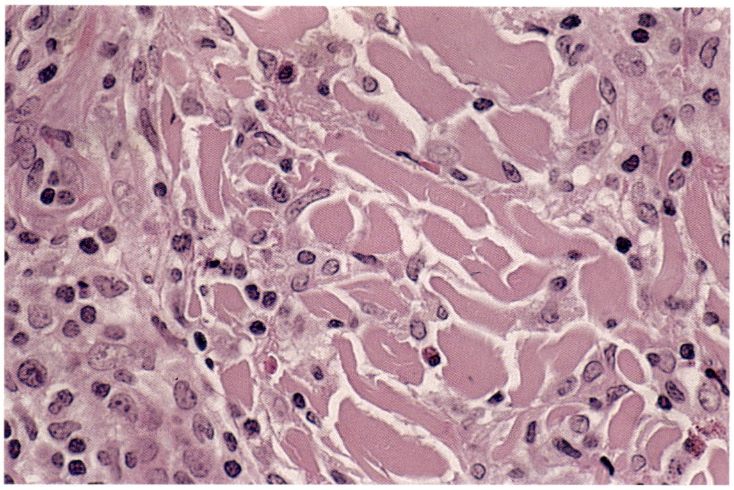

Figure 8–6. Granuloma annulare. Granulomatous infiltrate with characteristic splaying of collagen bundles by histiocytic cells.

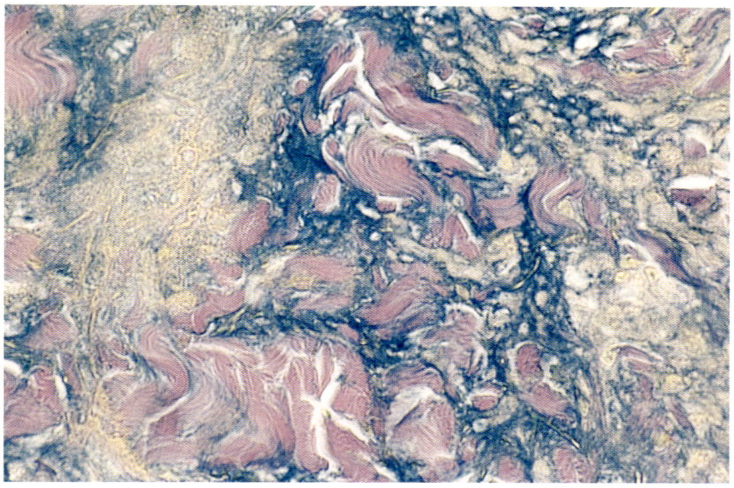

Figure 8–7. Granuloma annulare. Colloidal iron stains the mucin deposition between collagen bundles blue.

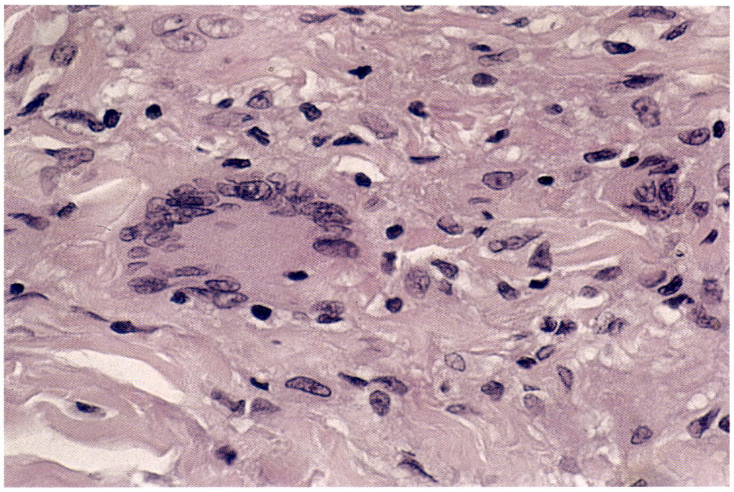

Figure 8–8. Granuloma annulare. Multinucleated histiocytic giant cells.

MIESCHER'S GRANULOMA

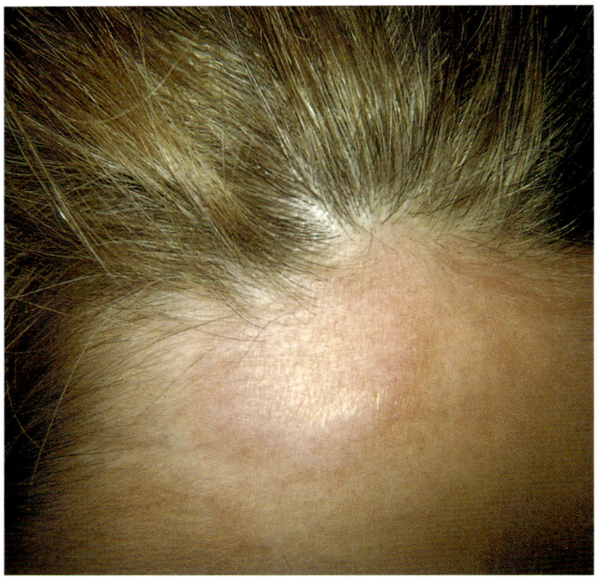

Figure 8–9. Miescher's granuloma. Erythematous annular plaque on forehead.

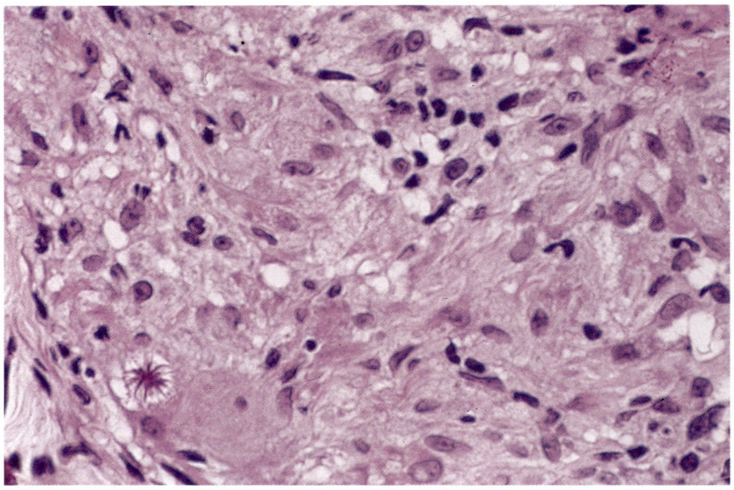

Figure 8–10. Miescher's granuloma. Granulomatous infiltrate with lymphocytes, histiocytic cells, and a multinucleated histiocytic giant cell containing an asteroid body.

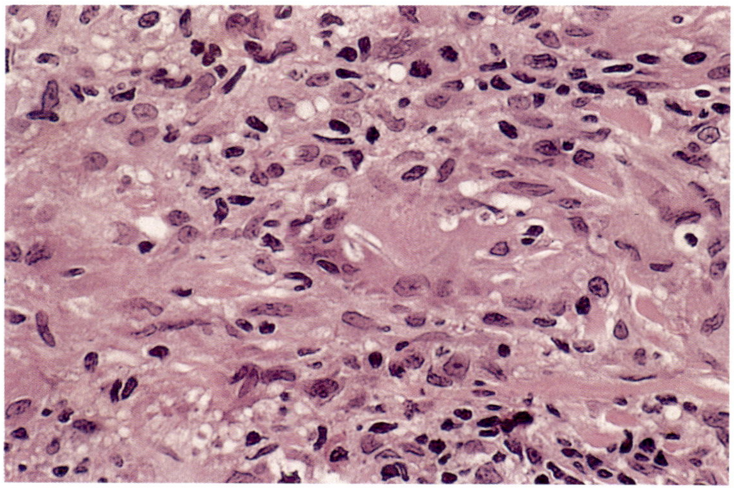

Figure 8–11. Miescher's granuloma. Granulomatous infiltrate with an elastic fiber within a multinucleated histiocytic giant cell.

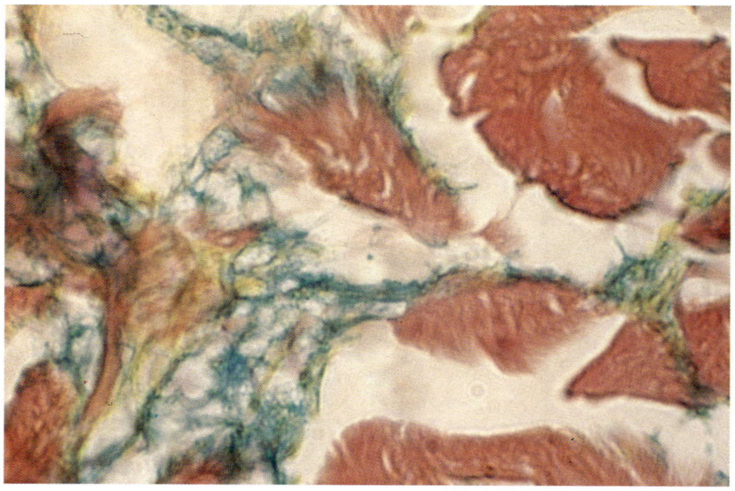

Figure 8–12. Miescher's granuloma. Colloidal iron stains the mucin deposited between collagen bundles blue.

NECROBIOSIS LIPOIDICA

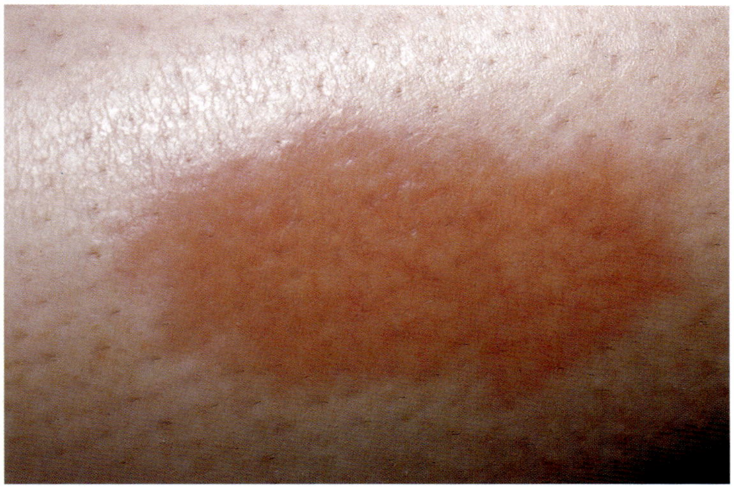

Figure 8–13. Necrobiosis lipoidica. Yellowish-red plaque on the lower leg.

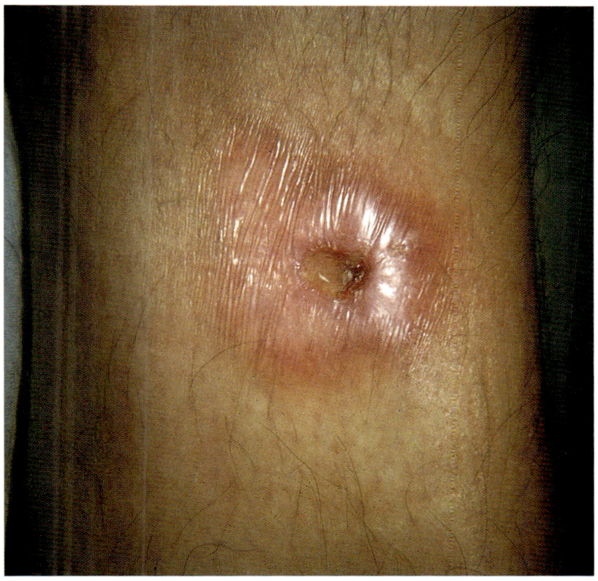

Figure 8–14. Necrobiosis lipoidica. Erythematous nodule with ulceration located on the lower leg.

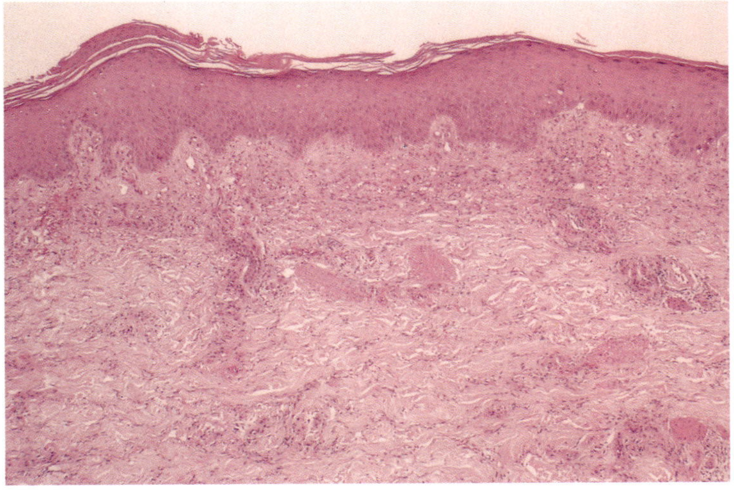

A

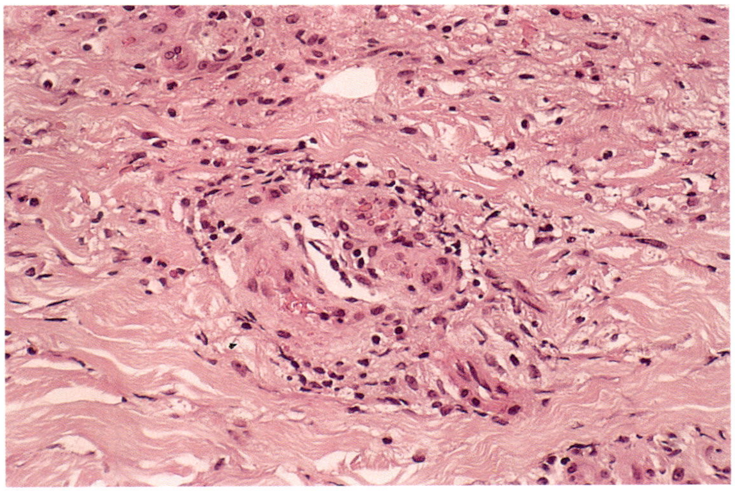

B

Figures 8–15A, 8–15B. Necrobiosis lipoidica, early stage. Patchy vascular and interstitial mixed-cell infiltrate loosely arranged around altered collagen. There is a leukocytoclastic and granulomatous vasculitis, with histiocytic cells, neutrophils, and fibrin within and around venules.

NECROBIOSIS LIPOIDICA

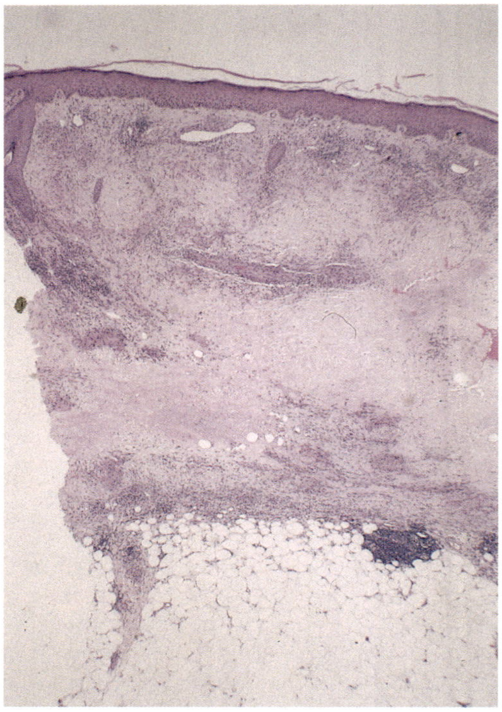

Figure 8–16. Necrobiosis lipoidica, Granulomatous infiltrate involving the reticular dermis and panniculus.

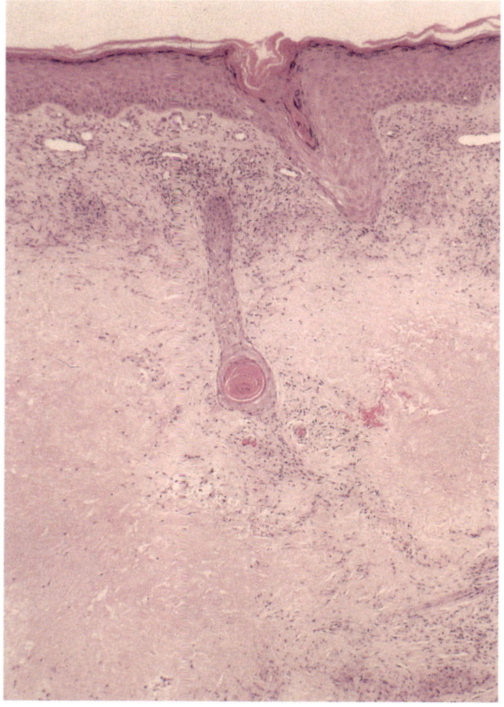

A

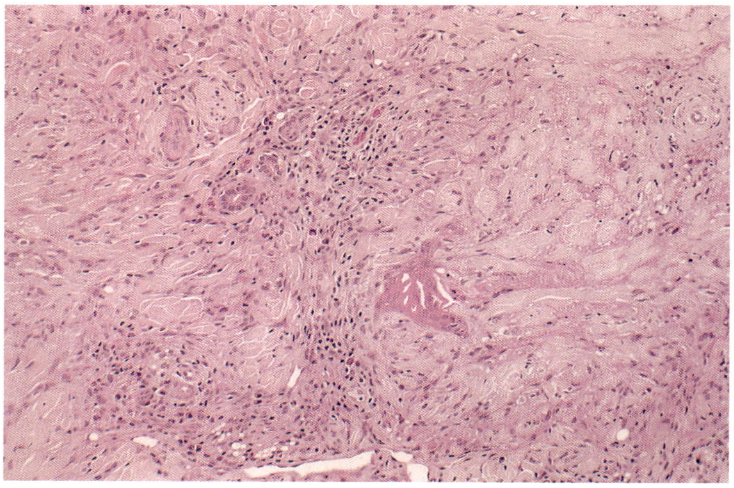

B

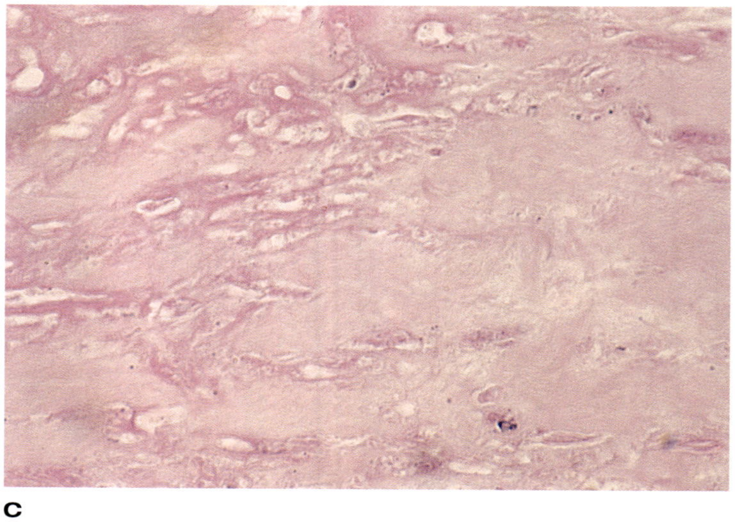

C

Figures 8–17A, 8–17B, 8–17C. Necrobiosis lipoidica. Granulomatous infiltrate around fibrotic, sclerotic, and degenerated collagen. There is necrosis of an eccrine duct.

NECROBIOSIS LIPOIDICA

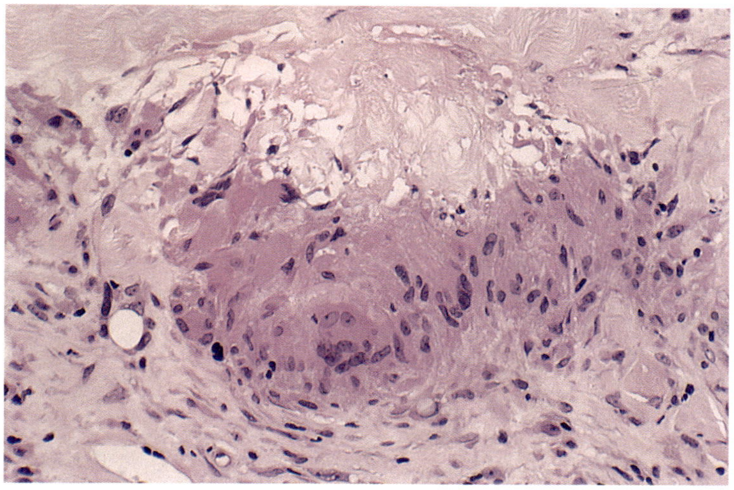

Figure 8–18. Necrobiosis lipoidica. Multinucleated histiocytic giant cells abutting sclerotic and degenerated collagen above, and fibroplasia below.

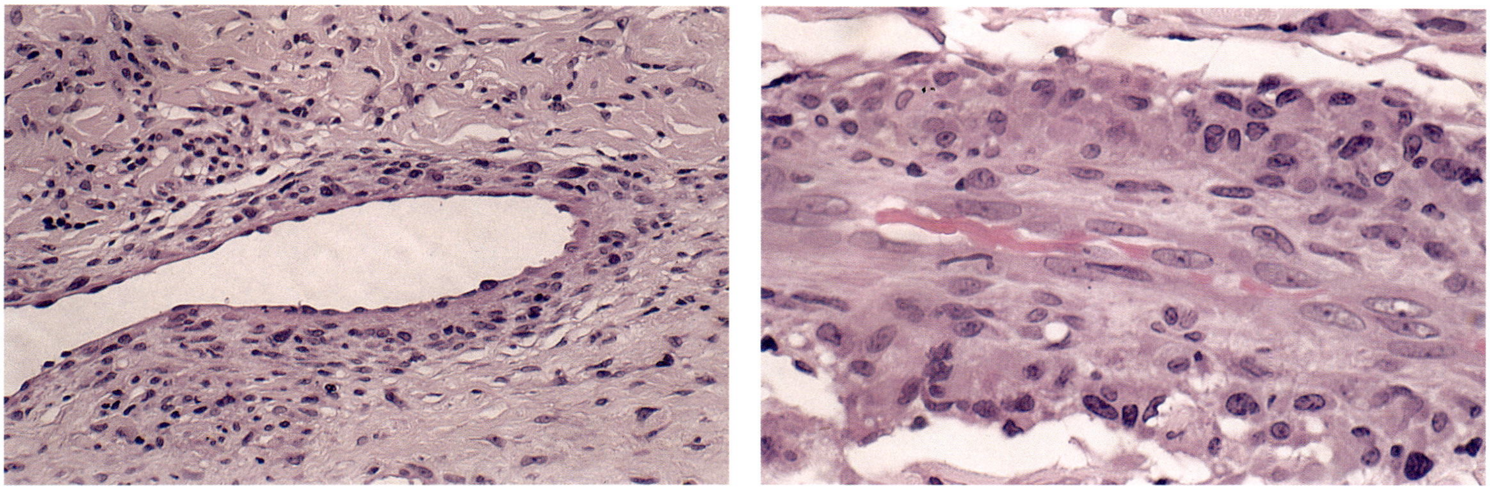

A B

Figures 8–19A, 8–19B. Necrobiosis lipoidica with granulomatous vasculitis. Lymphocytes and histiocytic cells involving the wall of a venule.

NECROBIOSIS LIPOIDICA

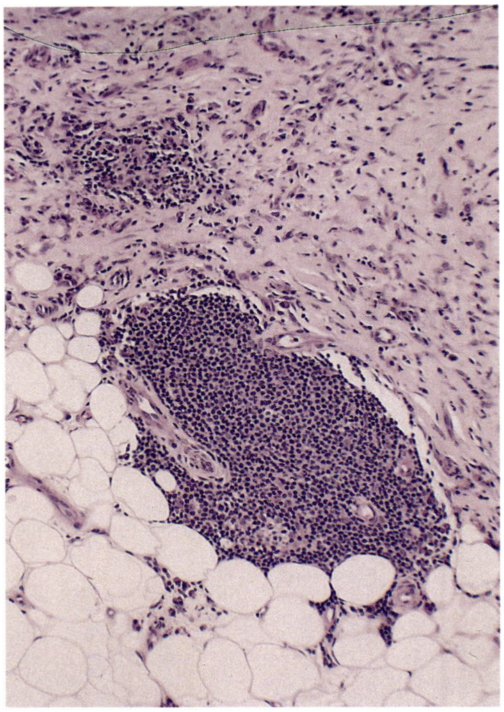

Figure 8–20. Necrobiosis lipoidica. Collection of lymphocytes, histiocytic cells, and plasma cells at the dermal-subcutaneous junction. This infiltrate is associated with dermal fibroplasia and extends into the subcutaneous tissue.

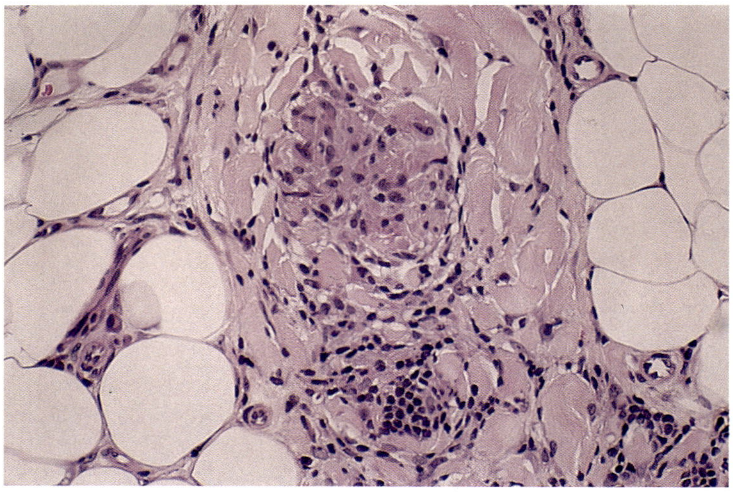

Figure 8–21. Necrobiosis lipoidica. Thickened fibrous septum in subcutaneous fat. There are fibrocytes, coarse collagen bundles, lymphocytes, histiocytic cells, and plasma cells.

NECROBIOTIC XANTHOGRANULOMA

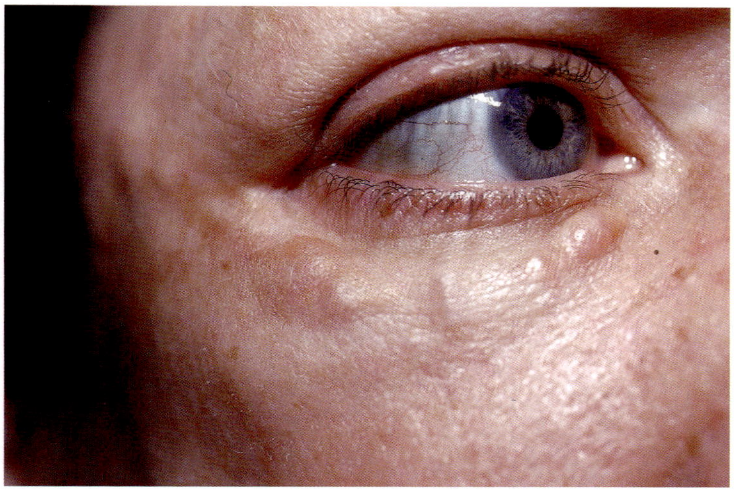

Figure 8–22. **Necrobiotic xanthogranuloma.** Periorbital skin-colored papules.

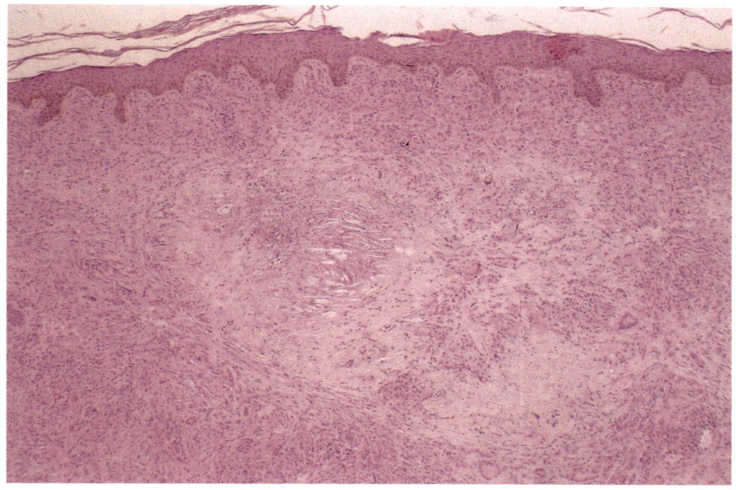

Figure 8–23. **Necrobiotic xanthogranuloma.** Dermal granulomatous infiltrate. There are areas with cholesterol clefts, multinucleated histiocytic giant cells, fibroplasia, and degenerated collagen.

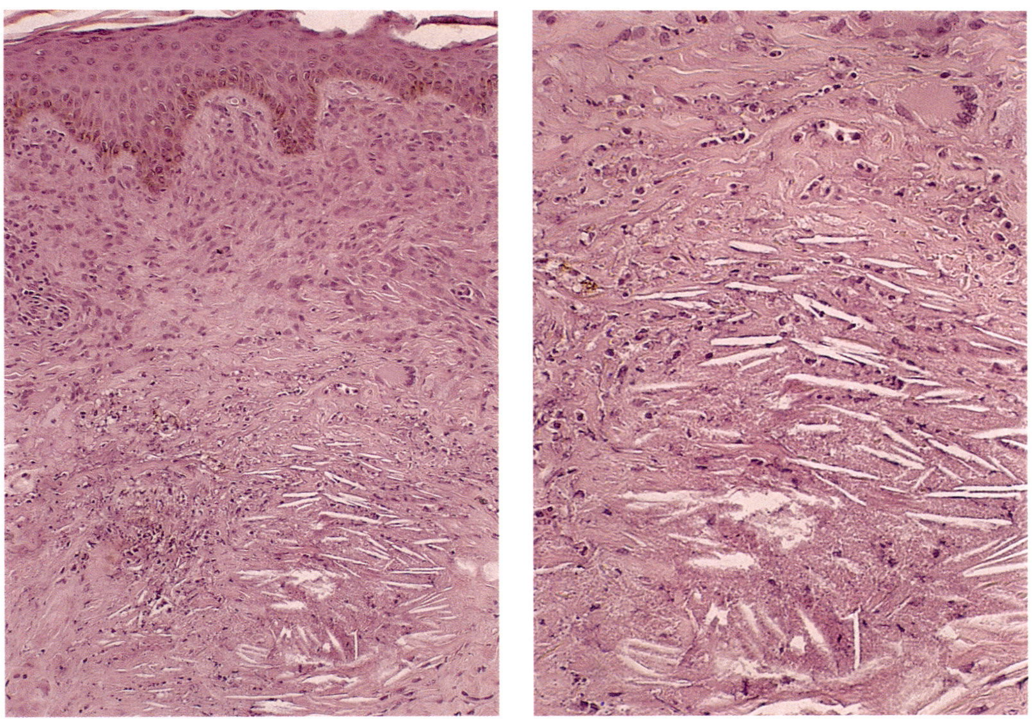

A B

Figures 8–24A, 8–24B. **Necrobiotic xanthogranuloma.** Multinucleated histiocytic giant cells, cholesterol clefts, siderophages, degenerated collagen with neutrophils, and nuclear debris.

NECROBIOTIC XANTHOGRANULOMA

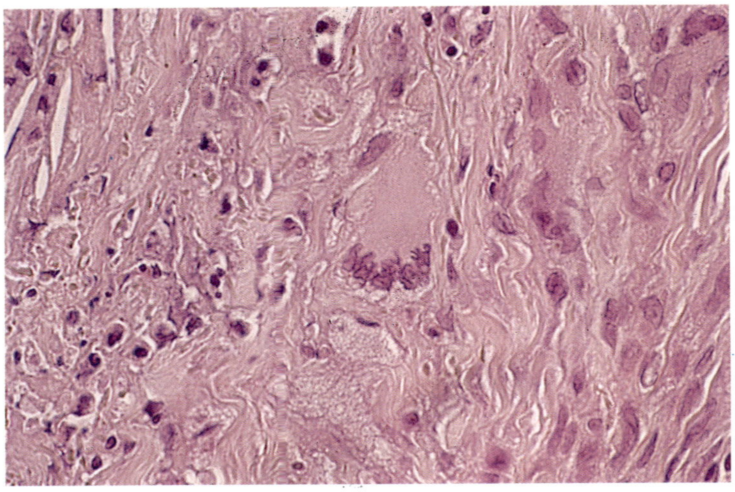

A

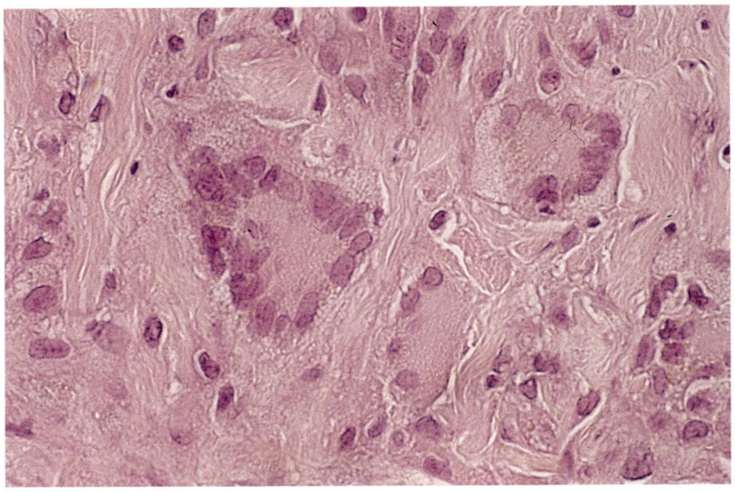

B

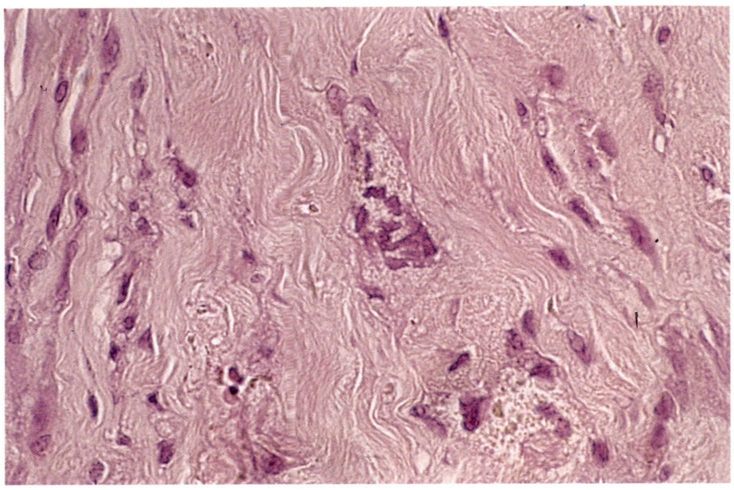

C

Figures 8–25A, 8–25B, 8–25C. Necrobiotic xanthogranuloma. Lipid-laden histiocytic cells, characteristic bizarre multinucleated histiocytic giant cells, degenerated collagen, and nuclear debris.

RHEUMATOID NODULE

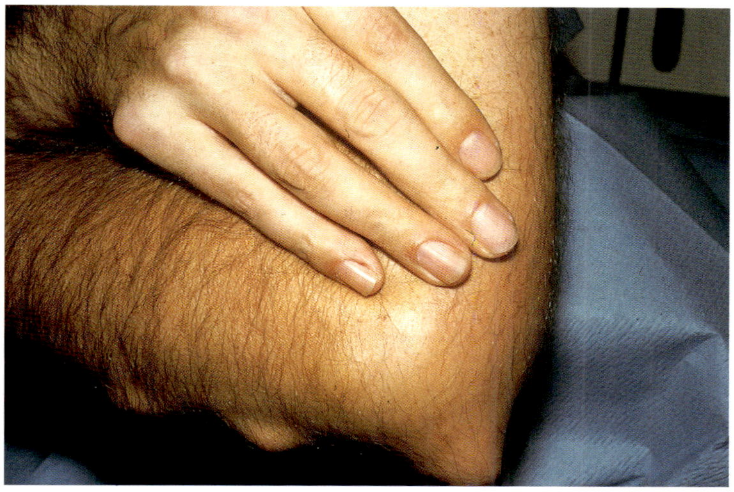

Figure 8–26. Rheumatoid nodule. Skin-colored nodules on the elbow and arm of a man with rheumatoid arthritis.

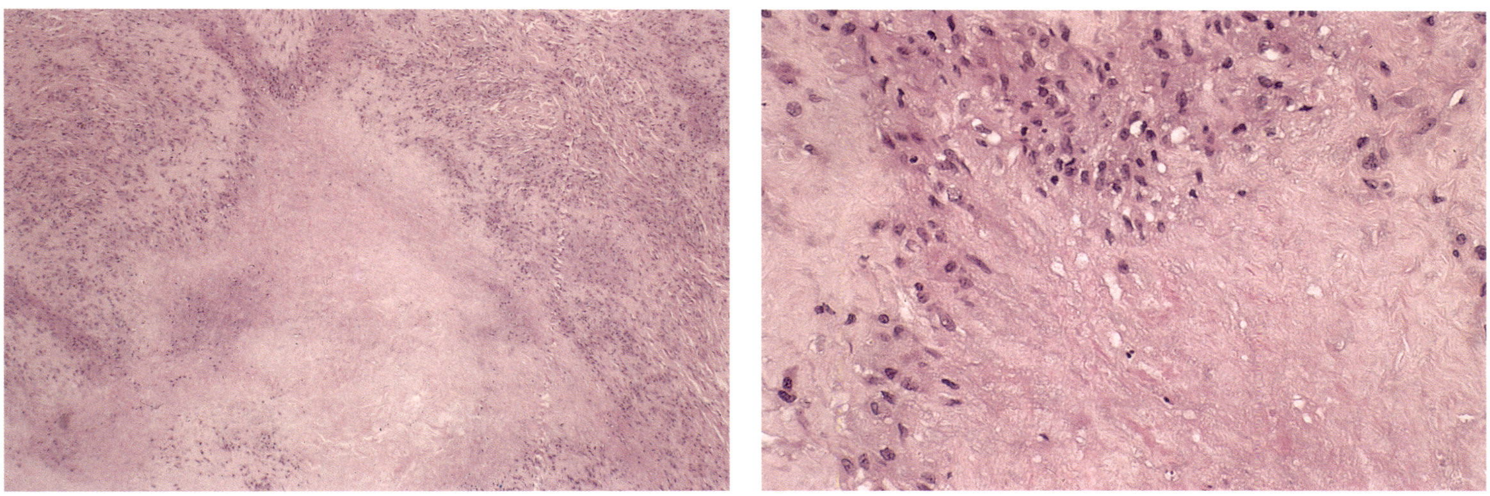

A B

Figures 8–27A, 8–27B. Rheumatoid nodule. Granulomatous infiltrate encircling large deposits of fibrin. Histiocytic cells predominate; characteristically, they are aligned in a palisade array.

SARCOIDOSIS

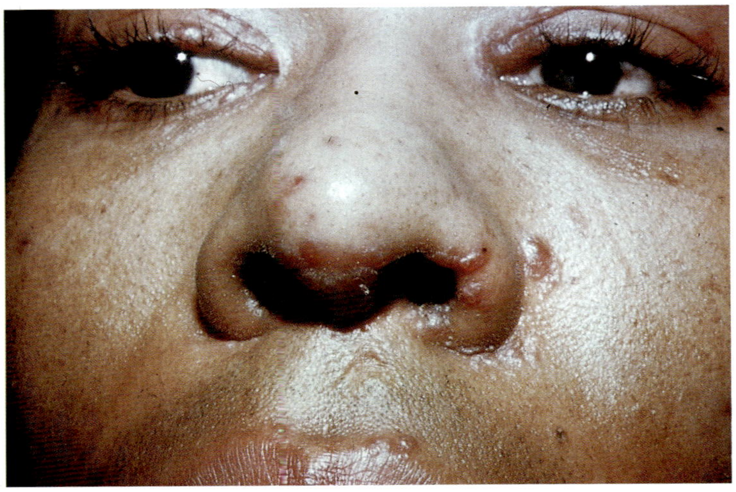

Figure 8–28. **Sarcoidosis.** Erythematous papules on the nose, lip, and cheek.

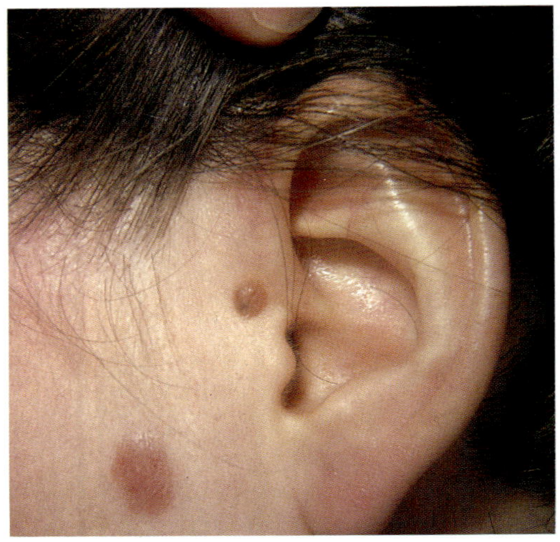

Figure 8–29. **Sarcoidosis.** Tan papule and plaque on the cheek.

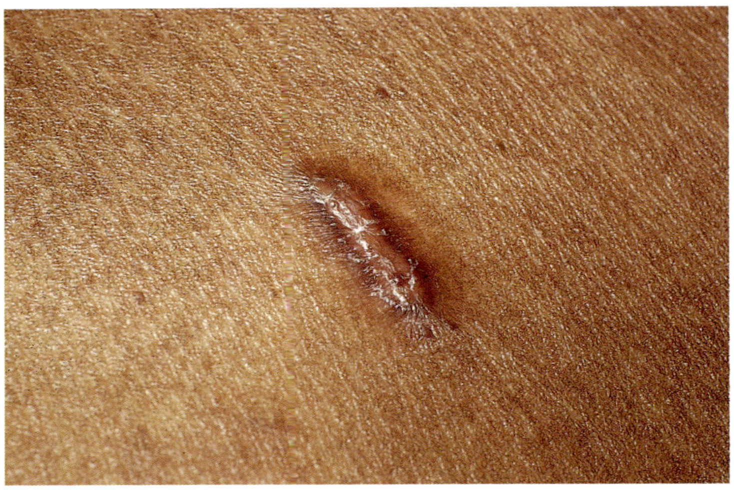

Figure 8–30. **Sarcoidcsis.** Elevation of a previously flat scar.

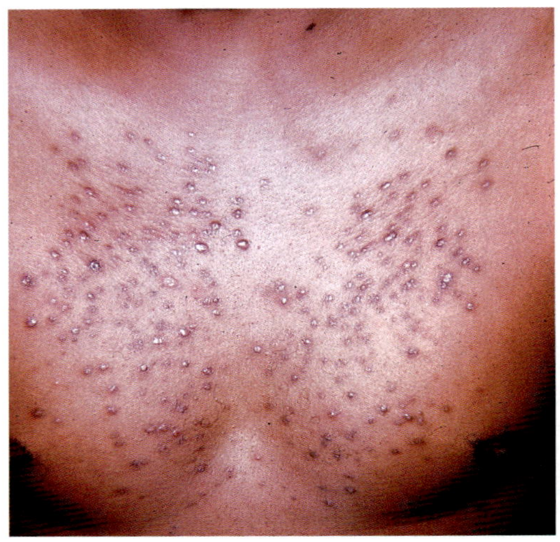

Figure 8–31. **Sarcoidosis.** Reddish-brown papules on the chest.

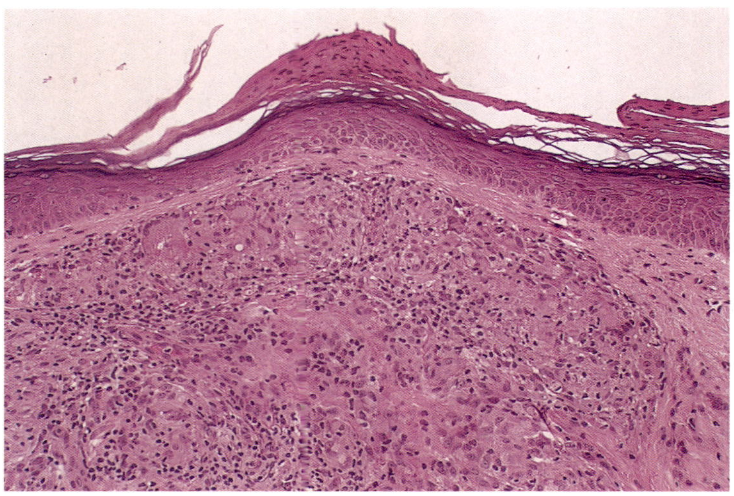

A

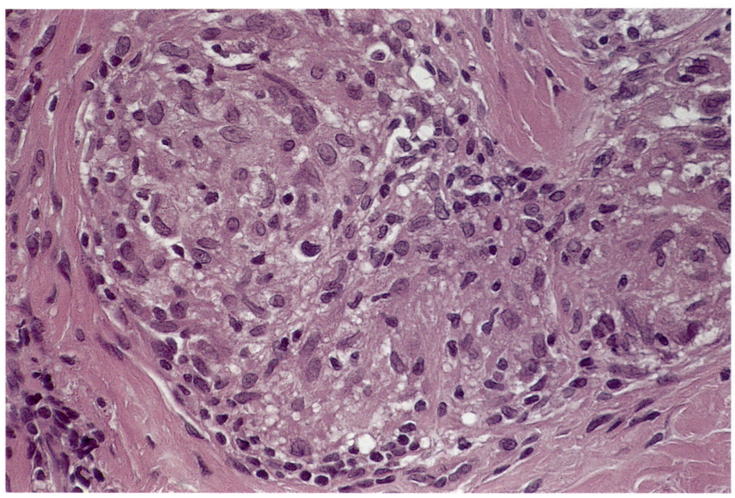

B

Figures 8–32A, 8–32B. **Sarcoidosis.** Granulomatous infiltrate with lymphocytes, histiocytic cells, and multinucleated histiocytic giant cells. There is a dermal granuloma with histiocytic cells and a paucity of lymphocytes.

CUTANEOUS CROHN'S DISEASE

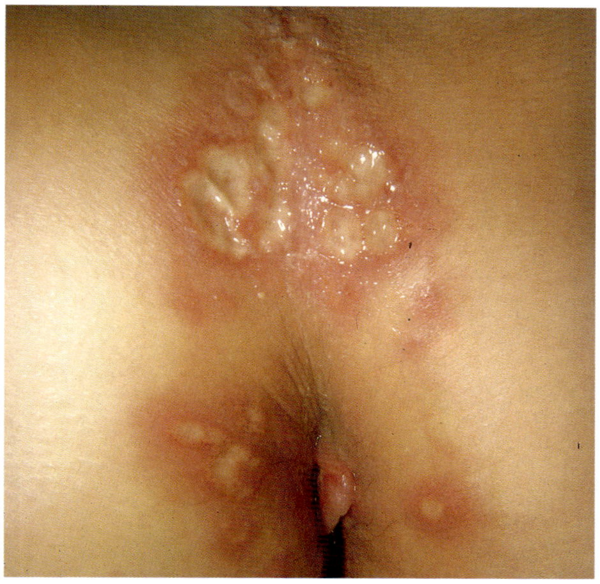

Figure 8–33. Cutaneous Crohn's disease. Perianal and sacral erythematous ulcerative papules and plaques in a young woman.

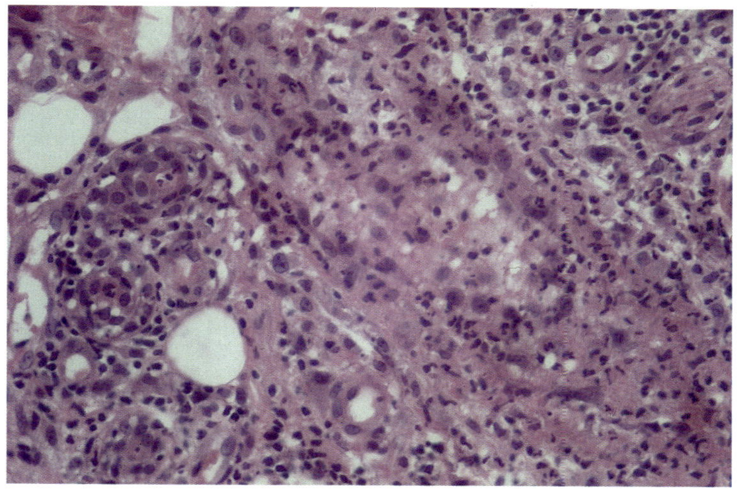

Figure 8–34. Cutaneous Crohn's disease. Mixed granulomatous dermal infiltrate. There are histiocytic cells, lymphocytes, and neutrophils.

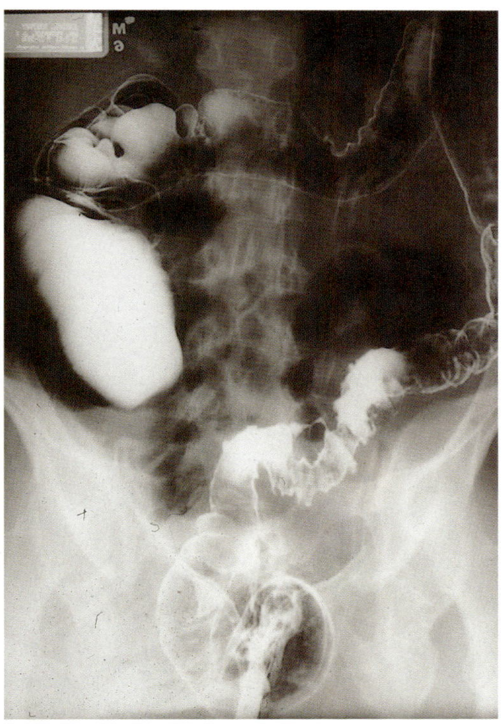

Figure 8–35. Crohn's disease. Barium radiograph. Changes seen are characteristic of Crohn's disease. There is segmented intestinal involvement where the walls are rigid and there is lumenal stenosis.

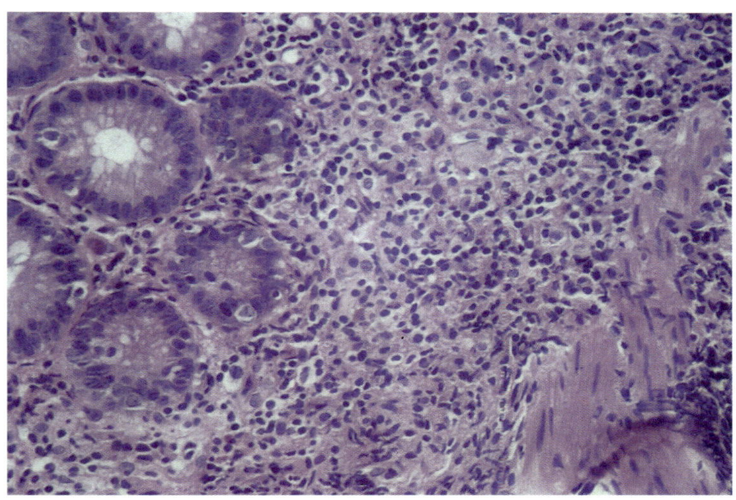

Figure 8–36. Crohn's disease. Bowel biopsy. Dense transmural granulomatous infiltrate involving mucosal crypts and muscularis mucosae. There are lymphocytes, plasma cells, histiocytic cells, and multinucleated histiocytic giant cells.

LICHEN NITIDUS

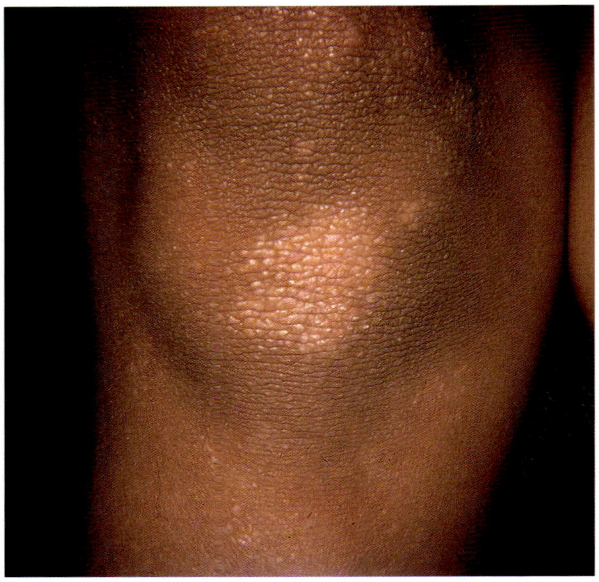

Figure 8–37. Lichen nitidus. Circumscribed collection of skin-colored papules on the knee of an adolescent.

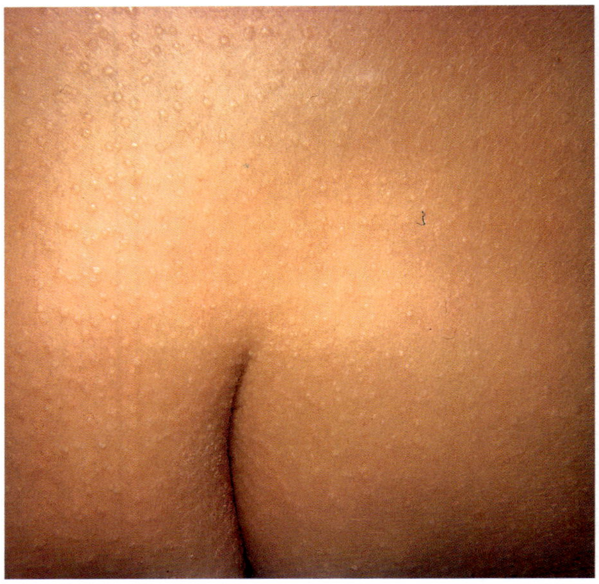

Figure 8–38. Lichen nitidus. Diffuse skin-colored papules on the back and buttocks of a young child.

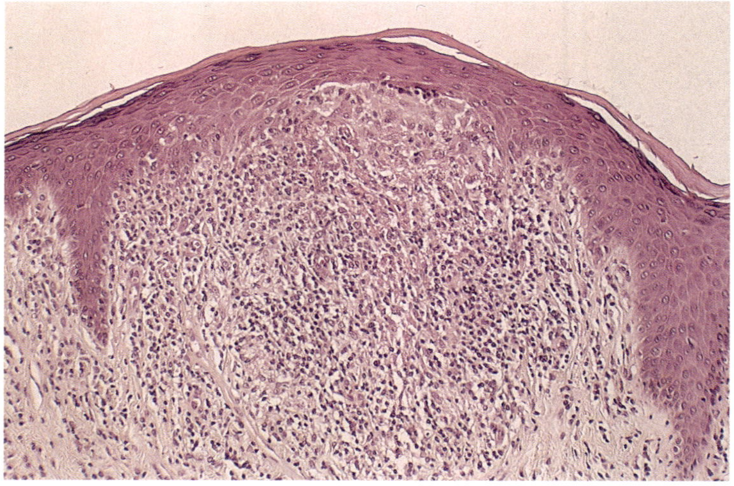

Figure 8–39. Lichen nitidus. Granulomatous infiltrate within a distended dermal papilla. Histiocytic cells and lymphocytes obscure the dermoepidermal junction.

RUPTURED FOLLICULAR CYST

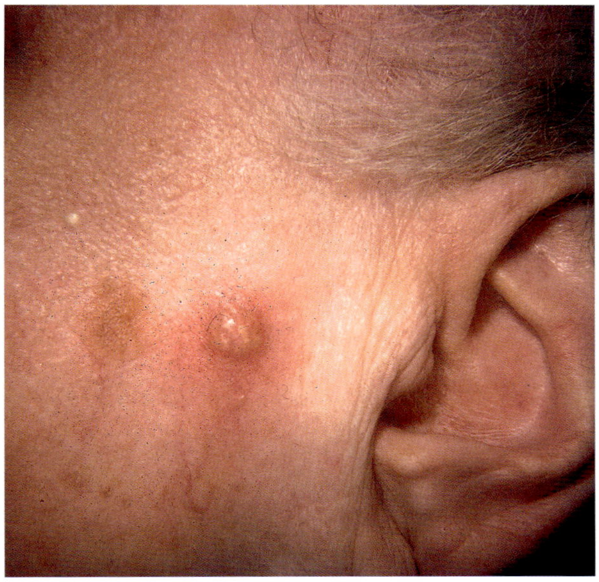
A

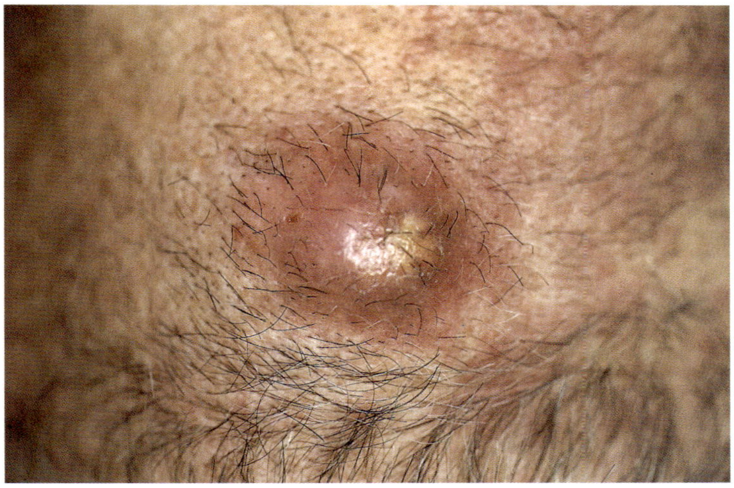
B

Figures 8–40A, 8–40B. Ruptured follicular cyst. Dome-shaped erythematous nodule with surrounding erythema.

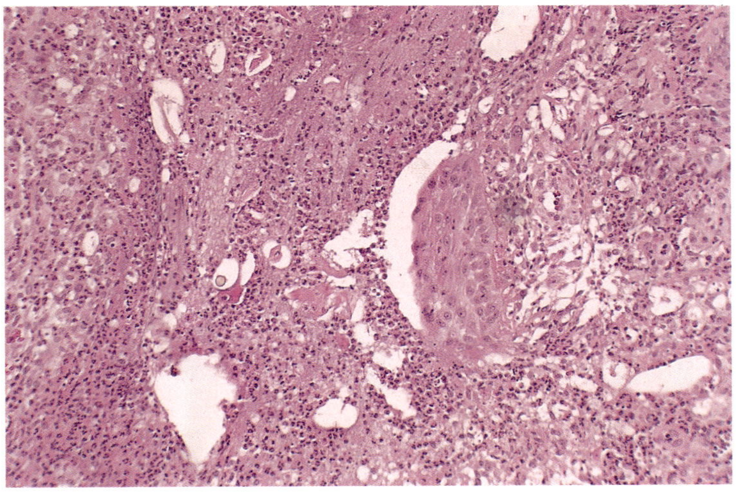

Figure 8–41. Ruptured follicular cyst. Infundibular fragments with a suppurative granulomatous infiltrate. There are hair-shaft fragments, squames (keratin debris), histiocytic cells, neutrophils, and multinucleated histiocytic giant cells.

9

HISTIOCYTIC AND LANGERHANS CELL REACTIONS

- Xanthogranuloma
- Reticulohistiocytoma
- Self-healing reticulohistiocytosis
- Xanthoma
- Langerhans cell histiocytosis
- Malignant histiocytosis

XANTHOGRANULOMA

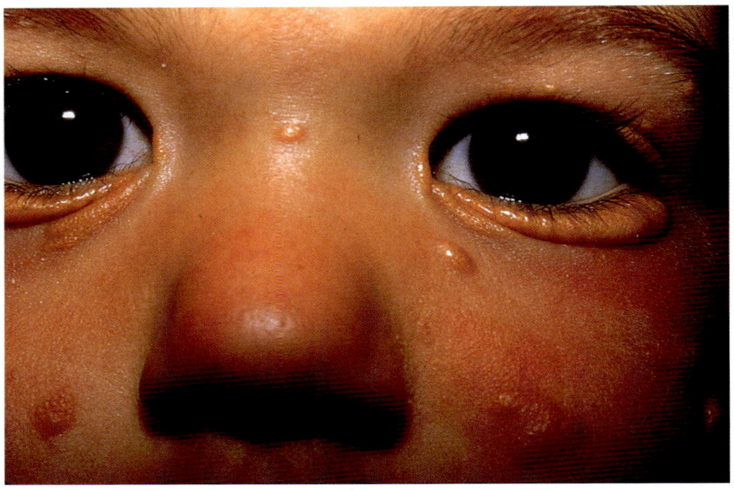

Figure 9–1. Xanthogranuloma. Multiple yellowish-red papules on the face of a child.

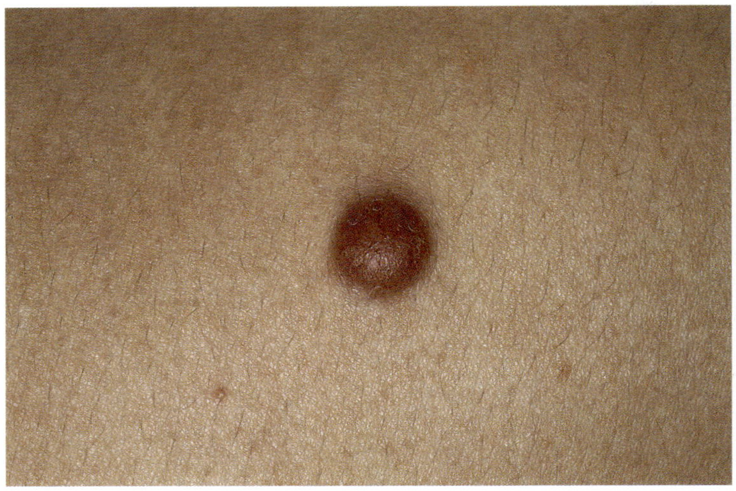

Figure 9–2. Xanthogranuloma. Solitary reddish-brown, dome-shaped nodule.

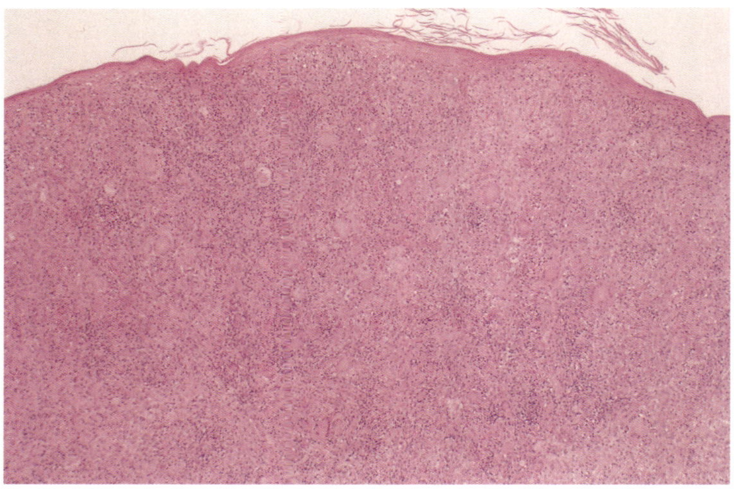

A

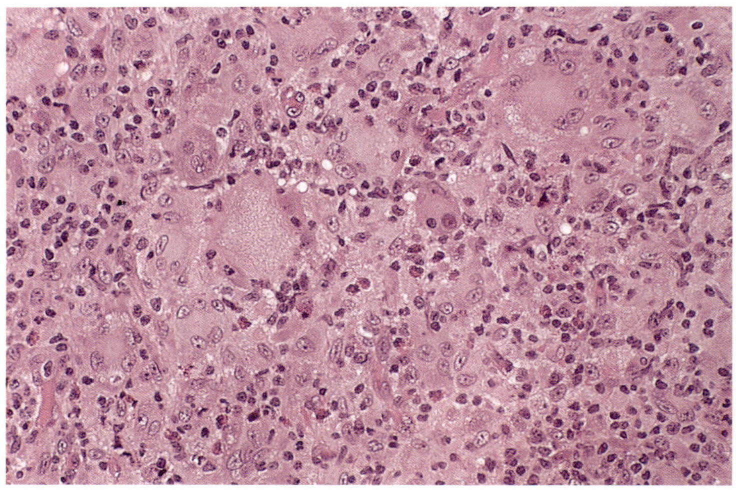

B

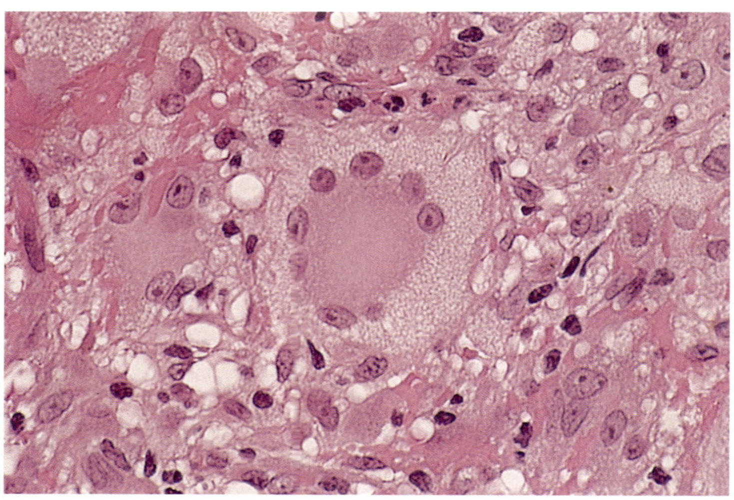

C

Figures 9–3A, 9–3B, 9–3C. Xanthogranuloma. Characteristic foamy, multinucleated histiocytic giant cells. There are eosinophils sprinkled among the histiocytic cells. Touton giant cell with a wreath of nuclei surrounded by lipid-laden cytoplasm.

RETICULOHISTIOCYTOMA

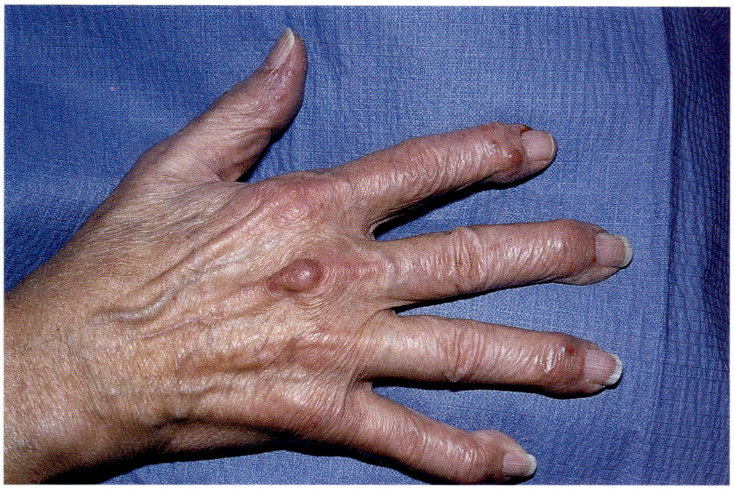

A

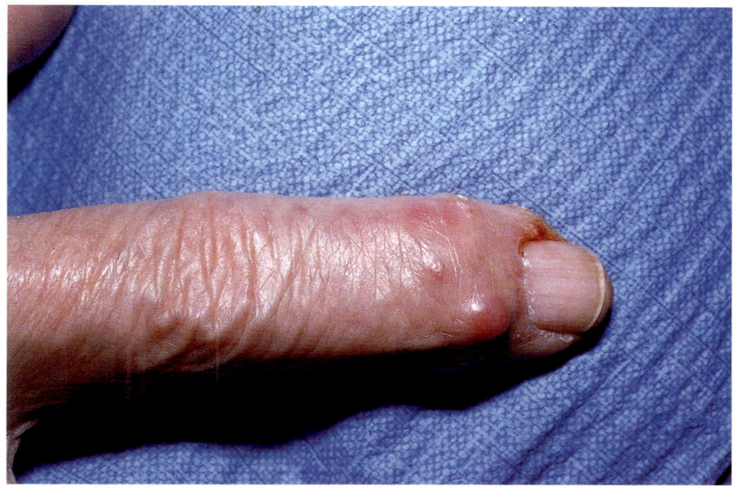

B

Figures 9–4A, 9–4B. Reticulohistiocytoma. Erythematous papules and nodules on the dorsum of hand and fingers, typically over the knuckle and interphalangeal joints.

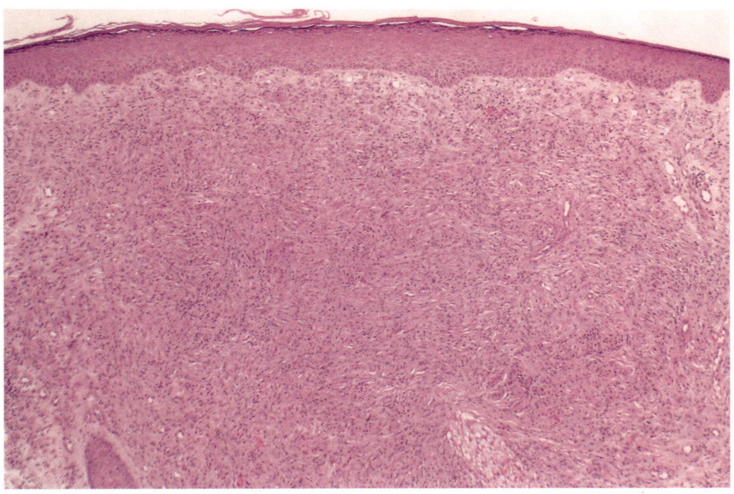

A

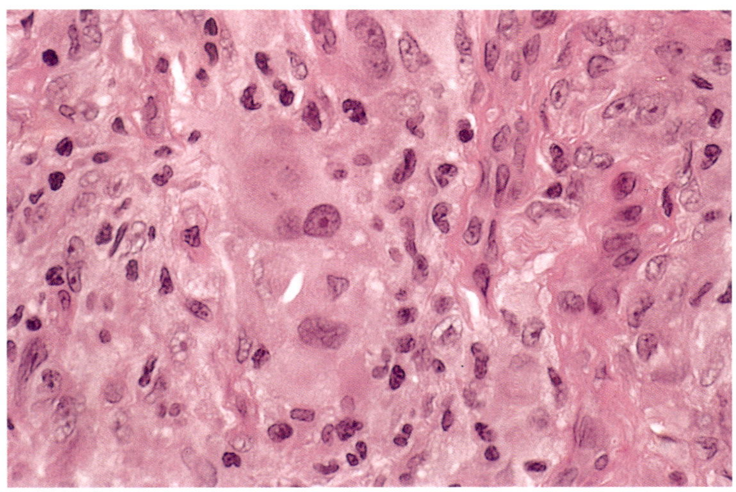

B

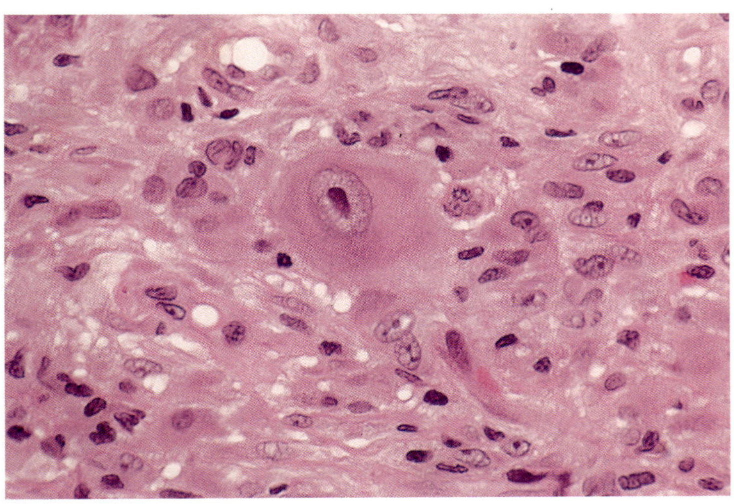

C

Figures 9–5A, 9–5B, 9–5C. Reticulohistiocytoma. Diffuse infiltrate of multinucleated histiocytic giant cells with characteristic ground-glass cytoplasms.

SELF-HEALING RETICULOHISTIOCYTOSIS

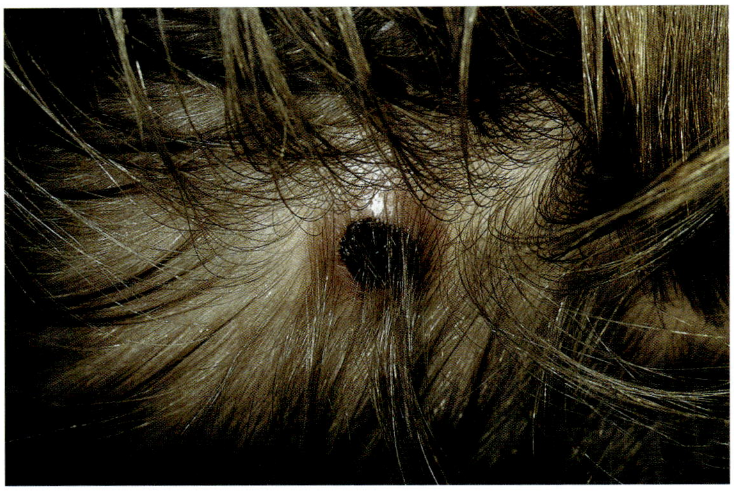

Figure 9–6. Self-healing reticulohistiocytosis. Scalp nodule with central ulceration in a three-year-old boy.

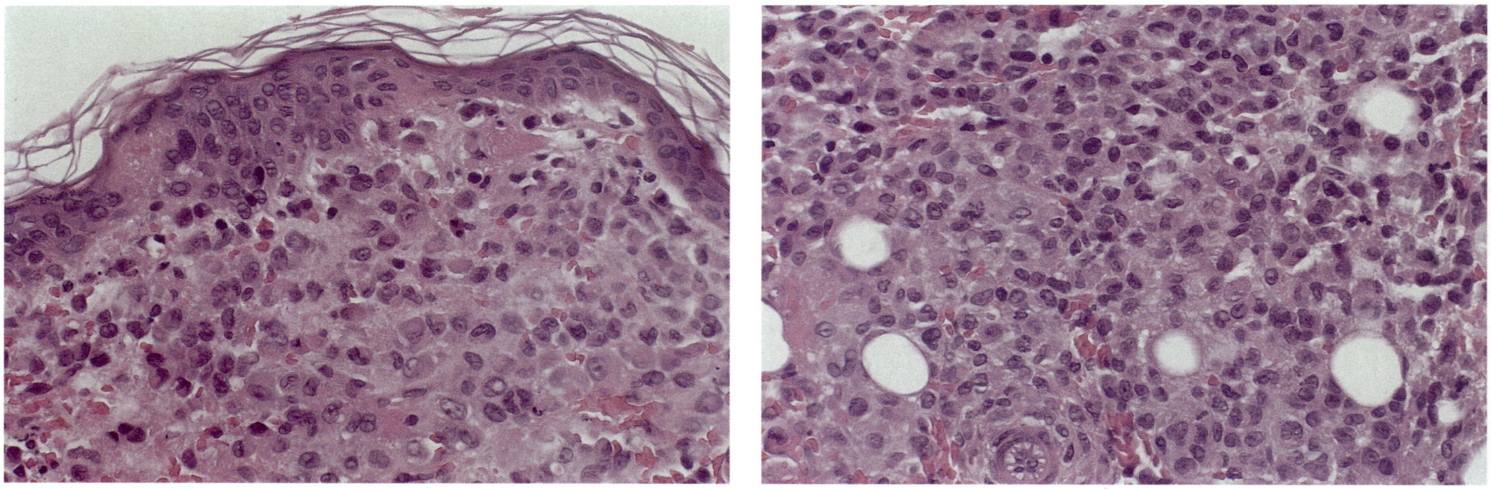

A B

Figures 9–7A, 9–7B. Self-healing reticulohistiocytosis. Histiocytic cells with large nuclei and amphophilic cytoplasm.

XANTHOMA

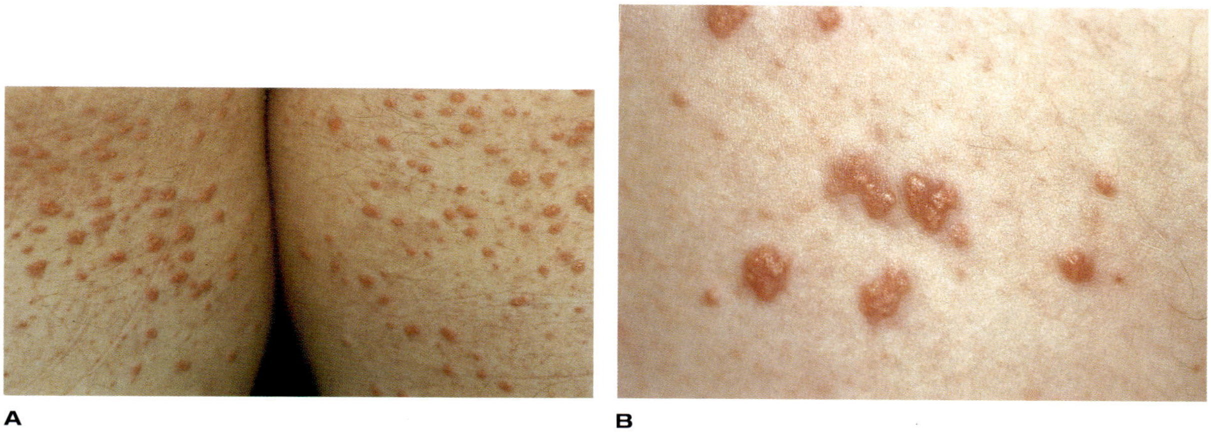

Figures 9–8A, 9–8B. **Xanthoma, eruptive type.** Reddish-yellow papules on the thighs of a woman with hyperlipidemia.

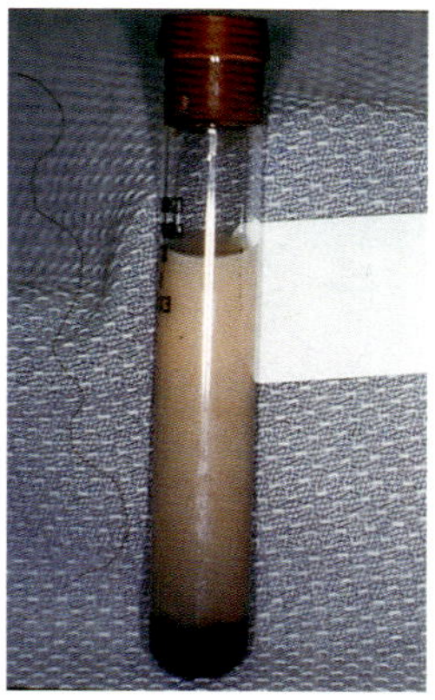

Figure 9–9. **Xanthoma, eruptive type.** Milky-colored serum taken from the hyperlipemic woman shown in Figures 9–8A and 9–8B.

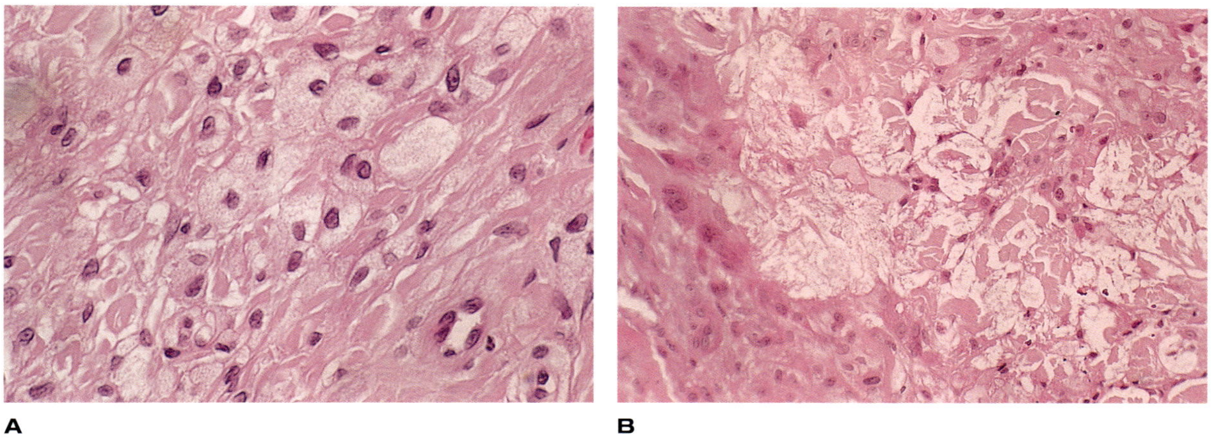

Figures 9–10A, 9–10B. **Xanthoma, eruptive type.** Histocytic cells with abundant foamy cytoplasm. There are extracellular deposits of lipid lying free in the dermis, which is characteristic of eruptive xanthoma, and a mixed-cell infiltrate.

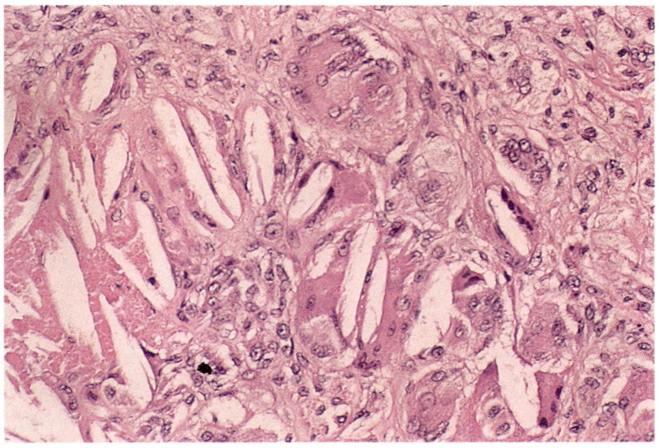

Figure 9–11. **Xanthoma, tuberous type.** Single and multinucleated histiocytic cells with abundant foamy cytoplasm. There are cholesterol clefts and a mixed-cell infiltrate in the dermis.

LANGERHANS CELL HISTIOCYTOSIS

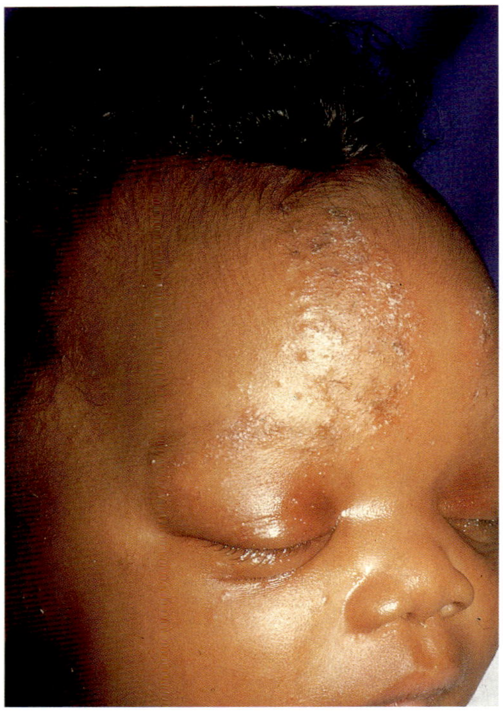

A

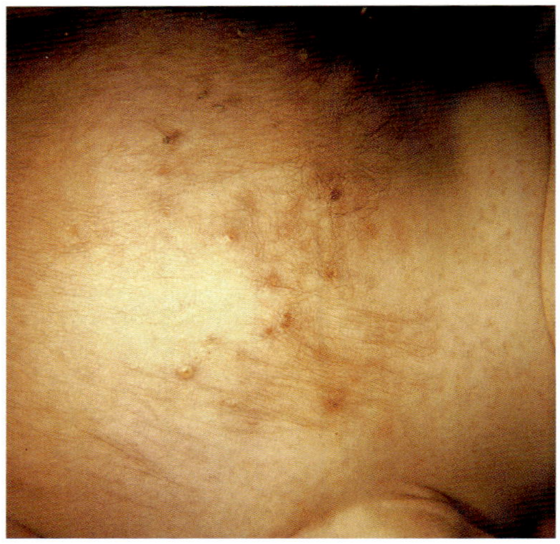

B

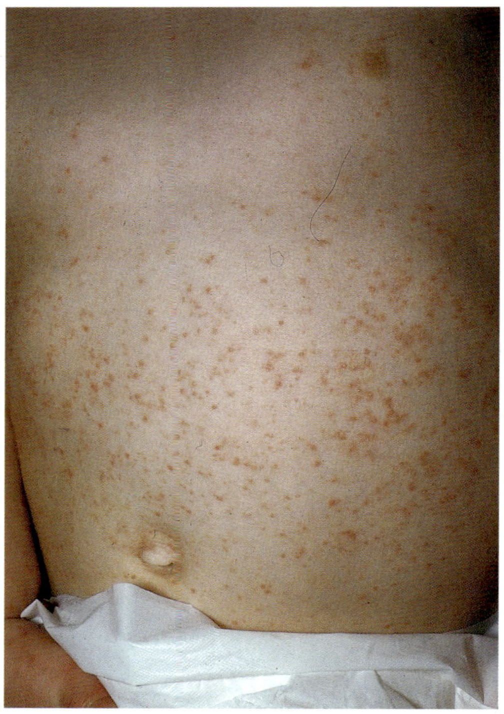

C

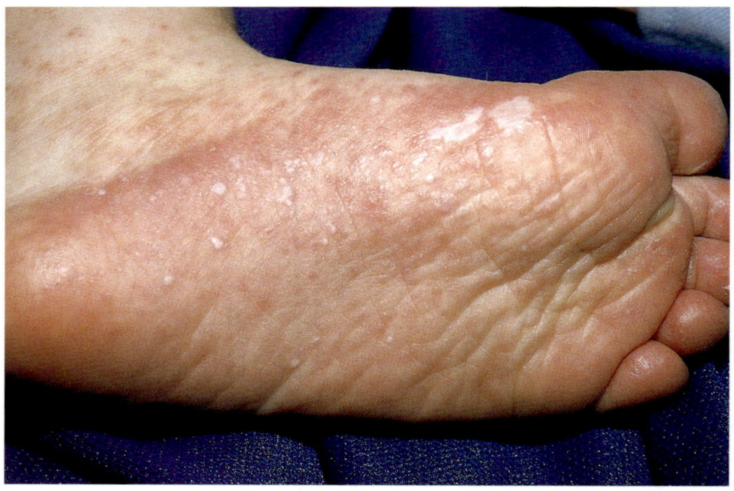

D

Figures 9–12A, 9–12B, 9–12C, 9–12D. Langerhans cell histiocytosis. Characteristic erythematous crusted papules on the face, scalp, trunk, and foot.

LANGERHANS CELL HISTIOCYTOSIS

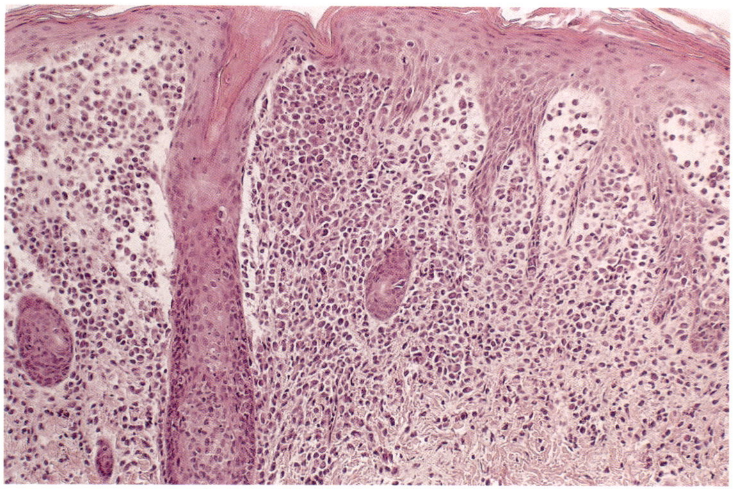

Figure 9–13. Langerhans cell histiocytosis. Diffuse dermal infiltrate of atypical mononuclear cells with cerebriform nuclei and eosinophilic cytoplasm, focally involving the epidermis.

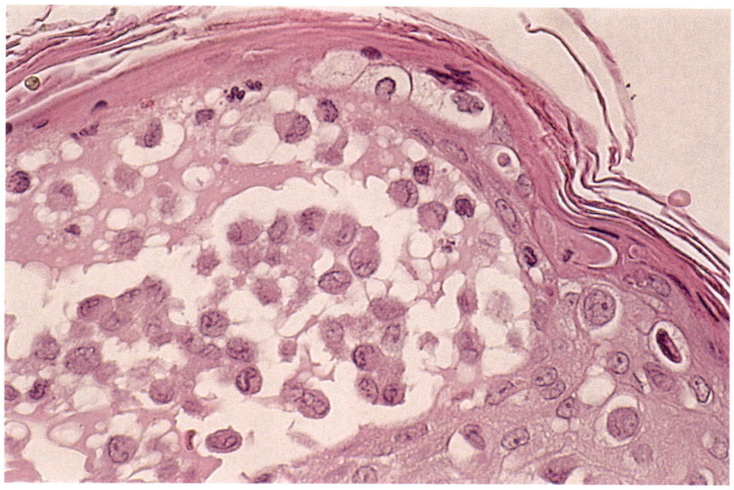

Figure 9–14. Langerhans cell histiocytosis. Atypical mononuclear cells with cerebrifrom nuclei and eosinophilic cytoplasm f lling the edematous papillary dermis and involving the spinous and granular layers of the epidermis.

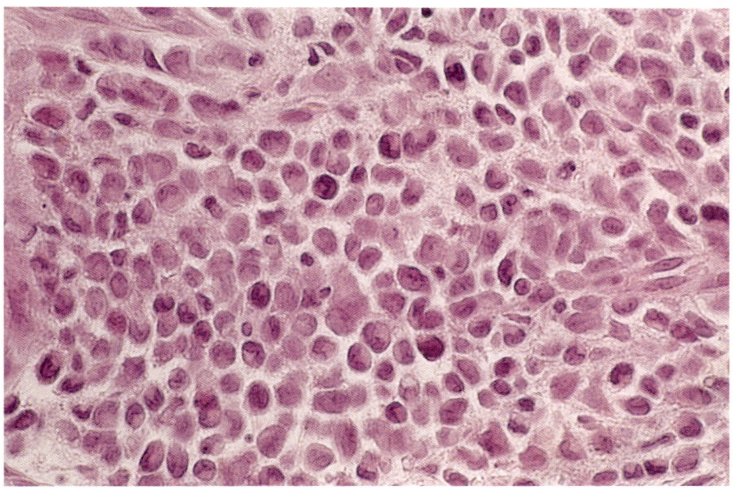

Figure 9–15. Langerhans cell histiocytosis. Sheet of atypical mononuclear cells with characteristic cerebriform nuclei and eosinophilic cytoplasm in the dermis.

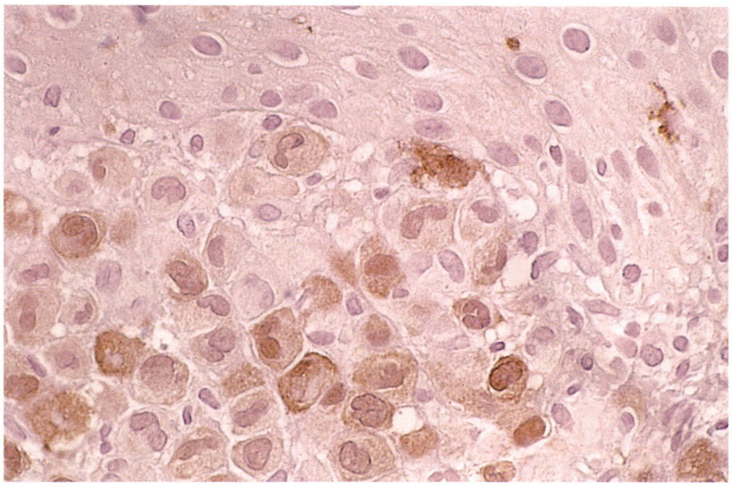

Figure 9–16. Langerhans cell histiocytosis. S-100 mmunoperoxidase staining of histiocytic cells in the epidermis and dermis.

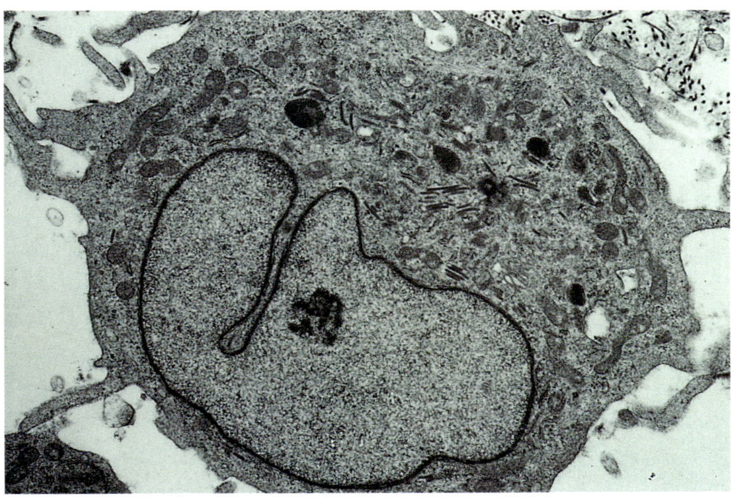

Figure 9–17. Langerhans cell histiocytosis. Electron-micrograph of a Langerhans cell with typical cytoplasmic Langerhans granules.

MALIGNANT H STIOCYTOSIS

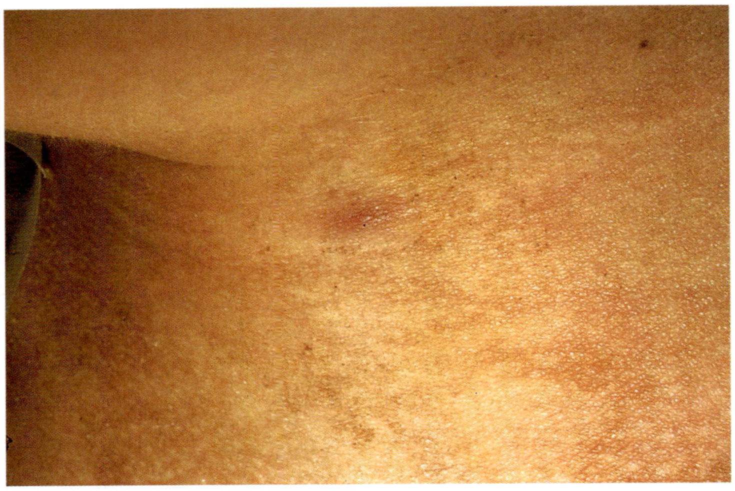

Figure 9–18. Malignant histiocytosis. Erythematous papule.

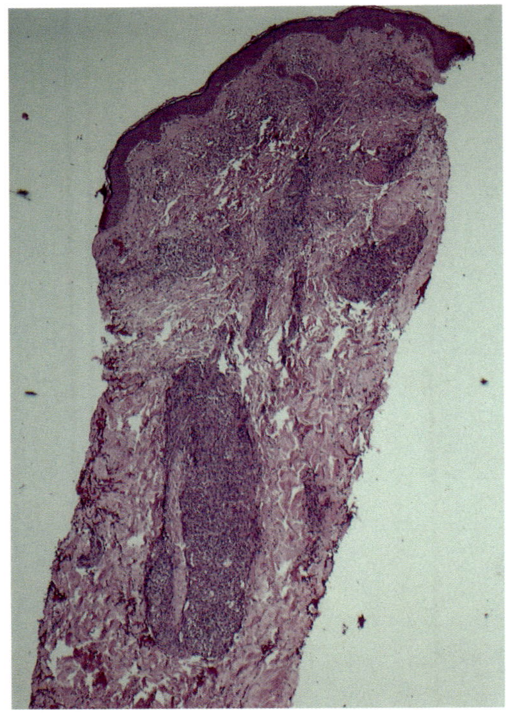

Figure 9–19. Malignant histiocytosis. Dense superficial and deep nodular infiltrate.

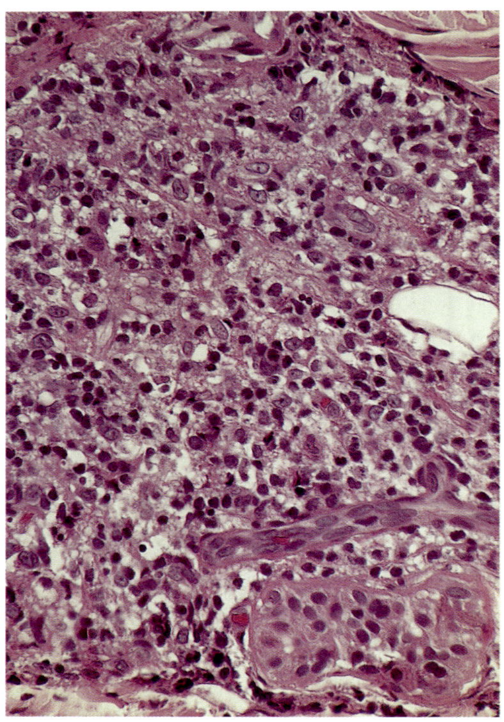

Figure 9–20. Malignant histiocytosis. Diffuse infiltrate of atypical mononuclear cells with pleomorphic, hyperchromatic, and vesicular nuclei and abundant, pale eosinophilic cytoplasm. Mitotic figures, karyorrhexis, and cytophagia are present.

10

PANNICULITIS

- Erythema nodosum
- Lupus erythematosus panniculitis (lupus profundus)
- Pancreatic panniculitis
- Subcutaneous fat necrosis
- Cytophagic histiocytic panniculitis
- Alpha 1-antitrypsin deficiency panniculitis
- Sclerosing panniculitis

ERYTHEMA NODOSUM

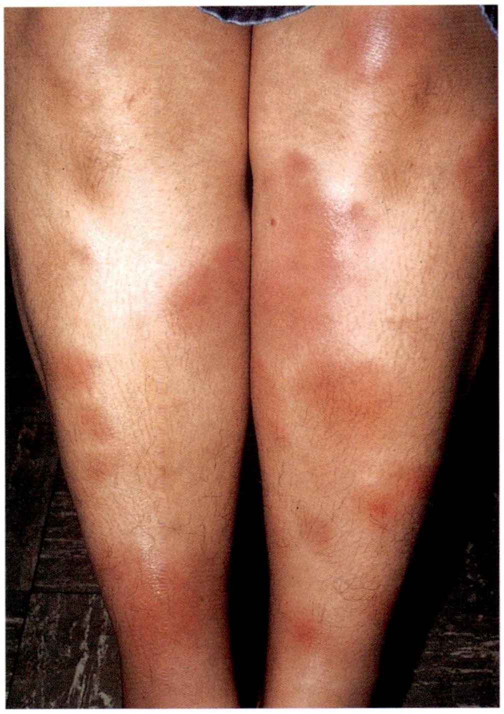

A

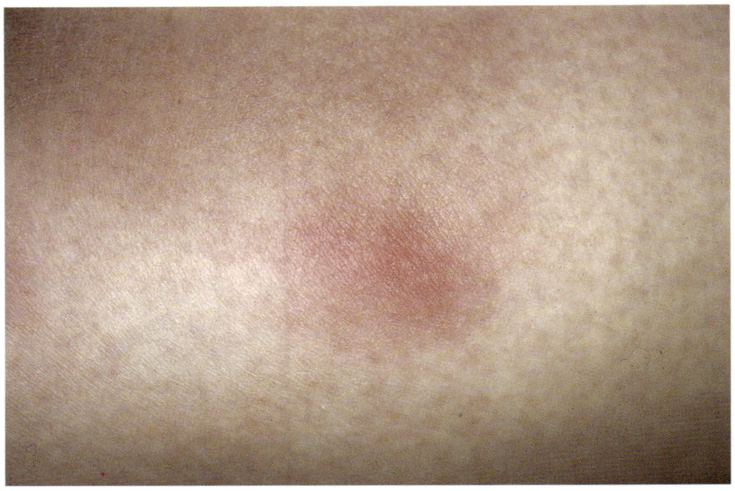

B

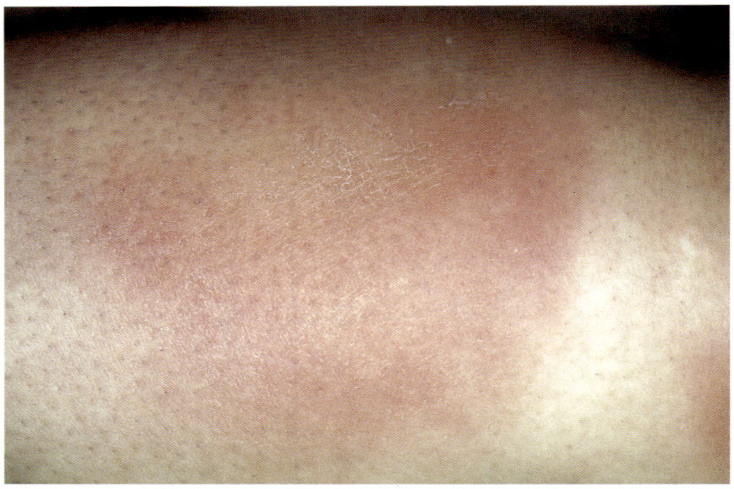

C

Figures 10–1A, 10–1B, 10–1C. **Erythema nodosum, evolving.** Painful, erythematous, indurated plaques and nodules on the lower legs of a woman.

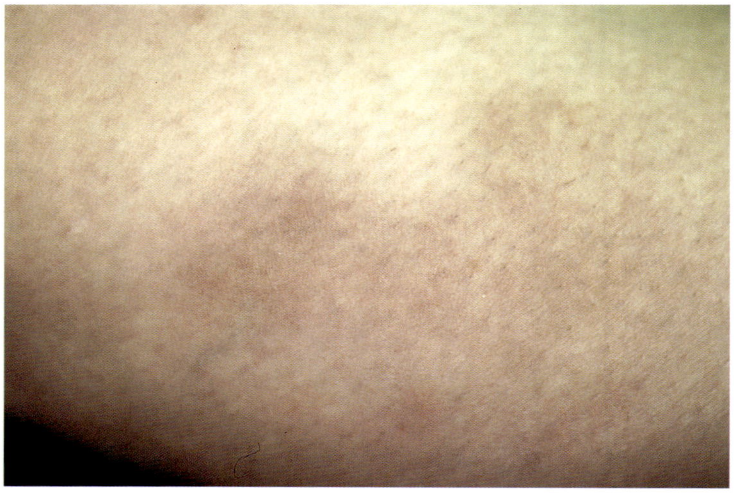

Figure 10–2. **Erythema nodosum, resolving.** Nonpainful, bluish-gray patches on the lower leg; this is known as erythema contusiformis.

ERYTHEMA NODOSUM

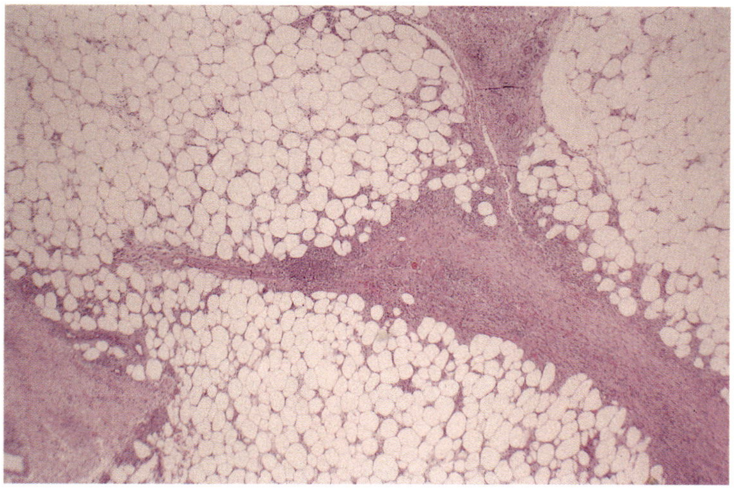

A

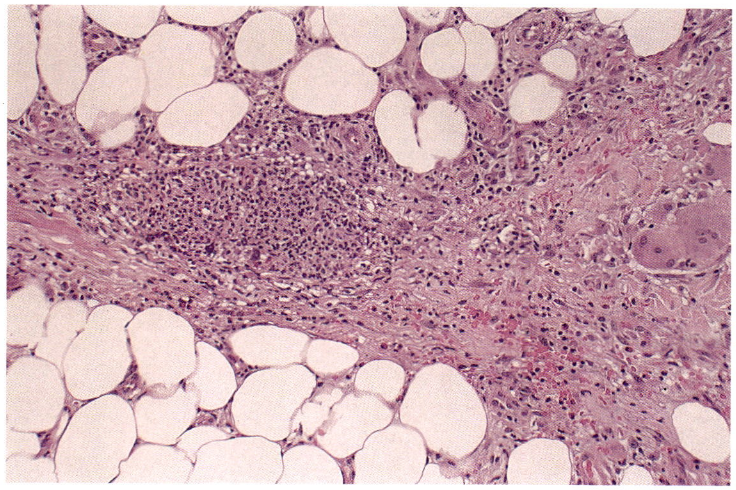

B

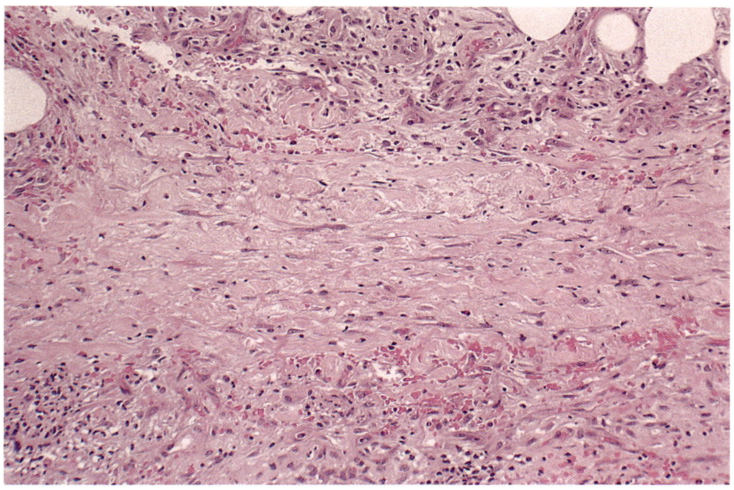

C

Figures 10–3A, 10–3B, 10–3C. Erythema nodosum. Thickened fibrous septum in the subcutaneous fat. There are fibrocytes, coarse collagen bundles, zones of neutrophils, and lymphohistiocytic cells.

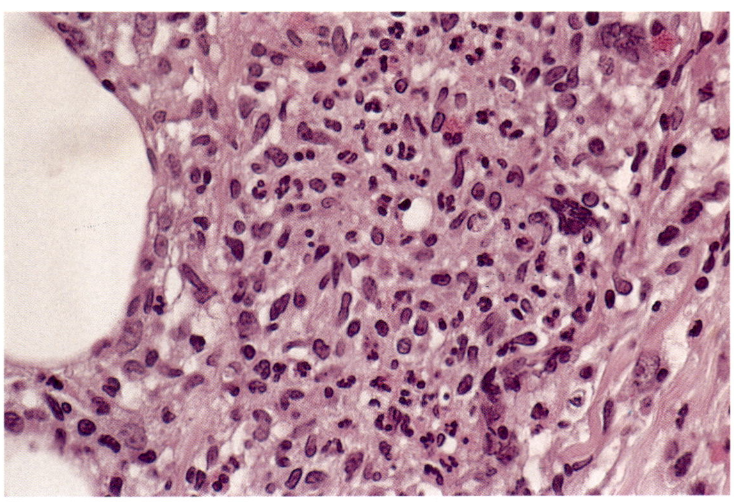

A

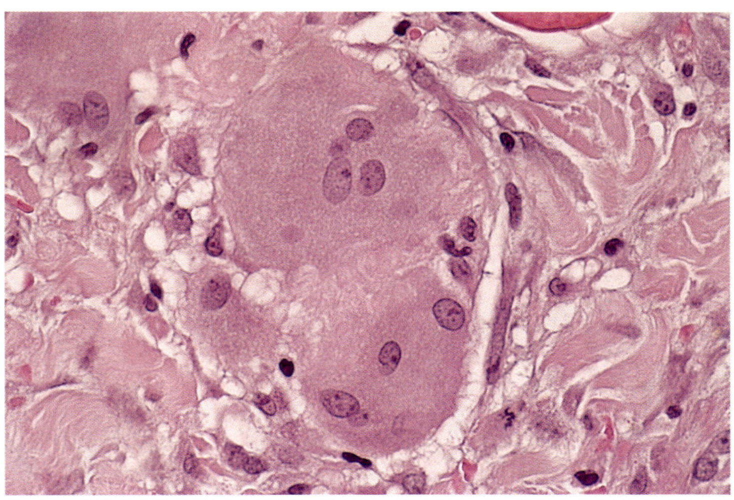

B

Figures 10–4A, 10–4B. Erythema nodosum. Thickened fibrous septum that is packed with a mixed-cell infiltrate containing sheets of neutrophils with lymphocytes and multinucleated histiocytic giant cells.

LUPUS ERYTHEMATOSUS PANNICULITIS (LUPUS PROFUNDUS)

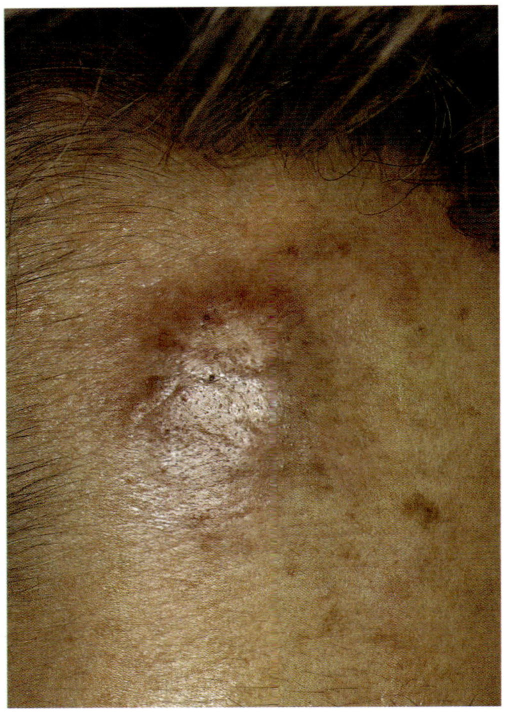

Figure 10–5. Lupus erythematosus panniculitis. Nontender erythematous nodule on the forehead.

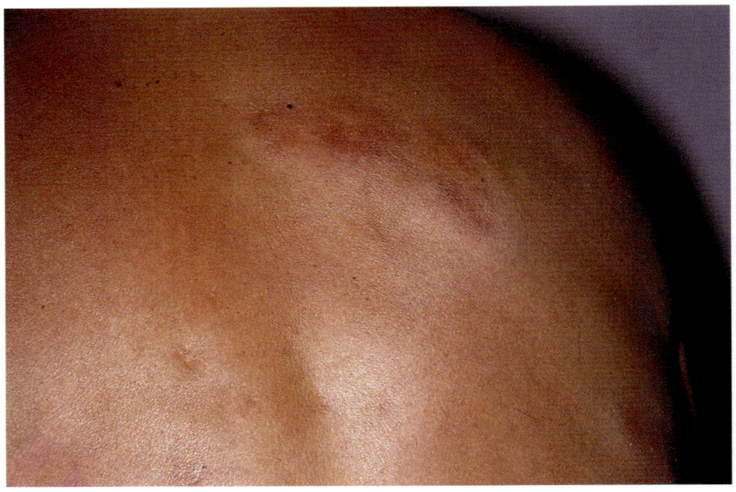

Figure 10–6. Lupus erythematosus panniculitis. Nontender erythematous plaques on the back.

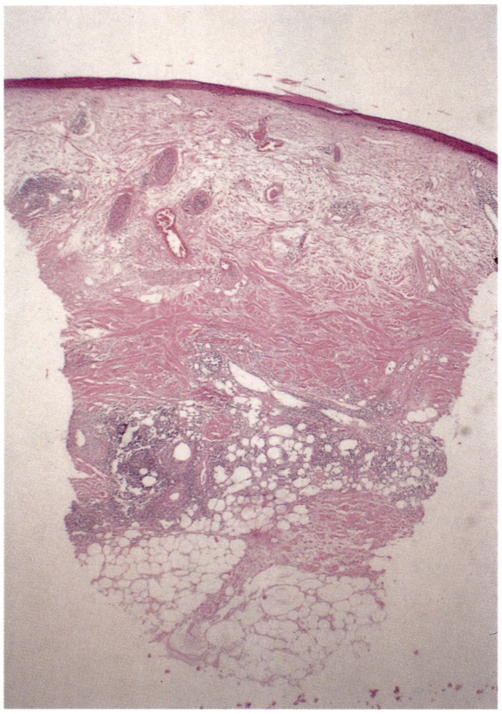

Figure 10–7. Lupus erythematosus panniculitis. Superficial and deep dermatitis and panniculitis.

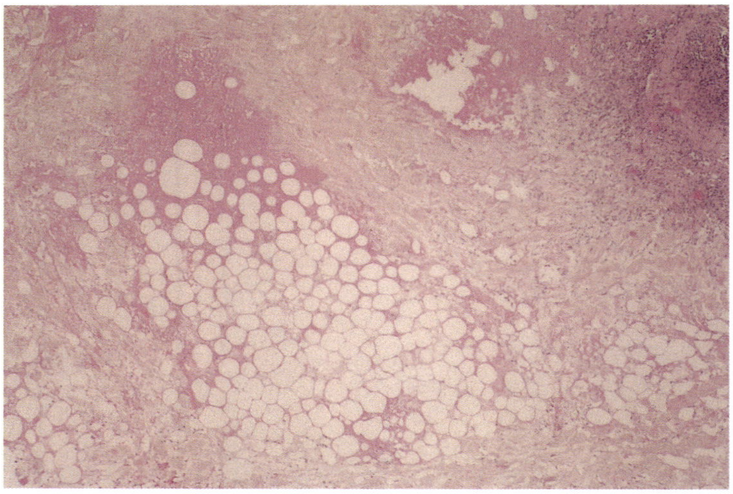

Figure 10–8. Lupus erythematosus panniculitis. Fat necrosis, sclerosis, and mucin deposition. There is a lymphoplasmacytic infiltrate, fat pseudocysts, and eosinophilic hyalinized sclerotic fat.

LUPUS ERYTHEMATOSUS PANNICULITIS (LUPUS PROFUNDUS)

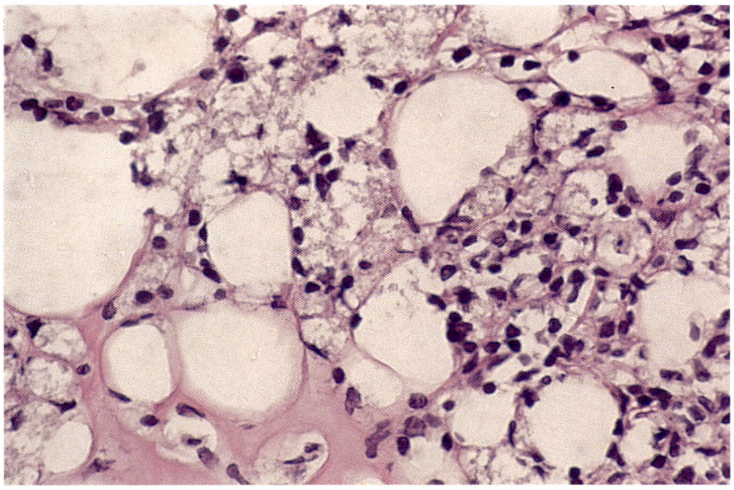

A

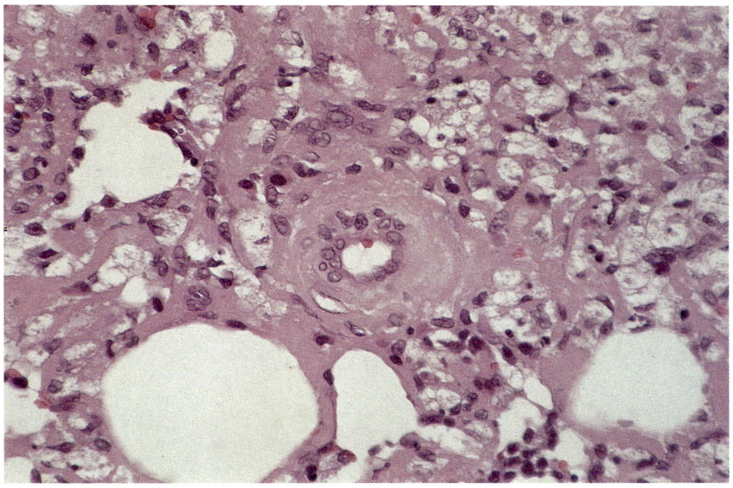

B

Figures 10–9A, 10–9B. Lupus erythematosus panniculitis. Fat necrosis and a lymphoplasmacytic infiltrate. There is eosinophilic hyalinized sclerotic fat and a blood vessel with a thickened hyalinized wall.

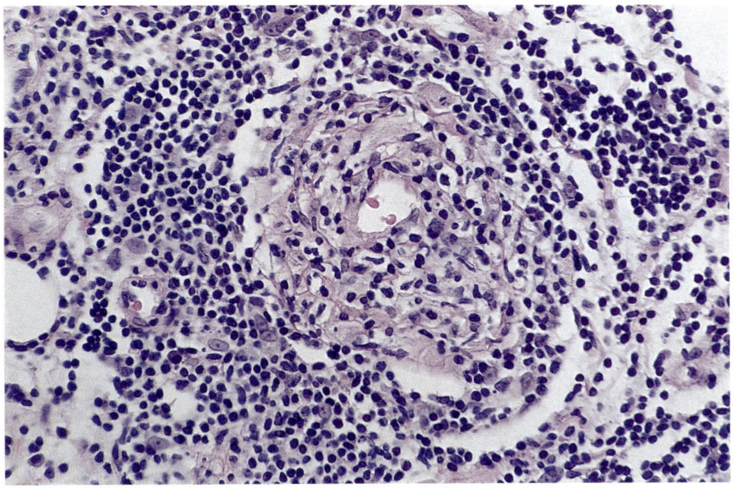

Figure 10–10. Lupus erythematosus panniculitis. Dense perivascular infiltrate of lymphocytes and plasma cells at the junction of the dermis and subcutis.

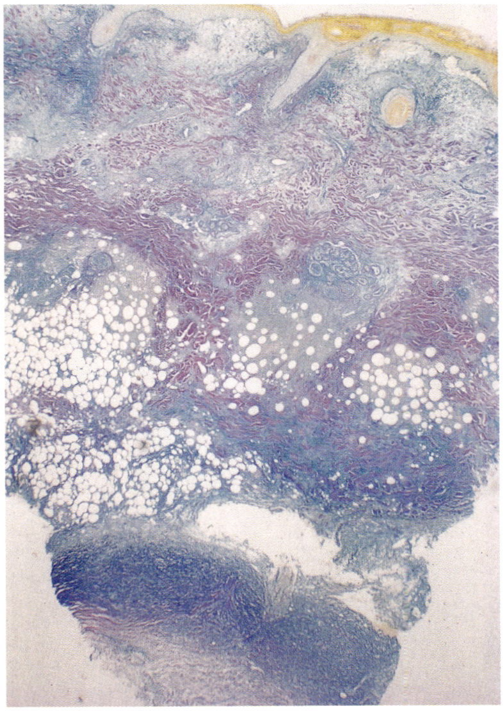

Figure 10–11. Lupus erythematosus panniculitis. Colloidal iron stain shows the blue mucin in the dermis and subcutaneous tissue.

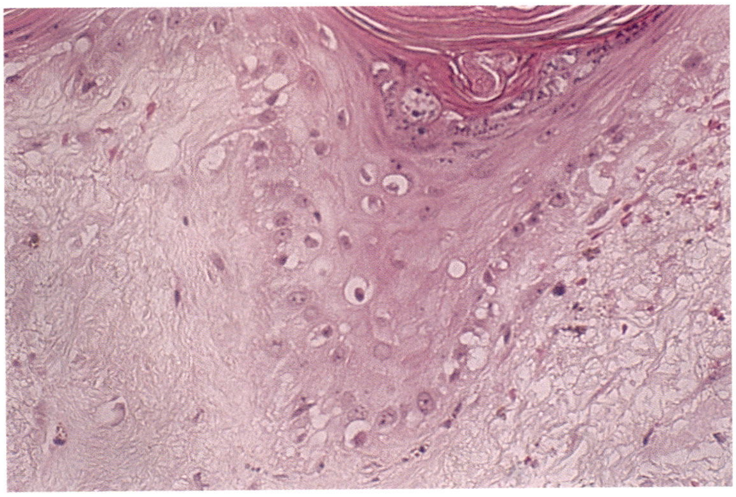

Figure 10–12. Lupus erythematosus panniculitis. Vacuolar alteration of the epidermis and adnexa. These characteristic epithelial changes of discoid lupus erythematosus may or may not be present.

PANCREATIC PANNICULITIS

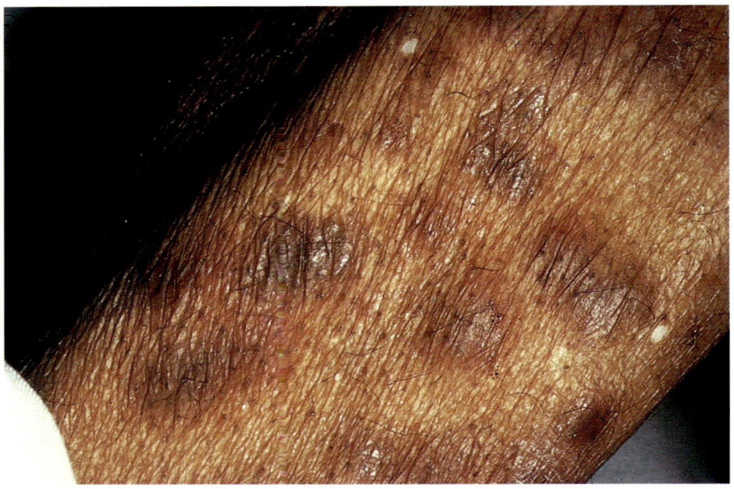

Figure 10–13. Pancreatic panniculitis. Tender reddish-purple nodules on an extremity.

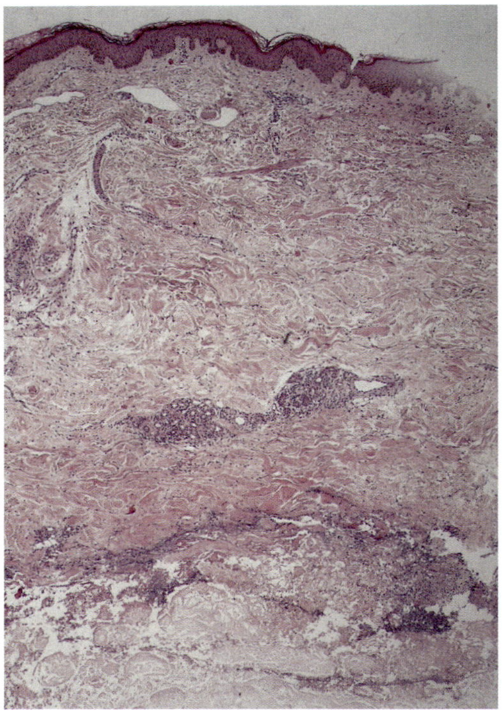

Figure 10–14. Pancreatic panniculitis. Lobular panniculitis and fat necrosis.

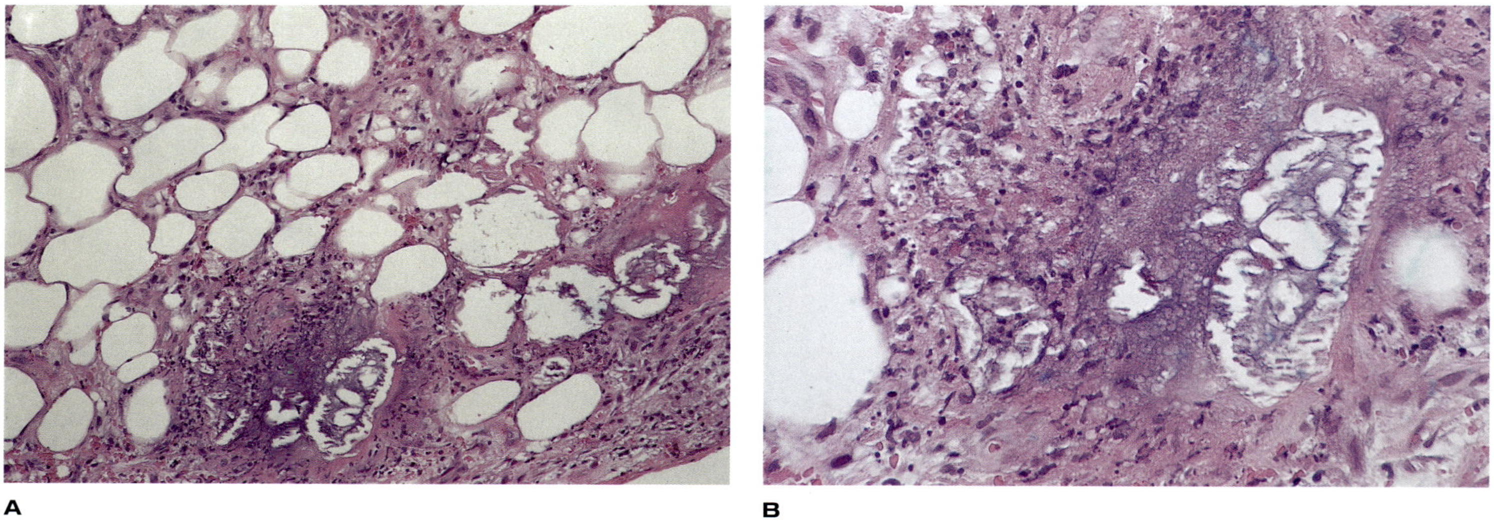

Figures 10–15A, 10–15B. Pancreatic panniculitis. Fat necrosis and calcification. There is a suppurative granulomatous infiltrate consisting of neutrophils, nuclear fragments, and histiocytic cells surrounding deposits of granular basophilic necrotic lipocytes and calcium. Additional signs of fat necrosis are present, which include foam cells and membranous fat necrosis.

SUBCUTANEOUS FAT NECROSIS

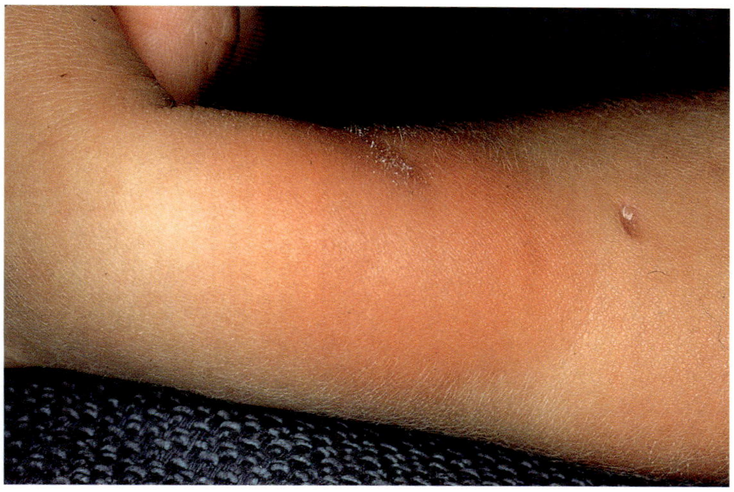

Figure 10–16. Subcutaneous fat necrosis. Erythematous plaque on lower leg of an infant.

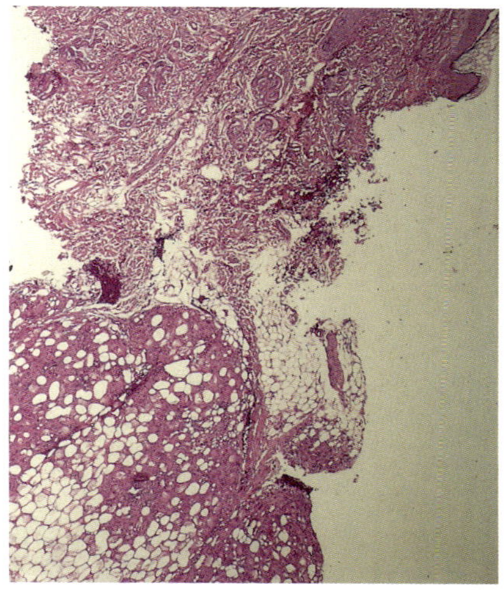

Figure 10–17. Subcutaneous fat necrosis. Granulomatous lobular panniculitis.

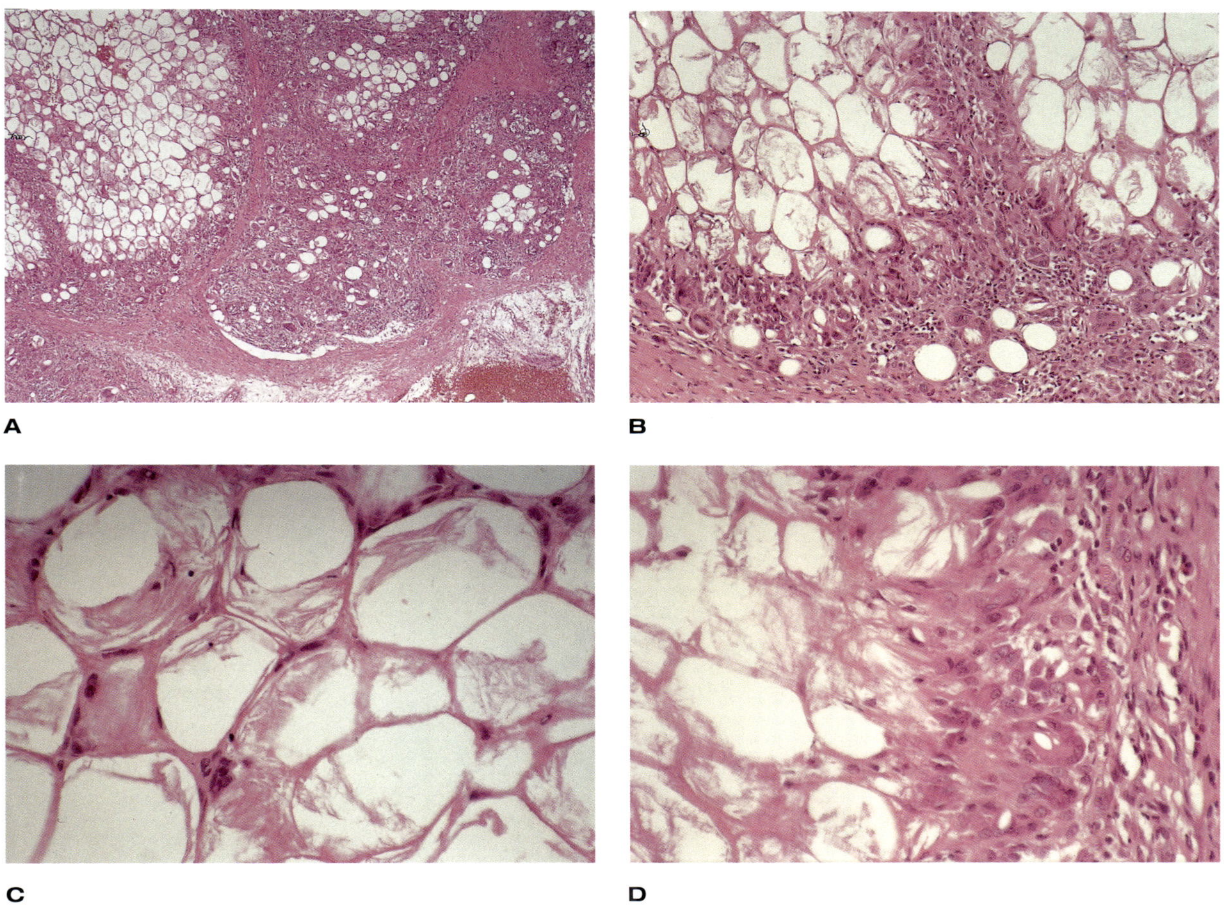

Figures 10–18A, 10–18B, 10–18C, 10–18D. Subcutaneous fat necrosis. Patchy, dense granulomatous infiltrate and fat necrosis. Feathery needle-shaped clefts are present within lipocytes and multinucleated histiocytic giant cells.

CYTOPHAGIC HISTIOCYTIC PANNICULITIS

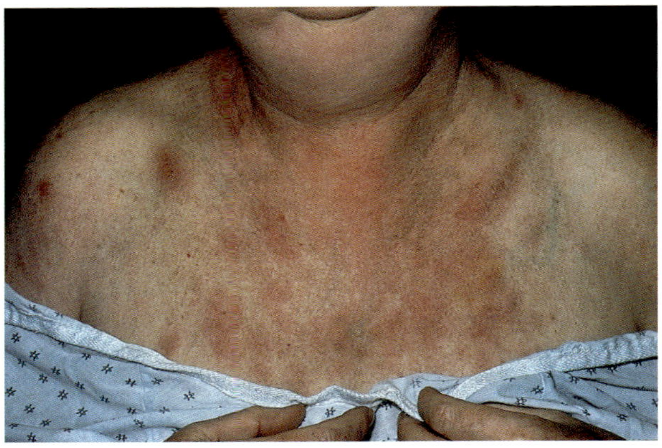

Figure 10–19. Cytophagic histiocytic panniculitis. Erythematous nodules and plaques on the chest, neck, and shoulder.

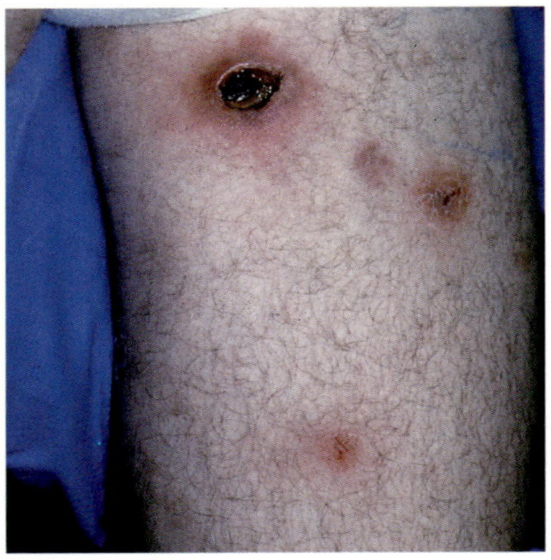

Figure 10–20. Cytophagic histiocytic panniculitis. Erythematous nodules, some with ulceration on the leg.

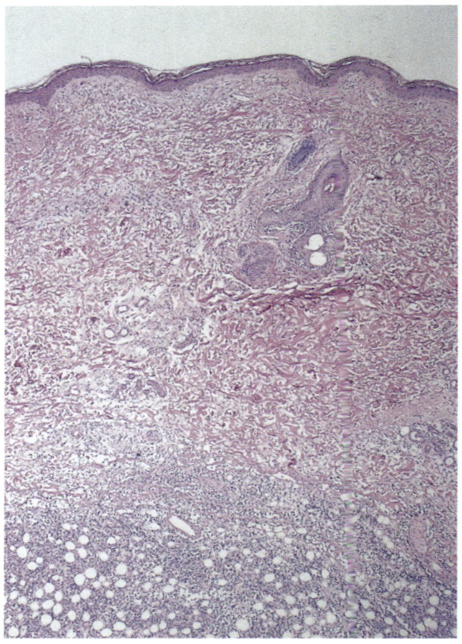

A

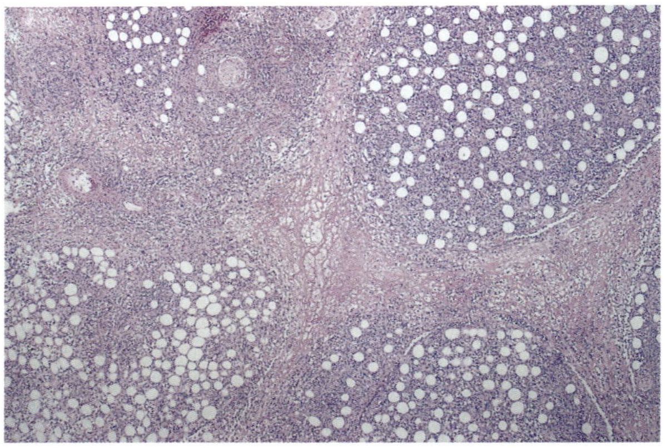

B

Figures 10–21A, 10–21B. Cytophagic histiocytic panniculitis. Diffuse and dense lobular and septal panniculitis.

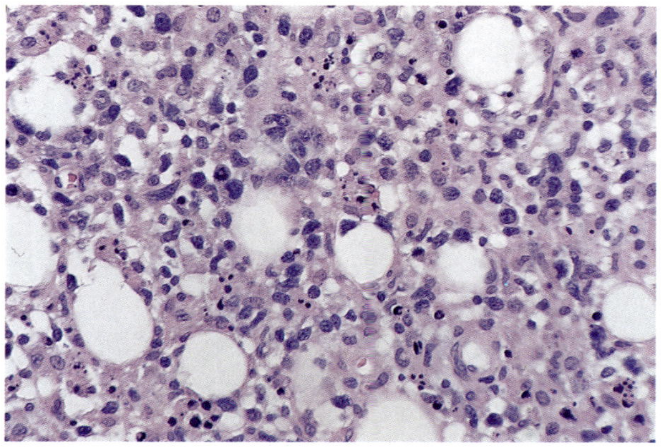

A

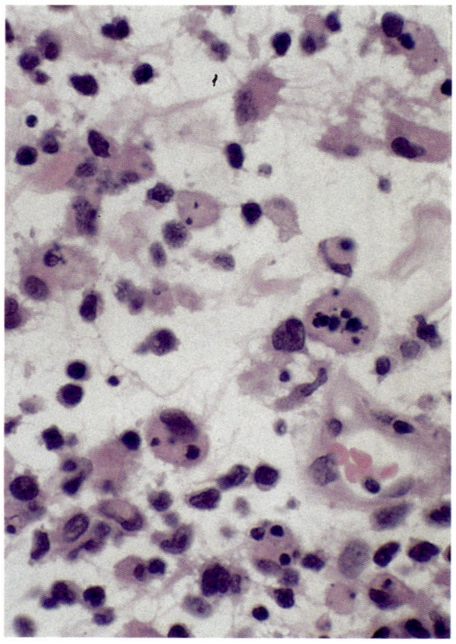

B

Figures 10–22A, 10–22B. Cytophagic histiocytic panniculitis. Atypical mononuclear cells with karyorrhexis. There are hyperchromatic mononuclear cells with pleomorphic nuclei, prominent nucleoli, abundant eosinophilic cytoplasm, mitotic figures, nuclear debris, and characteristic "bean bag" cells (lymphophagocytosis and erythrophagocytosis).

ALPHA 1-ANTITRYPSIN DEFICIENCY PANNICULITIS

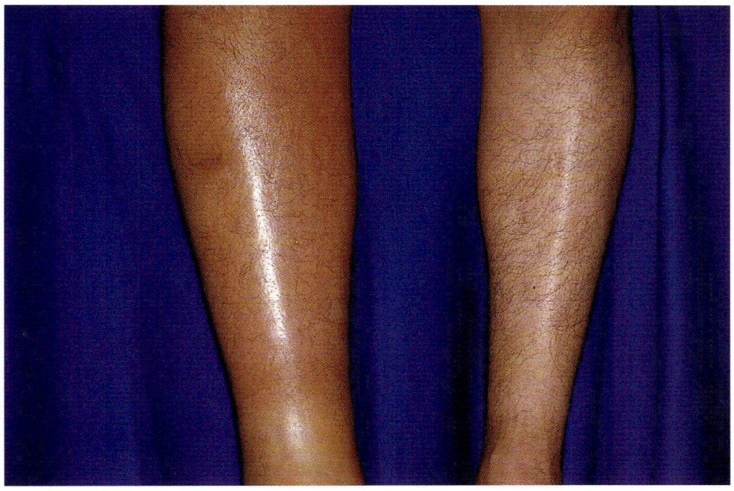

Figure 10–23. Alpha 1-antitrypsin deficiency panniculitis. Angioedema of the lower leg is a commonly associated finding.

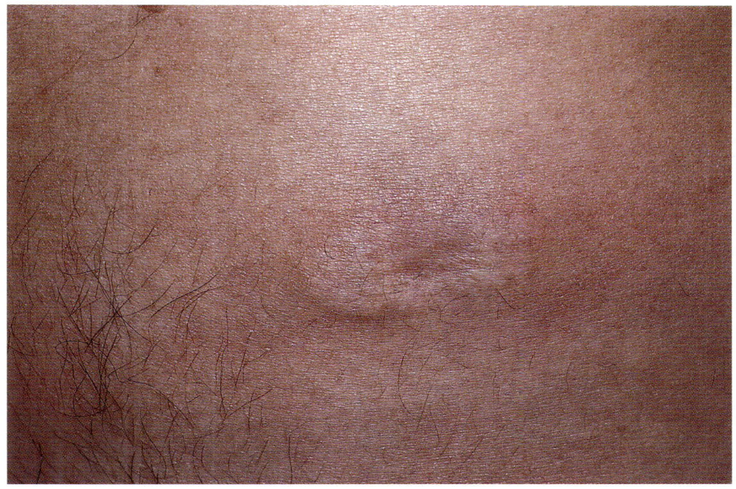

Figure 10–24. Alpha 1-antitrypsin deficiency pann culitis. Painful nodule on the back.

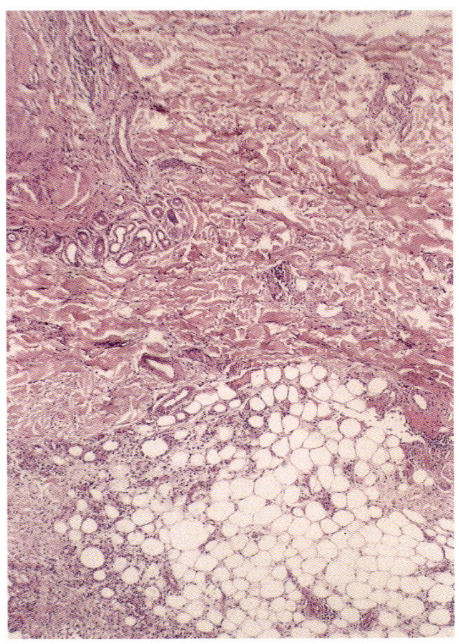

Figure 10–25. Alpha 1-antitrypsin deficiency panniculitis. Dermal and subcutaneous infiltrate with many neutrophils.

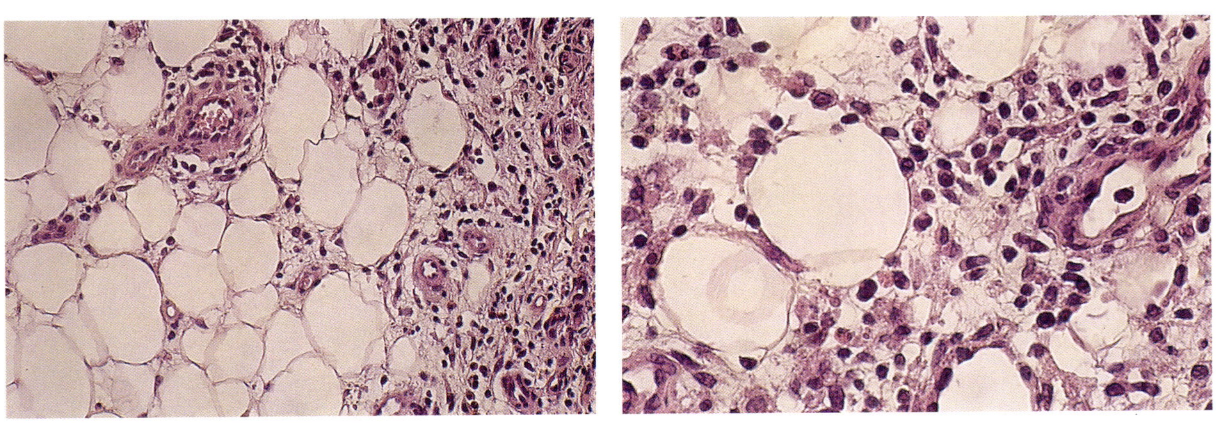

A B

Figures 10–26A, 10–26B. Alpha 1-antitrypsin deficiency panniculitis. Panniculitis with fat necrosis and a mixed-cell infiltrate with neutrophils.

SCLEROSING PANNICULITIS

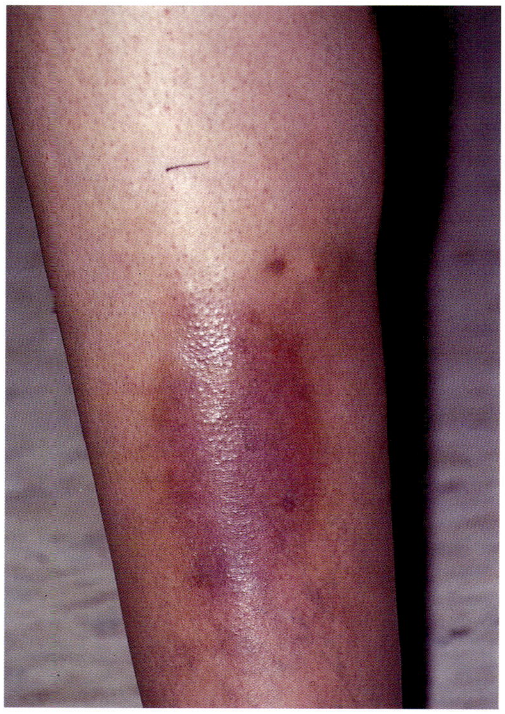

A

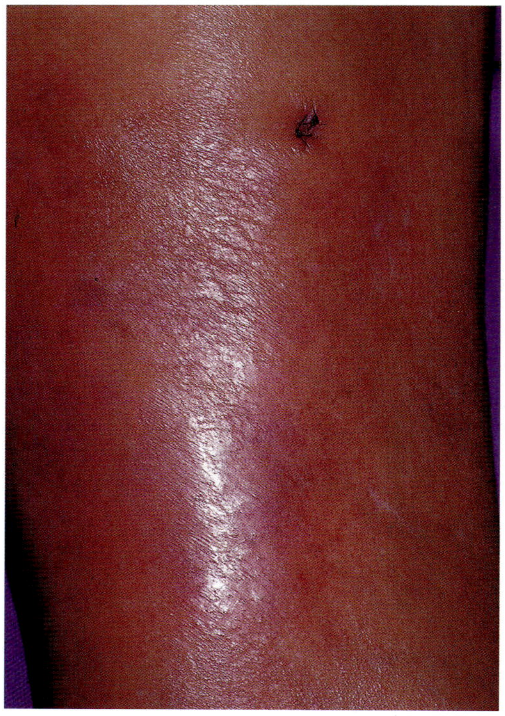

B

Figure 10–27A, 10–27B. Sclerosing panniculitis. Erythematous and violaceous plaques on the lower extremity.

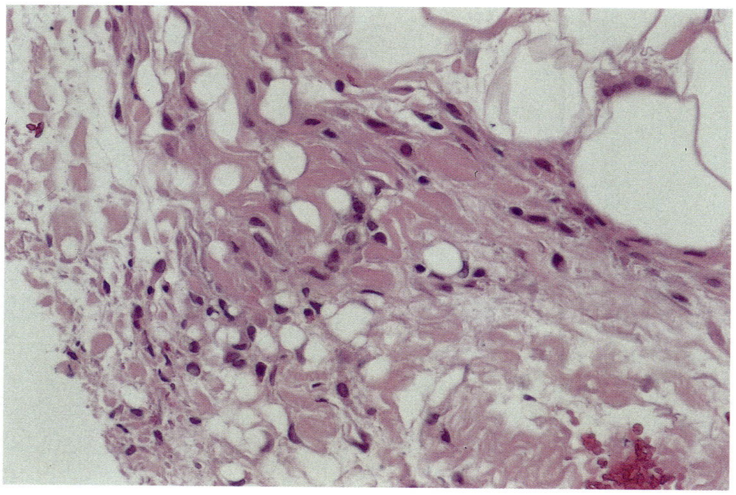

Figure 10–28. Sclerosing panniculitis. Septal fibrosis and inflammation.

11

VIRAL INFECTIONS

- Papular acrodermatitis of childhood (Gianotti-Crosti syndrome)
- Varicella and herpes zoster infections
- Herpes simplex infection
- Cytomegalovirus infection
- Viral exanthem
- Molluscum contagiosum
- Milker's nodule
- Coxsackie exanthem (hand, foot, and mouth disease)
- Verruca vulgaris
- Condyloma acuminatum
- Verruca plana
- Epidermodysplasia verruciformis
- Bowenoid papulosis
- Squamous-cell carcinoma in association with the human papilloma virus (HPV)

PAPULAR ACRODERMATITIS OF CHILDHOOD (GIANOTTI-CROSTI SYNDROME)

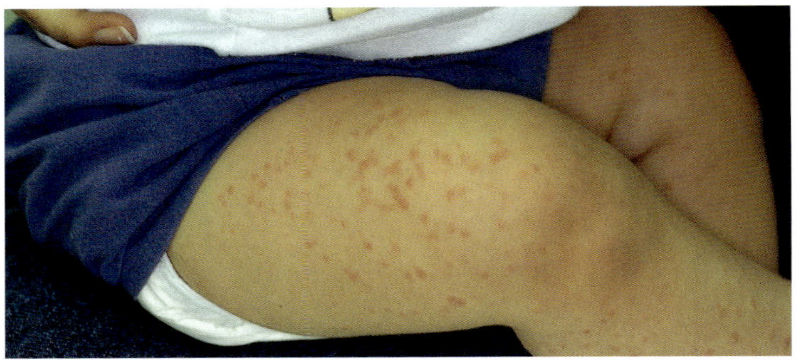

A

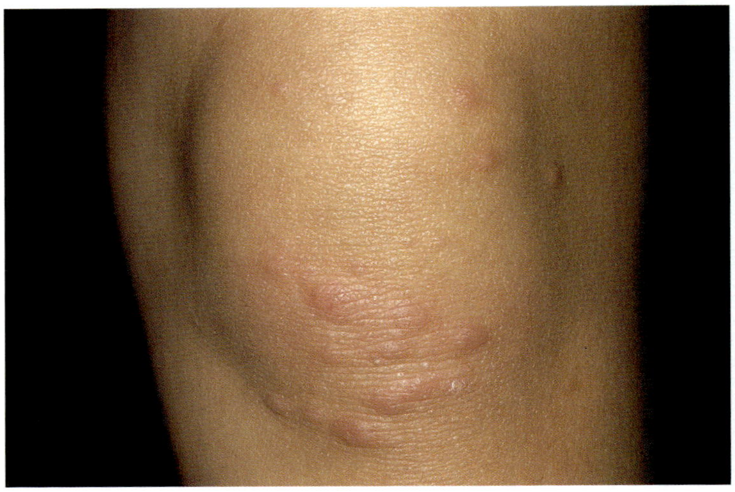

B

Figures 11–1A, 11–1B. Papular acrodermatitis of childhood. Erythematous papules on the lower legs of a child. There are prominent grouped papules on the knee.

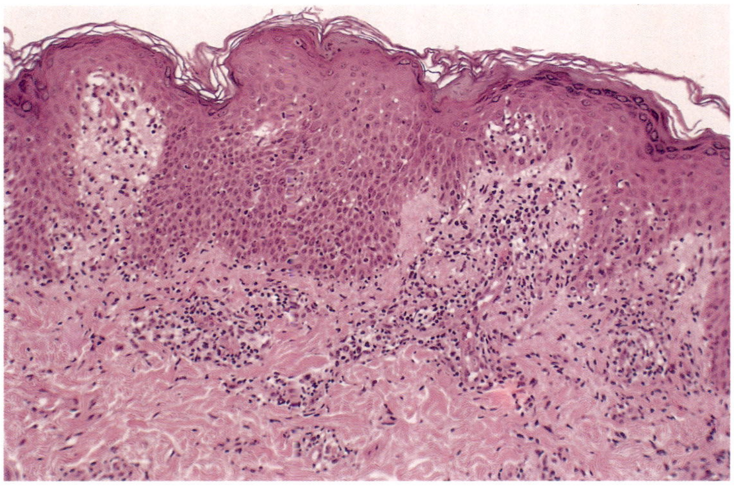

A

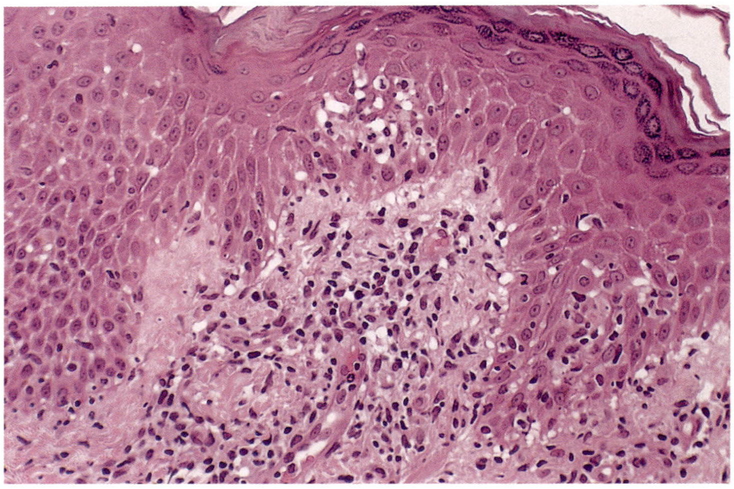

B

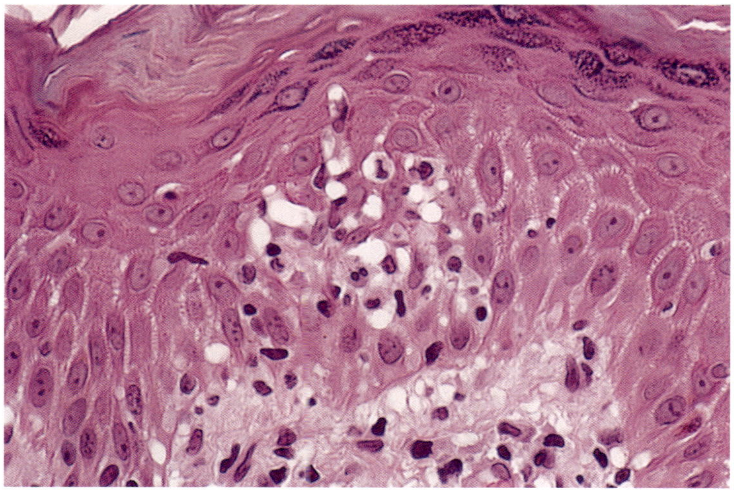

C

Figures 11–2A, 11–2B, 11–2C. Papular acrodermatitis of childhood. Epidermal hyperplasia and spongiosis. There is papillary dermal edema, dilated blood vessels, and a lymphohistiocytic infiltrate, which focally extends into the spongiotic epidermis.

VARICELLA AND HERPES ZOSTER INFECTIONS

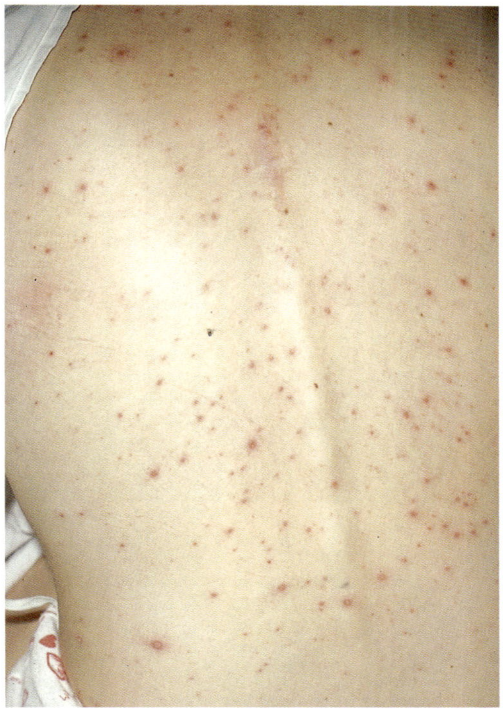

Figure 11–3. Varicella. Crusted vesiculopapules on the back of a child with chickenpox.

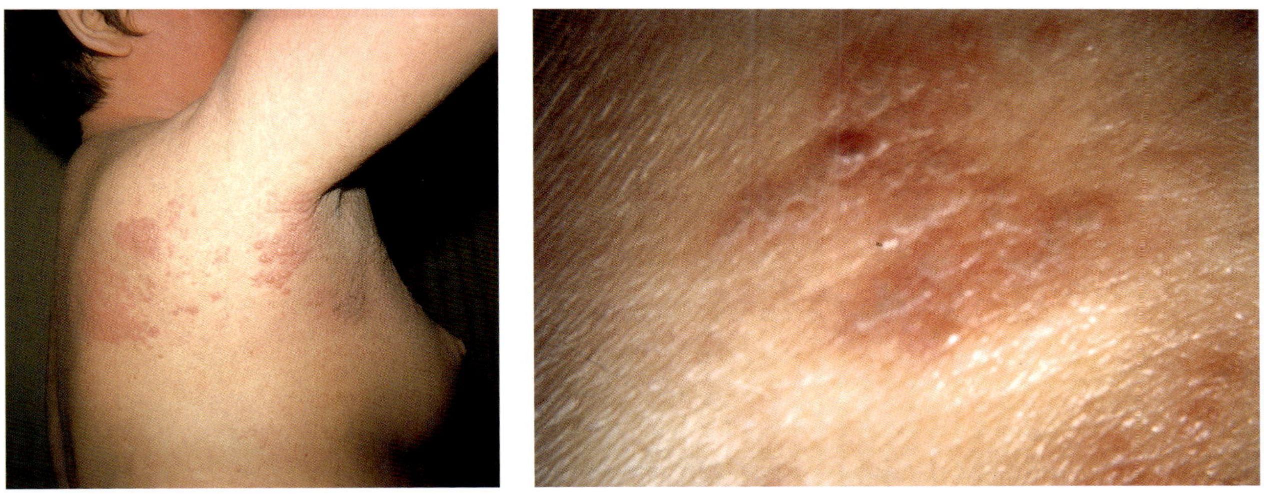

A **B**

Figures 11–4A, 11–4B. Herpes zoster infection, evolving lesions. Grouped vesicles on an erythematous base in a linear, dermatomal pattern involving the back, chest, and breast.

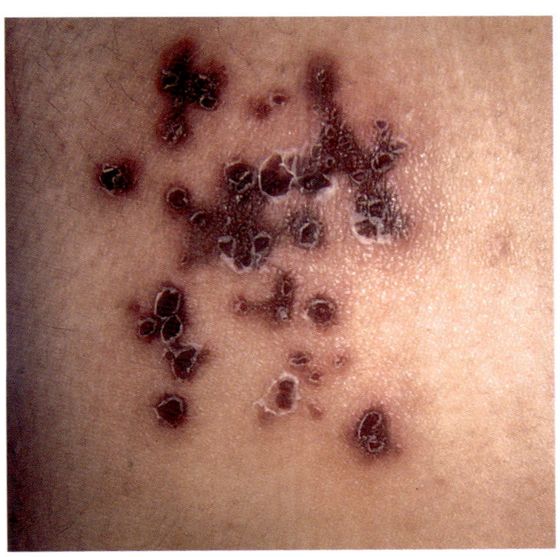

Figure 11–5. Herpes zoster infection, regressing lesions. Crusted papules following treatment on the buttocks of a man with Hodgkin's disease.

VARICELLA AND HERPES ZOSTER INFECTIONS

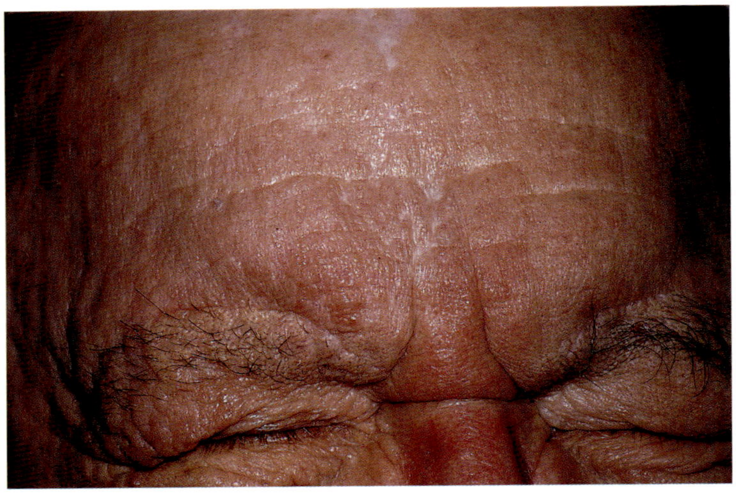

Figure 11–6. Herpes zoster infection. White atrophic scars are present over the forehead and eyebrow in areas of previous infection.

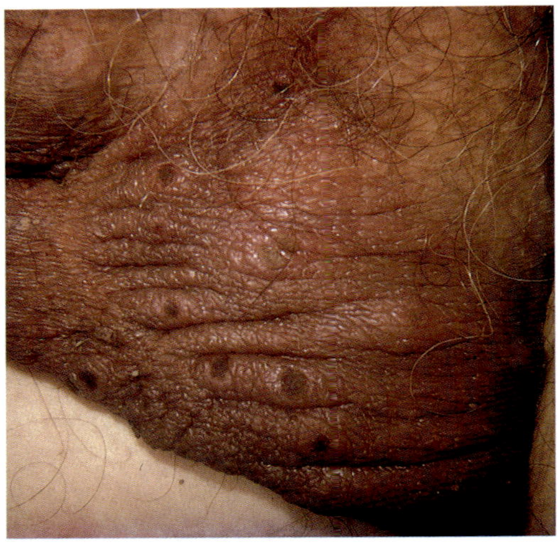

A

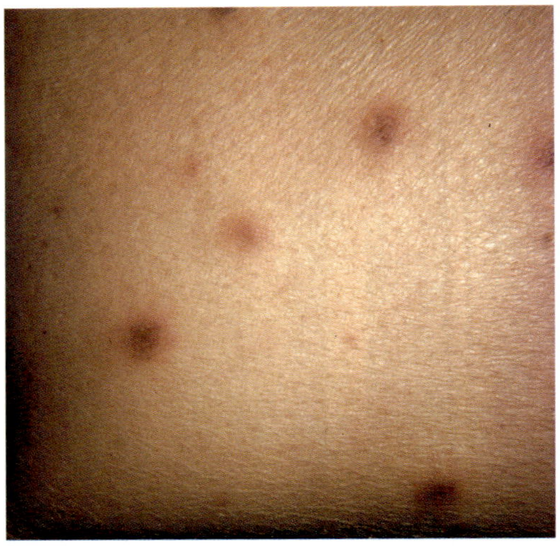

B

Figures 11–7A, 11–7B. Herpes zoster infection. Disseminated herpes zoster infection in an immunocompromised man involving the scrotum and thigh. There are umbilicated, crusted papules.

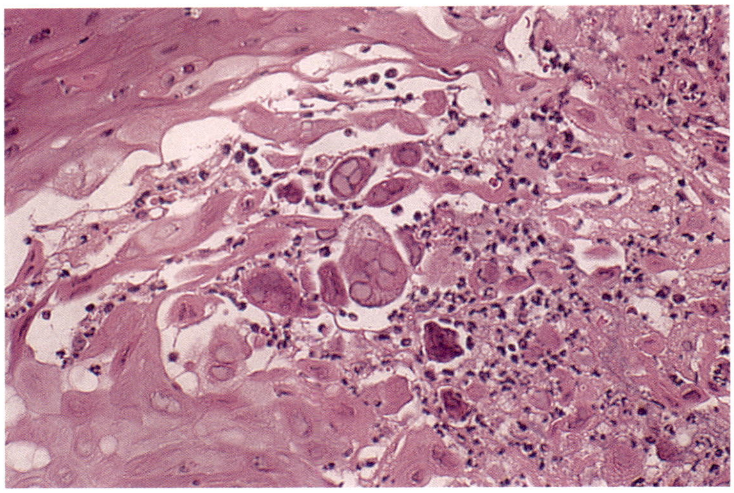

A

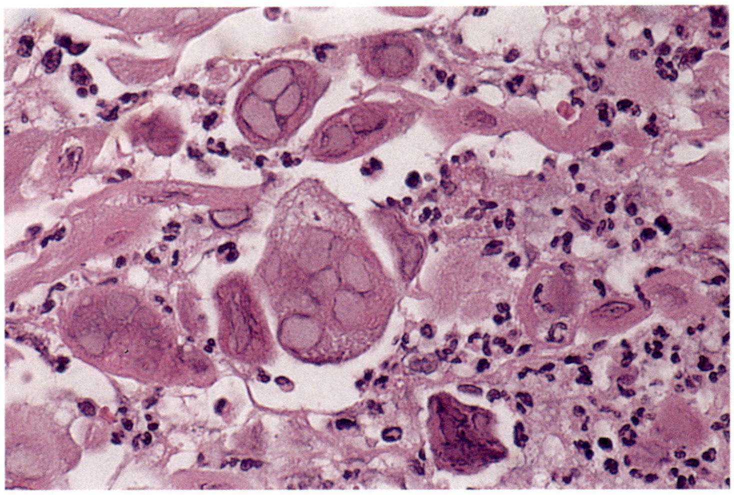

B

Figures 11–8A, 11–8B. Varicel a and herpes zoster infections. Acantholytic single and multinucleated epithelial giant cells with margination of their nucleoplasm at the periphery of the pale-gray-staining nuclei. One giant cell is necrotic with eosinophilic cytoplasm and pyknotic nuclei. There is a mixed-cell infiltrate present with neutrophils in the epidermis and dermis.

HERPES SIMPLEX INFECTION

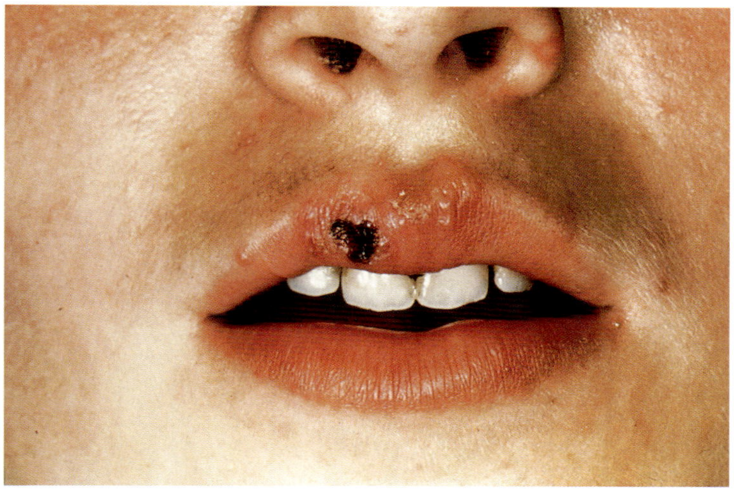

Figure 11–9. Herpes simplex infection. Grouped erythematous vesiculopapules with crust located on the vermillion of the upper lip and nose.

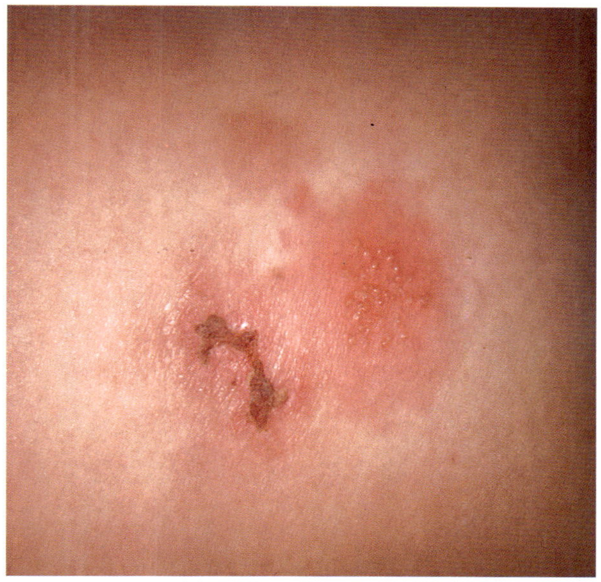

Figure 11–10. Herpes simplex infection. Agminated vesicles on an erythematous base adjacent to an eroded, crusted area of erythema.

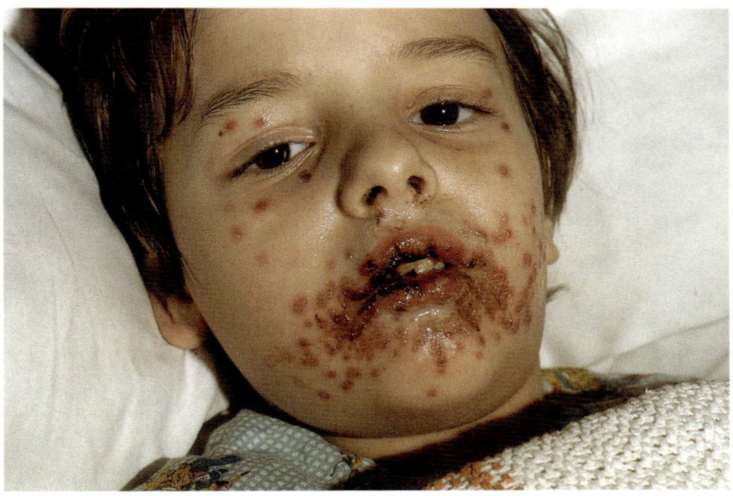

Figure 11–11. Herpes simplex infection. Primary herpes simplex infection with severe involvement of the oral mucosa and lips. Scattered lesions are present on the face. This presentation is not uncommon in the initial eruption of herpes simplex.

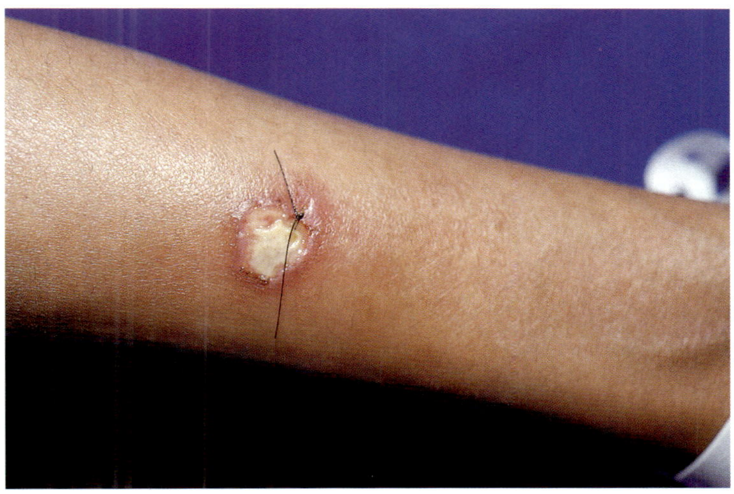

Figure 11–12. Herpes simplex infection. Long-standing ulcerated nodule in a patient who is HIV-positive.

HERPES SIMPLEX INFECTION

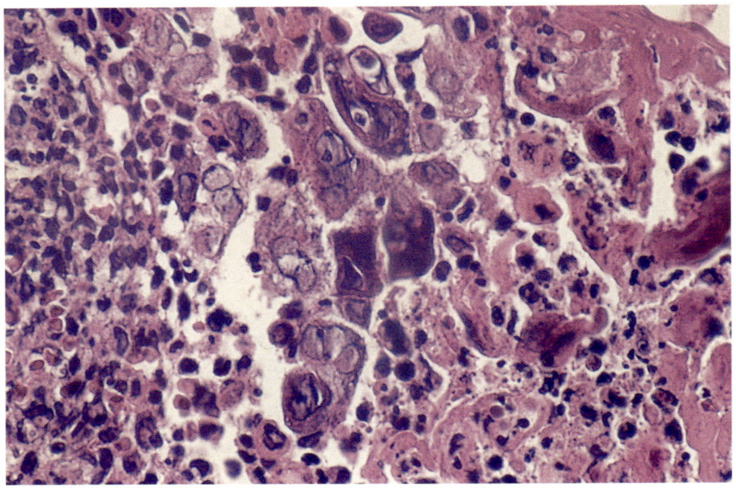

Figure 11–13. Herpes simplex infection. Sheets of single and multinucleated epithelial giant cells with margination of their nucleoplasm and pale-gray nuclei. Some of the cells are necrotic with eosinophilic cytoplasm and basophilic nuclei. A dense mixed-cell infiltrate is present.

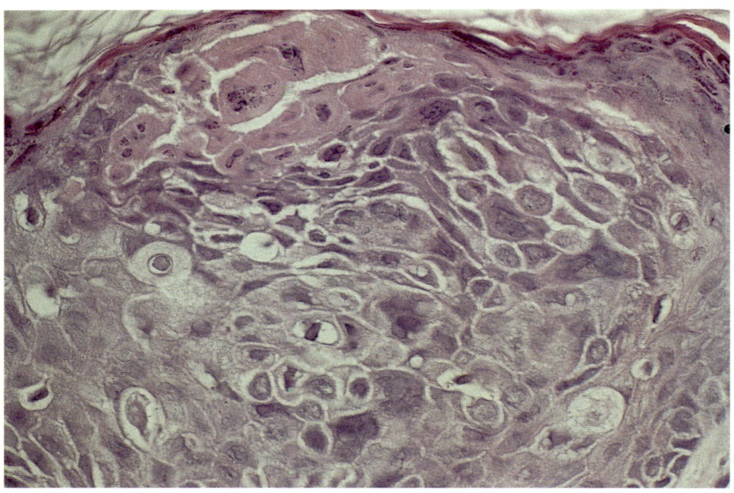

A

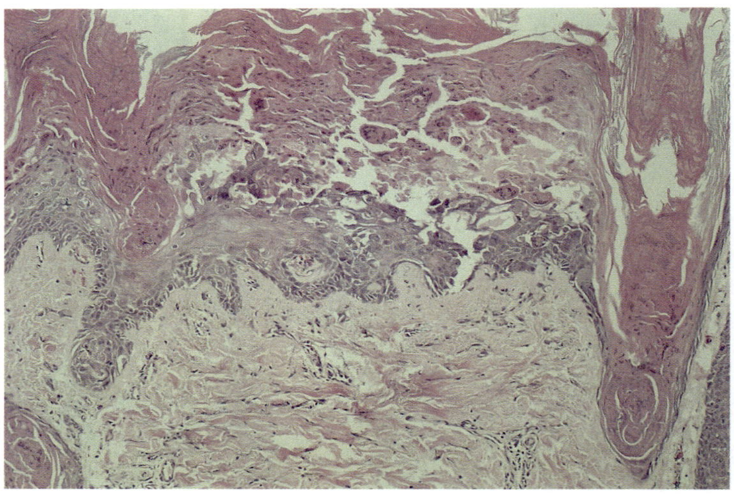

B

Figures 11–14A, 11–14B. Herpes simplex infection. Acantholytic multinucleated epithelial giant cells. Many of the giant cells are necrotic with basophilic, pyknotic nuclei and eosinophilic cytoplasms.

CYTOMEGALOVIRUS INFECTION

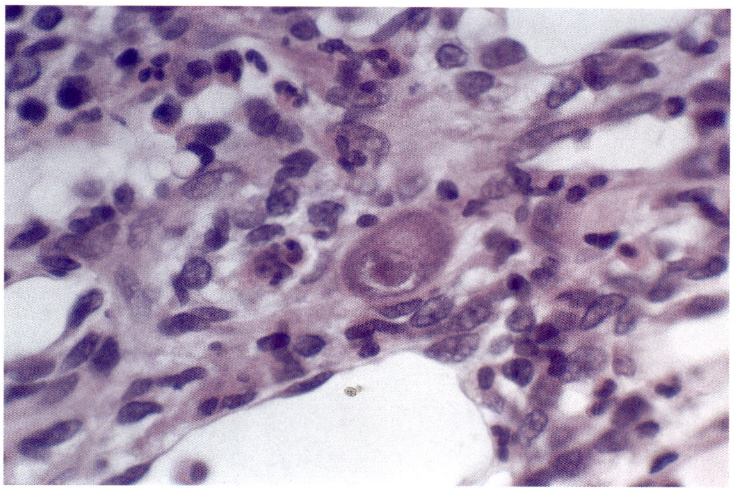

Figure 11–15. Cytomegalovirus infection. Enlarged cell with smudged cytoplasm, and a prominent amphophilic intranuclear inclusion surrounded by a perinuclear halo.

(owl's eye)

VIRAL EXANTHEM

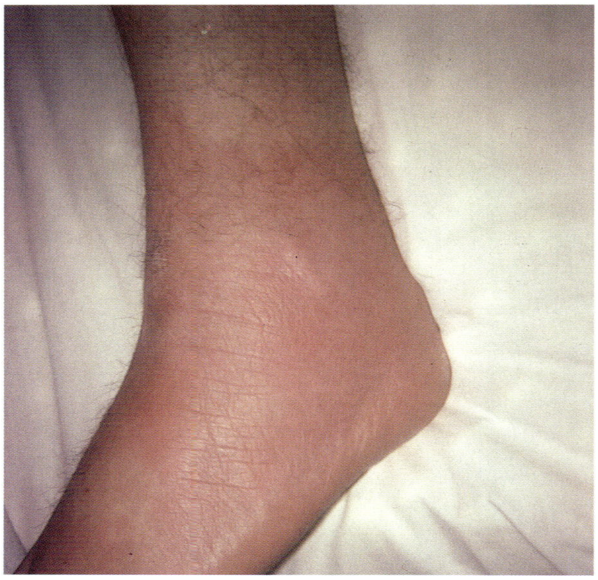

Figure 11–16. Viral exanthem, evolving. Macular erythema of the lower leg and foot.

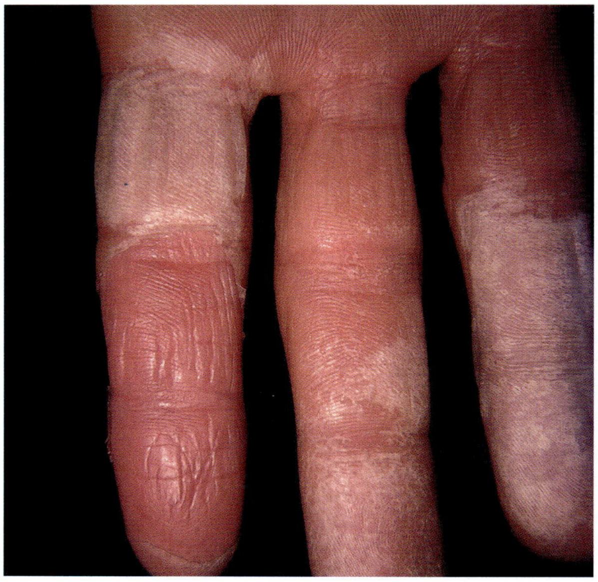

Figure 11–17. Viral exanthem, regressing. Erythema and desquamation of the palm and fingers.

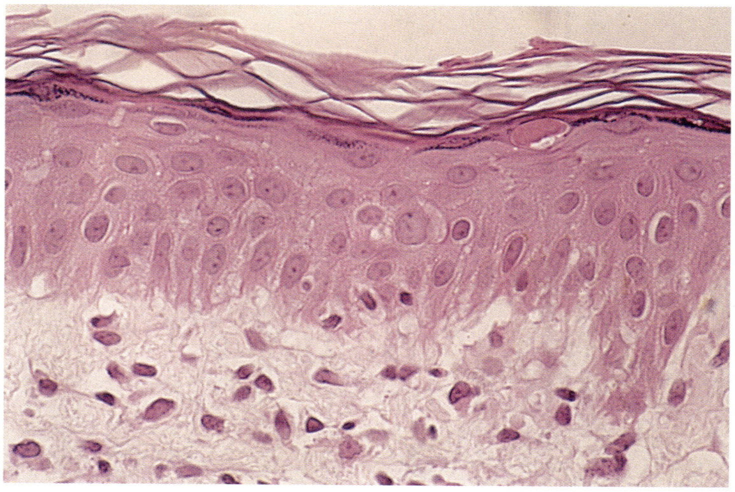

Figure 11–18. Viral exanthem. Vacuolar alteration and mild spongiosis. There is a mild perivascular lymphohistiocytic infiltrate.

MOLLUSCUM CONTAGIOSUM

(pox)

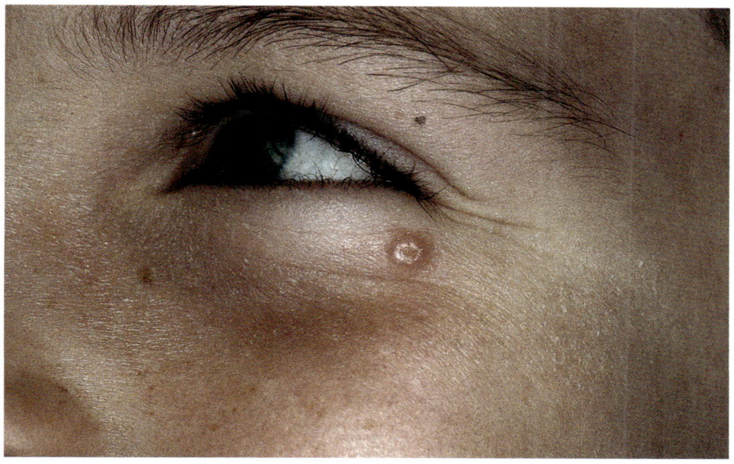

Figure 11–19. Molluscum contagiosum. Umbilicated erythematous papule on the eyelid of a child.

Ddx of molluscum in HIV:
paracocci
histo
blasto

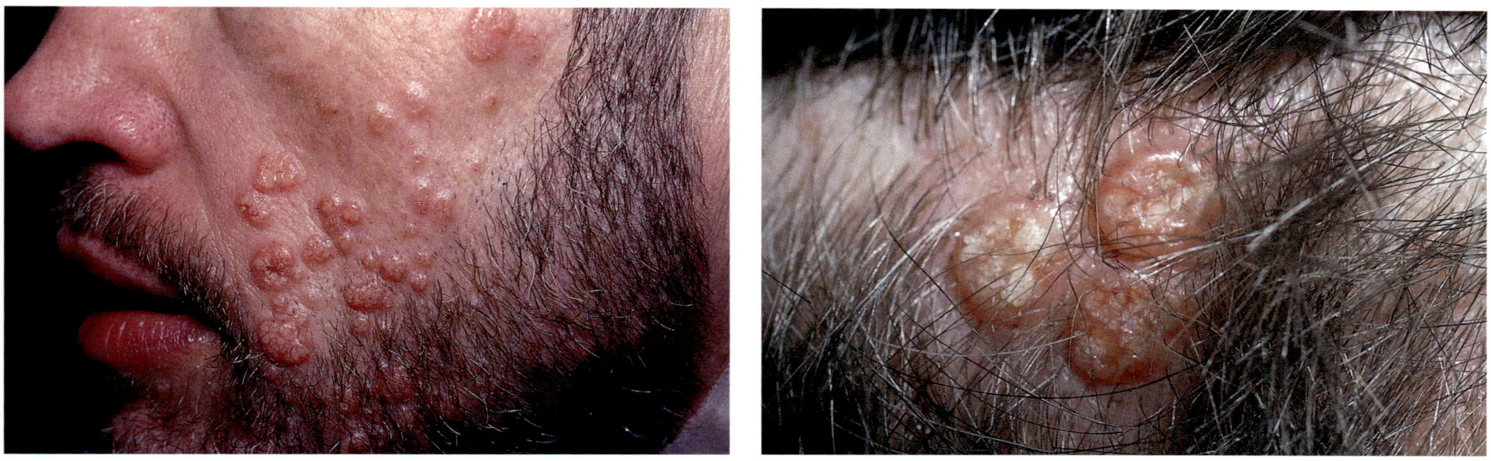

A B

Figures 11–20A, 11–20B. Molluscum contagiosum. Myriad of giant, pink and skin-colored, umbilicated, coalescing papules and nodules in the bearded cheek area of an HIV-infected man.

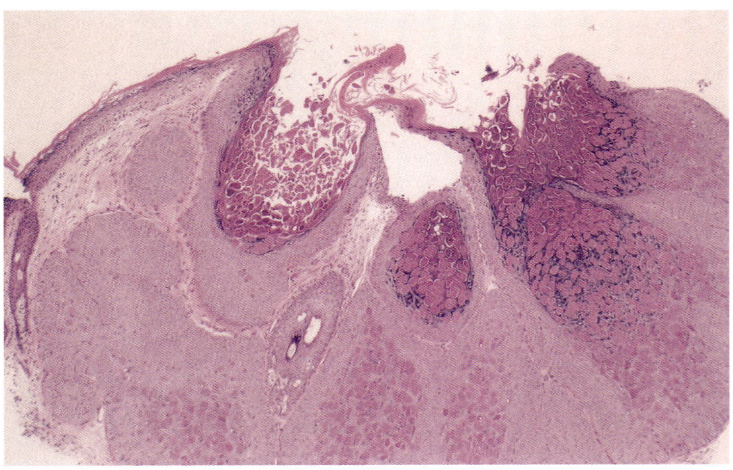

A

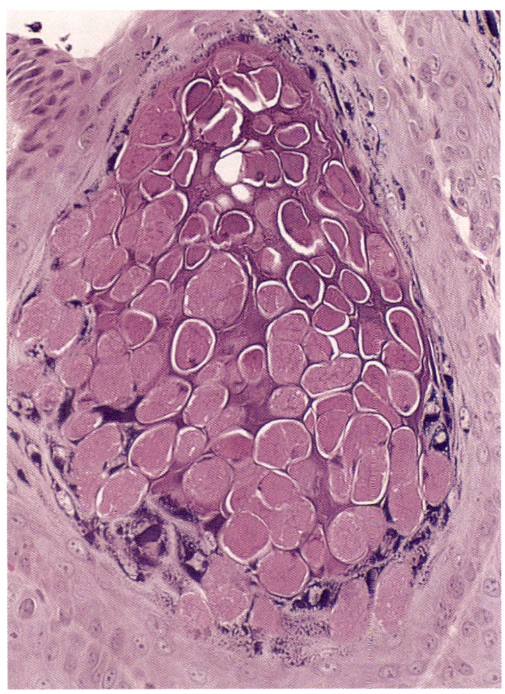

B

Figures 11–21A, 11–21B. Molluscum contagiosum. Molluscum bodies within the epidermis in what appears to be hyperplastic, epithelial adnexal structures. The distinctive intracytoplasmic molluscum bodies displace the nuclei to the periphery. The molluscum bodies vary in color from red to blue as they mature toward the skin surface.

MILKER'S NODULE

(pox virus)

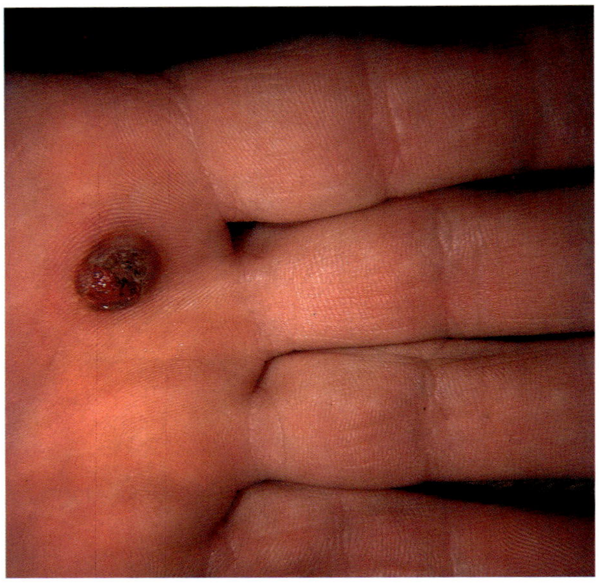

Figure 11–22. Milker's nodule. Exophytic, sharply circumscribed, ulcerated and crusted nodule on the palm of a dairy farmer.

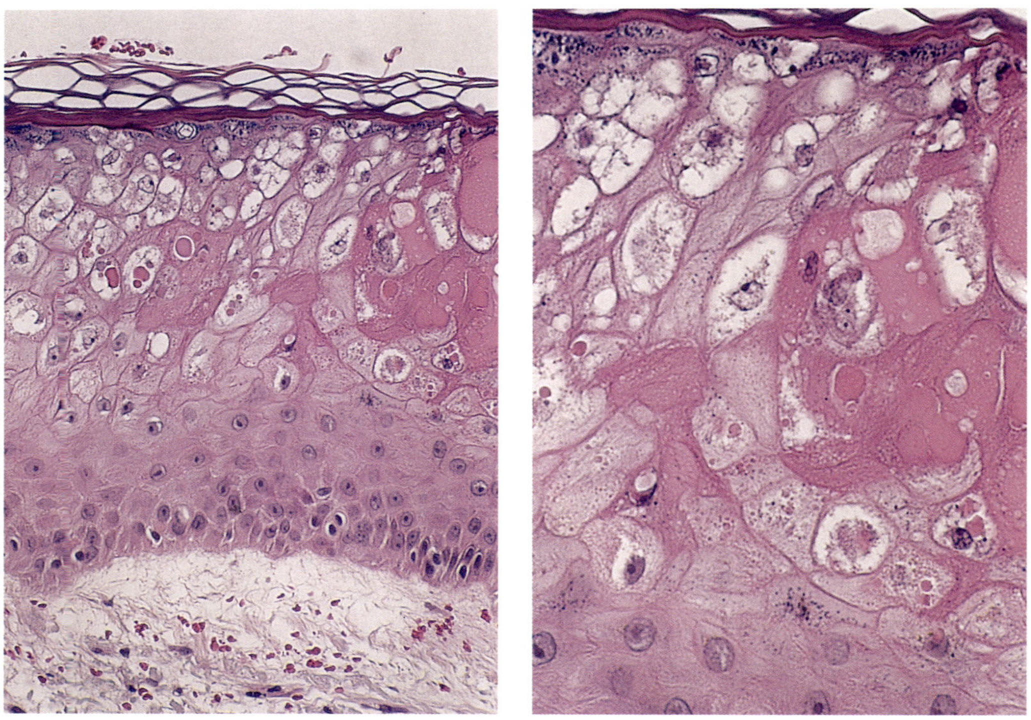

A B

Figures 11–23A, 11–23B. Milker's nodule. Epidermal hyperplasia with ballooned and necrotic keratinocytes. There is severe papillary edema and a mixed-cell infiltrate with neutrophils

COXSACKIE EXANTHEM (HAND, FOOT, AND MOUTH DISEASE)

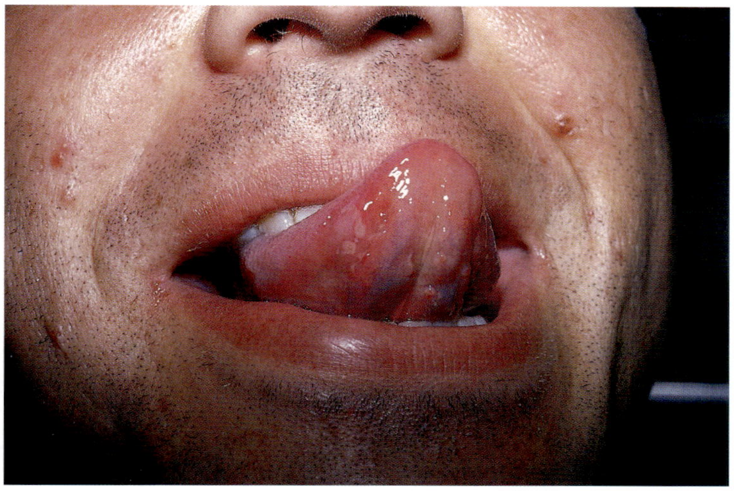

Figure 11–24. **Coxsackie exanthem.** Painful ulcers on the sides and tip of the tongue.

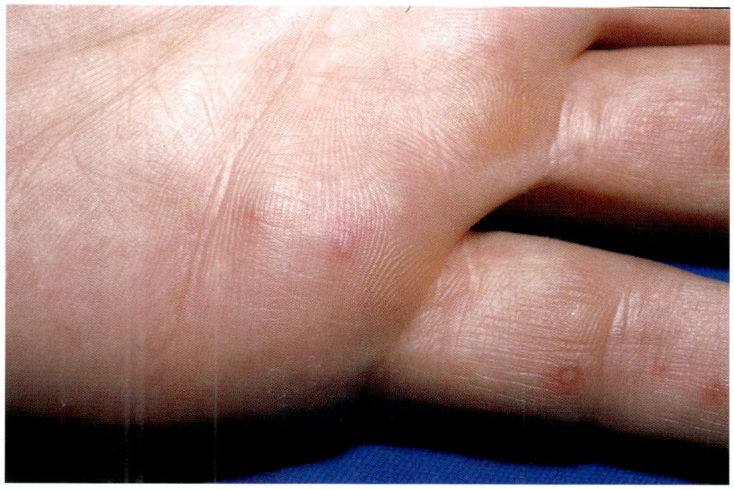

Figure 11–25. **Coxsackie exanthem.** Nonpainful vesicles on the palm and finger.

typical vesicular appearance (hand, foot, mouth)

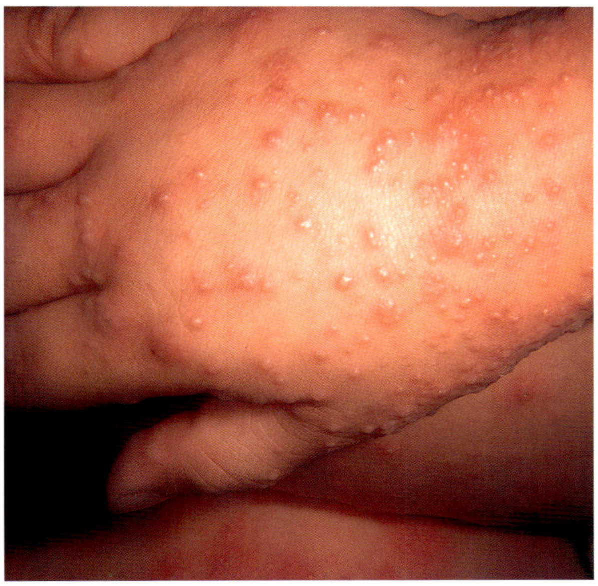

Figure 11–26. **Coxsackie exanthem.** Diffuse eruptive vesiculopapules on the hand of a 3-year-old child.

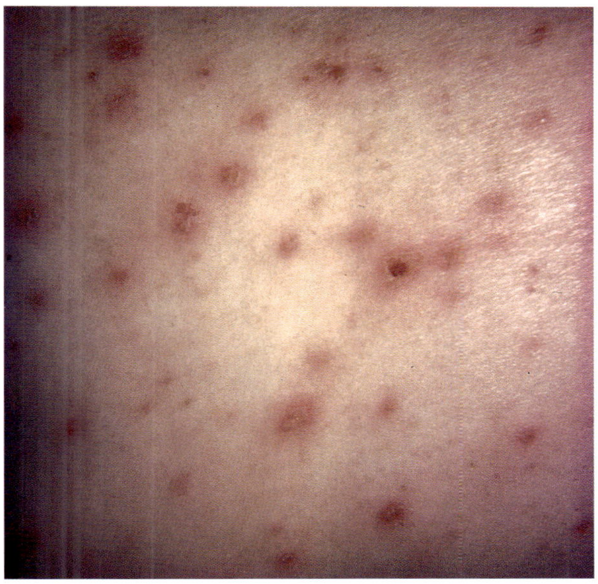

Figure 11–27. **Coxsackie exanthem.** Diffuse eruptive vesiculocrusted papules on the back of a man with generalized malaise, fever, arthralgias, and hepatosplenomegaly.

COXSACKIE EXANTHEM (HAND, FOOT, AND MOUTH DISEASE)

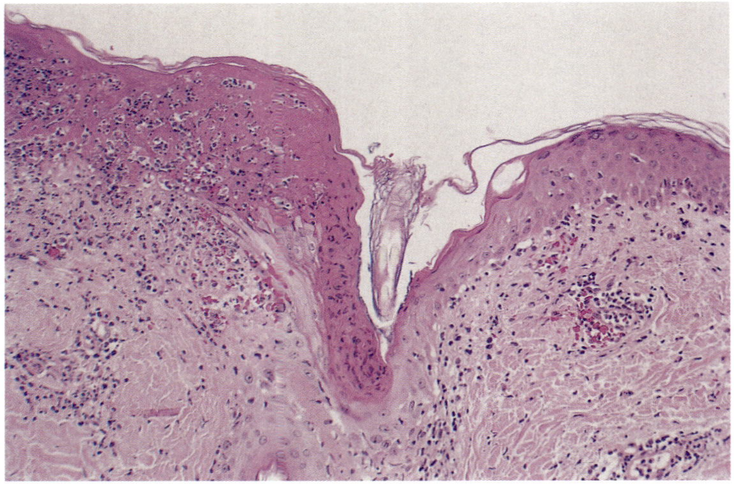

A

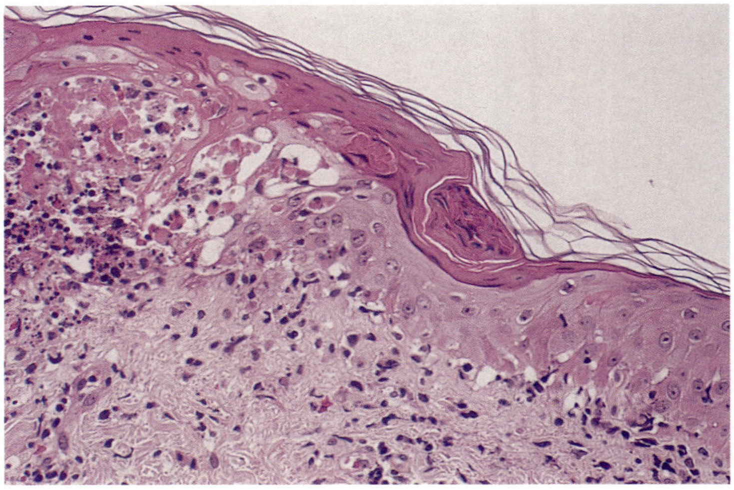

B

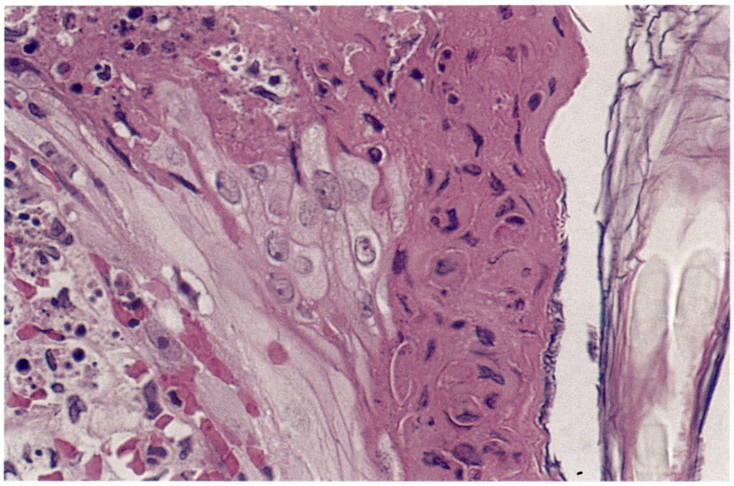

C

Figures 11–28A, 11–28B, 11–28C. Coxsackie exanthem. Epidermal and infundibular spongiosis, vacuolar alteration, ballooned and necrotic keratinocytes, and nuclear debris. There is papillary dermal edema and mixed-cell infiltrate with extravasated erythrocytes.

VERRUCA VULGARIS

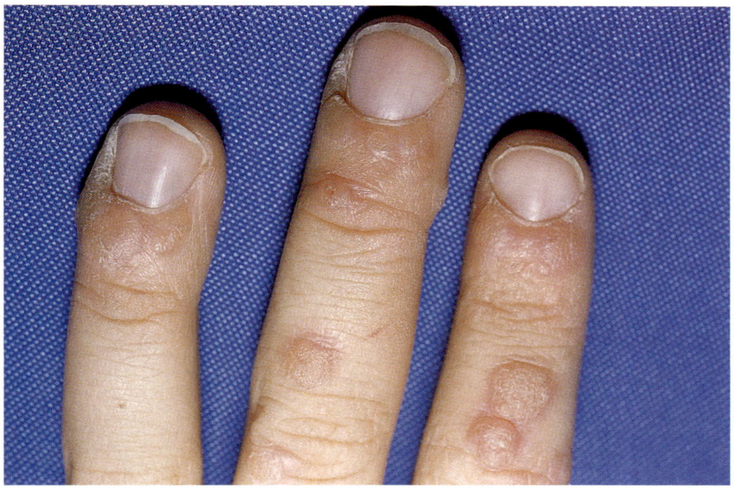

Figure 11–29. **Verruca vulgaris.** Paronychial and finger warts.

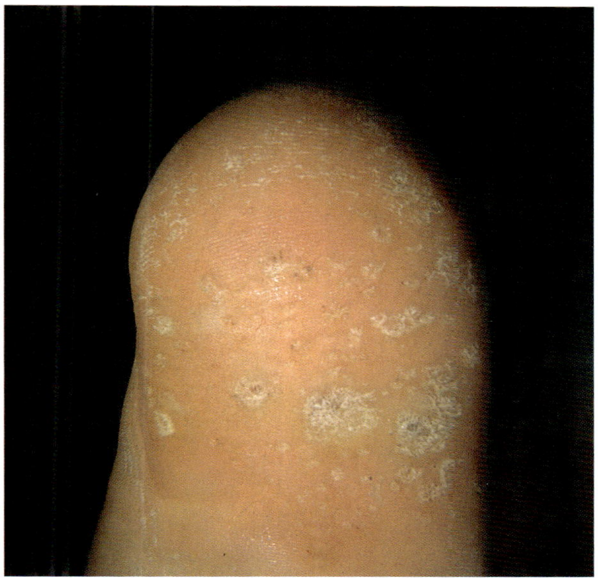

Figure 11–30. **Verruca vulgaris.** Recalcitrant, mosaic plantar warts on the heel present for many years. These lesions were unresponsive to a variety of topical and destructive treatment regimens.

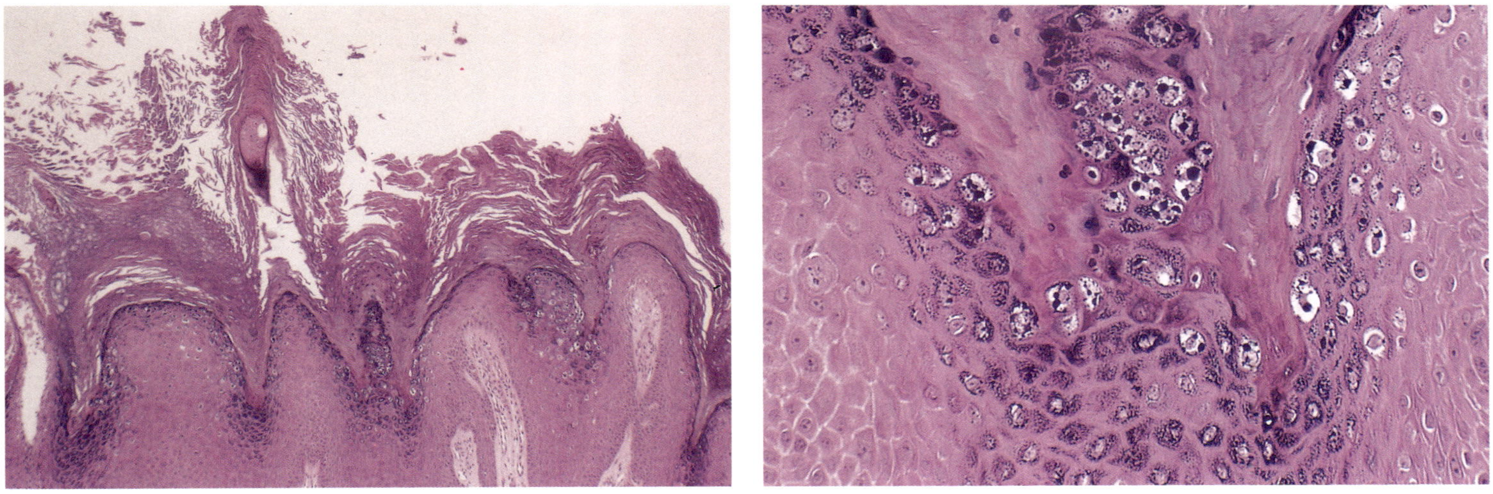

A

B

Figures 11–31A, 11–31B. **Verruca vulgaris.** Digitate epidermal hyperplasia with hypergranulosis, compact hyperkeratosis, and hyperparakeratosis in vertical spikes. There are vacuolated keratinocytes within the granular layer containing coarse keratohyalin granules.

VERRUCA VULGARIS

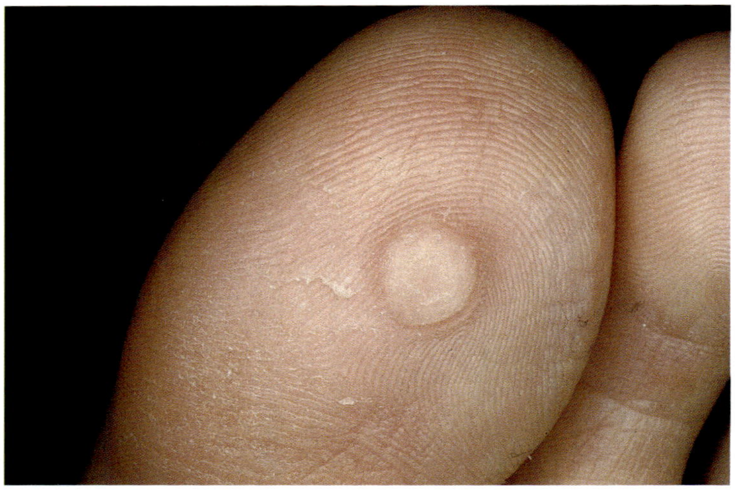

Figure 11–32. Verruca vulgaris. Regressed verruca vulgaris on the volar surface of the first toe. The solitary papule is dome-shaped and hyperkeratotic.

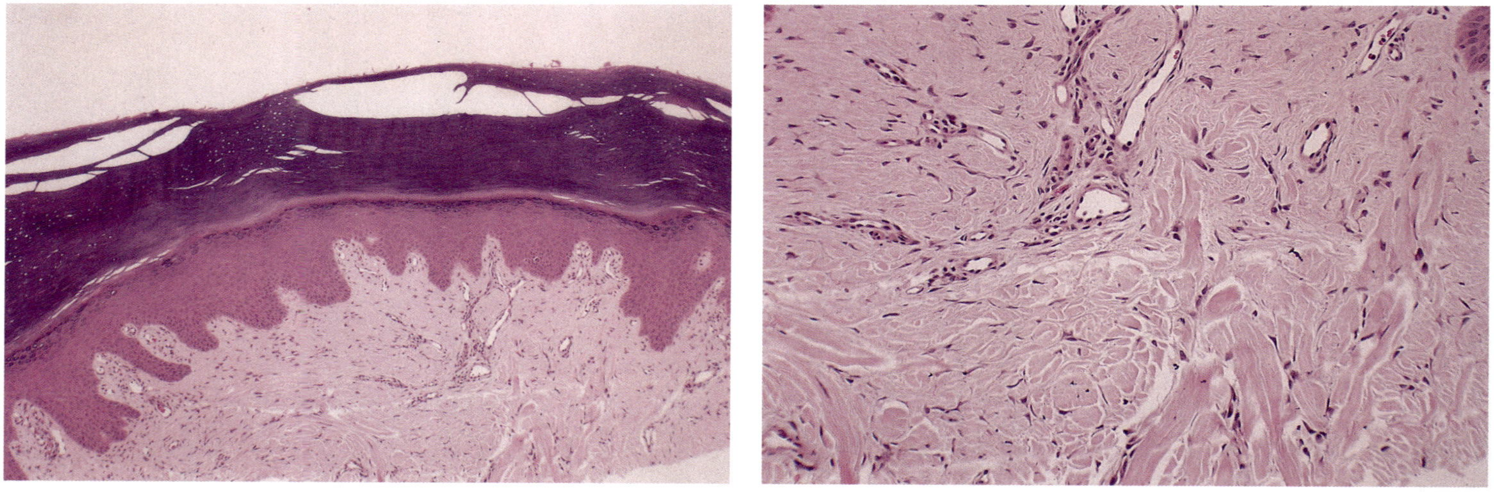

A B

Figures 11–33A, 11–33B. Verruca vulgaris. Regressed verruca vulgaris on the volar aspect of the first toe. There is compact orthokeratosis, epidermal hyperplasia, and conspicuous vascular ectasia with fibroplasia.

CONDYLOMA ACUMINATUM

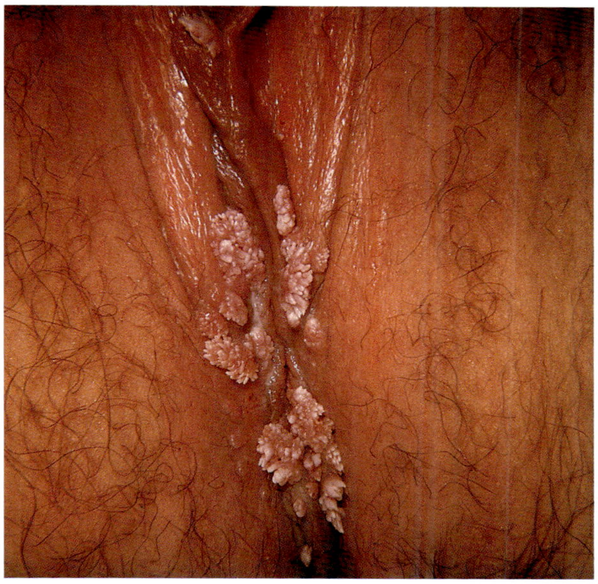

Figure 11–34. Condyloma acuminatum. Labial and perianal filiform pink-white warts.

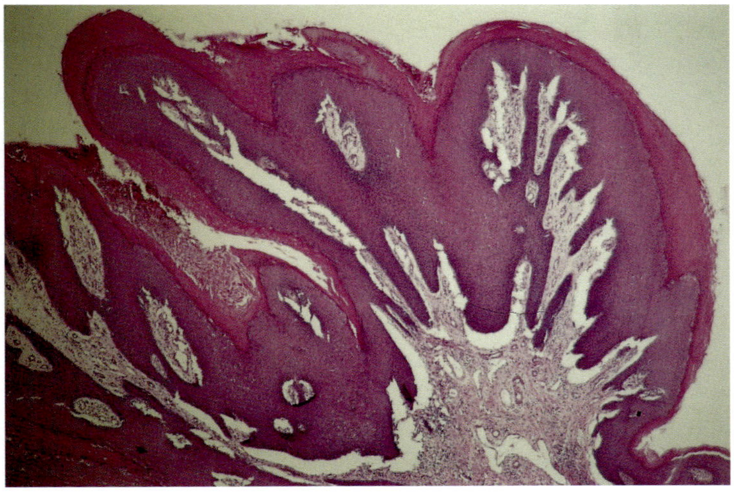

A

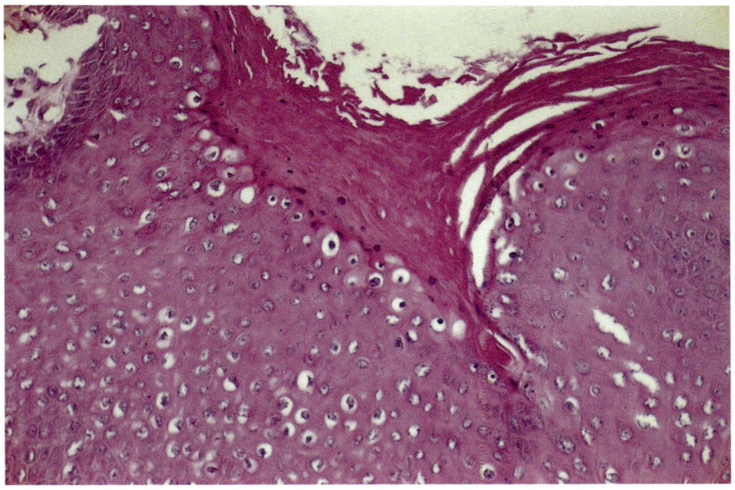

B

Figures 11–35A, 11–35B. Condyloma acuminatum. Polypoid, rounded growth with compact hyperkeratosis and dermal vascular ectasia. There are vacuolated keratinocytes within the upper spinous and granular layers. They contain shiny, basophilic globules that extend into the hyperkeratotic stratum corneum.

VERRUCA PLANA

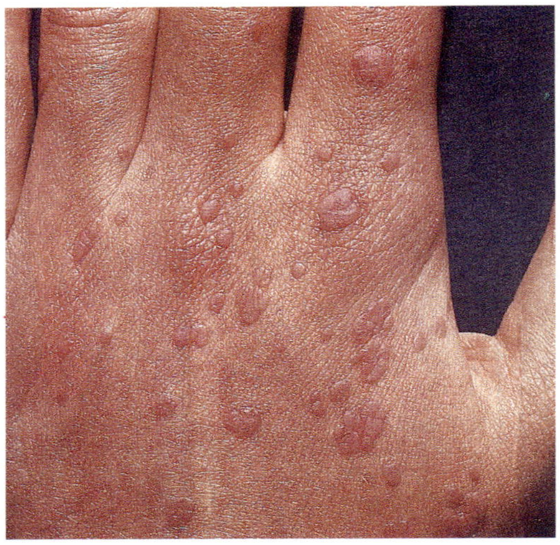

Figure 11–36. Verruca plana. Flat-topped, agminated, pink papules on the dorsum of the hand and fingers.

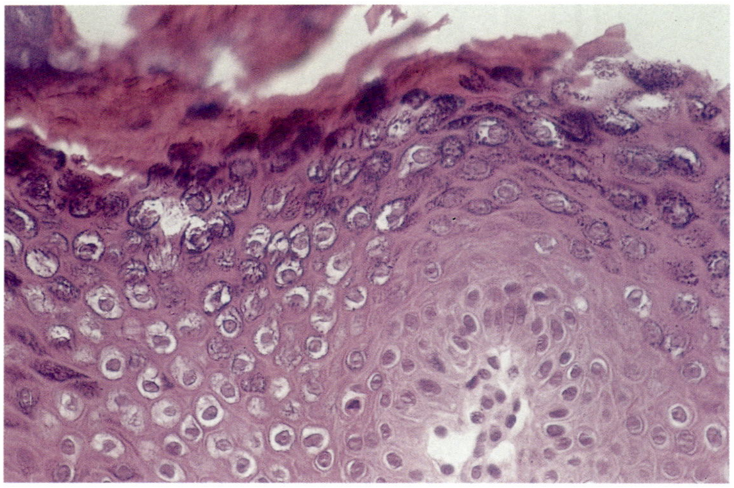

Figure 11–37. Verruca plana. Vacuolated keratinocytes with pyknotic nuclei present within the upper stratum spinosum and stratum granulosum. There is overlying mild hyperkeratosis.

EPIDERMODYSPLASIA VERRUCIFORMIS

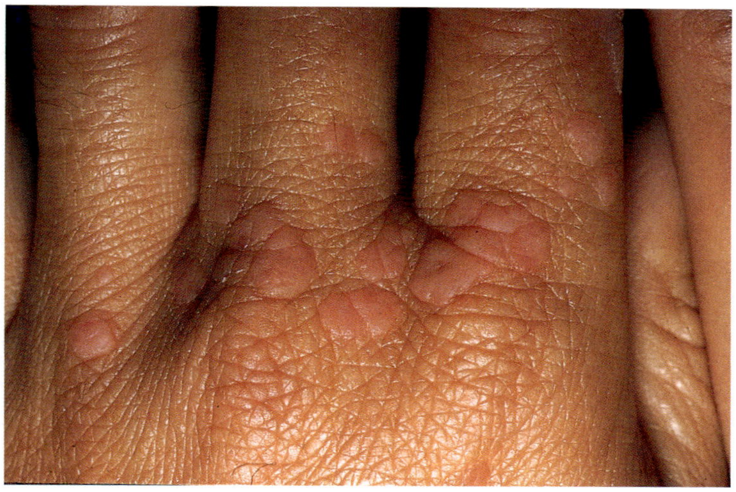

Figure 11–38. Epidermodysplasia verruciformis. Single and grouped pink keratotic papules on the dorsum of the hand and fingers.

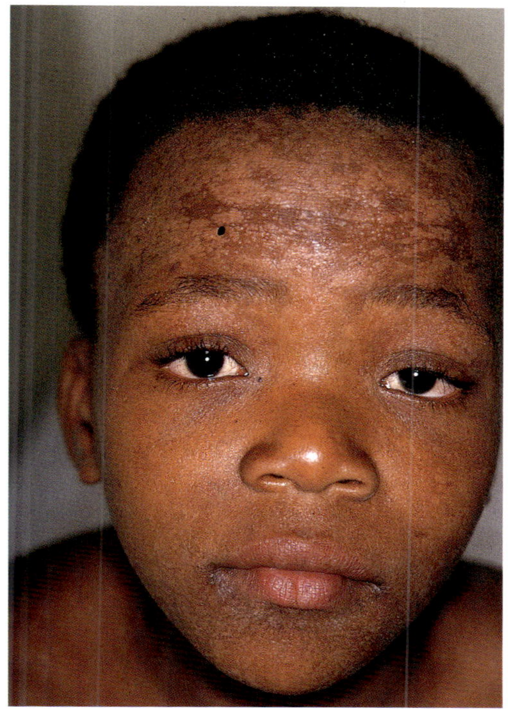

Figure 11–39. Epidermodysplasia verruciformis. Diffuse and confluent macules and papules on the face of a child.

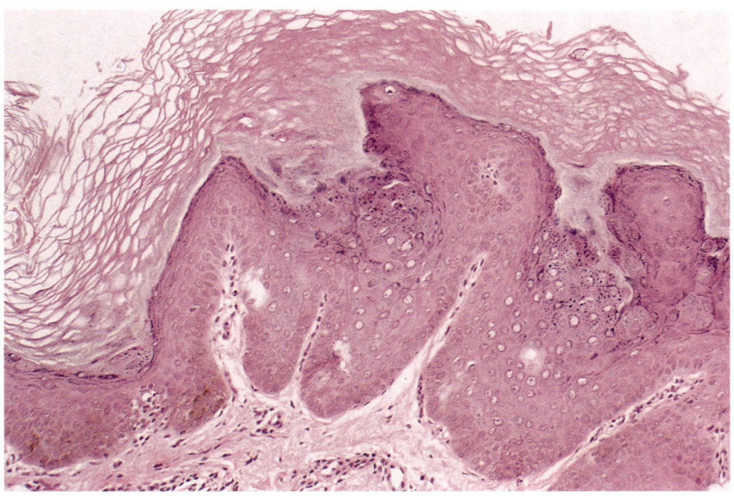

Figure 11–40. Epidermodysplasia verruciformis. Basket-weave hyperkeratosis, epidermal hyperplasia, and pale, vacuolated keratinocytes in the upper stratum malpighii.

BOWENOID PAPULOSIS

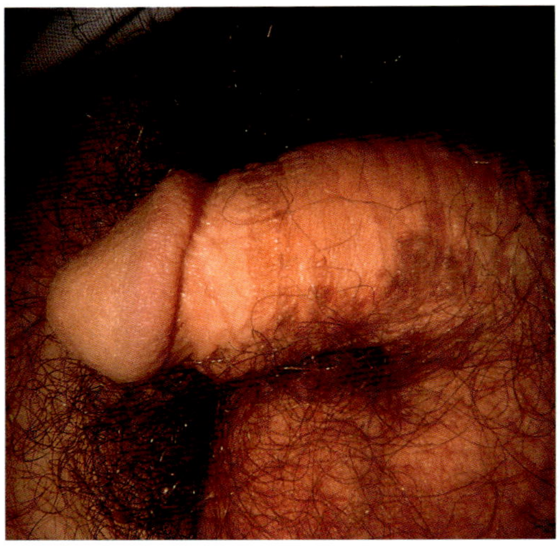

Figure 11–41. Bowenoid papulosis. Gray-brown verrucous papules on the shaft of a penis.

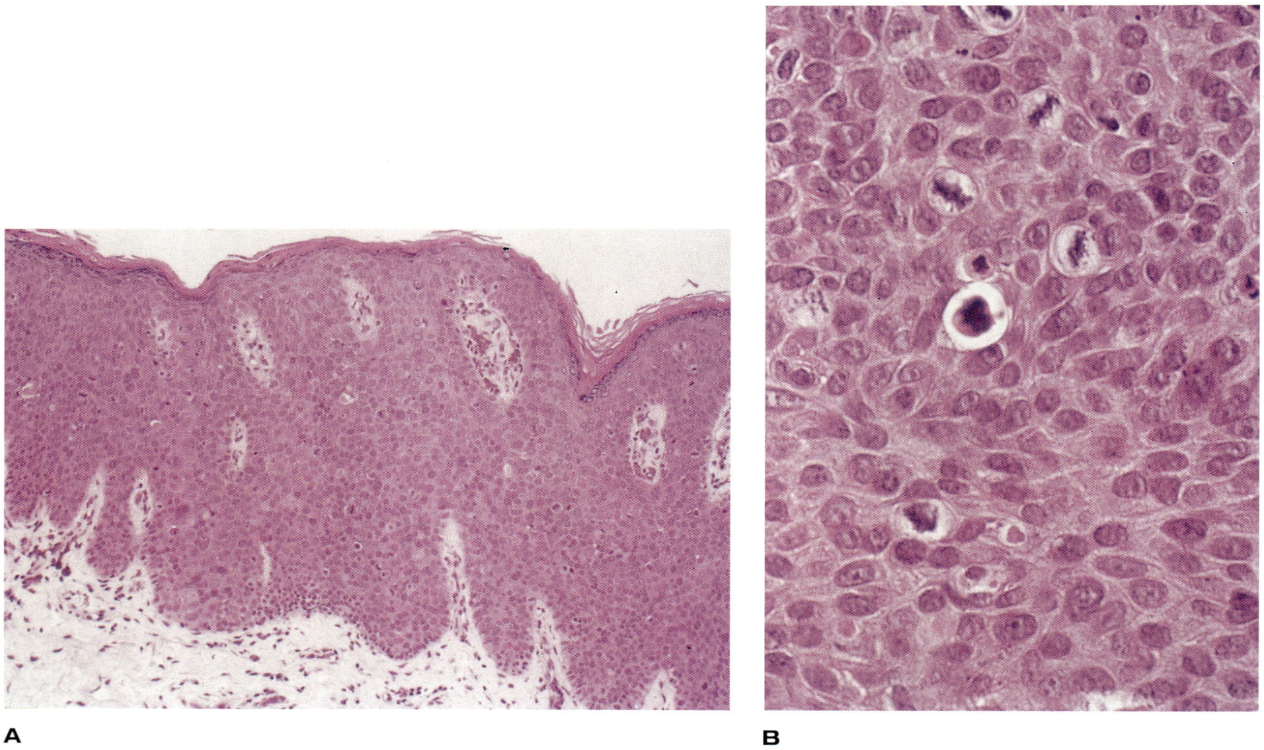

Figures 11–42A, 11–42B. Bowenoid papulosis. Epidermal hyperplasia with loss of normal maturation. There are atypical pleomorphic, mitotic, and necrotic keratinocytes at all levels of the epidermis.

SQUAMOUS-CELL CARCINOMA IN ASSOCIATION WITH THE HUMAN PAPILLOMA VIRUS (HPV)

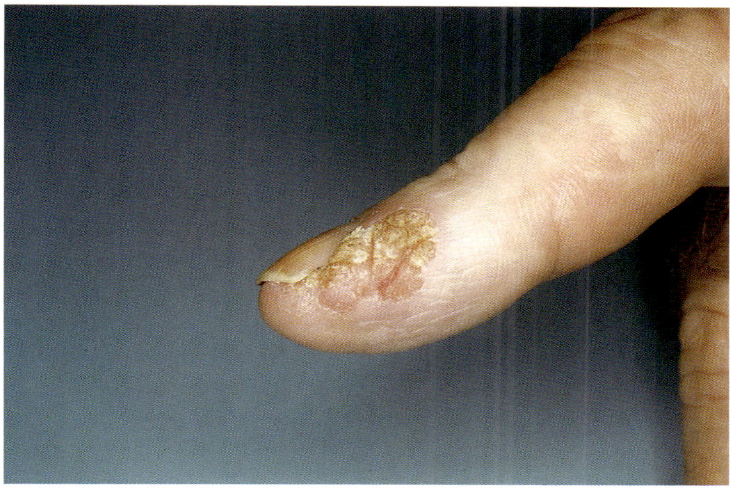

Figure 11–43. Squamous-cell carcinoma in association with HPV. Enlarging and recalcitrant paronychial verrucous growth on the index finger of a man for many years.

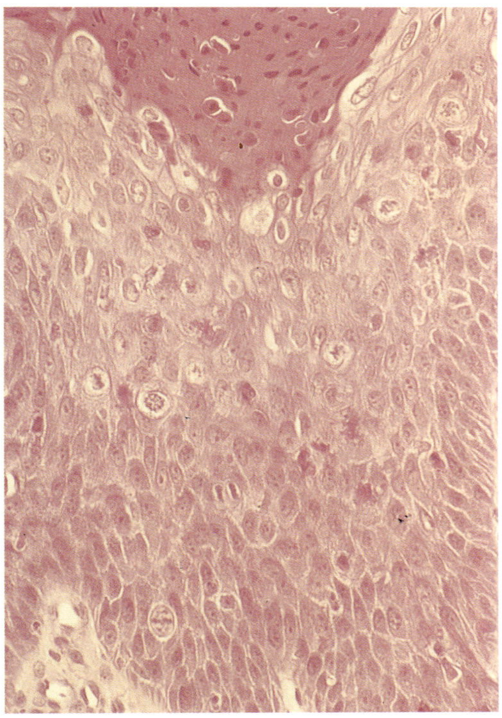

Figure 11–44. Squamous-cell carcinoma in association with HPV. Hyperkeratosis, parakeratosis, and epidermal hyperplasia with loss of normal cell maturation. There is full-thickness atypia with pleomorphic and necrotic keratinocytes and mitotic figures.

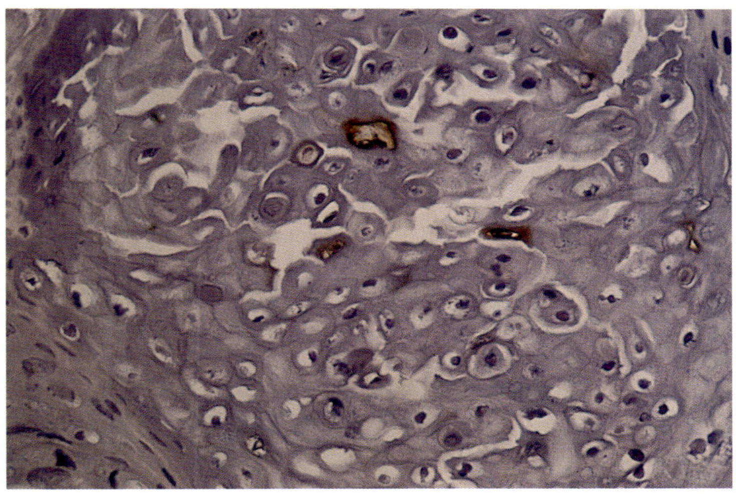

Figure 11–45. Squamous-cell carcinoma in association with HPV. Immunoperoxidase stain for HPV type 16. Many keratinocytes are staining positively (brown) for the virus.

12

Bacterial infections

- Actinomycosis
- Bacillary angiomatosis
- Chancroid
- Impetigo
- Staphylococcal scalded skin syndrome (SSSS)
- Toxic shock syndrome (TSS)
- Scarlet fever
- Bacterial cellulitis
- Erythrasma/pitted keratolysis
- Granuloma inguinale
- Localized septic vasculitis
- Systemic septic vasculitis

ACTINOMYCOSIS

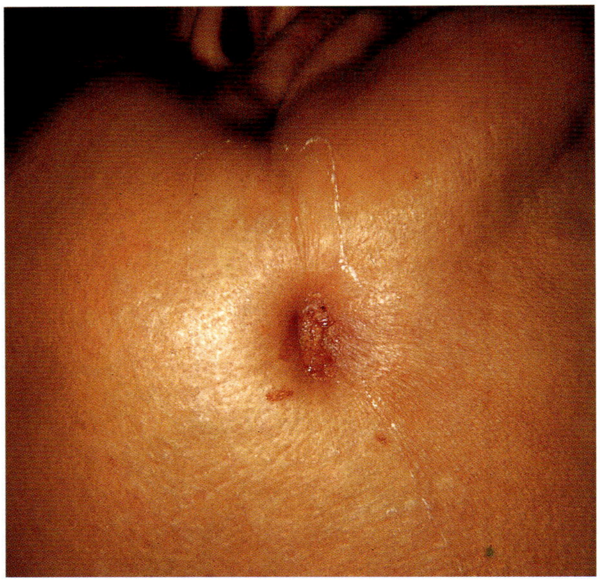

Figure 12–1. Actinomycosis. Draining sinus from an abscessed tooth.

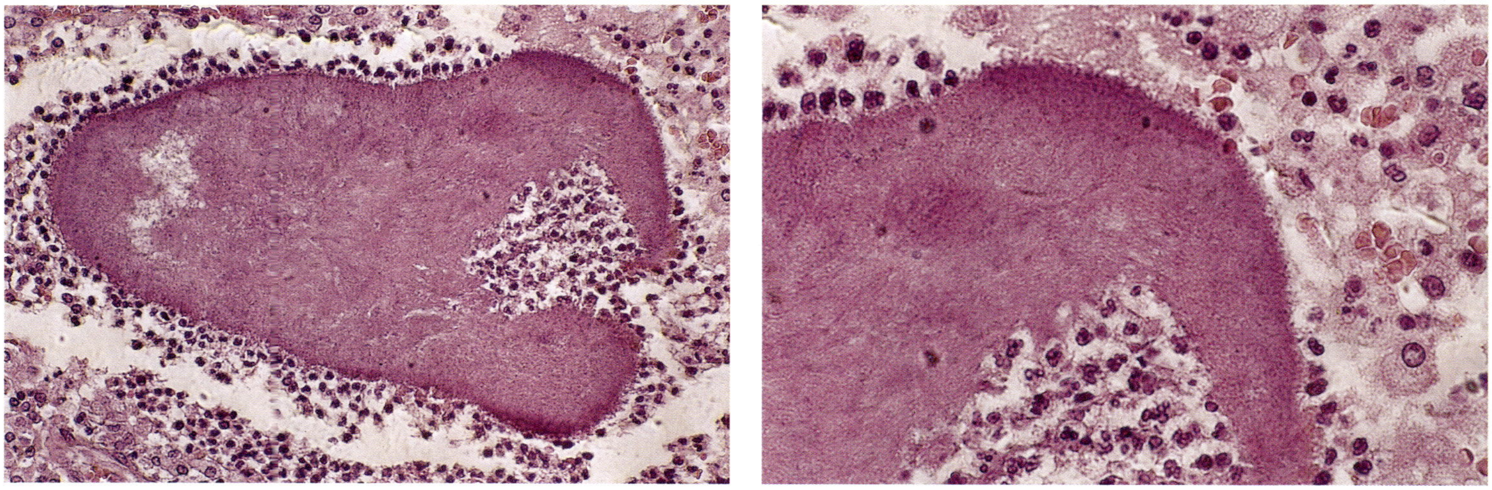

A B

Figures 12–2A, 12–2B. Actinomycosis. Sulfur granule within a neutrophilic dermal abscess. The sulfur granule is composed of clumped colonies of bacteria, which appear as peripheral radiating club-shaped filamentous bacteria, staining centrally pinkish and peripherally bluish with hematoxylin and eosin

BACILLARY ANGIOMATOSIS

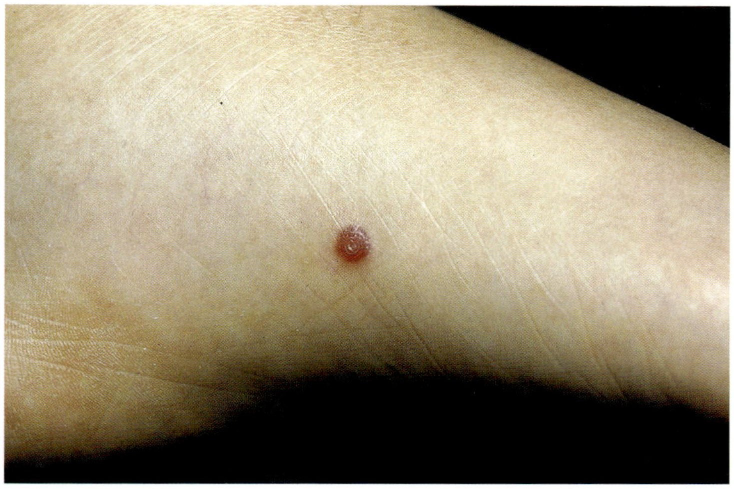

Figure 12–3. Bacillary angiomatosis. Solitary red papule resembling a hemangioma on the foot of an HIV-positive man.

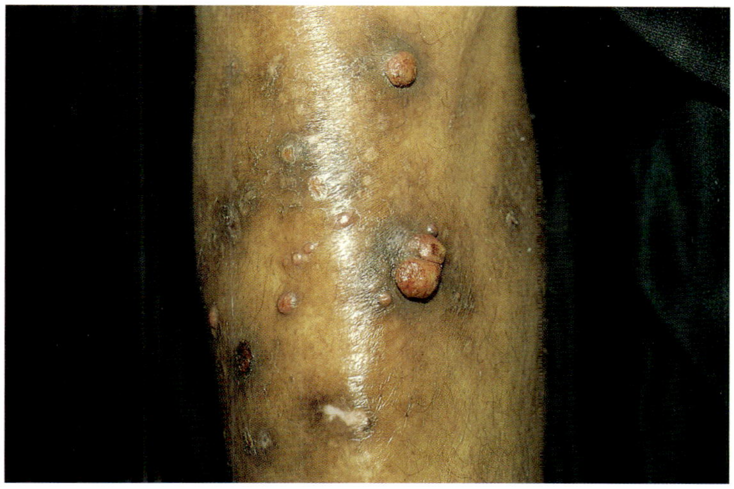

Figure 12–4. Bacillary angiomatosis. Erythematous papules and nodules on the lower leg. Some of the lesions have the appearance of "proud flesh," with exuberant granulation tissue.

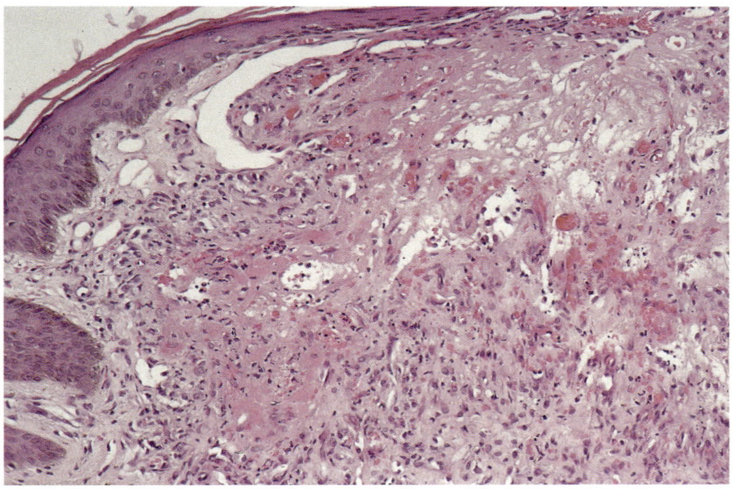

Figure 12–5. Bacillary angiomatosis. Dilated blood vessels and a mixed-cell infiltrate fill the dermis.

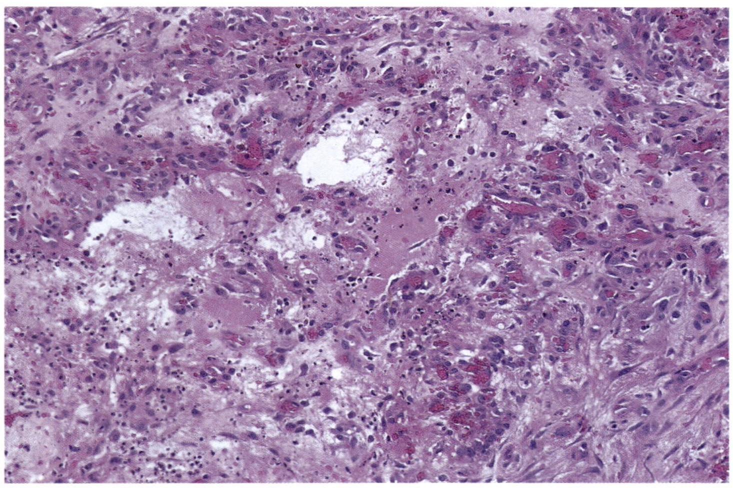

Figure 12–6. Bacillary angiomatosis. Deposition of eosinophilic granular material surrounded by a neutrophilic rich inflammatory infiltrate and dilated blood vessels.

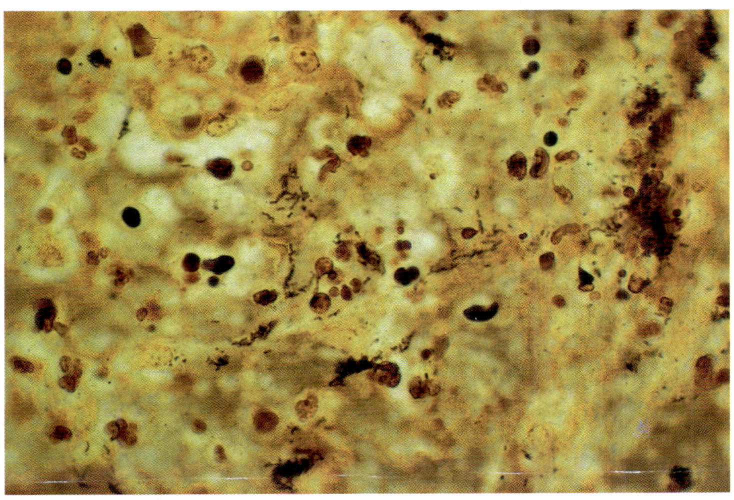

Figure 12–7. Bacillary angiomatosis. Silver stain showing clusters of rod-shaped organisms (*Bartonella henselae* and/or *quintana*) within the granular areas in the dermis.

CHANCROID

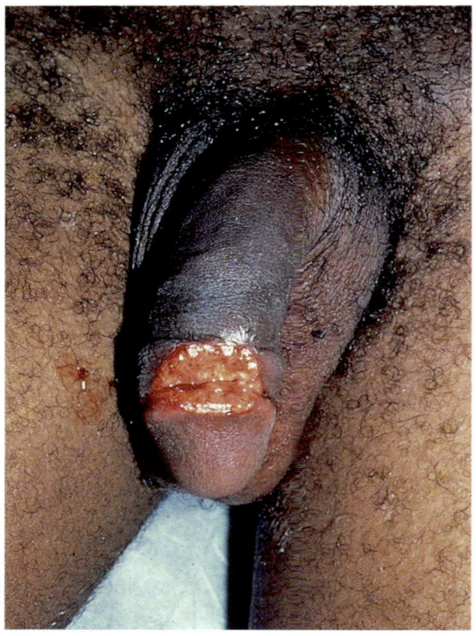

Figure 12–8. Chancroid. Large, painful ulcer on the penis with exuberant beefy-red granulation tissue.

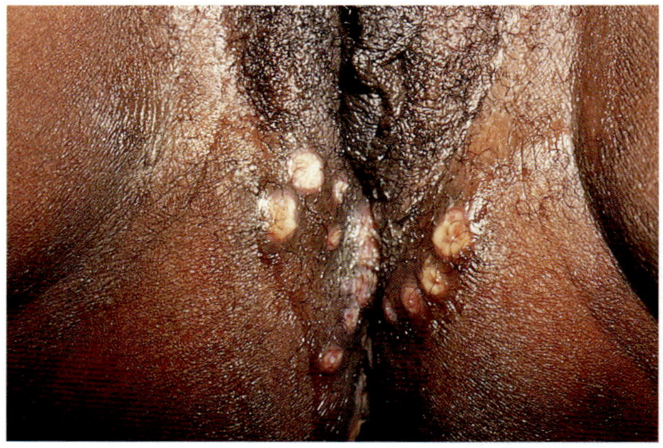

Figure 12–9. Chancroid. Multiple painful punched-out ulcers on the labia.

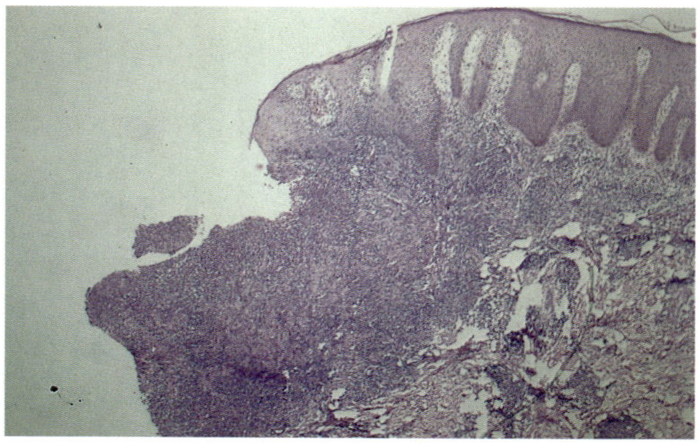

Figure 12–10. Chancroid. There is epidermal hyperplasia at the margin of the ulcer with a dense mixed-cell infiltrate subjacent to the ulcer.

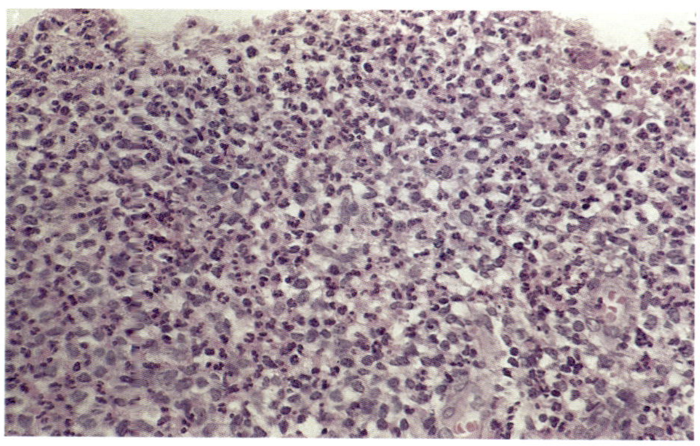

A

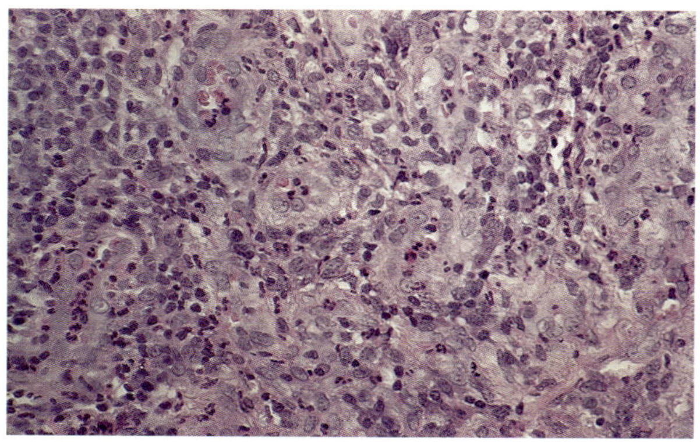

B

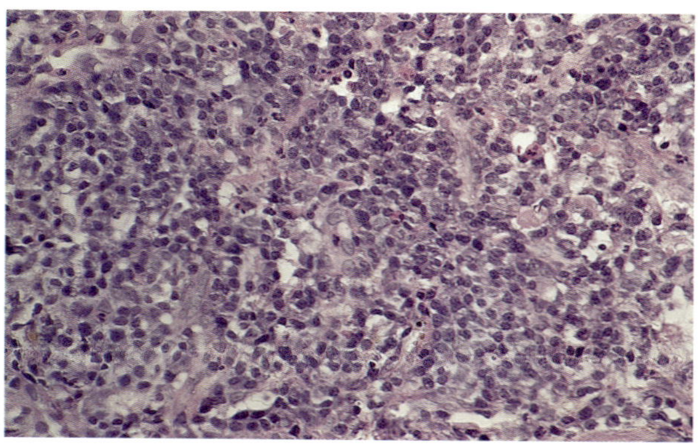

C

Figures 12–11A, 12–11B, 12–11C. Chancroid. The dermal infiltrate characteristically has a zonal pattern where neutrophils, dilated blood vessels, or a lymphoplasmocytic infiltrate predominate.

IMPETIGO

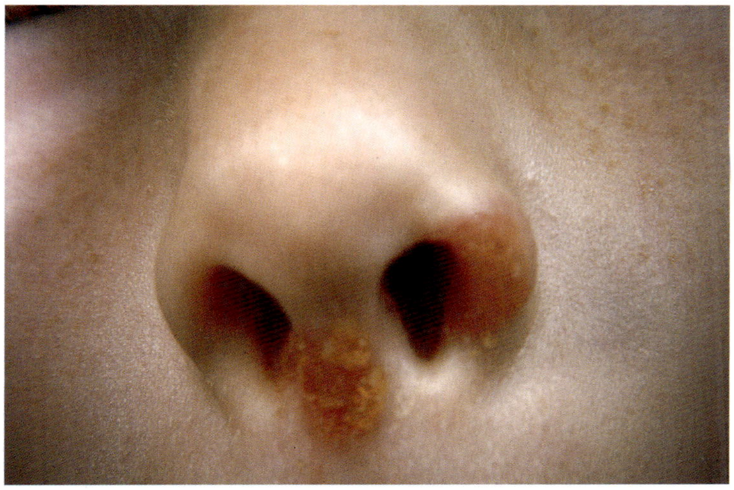

Figure 12–12. **Impetigo.** Yellow, crusted papules on the nose.

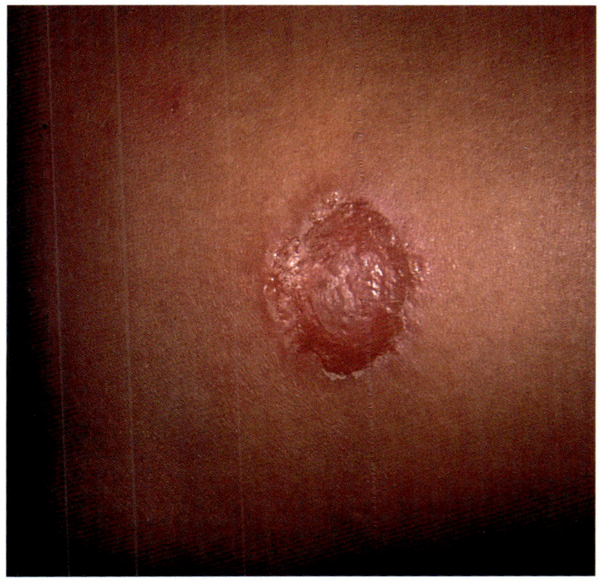

Figure 12–13. **Impetigo.** Ulcerated, crusted, oozing nodule on the thigh. This lesion is sometimes referred to as ecthyma.

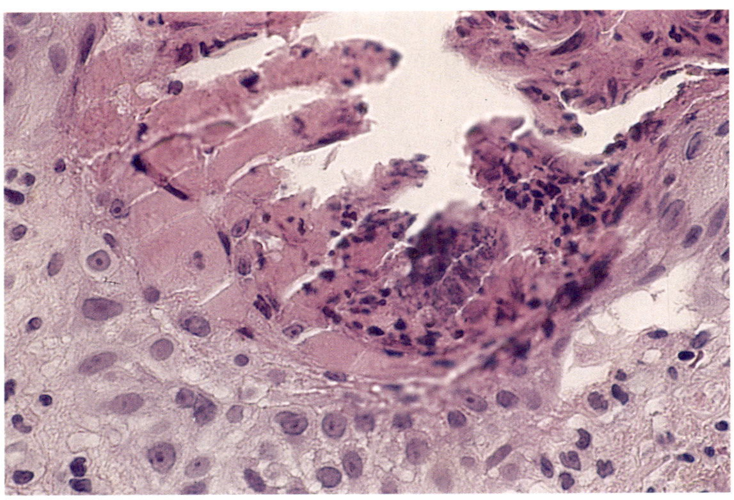

Figure 12–14. **Impetigo.** Subcorneal collection of necrotic keratinocytes, neutrophils, and bacterial organisms.

STAPHYLOCOCCAL SCALDED SKIN SYNDROME (SSSS)

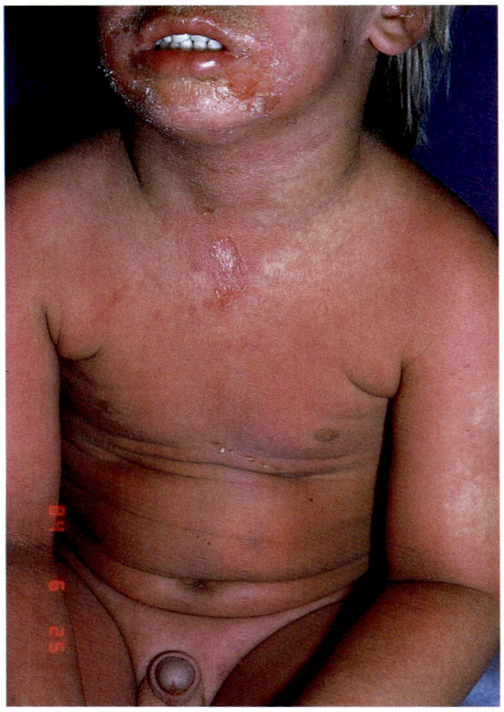

Figure 12–15. Staphylococcal scalded skin syndrome. Diffuse erythema, erosions, and stomatitis.

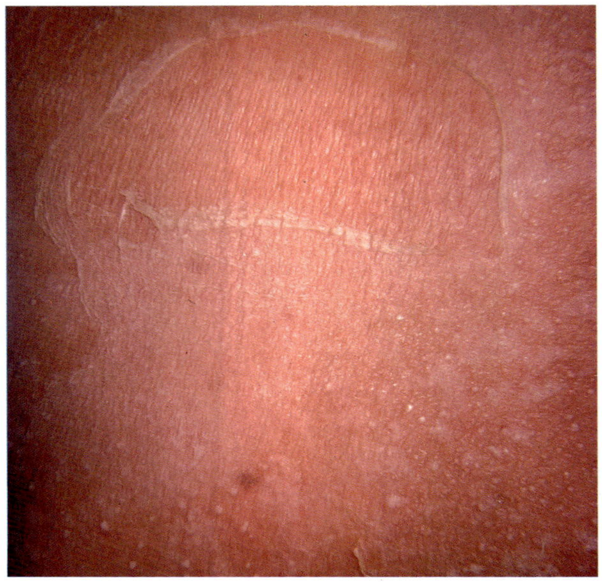

Figure 12–16. Staphylococcal scalded skin syndrome. Erythema, vesicles, and desquamation.

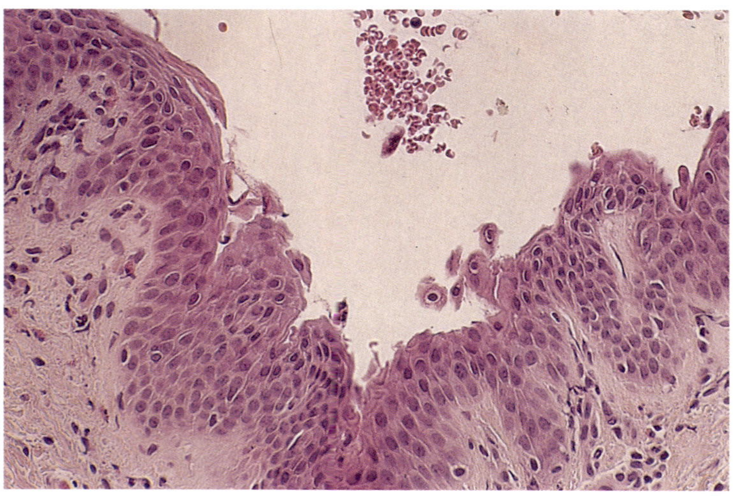

Figure 12–17. Staphylococcal scalded skin syndrome. Subcorneal layer separation with acantholytic keratinocytes and neutrophils. There is papillary dermal edema and a sparse mixed-cell infiltrate with neutrophils.

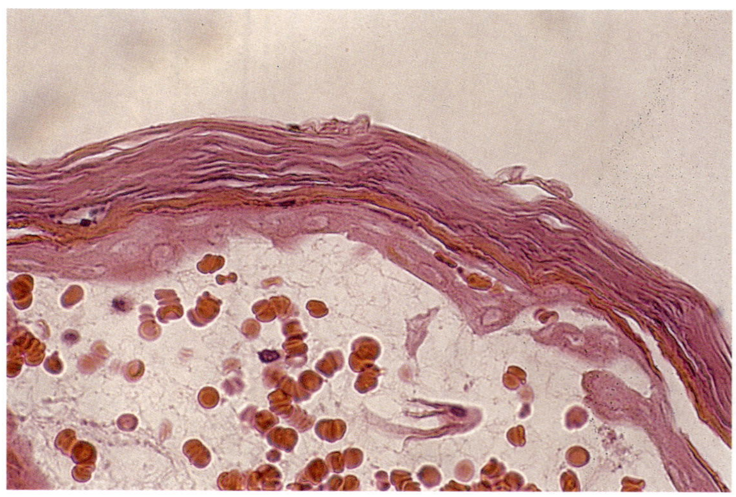

Figure 12–18. Staphylococcal scalded skin syndrome. Subgranular layer separation. There are necrotic keratinocytes, neutrophils, and erythrocytes.

TOXIC SHOCK SYNDROME (TSS)

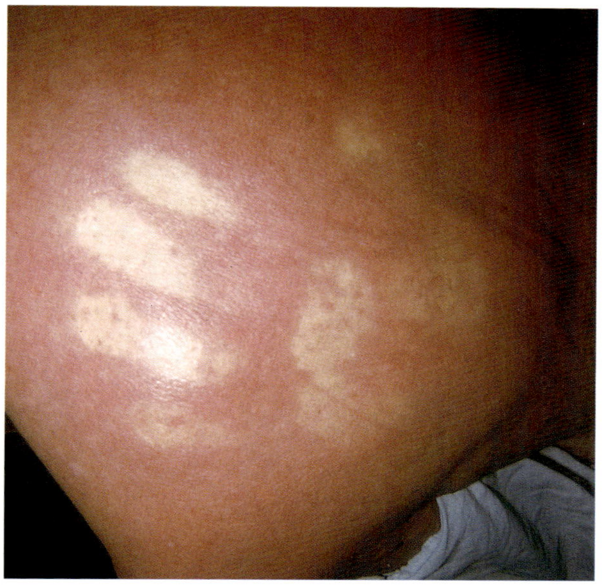

Figure 12–19. Toxic shock syndrome. Blanching hand imprint on the diffusely erythematous back of a woman with hypotension, nausea, vomiting, and fever. She had a vaginal discharge that grew *Staphylococcus aureus*.

Figure 12–20. Toxic shock syndrome. Diffuse and coalescing erythematous macular and papular lesions on the thigh of a woman with chronic renal failure. She had *Staphylococcus aureus* cultured from the tip of her peritoneal catheter.

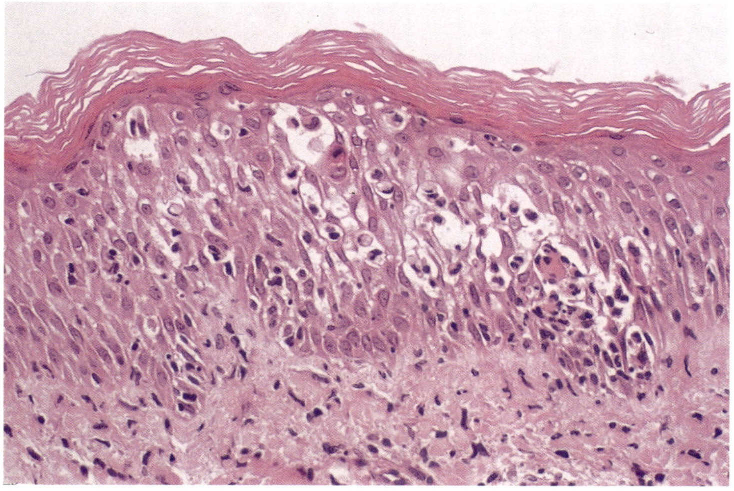

Figure 12–21. Toxic shock syndrome. Spongiosis, neutrophils, and necrotic keratinocytes. There is papillary dermal edema and a mixed-cell infiltrate with neutrophils.

SCARLET FEVER

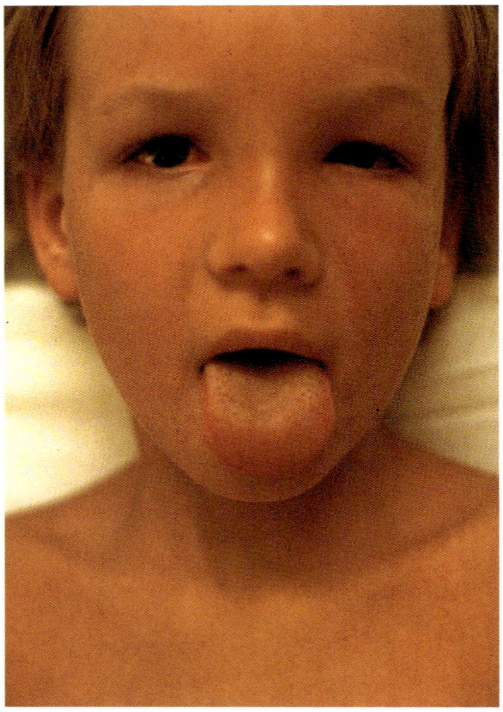

Figure 12–22. Scarlet fever. Dusky facial erythema, edema, and scaling that has a sandpaper quality to the touch. There is perioral pallor and a "strawberry" tongue.

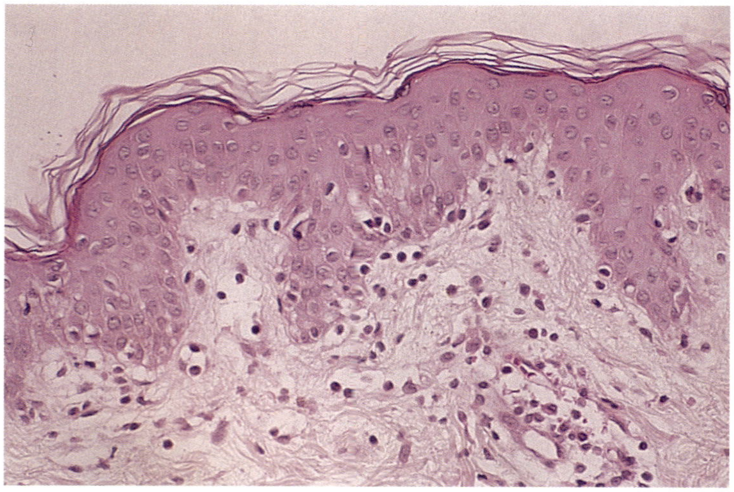

A

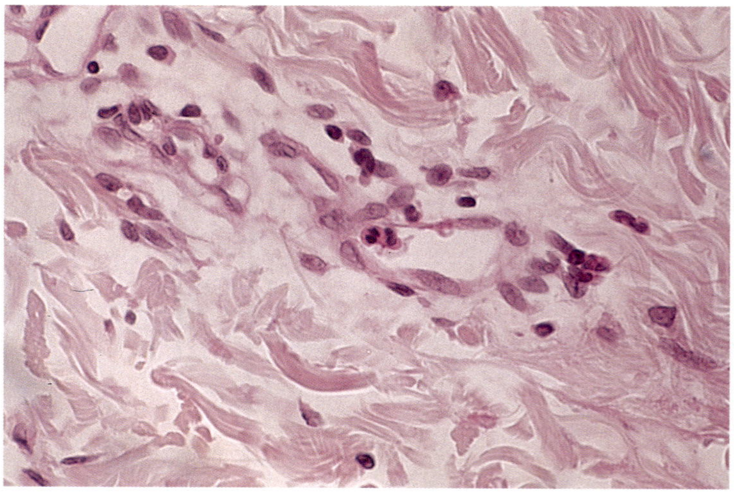

B

Figures 12–23A, 12–23B. Scarlet fever. Spongiosis, papillary dermal edema, dilated blood vessels, and a mild perivascular ar d interstitial mixed-cell infiltrate with neutrophils.

BACTERIAL CELLULITIS (Erysipelas)

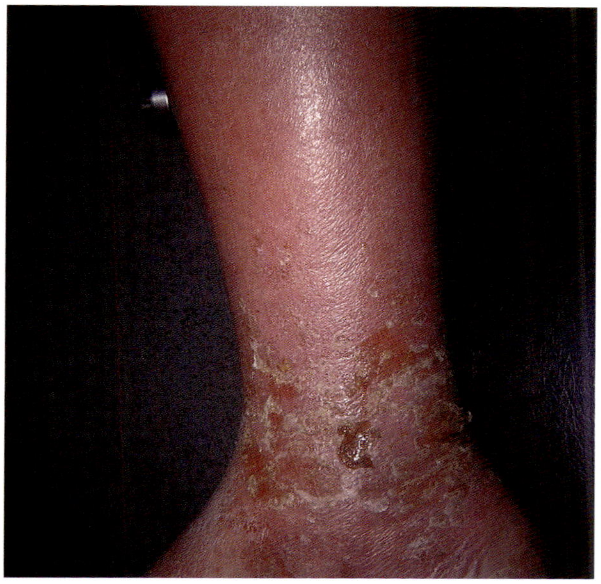

A

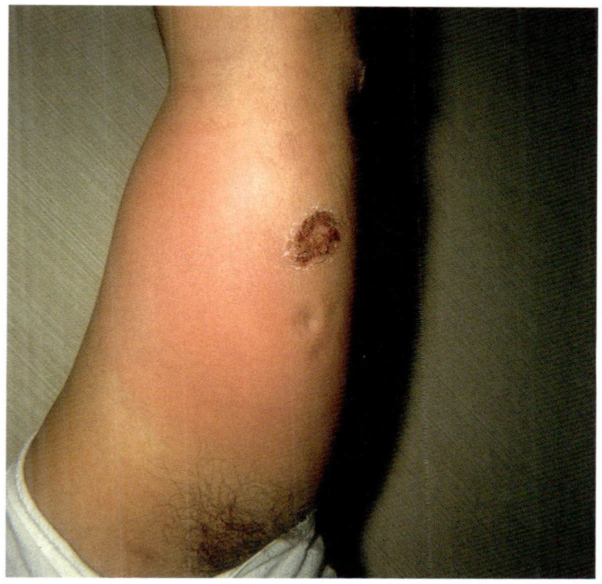

B

Figures 12–24A, 12–24B. Bacterial cellulitis. Staphylococcal infection of the arm. The extremities are warm, erythematous, and edematous, with oozing, crusted ulcers.

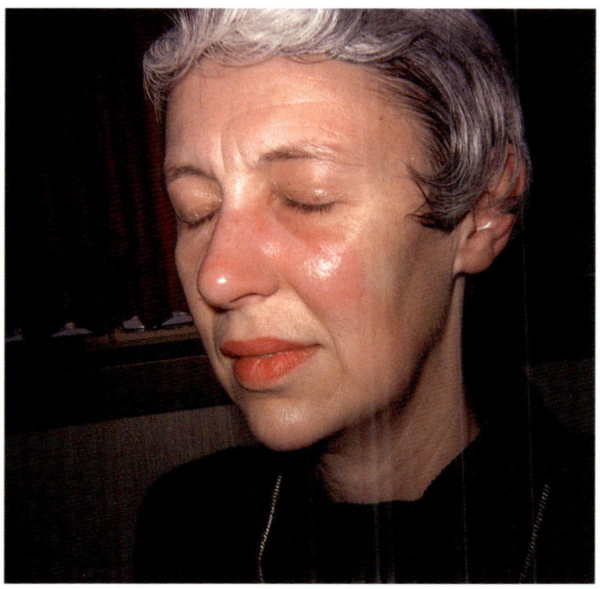

Erysipelas

Figure 12–25. Bacterial cellulitis. Streptococcal infection of the face, commonly referred to as erysipelas. Sharply marginated, warm, erythematous plaque on the face of a woman.

BACTERIAL CELLULITIS (Erysipelas)

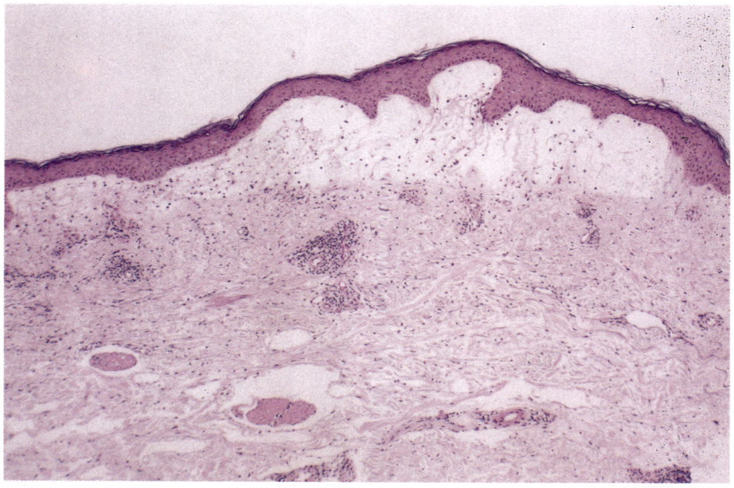

A

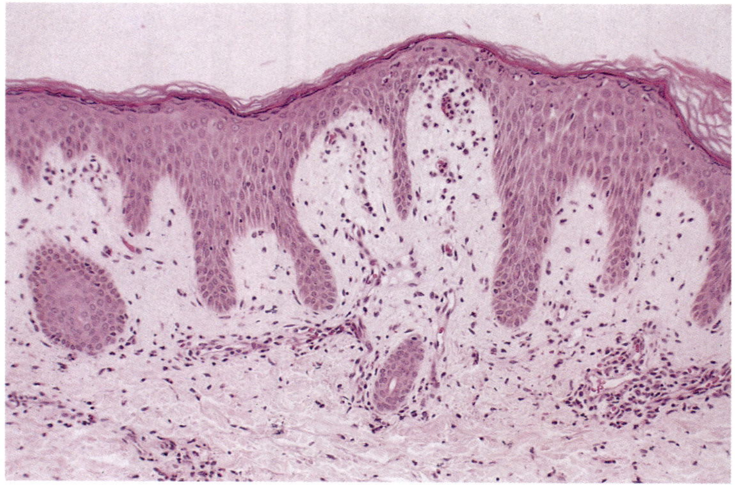

B

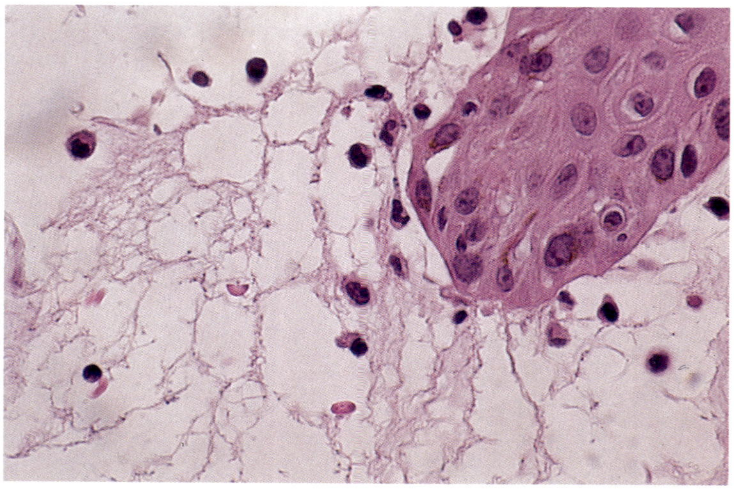

C

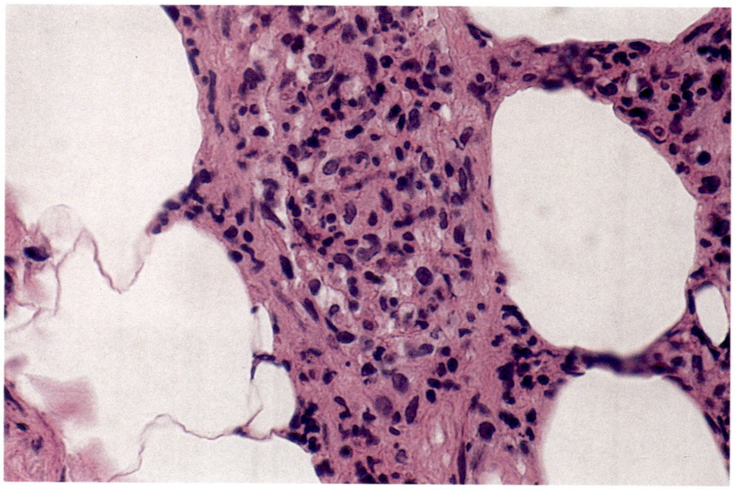

D

Figures 12–26A, 12–26B, 12–26C, 12–26D. Bacterial cellulitis. Severe papillary dermal edema with a superficial and deep perivascular and interstitial mixed-cell infiltrate containing neutrophils.

looks like Sweets but mixed infiltrate

ERYTHRASMA/PITTED KERATOLYSIS

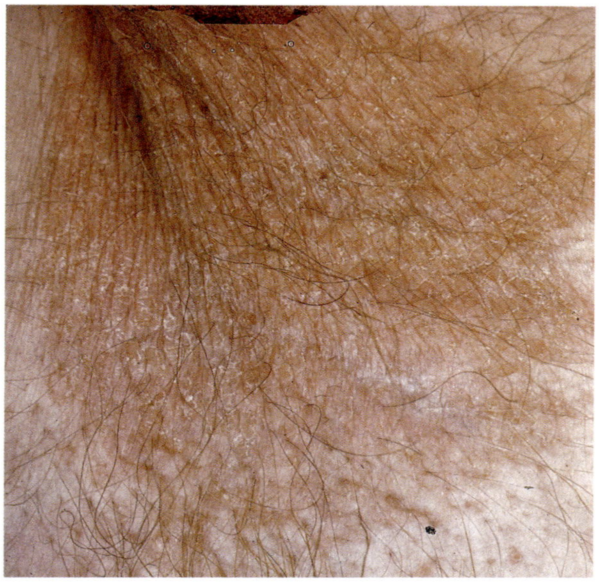

Figure 12–27. Erythrasma. Diffuse reddish-brown scaly patches in the axilla.

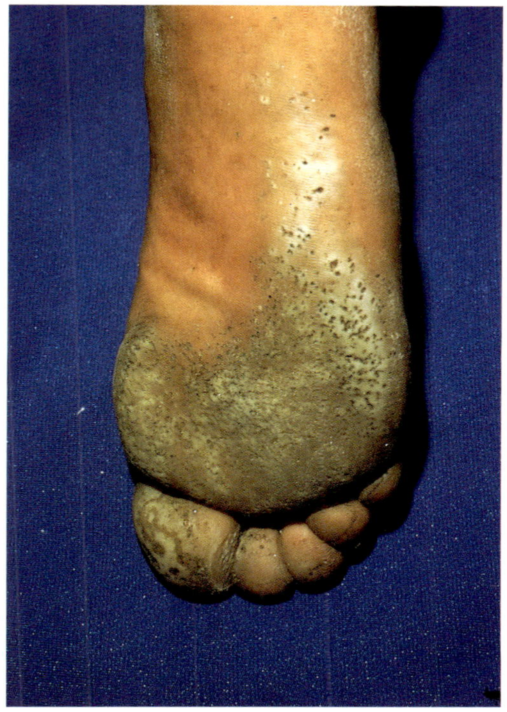

Figure 12–28. Pitted keratolysis. Hyperkeratotic pitted plaques on the sole of the foot.

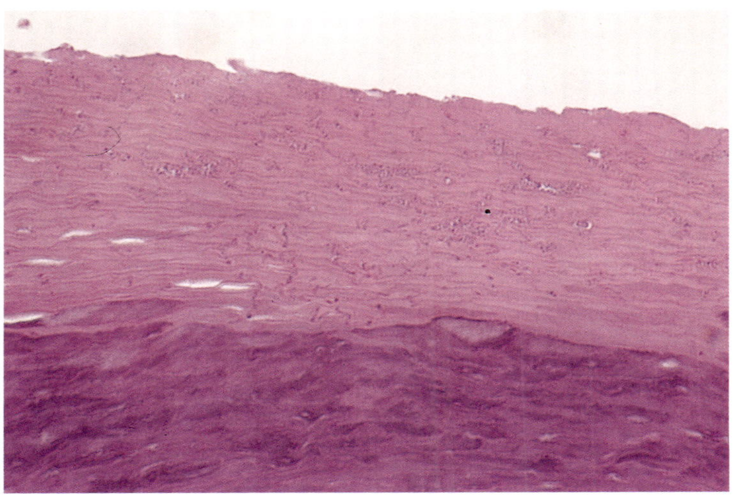

Figure 12–29. Pitted keratolysis. *Corynebacterium* in the cornified layer appear similar in both pitted keratolysis and erythrasma.

GRANULOMA INGUINALE

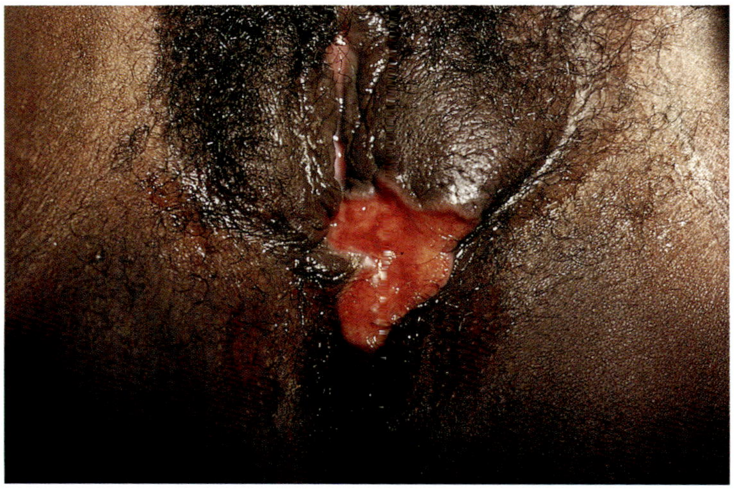

Figure 12–30. Granuloma inguinale. Genital ulcer with exuberant, beefy-red granulation tissue and raised irregular margins.

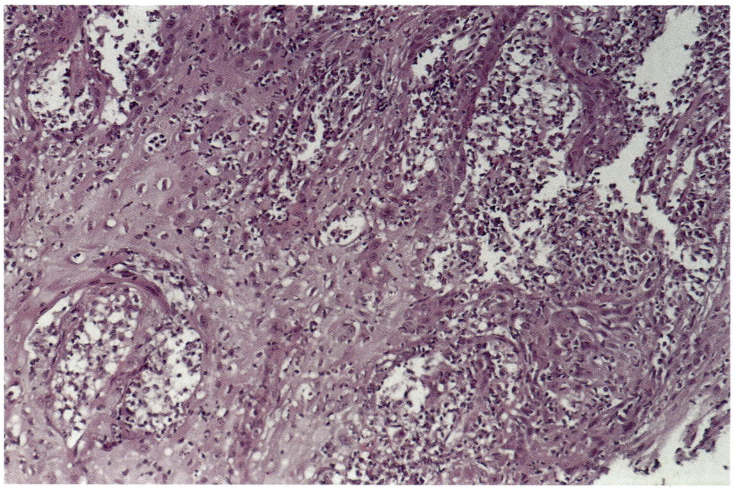

Figure 12–31. Granuloma inguinale. Mixed-cell infiltrate with lymphocytes, plasma cells, histiocytic cells, and neutrophils.

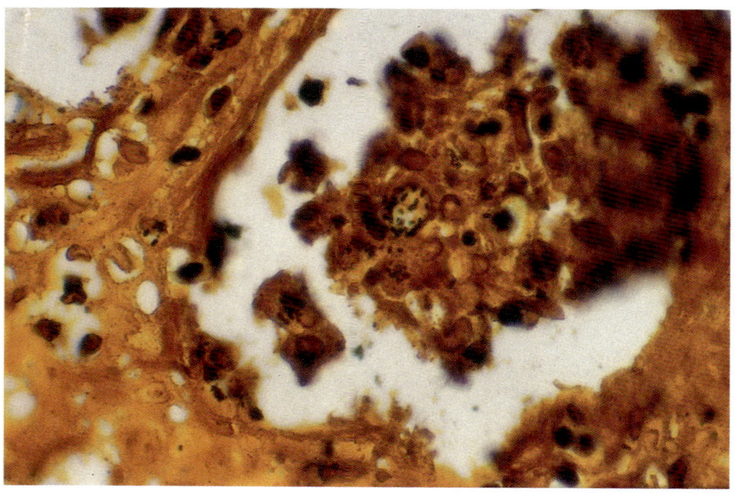

Figure 12–32. Granuloma inguinale. Silver stain shows the black, oval, intracytoplasmic bacilli (Donovan's bodies), resembling a safety pin.

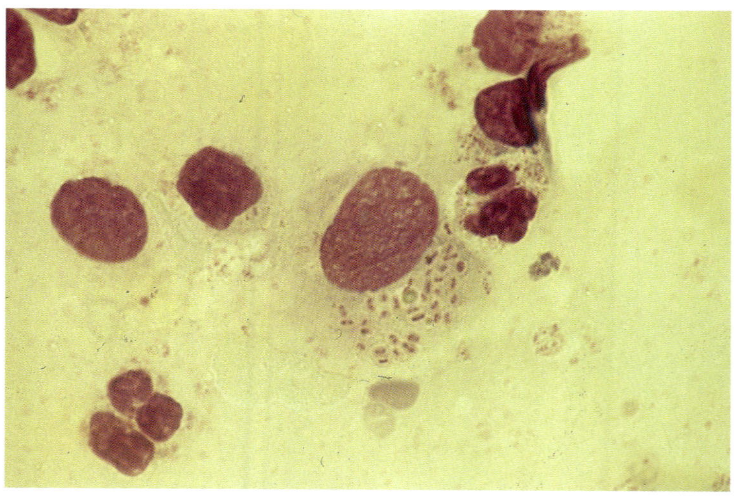

Figure 12–33. Granuloma inguinale. Giemsa stain shows the oval red intracytoplasmic bacilli (Donovan's bodies), resembling a safety pin.

LOCALIZED SEPTIC VASCULITIS

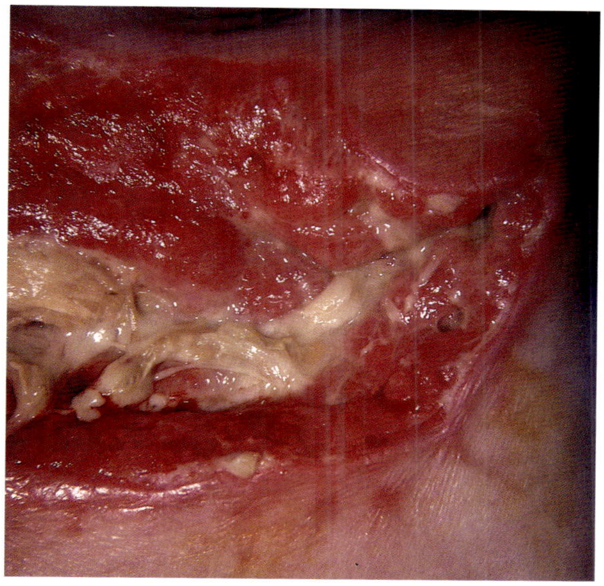

Figure 12–34. Localized septic vasculitis. Painful, recalcitrant, expanding ulcer in the groin. There is necrotic purulent debris centrally and beefy-red, undermined, raised margins peripherally. This lesion is referred to clinically as necrotic cellulitis and is caused by a persistent bacterial infection, usually a gram-negative rod.

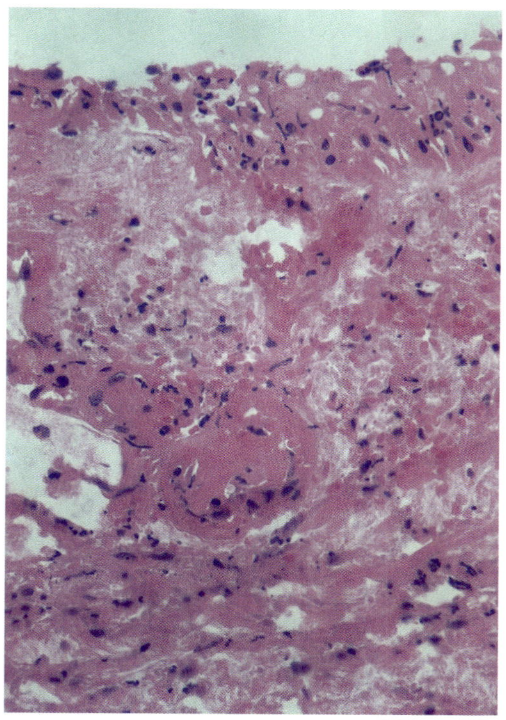

Figure 12–35. Localized septic vasculitis. There are altered dermal venules with fibrin thrombi, neutrophils, nuclear dust, and extravasated erythrocytes. This represents a form of septic vasculitis.

SYSTEMIC SEPTIC VASCULITIS

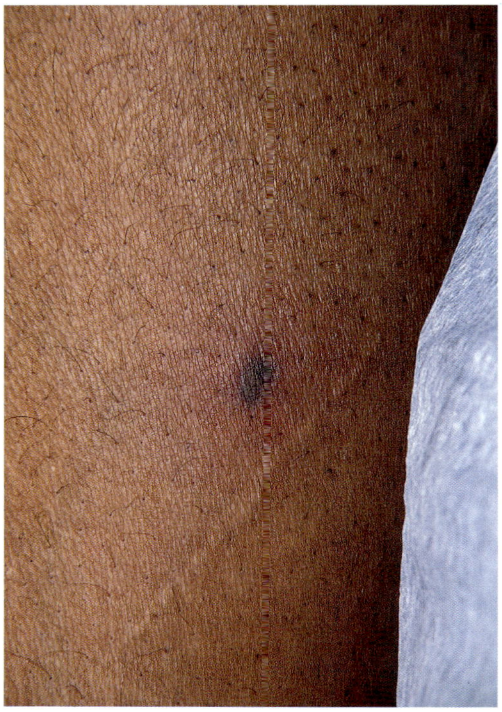

Figure 12–36. **Systemic septic vasculitis, gonococcemia.** There is a purpuric papule with surrounding erythema on the lower leg.

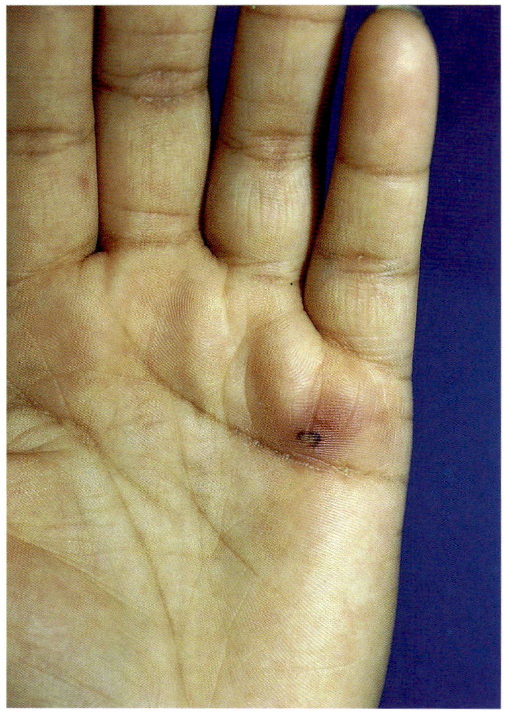

Figure 12–37. **Systemic septic vasculitis, gonococcemia.** On the palm there is a central gray violaceous macule with surrounding erythema.

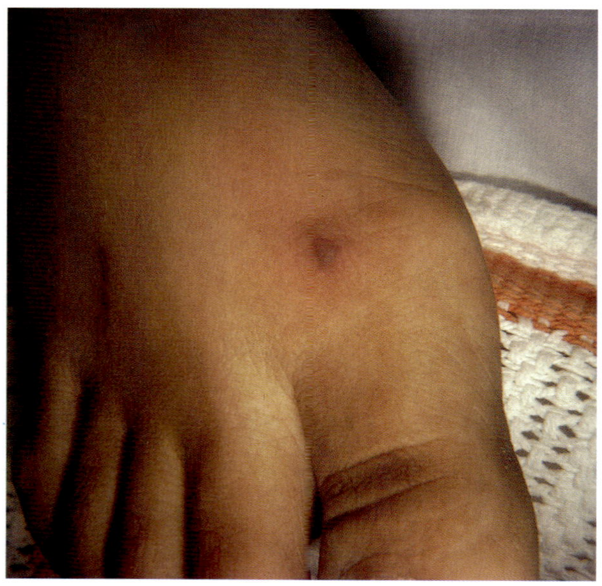

Figure 12–38. **Systemic septic vasculitis, meningococcemia.** Purpuric vesiculopapules on the toe.

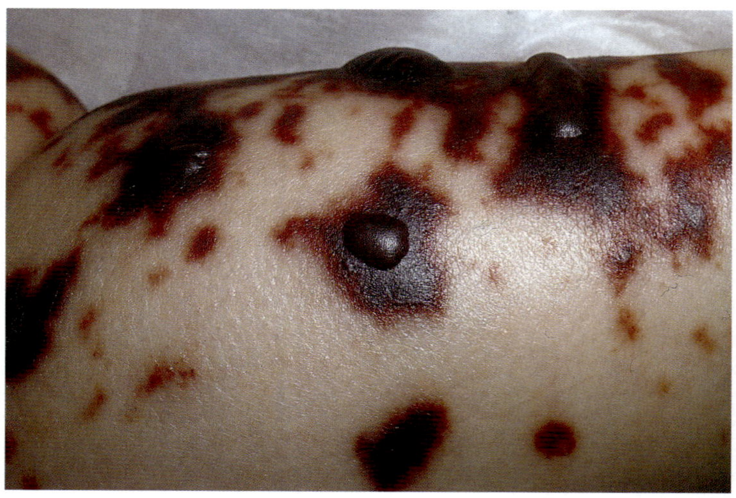

Figure 12–39. **Systemic septic vasculitis, meningococcemia.** Acute, generalized purpuric patches and hemorrhagic blisters in a child moribund with acute meningococcemia and disseminated intravascular coagulation.

SYSTEMIC SEPTIC VASCULITIS

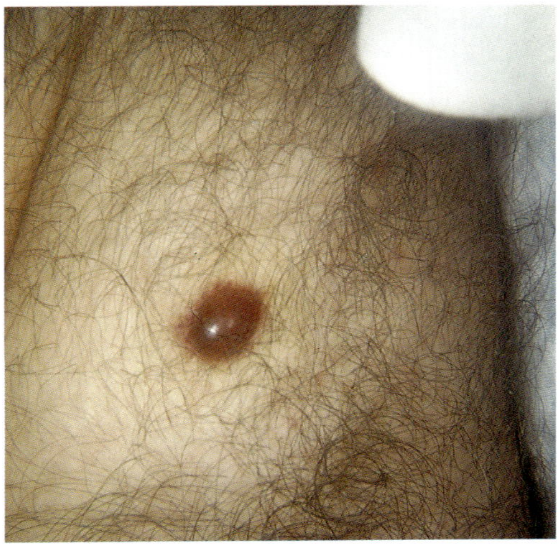

Figure 12–40. Systemic septic vasculitis, staphylococcal septicemia. Erythematous nodule on the arm of a man with a history of spiking fevers, chills, arthralgias, and myalgias.

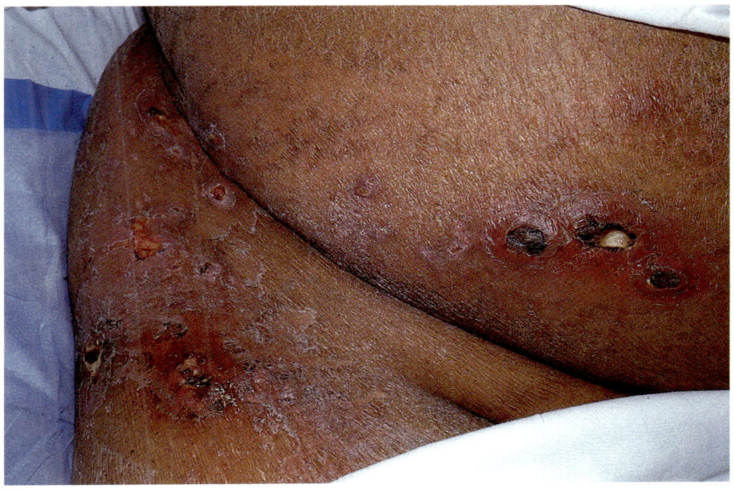

Figure 12–41. Systemic septic vasculitis, *Pseudomonas* septicemia. Multiple nodules on the buttocks with ulceration and purulent exudate. Some lesions have a thick, black crust with peripheral edematous, raised margins. This condition is commonly referred to as ecthyma gangrenosum.

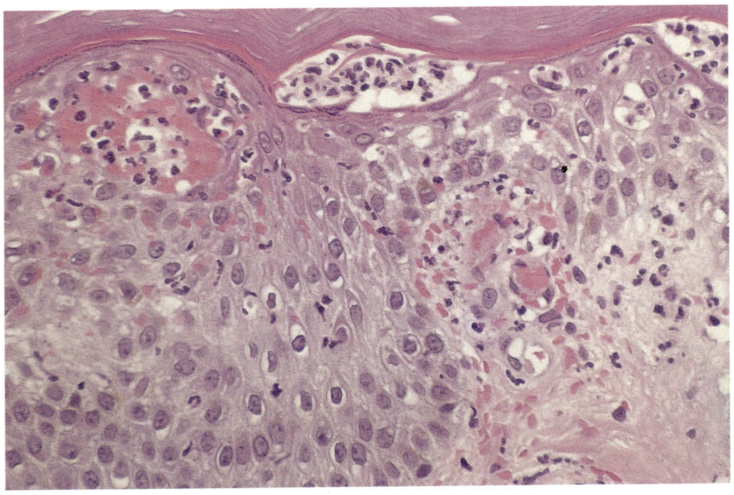

A

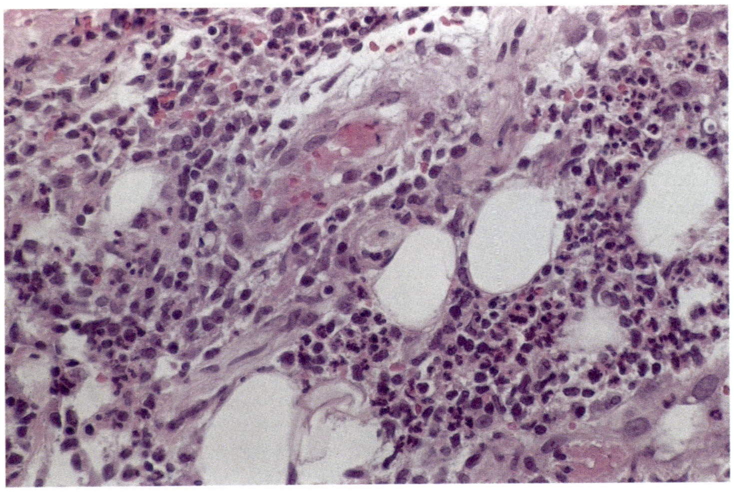

B

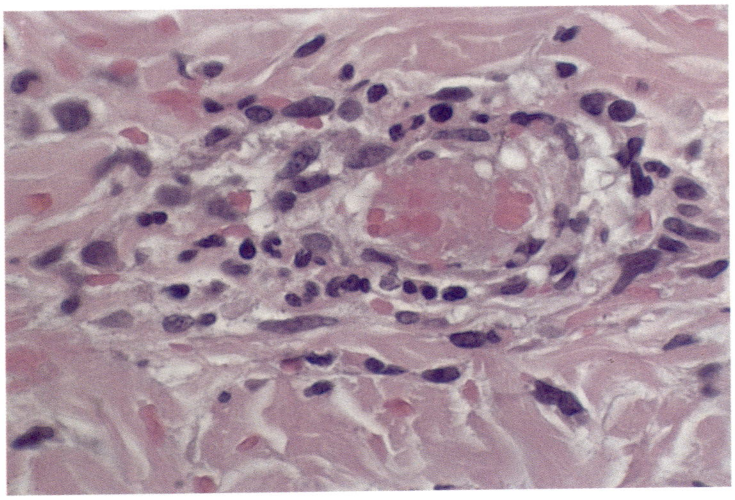

C

Figures 12–42A, 12–42B, 12–42C. Systemic septic vasculitis. Fibrin thrombi occlude superficial and deep dermal vessels. There is a diffuse dermal mixed-cell infiltrate with neutrophils, nuclear fragments, and extravasated erythrocytes. In the epidermis there is spongiosis, necrotic keratinocytes, neutrophils, and red blood cells.

13

Rickettsial and Chlamydial Infections

- African tick bite fever
- Lymphogranuloma venereum

AFRICAN TICK BITE FEVER

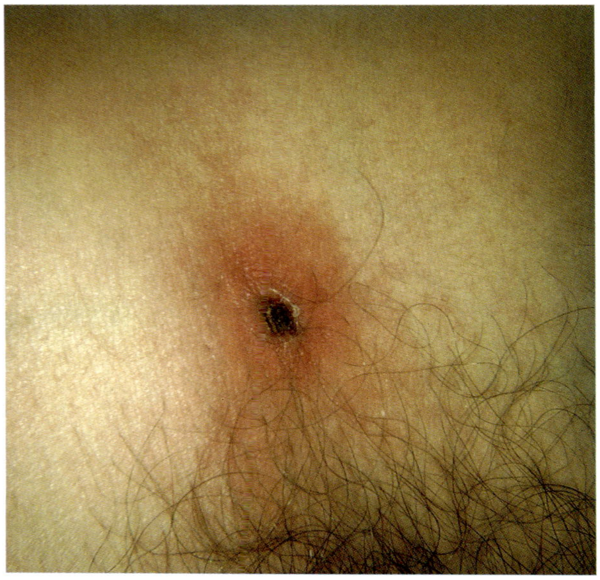

Figure 13–1. African tick bite fever. Crusted central ulceration with prominent surrounding erythema in the groin of a man with generalized malaise and fever. He was on safari in Africa, and had seen and had been bitten by ticks on many occasions.

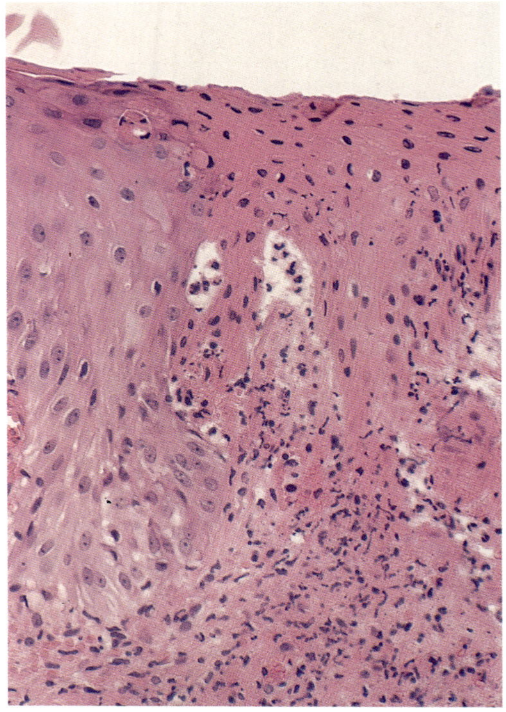

Figure 13–2. African tick bite fever. Epidermal ulceration and necrotic keratinocytes. Many neutrophils and nuclear fragments fill the subjacent dermis.

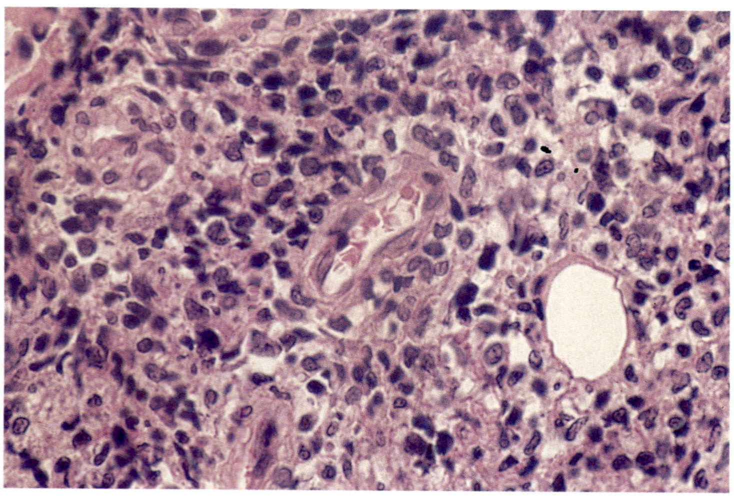

Figure 13–3. African tick bite fever. Blood vessel ectasia and a diffuse lymphohistiocytic infiltrate.

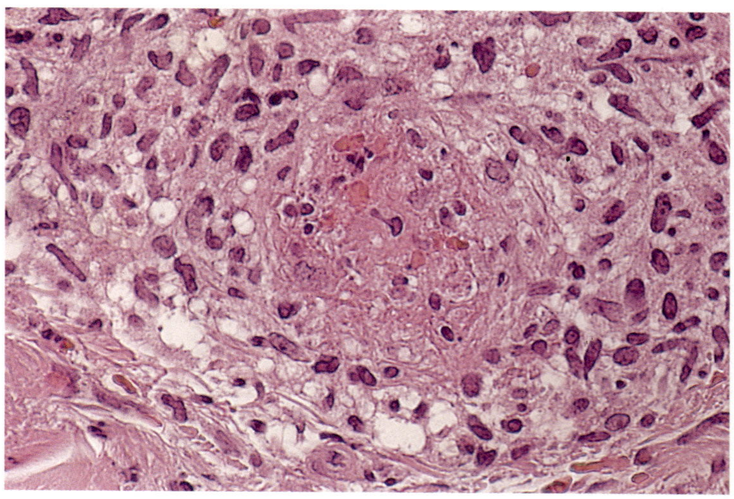

Figure 13–4. African tick bite fever, lymphocytic vasculitis. There is a fibrin thrombus in the lumen, fibrin within the wall of the venule, and a dense mononuclear cell infiltrate.

LYMPHOGRANULOMA VENEREUM

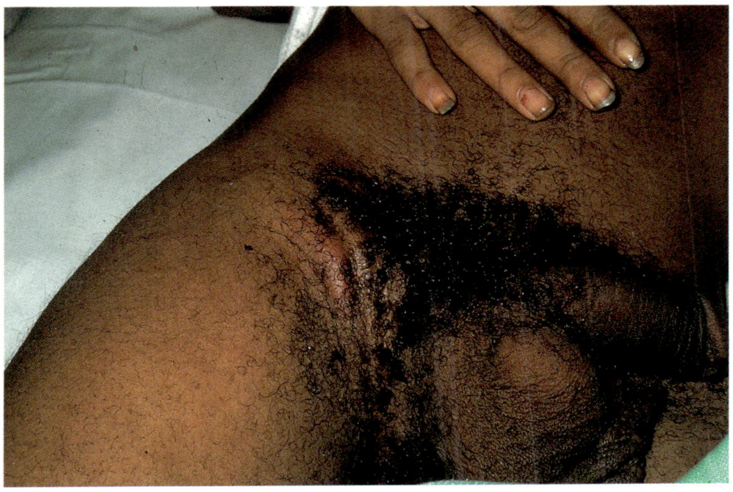

Figure 13–5. Lymphogranuloma venereum. Unilateral inguinal lymphadenopathy resulting in the so-called "grooves in the groin" lesion characteristic of this disease.

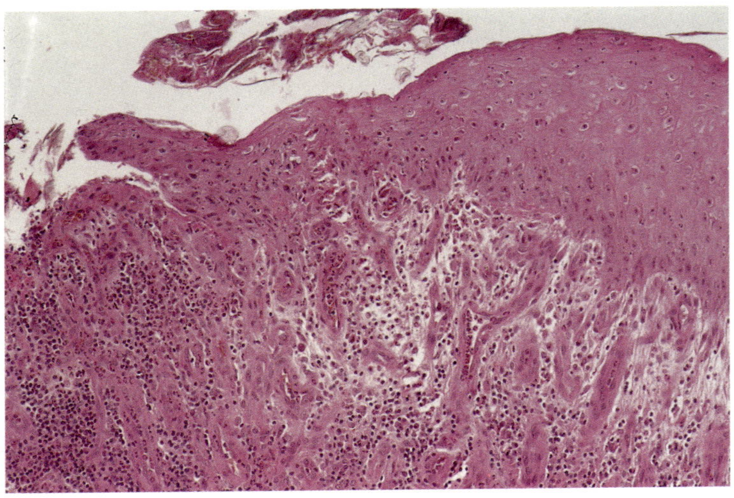

A

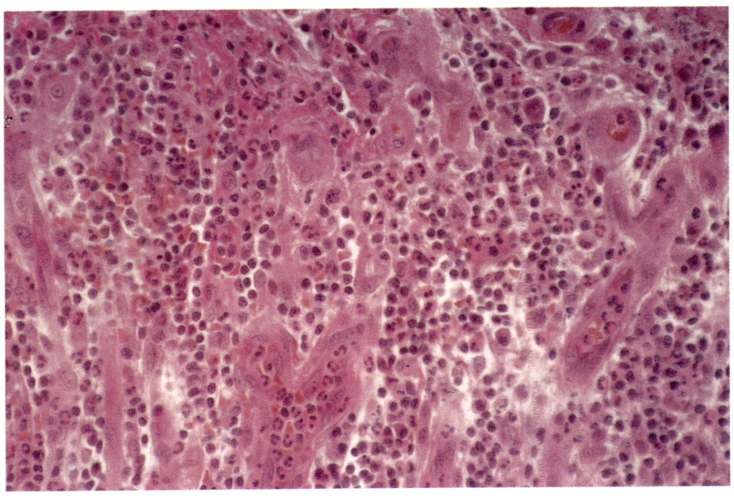

B

Figures 13–6A, 13–6B. Lymphogranuloma venereum. Epidermal ulceration, dilated blood vessels, and a mixed-cell infiltrate. There is a diffuse infiltrate of neutrophils, plasma cells, and mononuclear cells.

14

MYCOBACTERIAL INFECTIONS

- Tuberculosis
- Leprosy
- Atypical mycobacterial infections

TUBERCULOSIS

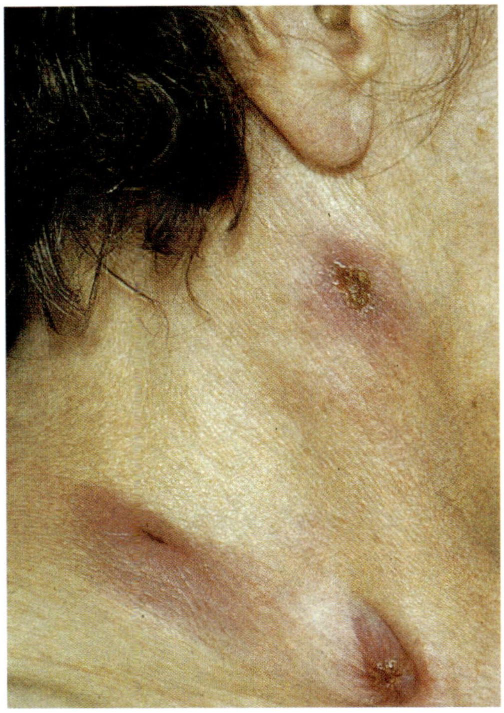

Figure 14–1. Scrofuloderma. Enlarged cervical lymph nodes with overlying erythema and draining sinus tracts.

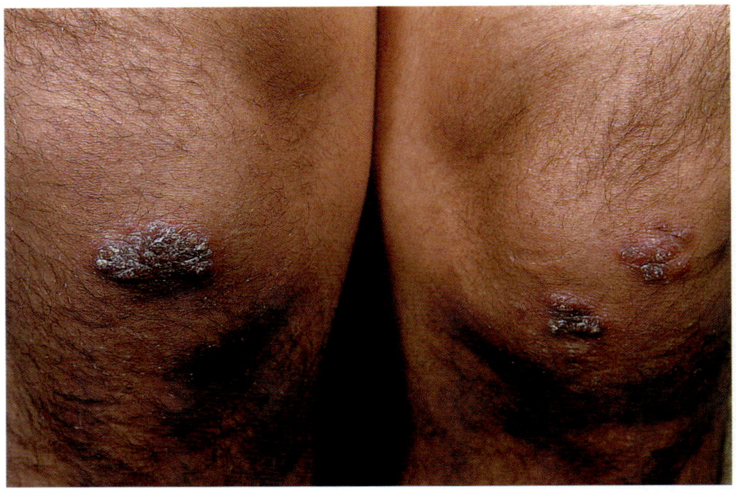

Figure 14–2. Tuberculosis verrucosa. Multiple verrucous nodules on the knees.

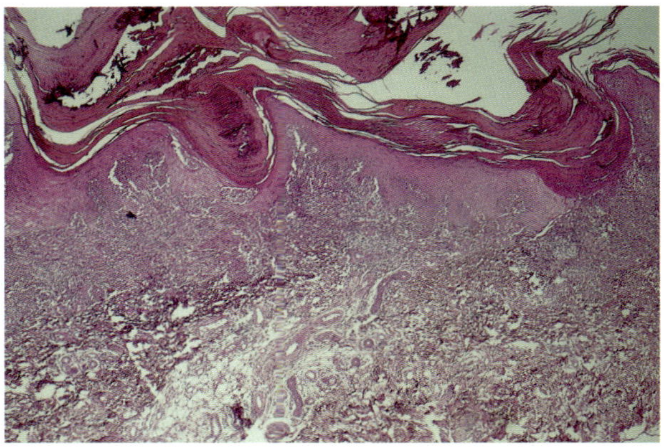

A

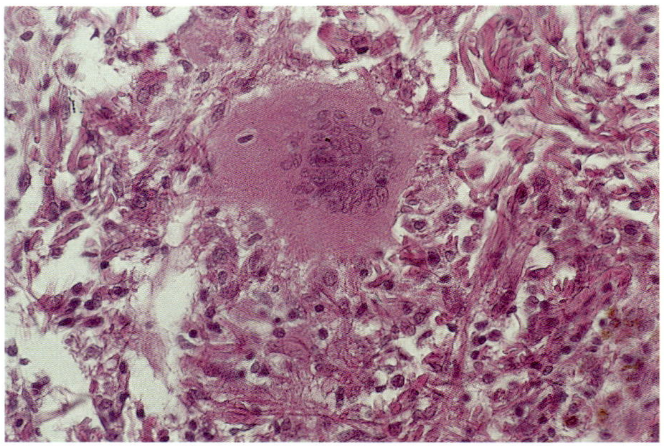

B

Figures 14–3A, 14–3B. Tuberculosis verrucosa. Epidermal hyperplasia, hyperkeratosis, and a granulomatous infiltrate. Multinucleated histiocytic giant cell is within the dermal tuberculoid granuloma.

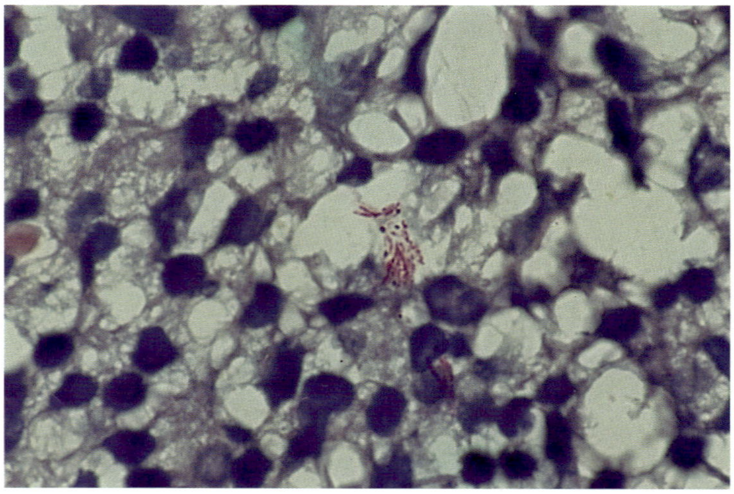

Figure 14–4. Tuberculosis. Ziehl-Neelsen acid-fast stain demonstrates slender, red bacilli within histiocytic cells.

LEPROSY

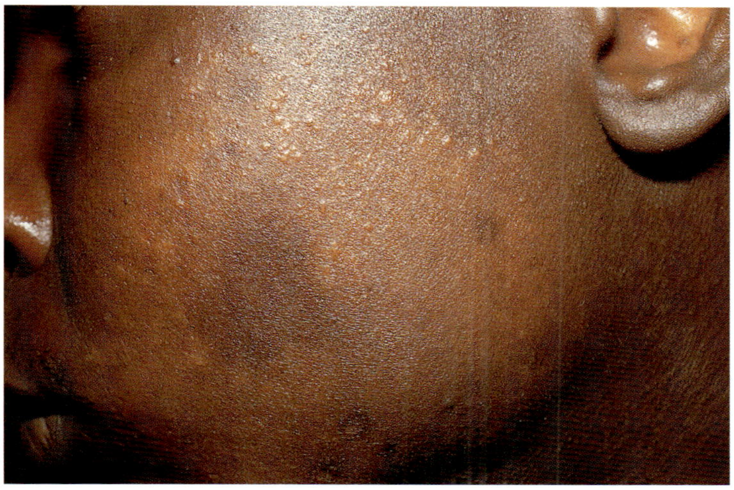

Figure 14–5. Tuberculoid leprosy. Anesthetic, scaly, hyperpigmented patch on the cheek of a man.

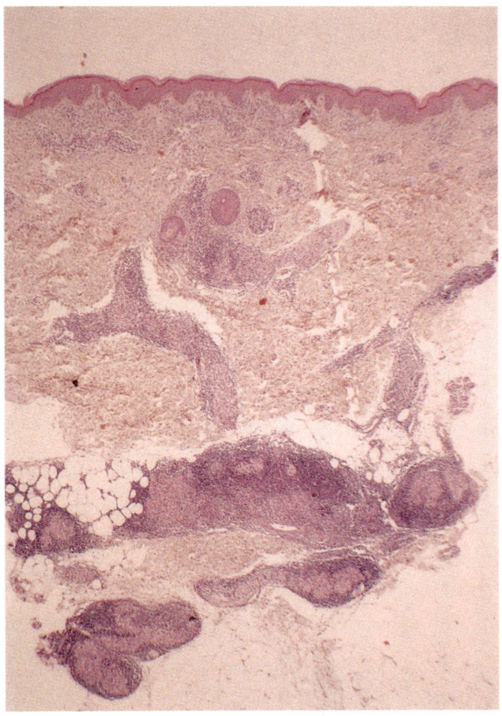

A

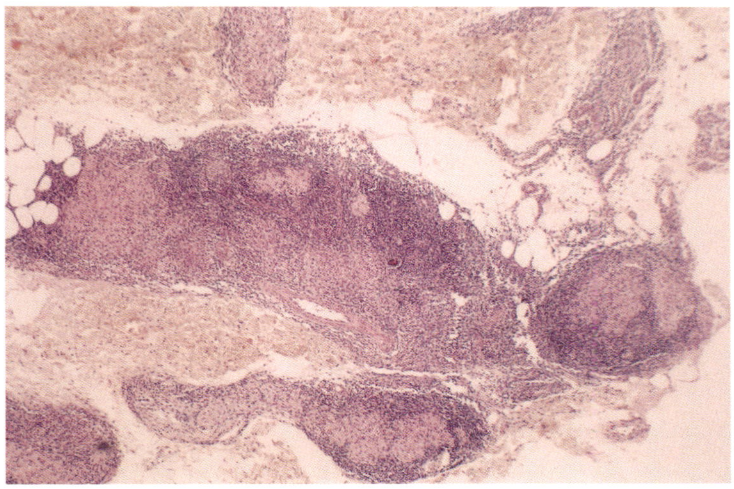

B

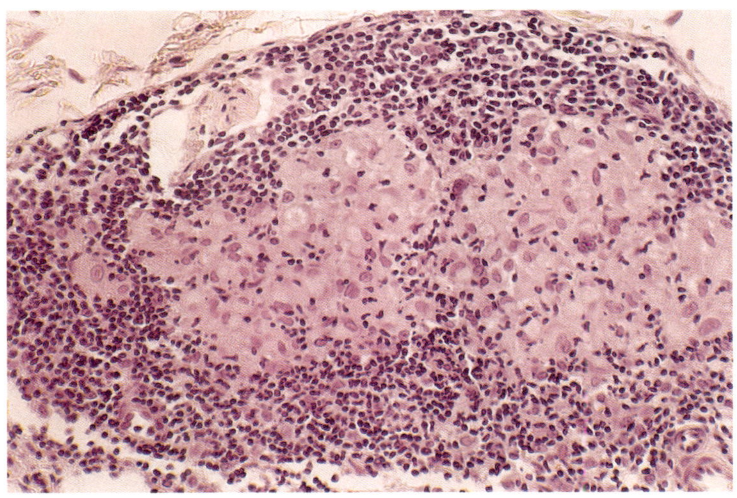

C

Figures 14–6A, 14–6B, 14–6C. Tuberculoid leprosy. Nodular granulomas surrounding nerve fascicles. Pale histiocytic cells clearly surrounded by numerous dark-staining lymphocytes involving a dermal nerve fascicle.

LEPROSY

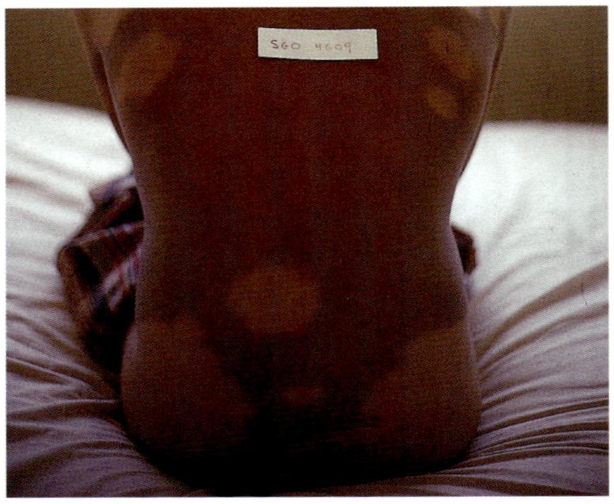

Figure 14–7. Borderline leprosy. Hypopigmented, anesthetic, irregular, circular scaly patches on the back and buttocks of a young boy.

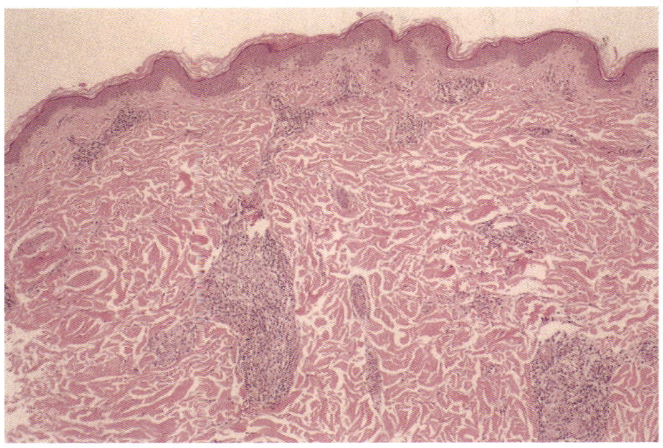

A

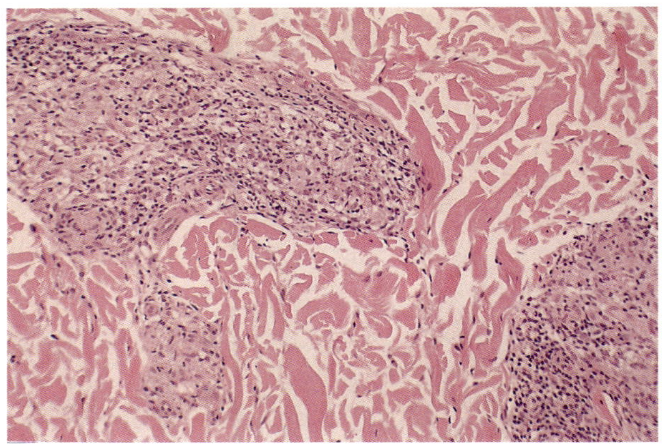

B

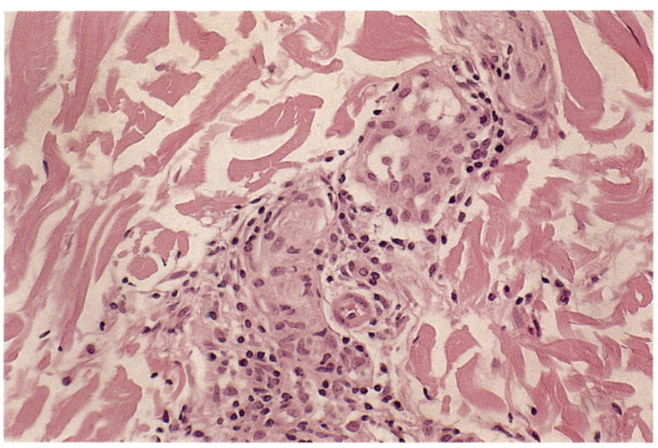

C

Figures 14–8A, 14–8B, 14–8C. Borderline leprosy. Elongated nodular granulomas in the dermis following nerve fascicles. There is a diffuse sprinkling of lymphocytes among the pale-staining histiocytic cells.

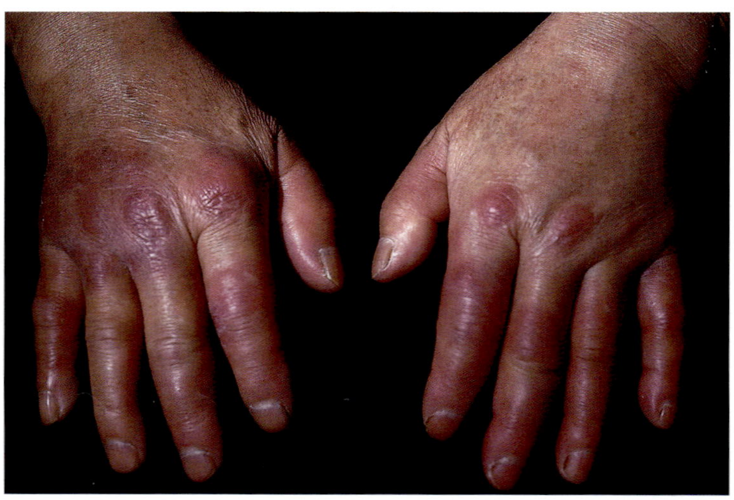

Figure 14–9. Lepromatous leprosy. Anesthetic, erythematous nodules and plaques on the dorsum of the hands, including the knuckles and fingers.

LEPROSY

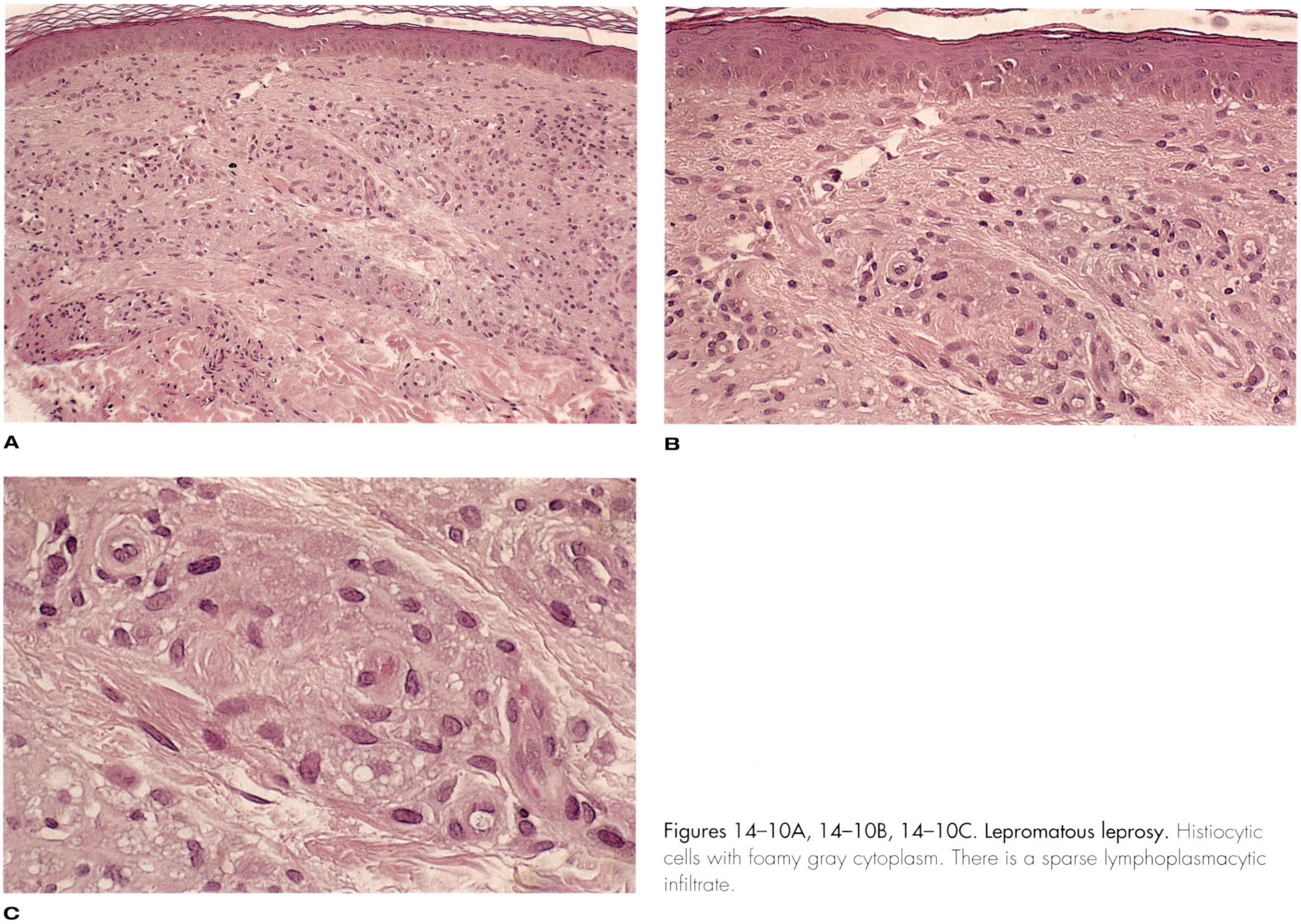

Figures 14–10A, 14–10B, 14–10C. **Lepromatous leprosy.** Histiocytic cells with foamy gray cytoplasm. There is a sparse lymphoplasmacytic infiltrate.

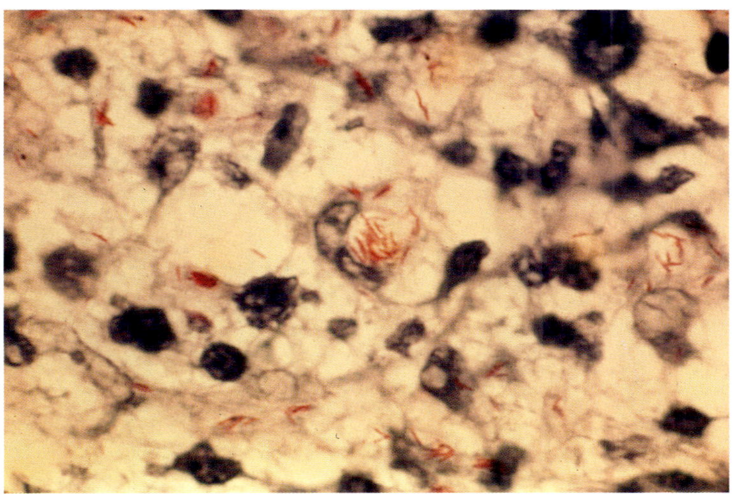

Figure 14–11. **Lepromatous leprosy.** Fite stain shows the leprosy bacilli within histiocytic cells.

ATYPICAL MYCOBACTERIAL INFECTIONS

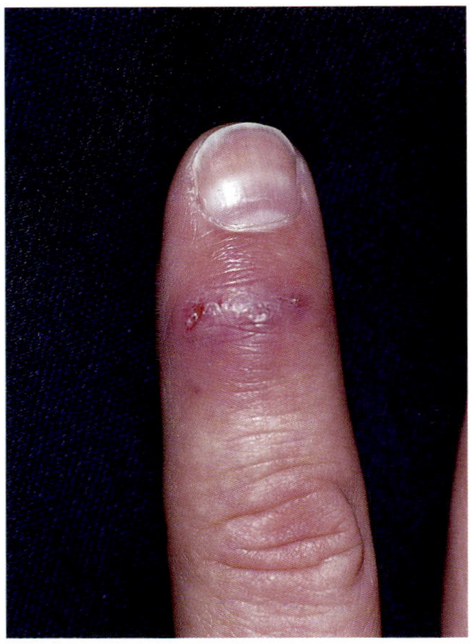

Figure 14–12. *Mycobacterium marinum* infection. Erythematous nodule with ulceration and crust on the finger. This atypical mycobacterial infection is also known as a swimming-pool granuloma.

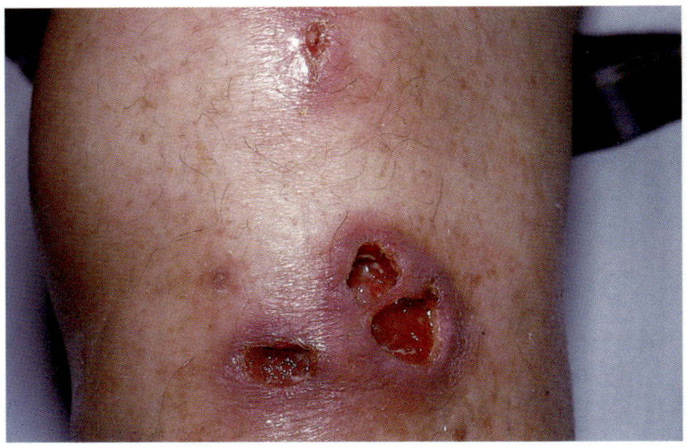

Figure 14–13. *Mycobacterium chelonei* infection. Erythematous, coalescing, deep noduloulcerative abscesses on the leg.

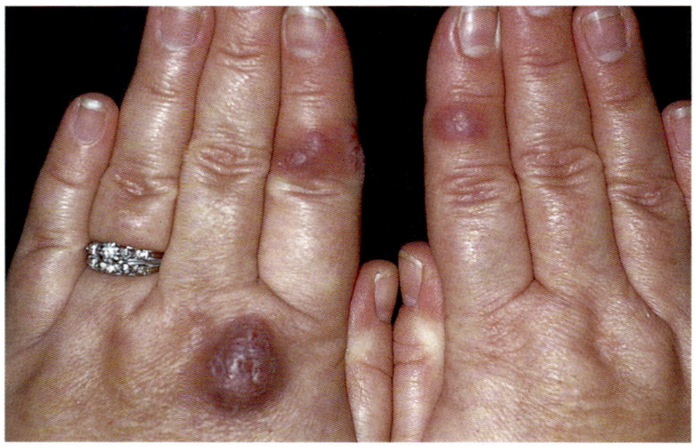

A

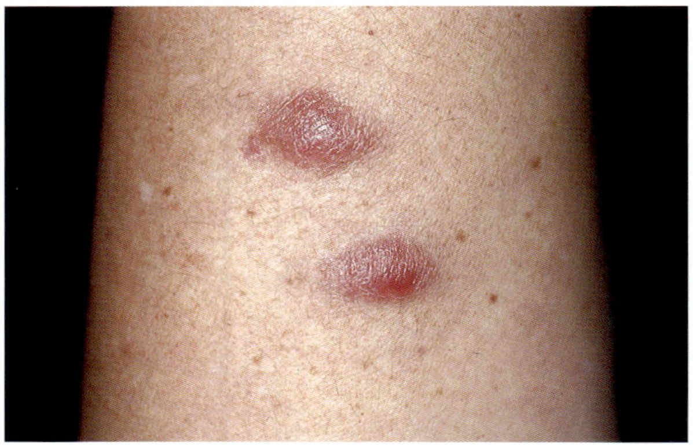

B

Figures 14–14A, 14–14B. *Mycobacterium kansasii* infection. Multiple dusky-red and erythematous papules and nodules on the hand, fingers, and arms.

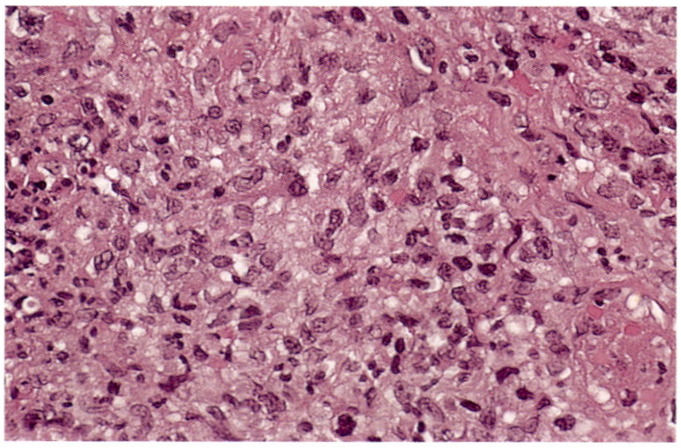

Figure 14–15. Atypical mycobacterial infection. Characteristic dense dermal mixed-cell infiltrate. There are neutrophils, lymphocytes and sheets of histiocytic cells with foamy gray cytoplasm.

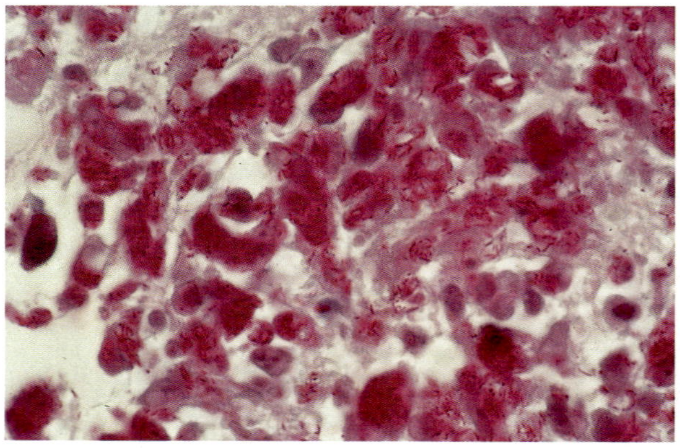

Figure 14–16. *Mycobacterium avium-intracellulare*. Ziehl-Neelsen acid-fast stain illustrates copious red bacilli in an immunocompromised patient with AIDS.

15

Spirochetal infections

- Syphilis
- Lyme disease

SYPHILIS

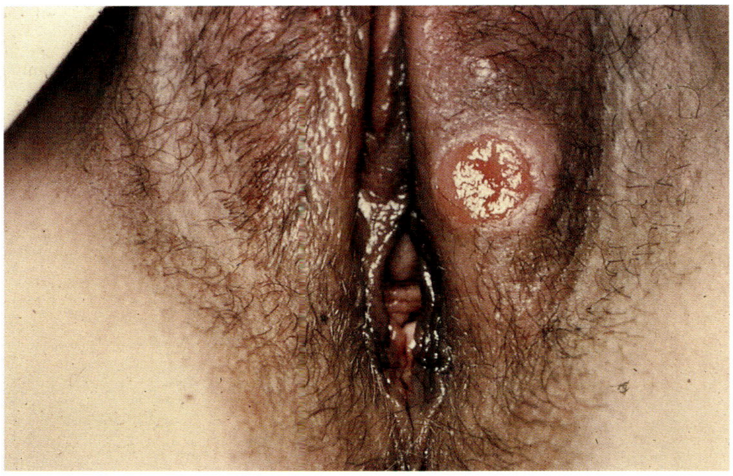

Figure 15–1. Primary syphilis Painless ulcerated nodule on the labia majora. This lesion is commonly referred to as a chancre and is usually teeming with spirochetes.

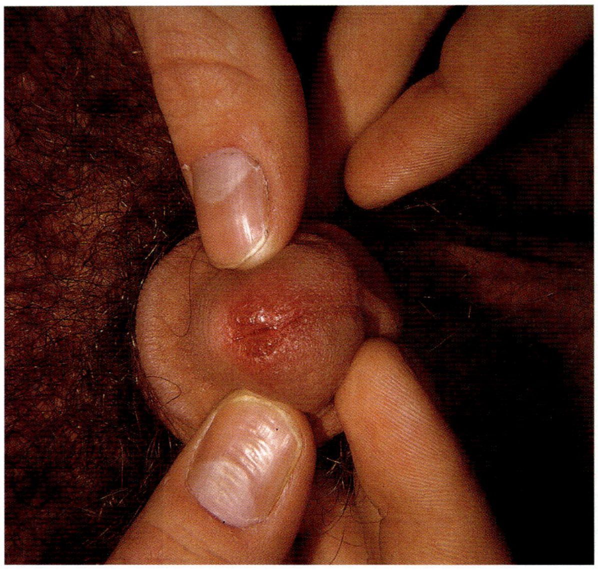

Figure 15–2. Primary syphilis. Painless ulcerated papule on the penis involving the urethral orifice.

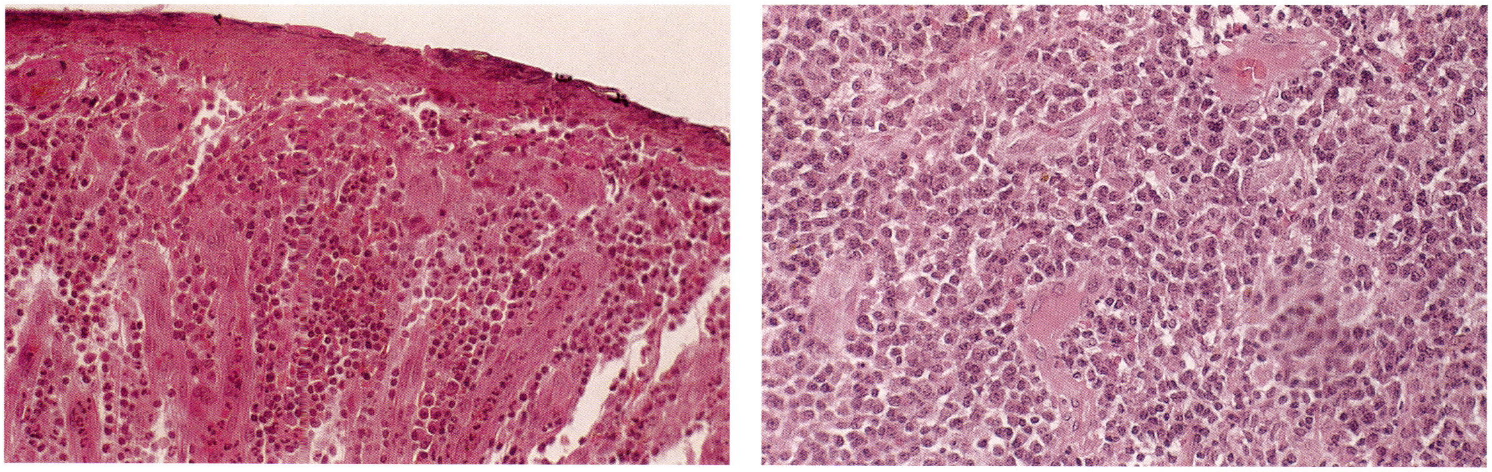

A

B

Figures 15–3A, 15–3B. Primary syphilis. Dense infiltrate of plasma cells and dilated blood vessels. There is epidermal ulceration with crust; neutrophils are present within the predominantly plasmocytic infiltrate.

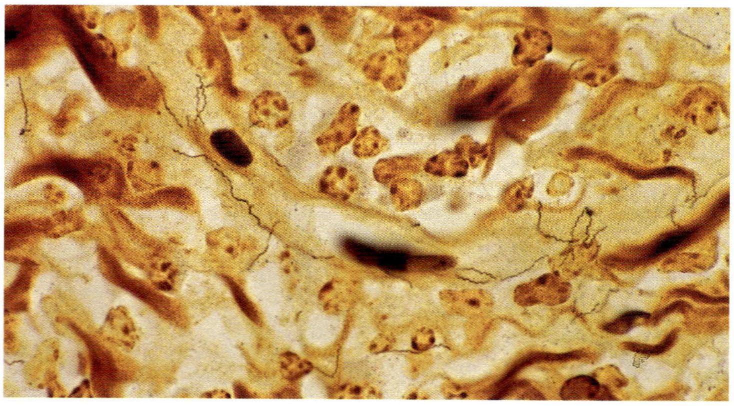

Figure 15–4. Primary syphilis. *Treponema pallidum* in the dermis. The Warthin-Starry stain colors the spirochetes black and emphasizes the spiral coils.

SYPHILIS

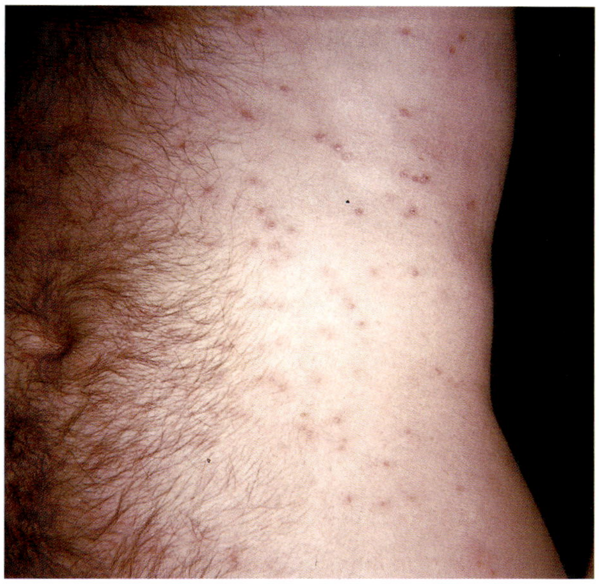

A

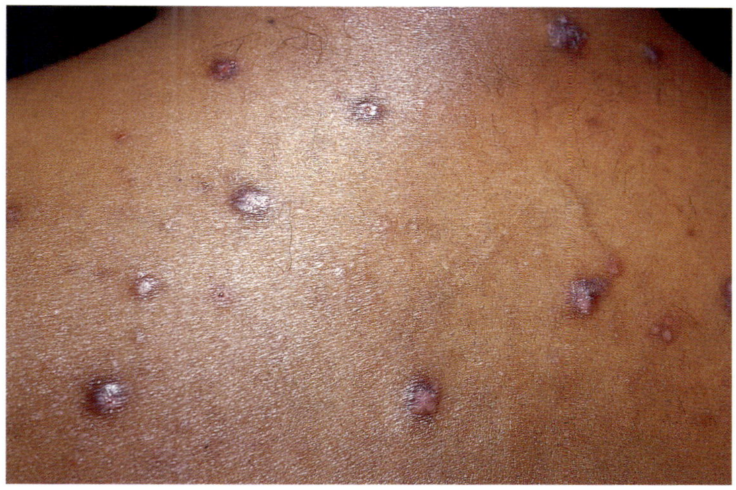

B

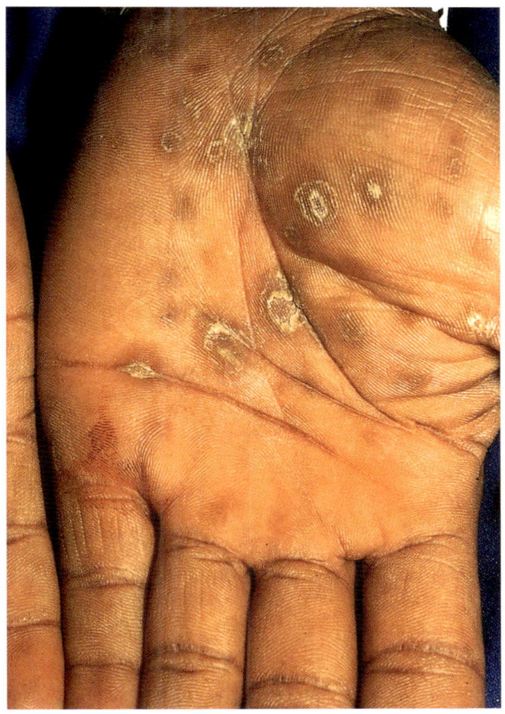

C

Figures 15–5A, 15–5B, 15–5C. Secondary syphilis. Scaly erythematous and hyperpigmented macules and papules on the trunk, back, and palm of the hand.

SYPHILIS

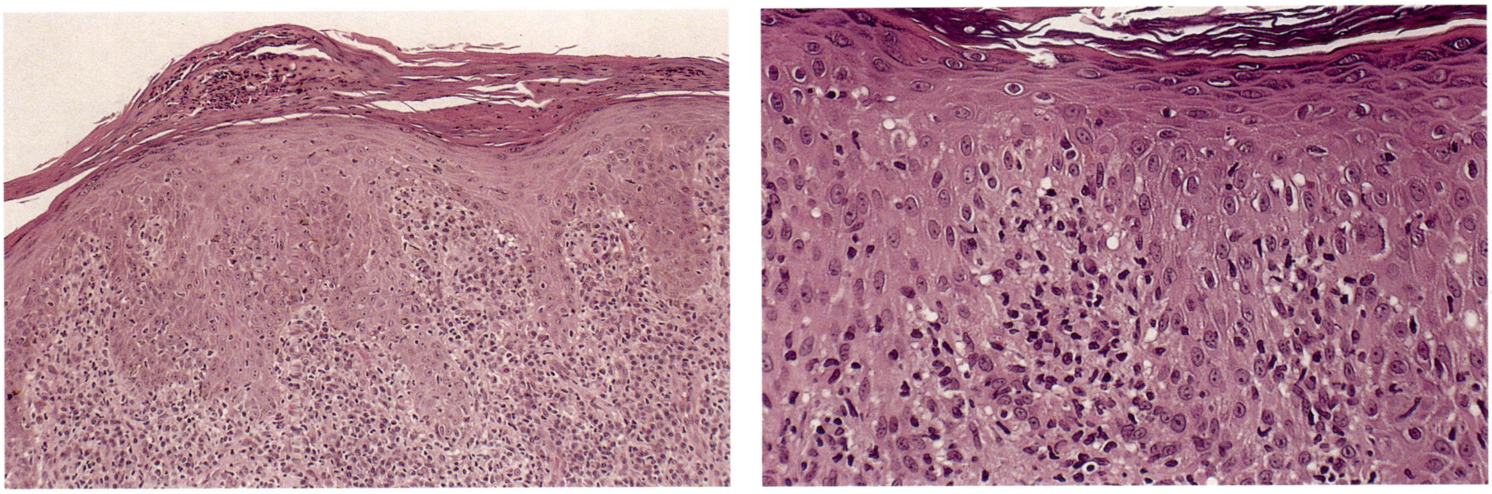

A B

Figures 15–6A, 15–6B. Secondary syphilis, early stage. Psoriasiform lichenoid dermatitis. There are neutrophils within the hyperplastic epidermis and parakeratotic stratum corneum. There is a predominance of pale histiocytic cells and plasma cells in a lichenoid array within the thickened papillary dermis.

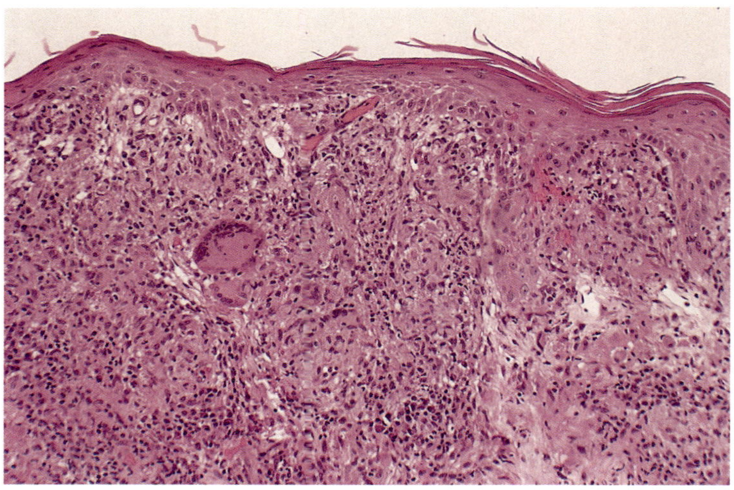

Figure 15–7. Secondary syphilis, later stage. Granulomatous dermatitis. There are collections of pale-staining histiocytic cells, multinucleated histiocytic giant cells, and plasma cells. These changes may be seen in tertiary syphilis as well.

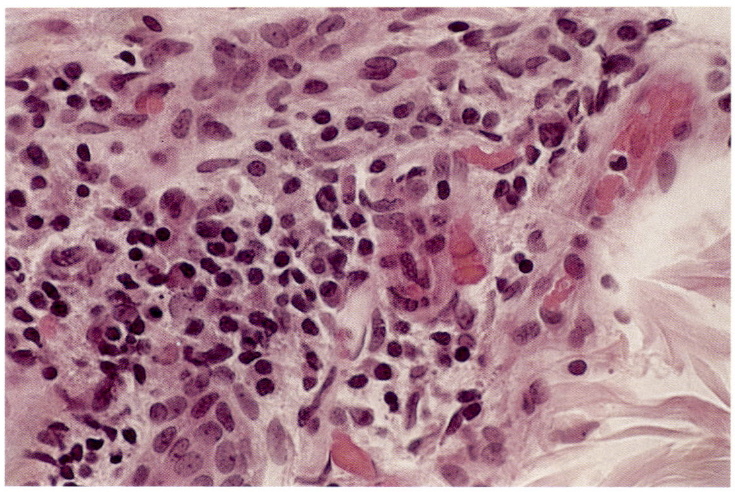

Figure 15–8. Secondary syphilis. Plasma cells, histiocytic cells, and congested blood vessels with plump endothelial cells.

SYPHILIS

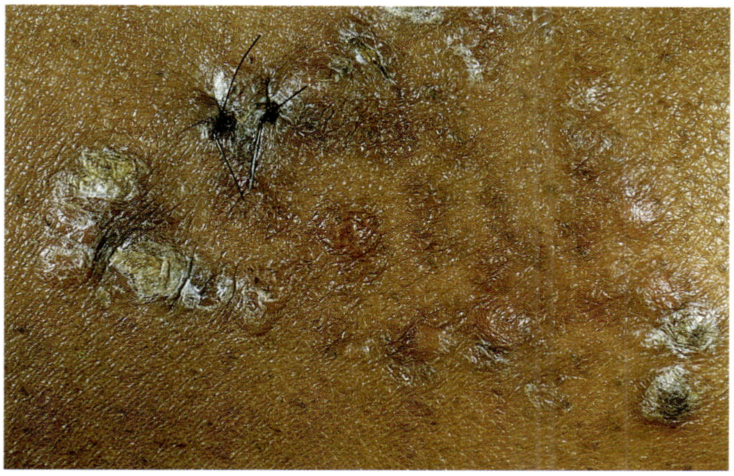

Figure 15–9. **Tertiary syphilis.** Irregular-shaped collection of hyperpigmented and reddish-brown scaly papules.

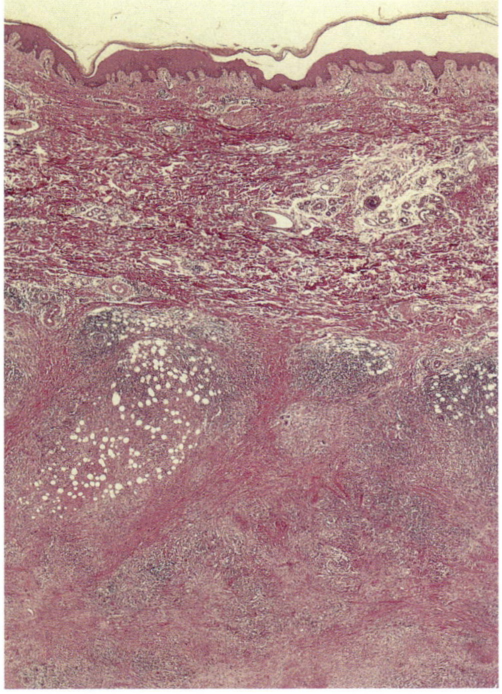

A

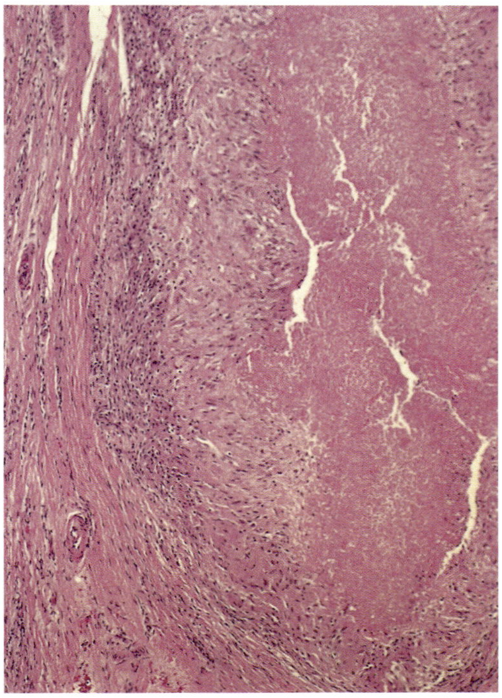

B

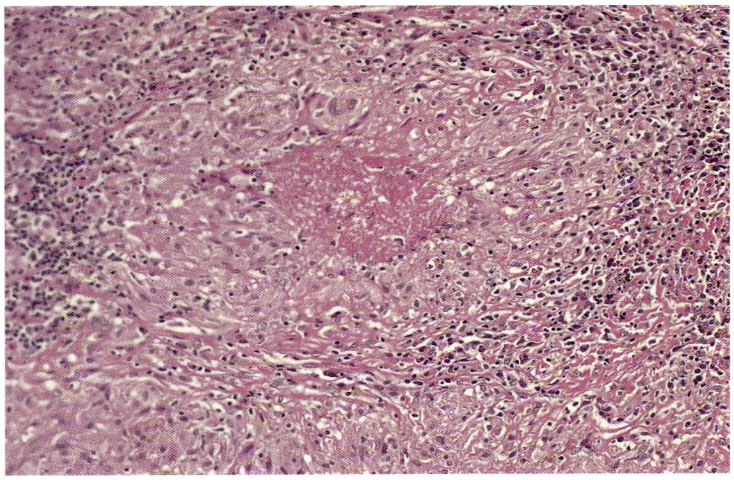

C

Figures 15–10A, 15–10B, 15–10C. **Tertiary syphilis.** Granulomatous and gummatous response. There are lymphocytes, plasma cells, histiocytic cells and multinucleated histiocytic giant cells, vascular ectasia, and fibroplasia positioned around eosinophilic-staining necrotic debris.

LYME DISEASE

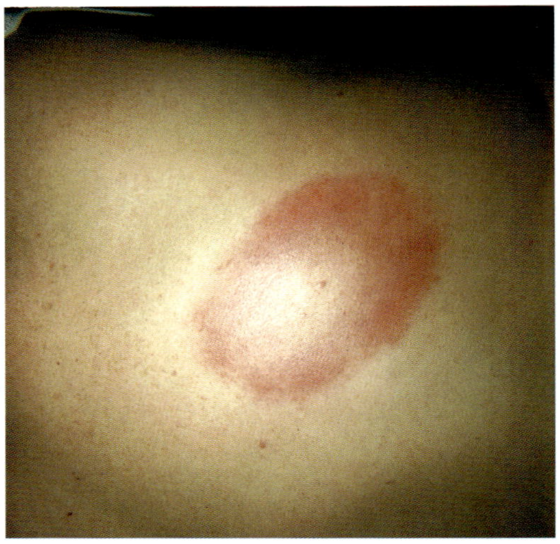

Figure 15–11. Lyme disease. Expanding erythematous plaque on the back of a woman who was bitten by a tick. There is central pallor and a raised puncta at the site of the tick bite. This lesion is commonly referred to as erythema chronica migrans.

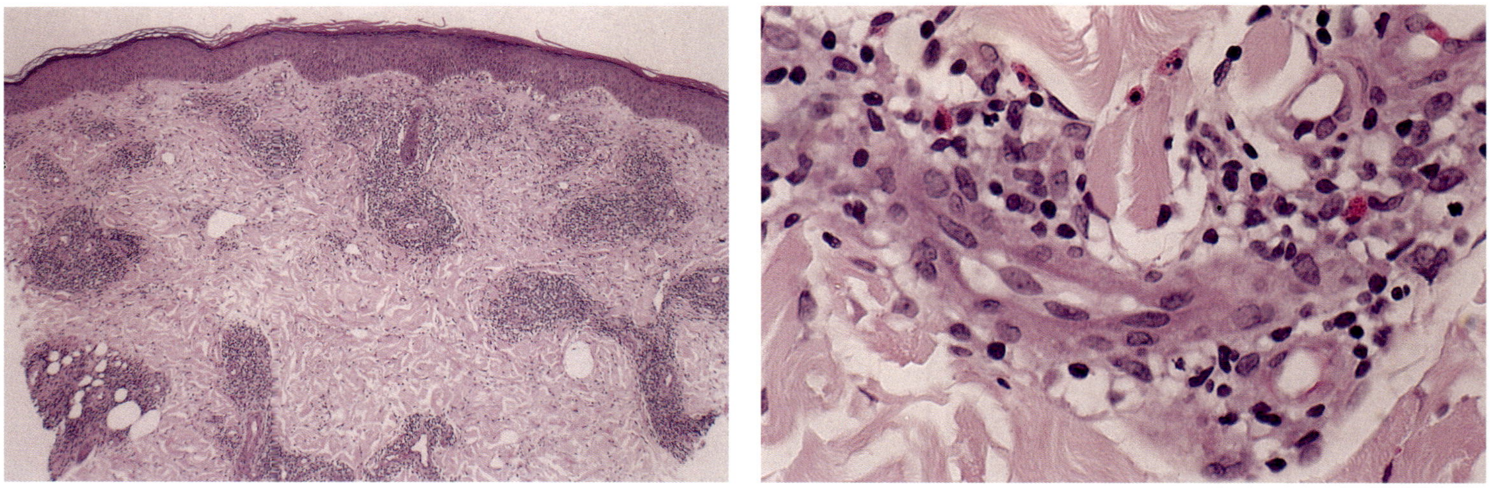

A B

Figures 15–12A, 15–12B. Lyme disease, tick bite site. Dense superficial and deep perivascular and interstitial mixed-cel infiltrate. There are lymphocytes, plasma and histiocytic cells, and eosinophils.

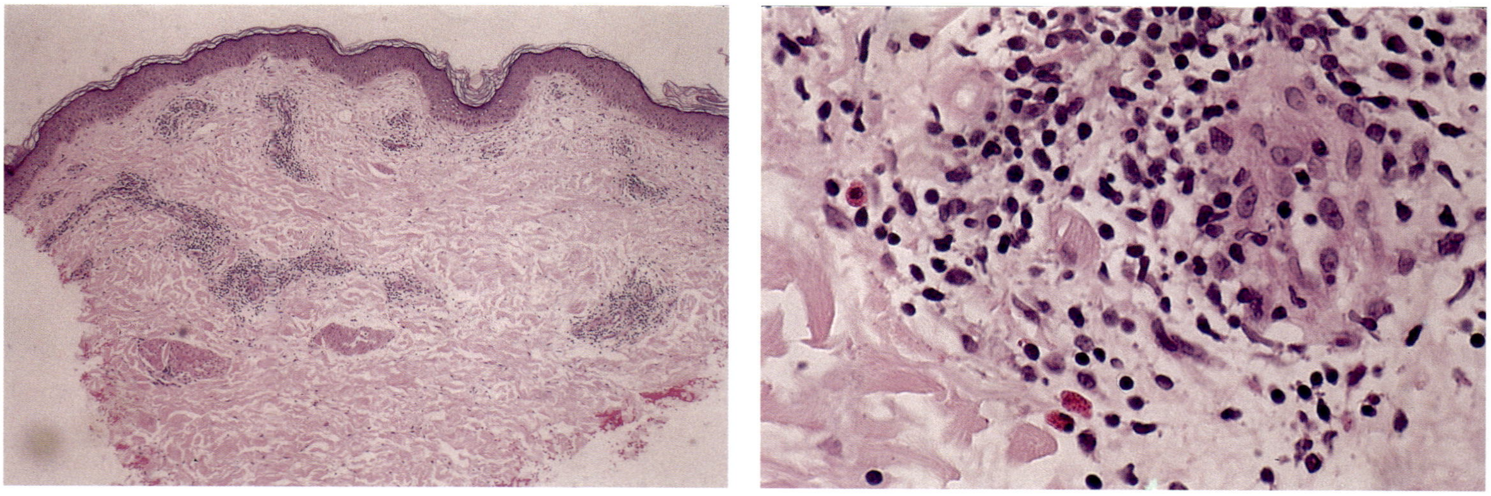

A B

Figures 15–13A, 15–13B. Lyme disease, area of peripheral erythema. Mild superficial and deep perivascular and intestitial mixed-cell infiltrate. There are lymphocytes, plasma and histiocytic cells, and eosinophils.

16

PROTOZOA, ALGAE, HELMINTH, AND MYIASIS INFECTIONS AND INFESTATIONS

- Leishmaniasis
- Protothecosis
- Cutanea larva migrans
- Onchocerciasis
- Myiasis

LEISHMANIASIS

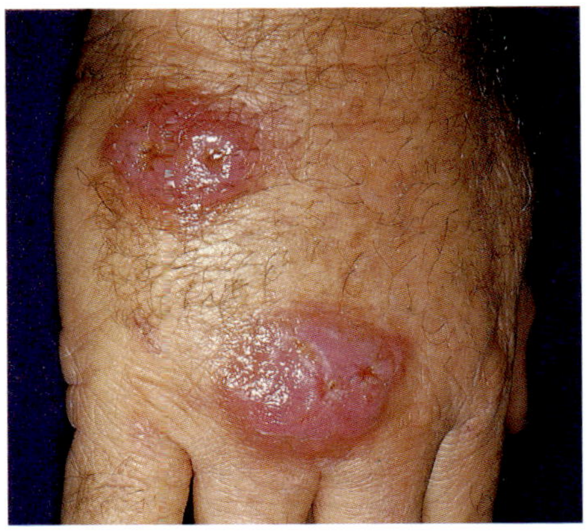

Figure 16–1. Leishmaniasis, cutaneous form, early lesion. Red nodules on the dorsum of the hand.

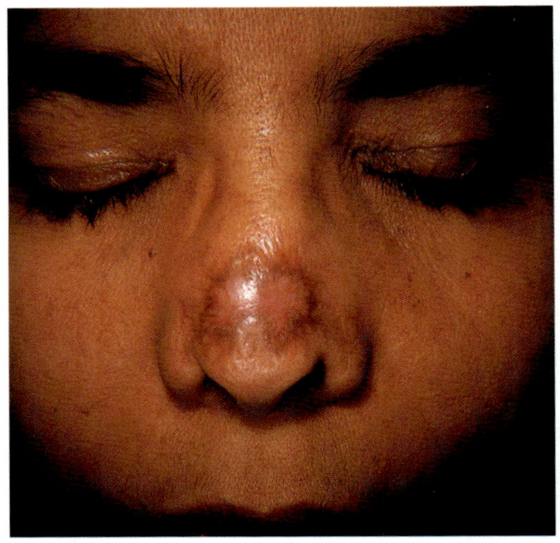

Figure 16–2. Leishmaniasis, cutaneous form, late lesion. Atrophic, pink, scarring plaque with peripheral hyperpigmentation on the nose of a woman from India.

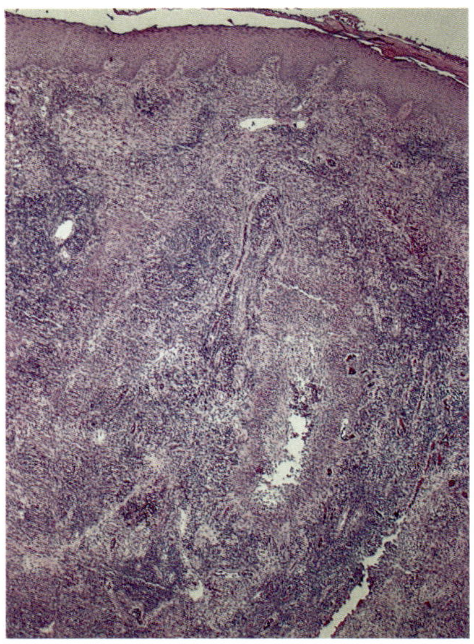

Figure 16–3. Leishmaniasis. Epidermal hyperplasia with a diffuse lymphohistiocytic dermal infiltrate.

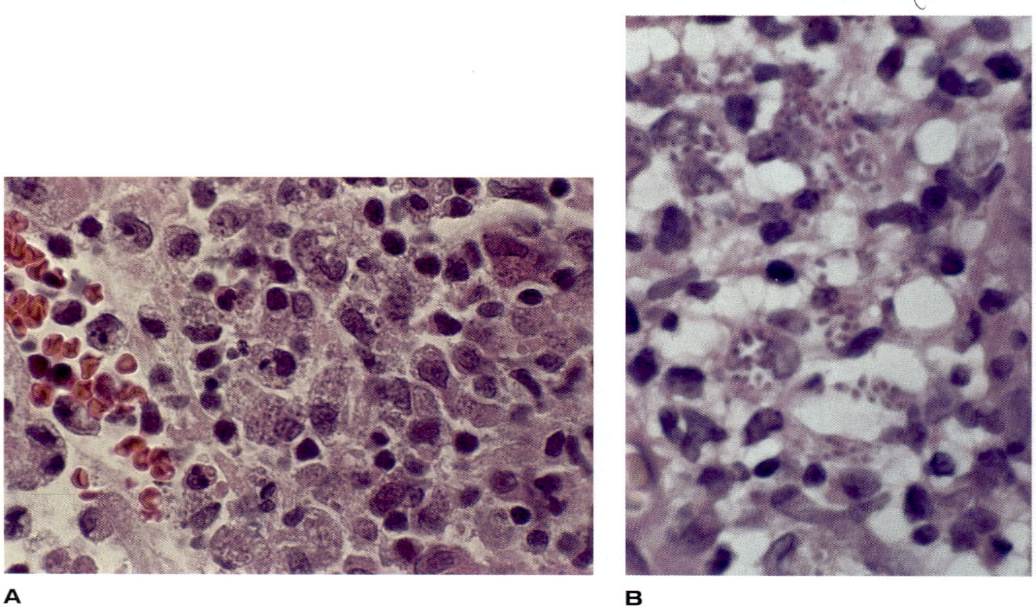

A B

Figures 16–4A, 16–4B. Leishmaniasis. Nonflagellated protozoa appear as gray-blue round-oval bodies within the cytoplasms of histiocytic cells stained with hematoxylin and eosin.

PROTOTHECOSIS

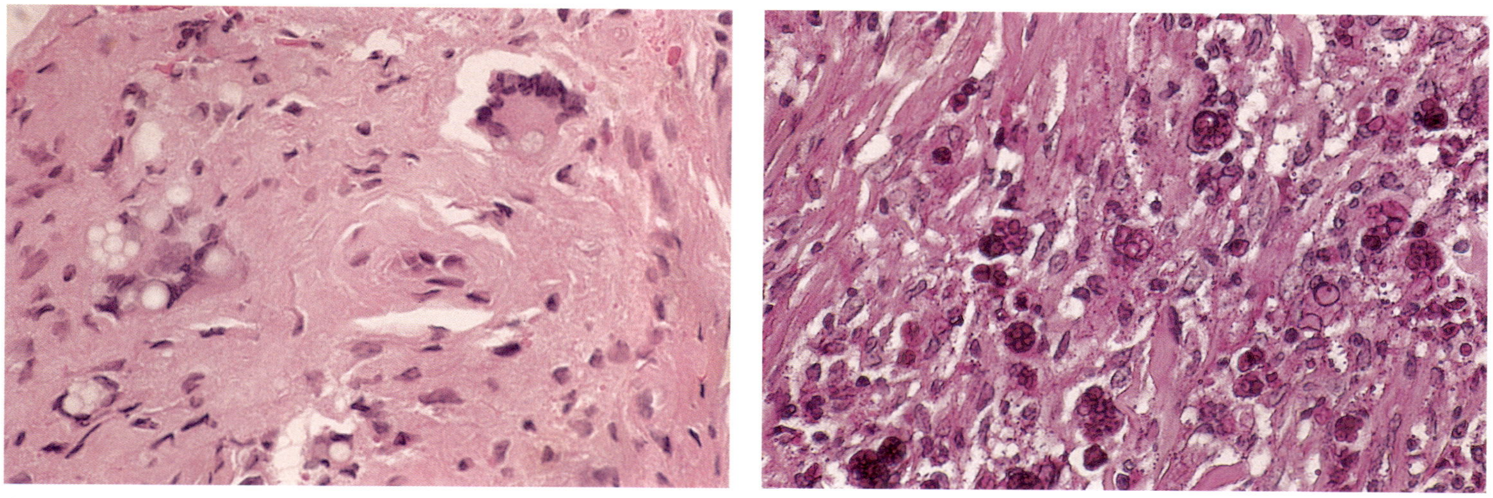

A **B**

Figures 16–5A, 16–5B. Protothecosis. Prototheca within the dermis and within multinucleated histiocytic giant cells. Characteristic morula are seen with hematoxylin-eosin and periodic acid-Schiff stains.

"soccer balls"

CUTANEA LARVA MIGRANS

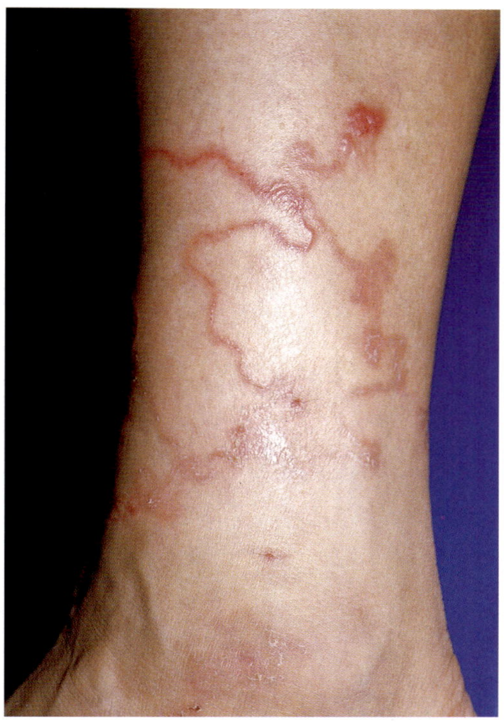

Figure 16–6. Cutanea larva migrans. Serpentine, erythematous, threadlike, vesicular, raised lesions on the lower leg.

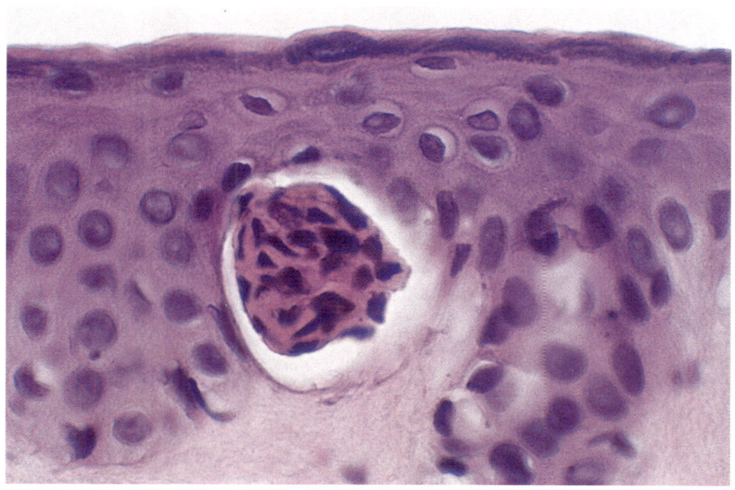

Figure 16–7. Cutanea larva migrans. Hookworm larva within the basal and lower spinous layer of the epidermis. Compressed keratinocytes surround the larva, which is contiguous with severe dermal papillary edema.

ONCHOCERCIASIS

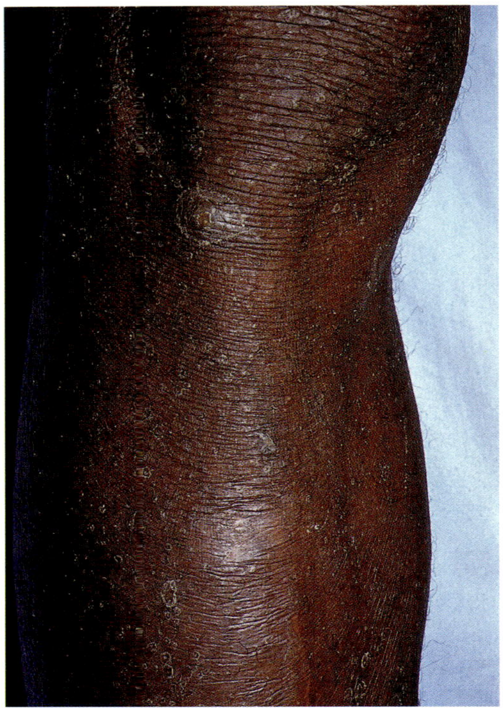

Figure 16–8. Onchocerciasis. Keratotic papules on the leg.

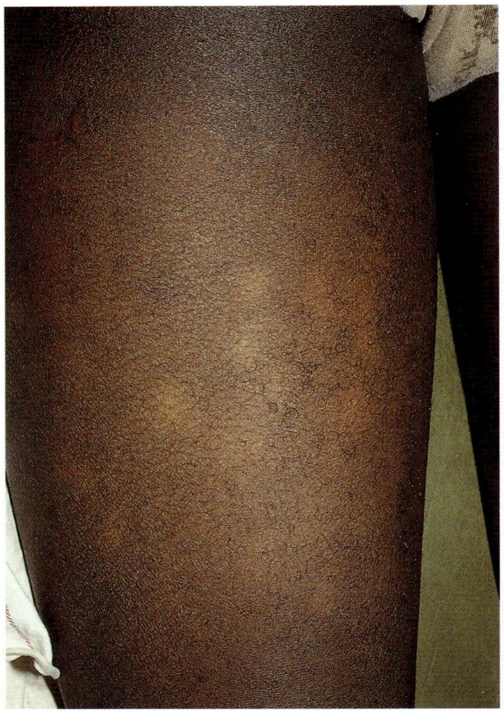

Figure 16–9. Onchocerciasis. Hypopigmented patches on the leg.

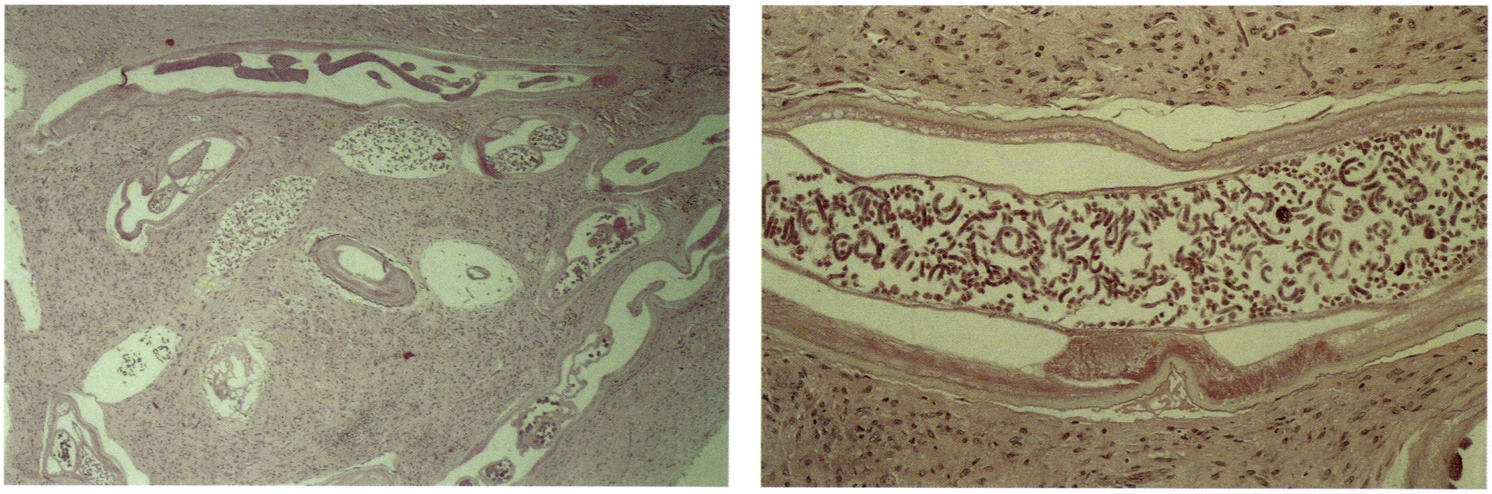

A **B**

Figures 16–10A, 16–10B. Onchocerciasis. Onchocercal nodule with adult worms. There is dermal fibroplasia and a dense mixed-cell infiltrate.

MYIASIS

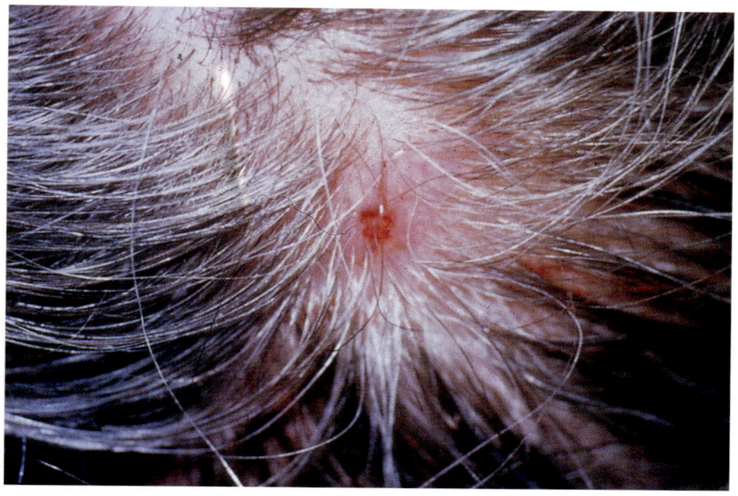

Figure 16–11. **Myiasis.** Ulcerated, erythematous papule in the scalp.

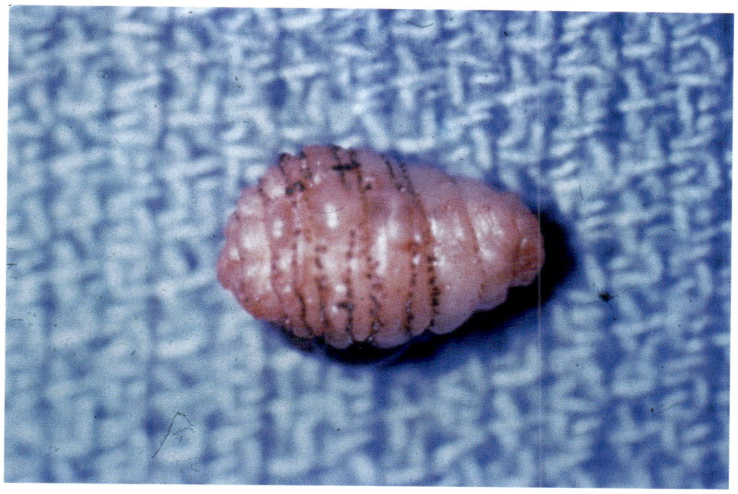

Figure 16–12. **Myiasis.** Larva "warble" with concentric rings and contiguous hyperpigmented spines.

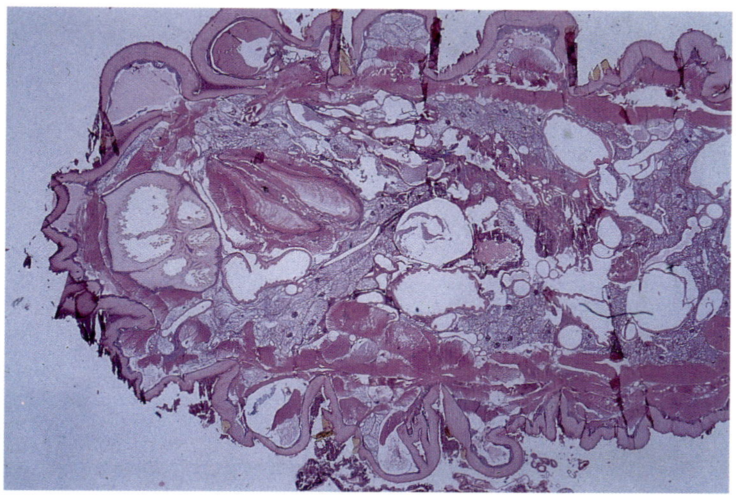

A

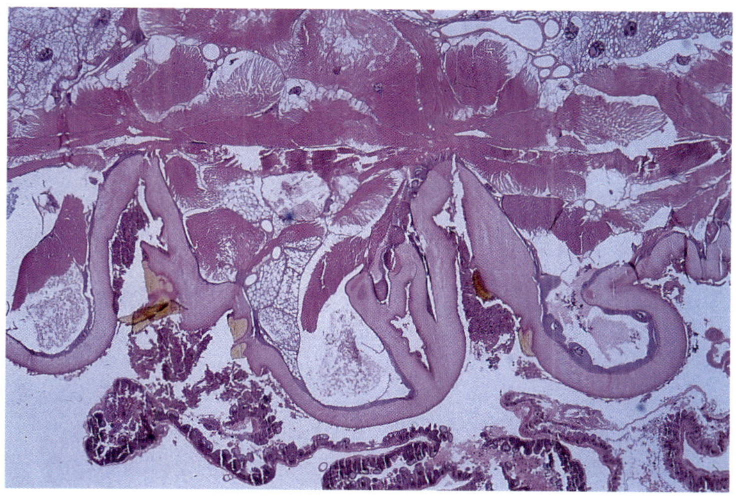

B

Figures 16–13A, 16–13B. **Myiasis.** Cross-sections through larva. Prominent spines along the central surface and oral hooks at one end help anchor the larva to the tissue.

17

FUNGAL INFECTIONS

- Dermatophytosis
- Pityriasis versicolor
- Candidiasis
- Sporotrichocosis
- Chromomycosis
- Lobomycosis
- Rhinosporidiosis
- Coccidioidomycosis
- Paracoccidioidomycosis (South American blastomycosis)
- Blastomycosis (North American blastomycosis)
- Histoplasmosis
- Cryptococcosis
- Aspergillosis
- Zygomycosis
- Alternariosis

DERMATOPHYTOSIS

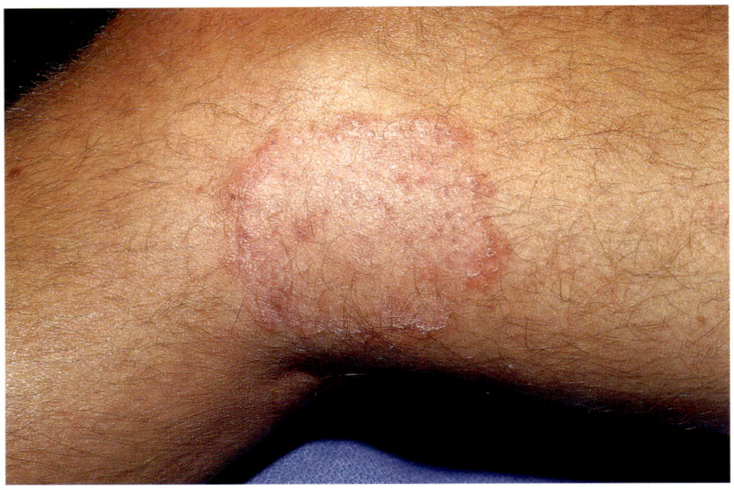

Figure 17–1. Dermatophytosis. Pruritic, circular, erythematous scaly patch with central clearing on the leg. This particular clinical presentation is commonly known as tinea or ringworm.

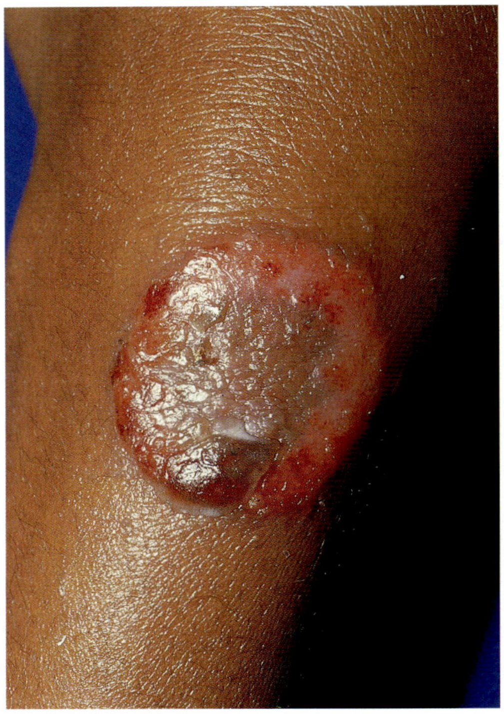

Figure 17–2. Dermatophytosis. Inflamed, oval-shaped, oozing, and crusted plaque on the leg.

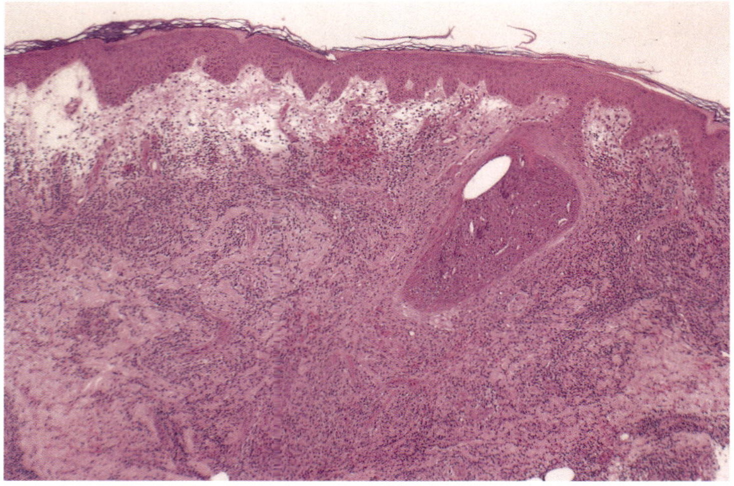

Figure 17–3. Dermatophytosis. Severe dermal papillary edema with a diffuse mixed-cell infiltrate. There is slight epidermal hyperplasia, alternating orthokeratosis and hyperkeratosis, and an infundibular abscess and folliculitis.

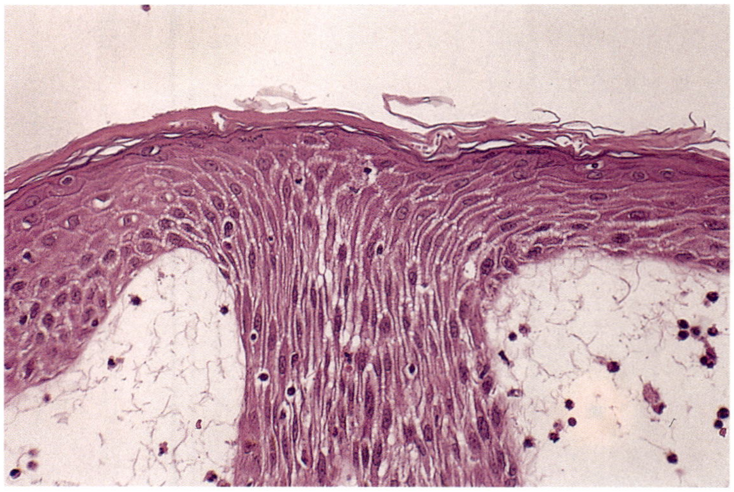

Figure 17–4. Dermatophytosis. Hyphal fragments within the stratum corneum, spongiosis, and severe papillary edema.

DERMATOPHYTOSIS

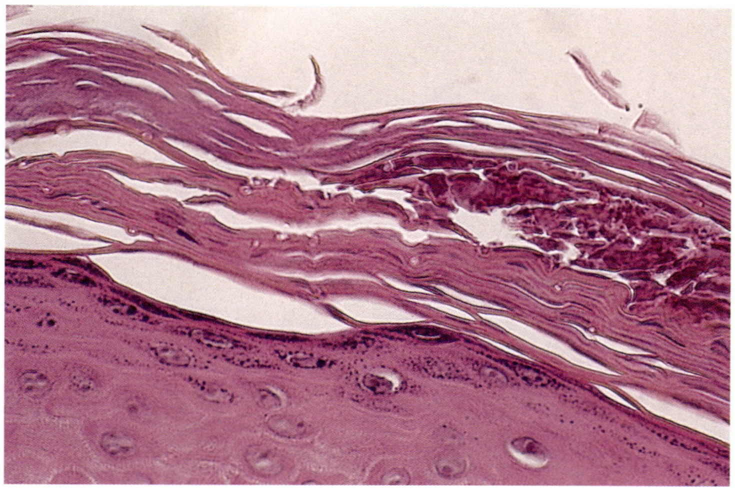

Figure 17–5. Dermatophytosis. Stratum corneum with numerous hyphae cut on cross-section associated with a collection of neutrophils.

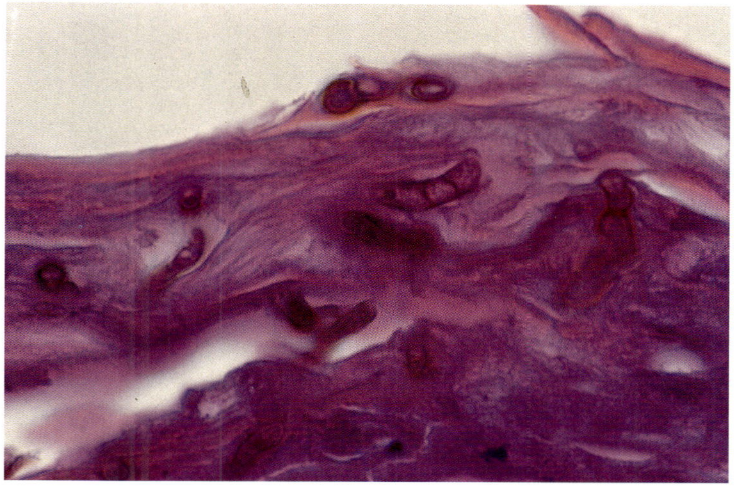

Figure 17–6. Tinea nigra. Brown, septate hyphae within the stratum corneum.

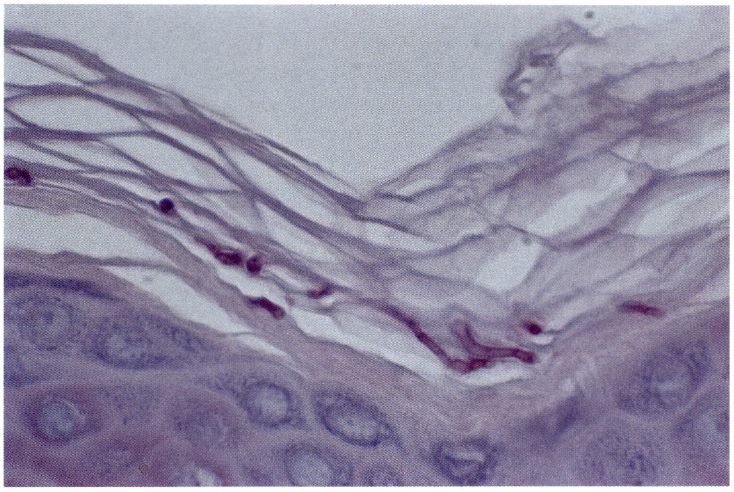

Figure 17–7. Dermatophytosis. Periodic acid-Schiff (PAS) stains the hyphae in the stratum corneum.

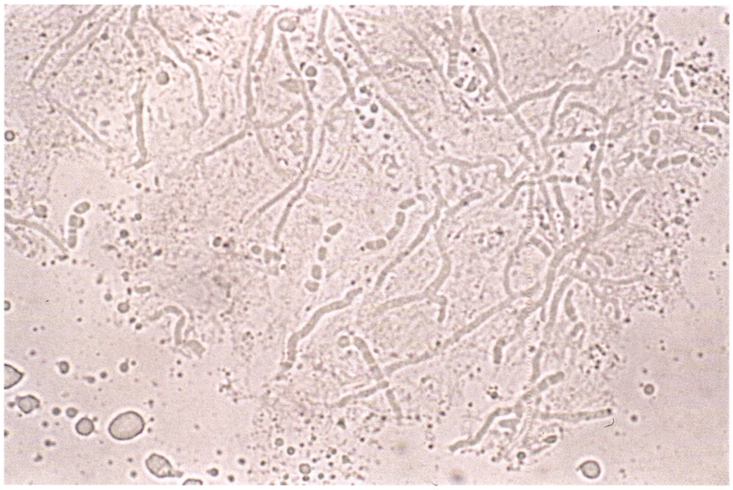

Figure 17–8. Dermatophytosis. Potassium hydroxide (KOH) preparation showing many branching, septate hyphae. Some hyphae are separated, and they have the appearance of box cars aligned in a row. This finding is characteristic of *Trichophyton verrucosum*.

PITYRIASIS VERSICOLOR

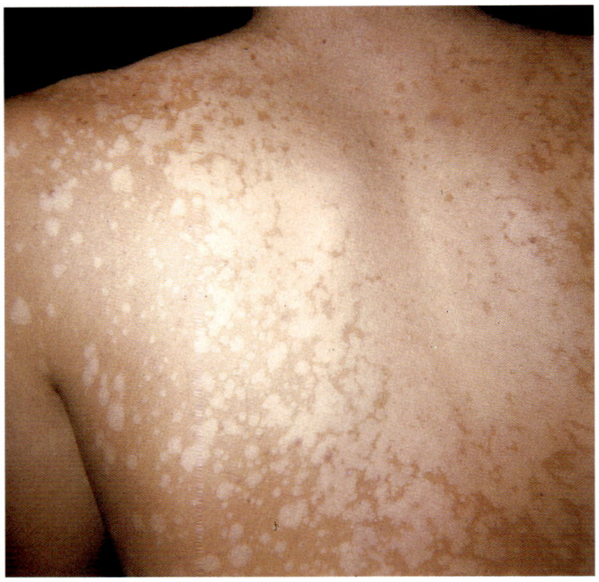

Figure 17–9. Pityriasis versicolor. Hyperpigmented and hypopigmented scaly patches on the back and shoulders. Formerly known as tinea versicolor.

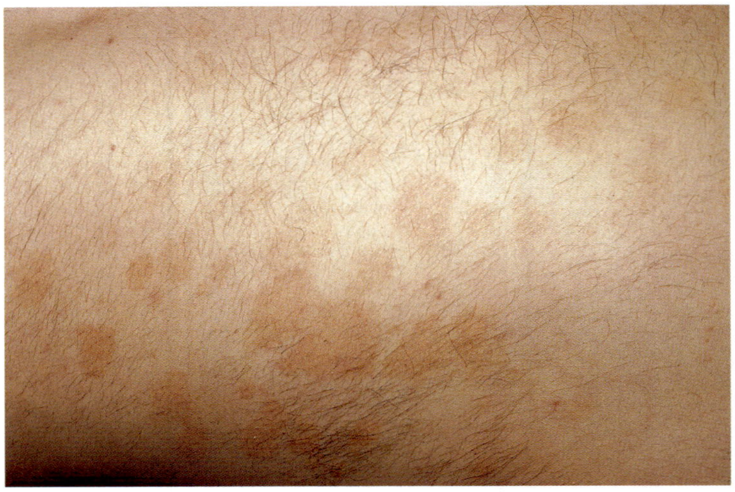

Figure 17–10. Pityriasis versicolor. Erythematous, scaly, circular patches involving the axilla, axillary folds, and arm.

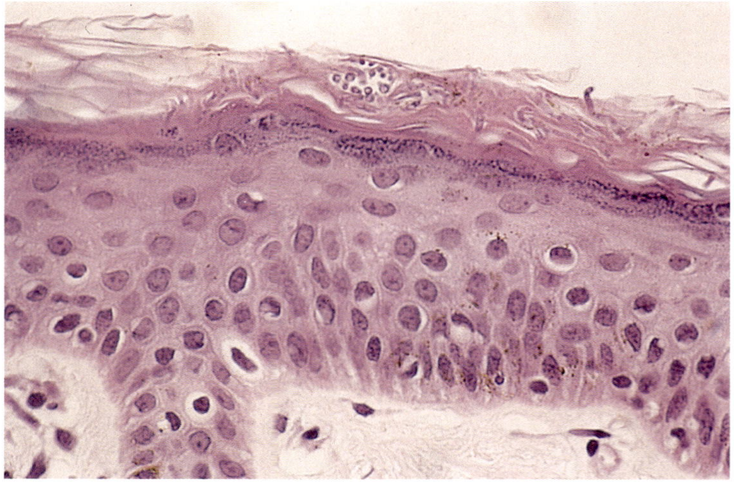

Figure 17–11. Pityriasis versicolor. Round spores and stubby pseudohyphae within the stratum corneum.

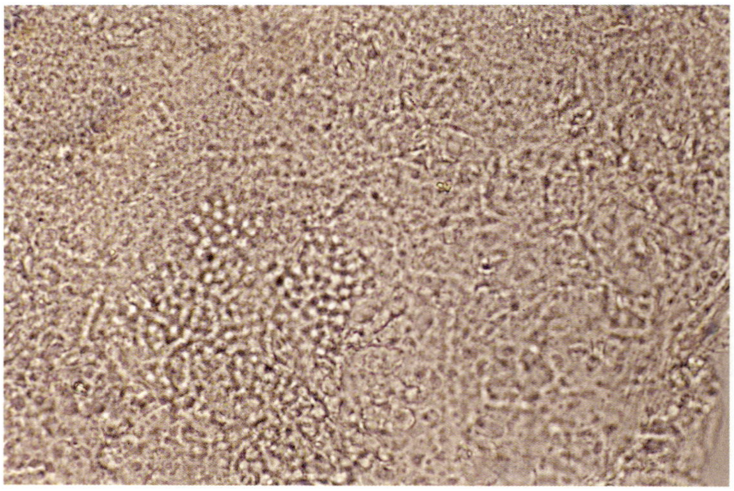

Figure 17–12. Pityriasis versicolor. Potassium hydroxide (KOH) preparation showing refractile round spores and stubby pseudohyphae.

CANDIDIASIS

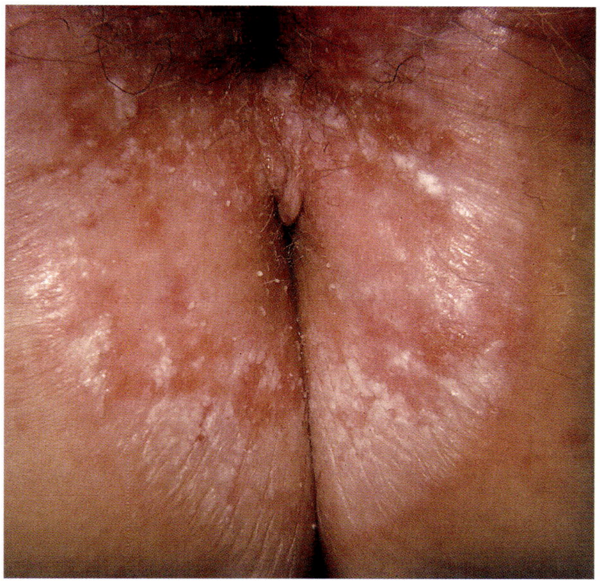

Figure 17–13. Candidiasis. Severely pruritic, erythematous, scaly patches on the buttocks and vulva. Shiny, lichenified areas attest to the chronic rubbing.

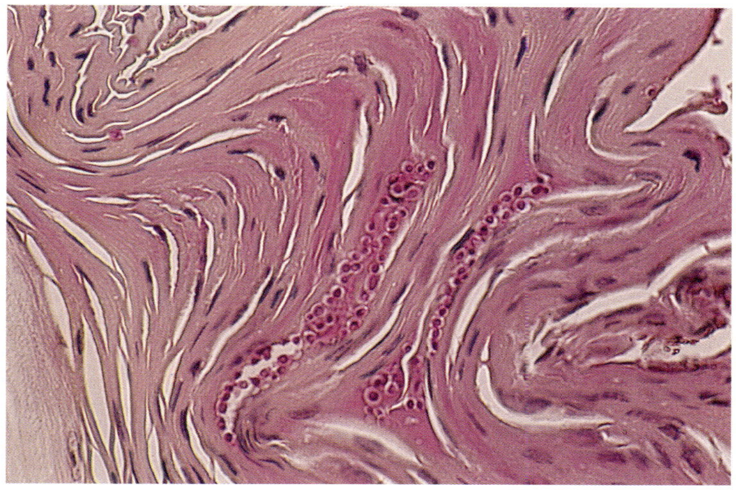

Figure 17–14. Candidiasis. Spores in chains within the parakeratotic stratum corneum. Periodic acid-Schiff (PAS) stains the spores red.

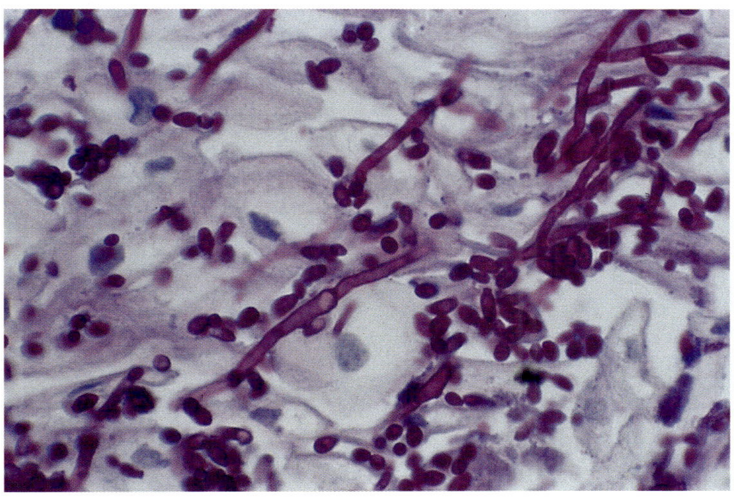

Figure 17–15. Candidiasis. Periodic acid-Schiff (PAS) stain shows spores and pseudohyphae.

CANDIDIASIS

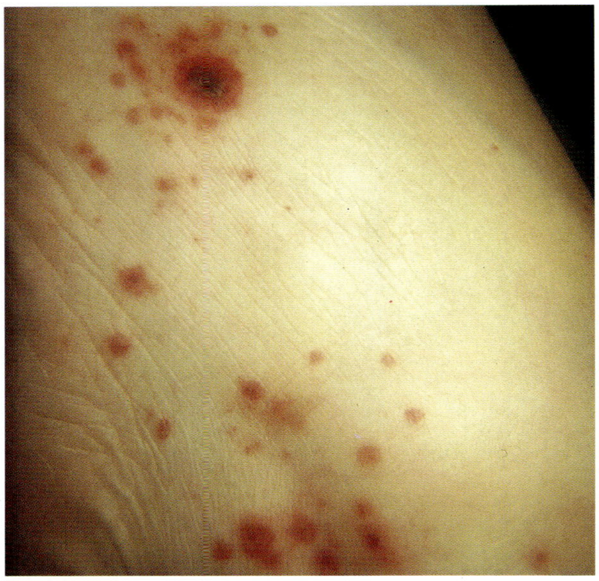

A

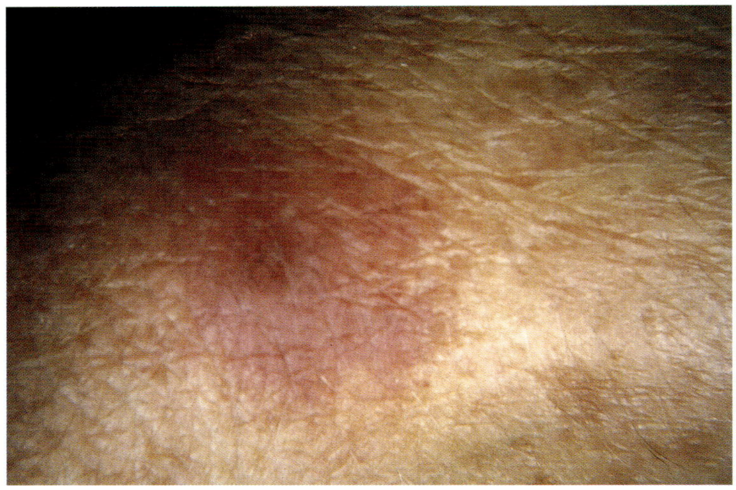

B

Figures 17–16A, 17–16B. *Candida* septicemia. Erythematous vesiculopapules on the leg. A central gray bulla is noted within some of the papules.

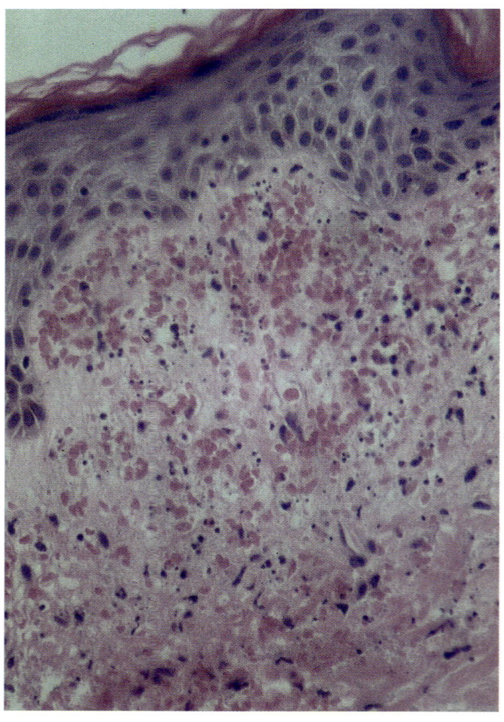

Figure 17–17. *Candida* septicemia. There is papillary dermal ecema, neutrophils, nuclear dust, and extravasated erythrocytes.

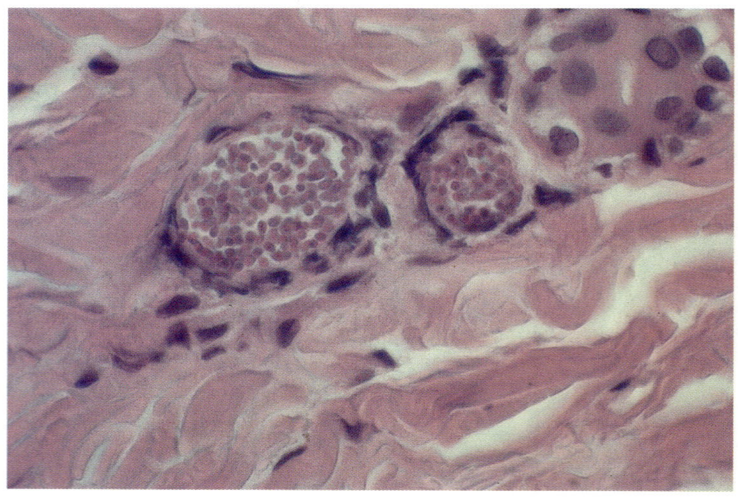

Figure 17–18. *Candida* septicemia. Dermal blood vessels filled with organisms.

SPOROTRICHOSIS

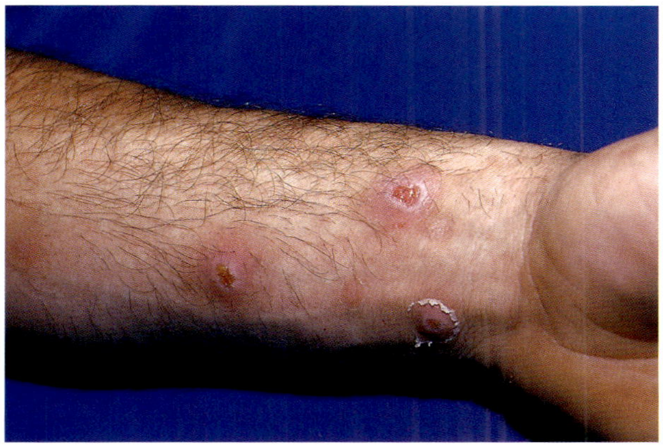

Figure 17–19. Sporotrichosis. Erythematous, crusted nodules in a linear array on the wrist and arm of an HIV-positive man.

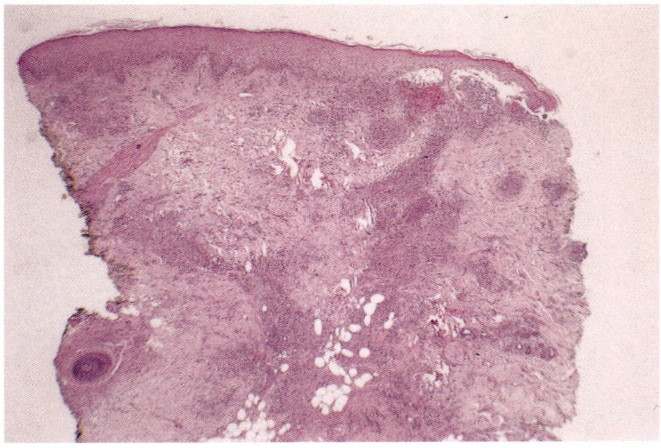

A

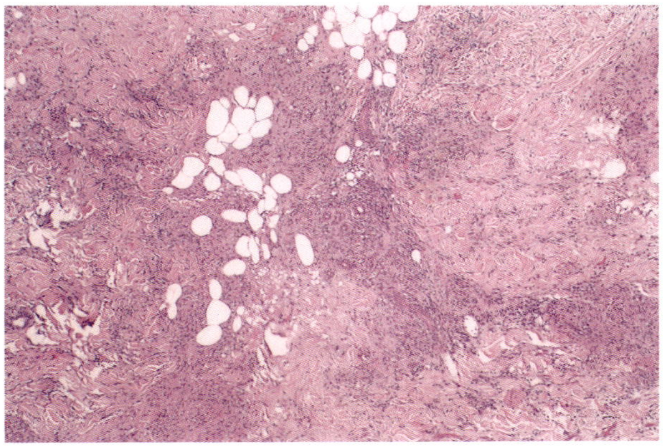

B

Figures 17–20A, 17–20B. Sporotrichosis. Nodular and diffuse mixed-cell infiltrate in the dermis and subcutaneous tissue.

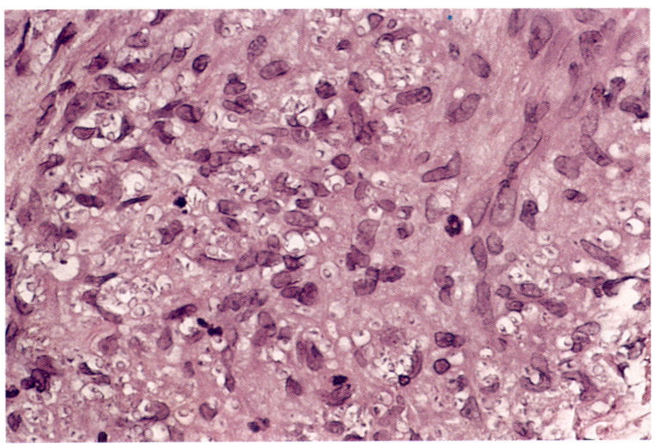

Figure 17–21. Sporotrichosis. Many single and multiple budding oval-round spores within histiocytic cells in a biopsy specimen from an immunocompromised patient.

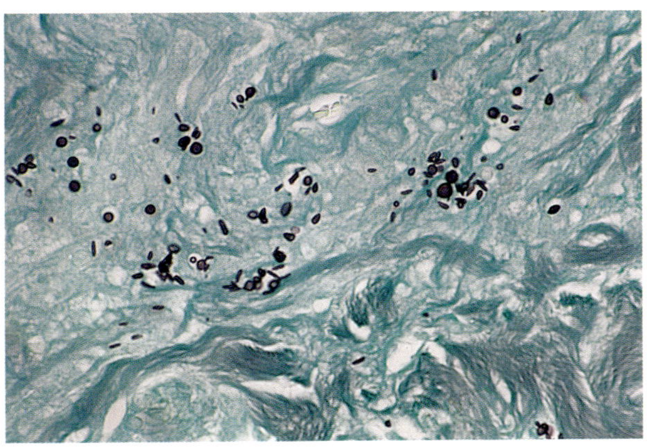

A

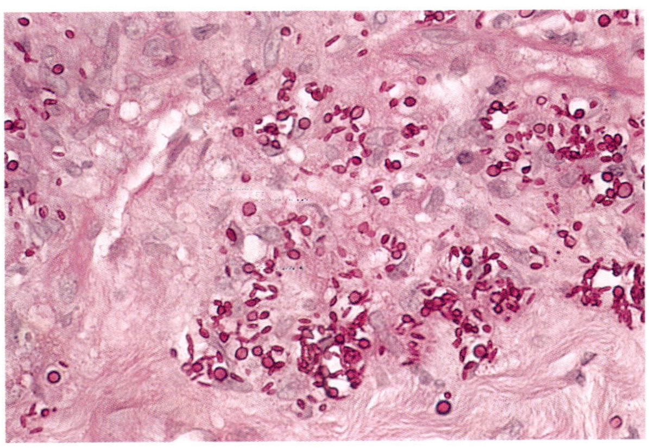

B

Figure 17–22. Sporotrichosis. Silver methenamine **(A)** and periodic acid-Schiff **(B)** stains show many round-oval, single, and multiple budding spores, and short hyphal forms (cigar bodies). This biopsy specimen was taken from an immunocompromised patient.

CHROMOMYCOSIS

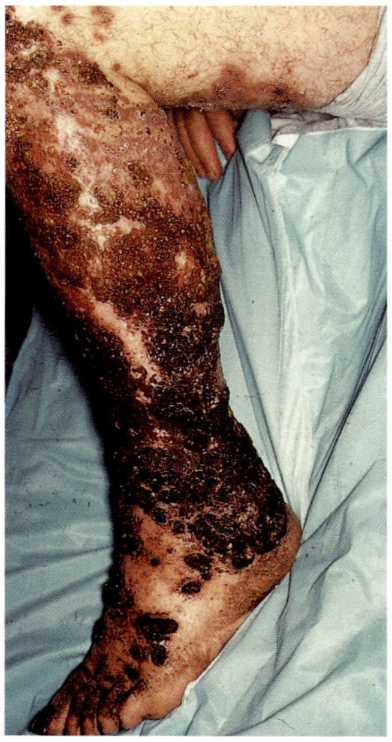

Figure 17–23. Chromomycosis. Confluent, hyperpigmented, verrucous papules, nodules, and plaques on the leg and foot.

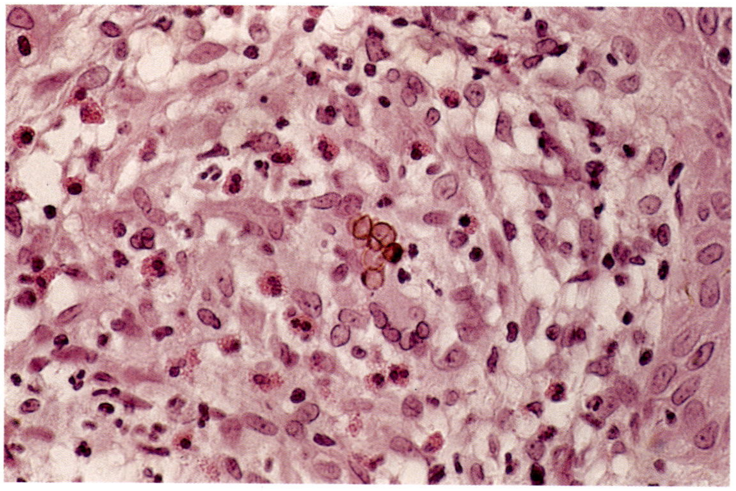

Figure 17–24. Chromomycosis. Bronze-colored, clustered, oval, septate spores within a multinucleated histiocytic giant cell. These sclerotic bodies that reproduce by cissiparity (planate-dividing) are also referred to as "copper pennies" or Medlar bodies.

LOBOMYCOSIS

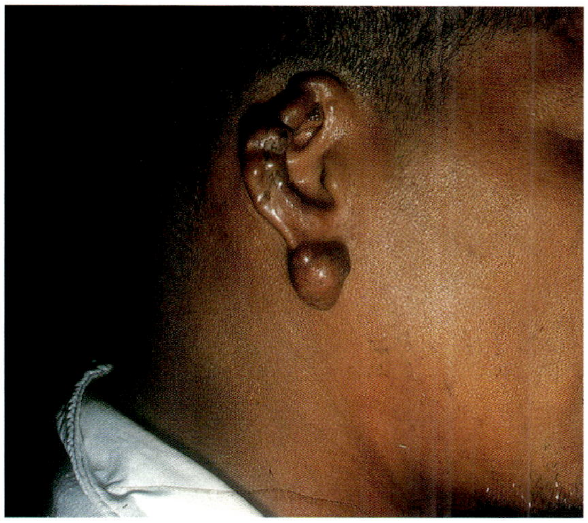

Figure 17–25. Lobomycosis. Hypertrophic, keloidal, and atrophic, smooth, hyperpigmented nodules on the ear.

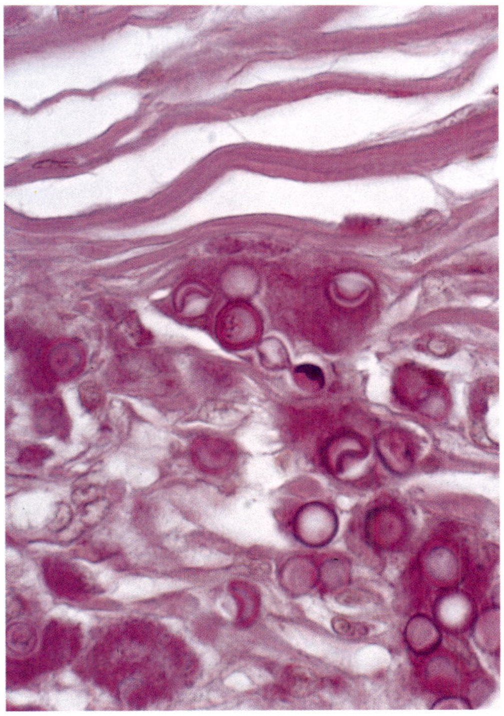

Figure 17–26. Lobomycosis. Periodic acid-Schiff (PAS) stains single budding, thick-walled, uniform-sized, round yeasts lying free, in chains and within multinucleated histiocytic giant cells.

RHINOSPORIDIOSIS

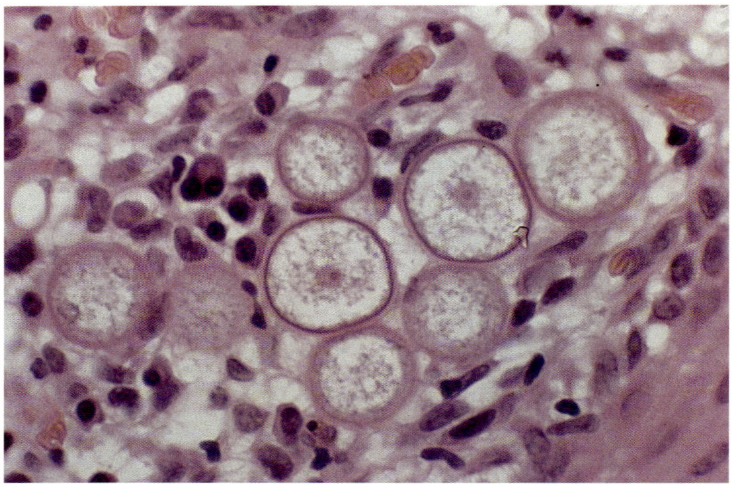

Figure 17–27. Rhinosporidiosis. Multiple cysts with surrounding mixed-cell infiltrate containing plasma cells.

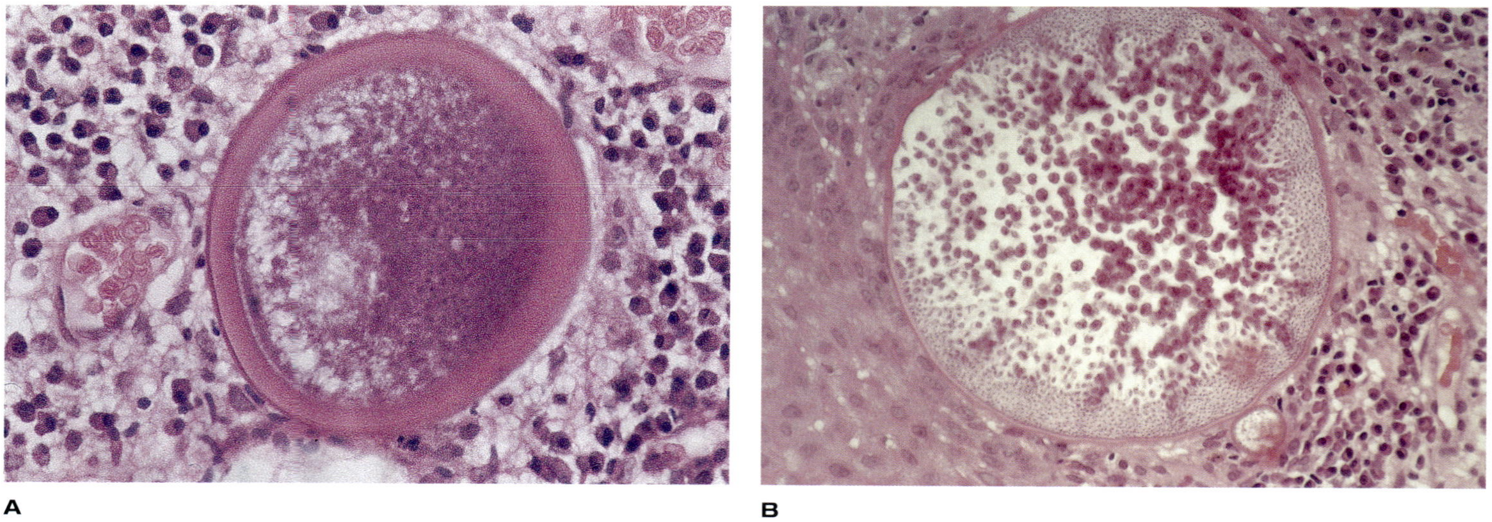

Figures 17–28A, 17–28B. Rhinosporidiosis. Large sporangium containing numerous spores.

COCCIDIOIDOMYCOSIS

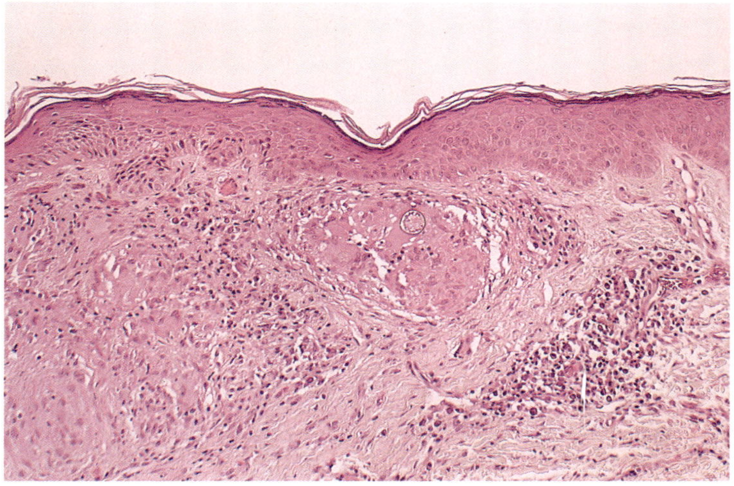

A

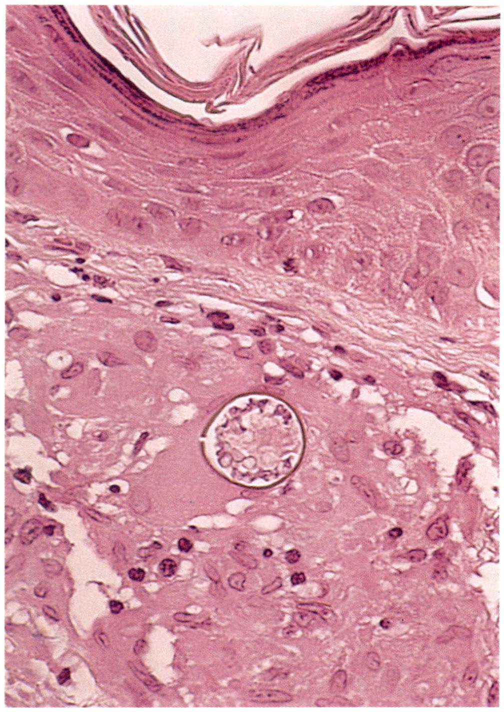

B

Figures 17–29A, 17–29B. Coccidioidomycosis. Spherule with endospores within dermal nodule. There are nodules containing multinucleated histiocytic giant cells and a dense inflammatory mixed-cell infiltrate with many plasma cells within the papillary and upper reticular dermis.

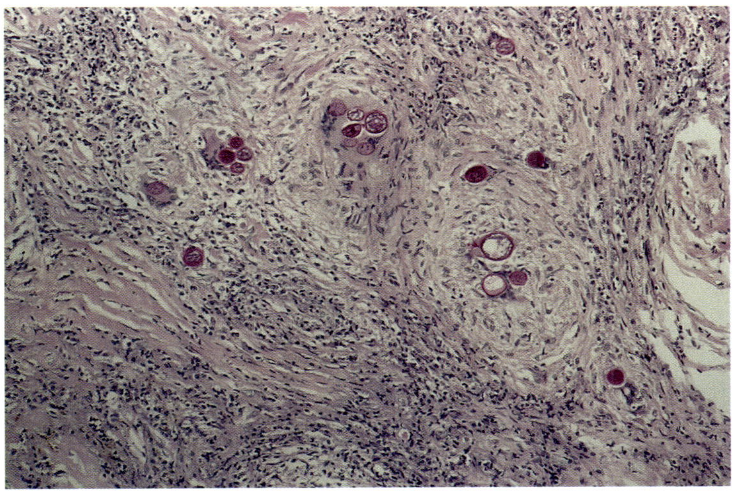

Figure 17–30. Coccidioidomycosis. Periodic acid-Schiff (PAS) stains numerous spherules red. Single or multiple sphericles that contain numerous endospores are found within multinucleated histiocytic giant cells or lying free in the dermis. The dermis contains a suppurative granulomatous infiltrate.

PARACOCCIDIOIDOMYCOSIS (SOUTH AMERICAN BLASTOMYCOSIS)

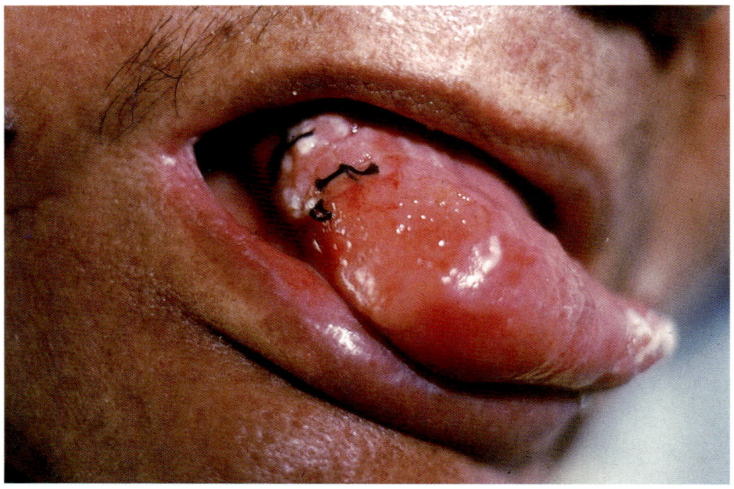

Figure 17–31. Paracoccidioidomycosis. Nodule with ulceration on the tongue.

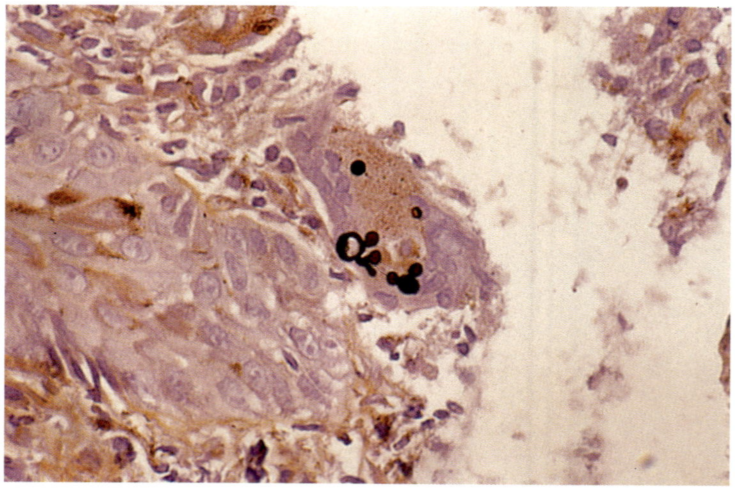

Figure 17–32. Paracoccidioidomycosis. Methenamine silver stains the variable-sized, round yeasts with multiple narrow-necked buds. The characteristic "Mickey Mouse" budding yeast form is seen.

BLASTOMYCOSIS (NORTH AMERICAN BLASTOMYCOSIS)

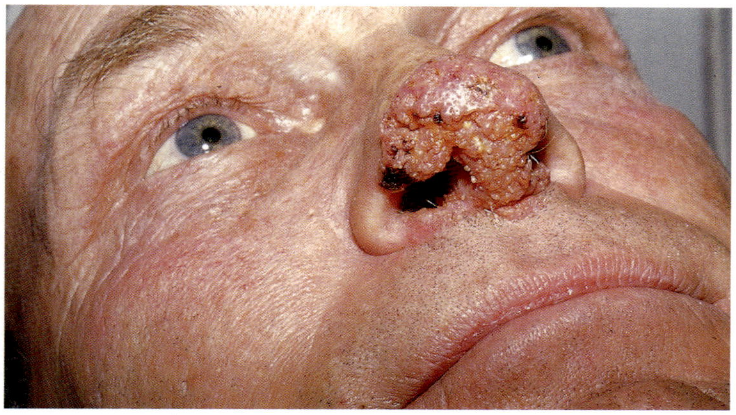

Figure 17–33. Blastomycosis. Verrucous nodule with ulcerations on the nasal tip, ala nasi, septum, and upper lip of a man.

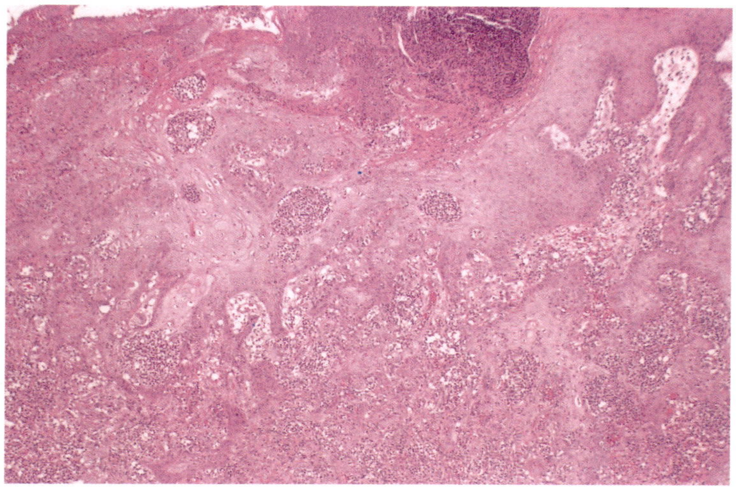

Figure 17–34. Blastomycosis. Pseudocarcinomatous hyperplasia with multiple intraepithelial neutrophilic abscesses. There s scale crust on the surface and a dense suppurative granulomatous infiltrate in the dermis.

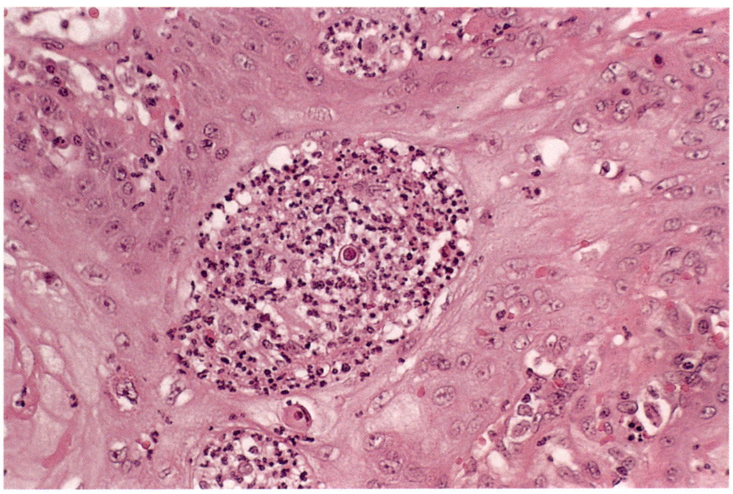

Figure 17–35. Blastomycosis. Neutrophilic microabscess containing encapsulated spore.

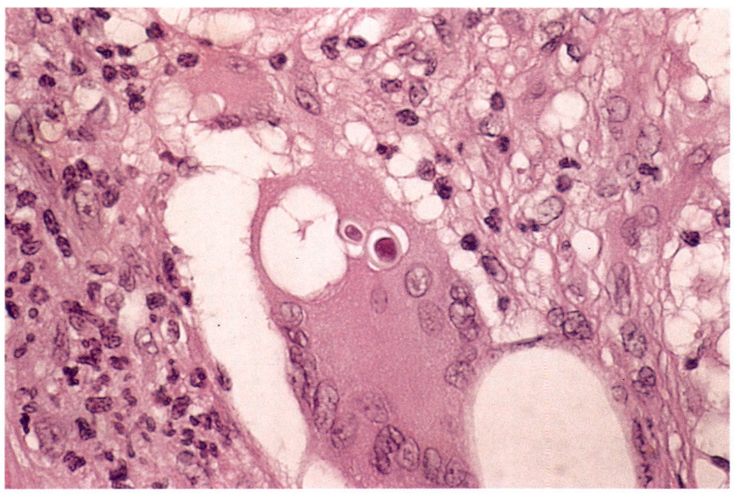

Figure 17–36. Blastomycosis. Broad-based budding spore characteristic of North American blastomycosis.

HISTOPLASMOSIS

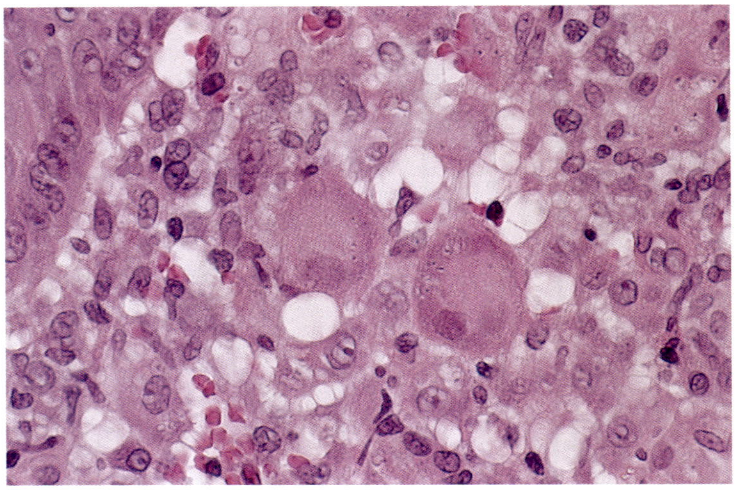

Figure 17–37. Histoplasmosis. Numerous uniform, small, dark-blue, thick-walled yeast spores within foamy histiocytic cells.

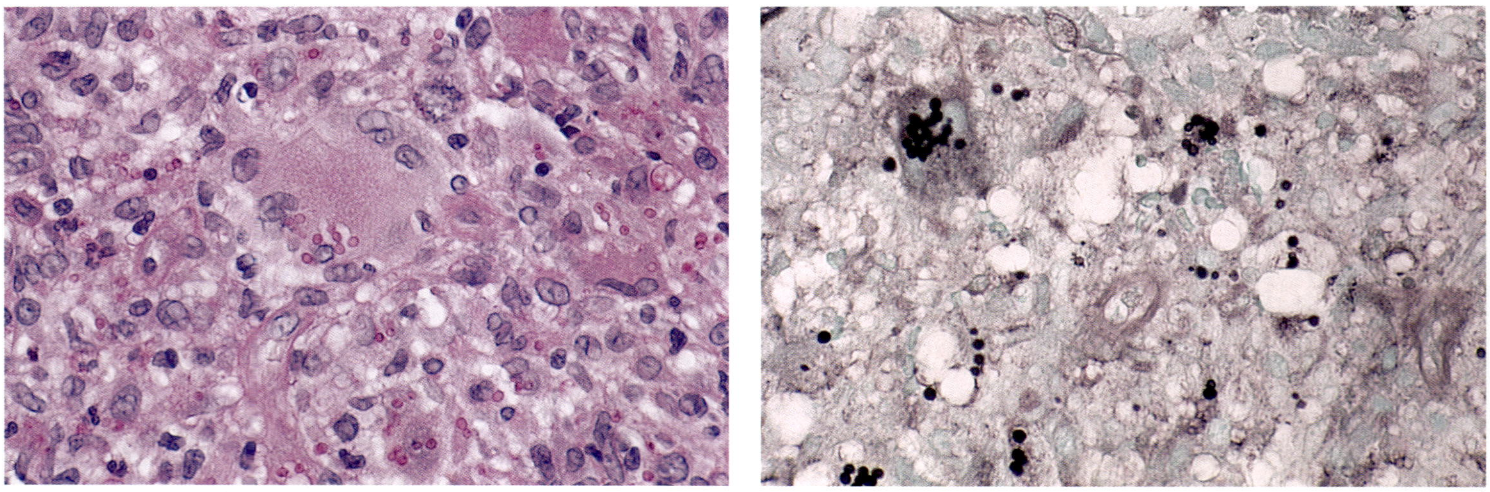

Figure 17–38. Histoplasmosis. Periodic acid-Schiff (PAS) **(A)** and methenamine silver **(B)** stains show numerous small spores within histiocytic cells in multinucleated histiocytic giant cells. Some of the spores are connected to one another by a narrow neck.

CRYPTOCOCCOSIS

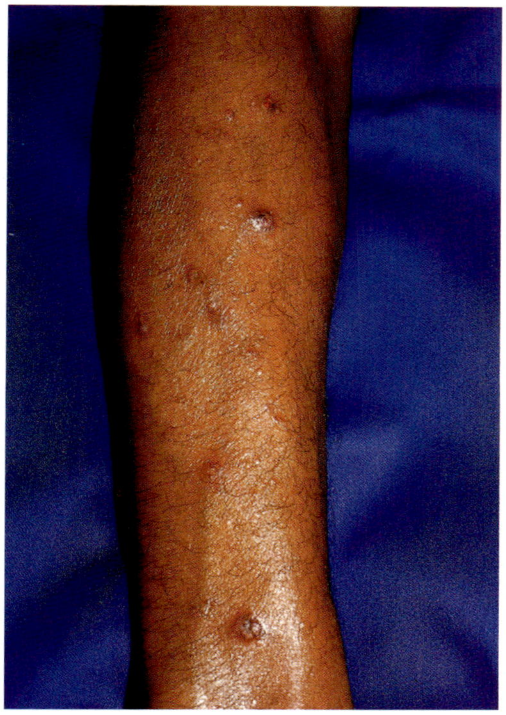

Figure 17–39. **Cryptococcosis.** Crusted papules and nodules on the arm of an immunocompromised patient.

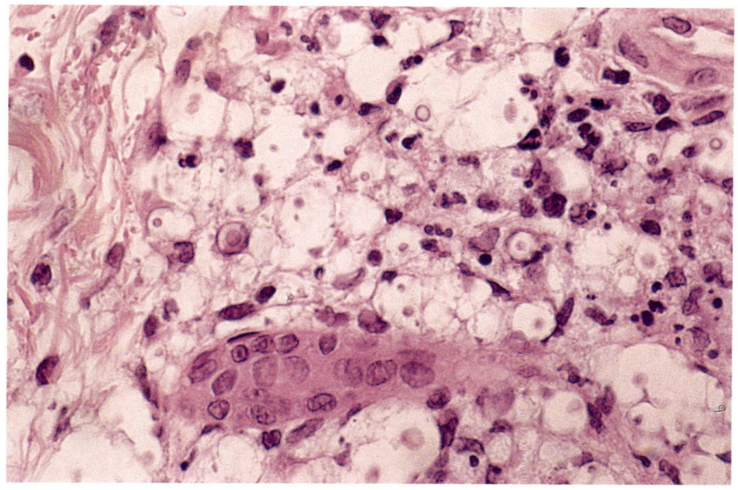

Figure 17–40. **Cryptococcosis, gelatinous pattern.** Masses of spores lying free in the dermis with a minimal inflammatory response.

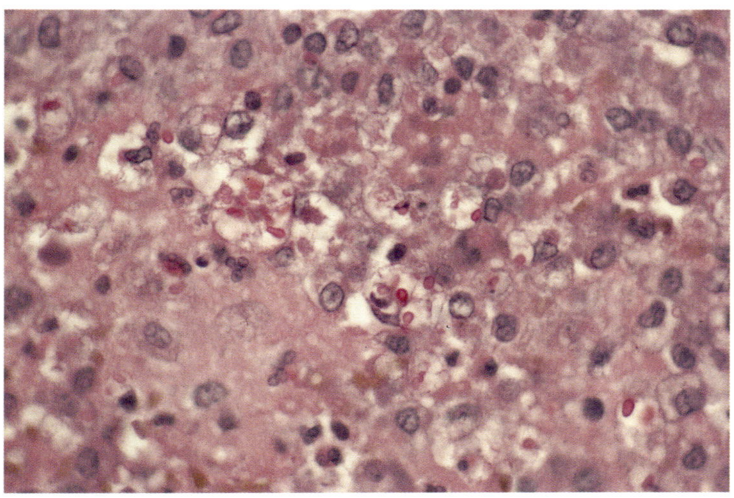

Figure 17–41. **Cryptococcosis, granulomatous pattern.** Mucicarmine stains the red, round, thick capsule of the spores within a dermal granulomatous and mixed-cell infiltrate.

ASPERGILLOSIS

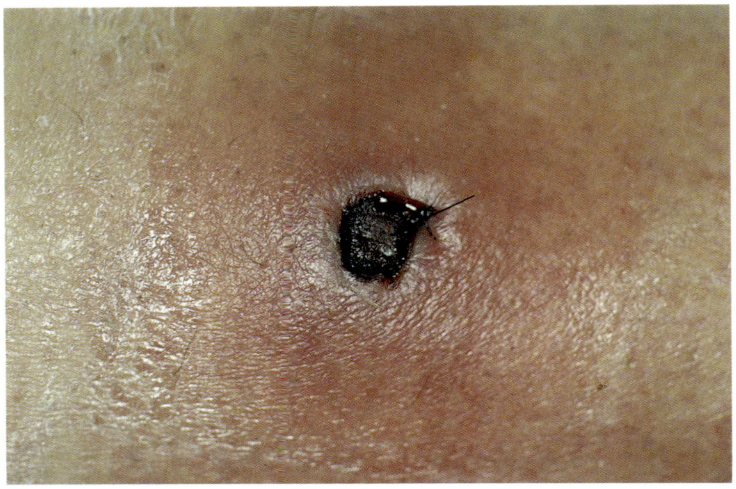

Figure 17–42. Aspergillosis. Erythematous plaque with a central black eschar in an immunocompromised patient.

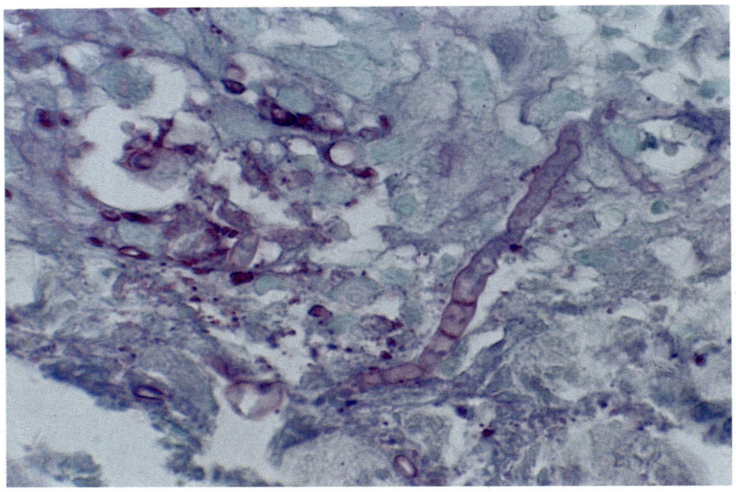

Figure 17–43. Aspergillosis. Periodic acid-Schiff (PAS) stains the irregular-shaped dichotomous, septate, acute-angle branching hyphae.

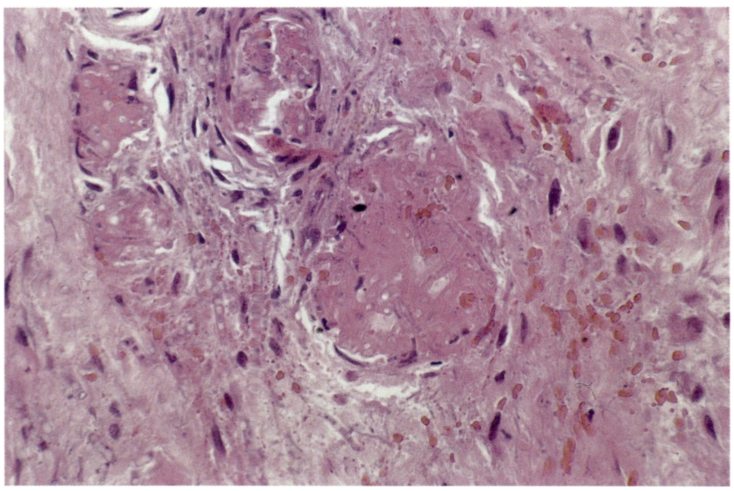

Figure 17–44. Aspergillosis. Blood vessel fibrin thrombus with numerous hyphal elements.

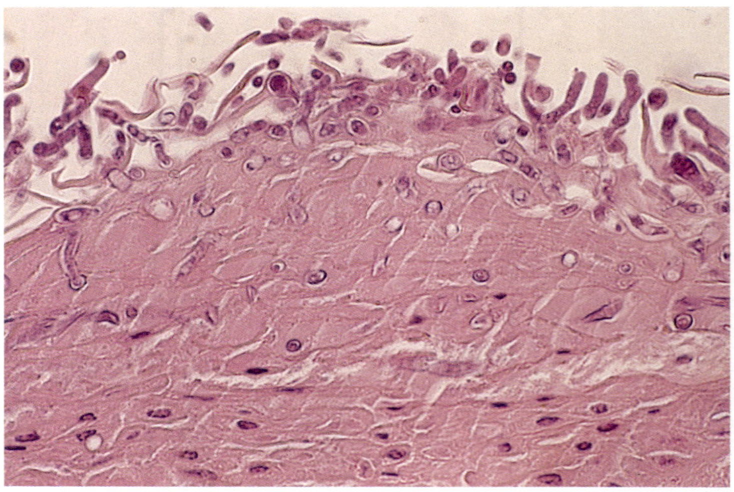

Figure 17–45. Aspergillosis. Dermis with numerous branching septate hyphae that vary in size and shape.

ZYGOMYCOSIS

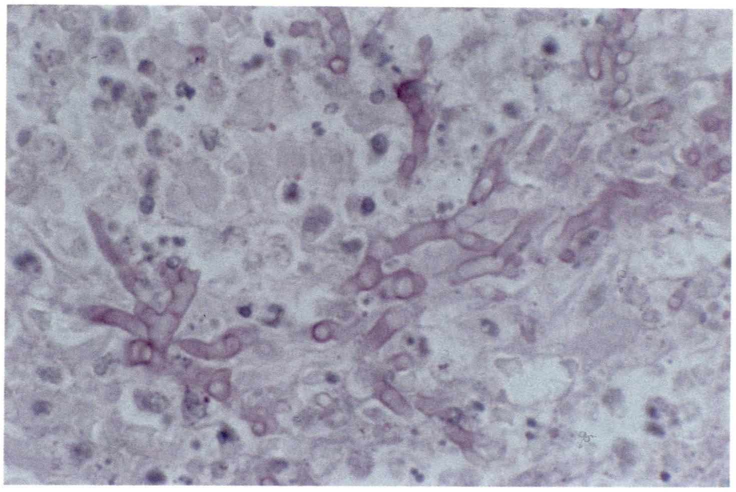

Figure 17–46. Mucormycosis. Periodic acid-Schiff (PAS) stains branching, predominantly nonseptate hyphae, which branch at odd intervals and at right angles. A few rounded structures resembling yeast forms are present.

ALTERNARIOSIS

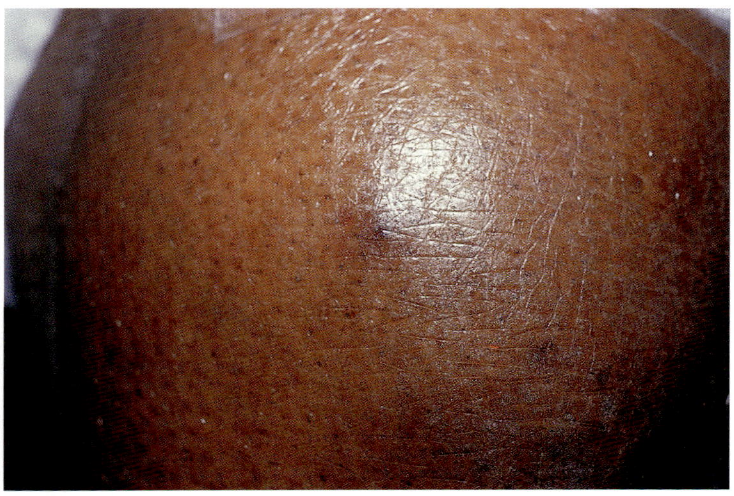

Figure 17–47. Alternariosis. Erythematous papule on the knee of an immunocompromised man.

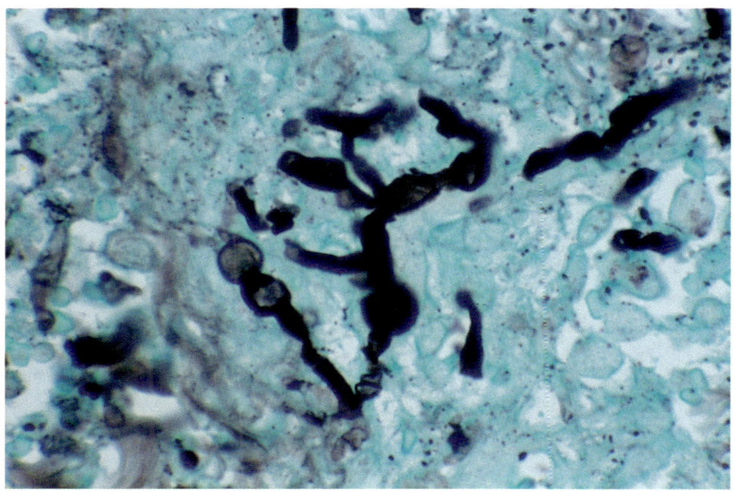

Figure 17–48. Alternariosis. Methenamine stain showing the irregular-shaped, thick-walled septate branching hyphae of varicble length. Acute right-angle branching is seen.

18

BITES AND INFESTATIONS

- Arthropod bite reactions
- Scabies
- Tick bite granuloma
- Brown recluse spider bite

ARTHROPOD BITE REACTIONS

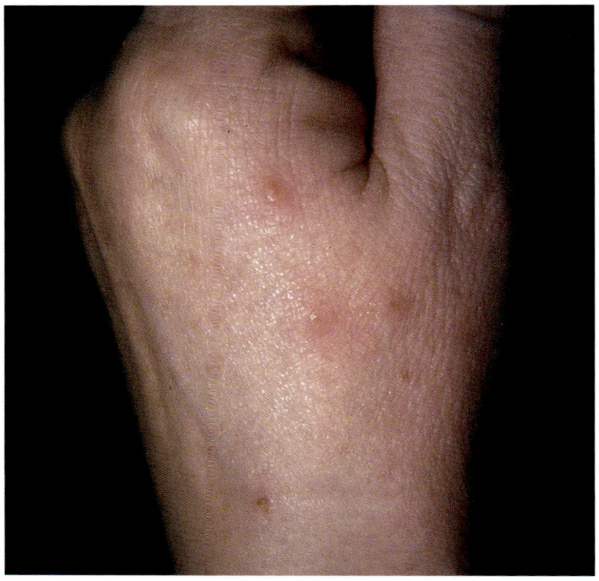

Figure 18–1. Flea bites. Erythematous papules with central puncta on the hand.

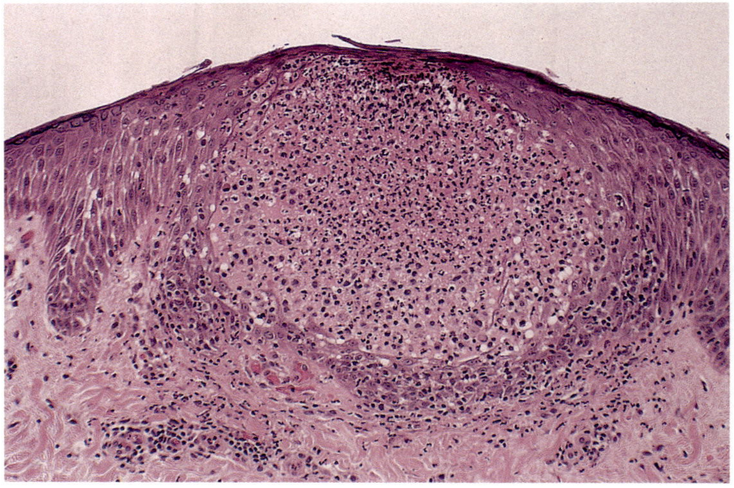

Figure 18–2. Flea bites. Intraepidermal abscess and spongiosis.

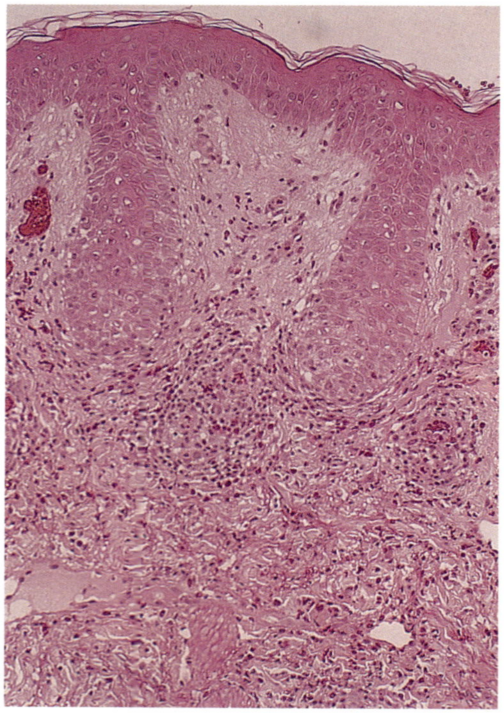

Figure 18–3. Flea bites. Severe papillary dermal edema, perivascular and interstitial inflammatory infiltrate with neutrophils and dilated blood vessels.

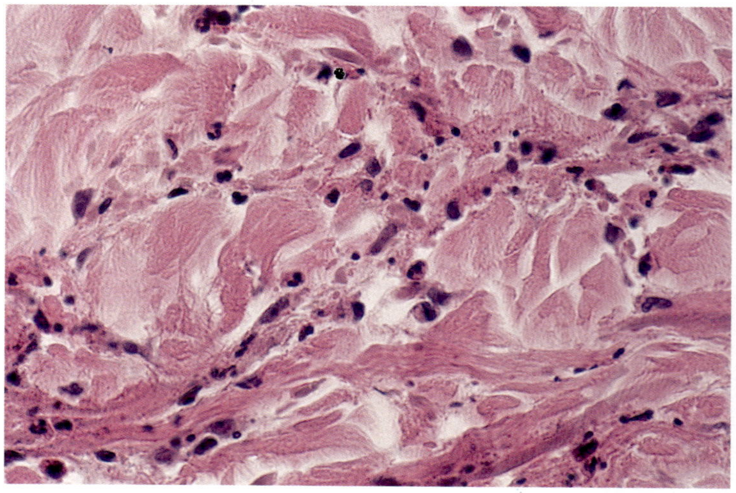

Figure 18–4. Flea bites. Neutrophils prevail among collagen bundles.

ARTHROPOD BITE REACTIONS

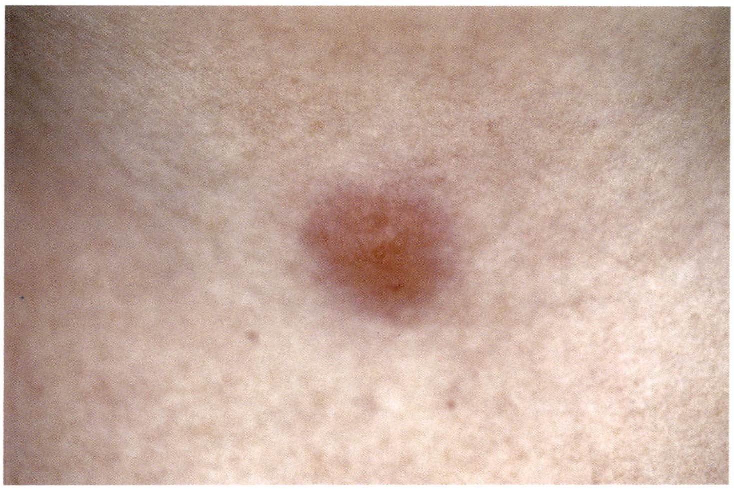

Figure 18–5. Insect bite. Erythematous, dome-shaped papule.

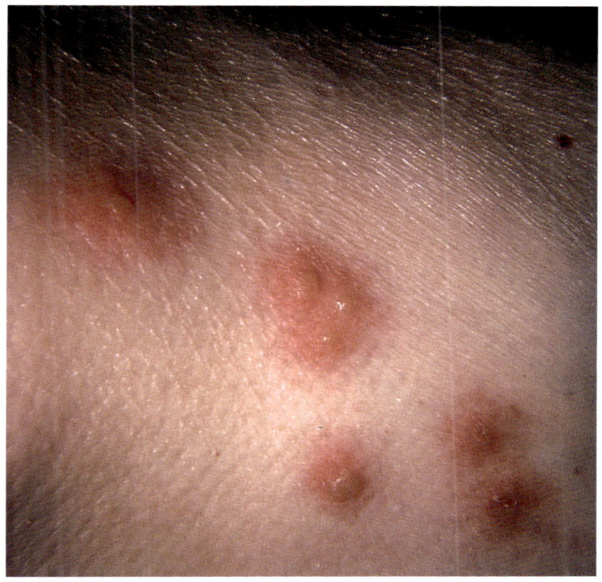

Figure 18–6. Insect bites. Grouped erythematous vesiculopapules on the leg.

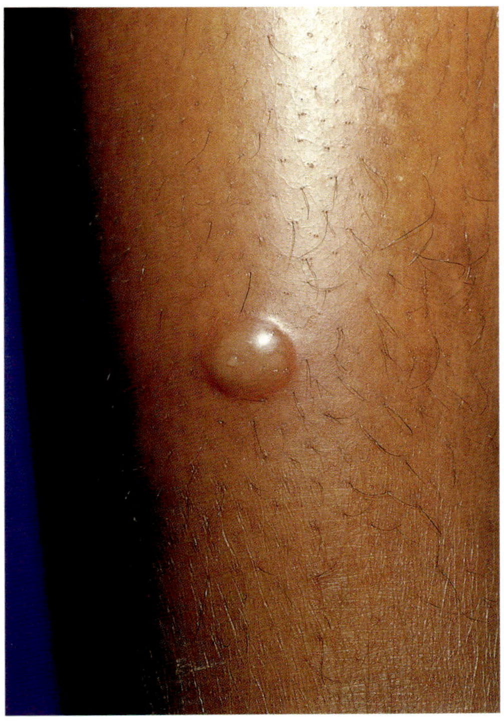

Figure 18–7. Insect bite. Bullous lesion with central puncta on the leg.

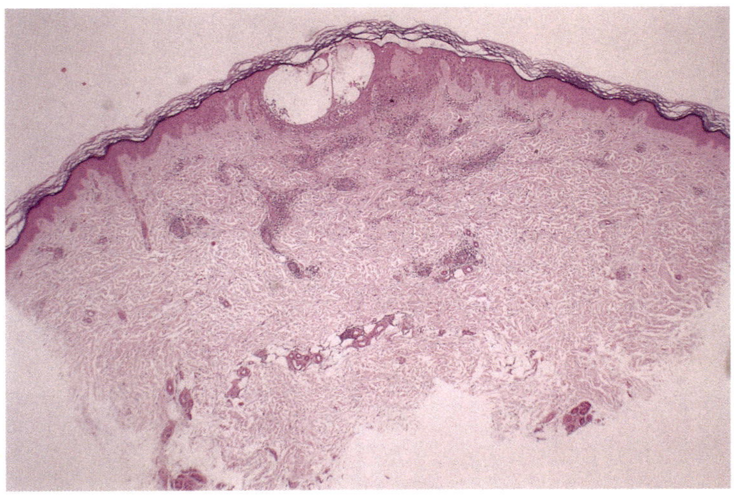

Figure 18–8. Insect bite. Centrally located intraepidermal vesicle with a dense perivascular and mild interstitial mixed-cell infiltrate.

ARTHROPOD BITE REACTIONS

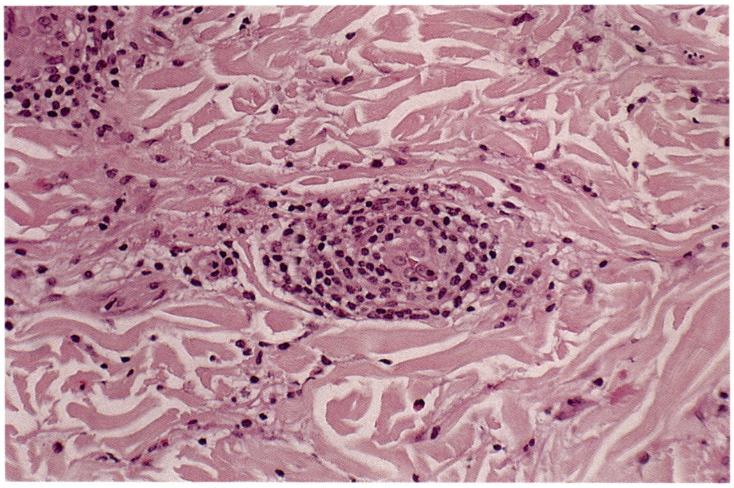

Figure 18–9. Insect bite. Perivascular and interstitial inflammatory infiltrate with numerous eosinophils.

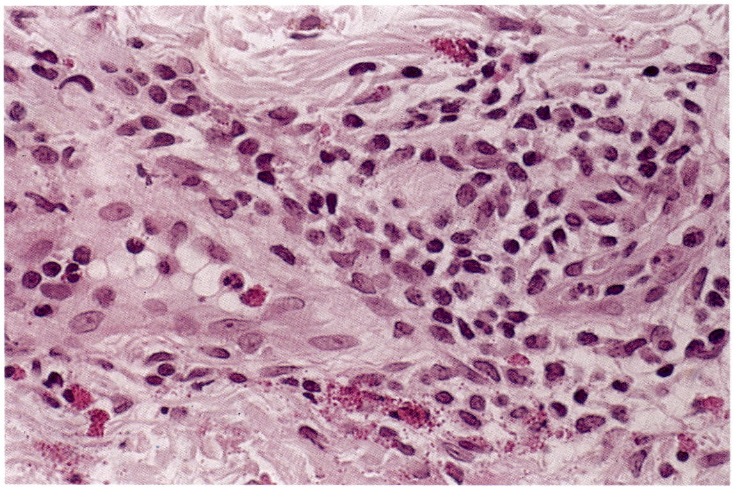

Figure 18–10. Insect bite. Focal areas with degranulation of eosinophils.

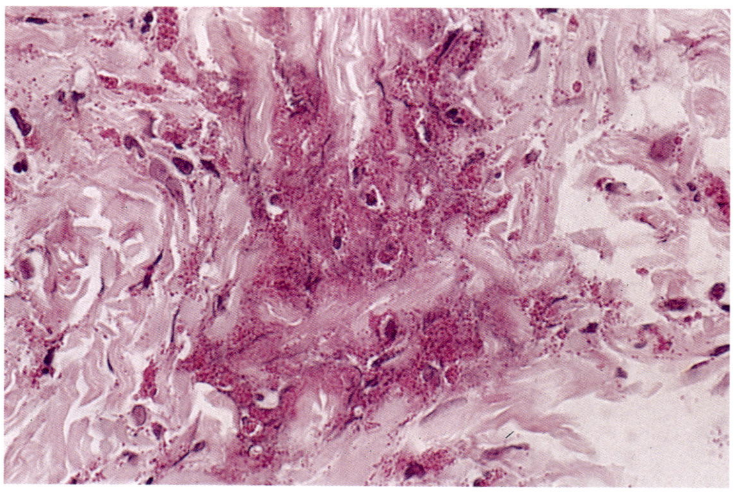

Figure 18–11. Insect bite. Collagen bundles with eosinophilic deposits from degranulated eosinophils. These areas are commonly referred to as "flame figures"; they are not pathognomonic for any specific disease.

SCABIES

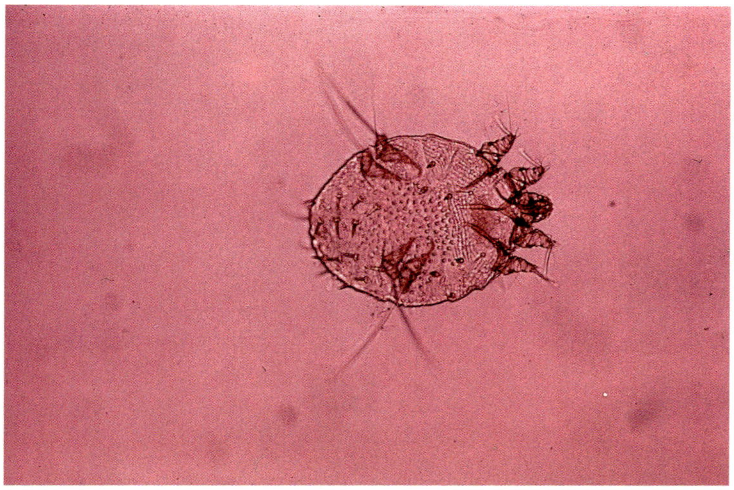

Figure 18–12. ***Sarcoptes scabiei,* adult mite.** Transverse corrugations, spines, and bristles. There are front legs with claw-shaped suckers, and rear legs that end in long, trailing bristles.

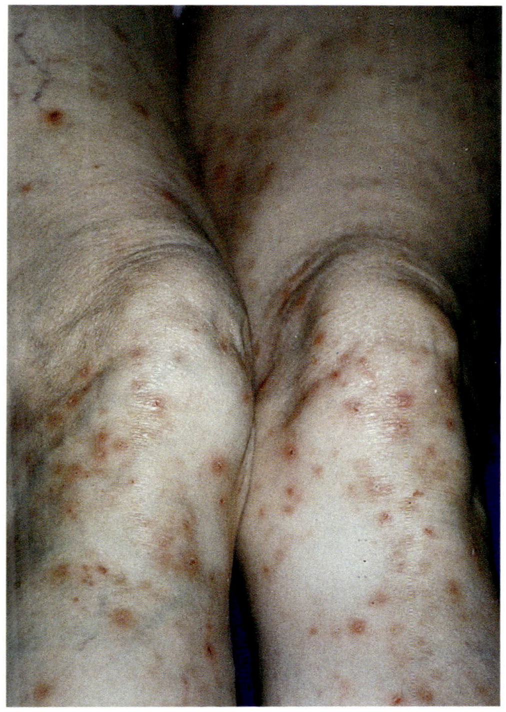

Figure 18–13. **Scabies.** Severely pruritic, excoriated erythematous papules on the legs.

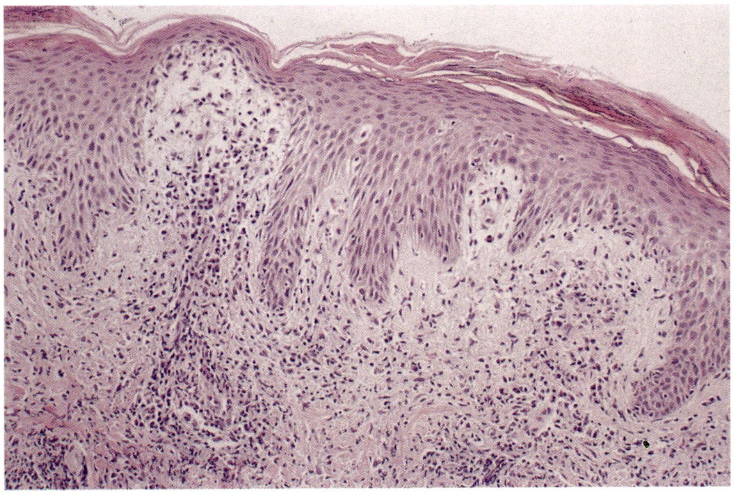

Figure 18–14. **Scabies.** Inflammatory infiltrate with scale-crust.

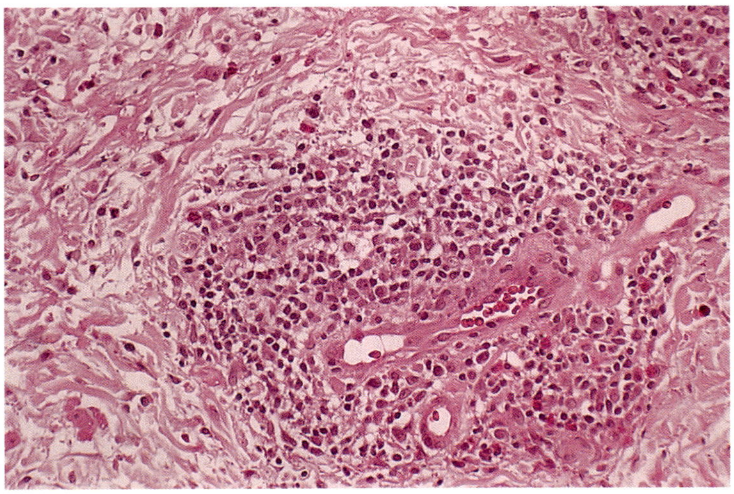

Figure 18–15. **Scabies.** Dermal mixed-cell infiltrate with numerous perivascular and interstitial eosinophils.

SCABIES

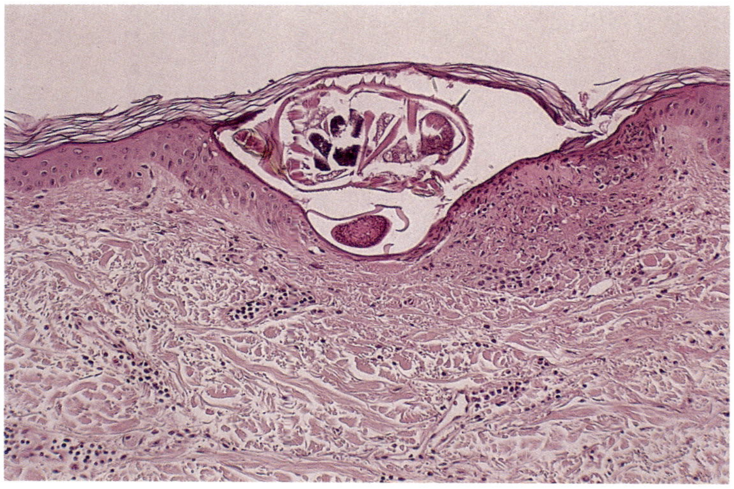

Figure 18–16. Scabies. Adult female mite with egg containing embryo within the epidermis.

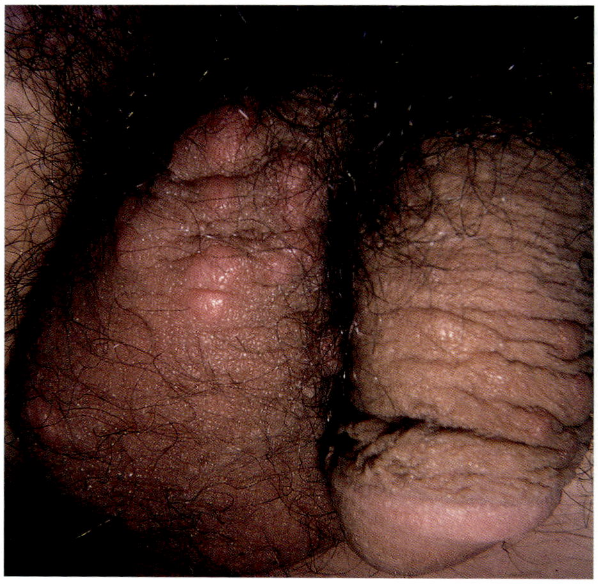

Figure 18–17. Nodular scabies. Pruritic papules on the scrotum and penis.

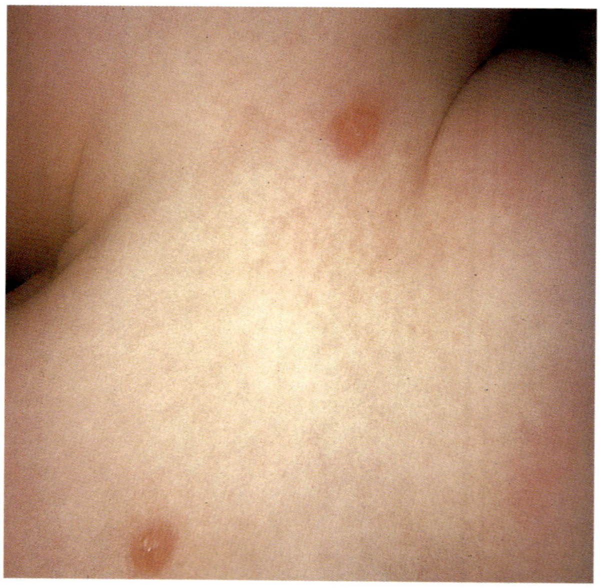

Figure 18–18. Nodular scabies. Pruritic erythematous papules on the neck and back of an infant.

SCABIES

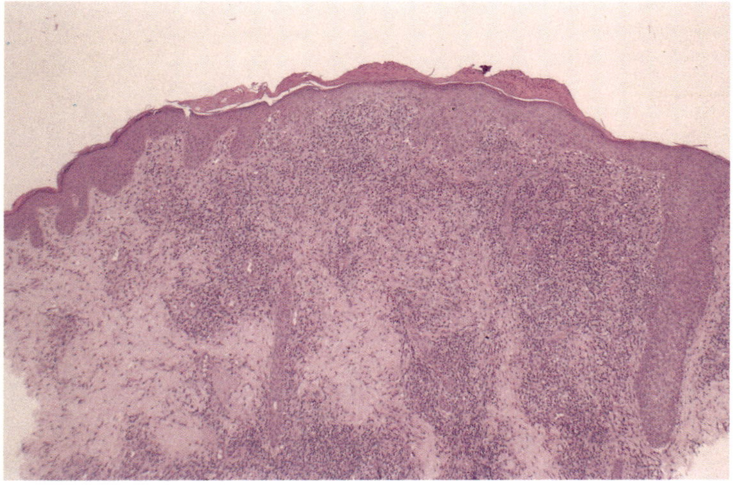

A

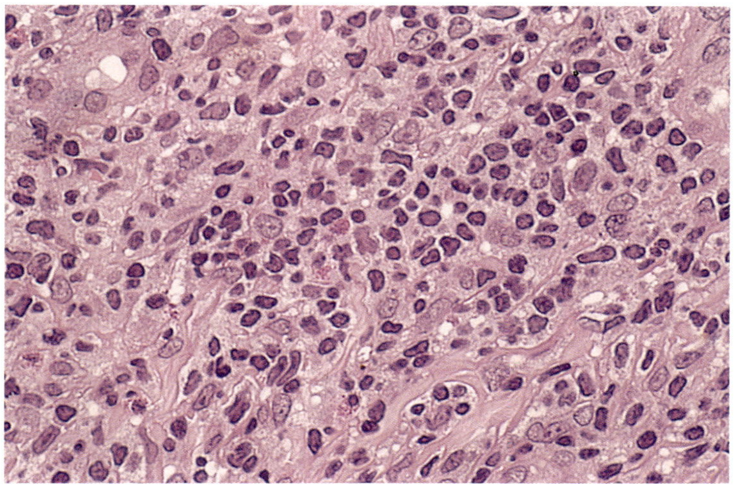

B

Figures 18–19A, 18–19B. Nodular scabies. Scale-crust, epidermal hyperplasia, and coarse collagen bundles. There is a dense dermal lymphohistiocytic infiltrate, eosinophils, and occasional mononuclear cell with atypia.

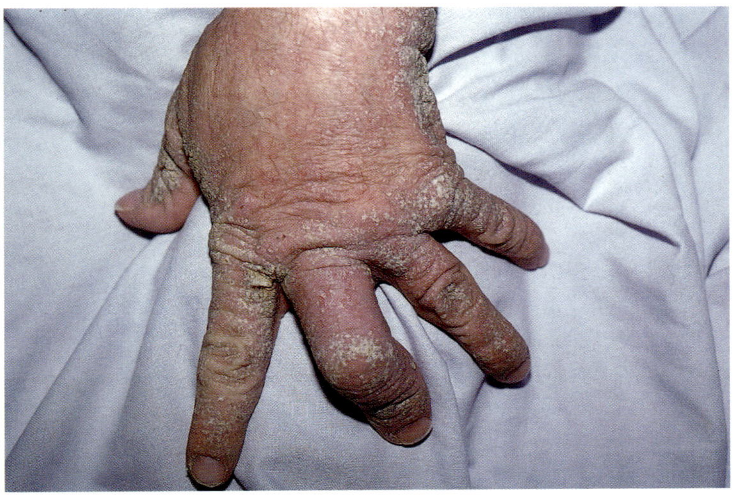

Figure 18–20. Norwegian scabies. Extensive hyperkeratosis of the arm, hand, and fingers.

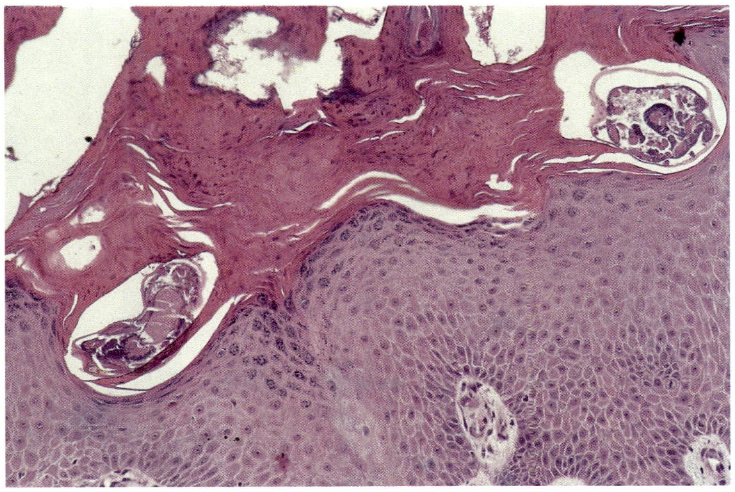

Figure 18–21. Norwegian scabies. Marked epidermal hyperplasia and hyperkeratosis with numerous mites within the cornified layer.

TICK BITE GRANULOMA

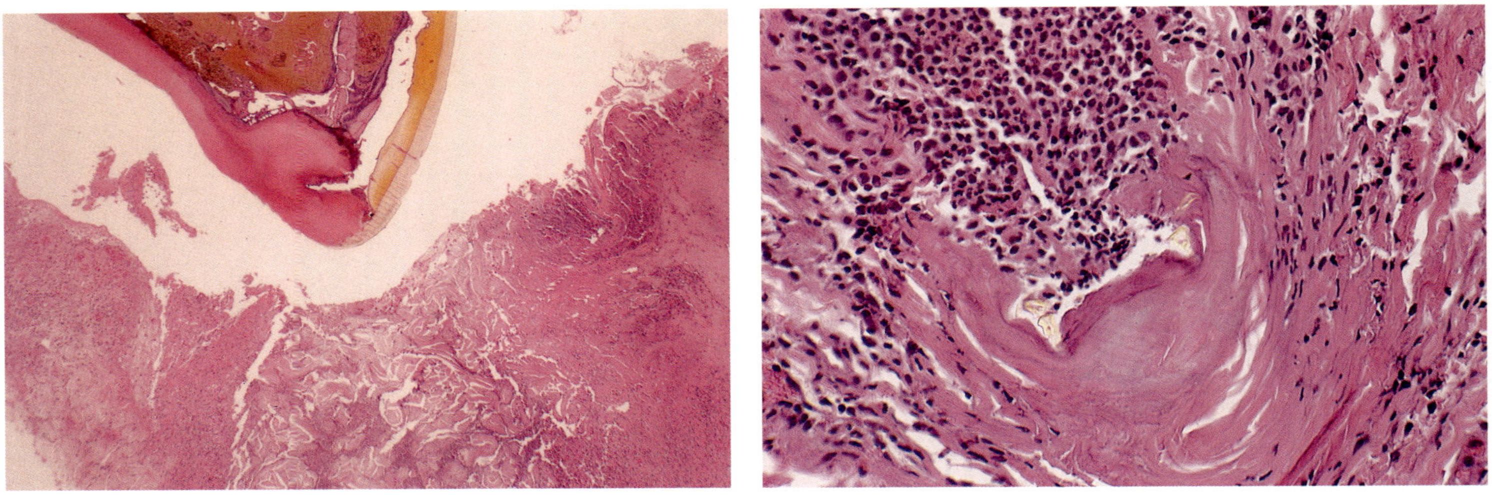

A B

Figures 18–22A, 18–22B. T ck bite granuloma. Proboscis of tick on the surface of the skin and within the dermis with a neutrophilic infiltrate.

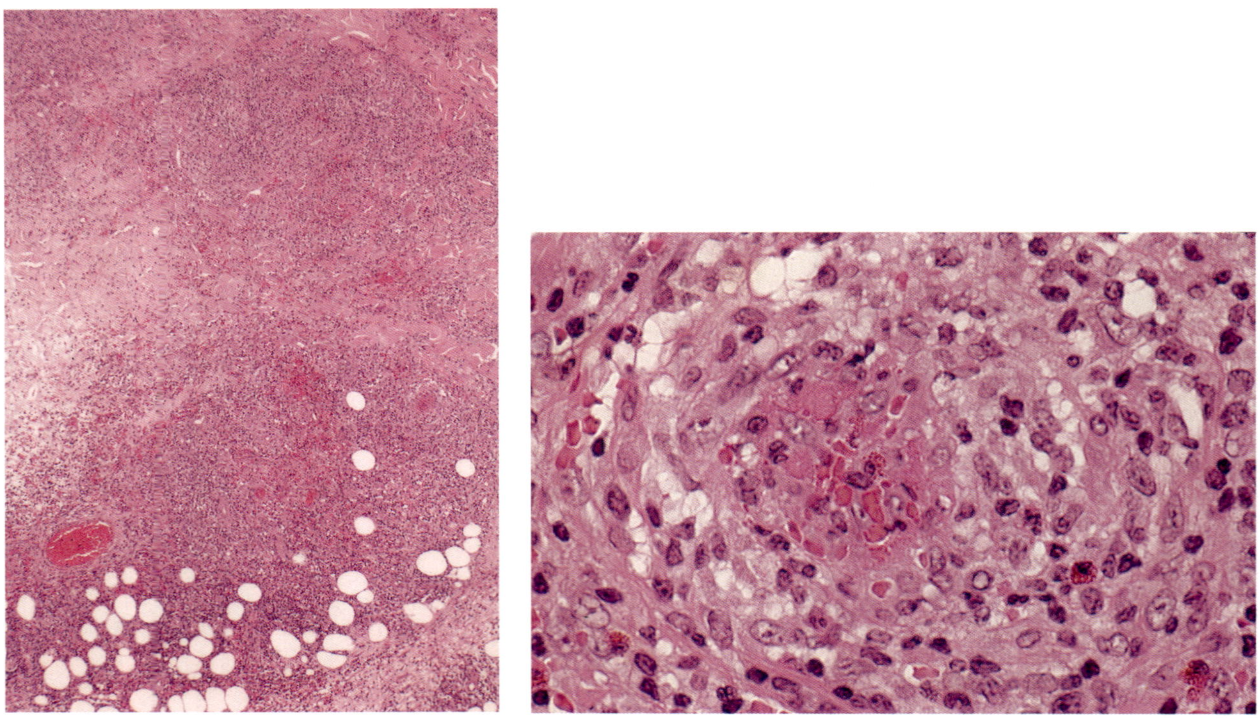

A B

Figures 18–23A, 18–23B. Tick bite granuloma. Dermal and subcutaneous suppurative granulomatous infiltrate. There are neutrophils, eosinophils, dilated and congested blood vessels with fibrin deposition and extravasated red blood cells, and focal leukocytoclastic vasculitis.

BROWN RECLUSE SPIDER BITE

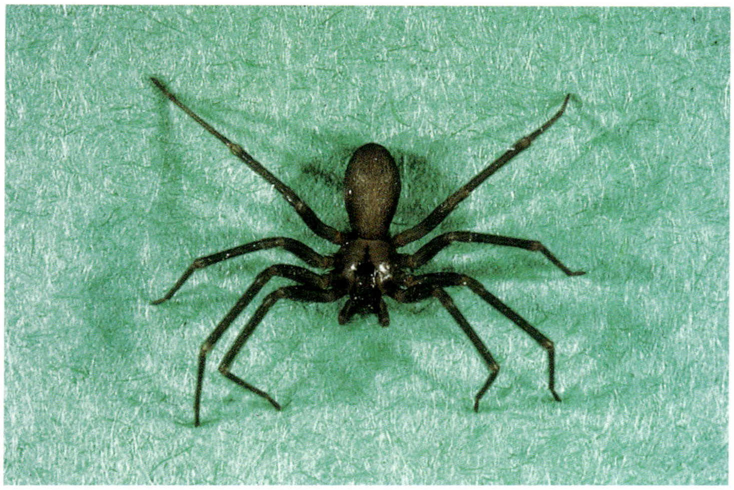

Figure 18–24. **Adult brown recluse spider, *Loxosceles reclusa*.** The cephalothorax bears the characteristic dark violin-shaped mark.

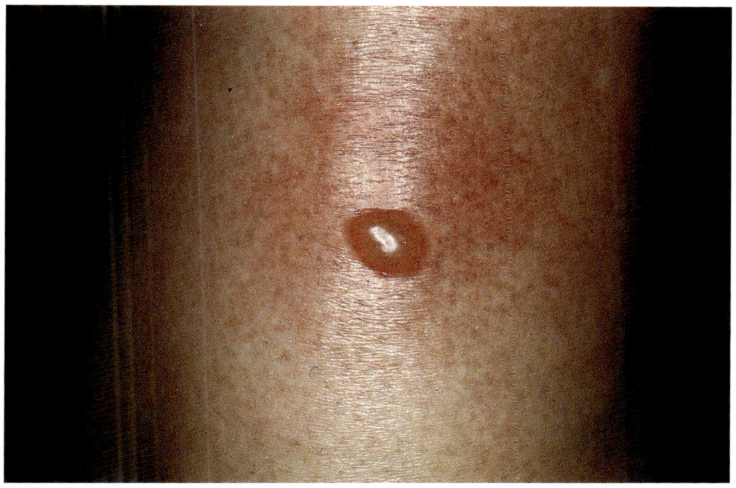

Figure 18–25. **Brown recluse spider bite, early evolving lesion.** Bulla with surrounding hemorrhagic erythema.

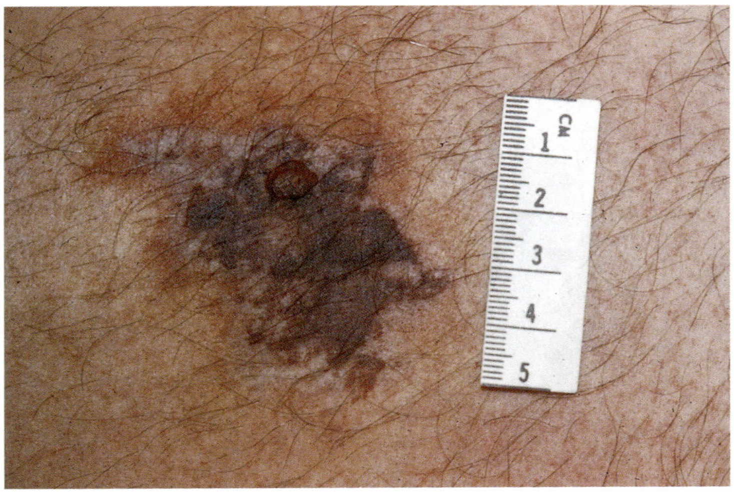

Figure 18–26. **Brown recluse spider bite, later lesion.** Central zone of bulla with hemorrhagic crusted midzone of surrounding pallor, and peripheral zone of hemorrhagic erythema.

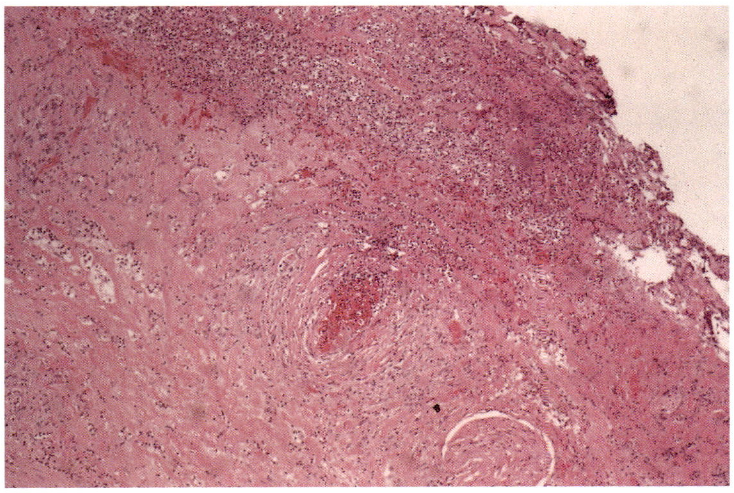

Figure 18–27. **Brown recluse spider bite.** Epidermal ulceration with a dense infiltrate of neutrophils. Venules are dilated, congested, and contain fibrin. Collagen degeneration is present with a mixed mononuclear and neutrophilic infiltrate.

19

Physical injuries

- Factitial dermatitis
- Traumatic intracorneal hemorrhage

FACTITIAL DERMATITIS

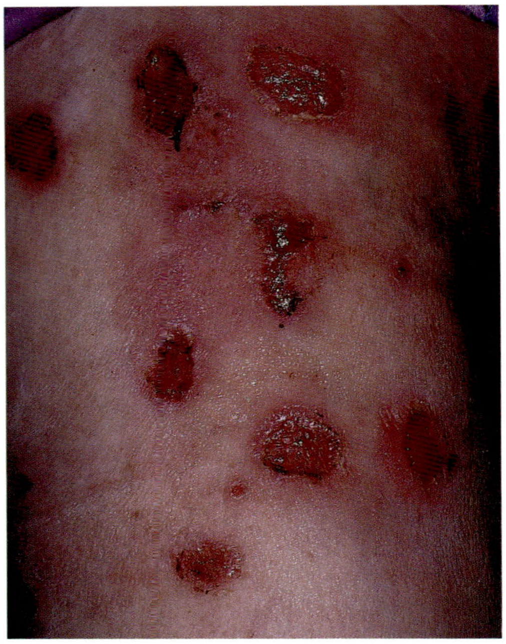

Figure 19–1. Factitial dermatitis. Oozing, erythematous, ulcerated plaques with sharp borders on the thigh of a woman.

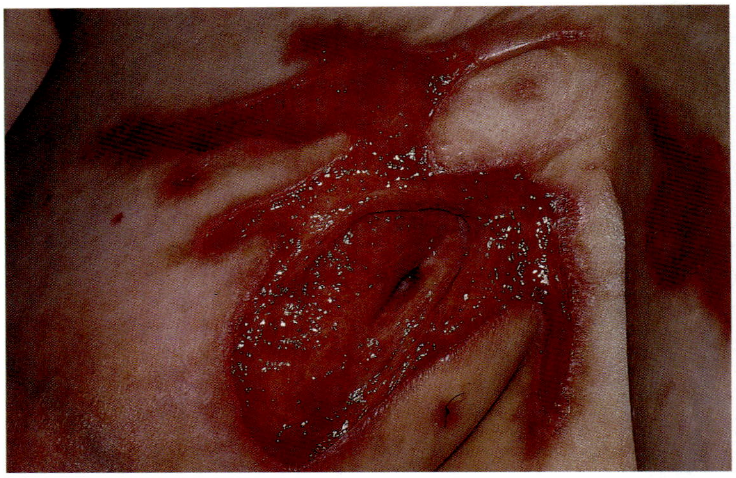

Figure 19–2. Factitial dermatitis. Bizarre-shaped sharply marginated erythematous, deeply ulcerated plaques on the chest and breast of a woman.

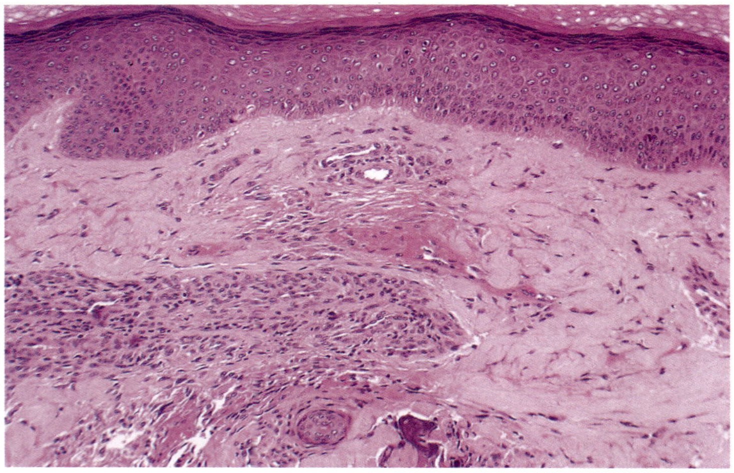

A

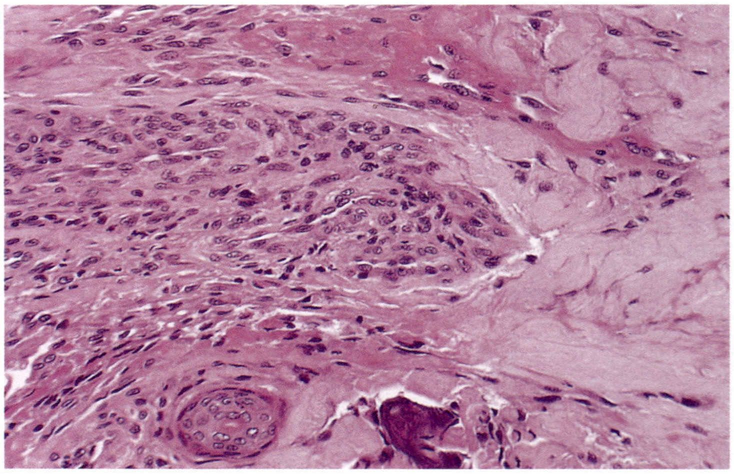

B

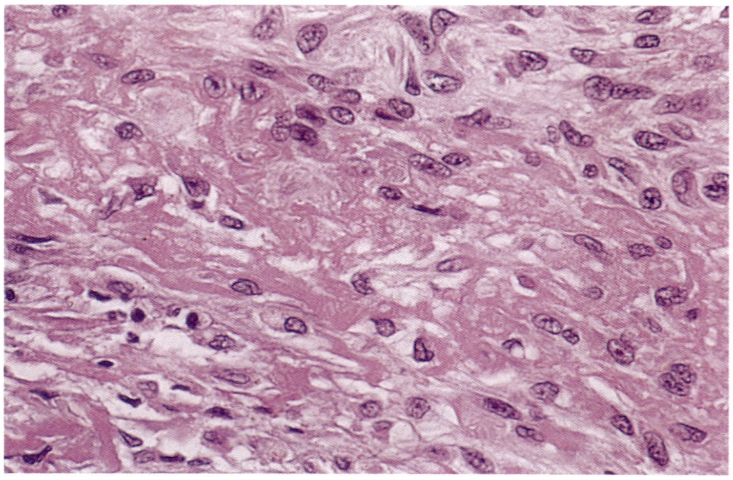

C

Figures 19–3A, 19–3B, 19–3C. Factitial dermatitis. Dermal fibrin deposits among altered collagen bundles and a mixed-cell infiltrate. There are atypical mononuclear cells.

TRAUMATIC INTRACORNEAL HEMORRHAGE

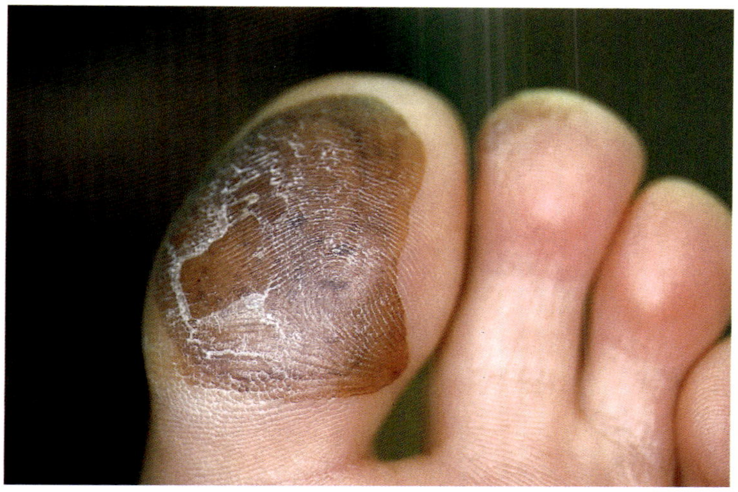

Figure 19–4. Traumatic intracorneal hemorrhage (tache noire). Nontender, sharply marginated, hyperpigmented scaly patch on the toe of a woman who plays tennis. This typically occurs on the heel, where it is referred to as "black heel."

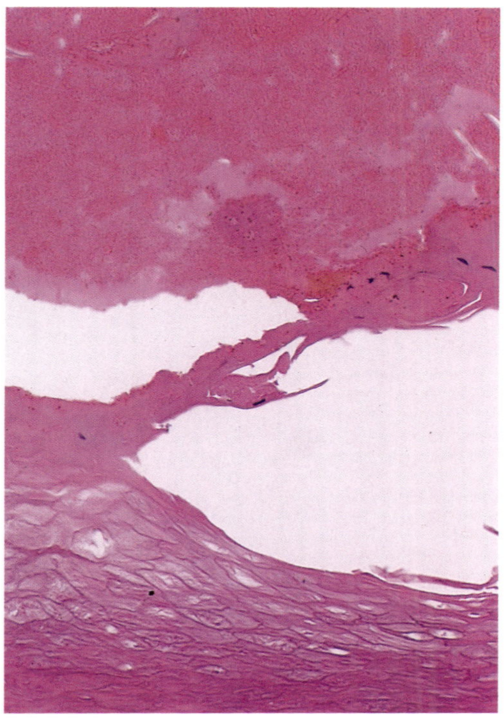

Figure 19–5. Traumatic intracorneal hemorrhage (tache noire). Scale-crust with erythrocytes within the thickened stratum corneum.

20

NONINFLAMMATORY DISORDERS

- Ichthyosis
- Punctate keratoderma
- Acanthosis nigricans
- Porokeratosis
- Necrolytic migratory erythema

ICHTHYOSIS

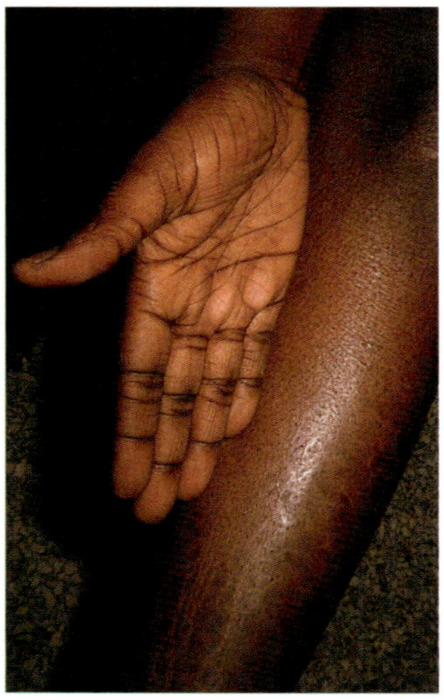

Figure 20–1. Ichthyosis vulgaris. Lower leg with fishlike scaling and follicular hyperkeratoses. Palm of hand with increased hyperpigmented creases.

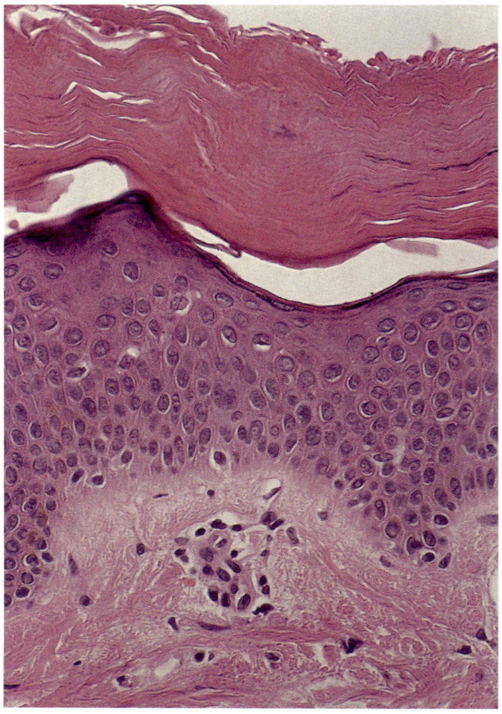

Figure 20–2. Ichthyosis vulgaris. Hyperkeratosis, slight epidermal hyperplasia, and hypogranulosis.

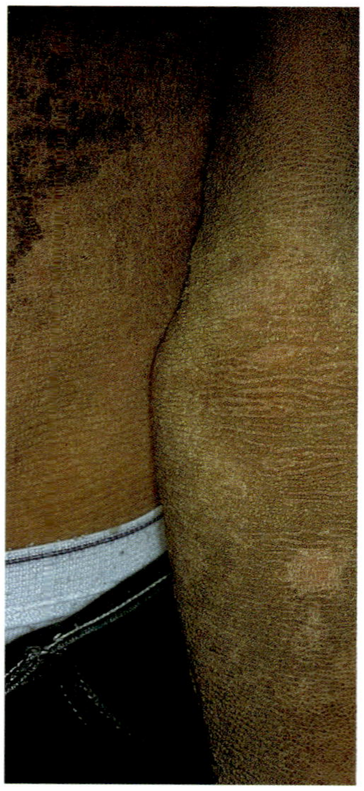

Figure 20–3. Lamellar ichthyosis. Extensive hyperkeratosis of the trunk and extremities.

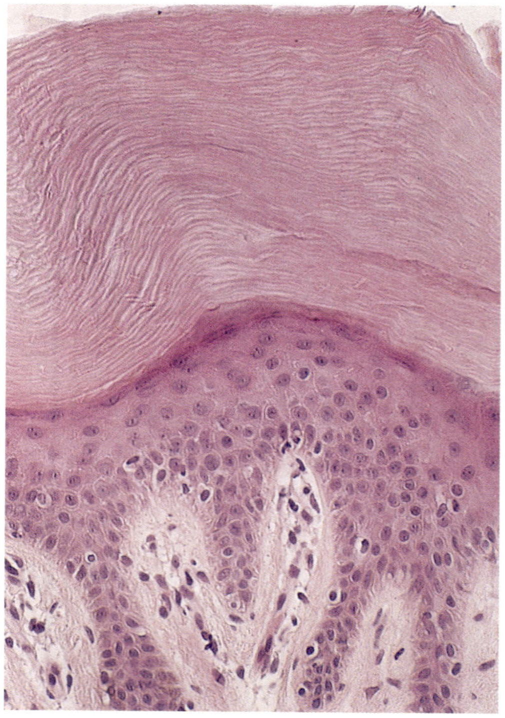

Figure 20–4. Lamellar ichthyosis. Markedly thickened stratum corneum with compact, laminated hyperkeratosis, hypergranulosis, and psoriasiform epidermal hyperplasia.

PUNCTATE KERATODERMA

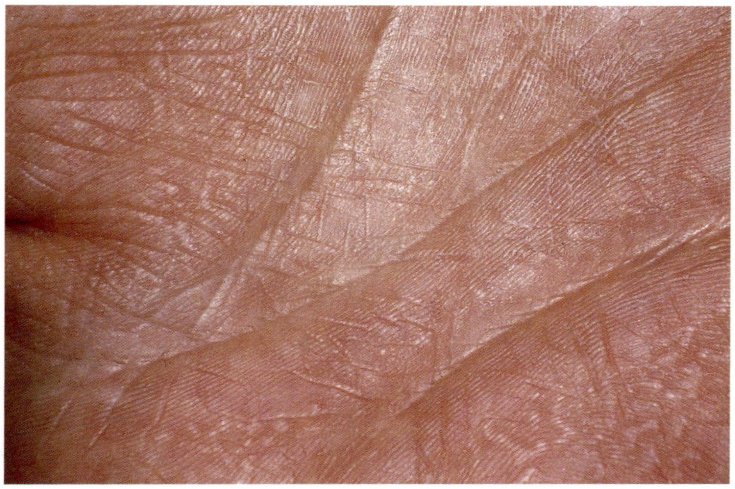

Figure 20–5. Punctate keratoderma. Keratotic papules on the palms of the hands.

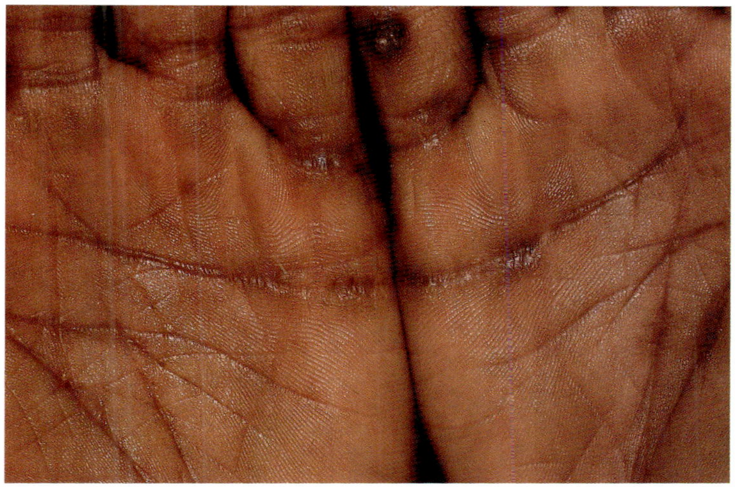

Figure 20–6. Punctate keratoderma. Depressed keratotic papules in linear array within finger and palmar creases.

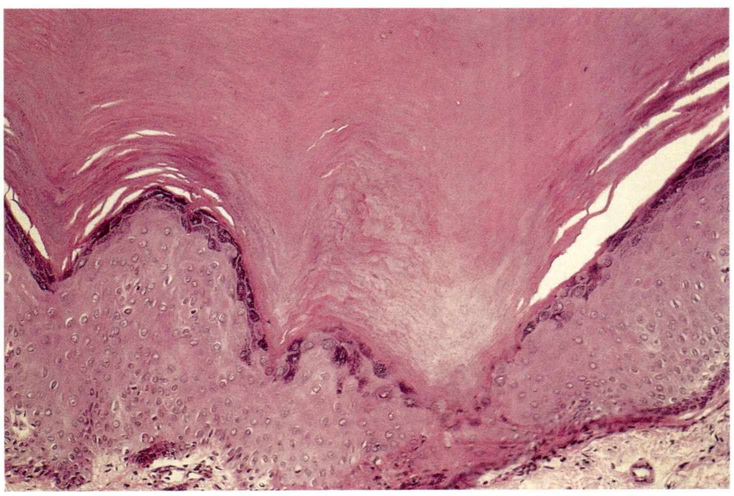

Figure 20–7. Punctate keratoderma. Markedly thickened stratum corneum with compact hyperkeratosis.

ACANTHOSIS NIGRICANS

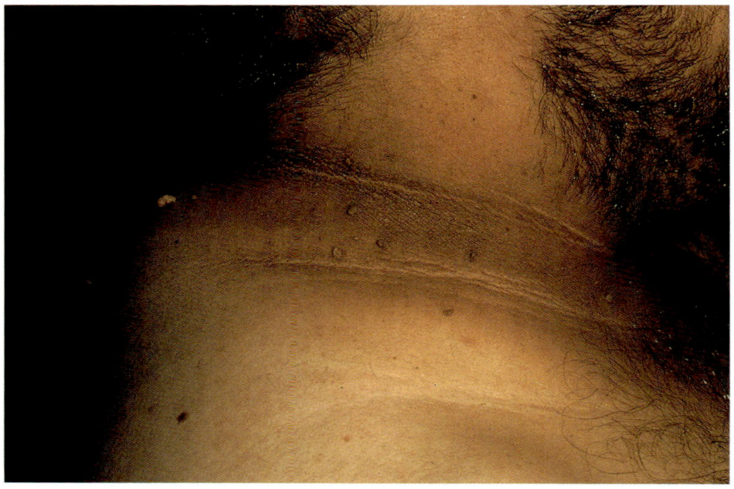

Figure 20–8. Acanthosis nigricans. Hyperpigmented, velvety plaques on the sides of the neck, a common location.

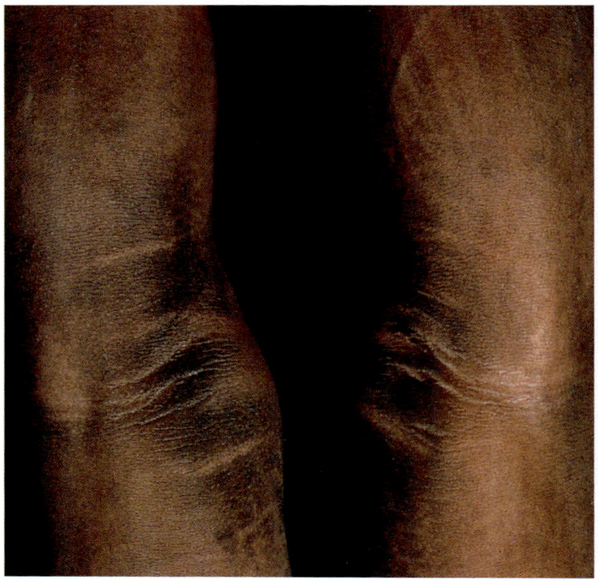

Figure 20–9. Acanthosis nigricans. Extensive hyperpigmented plaques on the arms in a patient with congenital lipodystrophy. This is an unusual distribution for acanthosis nigricans.

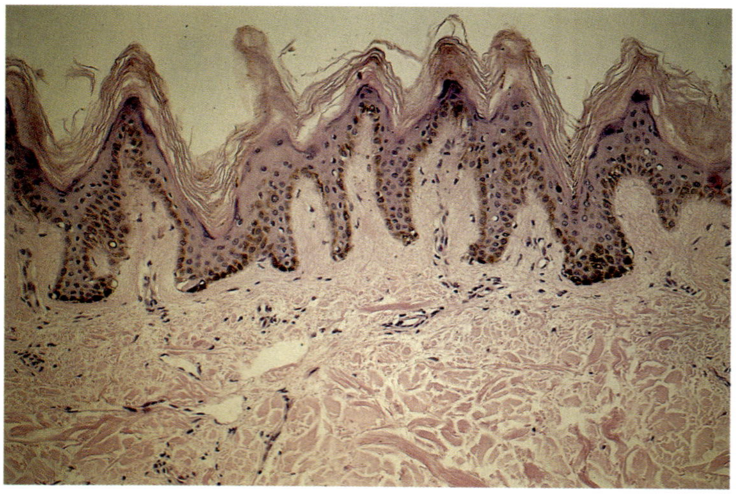

Figure 20–10. Acanthosis nigricans. Hyperkeratosis and papillomatosis.

POROKERATOSIS

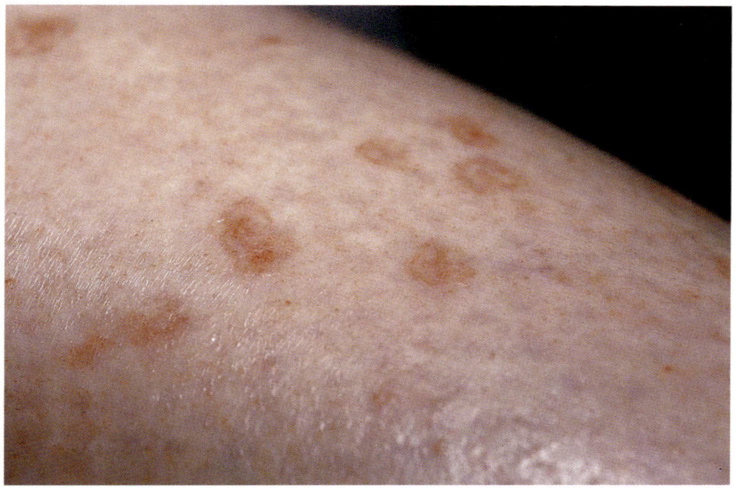

Figure 20–11. Disseminated actinic porokeratosis. Circular, erythematous patches with raised keratotic border.

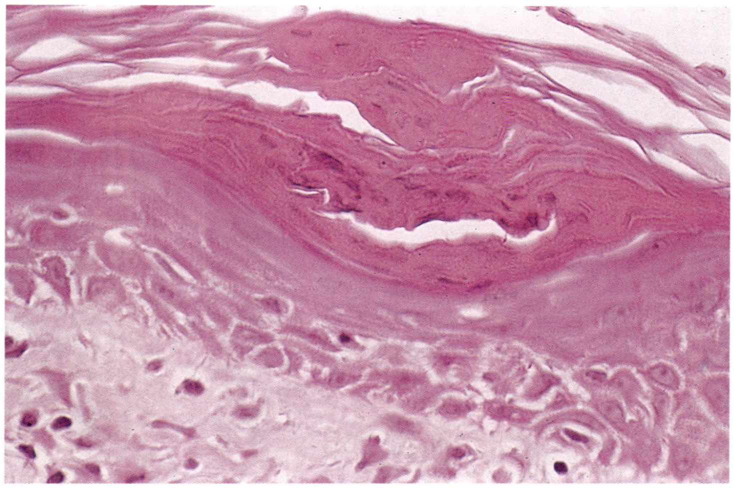

Figure 20–12. Disseminated actinic porokeratosis. Hyperkeratosis and vertical parakeratosis. There is hypogranulosis and cyskeratotic cells in the epidermis, and solar elastosis in the dermis.

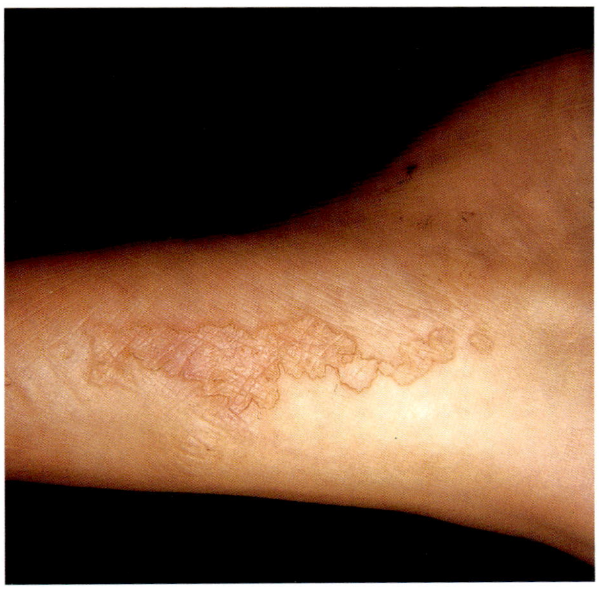

Figure 20–13. Porokeratosis of Mibelli. Annular erythematous plaque on the sole of the foot. There is a raised, irregular keratotic ridge at the periphery.

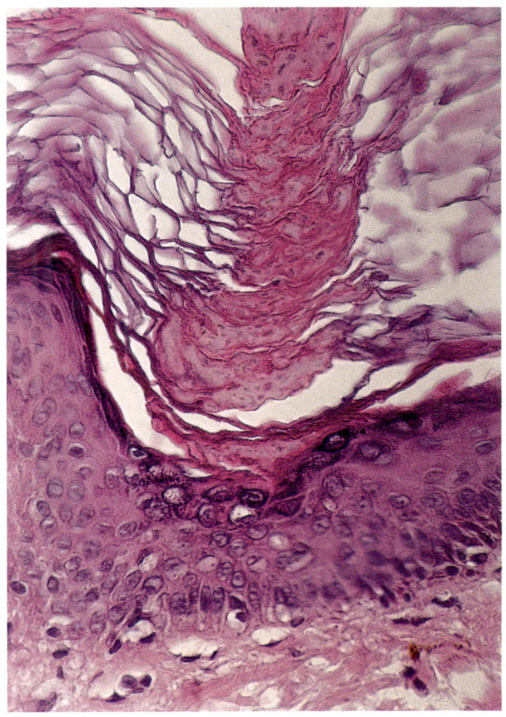

Figure 20–14. Porokeratosis. Thin, vertical column of parakeratotic cells commonly referred to as a coronoid lamella. Beneath the coronoic lamella, there is a focus of hypogranulosis and vacuolated and dyskeratotic cells.

NECROLYTIC MIGRATORY ERYTHEMA

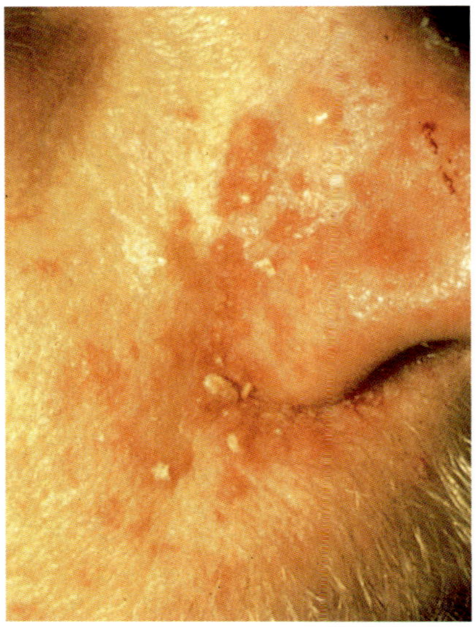

A

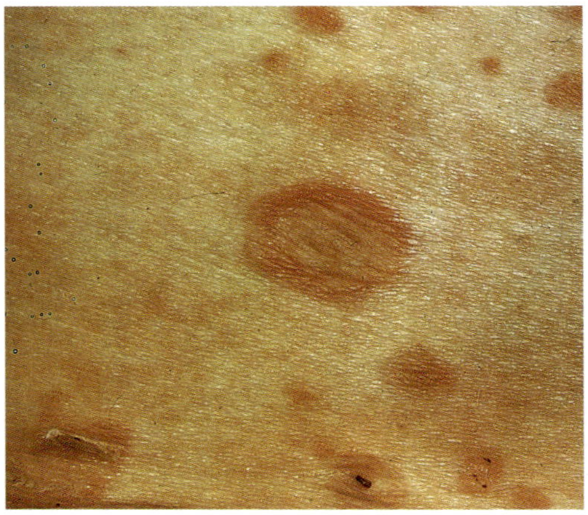

B

Figures 20–15A, 20–15B. Necrolytic migratory erythema. Erythematous, crusted patches in a man with glucagonoma syndrome.

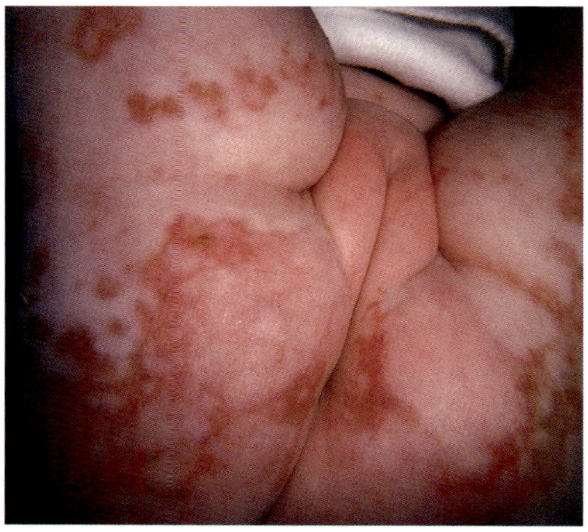

Figure 20–16. Necrolytic migratory erythema. Serpiginous, erythematous crusted patches and vesiculopapules in a child with zinc deficiency, which is known as acrodermatitis enteropathica. These changes may also occur in other vitamin or nutritional deficiencies, such as pellagra.

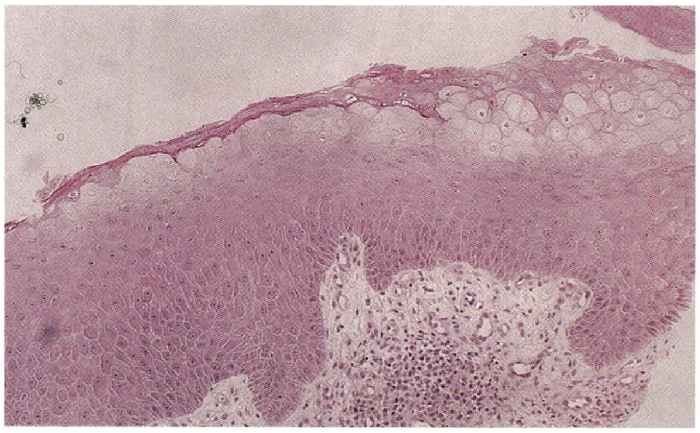

Figure 20–17. Necrolytic migratory erythema. Early changes are present in the upper spinous layers where there is extensive ballooning (intracellular edema), focal parakeratosis, and a mild dermal lymphohistiocytic infiltrate.

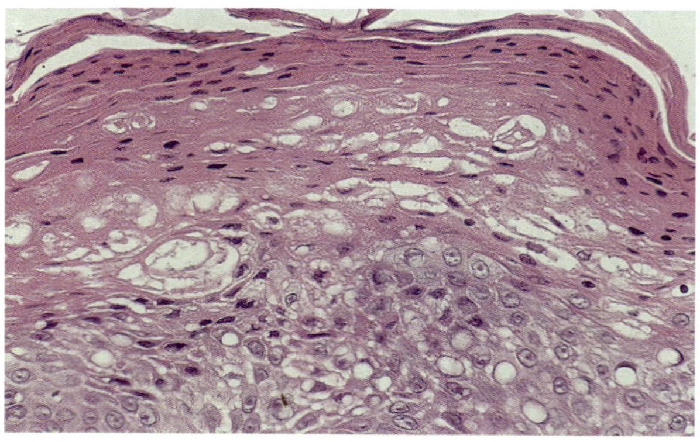

Figure 20–18. Necrolytic migratory erythema. Later changes in the epidermis are noted where there is widespread ballooning, spongiosis, dyskeratotic and parakeratotic spinous cells, and focal intraepidermal vesiculation.

21

FIBROUS TISSUE DISORDERS AND NEOPLASMS

- Lichen sclerosus et atrophicus/morphea
- Morphea and scleroderma
- Eosinophilic fasciitis
- Scleredema
- Solar elastosis
- Radiation dermatitis
- Stasis dermatitis
- Nodular fasciitis
- Fibromas
  - *A) Infantile digital fibromatosis*
  - *B) Acquired digital fibrokeratoma*
  - *C) Dermatofibroma*
  - *D) Pleomorphic fibroma*
  - *E) Sclerotic fibroma*
- Scar and keloid
- Fibroepithelial polyp
- Accessory nipple
- Focal dermal hypoplasia (Goltz syndrome)
- Angiofibroma (tuberous sclerosis)
- Nevus lipomatosis
- Fibrous hamartoma of infancy
- Connective tissue nevus
- Malignant neoplasms
  - *A) Dermatofibrosarcoma protuberans*
  - *B) Malignant fibrous histiocytoma/atypical fibroxanthoma*
  - *C) Fibrosarcoma*
  - *D) Epithelioid cell sarcoma*

LICHEN SCLEROSUS ET ATROPHICUS/MORPHEA

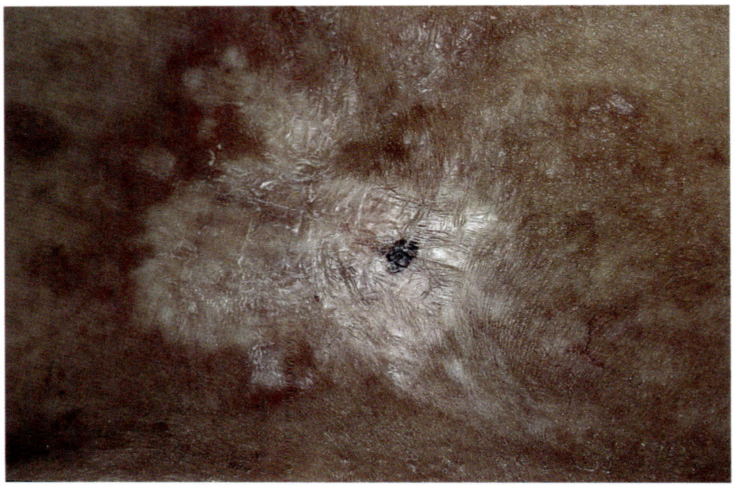

Figure 21–1. Lichen sclerosus et atrophicus/morphea. Indurated, hyperpigmented plaque with a central pale, waxy surface involving the inframammary area.

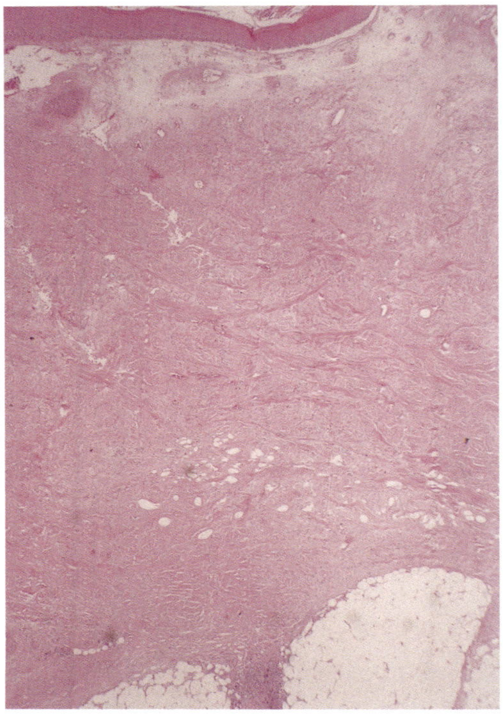

Figure 21–2. Lichen sclerosus et atrophicus/morphea. Effaced epidermis, marked papillary edema, and increased bundles of collagen in the thickened reticular dermis. There is a lymphoplasmacytic infiltrate at the dermal-subcutaneous junction, and the fibrous septum is thickened.

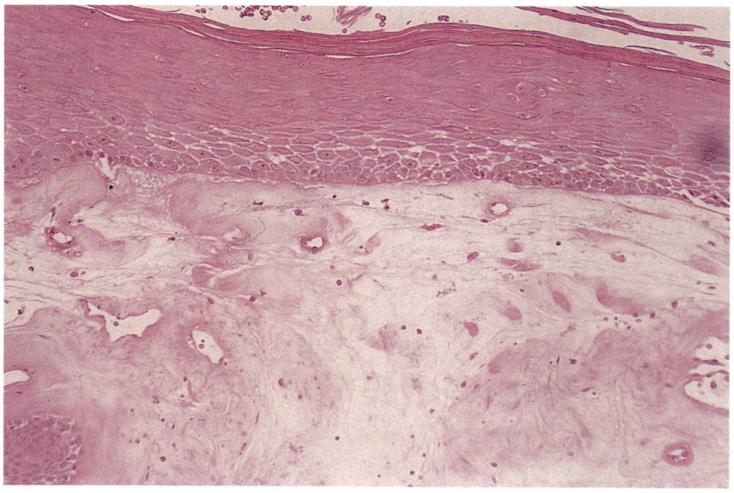

Figure 21–3. Lichen sclerosus et atrophicus. Characteristic changes with vacuolar alteration, and a thickened papillary dermis with edema, sclerosis, and telangiectases.

MORPHEA AND SCLERODERMA

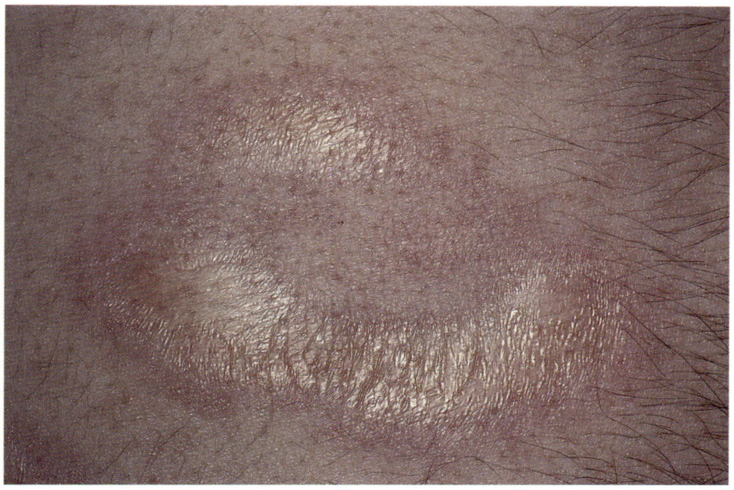

Figure 21–4. Morphea. Indurated plaque with peripheral erythema and central pallor.

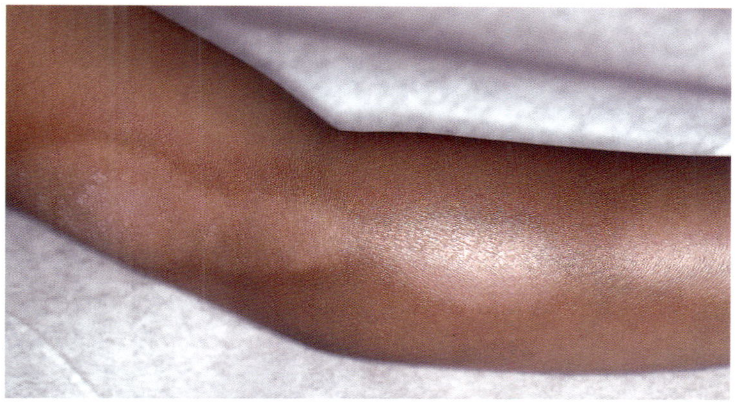

Figure 21–5. Morphea. Multiple, contiguous, linear, hypopigmented plaques with peripheral hyperpigmentation on the arm.

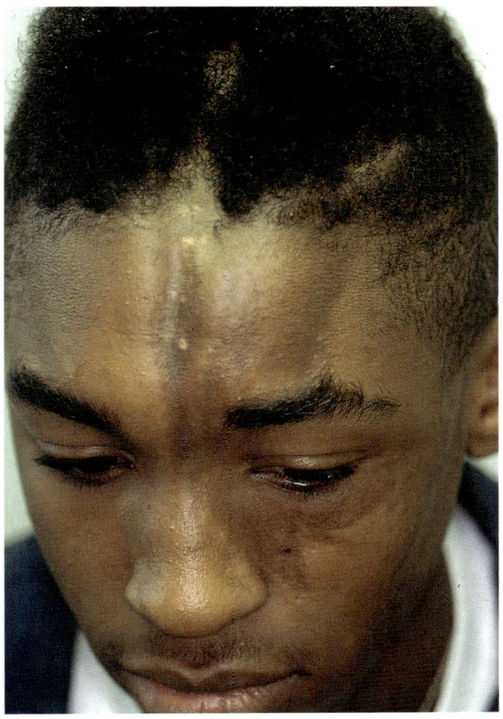

Figure 21–6. Morphea. Linear, hyperpigmented, atrophic lesion on the forehead and frontal scalp, where there is alopecia.

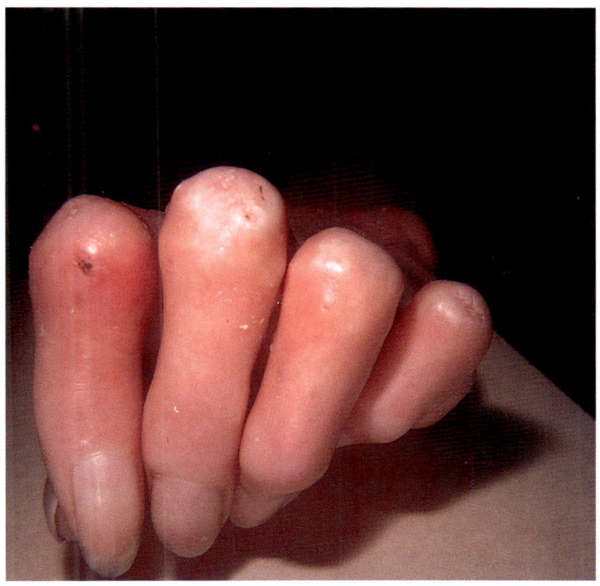

Figure 21–7. Scleroderma. Tapered, indurated fingers in a woman with progressive systemic sclerosis. There are calcified nodules and painful ulcers.

MORPHEA AND SCLERODERMA

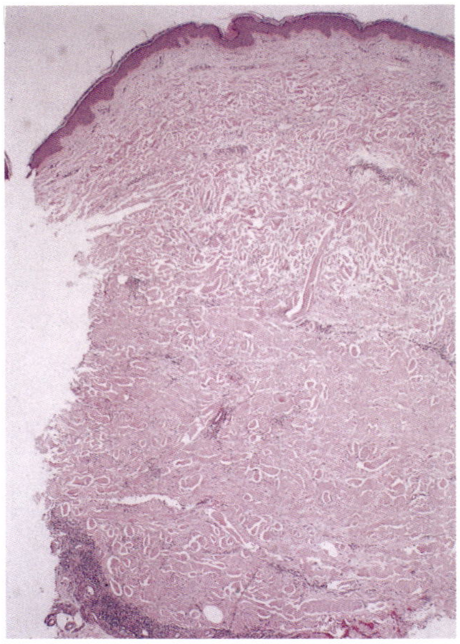

Figure 21–8. **Morphea and scleroderma.** Thickened reticular dermis with compressed collagen bundles and a lymphoplasmacytic infiltrate at the dermal-subcutaneous junction.

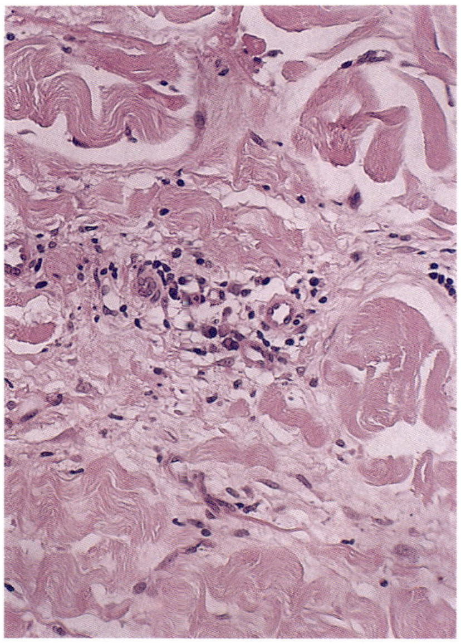

A

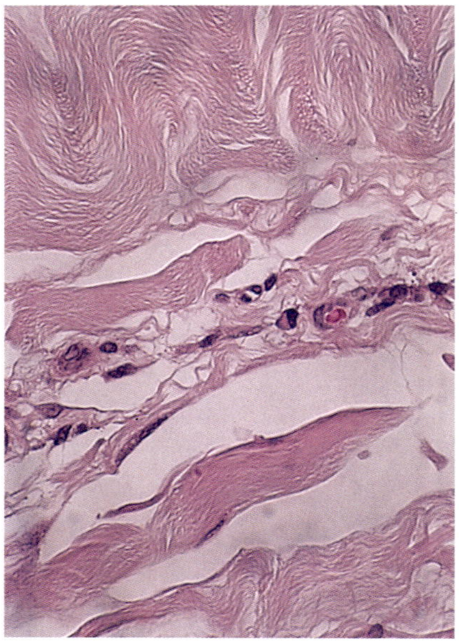

B

Figures 21–9A, 21–9B. **Morphea and scleroderma.** Thick collagen bundles and a lymphoplasmacytic perivascular and interstitial infiltrate.

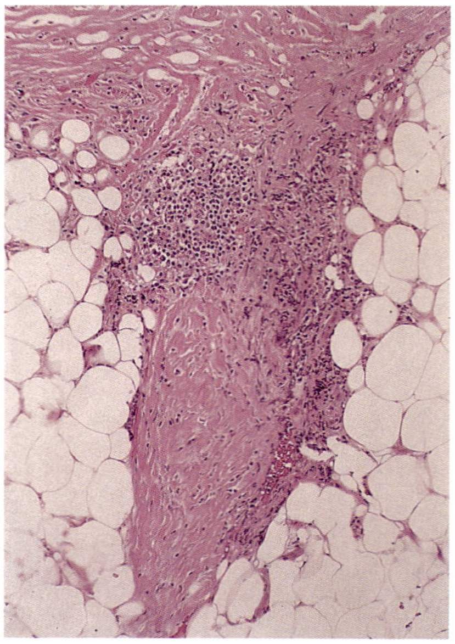

Figure 21–10. **Morphea and scleroderma.** Broad fibrous septum with thick bundles of collagen and a lymphoplasmacytic infiltrate.

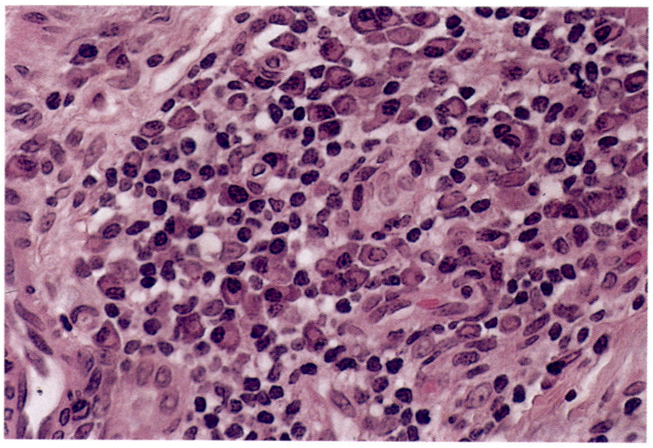

Figure 21–11. **Morphea and scleroderma.** Lymphoplasmacytic aggregation at the dermal-subcutaneous junction.

EOSINOPHILIC FASCIITIS

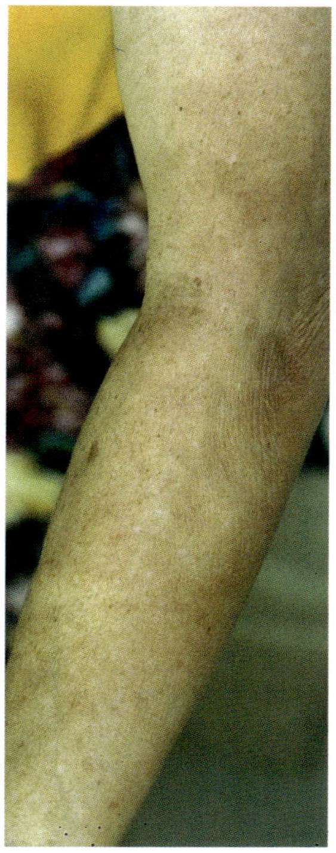

Figure 21–12. Eosinophilic fasciitis. Hard, tender, flesh-colored and pink nodules scattered over the dorsum of the upper and lower arm of a woman.

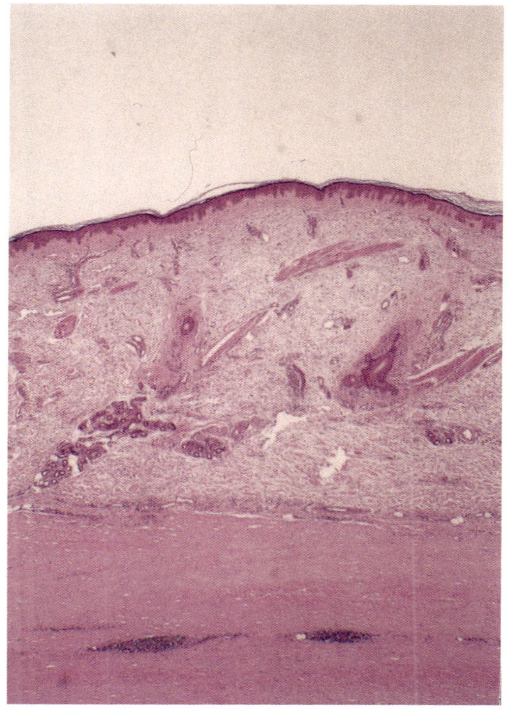

Figure 21–13. Eosinophilic fasciitis. Extensive thickening and sclerosis of the fascia and a mixed-cell infiltrate containing many plasma cells and a few eosinophils. The dermis does not appear to be involved.

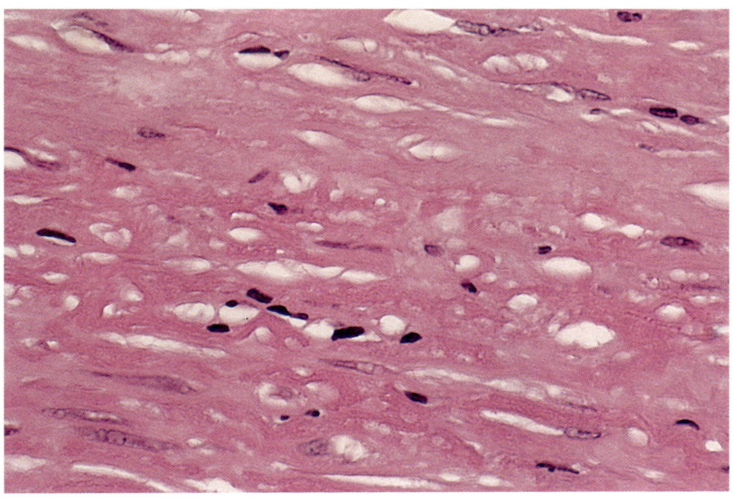

Figure 21–14. Eosinophilic fasciitis. Sclerosis of the fascia.

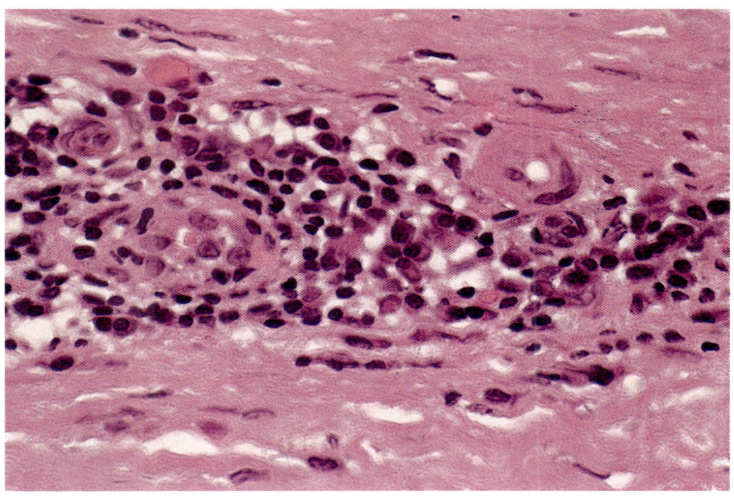

Figure 21–15. Eosinophilic fasciitis. Mixed-cell infiltrate with lymphocytes, plasma cells, and a few eosinophils.

SCLEREDEMA

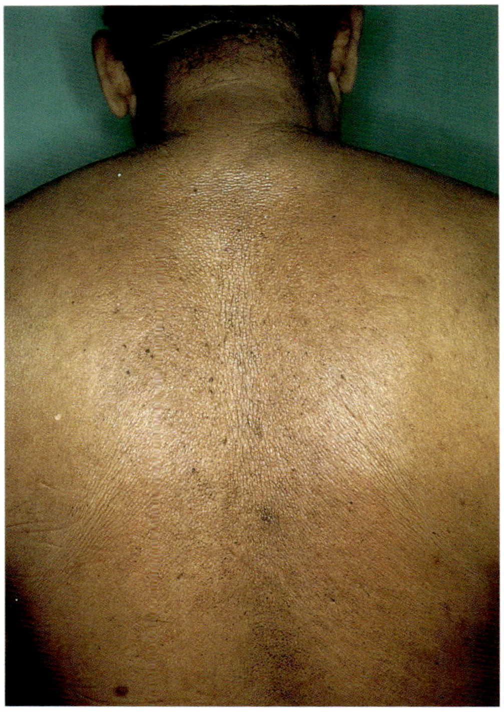

Figure 21–16. Scleredema. Induration and thickening of the sk n of the back and neck of a man.

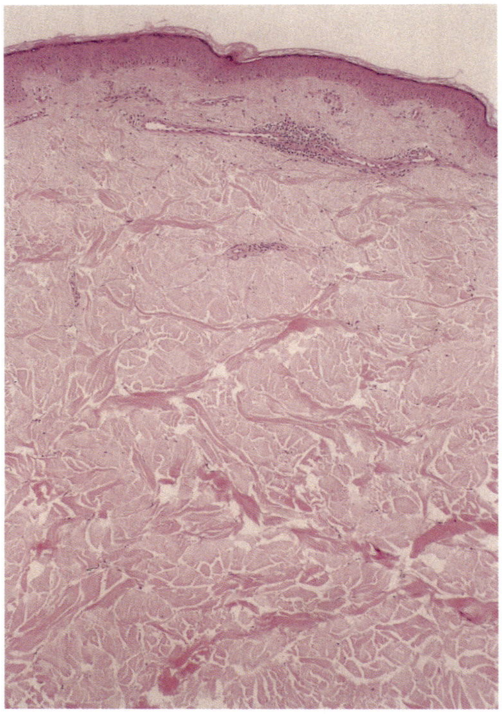

Figure 21–17. Scleredema. Extensive thickening of the reticular dermis. The collagen bundles are in a haphazard array, and there are prominent spaces between the bundles. Some collagen bundles are thickened, and there is a mild perivascular mononuclear cell infiltrate.

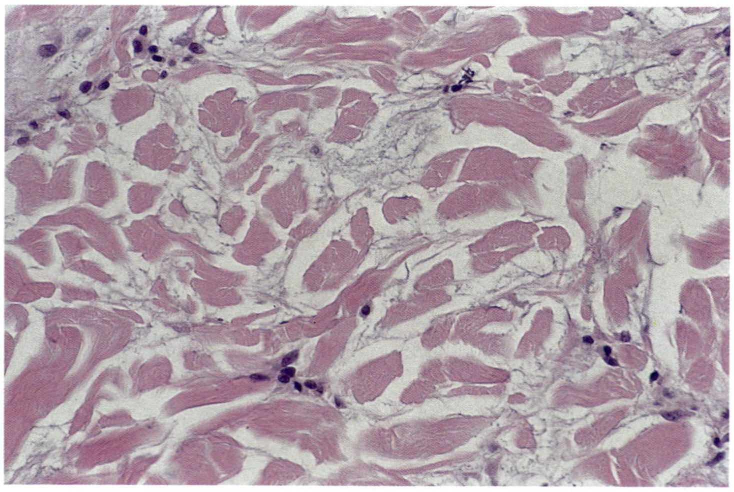

Figure 21–18. Scleredema. Grayish, granular, and feathery deposits of mucin are present within the spaces separating the collagen bundles.

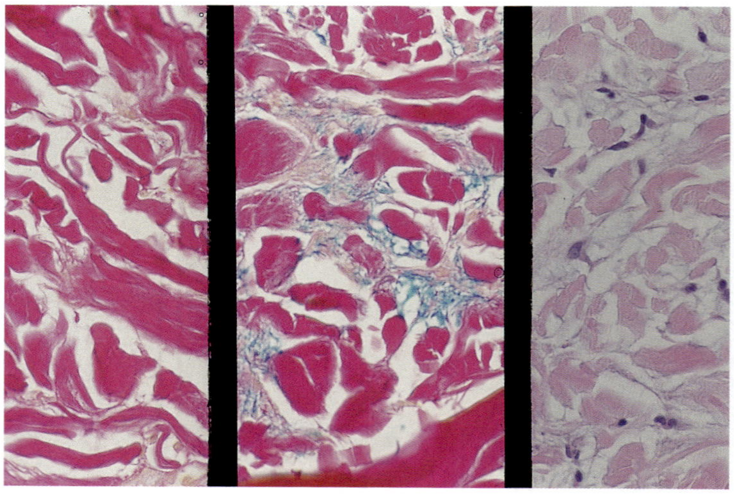

Figure 21–19. Scleredema. The left section is stained with hematoxylin and eosin and shows gray mucin deposits between collagen bundles; the middle section is stained with colloidal iron and shows blue mucin deposits between collagen bundles; the right section is stained with colloidal iron with hyaluronidase digestion, showing clear spaces between collagen bundles. Thus, the mucin present in scleredema is hyaluronidase.

SOLAR ELASTOSIS

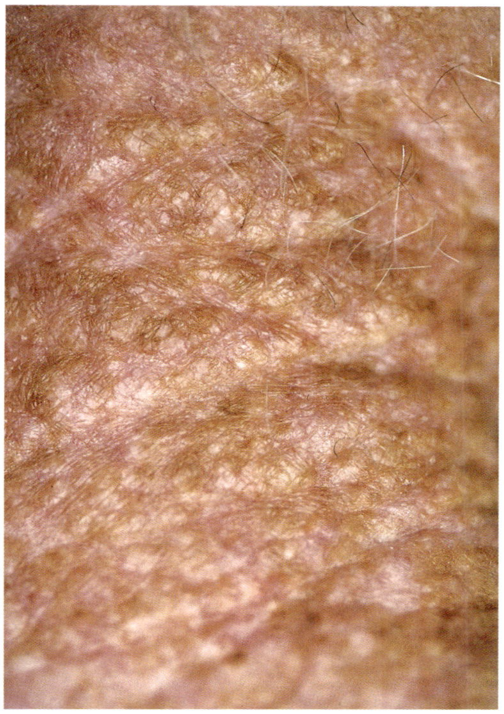

Figure 21–20. **Solar elastosis.** Sun-damaged skin on the posterior neck of a farmer. There is hyperpigmentation and hypopigmentation with many small, raised papules.

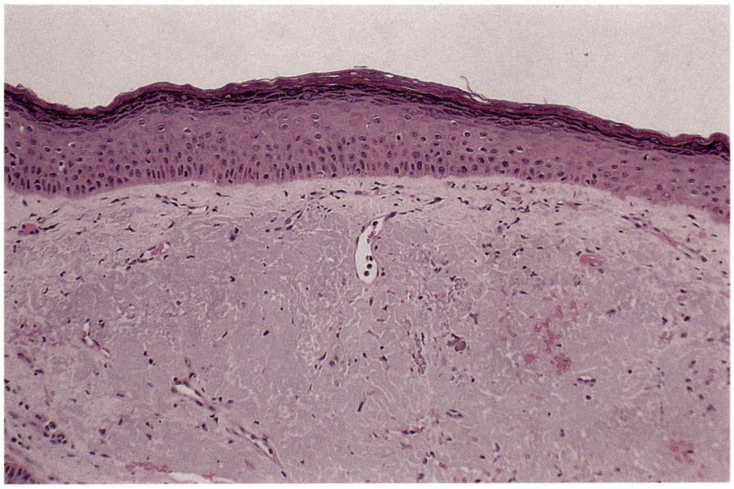

A

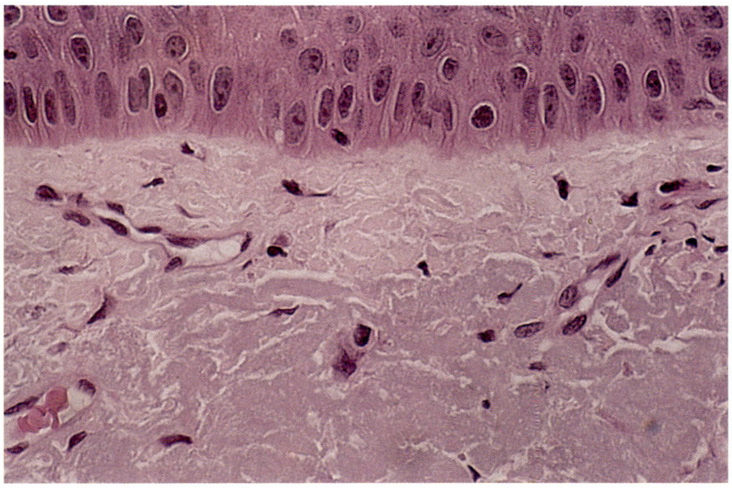

B

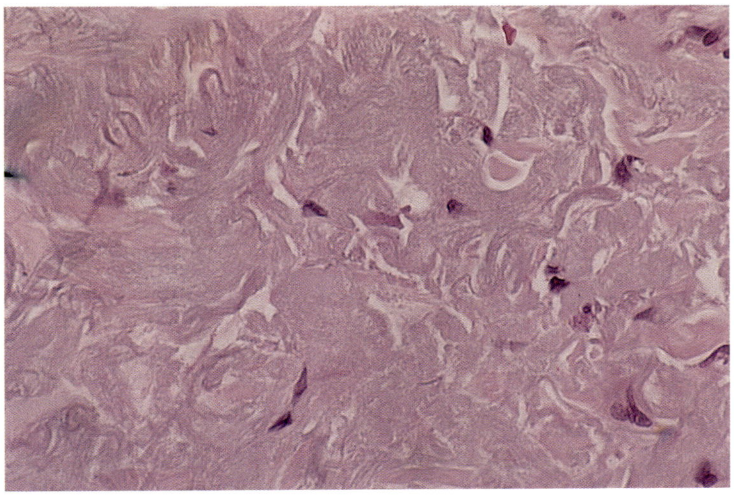

C

Figures 21–21A, 21–21B, 21–21C. **Solar elastosis.** The epidermis is effaced; the normal dermal collagen is replaced with bluish-gray-staining amorphous material; and there are dilated blood vessels.

RADIATION DERMATITIS

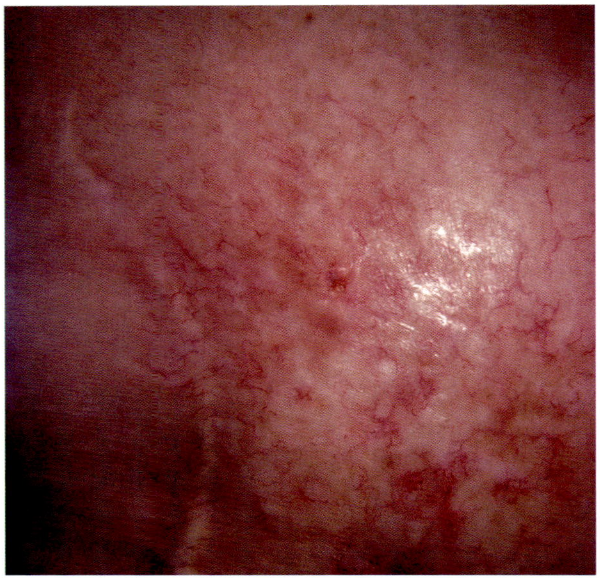

A

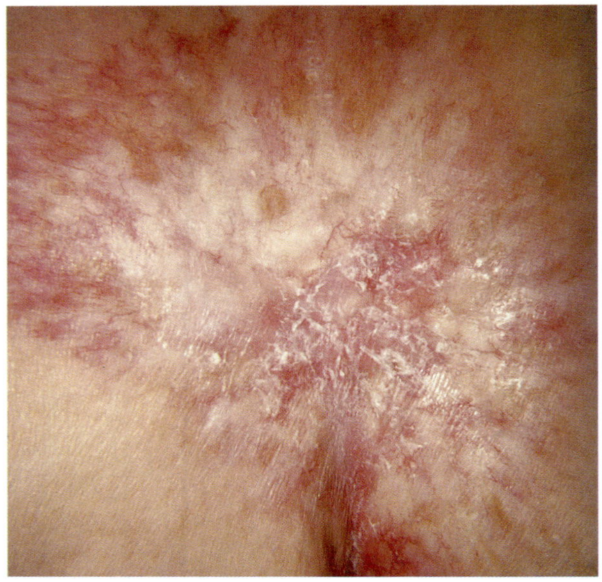

B

Figures 21–22A, 21–22B. Radiation dermatitis. Firm, shiny, hypopigmented plaques with telangiectases. The lesions developed many years after radiation therapy.

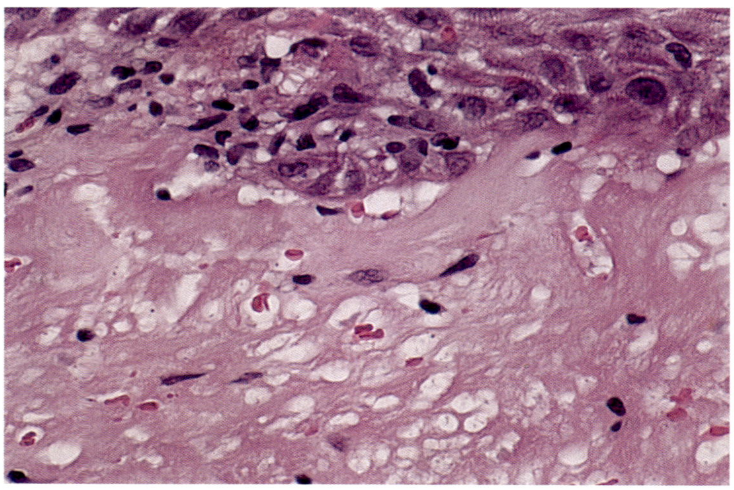

Figure 21–23. Radiation dermatitis. Sclerosis and telangiectases replace the normal papillary dermis. Atypical keratinocytes are present in the lower epidermis.

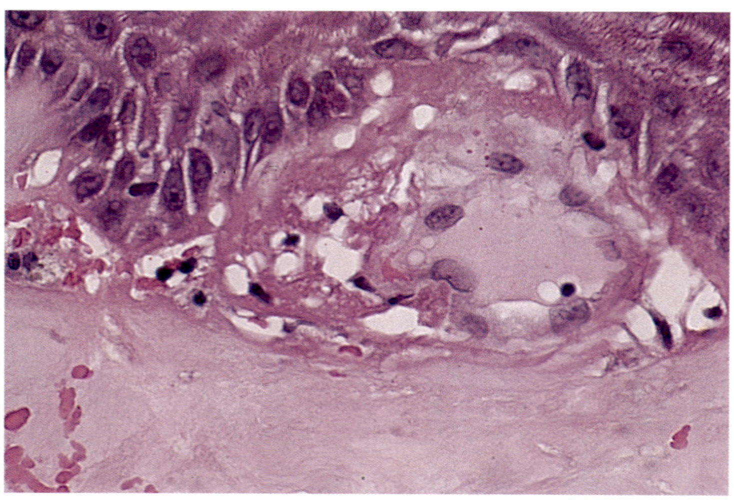

Figure 21–24. Radiation dermatitis. Dilated blood vessels with fibrin deposits within the sclerotic papillary dermis.

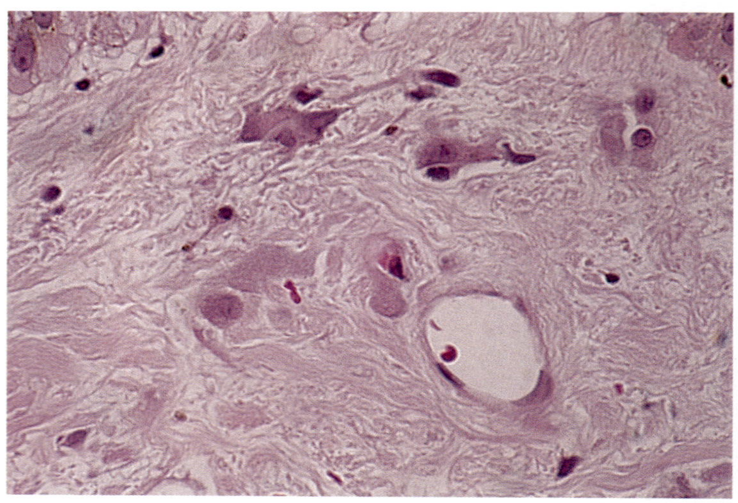

Figure 21–25. Radiation dermatitis. Characteristic bizarre-shaped, large single and multinucleated fibroblasts.

STASIS DERMATITIS

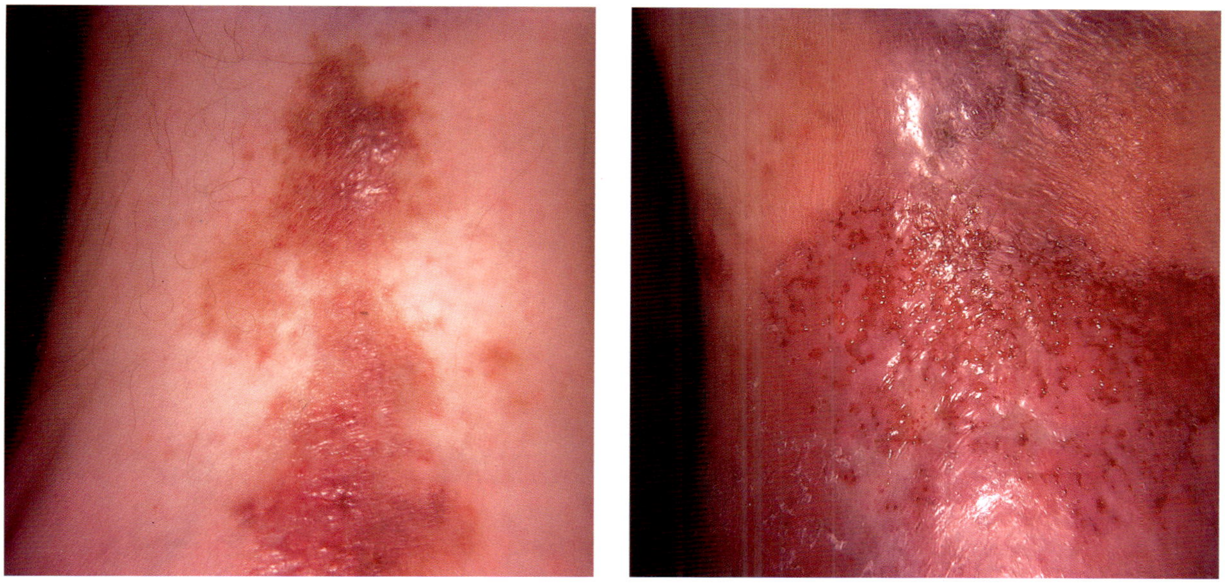

A B

Figures 21–26A, 21–26B. Stasis dermatitis. Erythematous, erosive papules and plaques on the lower leg.

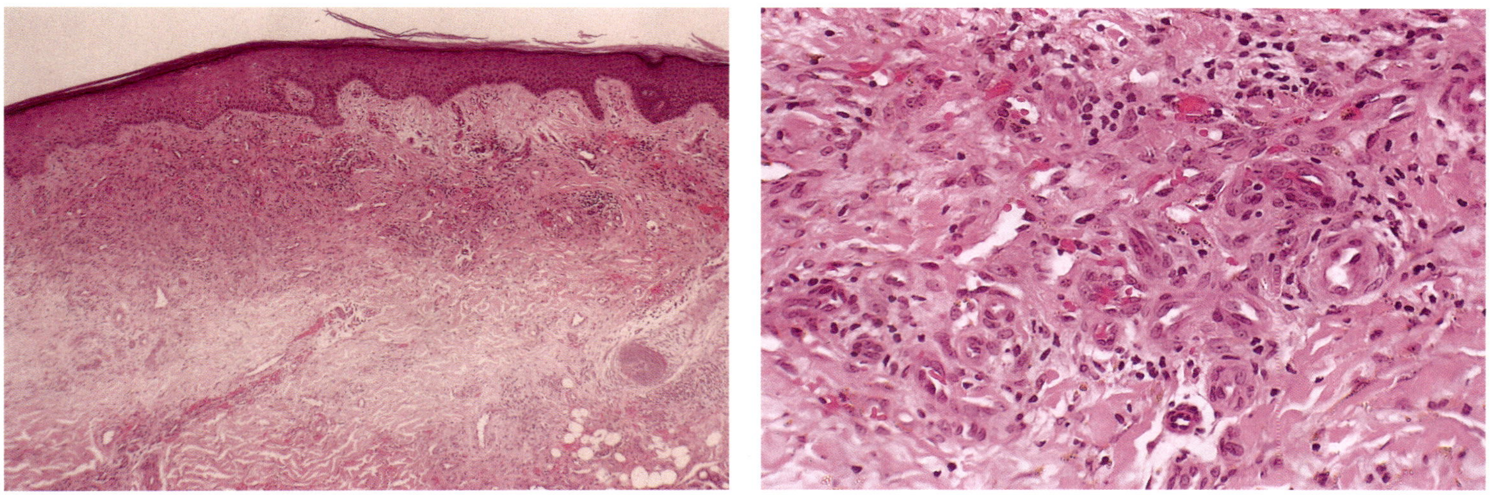

A B

Figures 21–27A, 21–27B. Stasis dermatitis. Thickened papillary dermis with coarse collagen bundles, dilated and thick-walled blood vessels, extravasated erythrocytes, and a mixed-cell infiltrate.

NODULAR FASCIITIS

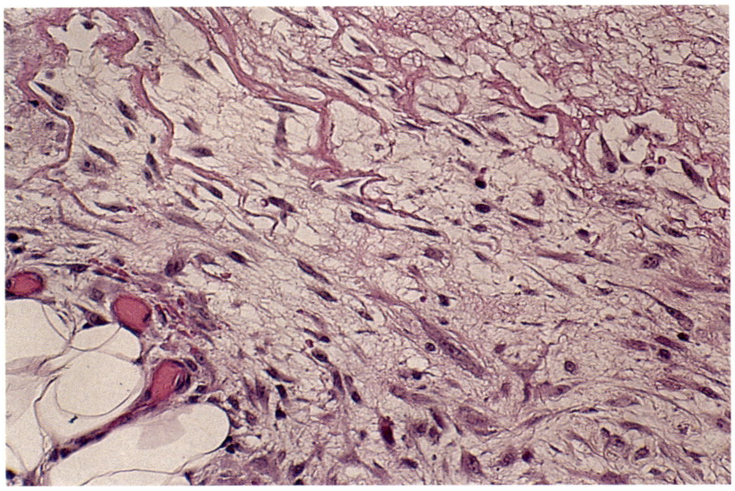

Figure 21–28. Nodular fasciitis. Haphazard array of spindle- and stellate-shaped fibroblasts in a myxomatous stroma with focal infiltration into the fat.

FIBROMAS

A) Infantile digital fibromatosis

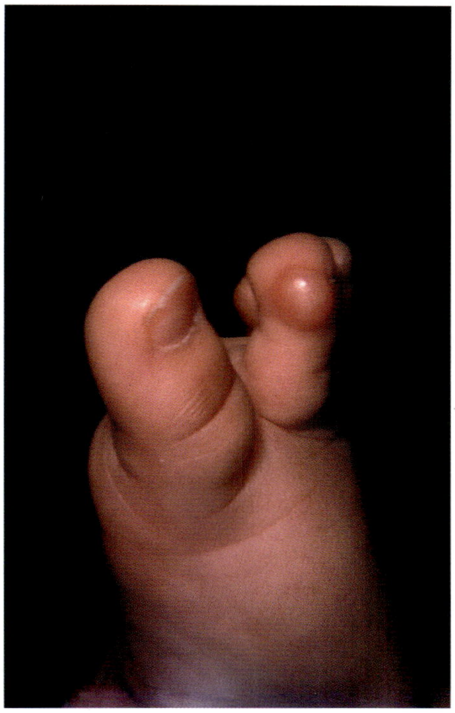

Figure 21–29. Infantile digital fibromatosis. Erythematous, well-circumscribed, shiny nodule on the toe of an infant.

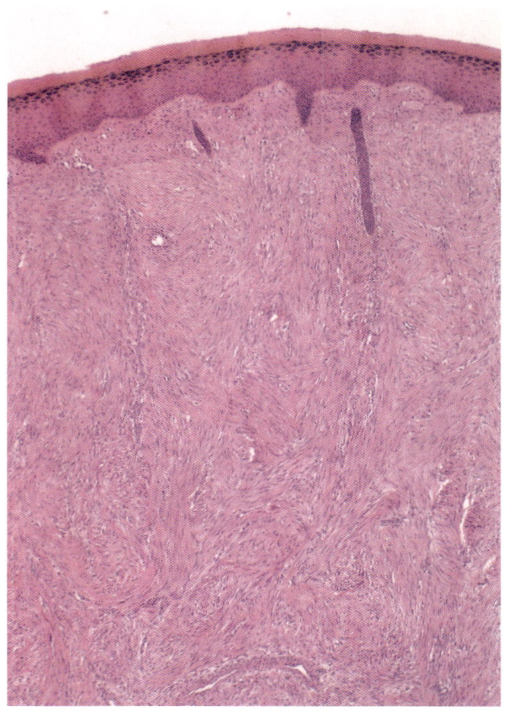

Figure 21–30. Infantile digital fibromatosis. Acral skin with intersecting fascicles of fibrocytes and collagen bundles.

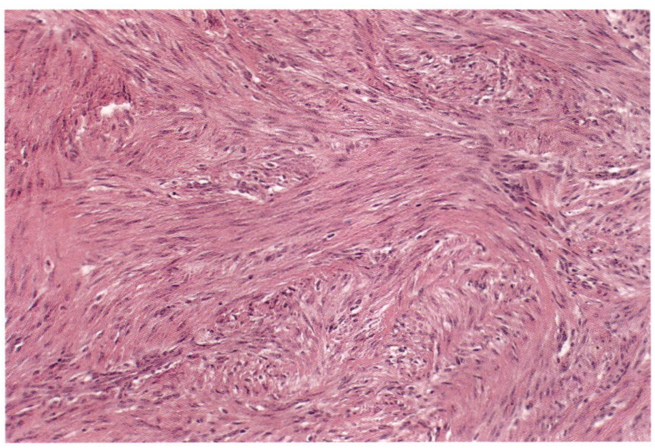

A

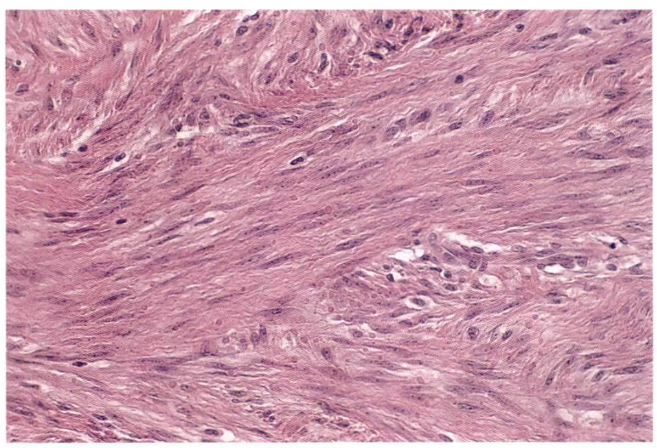

B

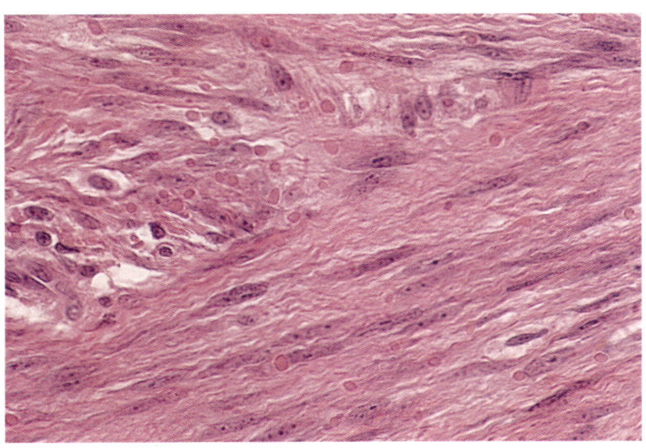

C

Figures 21–31A, 21–31B, 21–31C. Infantile digital fibromatosis. Fascicles of the fibroblasts with intracytoplasmic, round-oval, pink globules.

FIBROMAS

B) Acquired digital fibrokeratoma

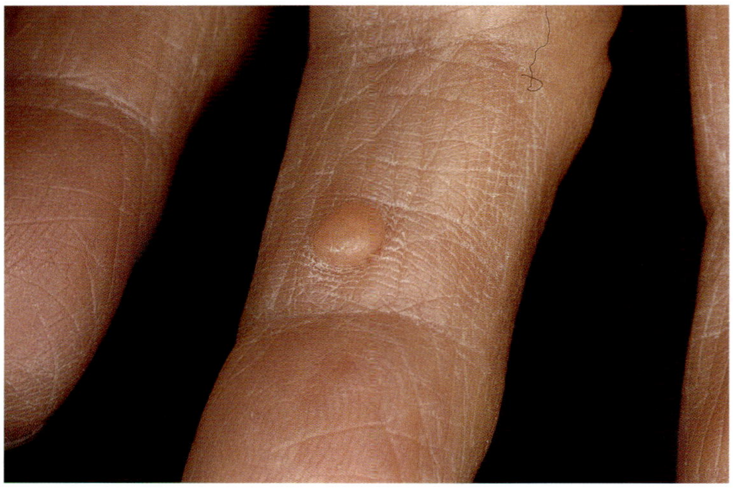

Figure 21–32. Acquired digital fibrokeratoma. Dome-shaped, keratotic, firm, flesh-colored nodule near the distal interphalangeal joint on the finger of a man.

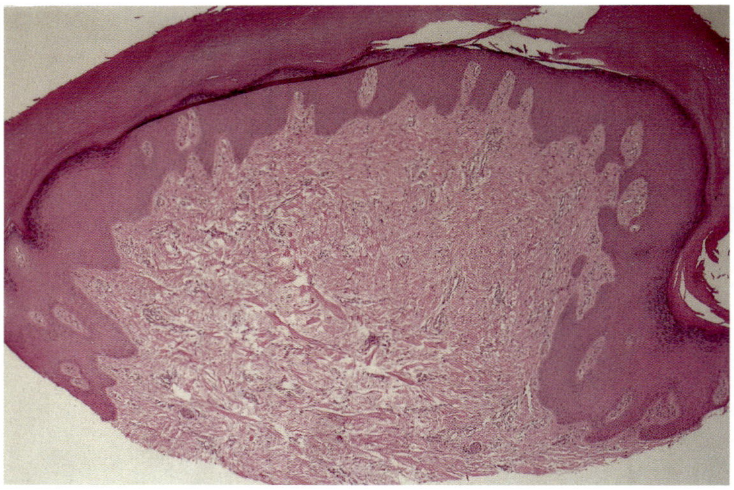

Figure 21–33. Acquired digital fibrokeratoma. Hyperkeratotic nodule with coarse and fibrillary collagen bundles and fibrocytes in disarray. There is an increased number of blood vessels.

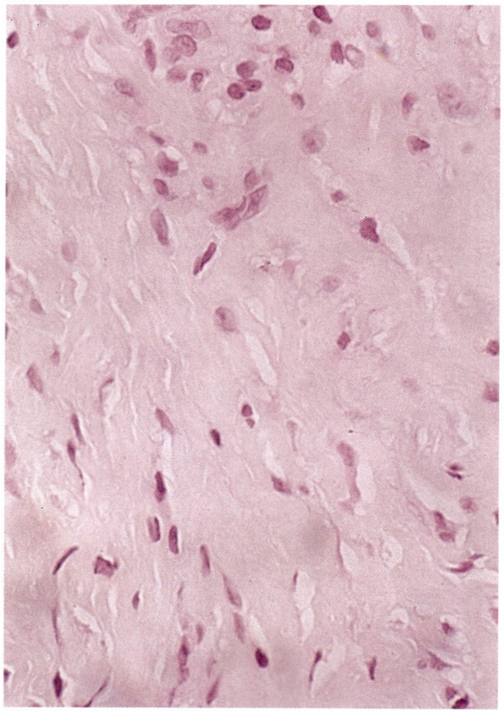

Figure 21–34. Acquired digital fibrokeratoma. Stellate fibrocytes and coarse collagen bundles.

FIBROMAS

C) Dermatofibroma

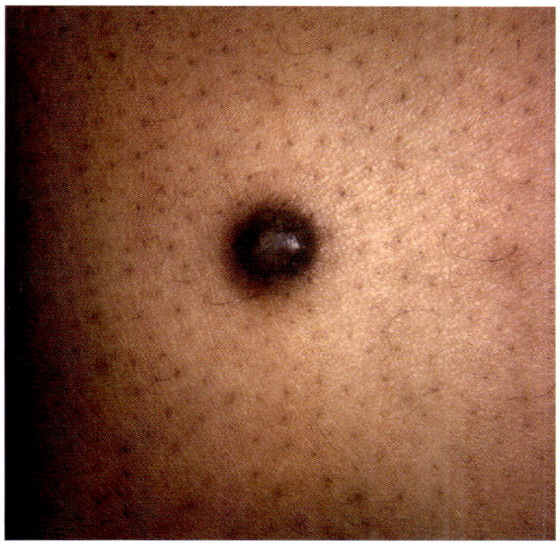

Figure 21–35. Dermatofibroma. Dome-shaped, well-circumscribed, black nodule on the arm.

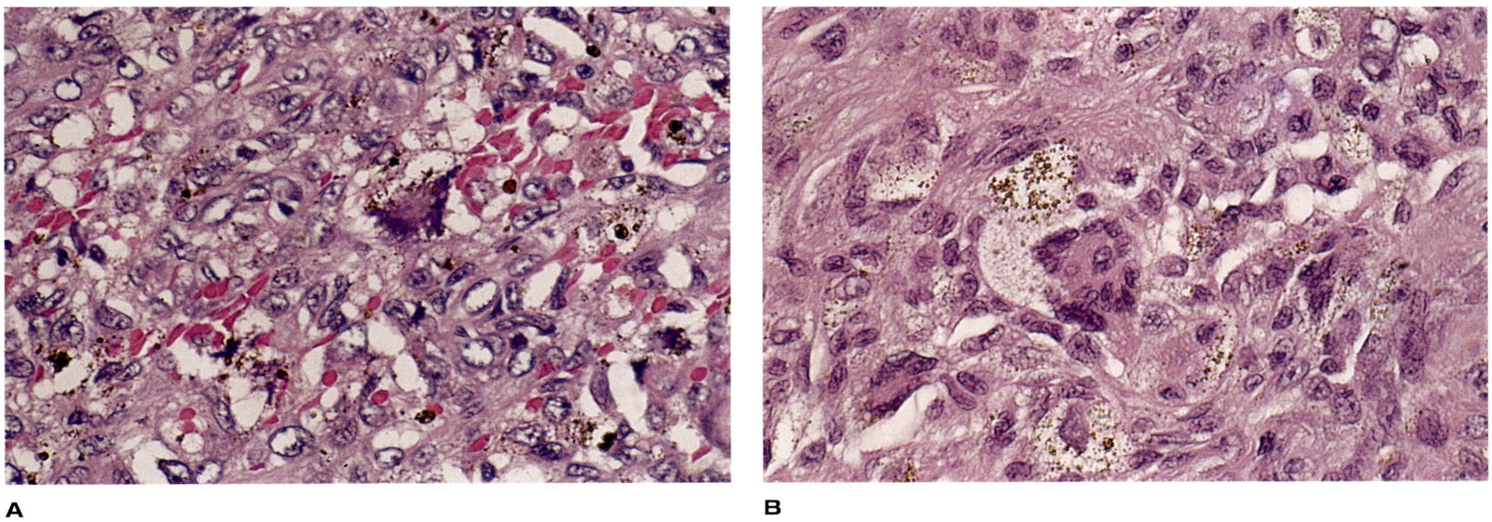

Figures 21–36A, 21–36B. Dermatofibroma. Histiocytic cells and fibrocytes in haphazard array. There are extravasated erythrocytes, siderophages, and multinucleated siderophages. This lesion in the past has been referred to as sclerosing hemangioma, and at times these changes may be seen in early evolving dermatofibromas.

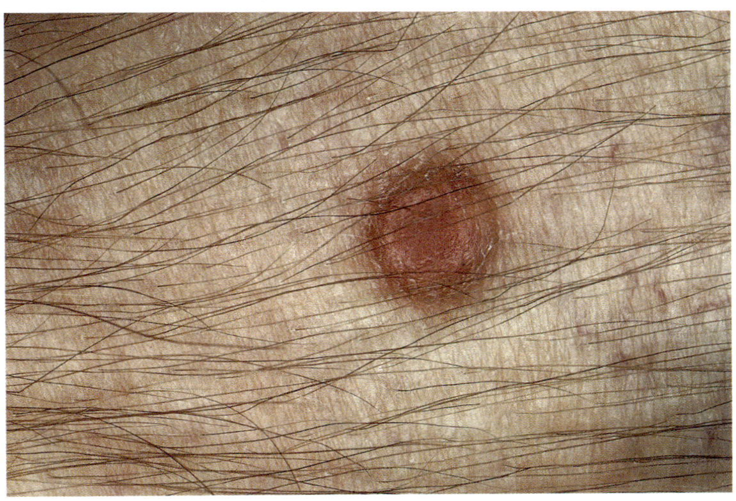

Figure 21–37. Dermatofibroma. Pink, firm, buttonlike nodule with a pale center and peripheral hyperpigmentation.

FIBROMAS

C) Dermatofibroma

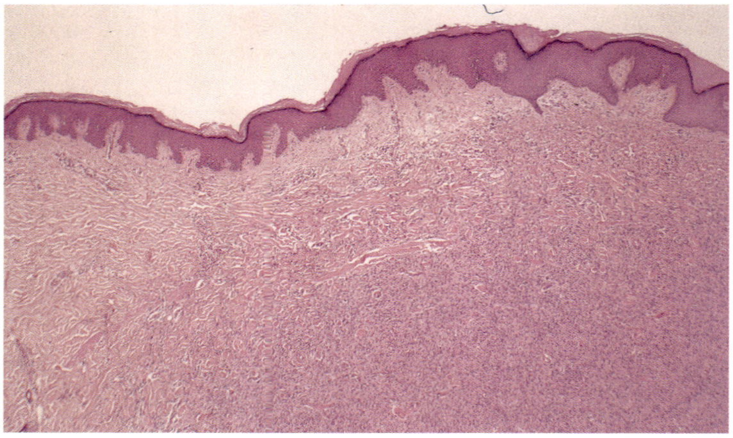

A

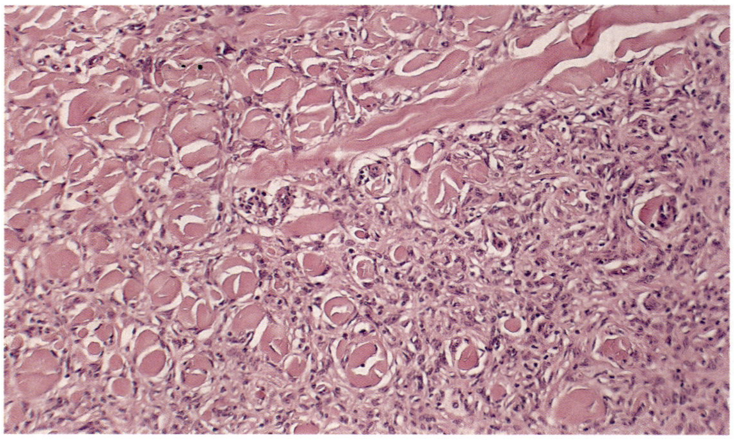

B

Figures 21–38A, 21–38B. Dermatofibroma. Epidermal hyperkeratosis, histiocytic cells, histiocytic giant cells, fibrocytes, and collagen bundles in disarray. There are thickened bundles of collagen in association with the cellular infiltrate.

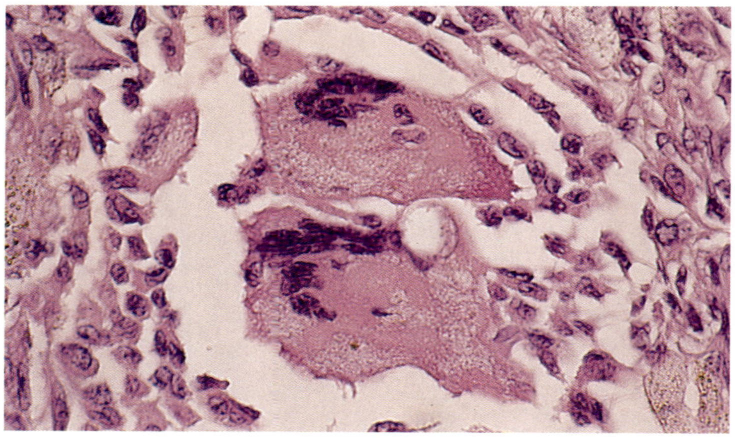

Figure 21–39. Dermatofibroma. Bizarre, very large, multinucleated histiocytic giant cells. Such large giant cells have been referred to as monster cells.

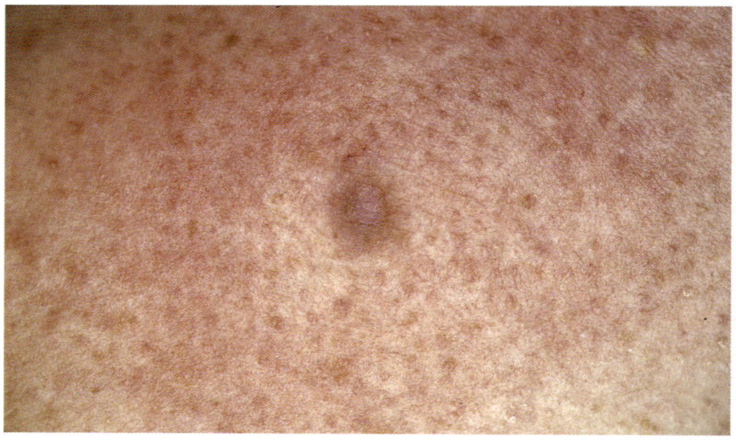

Figure 21–40. Dermatofibroma. Flat-topped, tan-colored papule.

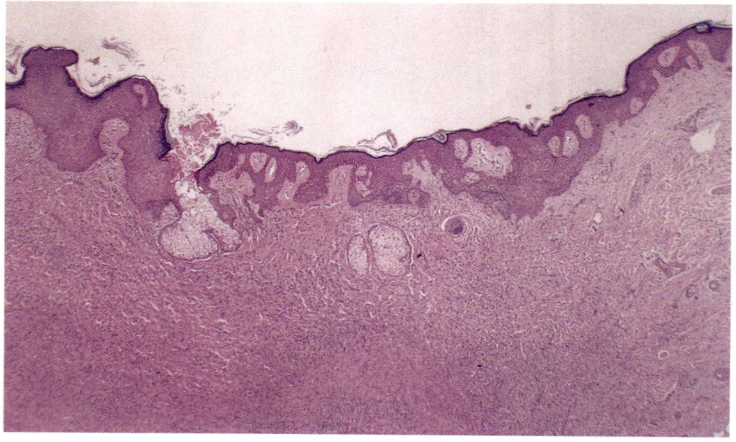

Figure 21–41. Dermatofibroma. Cellular infiltrate involves the upper dermis, where there is folliculosebaceous induction at the dermoepidermal junction.

FIBROMAS

D) Pleomorphic fibroma

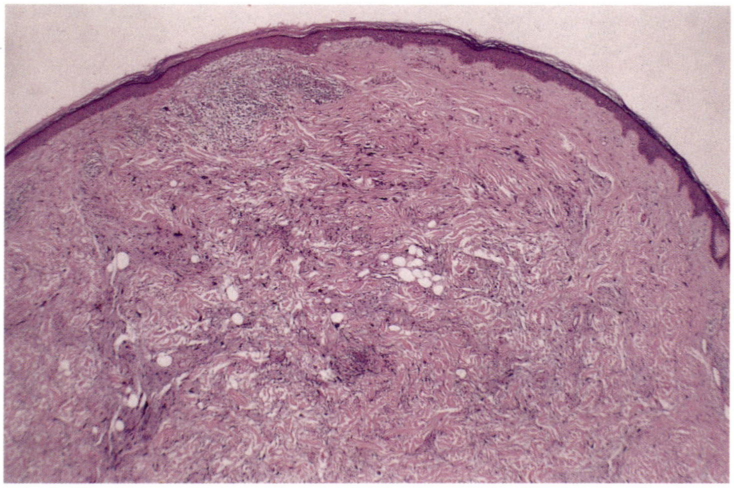

A

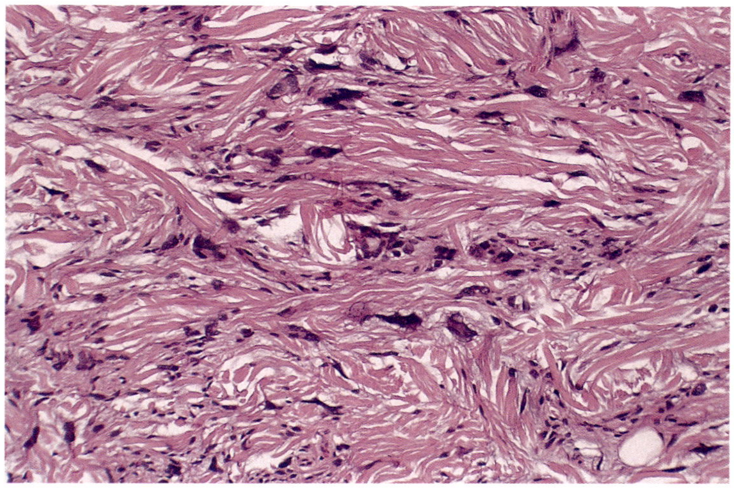

B

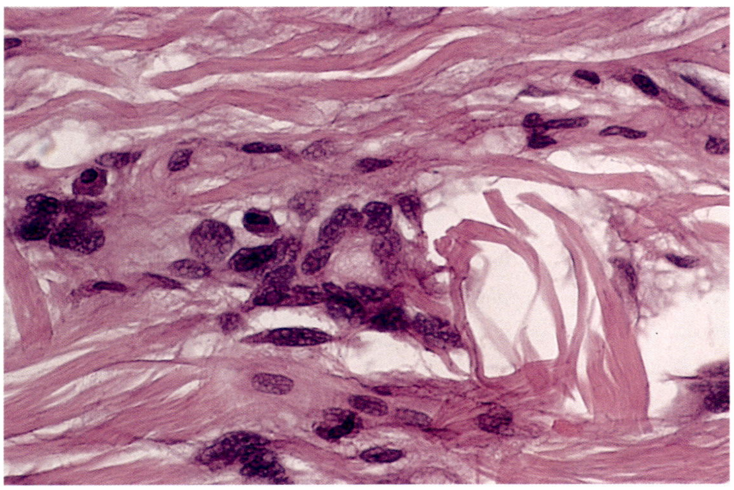

C

Figures 21–42A, 21–42B, 21–42C. Pleomorphic fibroma. Disarray of normal dermal architecture. There are coarse collagen bundles and bizarre, atypical multinucleated histiocytic giant cells.

FIBROMAS

E) Sclerotic fibroma

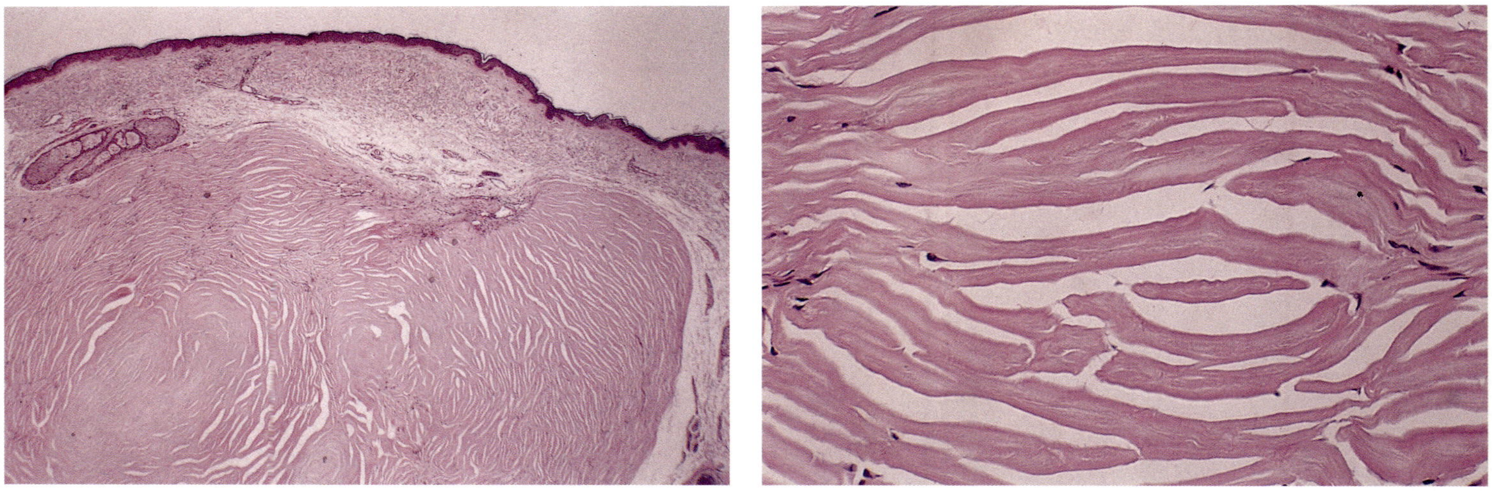

A B

Figures 21–43A, 21–43B. Sclerotic fibroma. Circumscribed deposit of eosinophilic, amorphous bands of collagen. There is a patchy mononuclear cell infiltrate, and fibroblasts are sparsely present.

SCAR AND KELOID

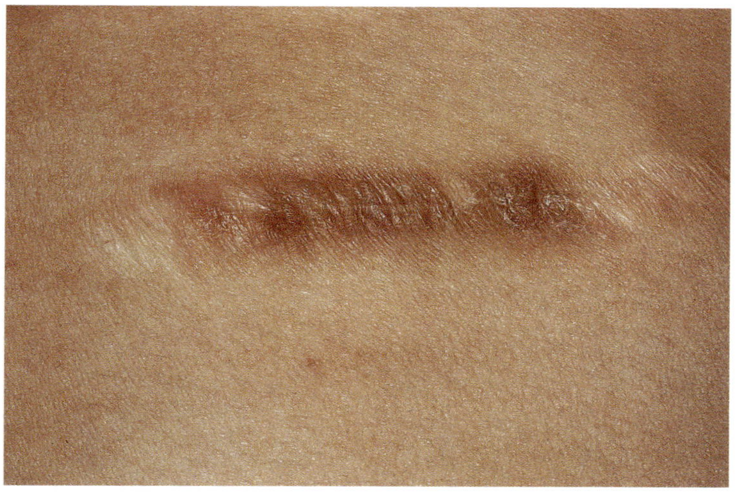

Figure 21–44. Scar. Raised, linear, hyper- and hypopigmented plaque in an area of previous surgery.

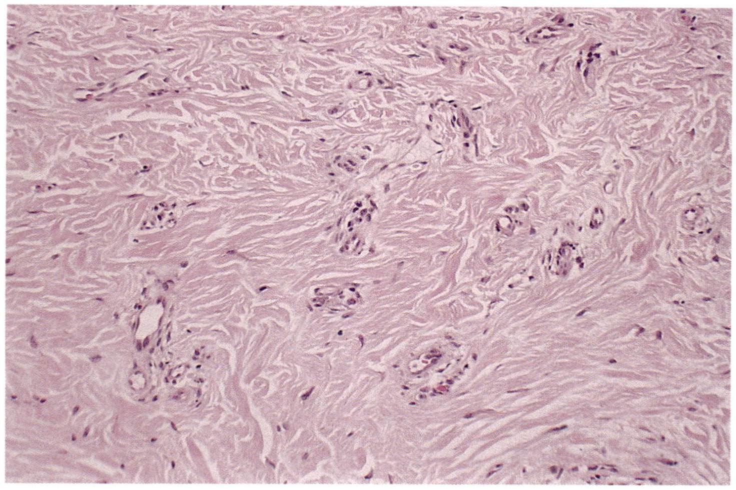

Figure 21–45. Scar. Collagen bundles are aligned horizontally, and blood vessels are directed vertically. There is a sparse inflammatory infiltrate and increased numbers of normal-appearing fibroblasts are present.

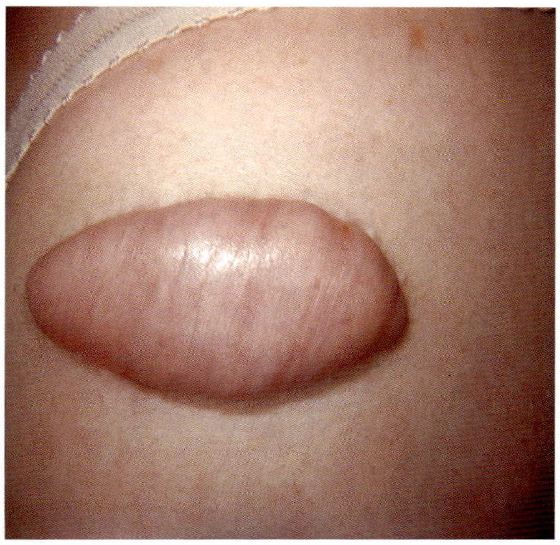

Figure 21–46. Keloid. Pedunculated, smooth, shiny nodule on the shoulder of a woman.

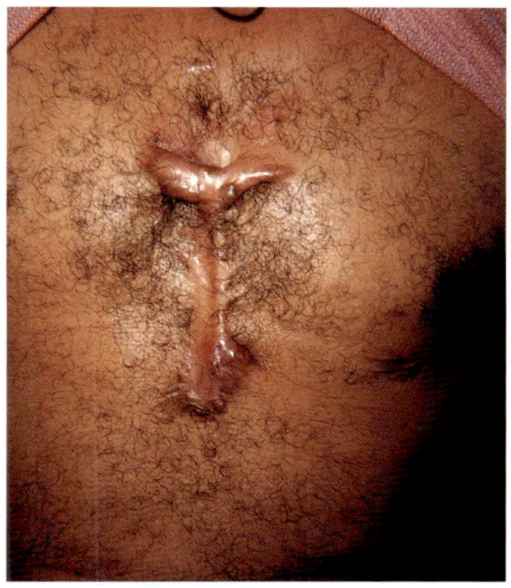

Figure 21–47. Keloid. Raised, vertical and horizontal, contiguous nodules on the chest of a man.

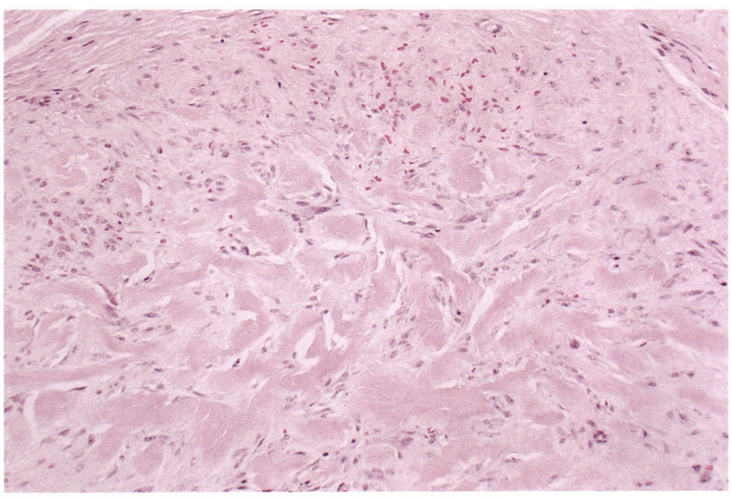

Figure 21–48. Keloid. Thick, eosinophilic collagen bundles with plump, vesicular, stellate fibroblasts.

FIBROEPITHELIAL POLYP

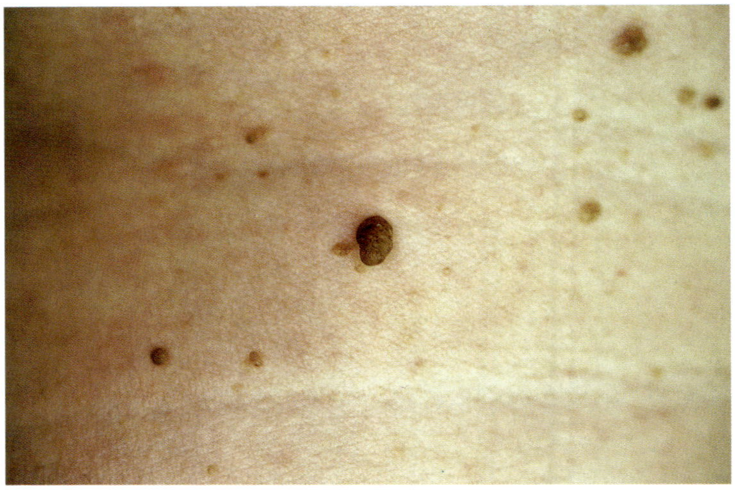

Figure 21–49. Fibroepithelial polyp. Hyperpigmented, sessile, soft papule.

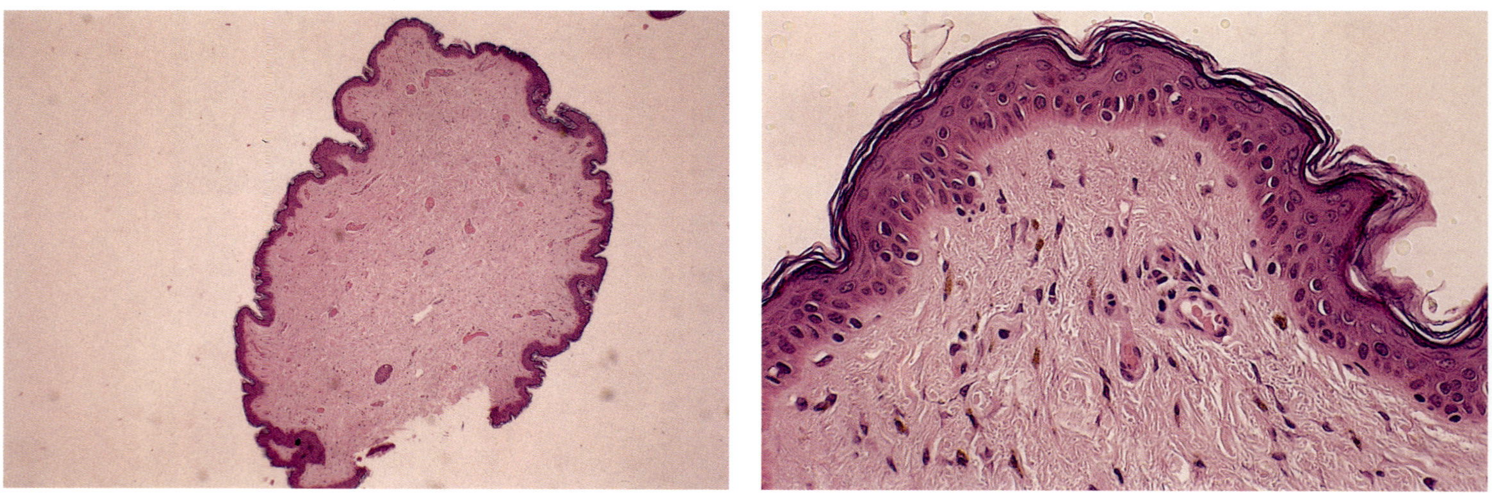

A B

Figures 21–50A, 21–50B. Fibroepithelial polyp. Pedunculated papule with fibrillary collagen and dilated blood vessels.

ACCESSORY NIPPLE

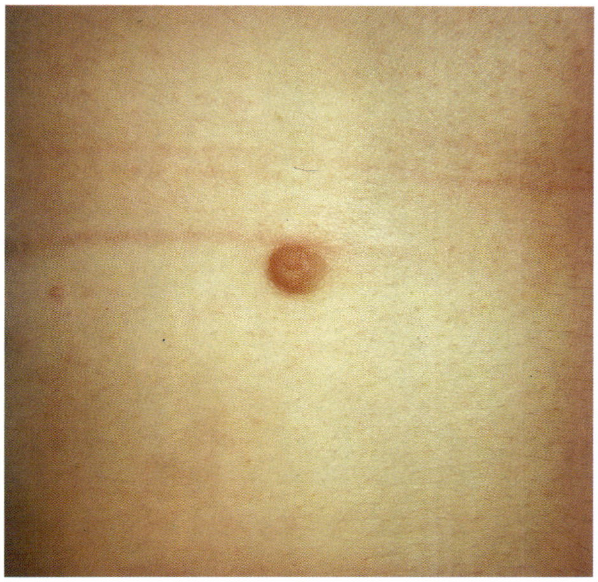

Figure 21–51. Accessory nipple. Life-long pink, sessile papule on the inframammary chest wall of a woman. The papule becomes firm when rubbed.

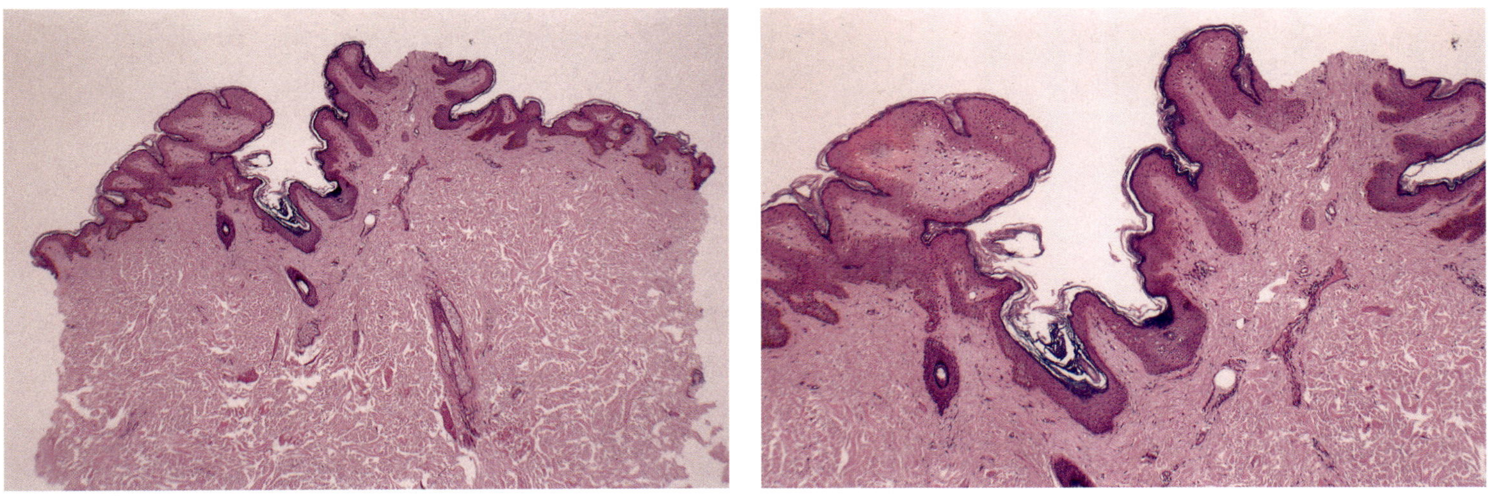

A B

Figures 21–52A, 21–52B. Accessory nipple. Hyperkeratosis, papillomatosis, and sebaceous glands (Montgomery tubercles) within the epidermis and dermis. There are muscle bundles and dilated blood vessels in the dermis.

FOCAL DERMAL HYPOPLASIA (GOLTZ SYNDROME)

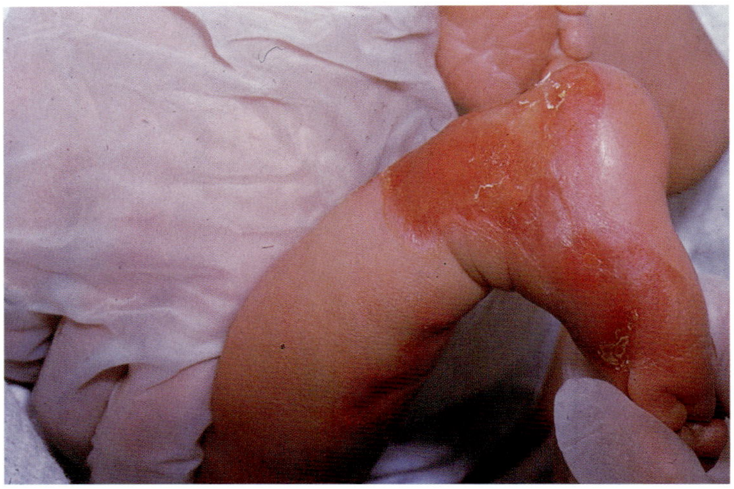

Figure 21–53. Focal dermal hypoplasia. Confluent, erythematous, linear and circular, depressed patches on the lower leg and foot of a female infant. Areas of scale-crust and scaling are present.

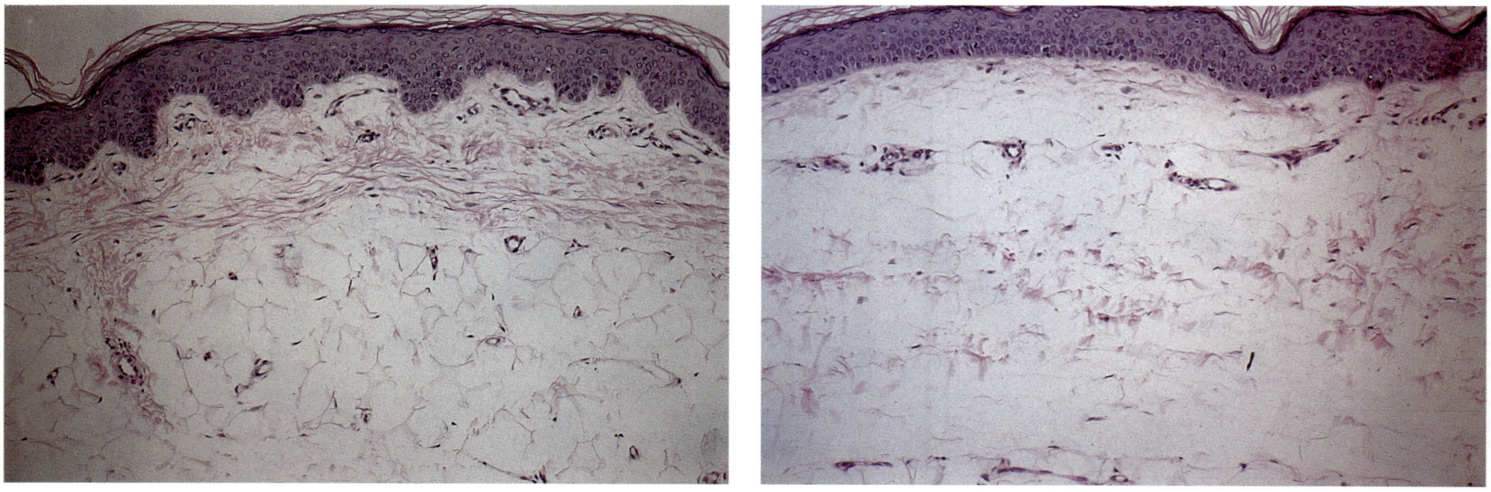

A B

Figures 21–54A, 21–54B. Focal dermal hypoplasia. Dermal atrophy with residual strands of fibrillary collagen and dilated blood vessels. Subcutaneous fat progressively replaces the dermis, where it approaches and becomes contiguous with the unaltered epidermis.

ANGIOFIBROMA (TUBEROUS SCLEROSIS)

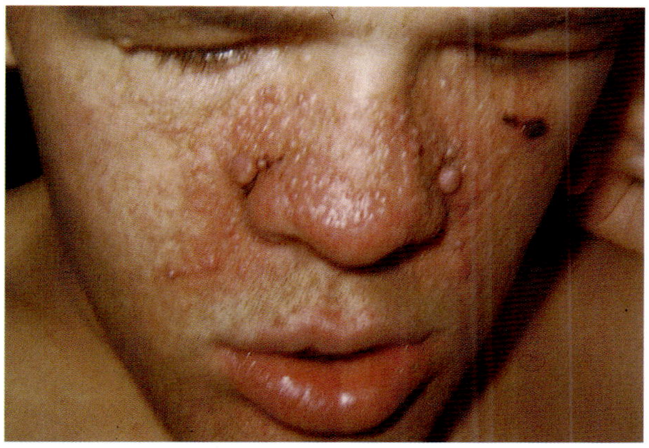

Figure 21–55. Angiofibroma. Erythematous perinasal papules and polyps in a boy with tuberous sclerosis.

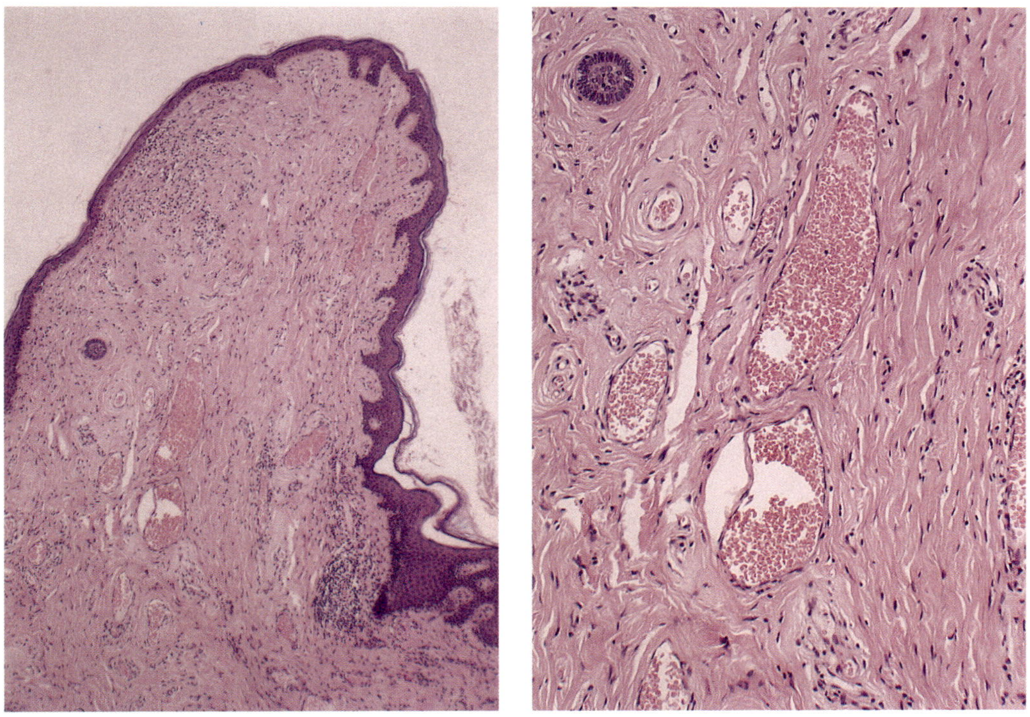

A B

Figures 21–56A, 21–56B. Angiofibroma. Dilated blood vessels, fibroplasia, and a patchy lymphohistiocytic infiltrate. Concentric bundles of collagen with plump and stellate fibroblasts are present around blood vessels and structures of adnexa.

NEVUS LIPOMATOSIS

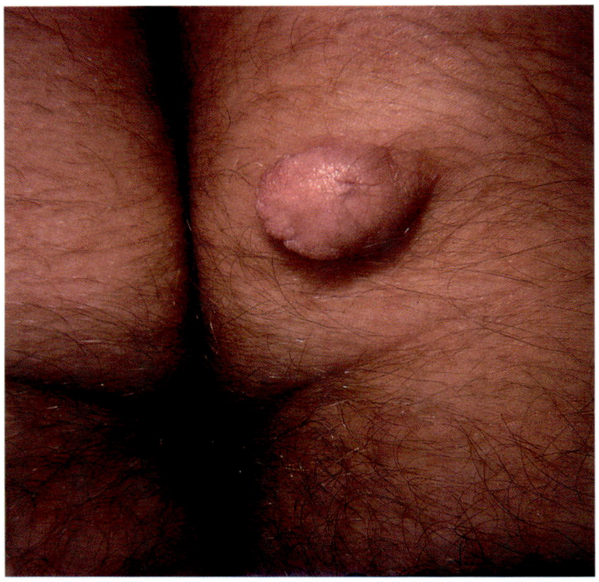

Figure 21–57. Nevus lipomatosis. Pedunculated, pink, pebbly nodule on the buttocks.

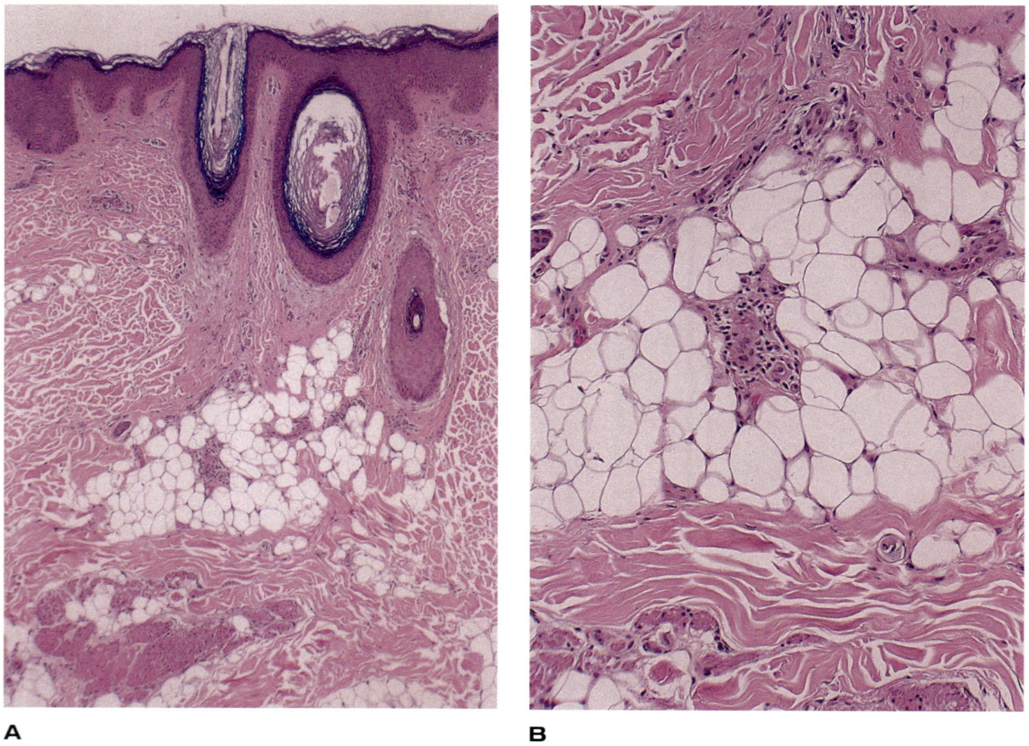

Figures 21–58A, 21–58B. Nevus lipomatosis. Fat lobules in a patchy distribution throughout the reticular dermis.

FIBROUS HAMARTOMA OF INFANCY

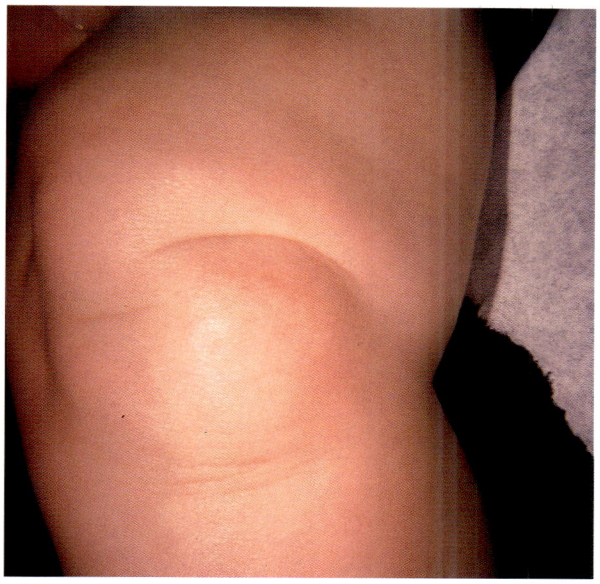

Figure 21–59. Fibrous hamartoma of infancy. Rapid swelling of the knee in a six-month-old boy.

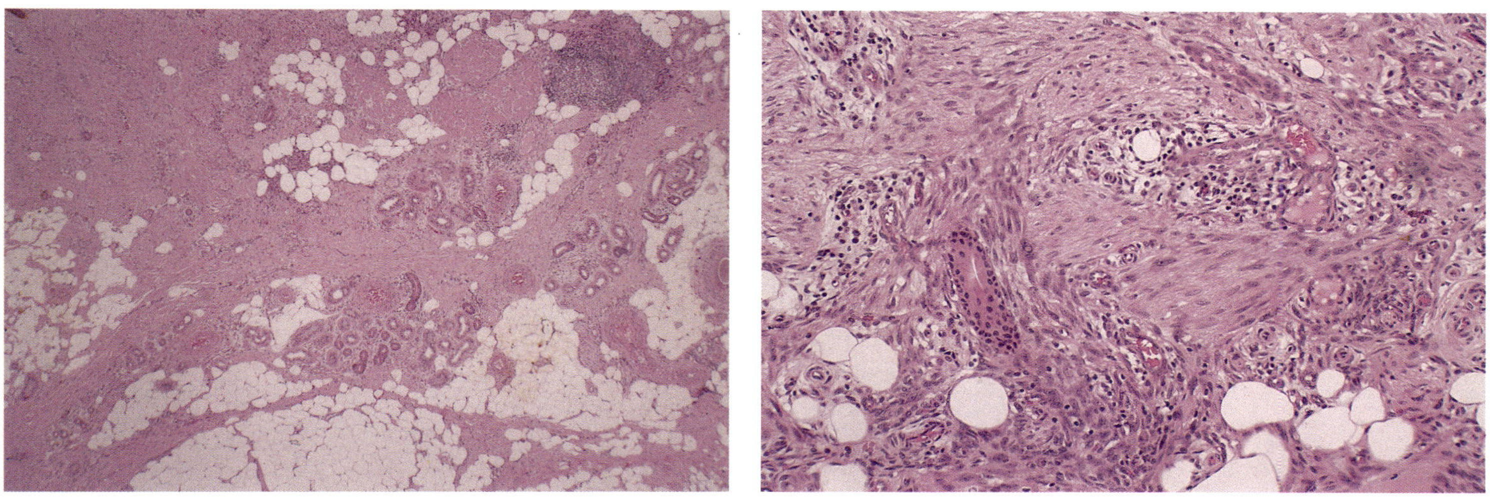

A B

Figures 21–60A, 21–60B. Fibrous hamartoma of infancy. Fibroplasia with fascicles of plump, spindle-shaped fibrocytes interlacing with bundles of collagen admixed with numerous dispersed fat lobules. There are dilated blood vessels and a patchy lymphohistiocytic infiltrate.

CONNECTIVE TISSUE NEVUS

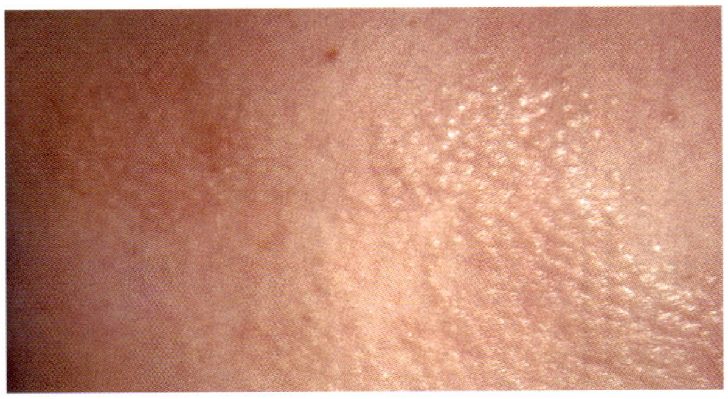

Figure 21–61. Connective tissue nevus. Firm plaque with flesh-colored papules having a cobblestone appearance.

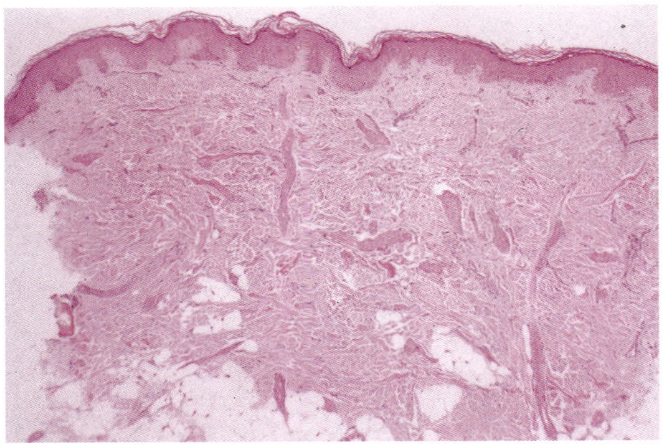

A

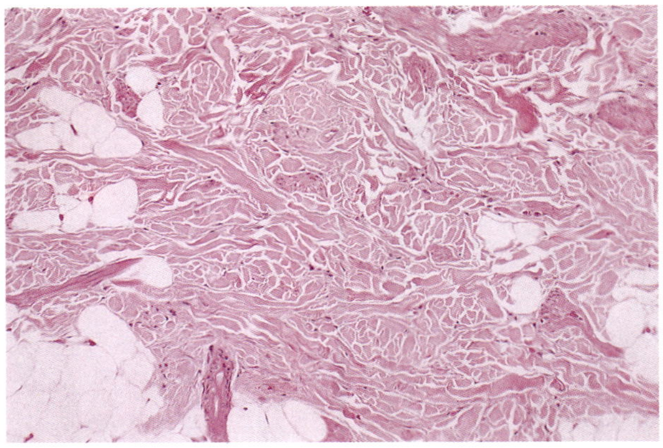

B

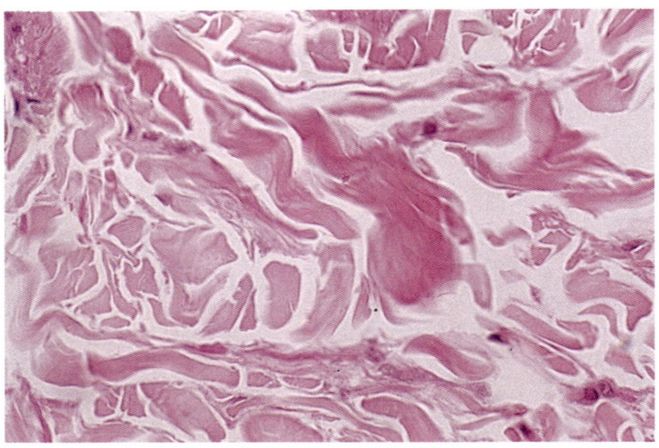

C

Figures 21–62A, 21–62B, 21–62C. Connective tissue nevus, collagen type. Dermal thickening with coarse collagen bundles in disarray. In some foci, fibroblasts are diminished.

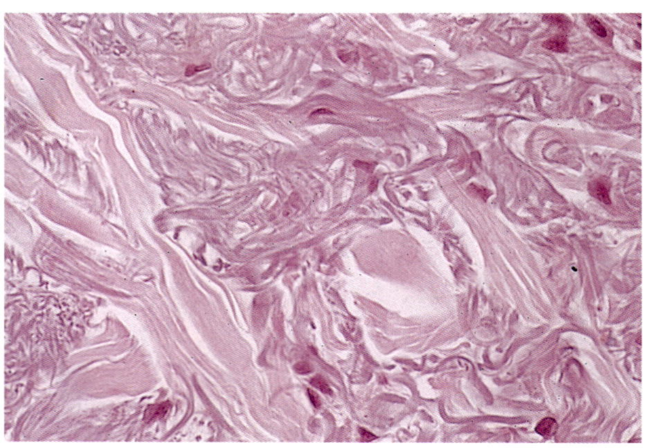

Figure 21–63. Connective tissue nevus, elastic tissue type. Broad bands of hyperplastic elastic tissue fibers and clumps of fragmented elastic tissue fibers are admixed with thick collagen bundles. Fibrocytes are sparse, giving the tissue an acellular appearance.

MALIGNANT NEOPLASMS

A) Dermatofibrosarcoma protuberans

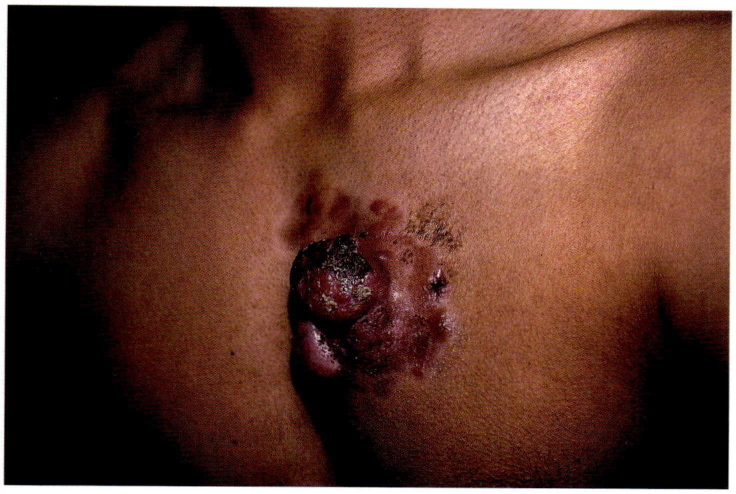

Figure 21–64. Dermatofibrosarcoma protuberans. Irregular, reddish-brown, indurated, multilobular and nodular crusted lesion on the chest of a man.

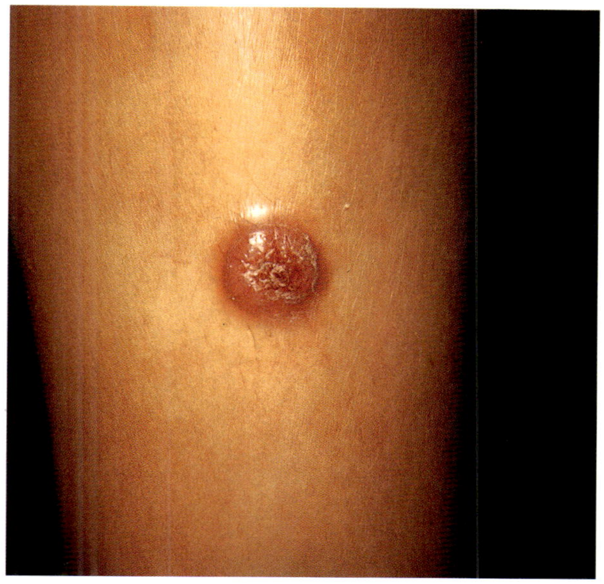

Figure 21–65. Dermatofibrosarcoma protuberans. Erythematous, ulcerated, round nodule on the arm.

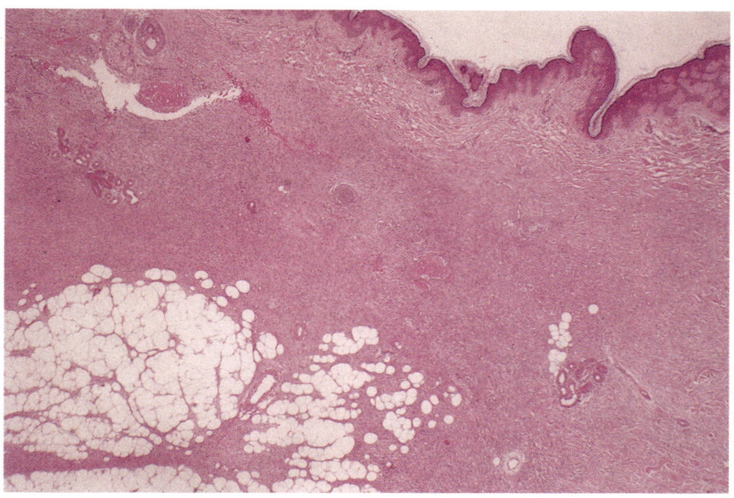

Figure 21–66. Dermatofibrosarcoma protuberans. Interweaving fascicles of spindle-shaped cells involving the dermis and subcutaneous fat.

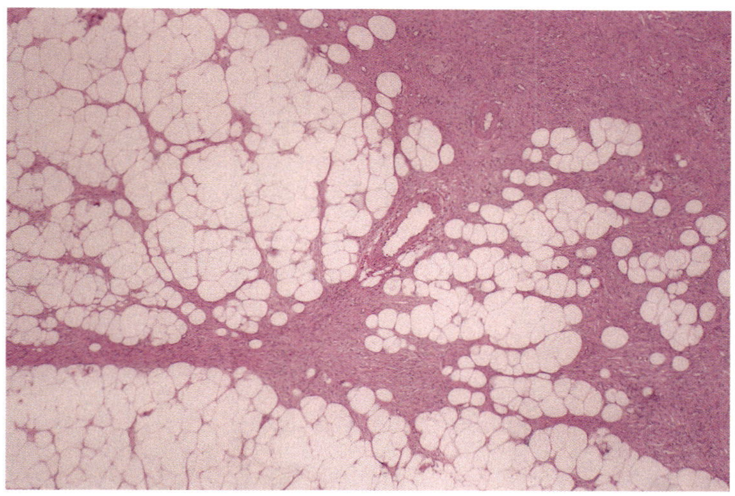

Figure 21–67. Dermatofibrosarcoma protuberans. Fascicles of neoplastic cells involve the dermis, form fibrous septa, encircle adipocytes, and relentlessly replace the normal fat lobules.

MALIGNANT NEOPLASMS

A) Dermatofibrosarcoma protuberans

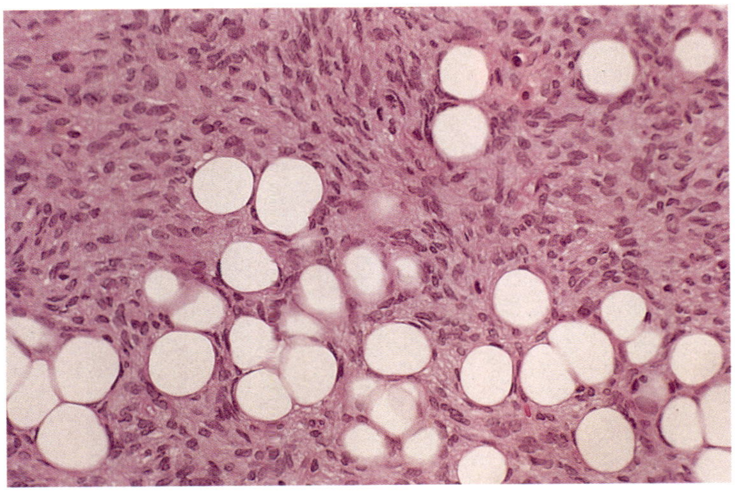

A

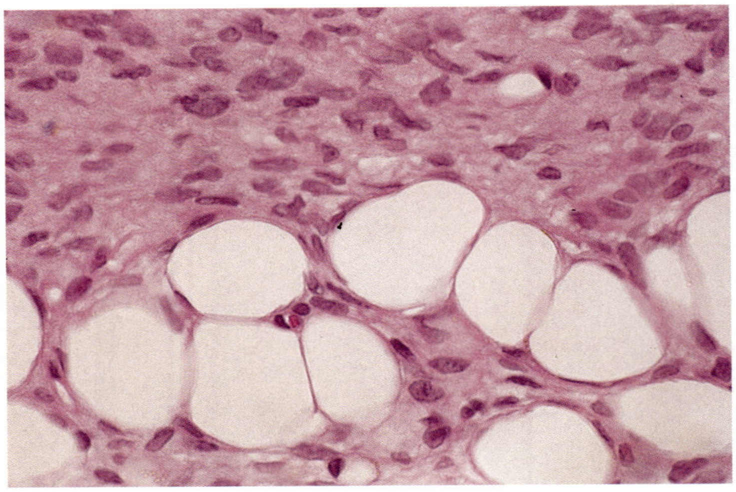

B

Figures 21–68A, 21–68B. Dermatofibrosarcoma protuberans. Oval, spindle, and wavy neoplastic cells form interweaving fascicles that surround and replace individual adipocytes. Only an occasional mitotic neoplastic cell is present.

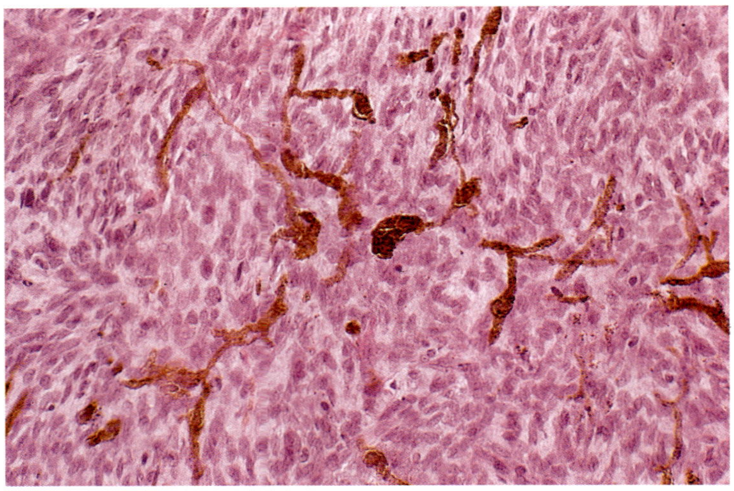

Figure 21–69. Pigmented dermatofibrosarcoma protuberans (Bednar tumor). Markedly hyperpigmented dendritic melanocytes among spindle-shaped neoplastic cells.

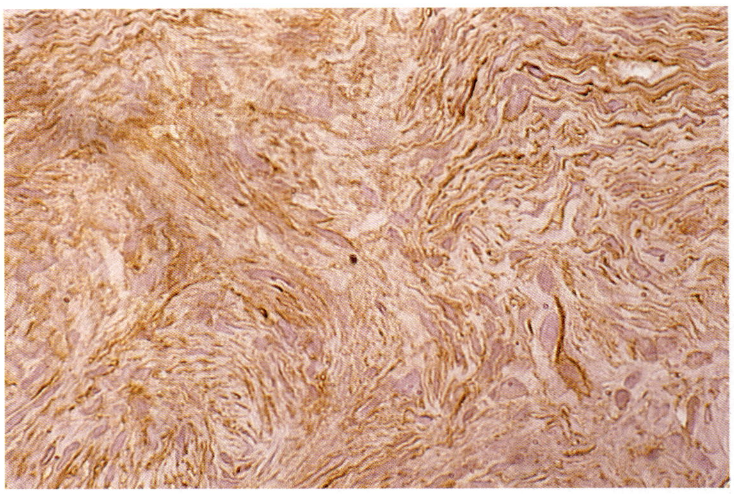

Figure 21–70. Dermatofibrosarcoma protuberans. CD-34 positive staining of spindle cells.

MALIGNANT NEOPLASMS

B) Malignant fibrous histiocytoma/atypical fibroxanthoma

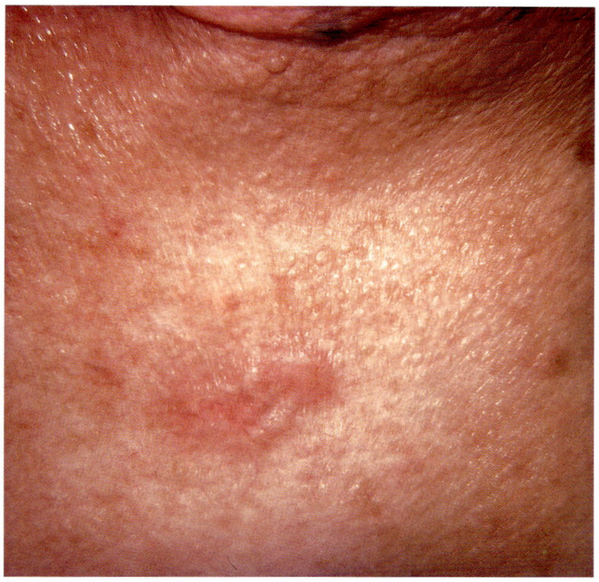

Figure 21–71. Malignant fibrous histiocytoma. Erythematous nodule on the chest of a man with severely sun-damaged skin.

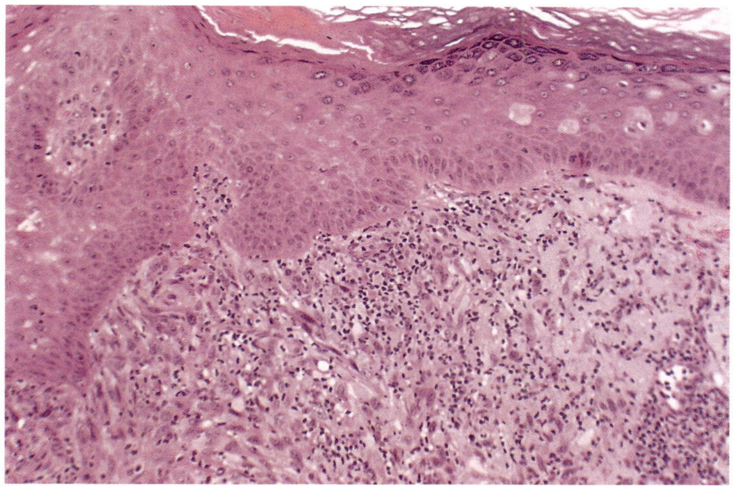

Figure 21–72. Malignant fibrous histiocytoma. Severe solar elastosis, pleomorphic oval and spindle-shaped neoplastic cells, and a lymphoplasmacytic infiltrate fill the thickened papillary dermis.

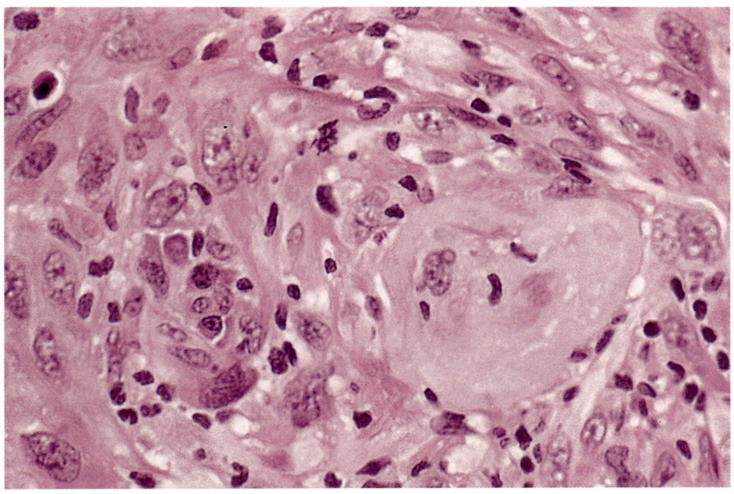

A

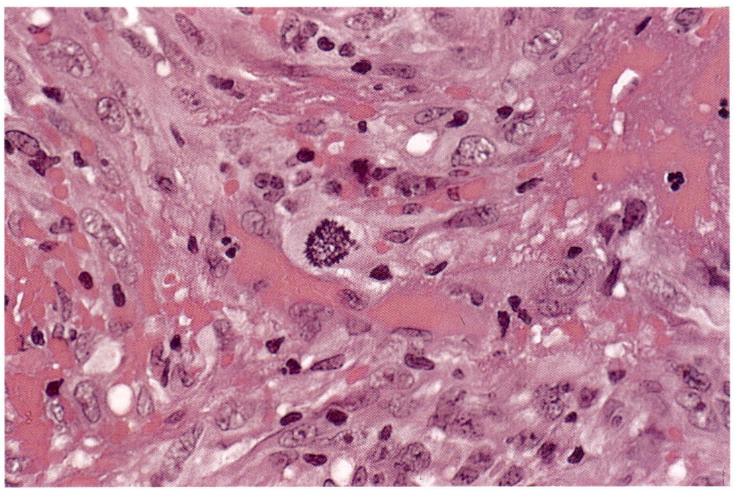

B

Figures 21–73A, 21–73B. Malignant fibrous histiocytoma. Atypical and pleomorphic neoplastic cells with vesicular nuclei and prominent nucleoli. Characteristic, atypical, bizarre neoplastic foam cells, giant cells, and mitotic cells are present in association with a lymphoplasmacytic infiltrate and severe solar elastosis.

MALIGNANT NEOPLASMS

C) Fibrosarcoma

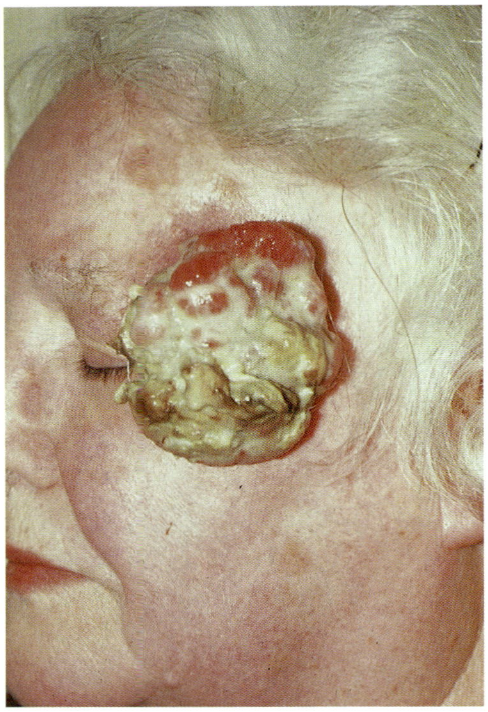

Figure 21–74. Fibrosarcoma. Massive exophytic, ulcerated, crusted tumor on the temple of a woman.

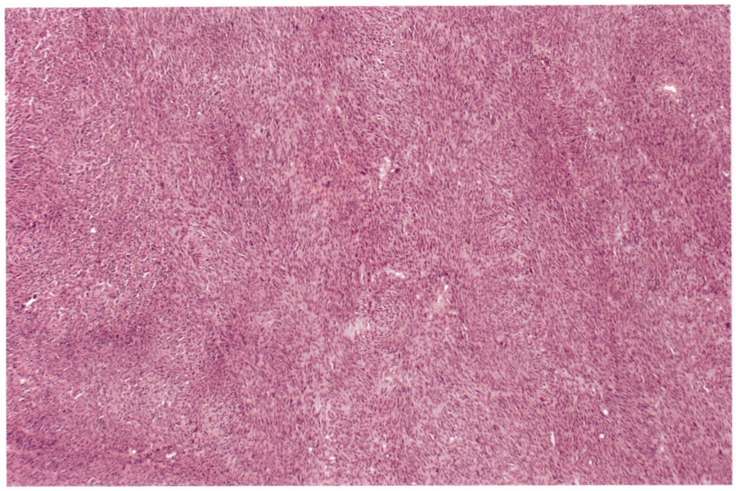

Figure 21–75. Fibrosarcoma. Confluent interweaving fascicles of spindle-shaped neoplastic cells.

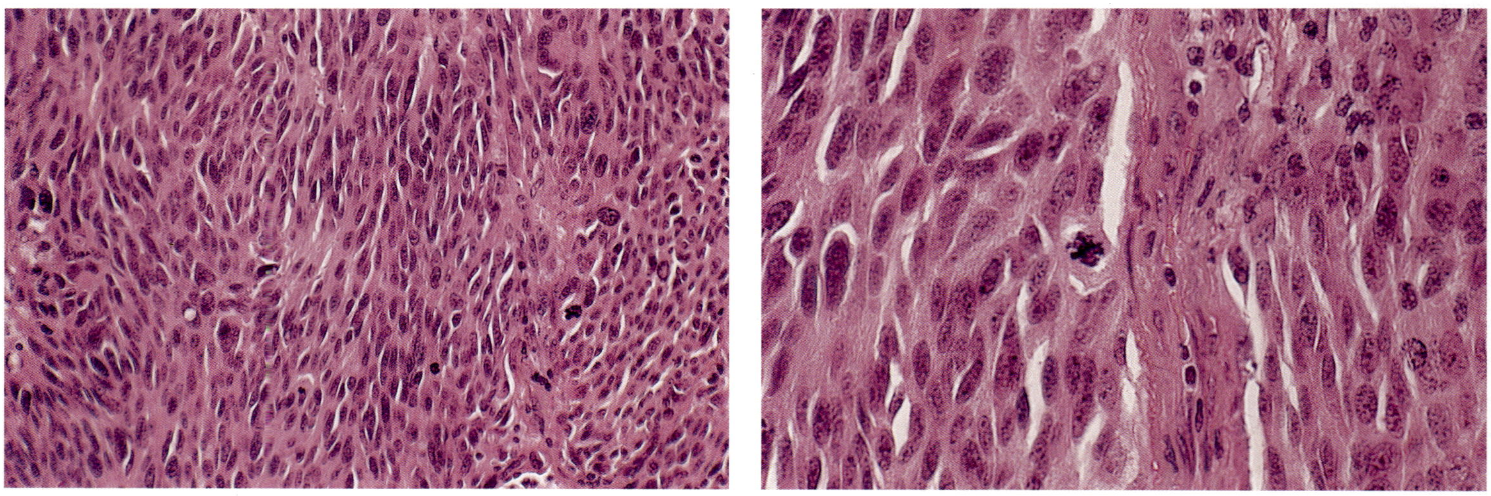

A B

Figures 21–76A, 21–76B. Fibrosarcoma. Sheets of atypical and pleomorphic spindle- and oval-shaped neoplastic cells. There are numerous mitotic figures including atypical forms.

MALIGNANT NEOPLASMS

D) Epithelioid cell sarcoma

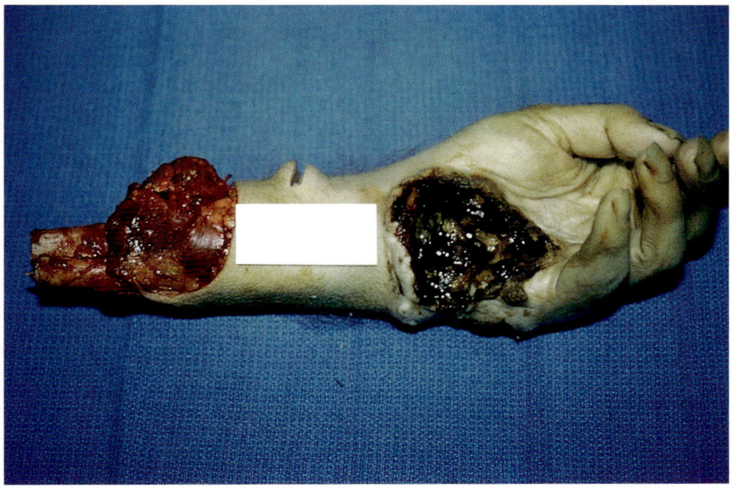

Figure 21–77. Epithelioid cell sarcoma. Amputation of the hand and distal arm. Fungating tumor on the palm and metastatic nodule on the arm.

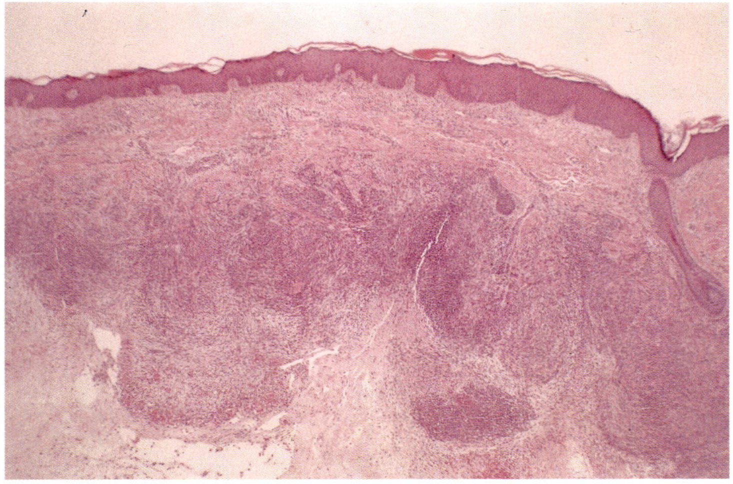

Figure 21–78. Epithelioid cell sarcoma. Multiple dermal nodules with central necrosis, a characteristic pattern for this neoplasm.

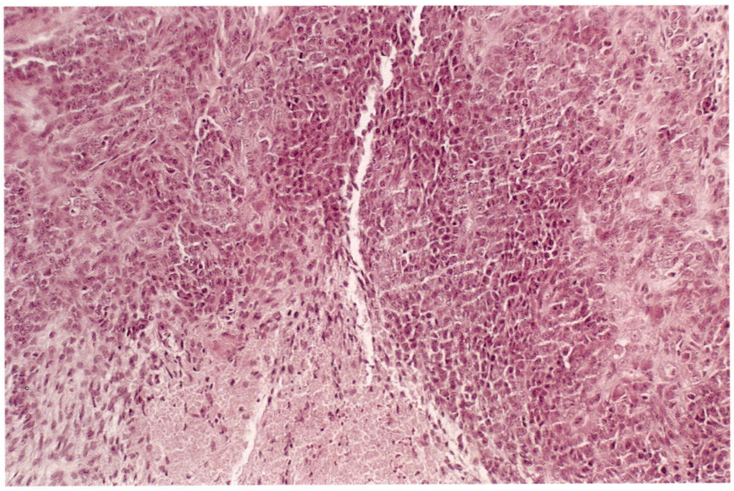

A

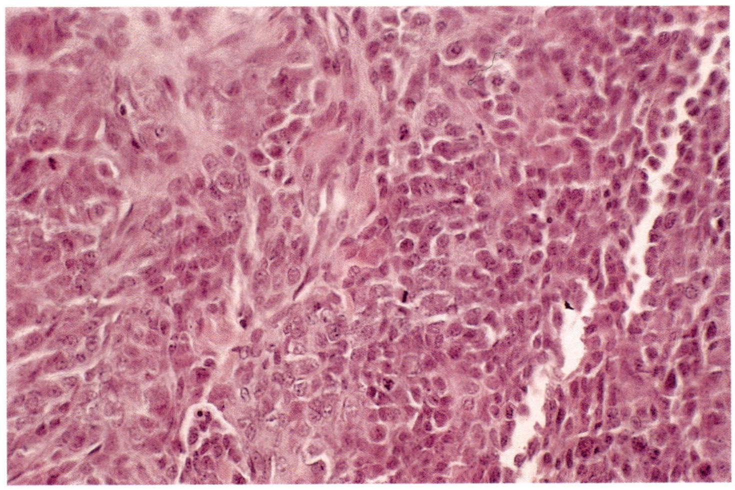

B

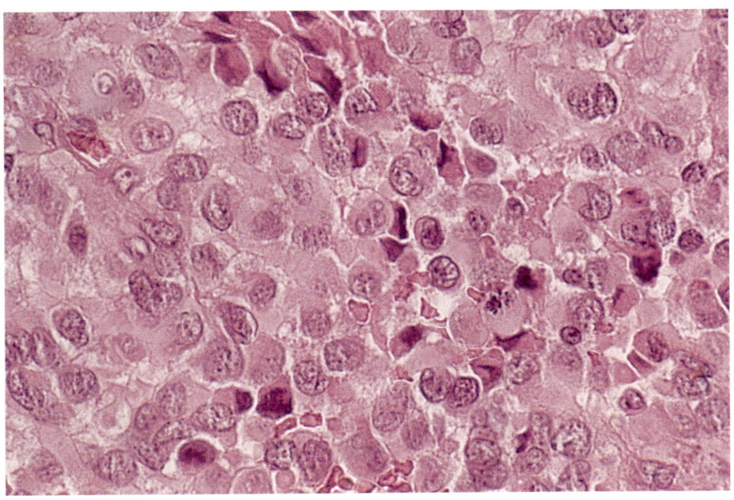

C

Figures 21–79A, 21–79B, 21–79C. Epithelioid cell sarcoma. Nodule composed of polygonal cells with eosinophilic cytoplasm and plump spindle cells surrounding a central area of necrosis. Neoplastic cells have an epithelioid appearance, and there are many necrotic cells and mitotic figures within tumor cells.

22

Elastic tissue disorders

- Striae distensae
- Cutis laxa
- Pseudoxanthoma elasticum
- Elastosis perforans serpiginosa
- Anetoderma

STRIAE DISTENSAE

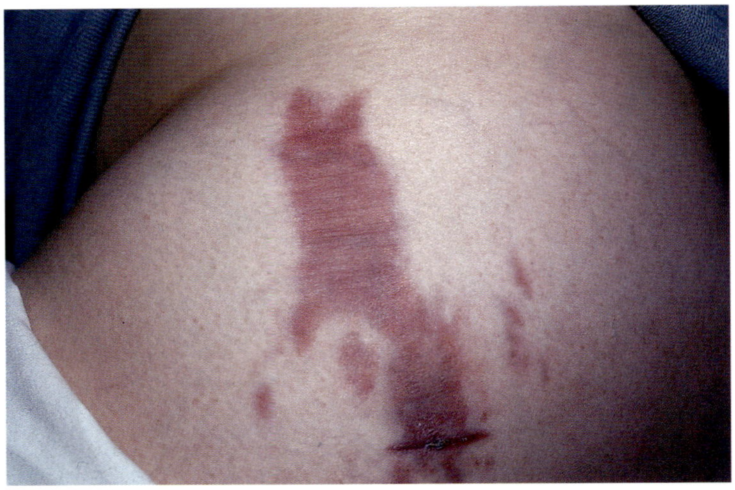

A

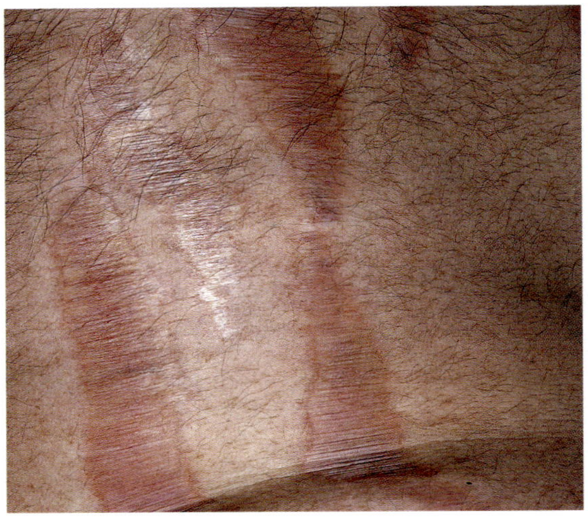

B

Figures 22–1A, 22–1B. Striae distensae. Broad, erythematous, linear lesions on the thigh and abdomen.

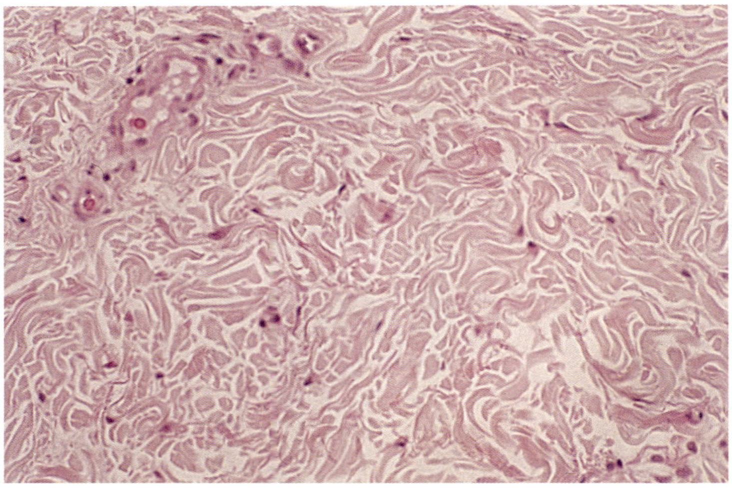

Figure 22–2. Striae distensae. Dilated venules and edema of the reticular dermis.

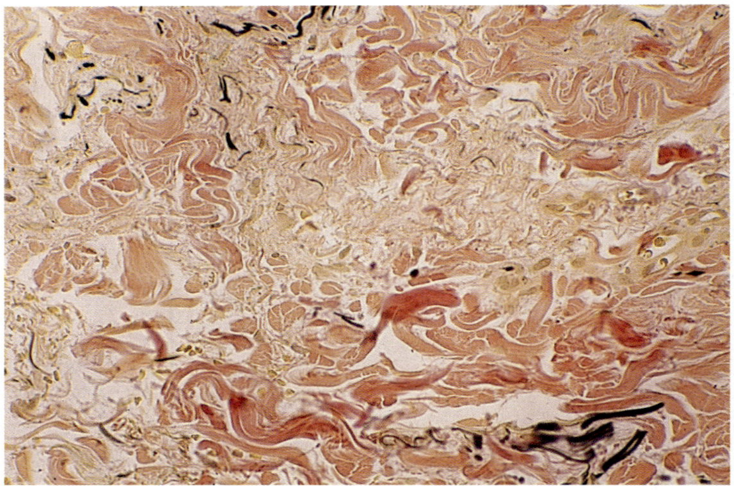

Figure 22–3. Striae distensae. Elastic stain shows fragmented, short, stubby, elastic fibers.

CUTIS LAXA

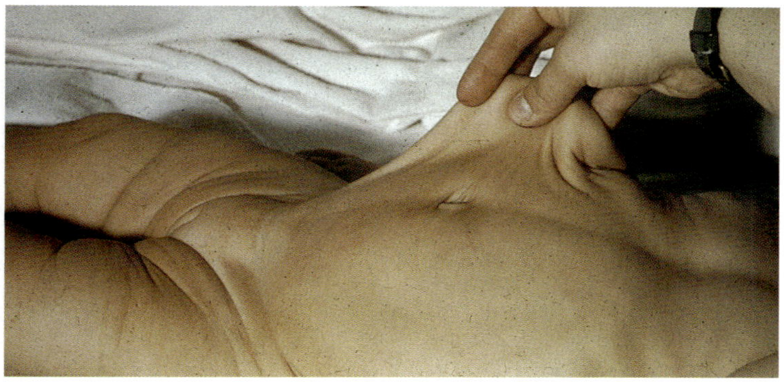

A

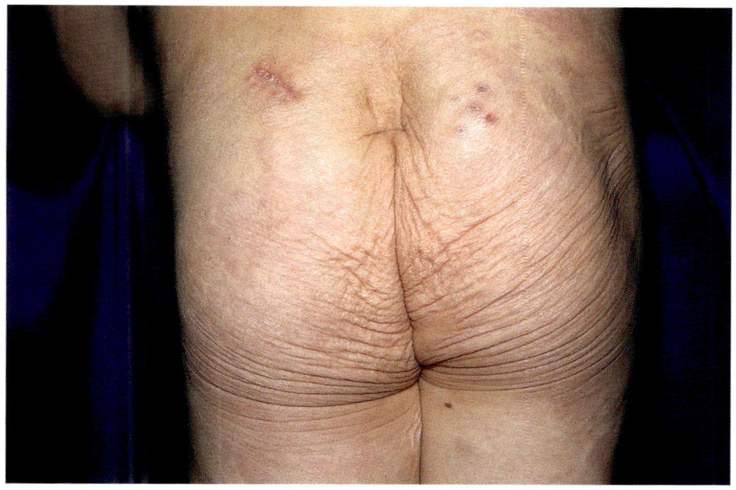

B

Figures 22–4A, 22–4B. **Cutis laxa.** Redundant, wrinkled, and folded skin in a young patient.

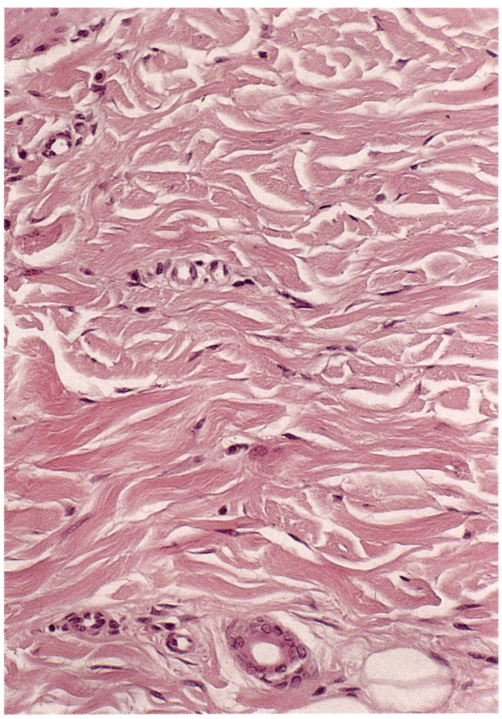

Figure 22–5. **Cutis laxa.** Normal-appearing reticular dermis, hematoxylin and eosin stain.

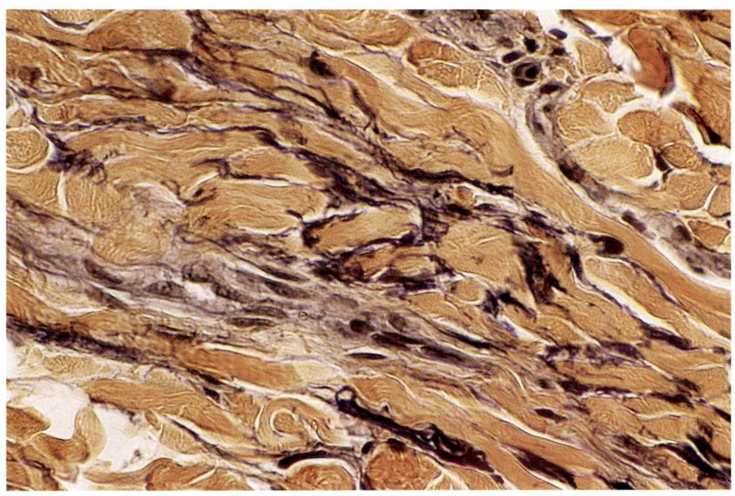

Figure 22–6. **Cutis laxa.** Elastic stain shows abnormal granular and fragmented elastic fibers.

PSEUDOXANTHOMA ELASTICUM

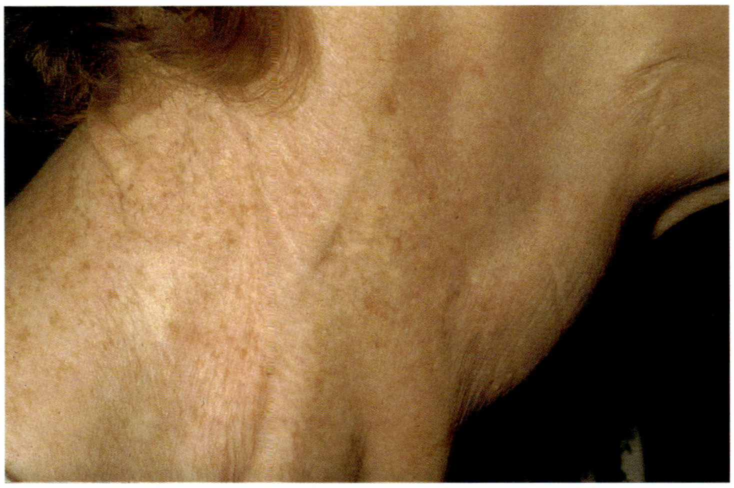

A

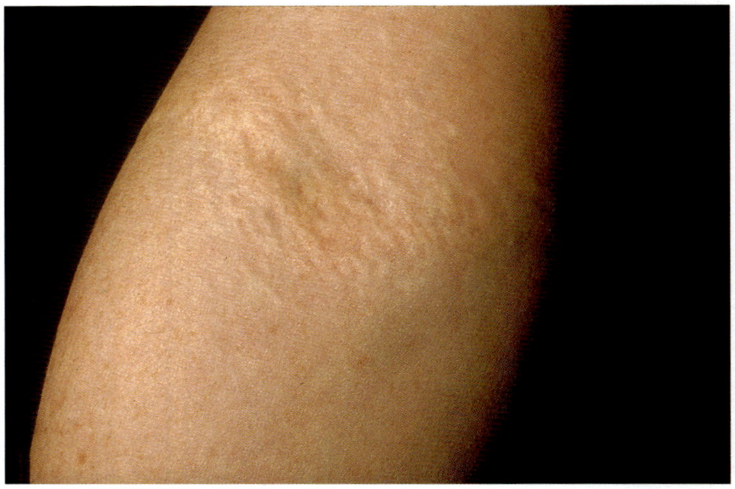

B

Figures 22–7A, 22–7B. Pseudoxanthoma elasticum. Pebbly, yellow papules involve the side of the neck and antecubital fossa.

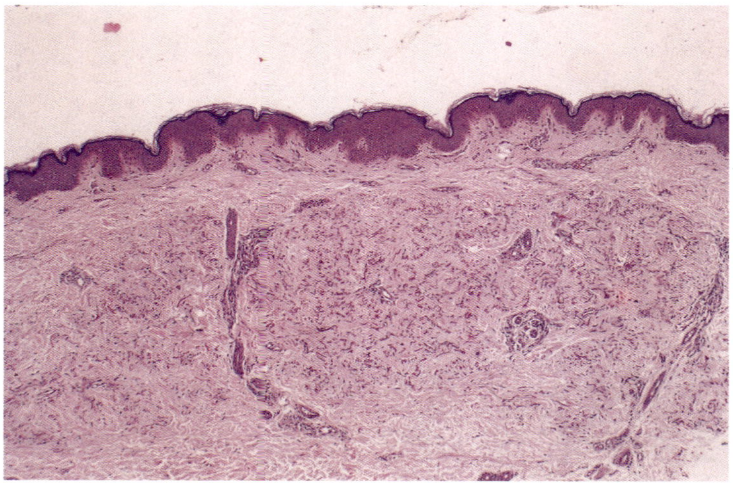

A

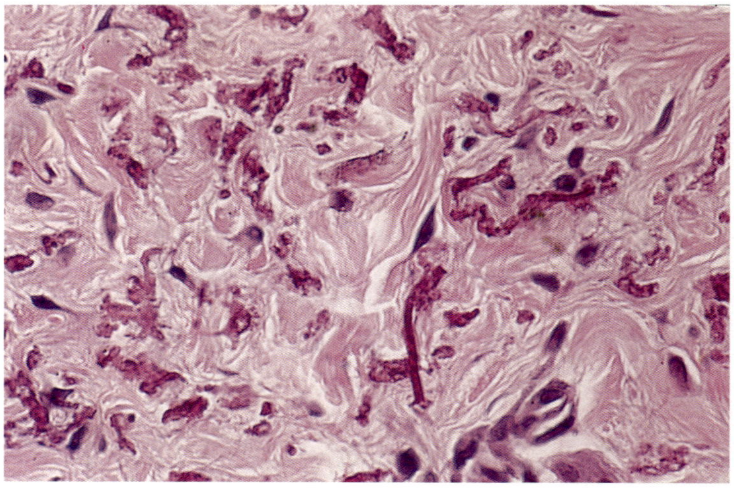

B

Figures 22–8A, 22–8B. Pseudoxanthoma elasticum. Fragmented, coarse, granular, wavy, amphophilic, elastic fibers in the mid-reticular dermis.

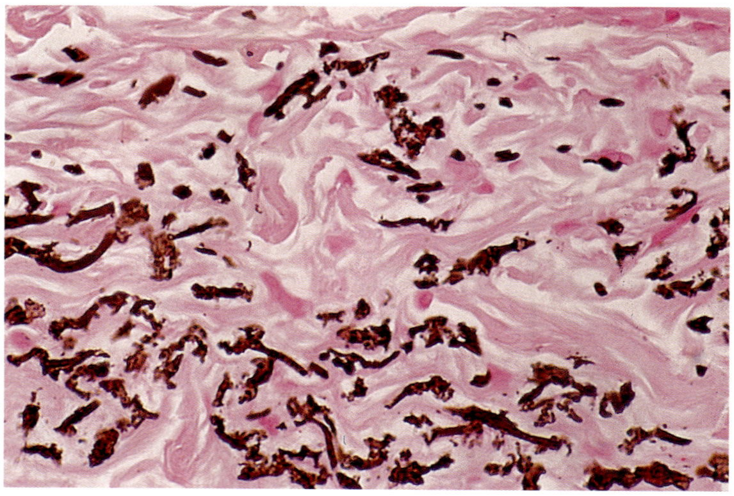

Figure 22–9. Pseudoxanthoma elasticum. VonKossa calcium stain illustrates calcium deposition within the altered elastic fibers.

ELASTOSIS PERFORANS SERPIGINOSA

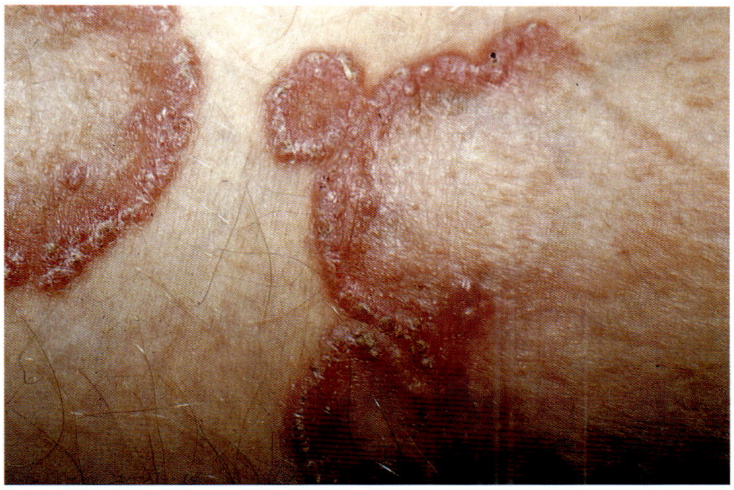

Figure 22–10. Elastosis perforans serpiginosa. Erythematous, keratotic papules arranged in a serpiginous pattern.

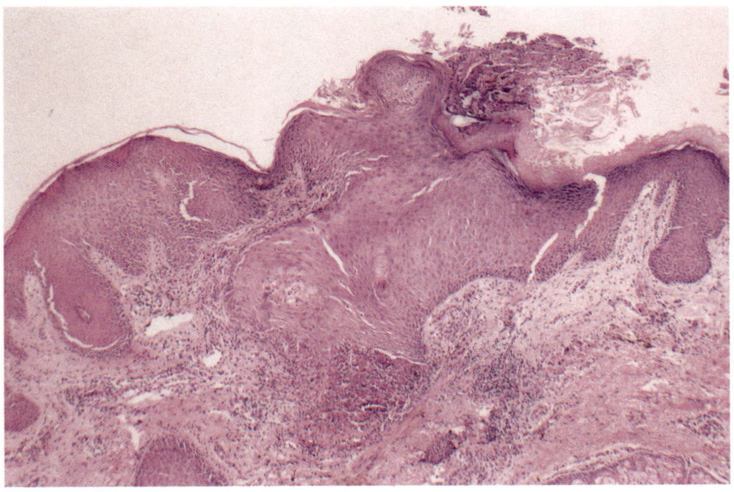

A

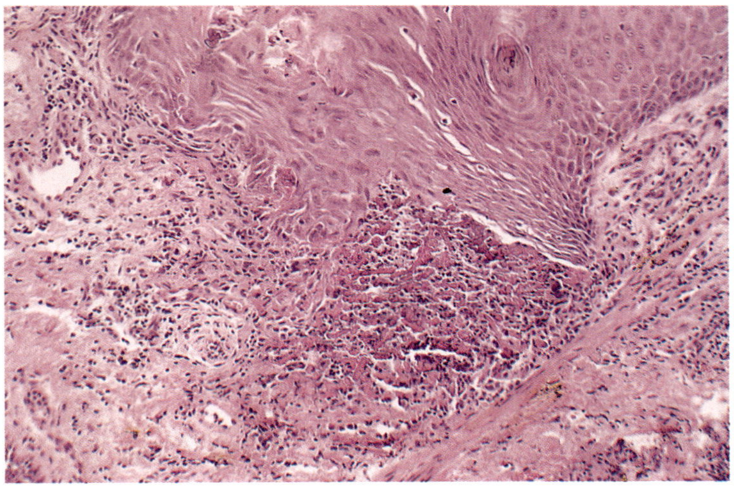

B

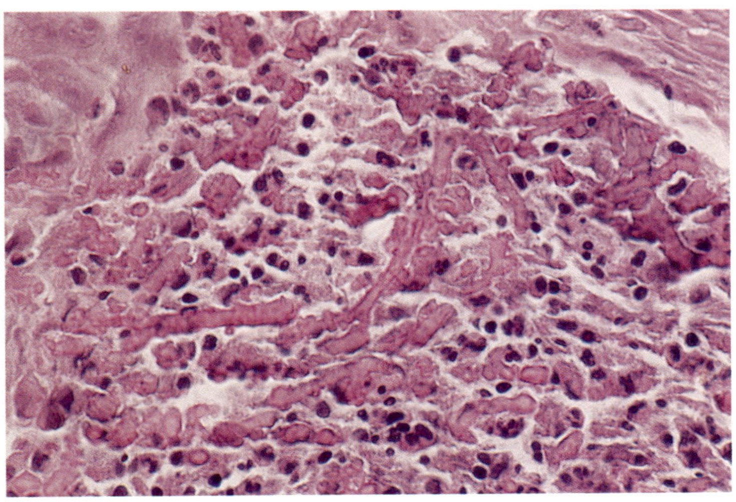

C

Figures 22–11A, 22–11B, 22–11C. Elastosis perforans serpiginosa. Epithelial hyperplasia with scale-crust. There is a collection of neutrophils, nuclear debris, and thickened, eosinophilic, elastic fibers in the papillary dermis, which extend into the overlying epithelium forming a narrow channel. These changes may occur in the epidermis or structures of adnexa (i.e., infundibulum).

ANETODERMA

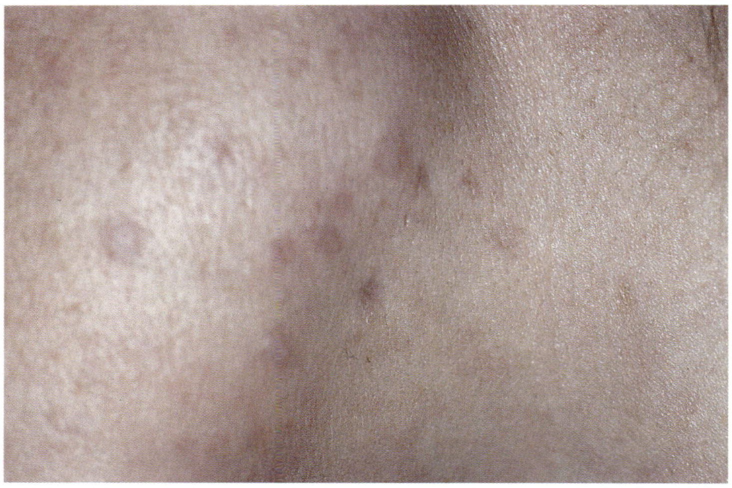

Figure 22–12. Anetoderma. Thin, macular, round-oval, depressed areas on the abdomen of a woman.

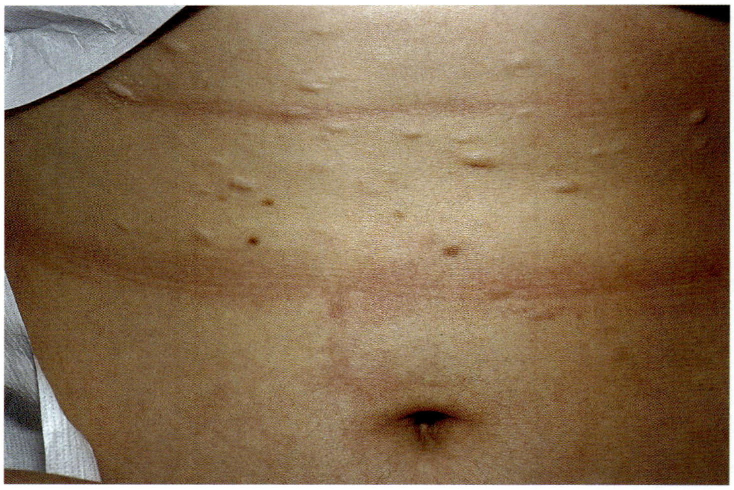

Figure 22–13. Anetoderma. Characteristic "outpouchings" of round, atrophic macules.

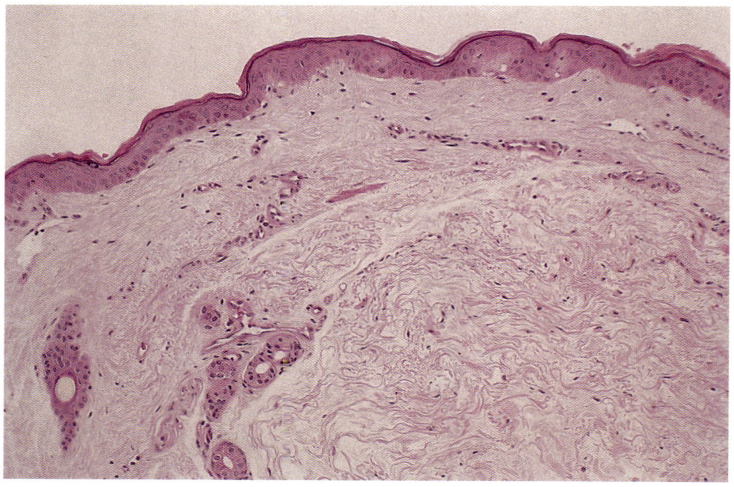

A

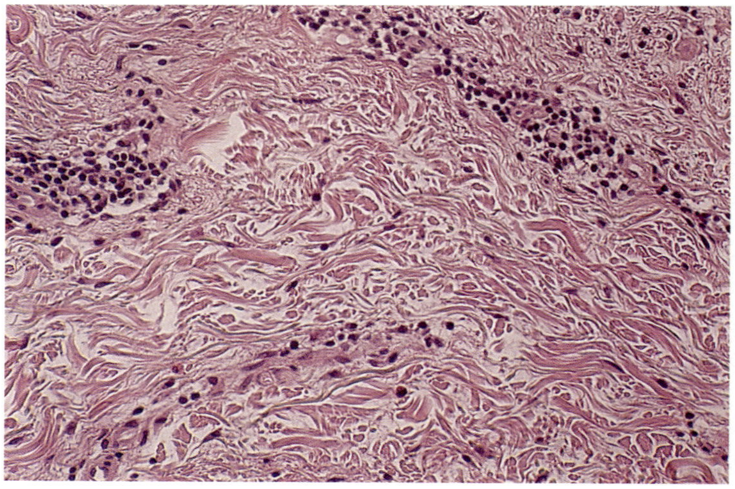

B

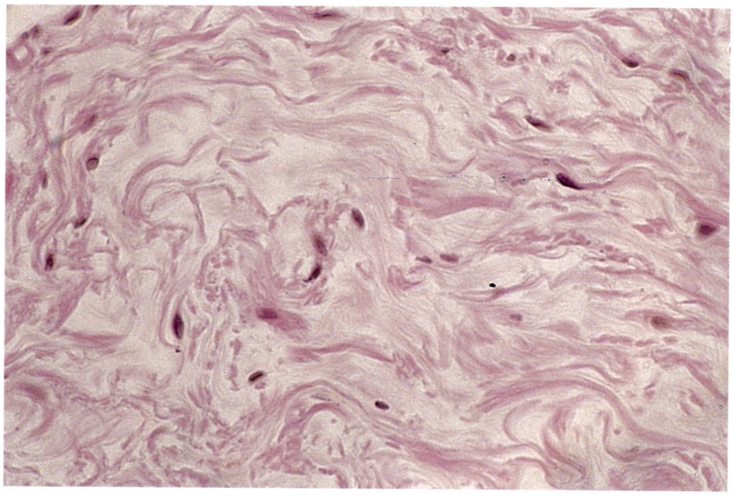

C

Figures 22–14A, 22–14B, 22–14C. Anetoderma. Thin, reticular dermis. There is fibrillary collagen and a mild perivascular mononuclear cell infiltrate.

ANETODERMA

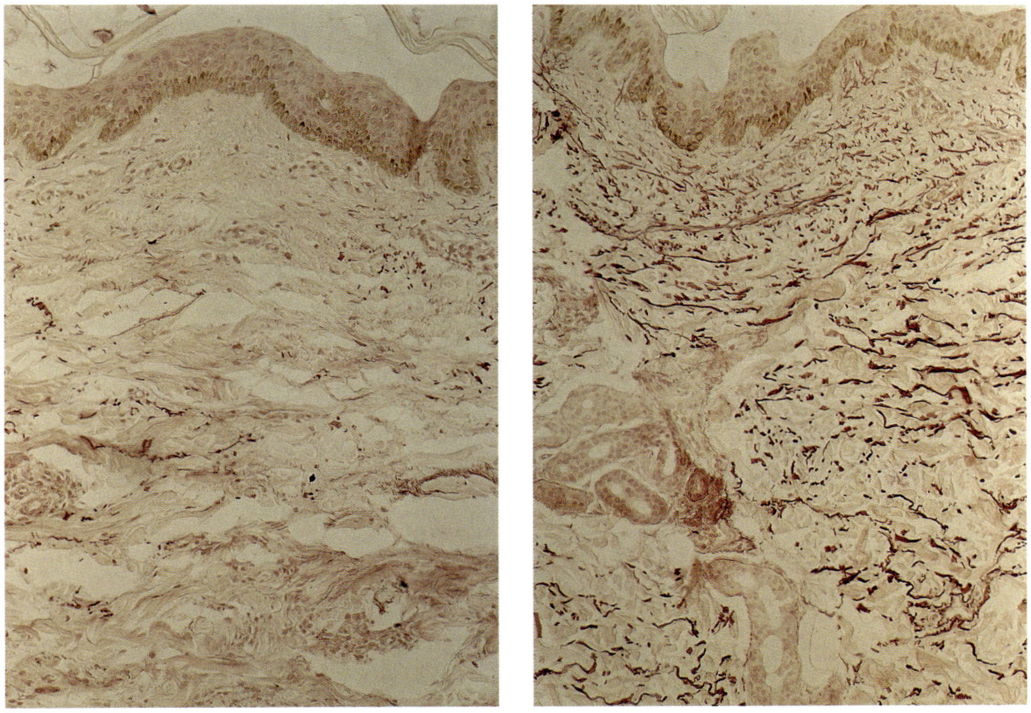

A B

Figures 22–15A, 22–15B. Anetoderma. Elastic stain shows absence of elastic fibers (Fig. 22–15A) in a biopsy specimen of anetoderma compared to the patient's adjacent normal skin (Fig. 22–15B), where elastic fibers are present.

23

Cutaneous deposits

- Calciphylaxis
- Calcinosis cutis
- Osteoma cutis
- Steroid deposits
- Gouty tophus
- Tattoo reaction
- Papular mucinosis/scleromyxedema
- Porphyrias
- Lipoid proteinosis
- Amyloidosis
- Pretibial myxedema
- Focal mucocutaneous mucinosis
- Colloid milium
- Ochronosis

CALCIPHYLAXIS

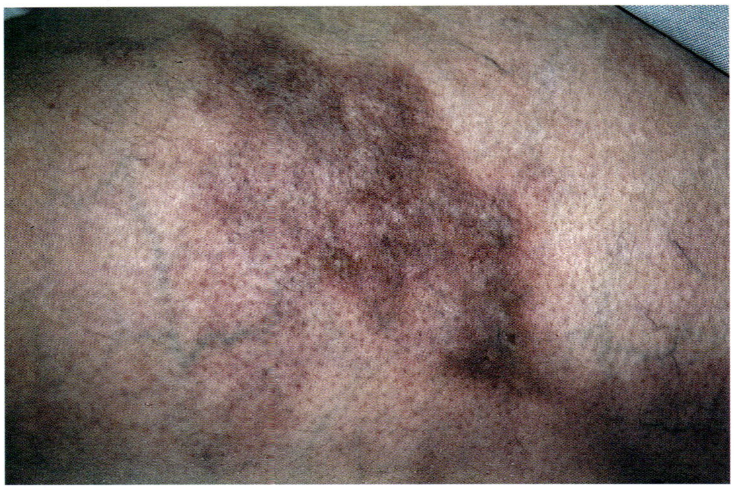

Figure 23–1. Calciphylaxis, early. Mottled bluish-gray and white, irregular patch with peripheral erythema on the leg of a woman.

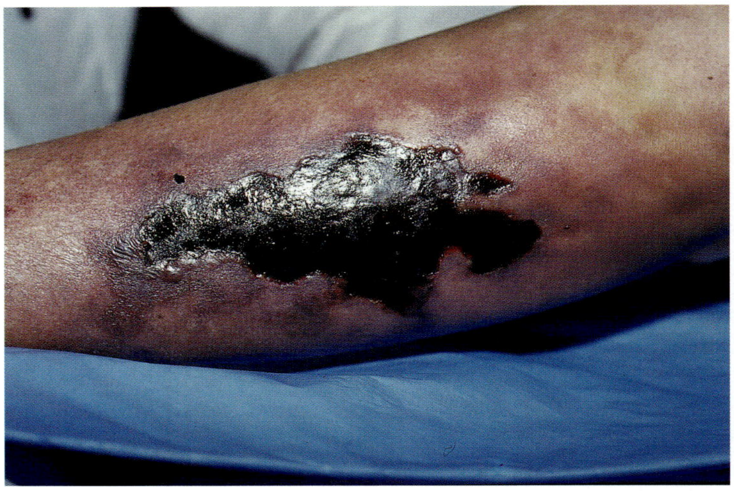

Figure 23–2. Calciphylaxis, late. Thick black eschar with surrounding vesicles and bluish-gray discoloration.

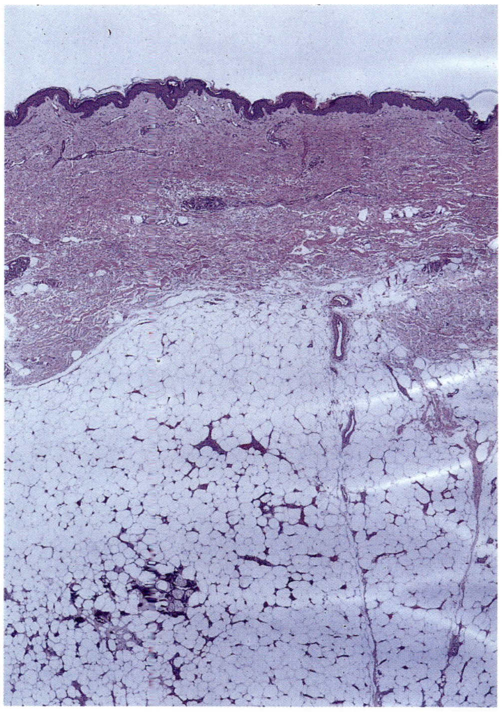

A

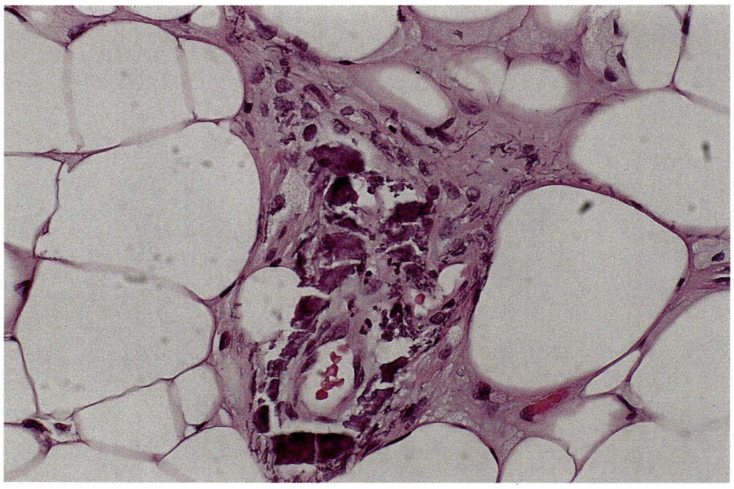

B

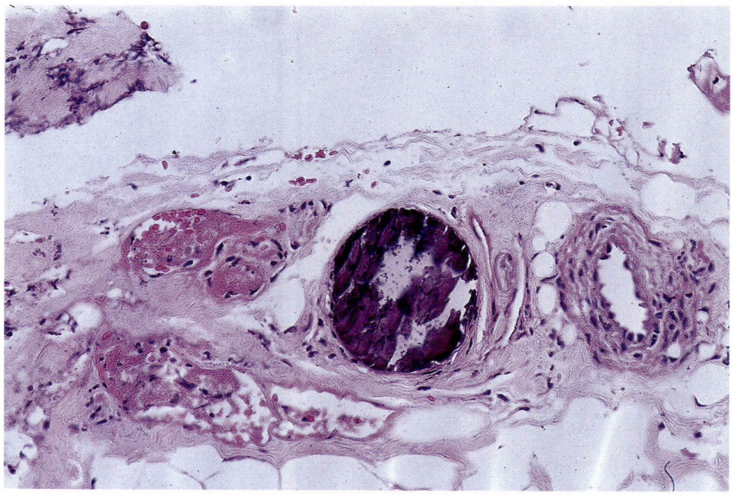

C

Figures 23–3A, 23–3B, 23–3C. Calciphylaxis. Calcium deposits within the lumen of blood vessels and in blood vessel walls in the subcutaneous tissue.

CALCINOSIS CUTIS

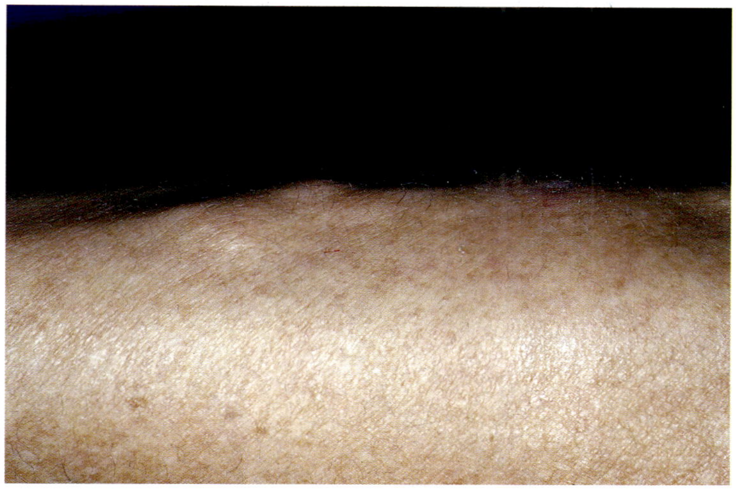

Figure 23–4. Calcinosis cutis. Hard, skin-colored nodules on the arm.

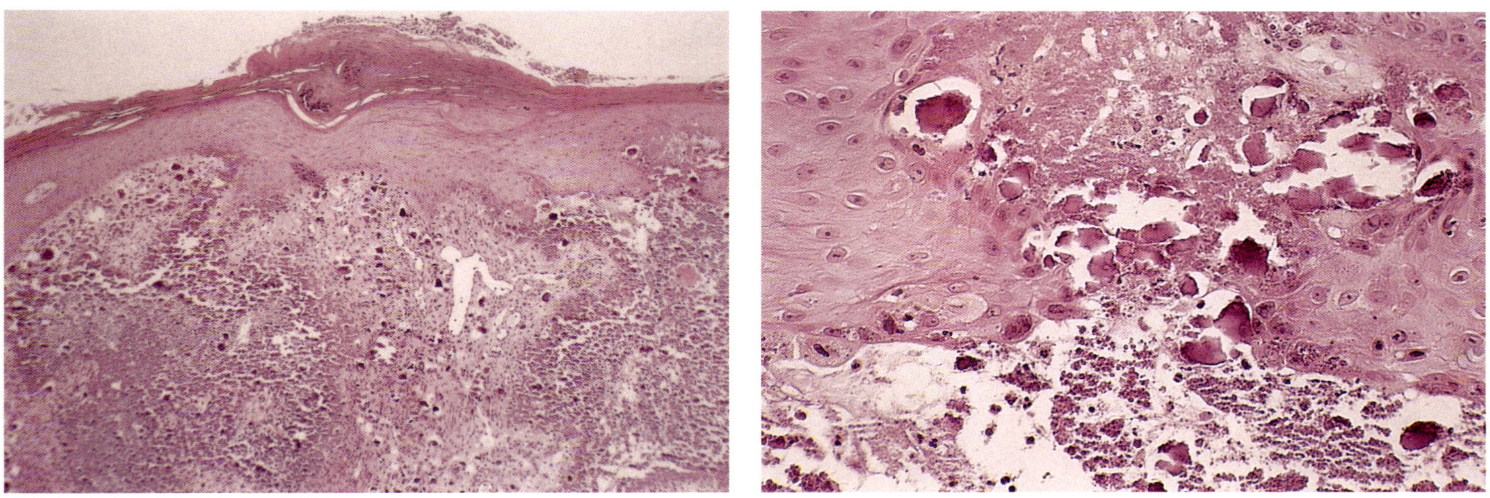

A B

Figures 23–5A, 23–5B. Calcinosis cutis. Dermal amphophilic calcium deposits that vary in size and shape.

OSTEOMA CUTIS

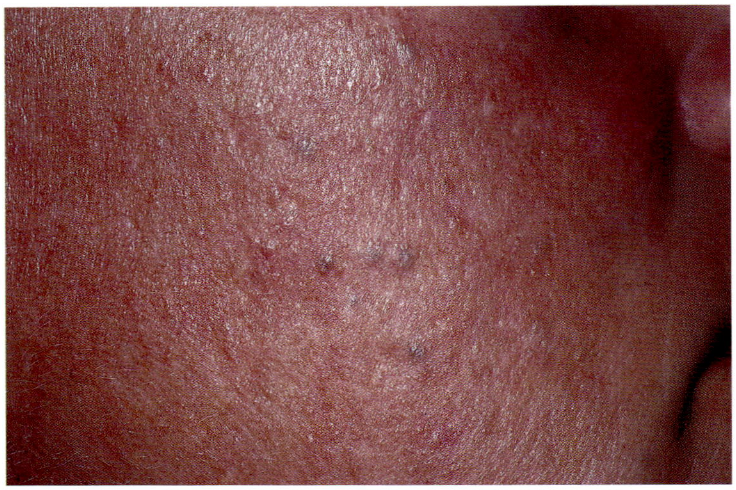

Figure 23–6. Osteoma cutis. Hard, bluish papules on the cheek of a woman with acne vulgaris.

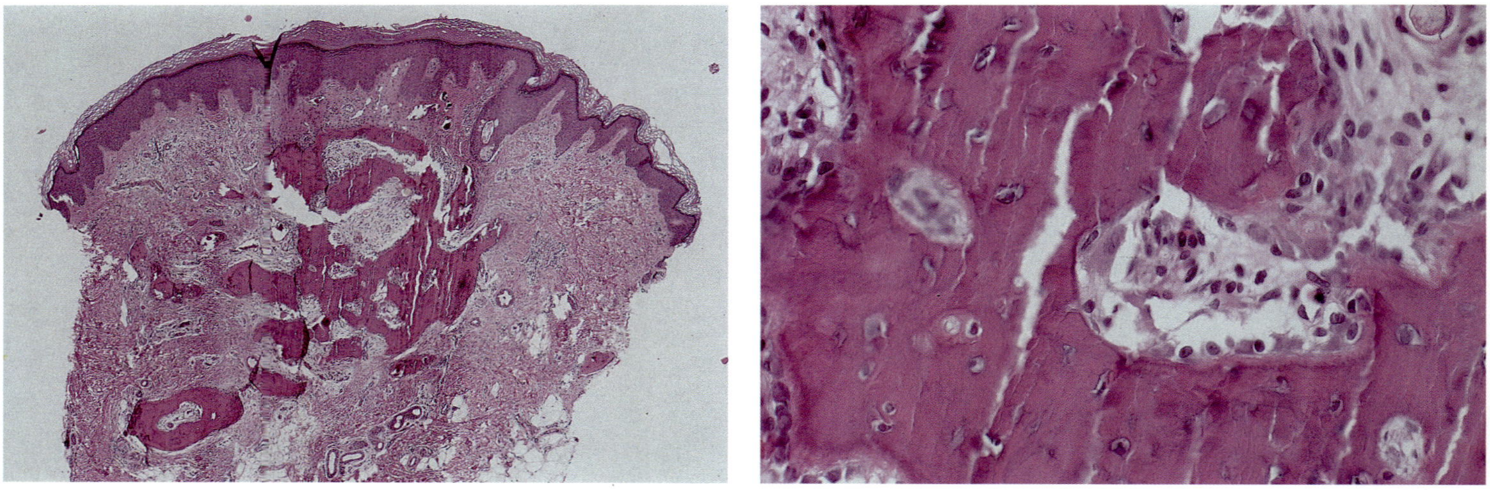

A B

Figures 23–7A, 23–7B. Osteoma cutis. Eosinophilic, bony trabeculae. There are small, spindle-shaped osteocytes in lacunae, and columnar-shaped osteoblasts along the surface of the bony trabecula.

STEROID DEPOSITS

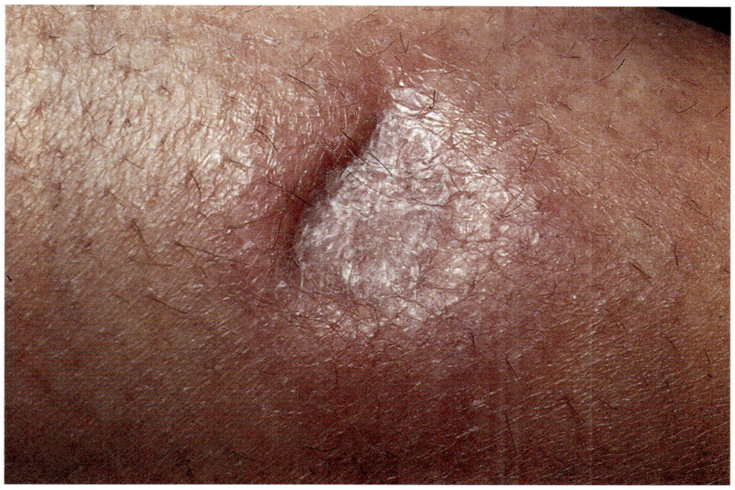

Figure 23–8. Steroid deposits. Localized, cutaneous atrophy from steroid administration.

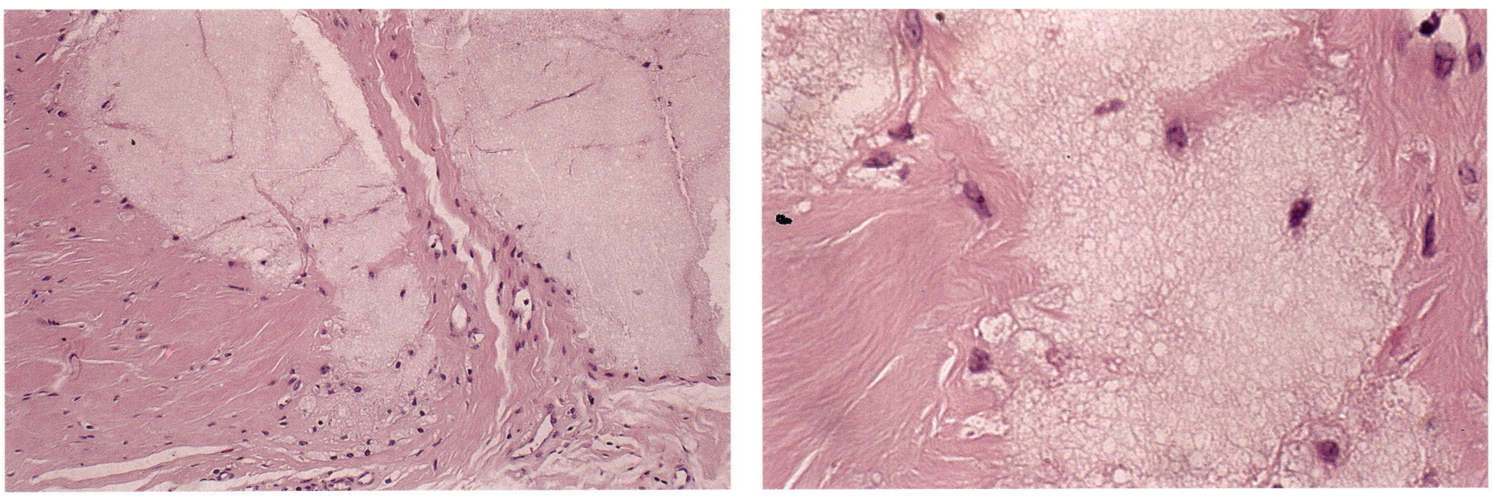

A B

Figures 23–9A, 23–9B. Steroid deposits. Foamy, gray material within an area of fibroplasia.

GOUTY TOPHUS

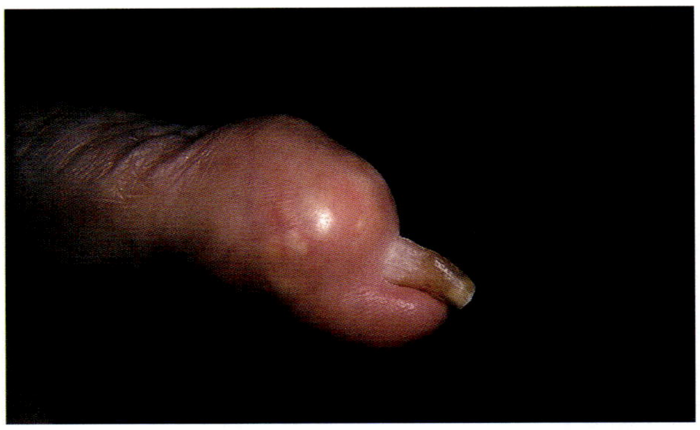

Figure 23–10. Gouty tophus. Firm, erythematous nodule near the distal, interphalangeal joint of the finger.

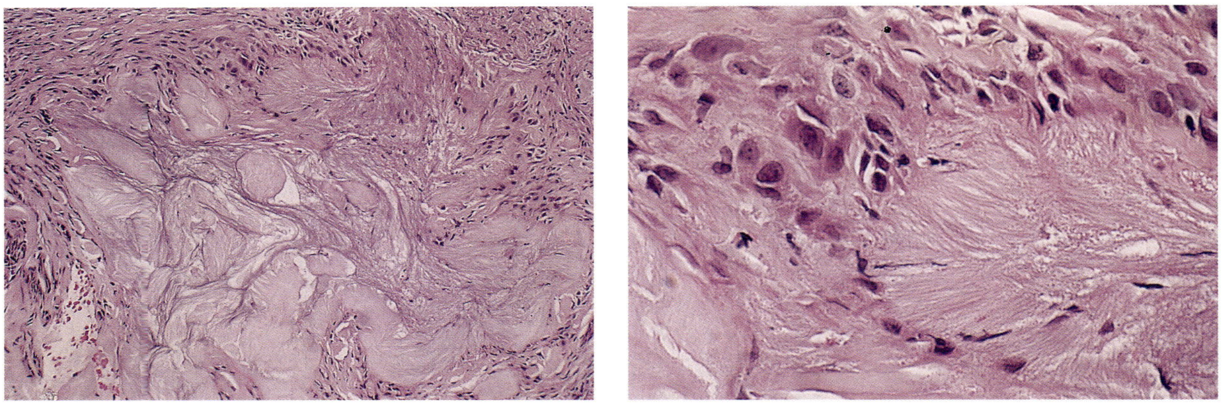

A **B**

Figures 23–11A, 23–11B. Gouty tophus. Feathery, basophilic material with needle-shaped clefts, representing dissolved sodium urate crystals. There is a granulomatous infiltrate in palisaded array.

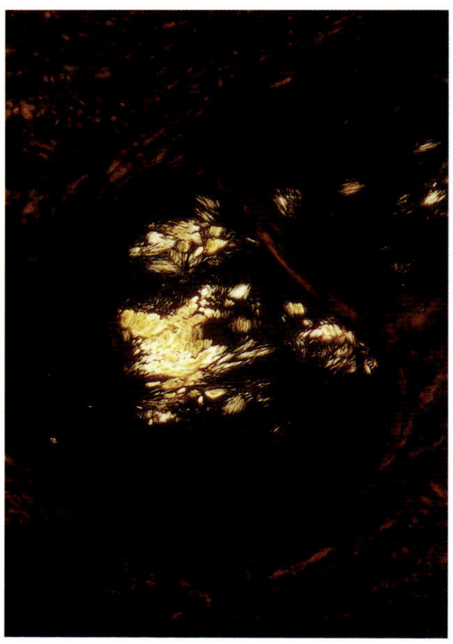

Figure 23–12. Gouty tophus. Refractile, monosodium urate crystals are seen with polarized light.

TATTOO REACTION

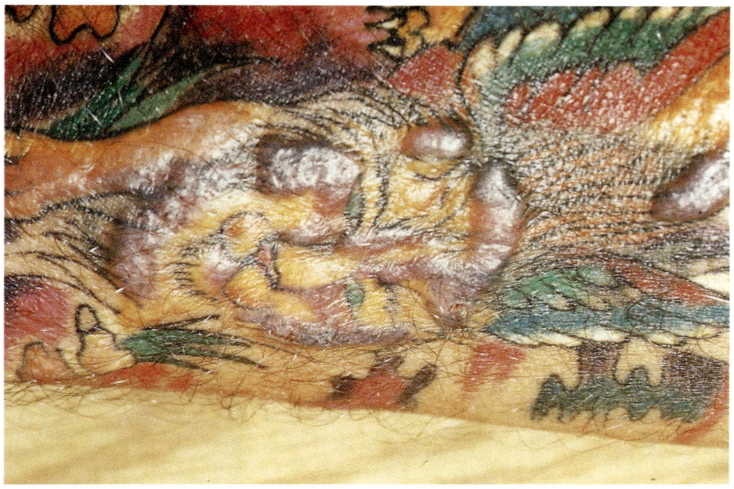

Figure 23–13. Tattoo reaction. Firm, irregularly shaped papules within a professional, multicolored tattoo.

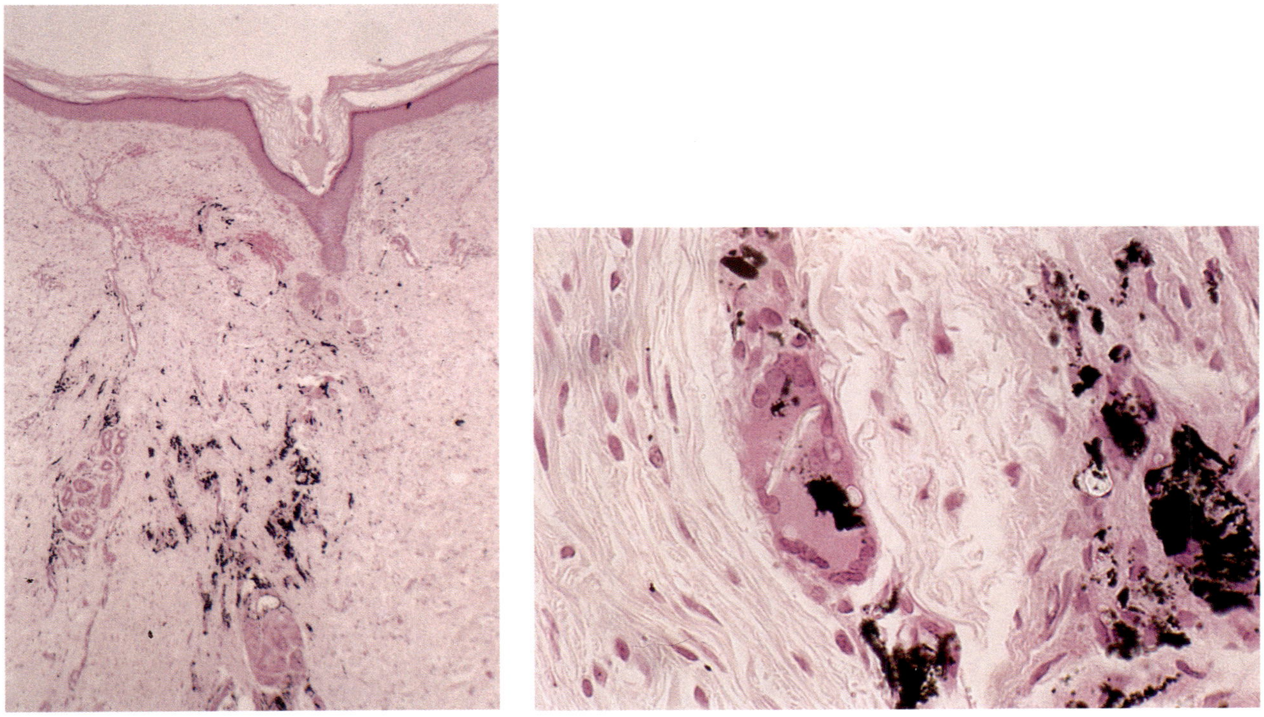

A B

Figures 23–14A, 23–14B. Tattoo reaction. Multinucleated, histiocytic, giant cells containing black particles of dye.

PAPULAR MUCINOSIS/SCLEROMYXEDEMA

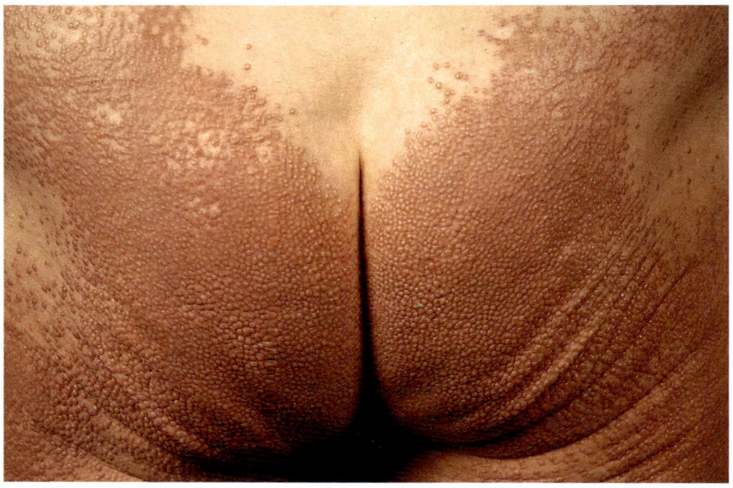

Figure 23–15. Papular mucinosis/scleromyxedema. Confluent, erythematous papules on the buttocks.

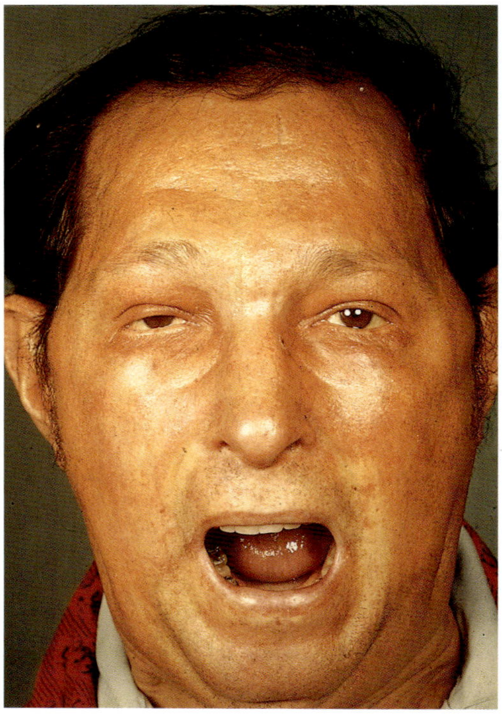

Figure 23–16. Papular mucinosis/scleromyxedema. Sclerodermoid facial features.

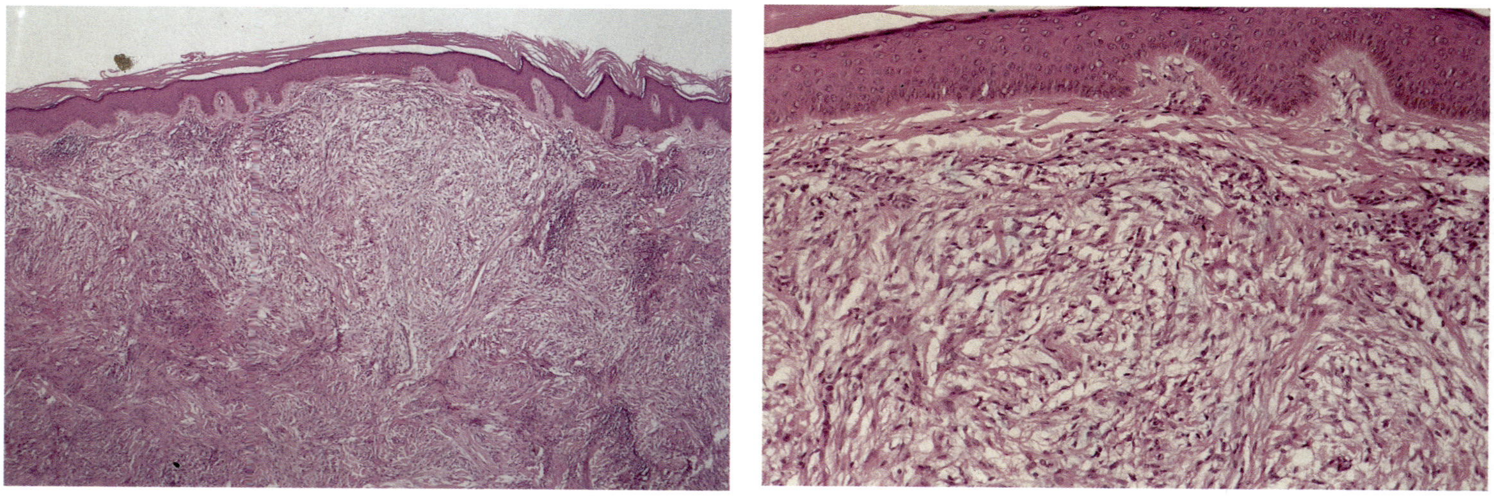

A B

Figures 23–17A, 23–17B. Papular mucinosis/scleromyxedema. Increased number of fibrocytes; mucin; and a patchy, lymphohistiocytic infiltrate throughout the reticular dermis.

PAPULAR MUCINOSIS/SCLEROMYXEDEMA

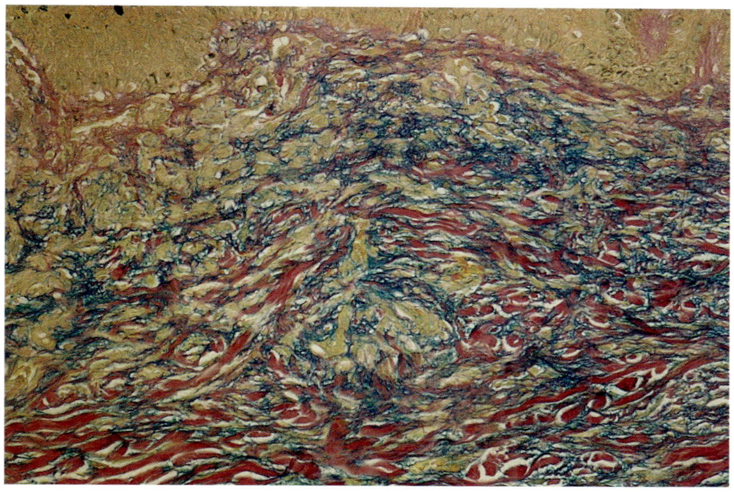

Figure 23–18. Papular mucinosis/scleromyxedema. Colloidal iron stains blue the mucin deposited between collagen bundles.

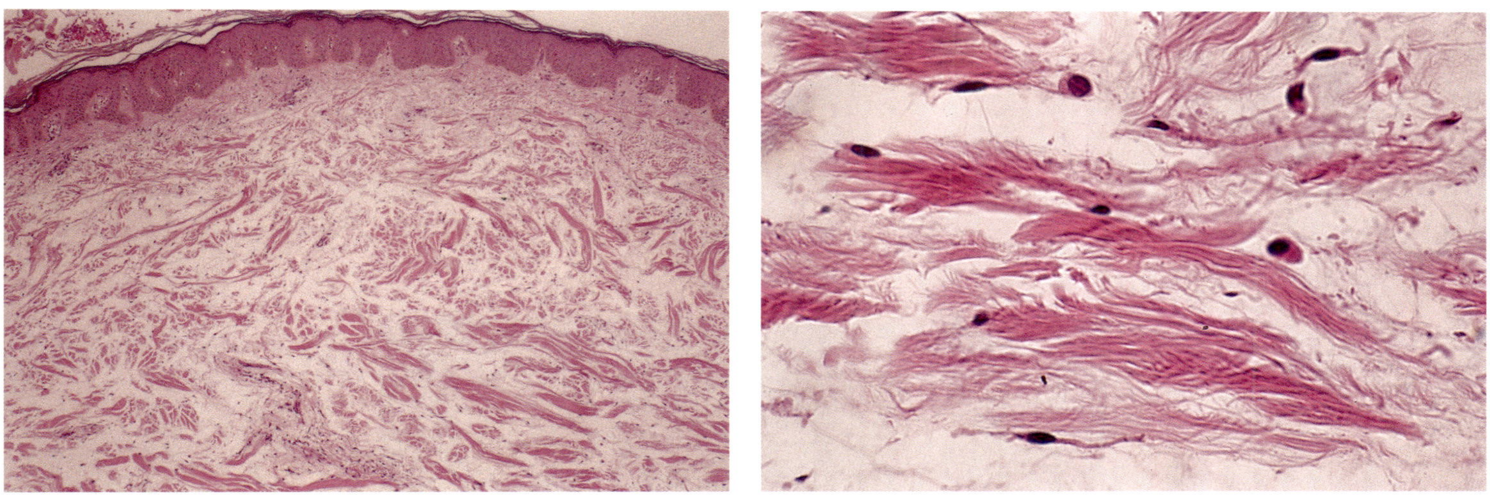

A B

Figures 23–19A, 23–19B. Papular mucinosis/scleromyxedema. Mucin deposition produces separation and disarray of collagen bundles.

PORPHYRIAS

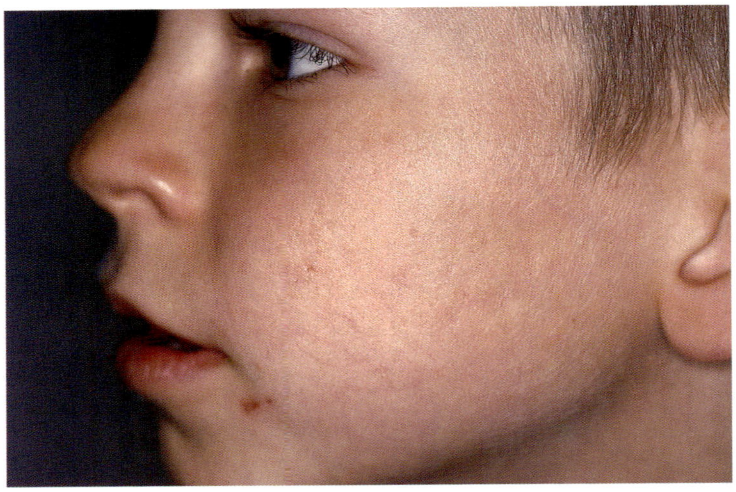

Figure 23–20. Erythropoietic protoporphyria. Subtle, pitted scars on the cheeks of a young boy.

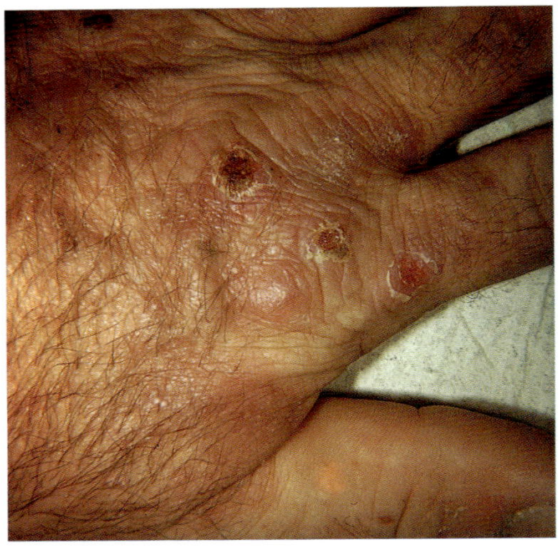

Figure 23–21. Porphyria cutanea tarda. Vesicles, erosions, crusts, and milia on the dorsum of the hand and fingers.

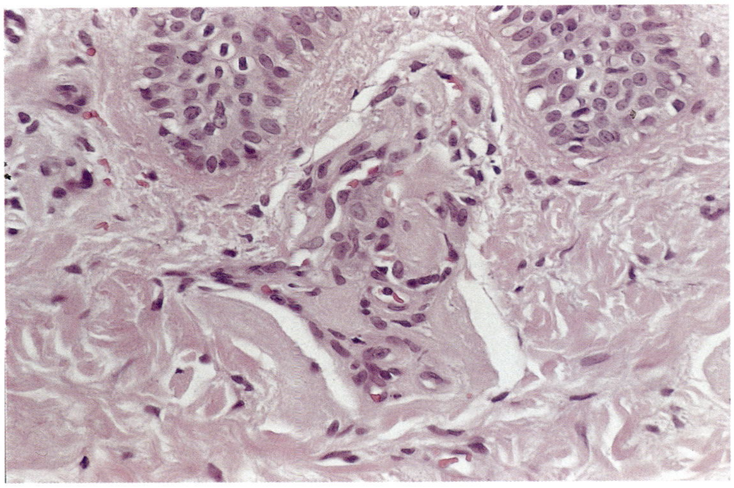

Figure 23–22. Porphyria. Eosinophilic, homogeneous, hyalin-like material in and around blood vessel walls of the upper dermis.

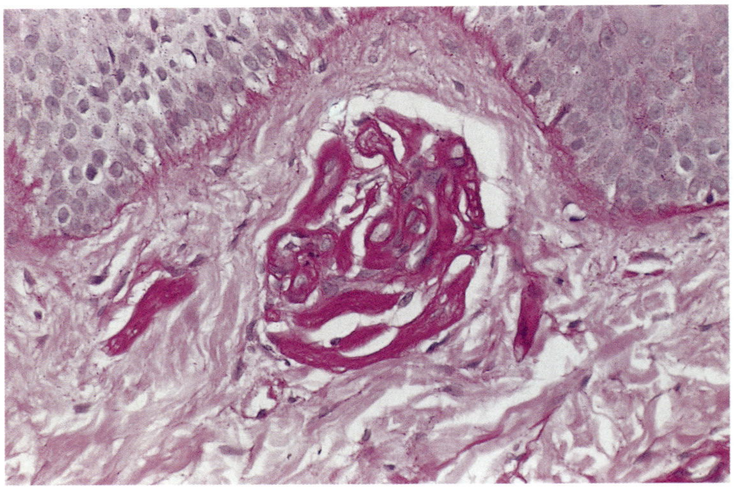

Figure 23–23. Porphyria. Periodic acid-Schiff (PAS) stains blood vessel hyalin-like material.

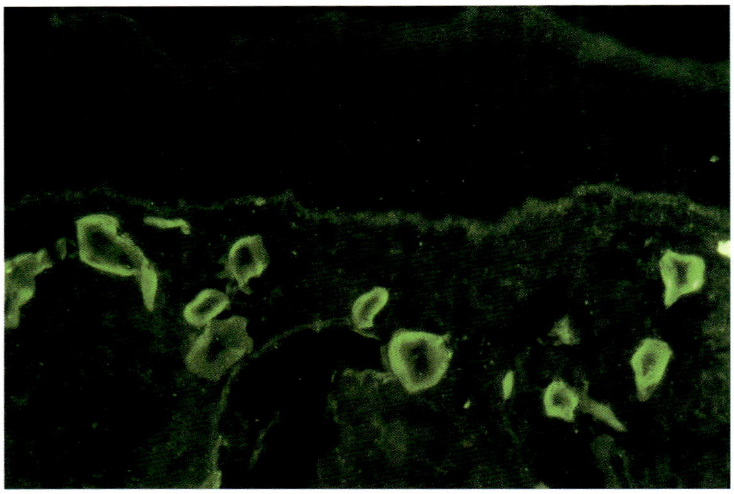

Figure 23–24. Porphyria. Direct immunofluorescence of a lesion from a patient with erythropoietic protoporphyria. Note homogeneous deposition of IgG within the walls of blood vessels and along the basement membrane zone.

LIPOID PROTEINOSIS

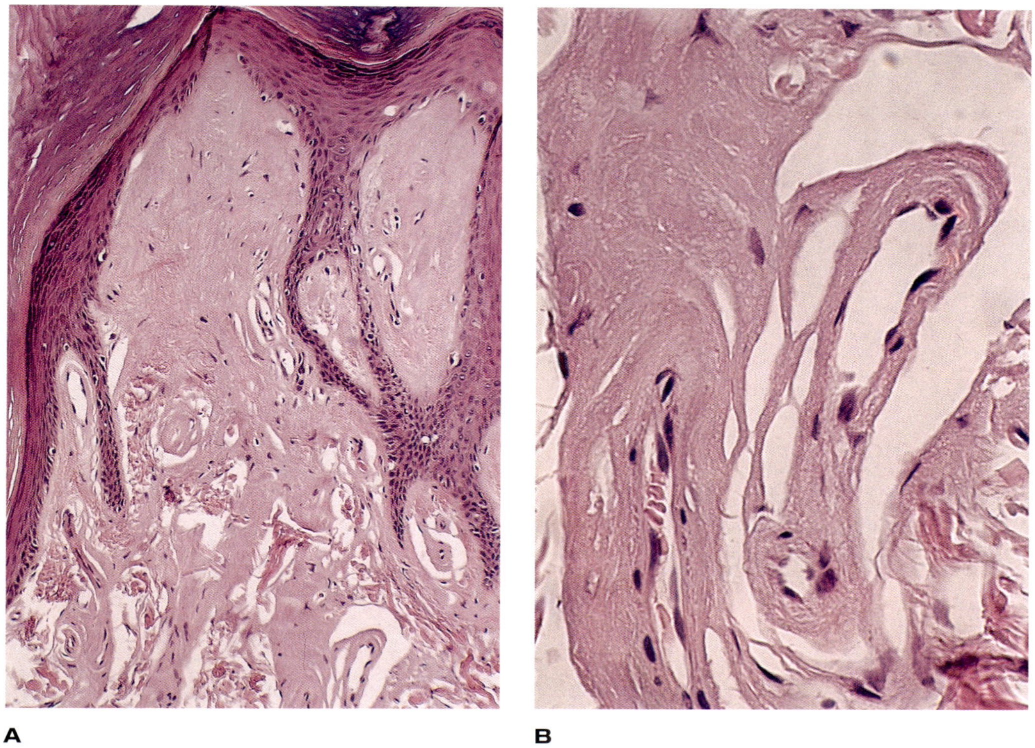

Figures 23–25A, 23–25B. Lipoid proteinosis. Pink, hyalin-like material within the thickened, papillated dermis. Characteristic deposits of hyalinized material are present around blood vessel walls of the superficial plexus.

AMYLOIDOSIS

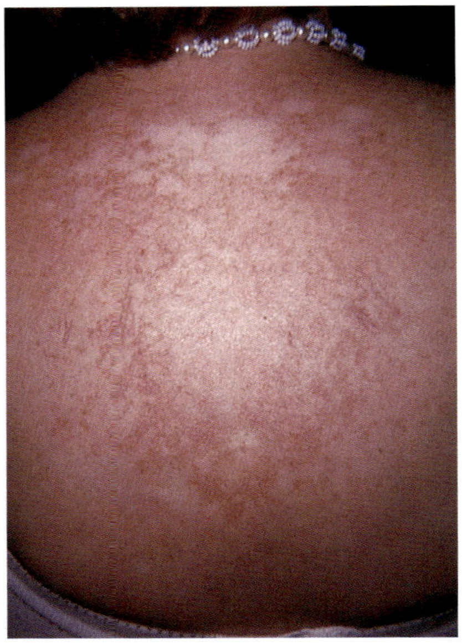

Figure 23–26. Macular amyloidosis. Pruritic, hypo- and hyperpigmented patches in the interscapular area.

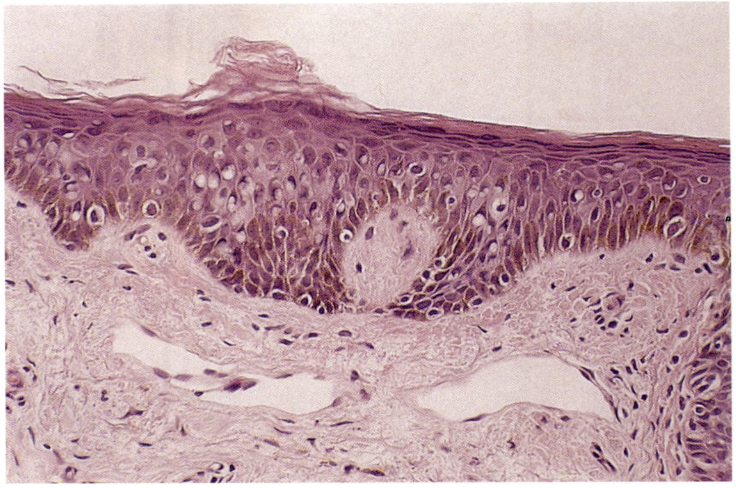

Figure 23–27. Macular amyloidosis. Widened, dermal papilla with homogeneous eosinophilic globules. The dermis has dilated blood vessels, melanophages, and stellate fibroblasts.

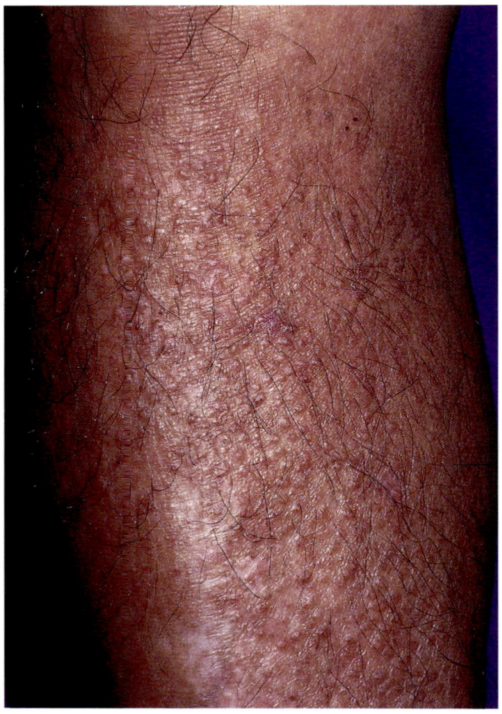

Figure 23–28. Lichen amyloidosis. Confluent, red-brown, keratotic papules over the pretibial surface of the leg.

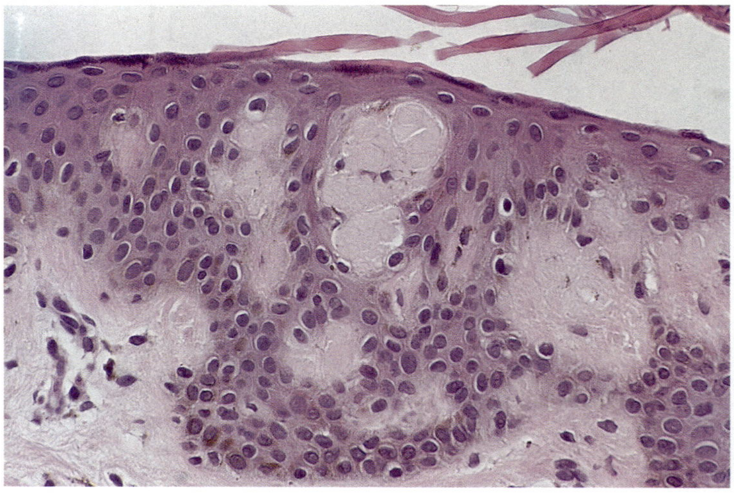

Figure 23–29. Lichen amyloidosis. Hyperplastic epidermis surrounds deposits of homogeneous, eosinophilic globules within the thickened papillary dermis. The dermis contains melanophages, dilated blood vessels, and stellate fibrocytes.

AMYLOIDOSIS

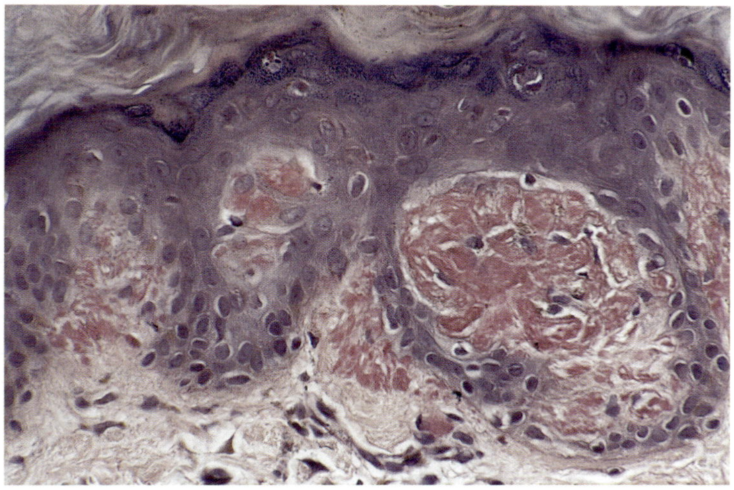

Figure 23–30. **Lichen amyloidosis.** Congo red stains the amyloid globules in the thickened papillary dermis.

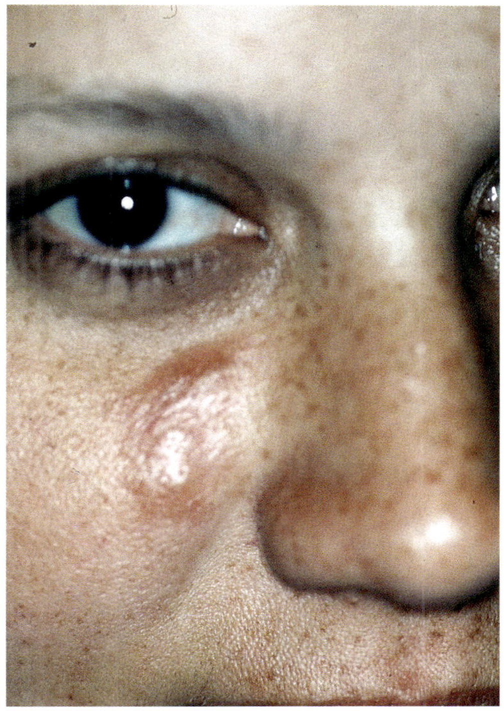

Figure 23–31. **Nodular amyloidosis.** Firm, erythematous nodule on the cheek of a young woman.

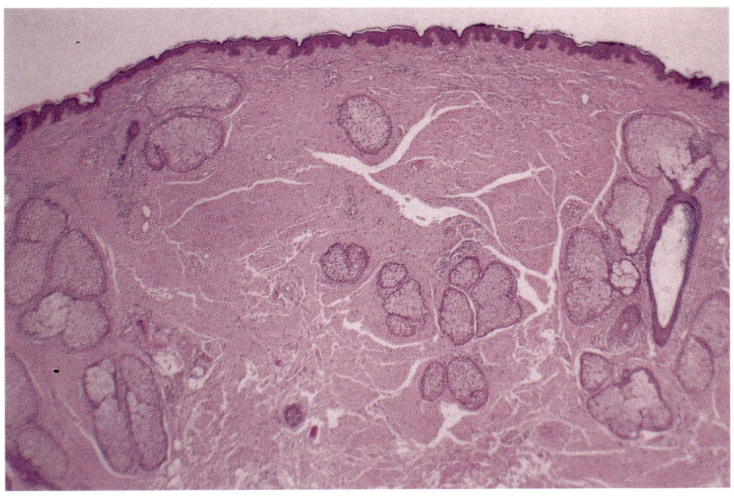

A

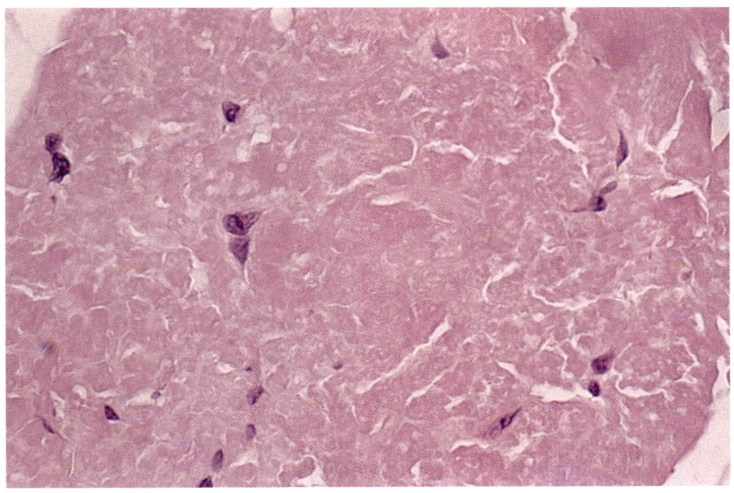

B

Figures 23–32A, 23–32B. **Nodular amyloidosis.** Demarcated, nodular deposits of eosinophilic, amorphous material throughout the reticular dermis. There is a patchy lymphoplasmacytic infiltrate and stellate fibroblasts.

AMYLOIDOSIS

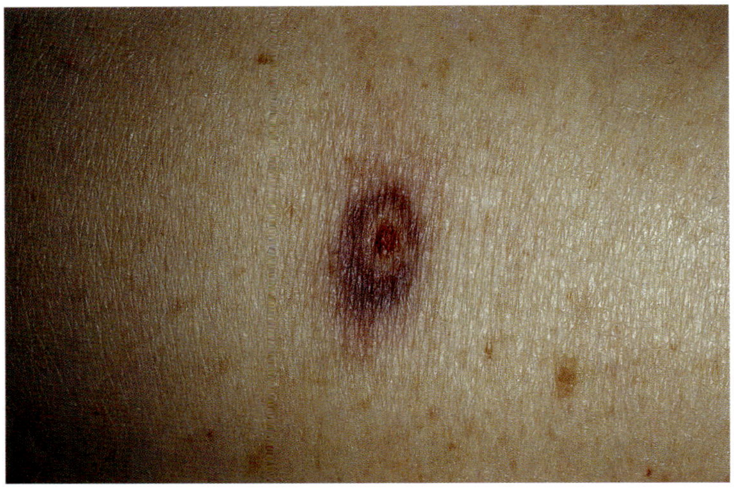

Figure 23–33. Systemic amyloidosis. Erythematous papule with surrounding purpura.

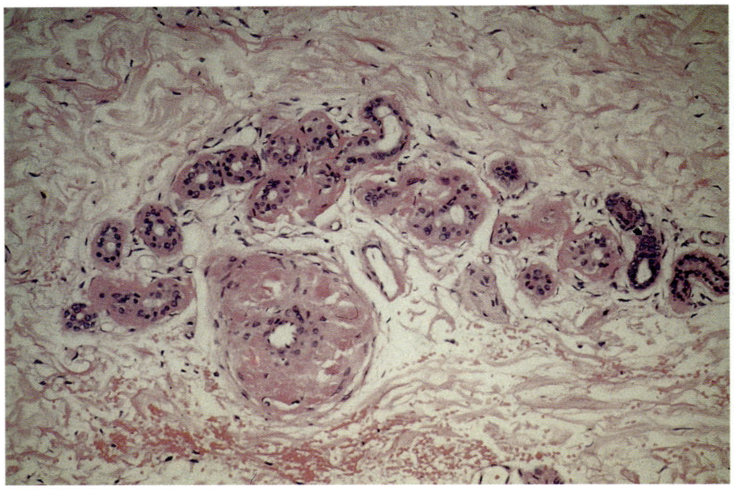

Figure 23–34. Systemic amyloidosis. Eosinophilic, amorphous deposits within the wall of blood vessels, eccrine glands, and eccrine ducts.

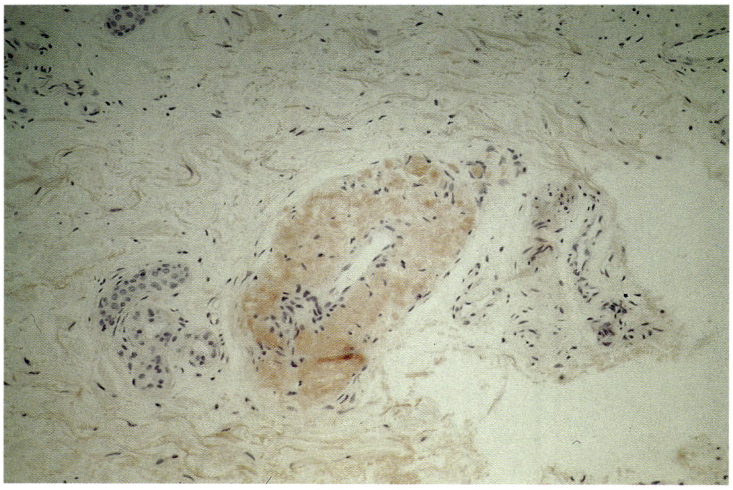

Figure 23–35. Systemic amyloidosis. Congo red stains amyloid deposits within the blood vessel walls.

PRETIBIAL MYXEDEMA

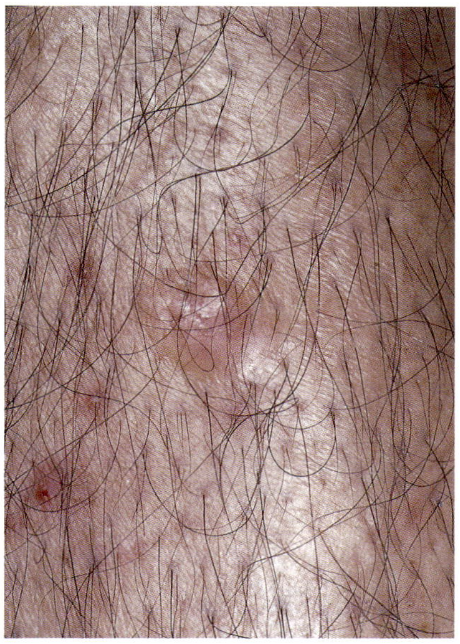

Figure 23–36. Pretibial myxedema. Firm, tender, pink nodule on the lower leg of a man with exophthalmos. Both conditions occurred following treatment for hyperthyroidism.

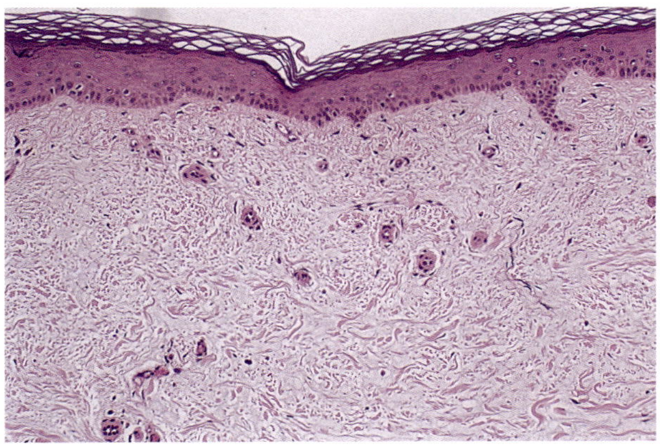

A

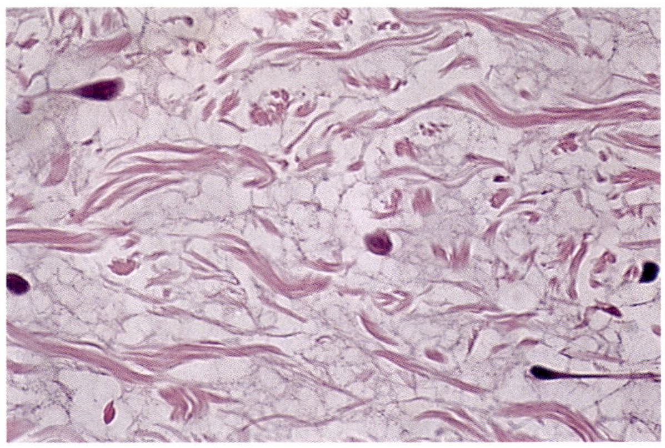

B

Figures 23–37A, 23–37B. Pretibial myxedema. Mucin separates collagen bundles. There are deposits of gray, finely, granular mucin between collagen bundles and stellate fibrocytes.

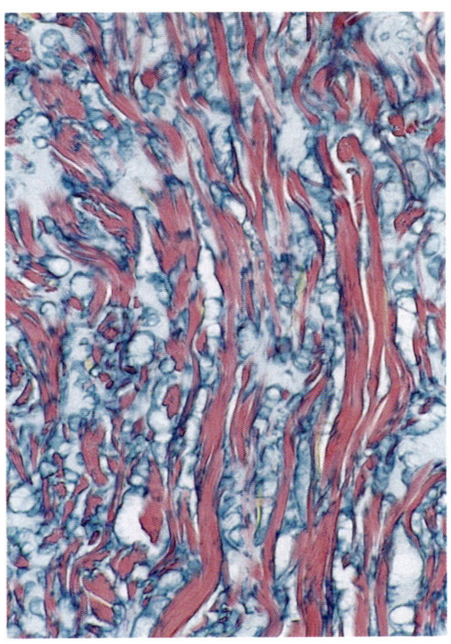

Figure 23–38. Pretibial myxedema. Mucin between collagen bundles stains blue with colloidal iron.

FOCAL MUCOCUTANEOUS MUCINOSIS

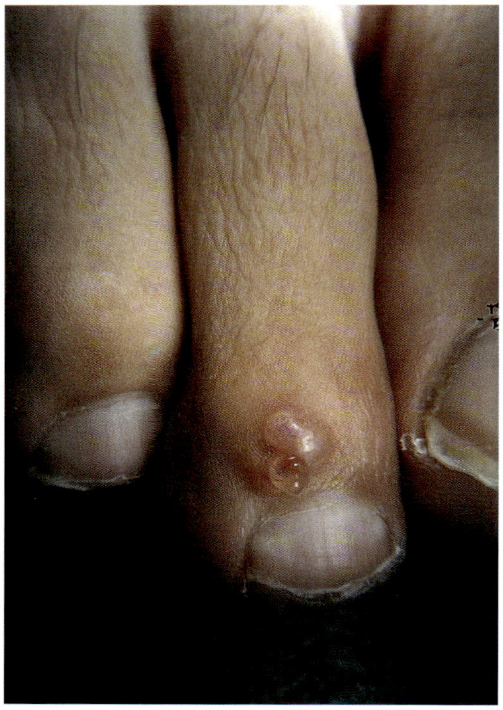

Figure 23–39. Myxoid cyst. Pink, translucent papule on the dorsum of the distal interphalangeal joint of the toe. There is drop of mucin oozing onto the surface.

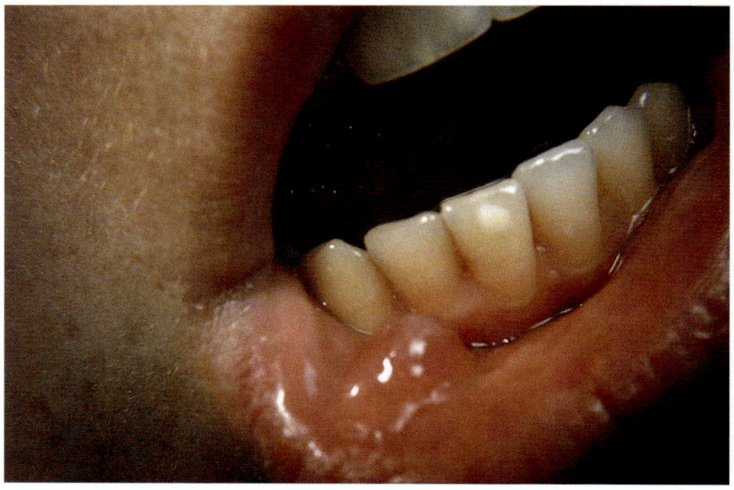

Figure 23–40. Mucocele. Pink, clear, dome-shaped papule on the mucosal surface of the lower lip.

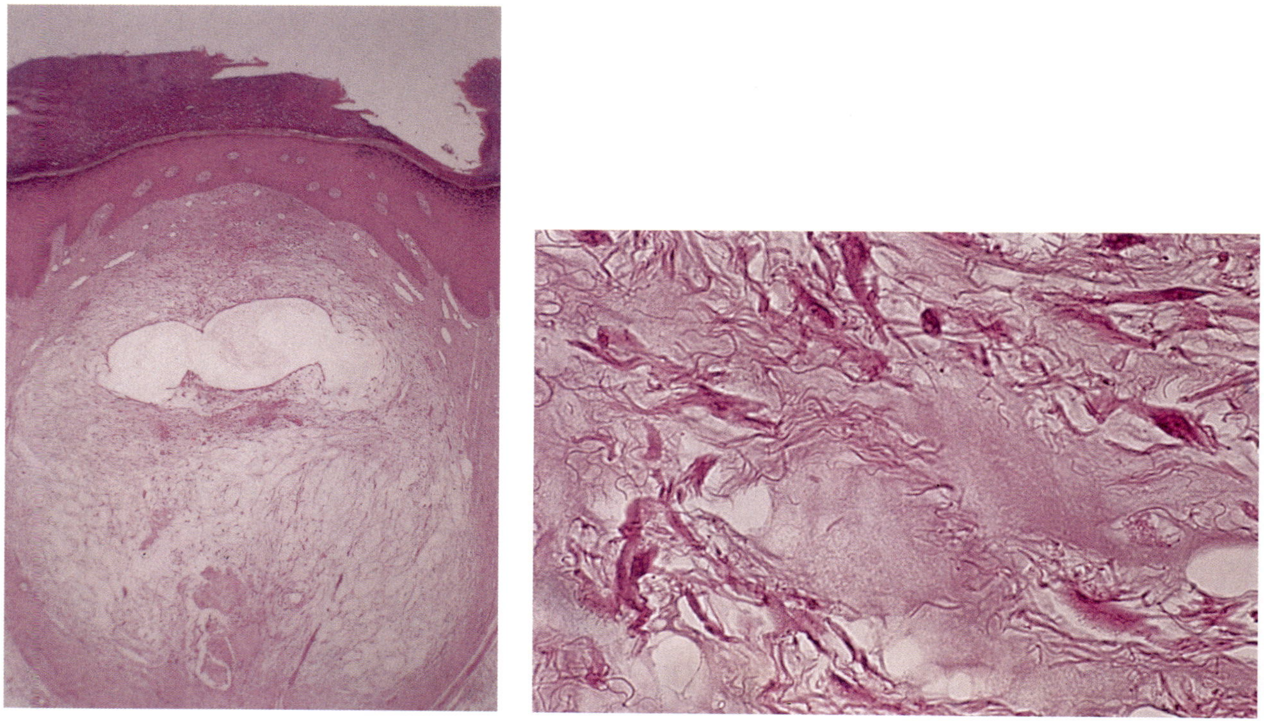

A **B**

Figures 23–41A, 23–41B. Myxoid cyst. Large deposits of mucin in the dermis. There is epidermal hyperkeratosis and hyperplasia, and dermal amphophilic granular deposits of mucin widely separating the collagen bundles.

COLLOID MILIUM

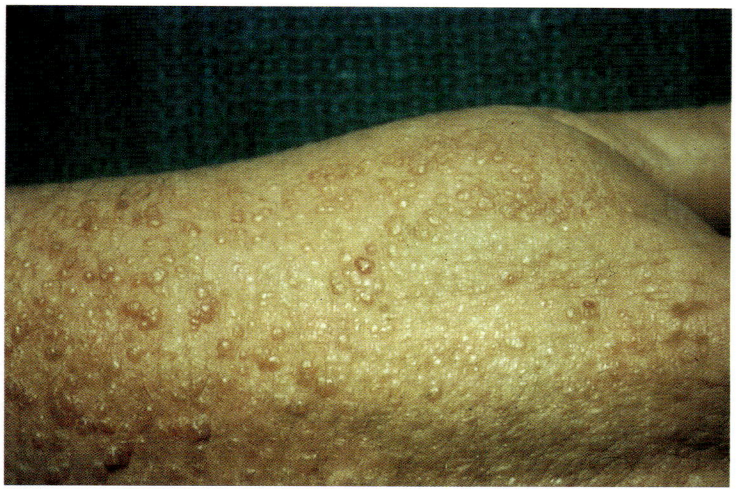

Figure 23–42. Colloid milium. Smooth, firm, translucent papules on sun-damaged skin of the hand.

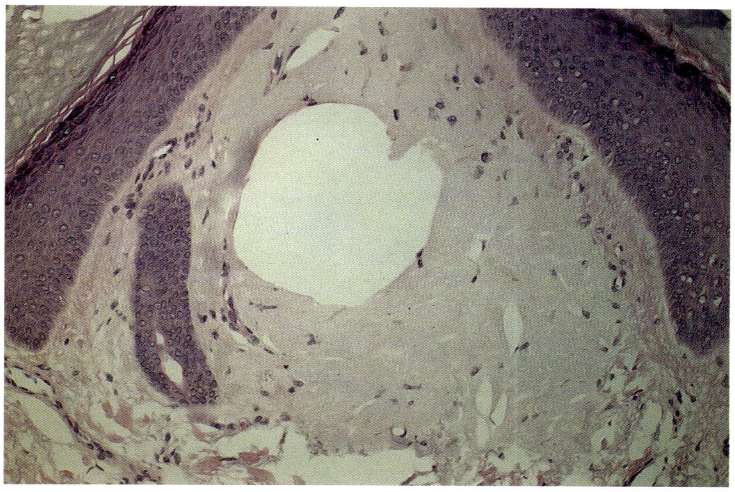

Figure 23–43. Colloid milium. Large deposits of amphophilic, homogeneous material in the dome-shaped dermis. There are dilated blood vessels and fibrocytes.

OCHRONOSIS

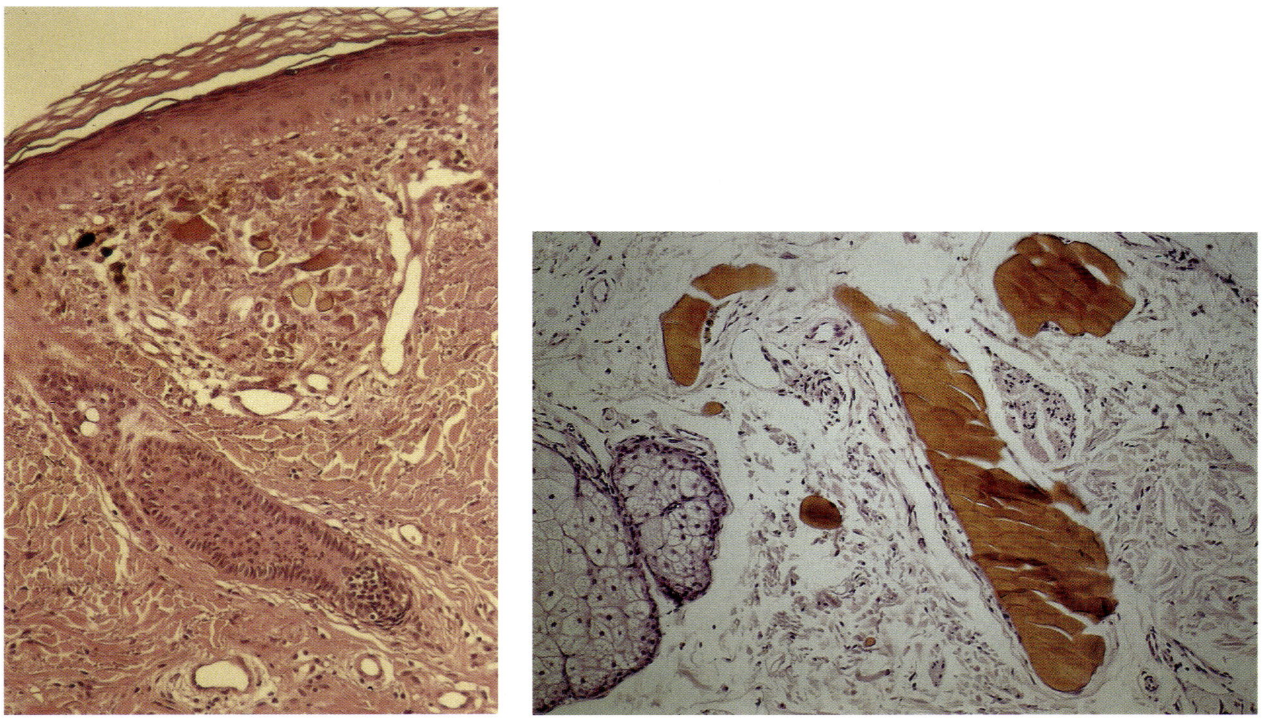

A

B

Figures 23–44A, 23–44B. Ochronosis. Large, yellow-brown, irregularly shaped deposits of homogentisic acid in the dermis. They are found free in the dermis, or may be associated with collagen, vascular, and adnexal structures.

24

Perforating disorders

- Reactive perforating collagenosis
- Hyperkeratosis follicularis et parafollicularis in cutem penetrans (Kyrle's disease)

REACTIVE PERFORATING COLLAGENOSIS

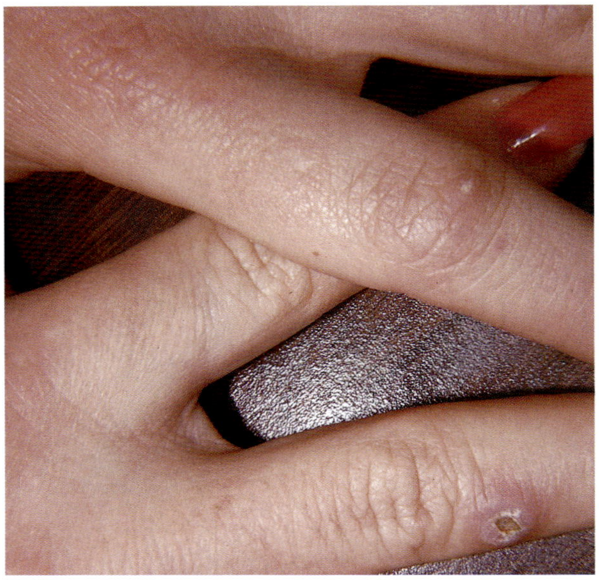

Figure 24–1. Reactive perforating collagenosis. Ulcerated, crusted papule on the finger of a patient with a history of recurrent lesions for many years. There is also a keratotic papule on the proximal interphalangeal joint of the left hand.

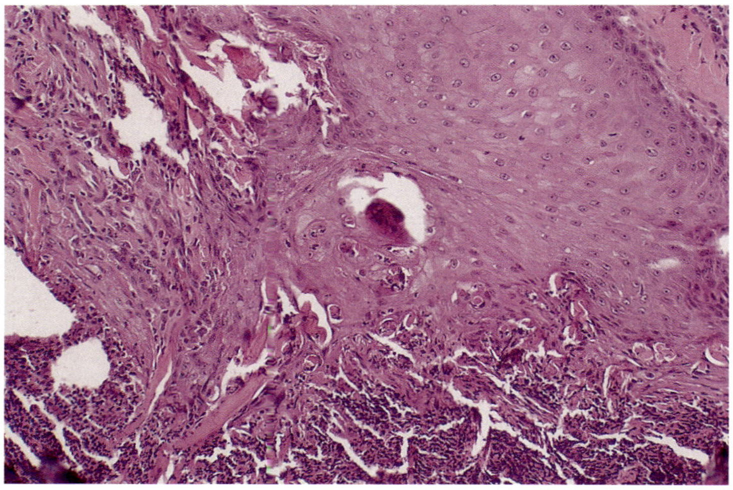

A

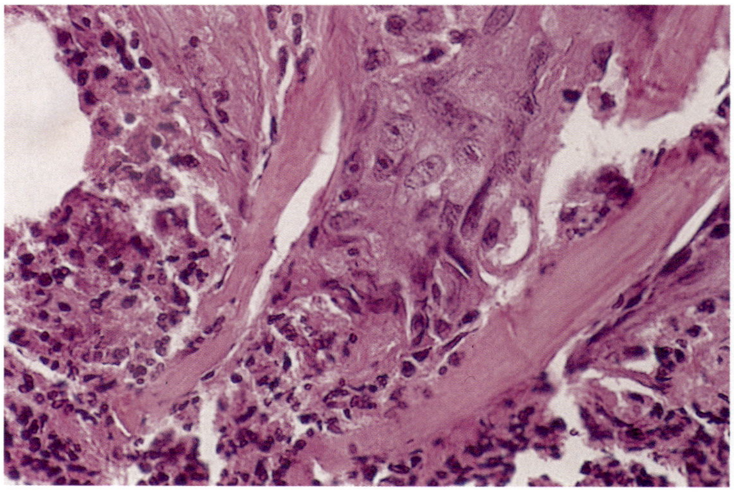

B

Figures 24–2A, 24–2B. Reactive perforating collagenosis. Collagen bundles within the hyperplastic epithelium associated with numerous neutrophils. These changes are not specific and may be found in any ulcerated lesion that involves the dermis, such as perforating folliculitis.

HYPERKERATOSIS FOLLICULARIS ET PARAFOLLICULARIS IN CUTEM PENETRANS (KYRLE'S DISEASE)

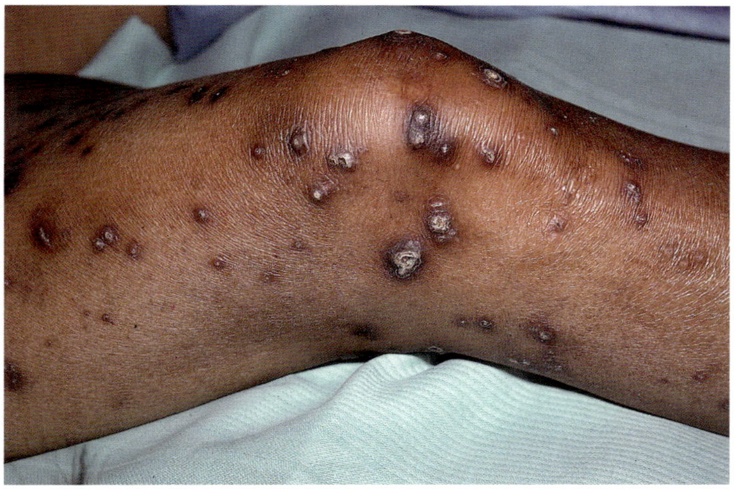

Figure 24–3. Kyrle's disease. Numerous keratotic papules on the leg of a man with chronic renal failure undergoing hemodialysis.

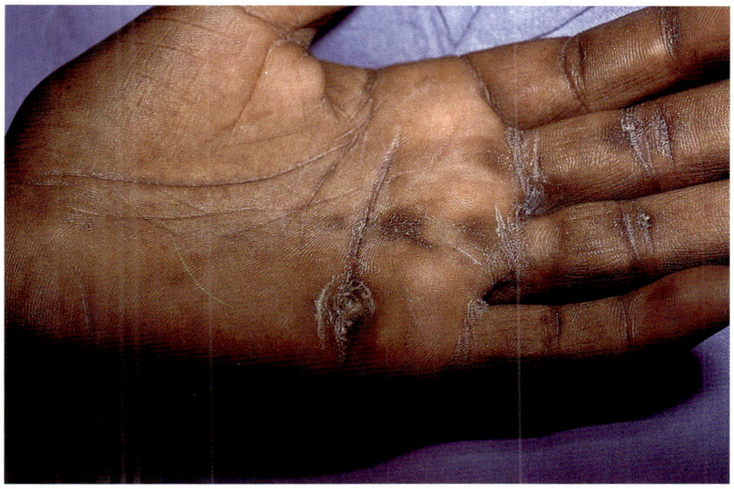

Figure 24–4. Kyrle's disease. Keratotic papule on the palm of the man seen in Figure 24–3.

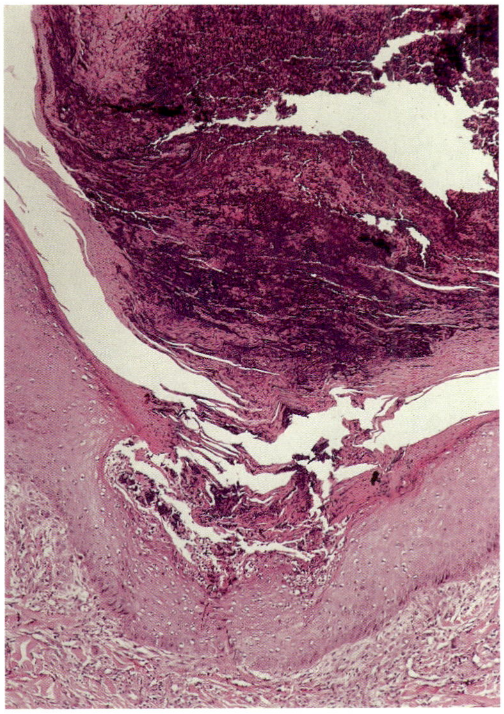

Figure 24–5. Kyrle's disease. Wedge-shaped hyperkeratosis with crust, and epithelial hyperplasia with ulceration. There is a subjacent dermal mixed-cell infiltrate. These are the characteristic changes described for this condition (i.e., hyperkeratosis follicularis et parafollicularis in cutem penetrans) and in actuality represent adnexal involvement, such as the infundibulum or acrosyringium.

25

ALTERATIONS IN PIGMENTATION

- Freckle
- Café-au-lait
- Chloasma
- Becker's nevus
- Labial melanosis (oral and genital)
- Post-inflammatory hyperpigmentation
- Vitiligo

FRECKLE

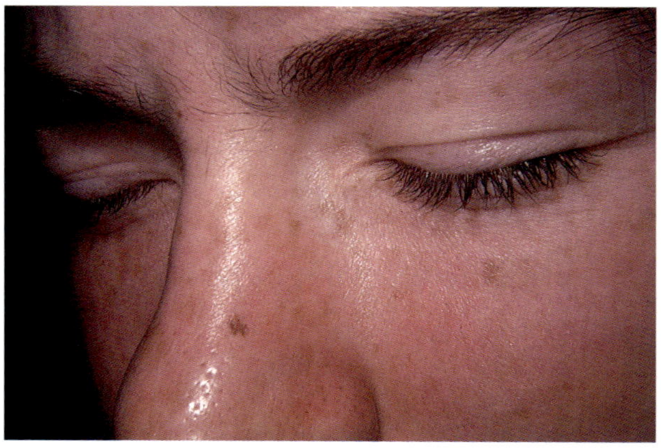

Figure 25–1. Freckle. Uniformly hyperpigmented macules with irregular margins.

CAFÉ-AU-LAIT

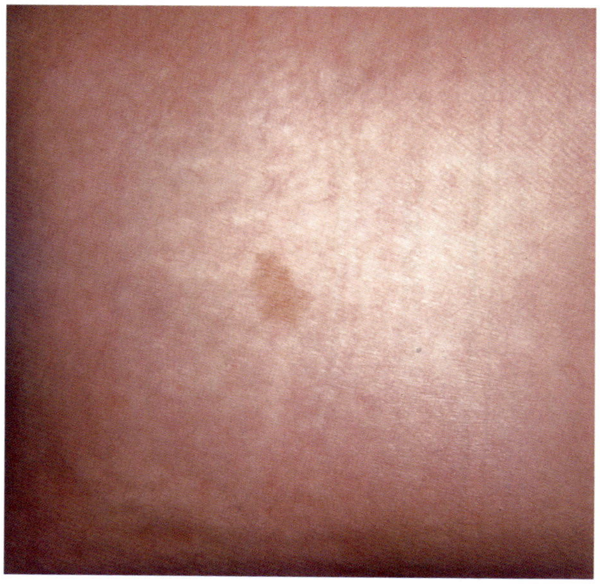

Figure 25–2. Café-au-lait. Tan, coffee-with-milk colored macule with slightly irregular margins.

CHLOASMA

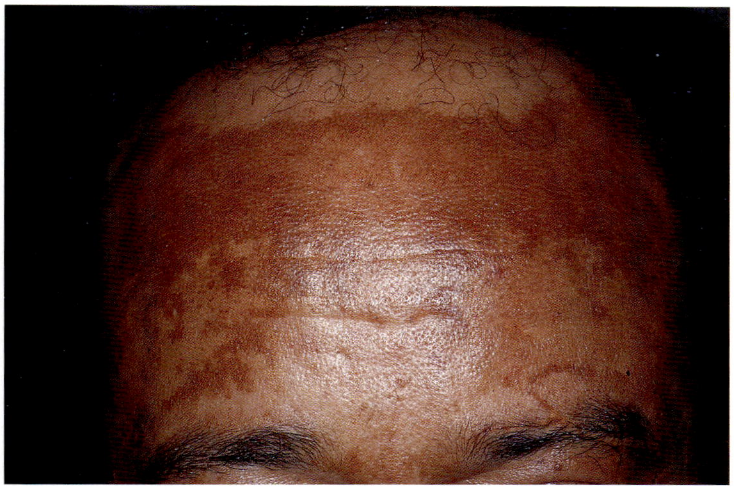

Figure 25–3. **Chloasma.** Hyperpigmented patches on the forehead.

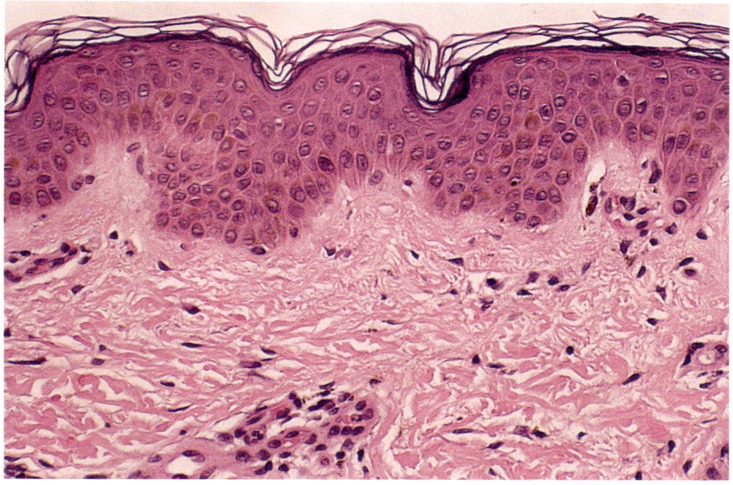

Figure 25–4. **Freckle, café-au-lait, and chloasma.** Increased melanin in keratinocytes and in melanophages in the dermis. Similar, histopathologic findings are seen in all three conditions.

BECKER'S NEVUS

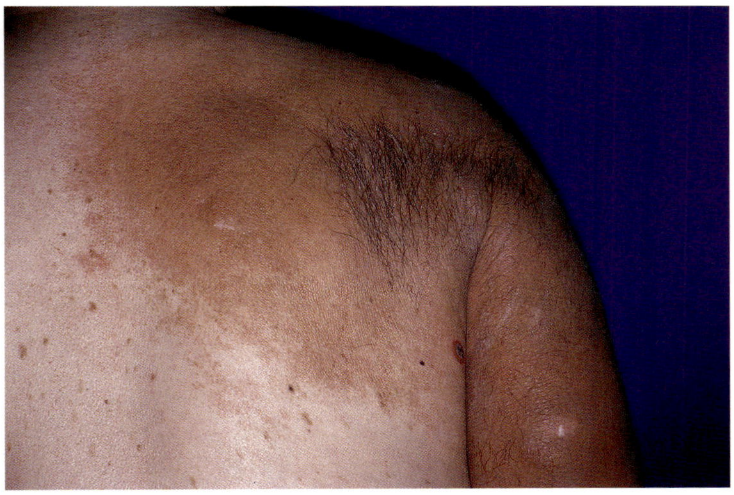

Figure 25–5. **Becker's nevus.** Hyperpigmented patch on the upper back. There is the characteristic associated hypertrichosis.

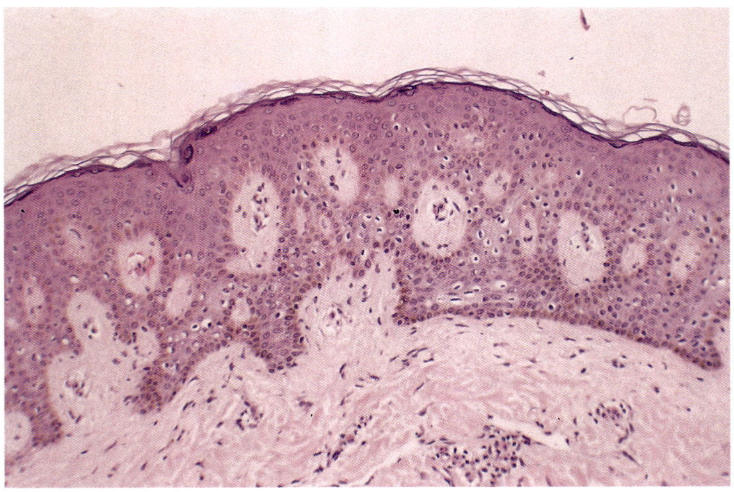

Figure 25–6. **Becker's nevus.** Epidermal hyperplasia and hyperpigmentation. There are scattered melanophages in the dermis.

LABIAL MELANOSIS (ORAL AND GENITAL)

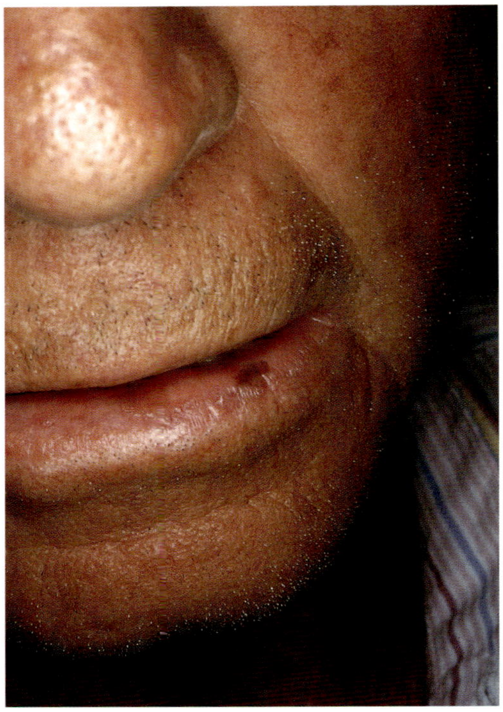

Figure 25–7. Labial melanosis. Hyperpigmented macule on the lower lip.

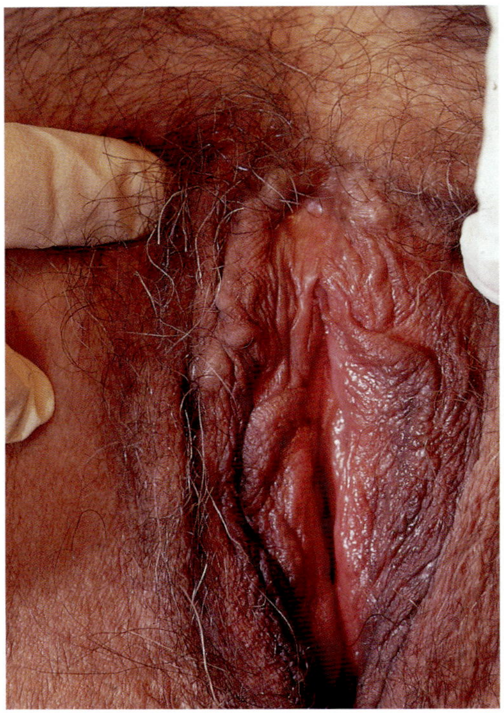

Figure 25–8. Labial melanosis. Hyperpigmented patch on the lower left labia majora.

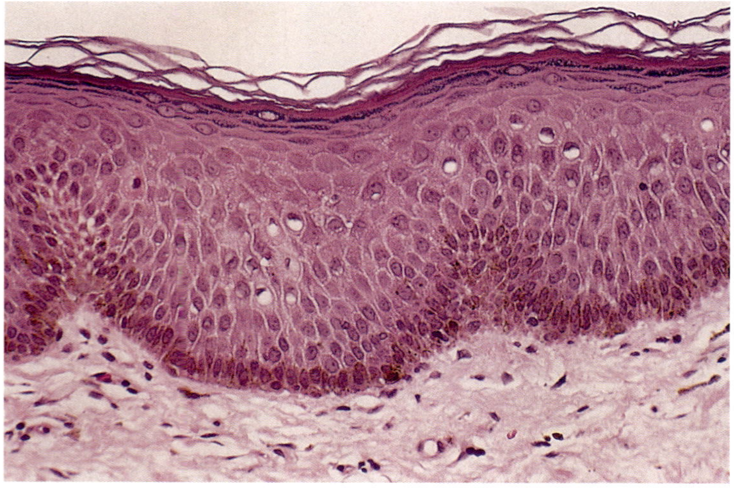

A

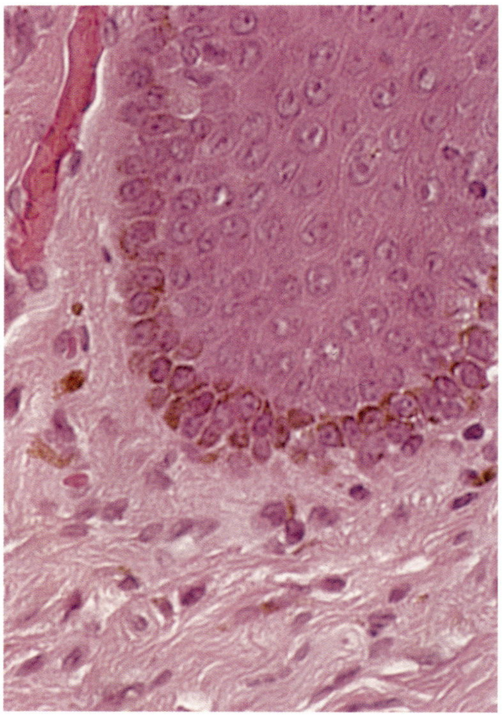

B

Figures 25–9A, 25–9B. Labial melanosis. There is epidermal hyperplasia with increased melanin deposition within the lower epidermis, mostly the basal cell layer. Melanocytes appear normal in number and size, and a few short dendrites are present. Melanophages are scattered in the dermis.

POST-INFLAMMATORY HYPERPIGMENTATION

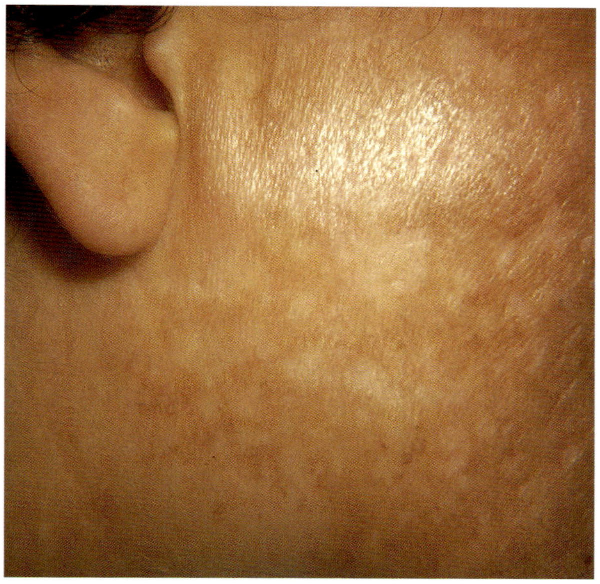

Figure 25–10. **Post-inflammatory hyperpigmentation.** Mottled hypo- and hyperpigmentation on the cheek of a man.

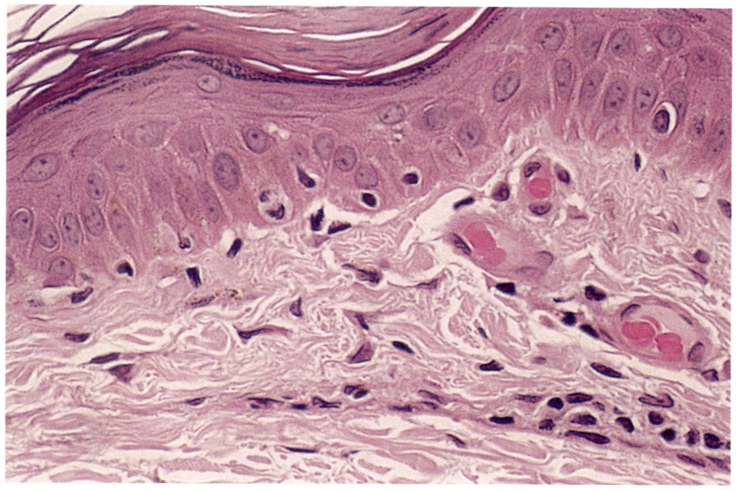

Figure 25–11. **Post-inflammatory hyperpigmentation.** Melanophages, stellate fibrocytes, fibroplasia, and dilated blood vessels.

VITILIGO

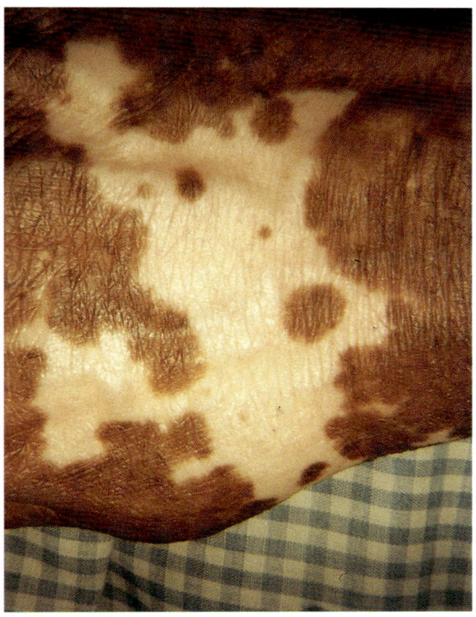

Figure 25–12. **Vitiligo.** Hypopigmented, sharply demarcated patches on the dorsum of the hand in a black individual.

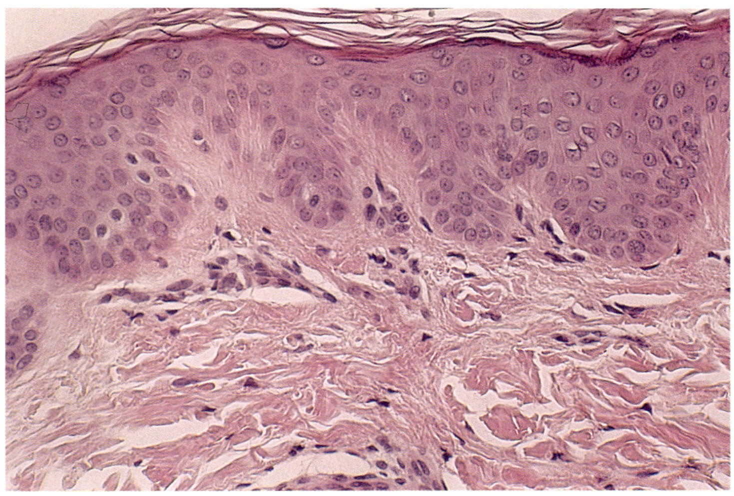

Figure 25–13. **Vitiligo.** Complete absence of melanocytes and melanin granules in the epidermis.

26

Inflammatory Reactions of the Folliculosebaceous Unit

- Acne vulgaris
- Steroid acne
- Perioral/periocular dermatitis
- Rosacea
- Keratosis pilaris/lichen spinulosus
- Eosinophilic folliculitis
- Staphylococcal folliculitis
- Dermatophyte folliculitis
- *Pityrosporum* folliculitis
- Herpes simplex folliculitis
- Molluscum folliculitis
- Follicular occlusion tetrad
- Perforating folliculitis of chronic renal disease
- Painful papule of the ear (chondrodermatitis nodularis)
- Pyoderma gangrenosum

ACNE VULGARIS

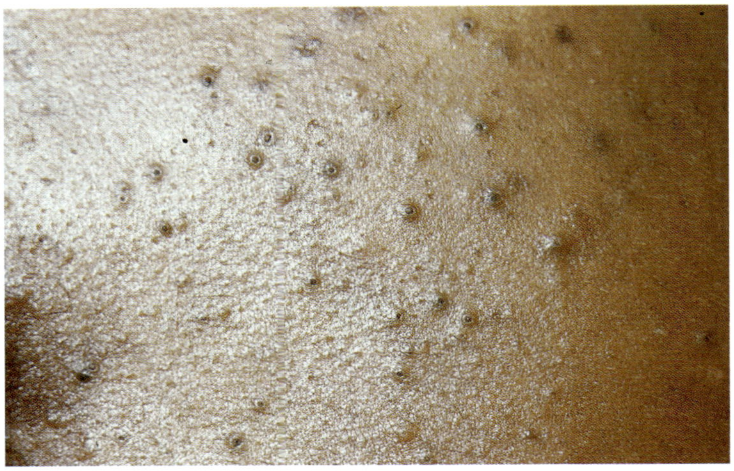

Figure 26–1. Acne vulgaris Comedones: skin-colored papules with black, keratotic plugs.

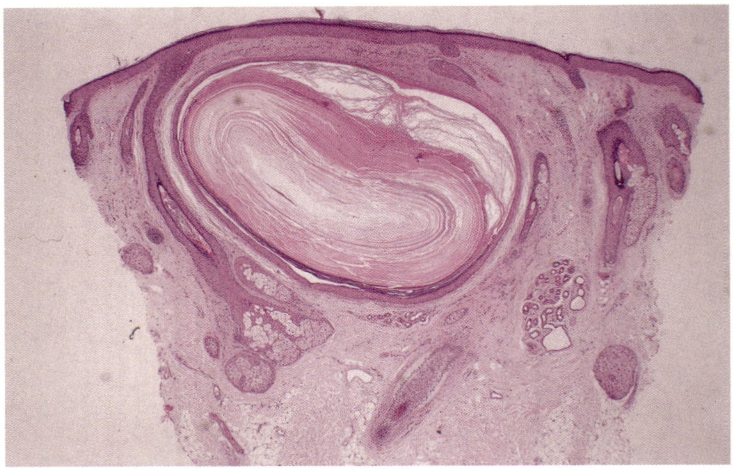

Figure 26–2. Acne vulgaris. Dilated infundibulum and compact, eosinophilic staining keratin.

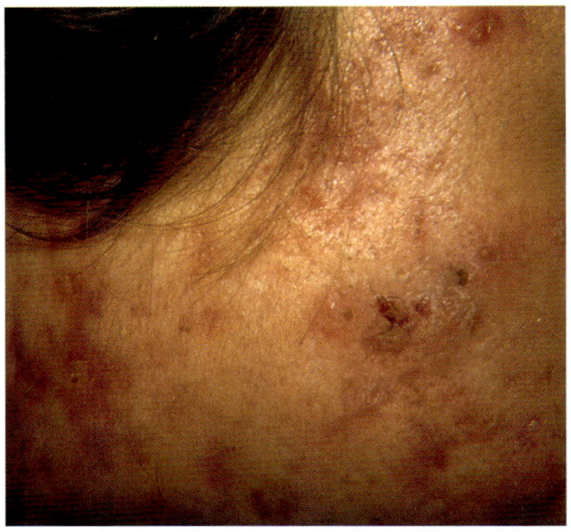

Figure 26–3. Acne vulgaris. Erythematous, crusted papules and nodules and occasional comedones. Scarring is present peripheral to some of the inflammatory lesions.

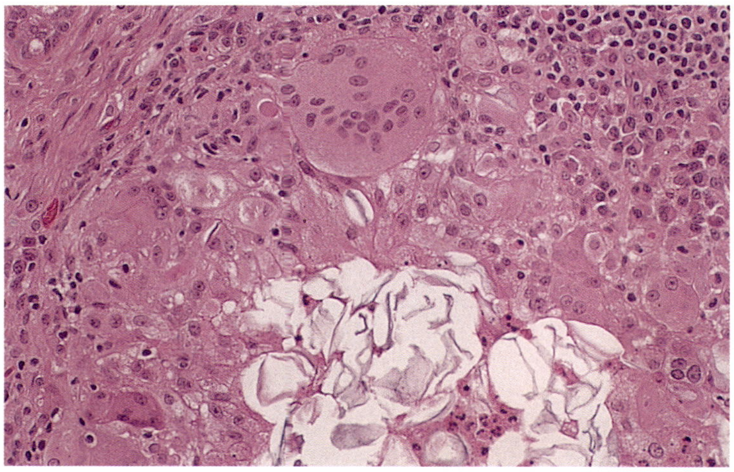

A

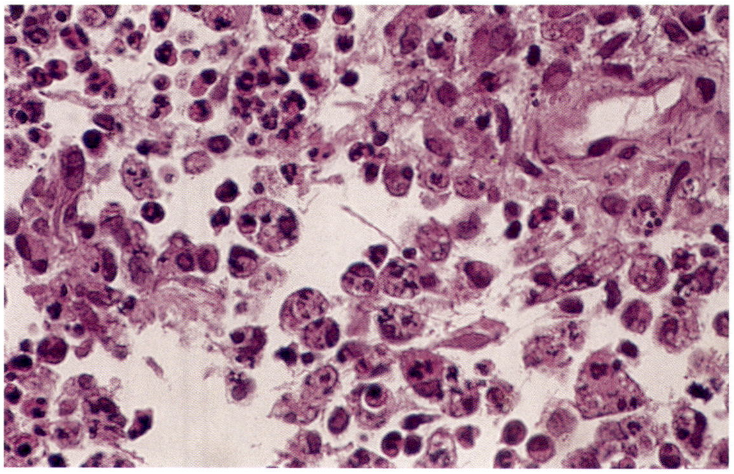

B

Figures 26–4A, 26–4B. Acne vulgaris. Suppurative granulomatous infiltrate and squames (cornified cells). Squames lie among neutrophils and within histiocytic giant cells in the dermis.

STEROID ACNE

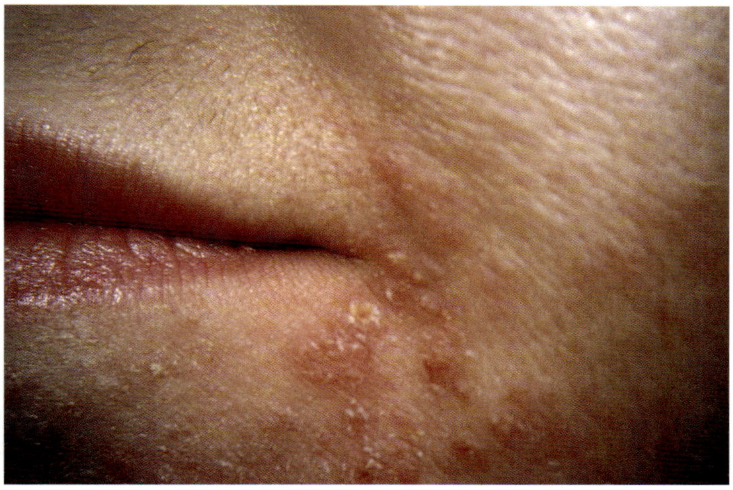

Figure 26–5. Steroid acne. Steroid acne from topical application of corticosteroids. Erythematous, scaly papules and pustules on the upper and lower lips that occurred after applying a corticosteroid cream to the area for many months.

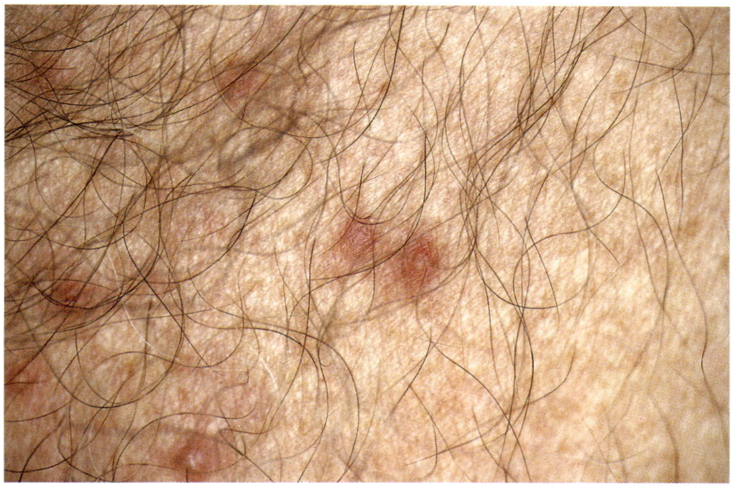

Figure 26–6. Steroid acne. Steroid acne from systemic administration of prednisone. Recent onset of erythematous papules and pustules on the chest of a man with Crohn's disease being treated with systemic prednisone.

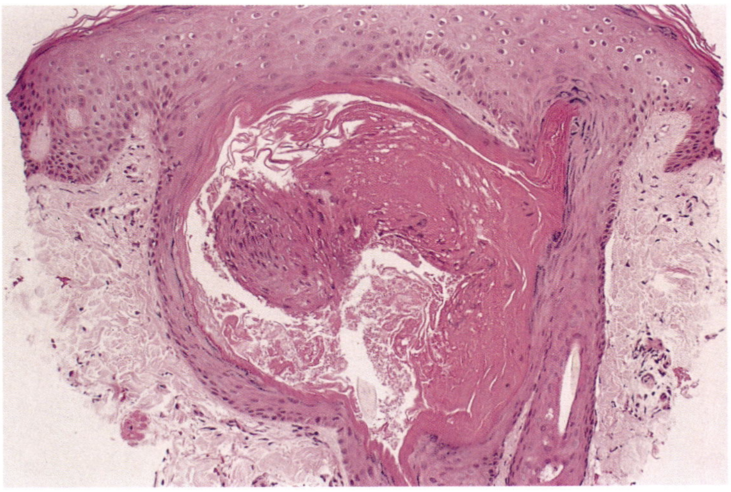

Figure 26–7. Steroid acne. Distended infundibulum packed with cornified cells (microcomedone).

PERIORAL/PERIOCULAR DERMATITIS

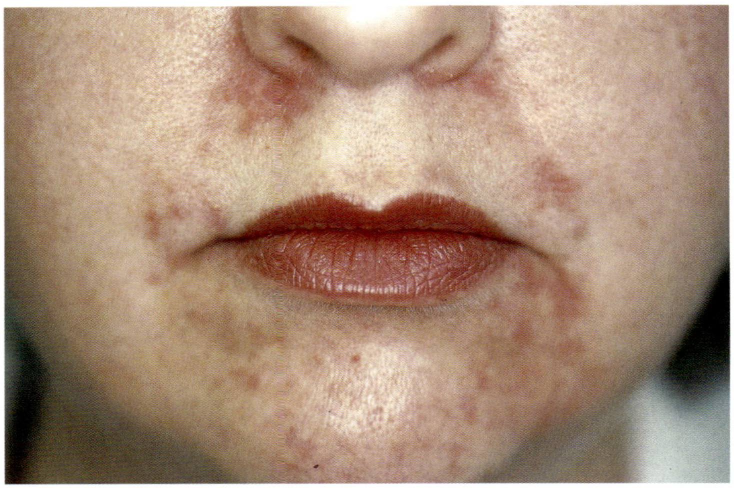

Figure 26–8. Perioral dermatitis. Erythematous papules and pustules on the upper and lower lips, sparing the vermilion edge.

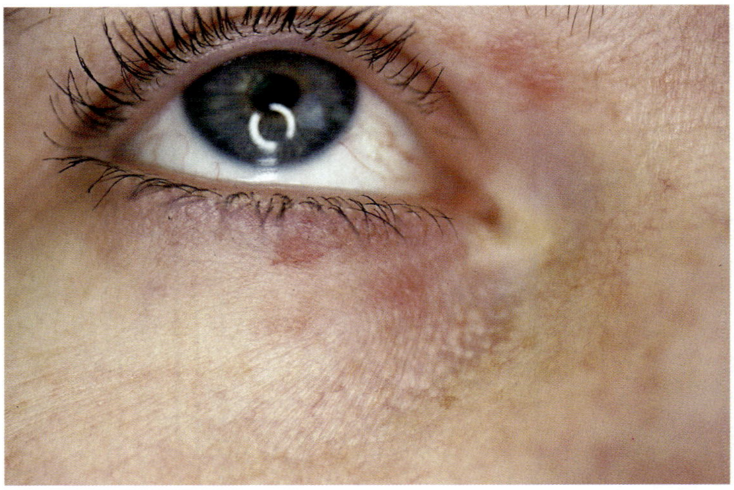

Figure 26–9. Periocular dermatitis. Erythematous papules involving the upper and lower eyelid.

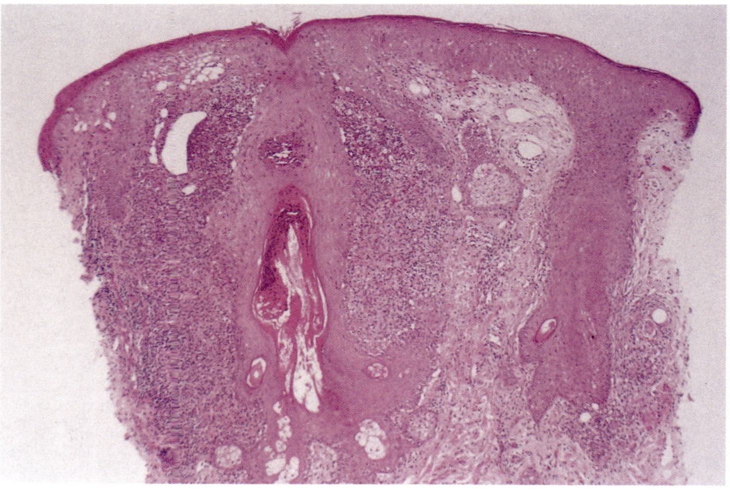

A

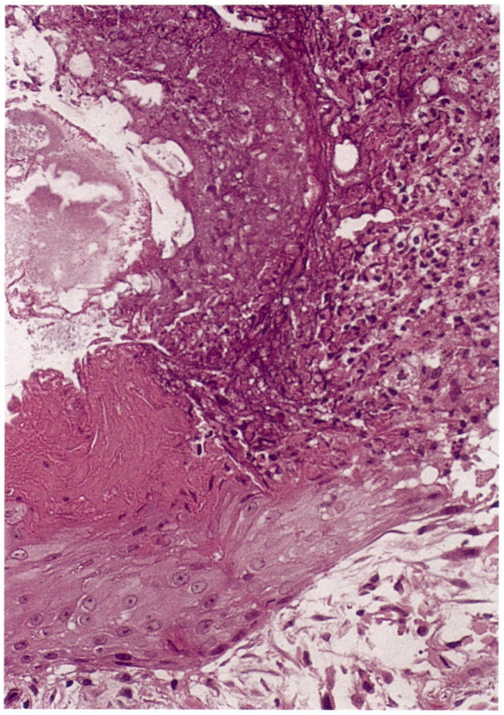

B

Figures 26–10A, 26–10B. Perioral dermatitis. Severe perifollicular and intrafollicular suppurative granulomatous inflammation. There is rupture of the infundibular wall with spillage of keratinous debris into the dermis.

ROSACEA

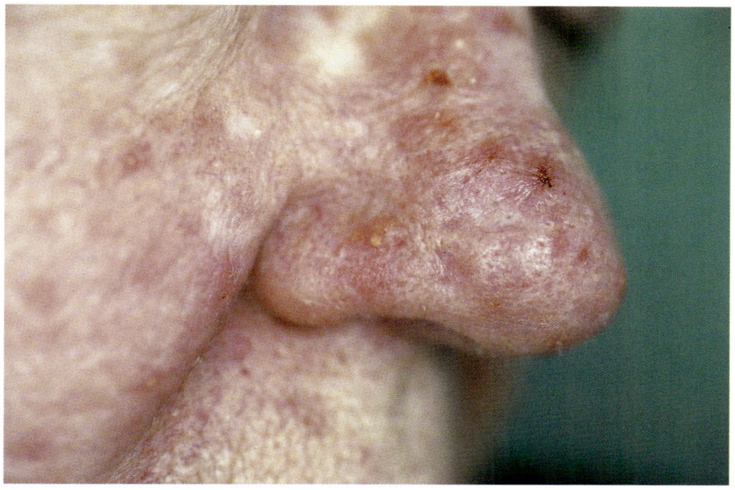

Figure 26–11. Rosacea. Erythematous papules, pustules, and telangiectases.

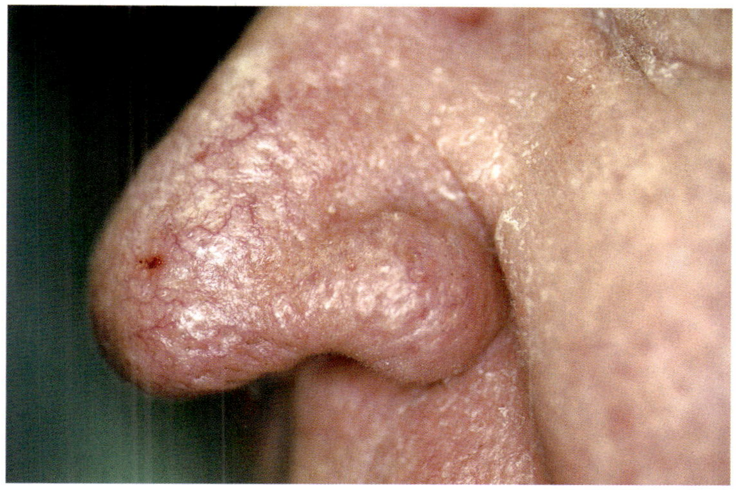

Figure 26–12. Rosacea, later stage. Distal enlargement of the nose (rhinophyma) with erythematous papules, pustules, and extensive telangiectases.

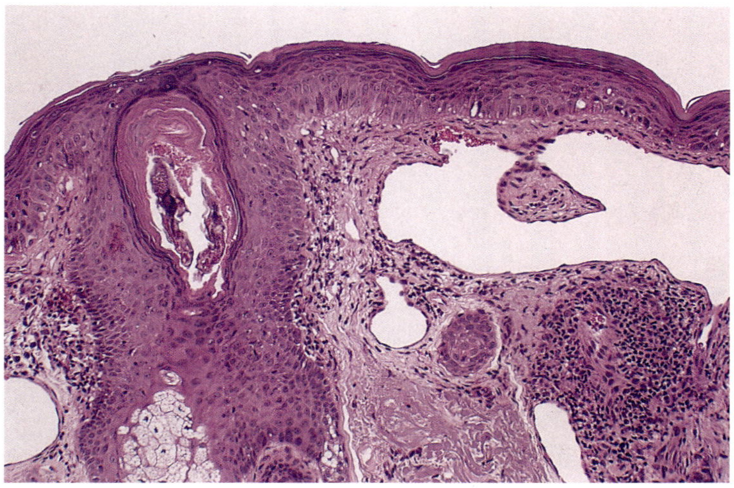

Figure 26–13. Rosacea. Perifollicular and perivascular mononuclear cell dermal infiltrate and markedly dilated blood vessels.

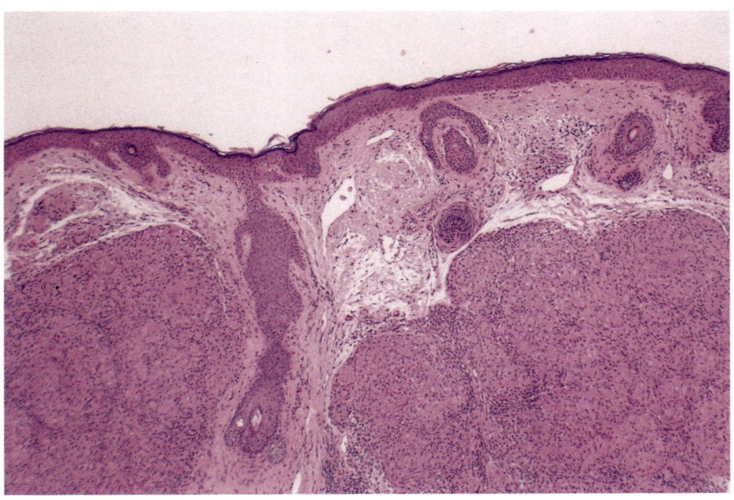

A

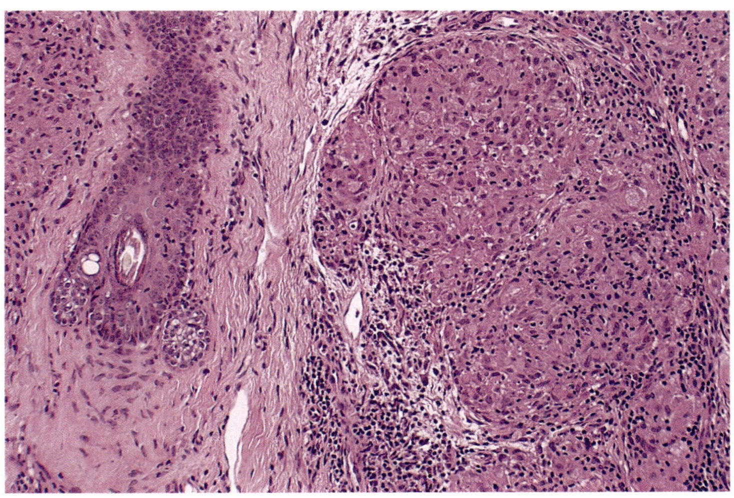

B

Figures 26–14A, 26–14B. Rosacea. Perifollicular sarcoidal granulomas and dilated blood vessels on sun-damaged skin. There is dermal fibroplasia, and a mixture of lymphocytes and histiocytic cells.

KERATOSIS PILARIS/LICHEN SPINULOSUS

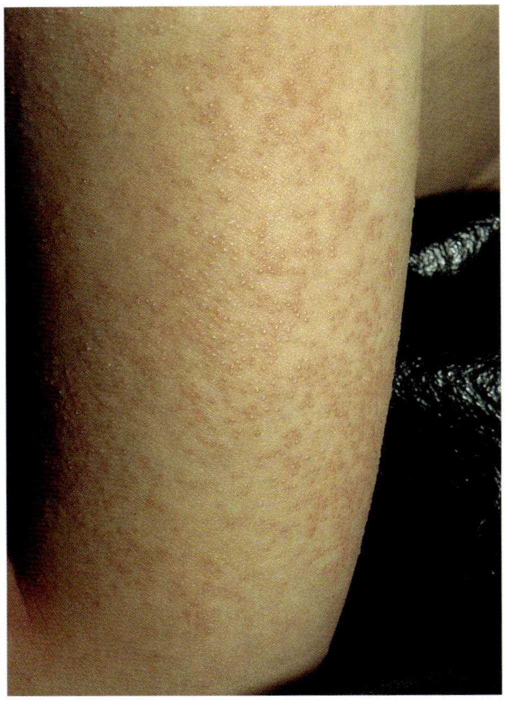

Figure 26–15. Keratosis pilaris. Erythematous, tiny, keratotic papules on the upper and lateral arm of an atopic woman.

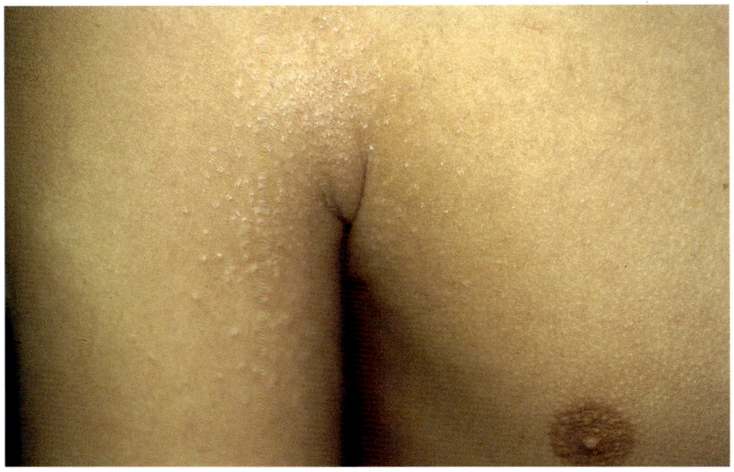

A

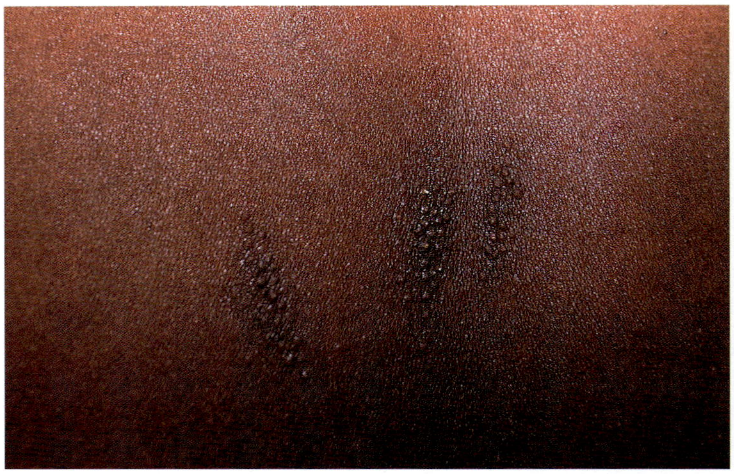

B

Figures 26–16A, 26–16B. Lichen spinulosus. Skin-colored, tiny, agminated papules on the arm and chest of a boy and on the back of a woman.

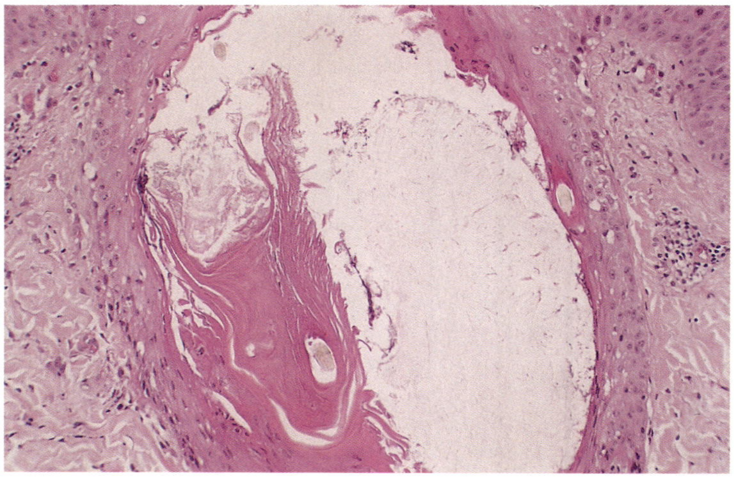

Figure 26–17. Keratosis pilaris/lichen spinulosus. Dilated infundibulum with compact eosinophilic keratinous debris and hair shaft fragments. There is a mild perifollicular infiltrate of lymphocytes.

EOSINOPHILIC FOLLICULITIS

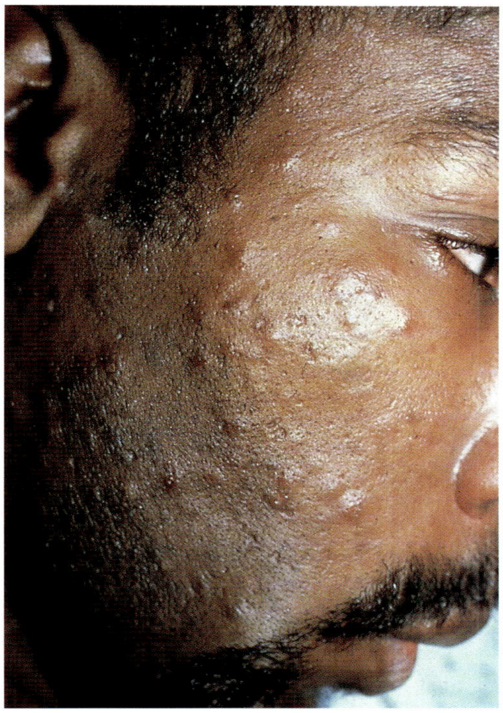

Figure 26–18. Eosinophilic folliculitis. Follicular papules on the face of an HIV-positive man.

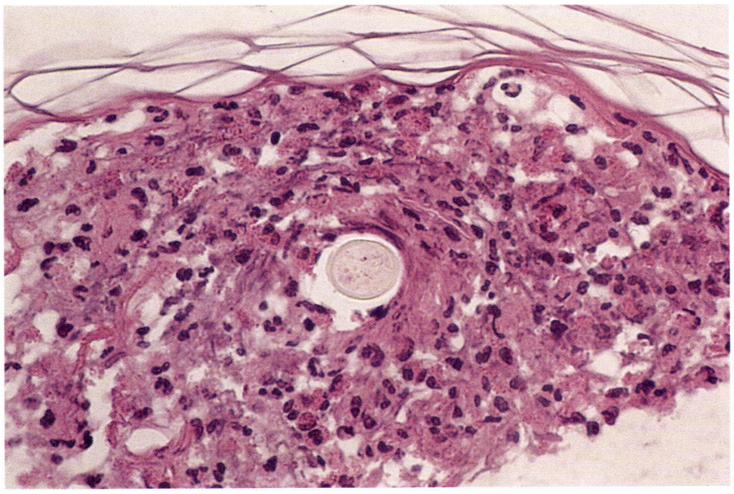

Figure 26–19. Eosinophilic folliculitis. Numerous eosinophils and neutrophils surround a hair shaft in a dilated infundibulum.

STAPHYLOCOCCAL FOLLICULITIS

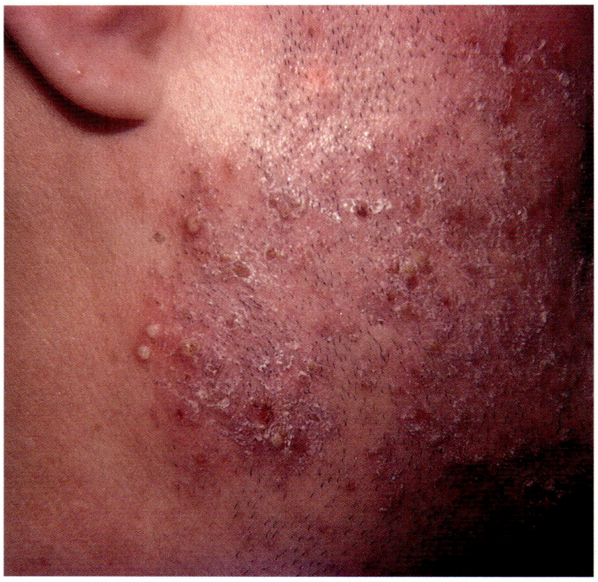

Figure 26–20. Staphylococcal folliculitis. Erythematous pustules and crusted papules on the cheek and neck.

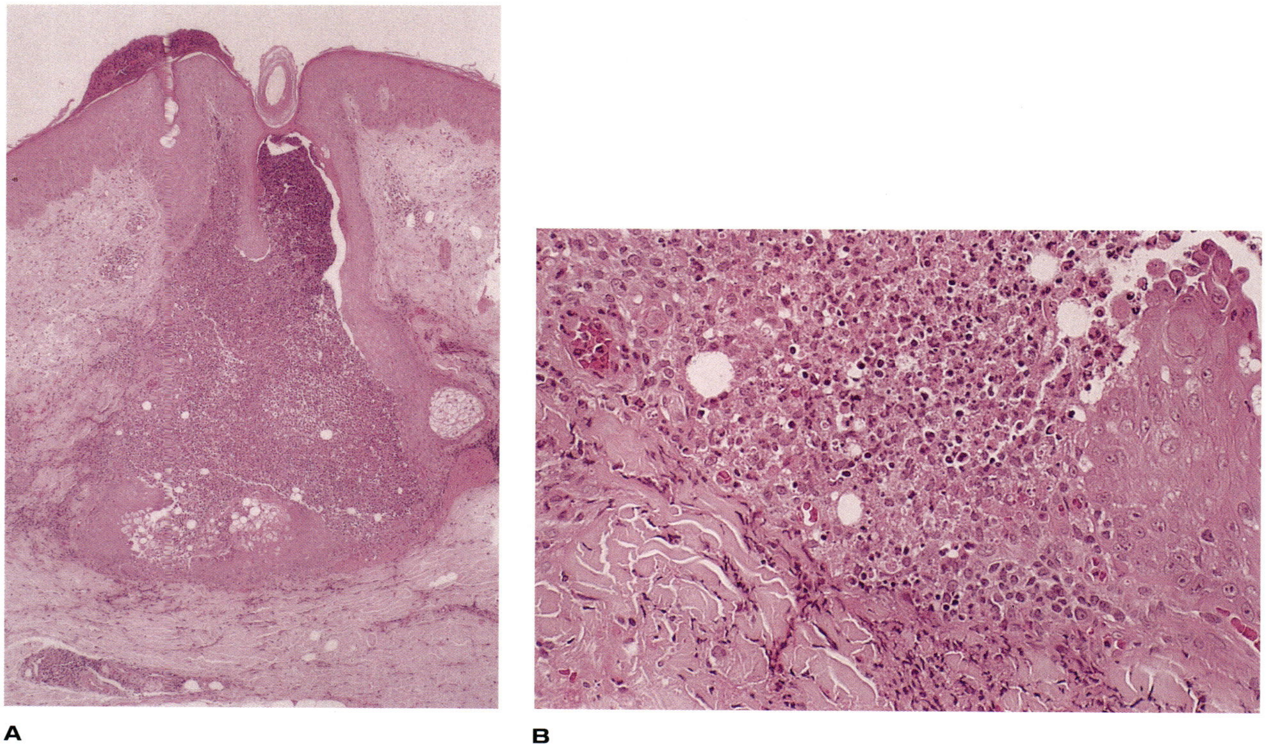

Figures 26–21A, 26–21B. Staphylococcal folliculitis. Distended and ruptured infundibulum with a copious infiltrate of neutrophils. Organisms are often seen with or without special stains.

DERMATOPHYTE FOLLICULITIS

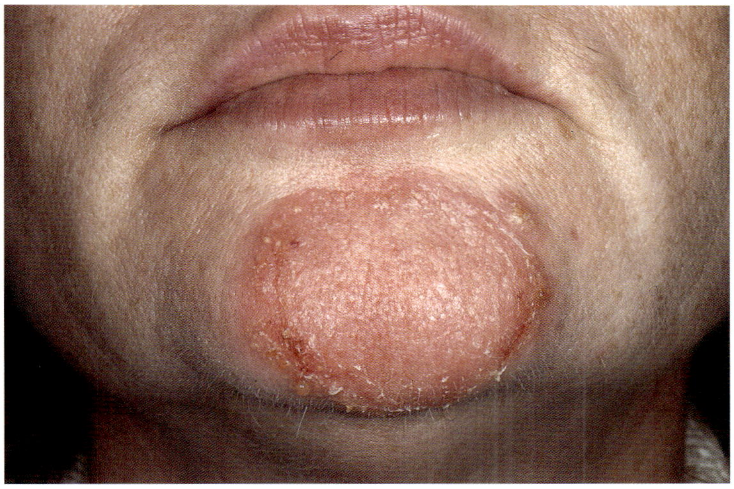

Figure 26–22. Dermatophyte folliculitis. Pruritic, enlarging, annular, scaly, erythematous patch on the chin of a woman.

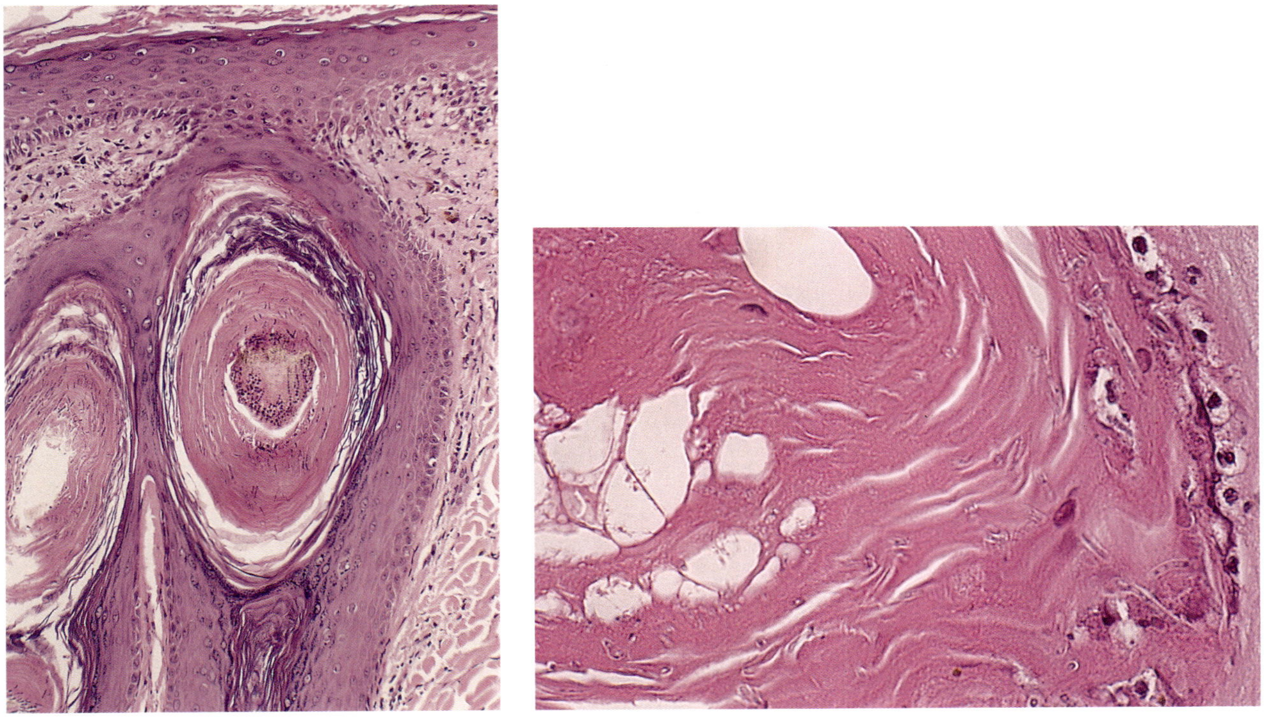

A B

Figures 26–23A, 26–23B. Dermatophyte folliculitis. Hyphal elements and spores within the hair shaft (endothrix) and within cornified cells of the infundibulum.

PITYROSPORUM FOLLICULITIS

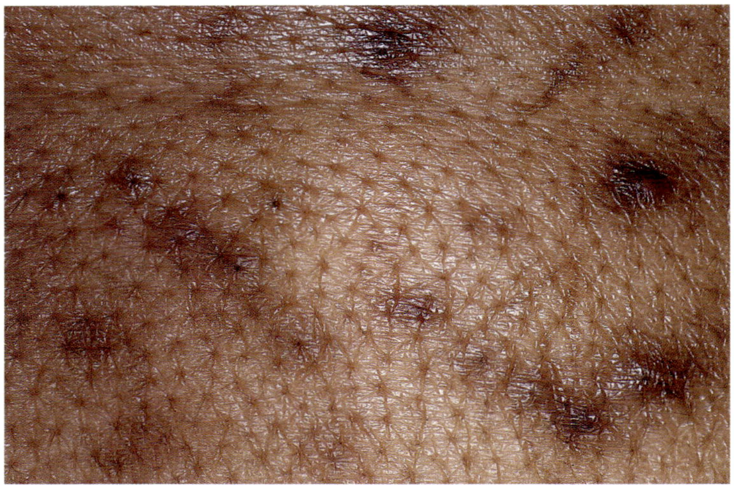

Figure 26–24. ***Pityrosporum*** **folliculitis.** Hyperpigmented follicular papules.

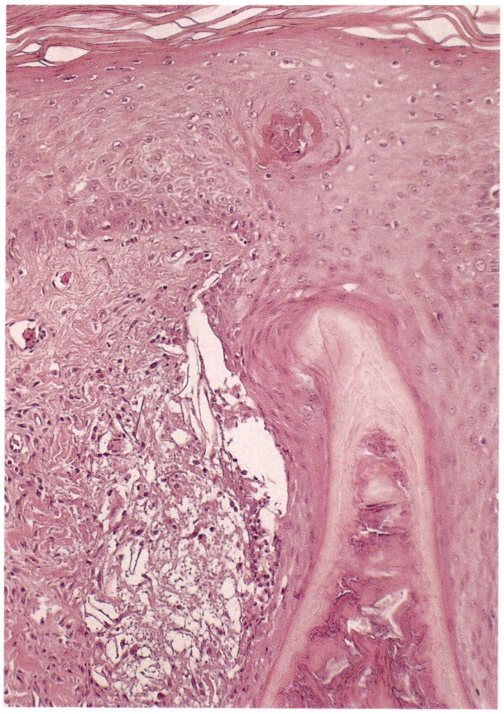

Figure 26–25. ***Pityrosporum*** **folliculitis.** Ruptured infundibular wall with numerous cornified cells and spores in the perifollicular dermis.

HERPES SIMPLEX FOLLICULITIS

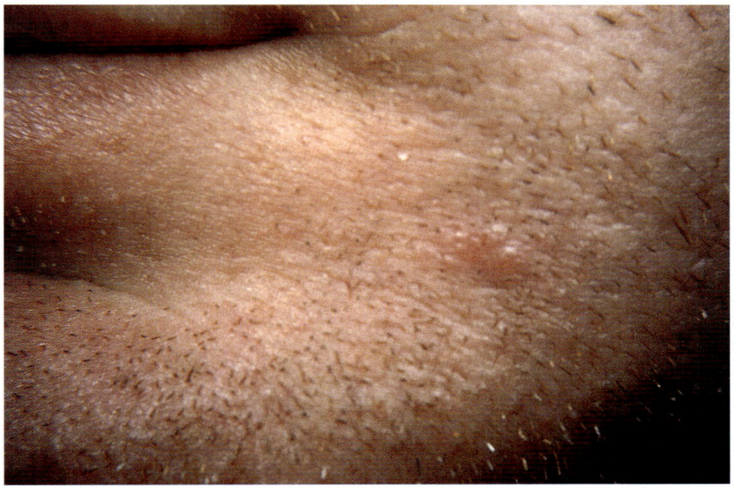

Figure 26–26. Herpes simplex folliculitis, early. Grouped, erythematous papulovesicles on the cheek of a man.

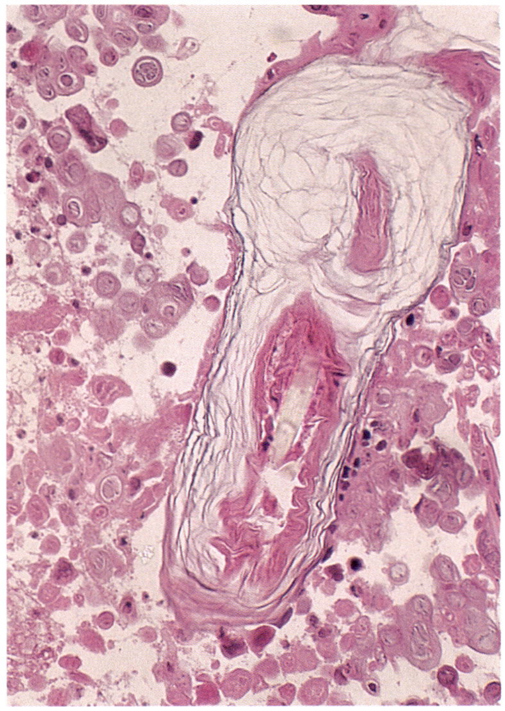

Figure 26–27. Herpes simplex folliculitis, early. Acantholytic, solitary, and multinucleated infundibular keratinocytes surround a hair shaft. Infected cells have characteristic pale-gray-staining nuclei with marginated nucleoplasm.

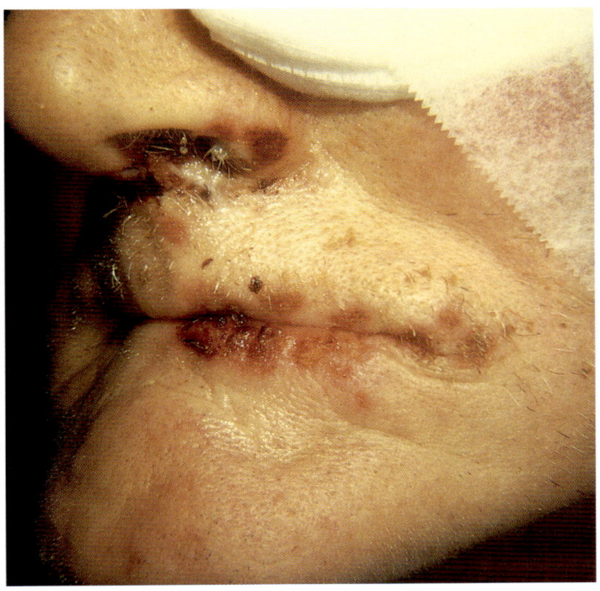

Figure 26–28. Herpes simplex, late. Lesions involve hair-bearing and non-hair-bearing skin.

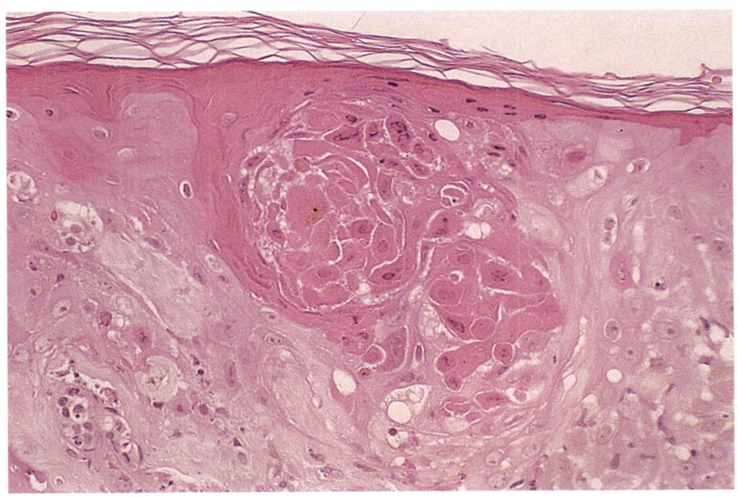

Figure 26–29. Herpes simplex, late. Acantholytic, necrotic, single, and multinucleated infundibular keratinocytes with brightly eosinophilic cytoplasm and fragmented basophilic nuclei.

MOLLUSCUM FOLLICULITIS

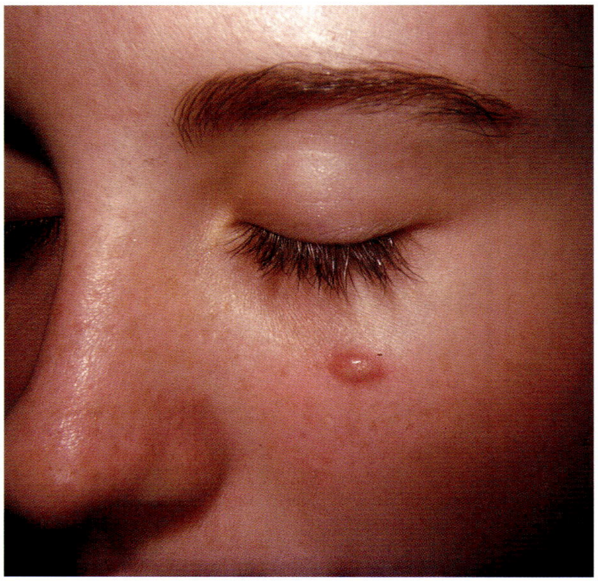

Figure 26–30. Molluscum folliculitis. Tender, dome-shaped, erythematous papule on the cheek of a woman.

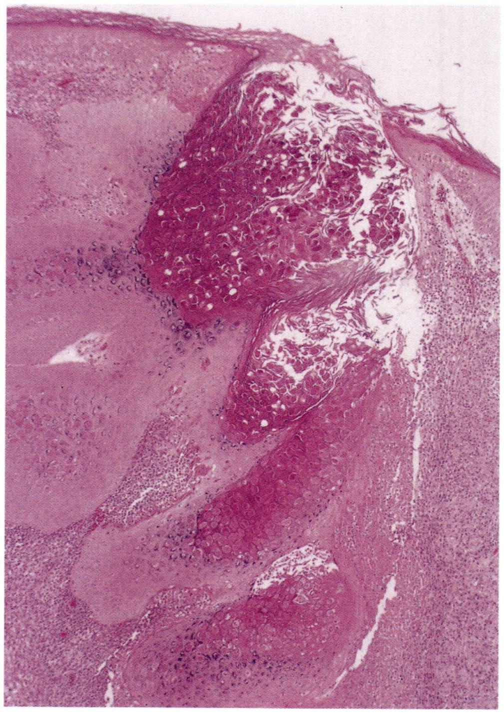

Figure 26–31. Molluscum folliculitis. Dilated and ruptured infundibulum is packed with eosinophilic and amphophilic molluscum bodies. A dense, dermal, suppurative granulomatous infiltrate surrounds the site of infundibular perforation.

FOLLICULAR OCCLUSION TETRAD

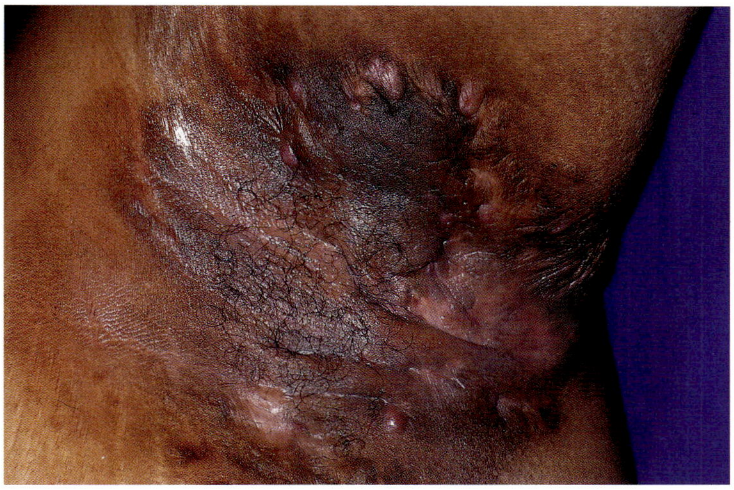

Figure 26–32. Hidradenitis suppurativa. Recurrent, painful, draining, confluent nodules in the axilla of a woman.

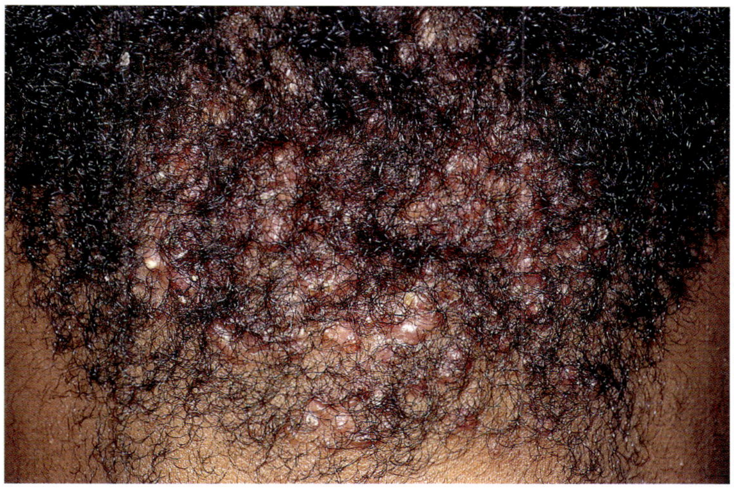

Figure 26–33. Acne keloidalis. Recalcitrant aggregate of oozing, tender nodules on the posterior scalp and neck of a man.

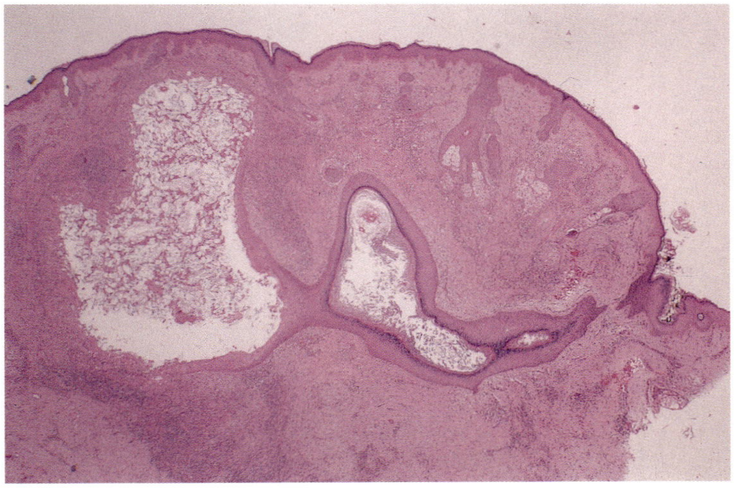

A

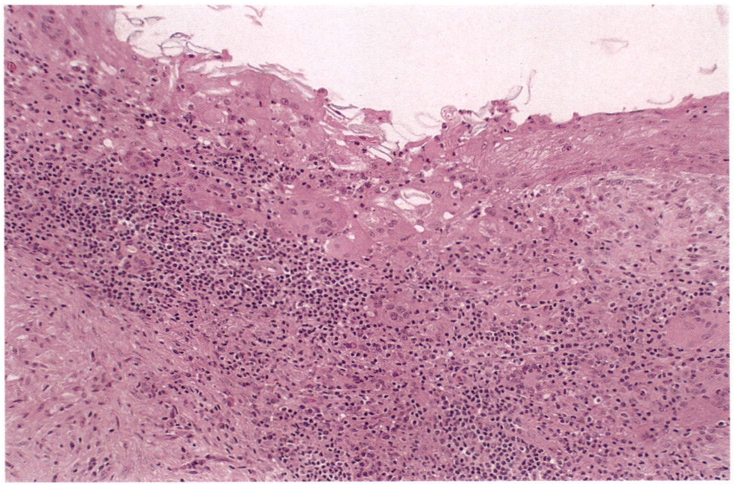

B

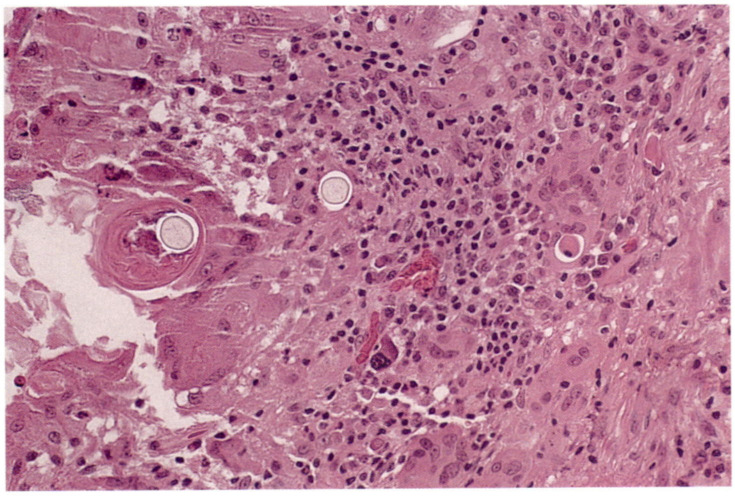

C

Figures 26–34A, 26–34B, 26–34C. Follicular occlusion tetrad. Tortuous, dilated, and ruptured infundibulum with a dense dermal suppurative granulomatous infiltrate with accompanying fibroplasia. Many multinucleated histiocytic giant cells have engulfed cornified cells and hair shaft fragments.

PERFORATING FOLLICULITIS OF CHRONIC RENAL DISEASE

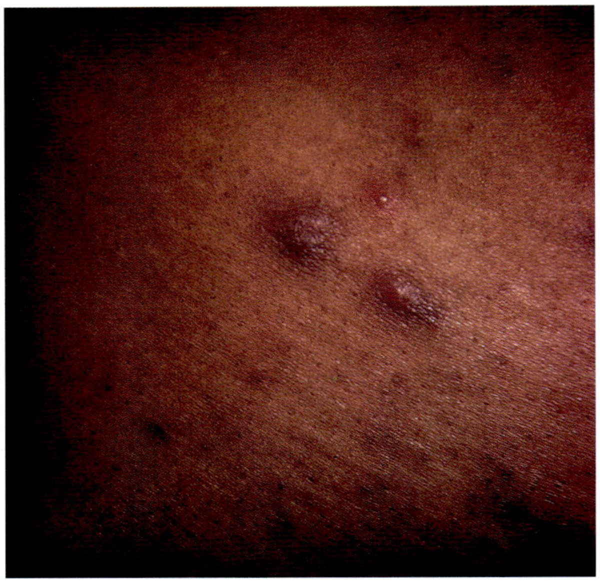

Figure 26–35. Perforating folliculitis of chronic renal disease. Pustule and dome-shaped keratotic papules represent the evolution of early and late lesions, respectively.

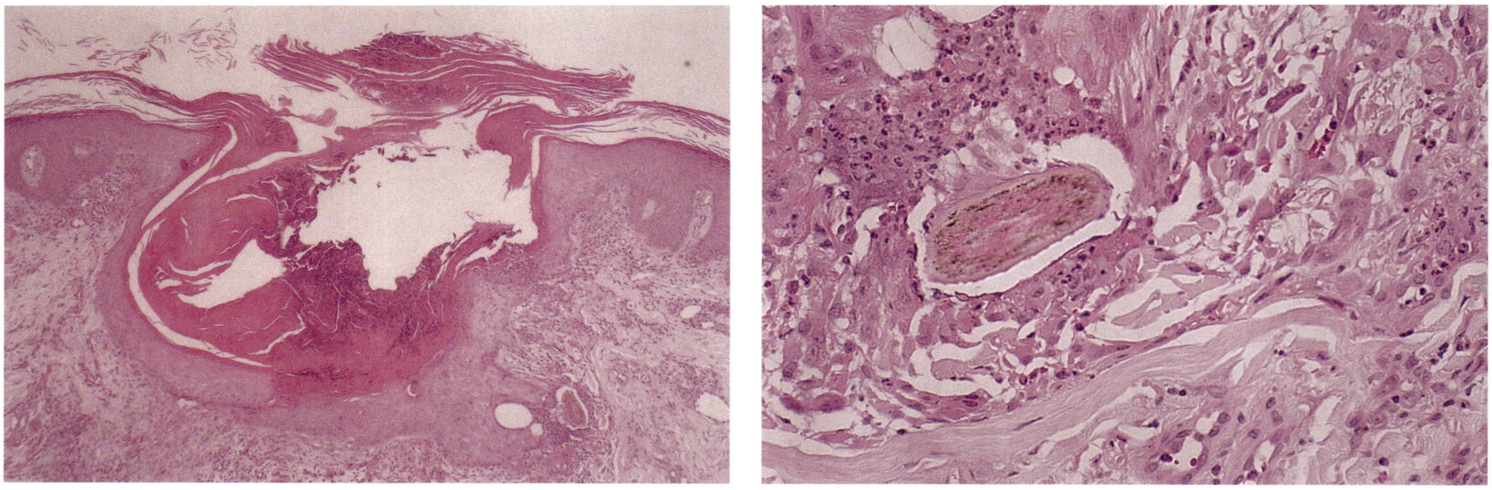

A B

Figures 26–36A, 26–36B. Perforating folliculitis of chronic renal disease. Dilated, plugged, and ruptured infundibulum. There is a large contiguous hair shaft fragment with a suppurative-granulomatous and fibrosing perifollicular dermatitis.

PAINFUL PAPULE OF THE EAR (CHONDRODERMATITIS NODULARIS)

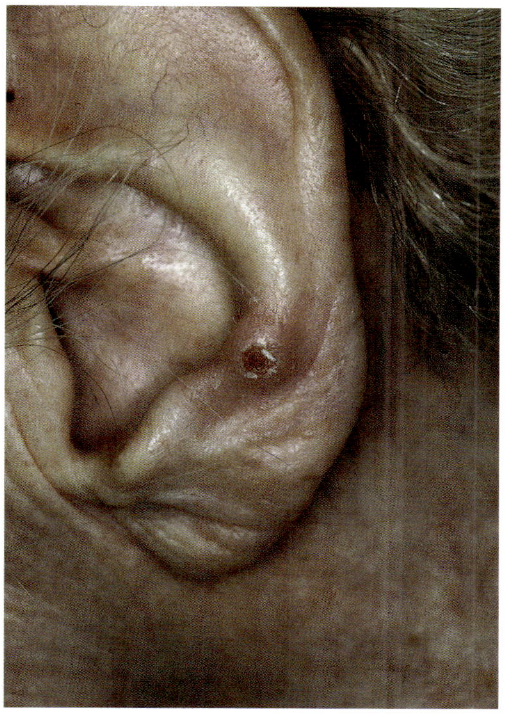

Figure 26–37. Painful papule of the ear. Exquisitely tender, erythematous, crusted papule on the antihelix of the ear.

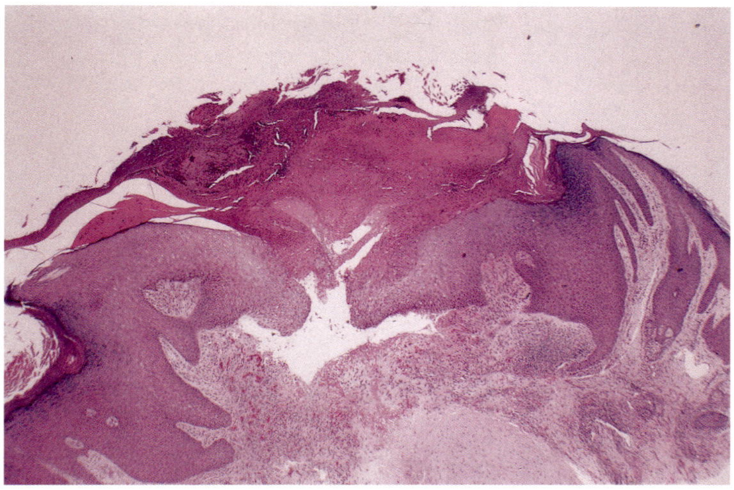

A

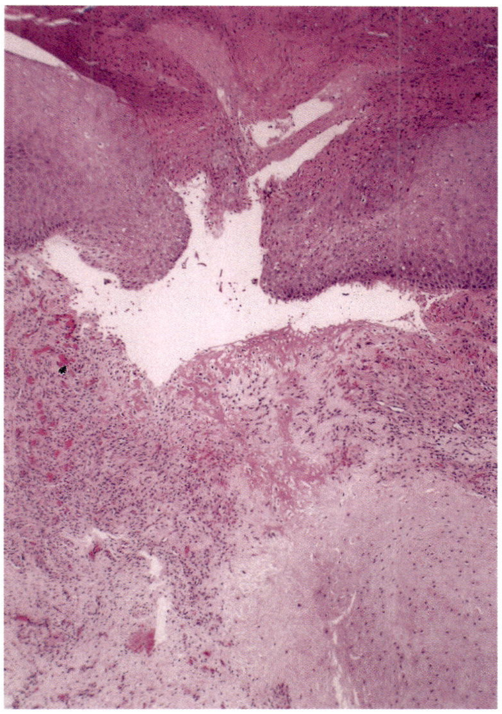

B

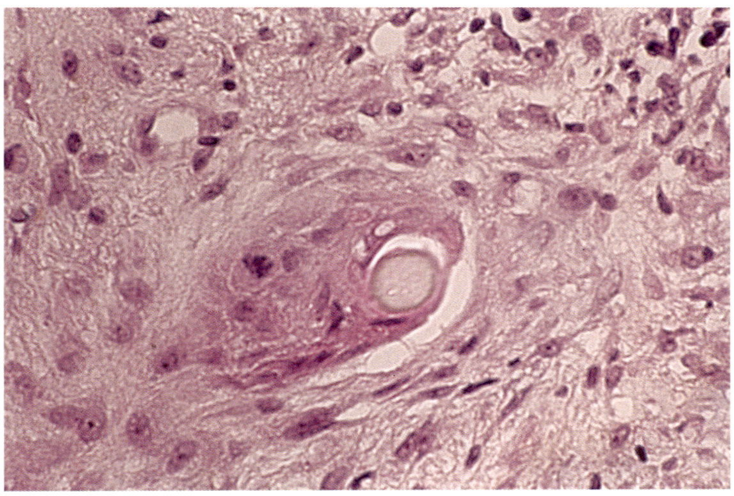

C

Figures 26–38A, 26–38B, 26–38C. Painful papule of the ear. Infundibular hyperplasia with a wedge-shaped, keratotic perforating plug. There is fibrin deposited immediately subjacent to the ulcer. Granulation tissue, fibroplasia, and a granulomatous infiltrate fill the thickened papillary dermis. Cartilage is present at the base of the biopsy specimen, and within the dermis a hair shaft has been engulfed by a multinucleated histiocytic giant cell.

PYODERMA GANGRENOSUM

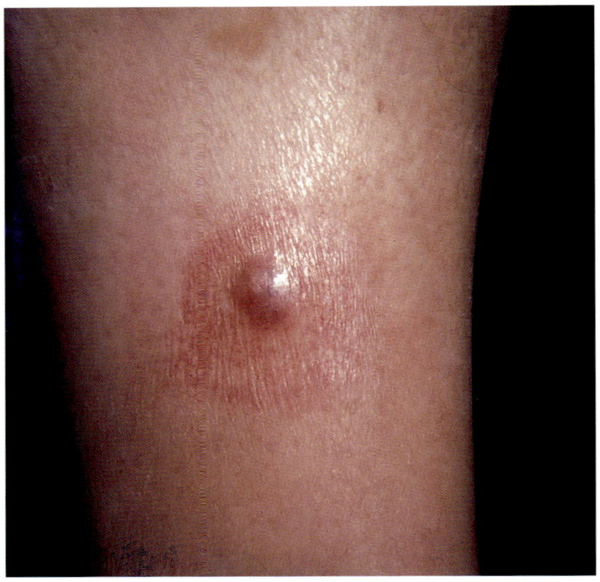

Figure 26–39. Pyoderma gangrenosum, evolving lesion. Erythematous, dome-shaped nodule on the lower leg of a woman with Crohn's disease.

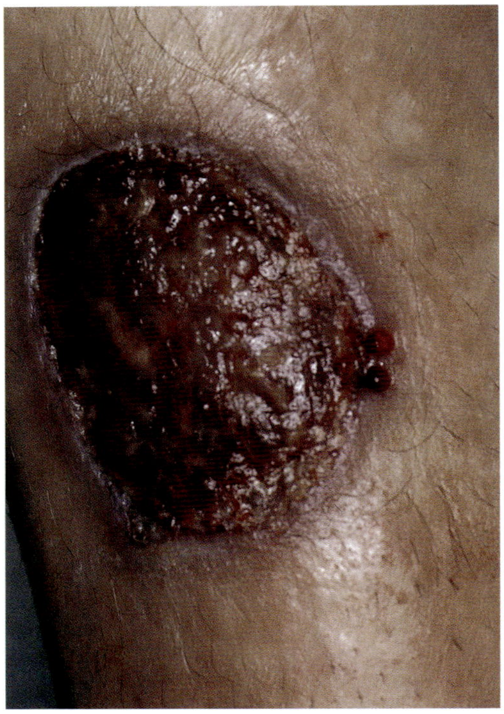

Figure 26–40. Pyoderma gangrenosum, fully developed lesion. Ulcerated plaque with a raised, undermined, purpuric border on the lower leg.

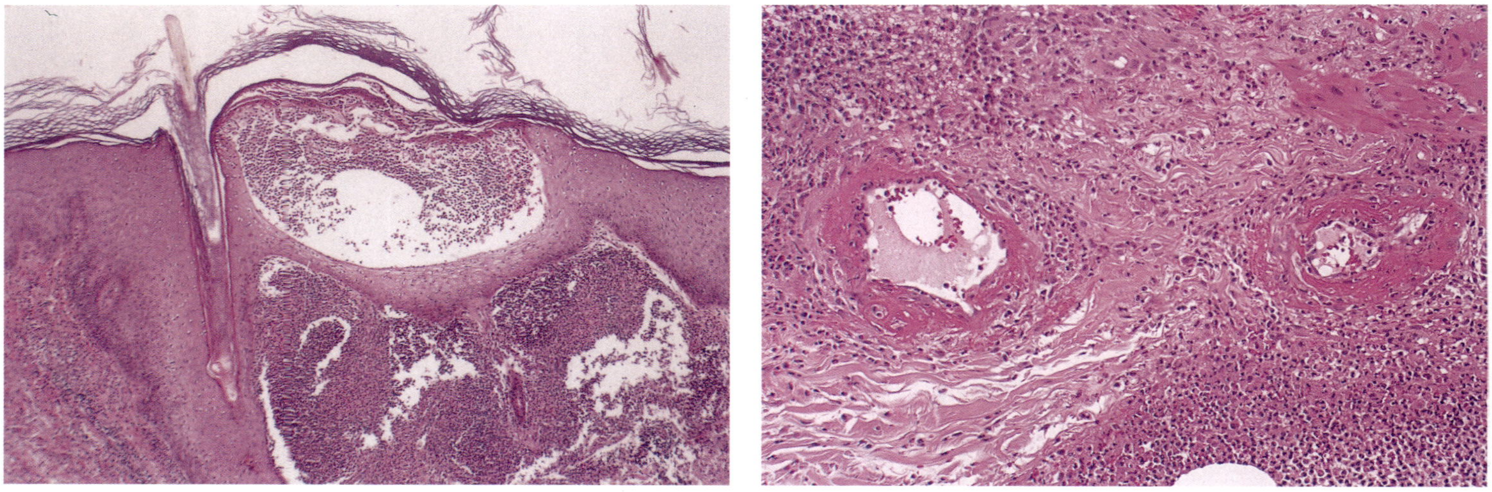

A B

Figures 26–41A, 26–41B. Pyoderma gangrenosum. Folliculosebaceous unit replete with neutrophils. There is rupture of the follicular wall with extensive inflammation spilling into the adjacent dermis. Leukocytoclastic vasculitis is secondary to the intense neutrophilic infiltrate.

27

ALOPECIAS

- Follicular mucinosis
- Telogen effluvium
- Pseudopalade
- Lichen planopilaris
- Alopecia areata
- Trichotillomania
- Discoid lupus erythematosus

FOLLICULAR MUCINOSIS

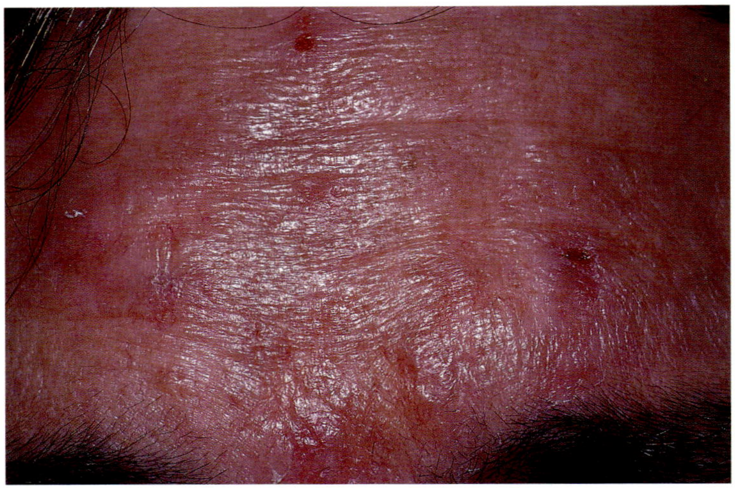

Figure 27–1. Follicular mucinosis. Erythematous, boggy plaque with prominent follicular ostia on the forehead of a man.

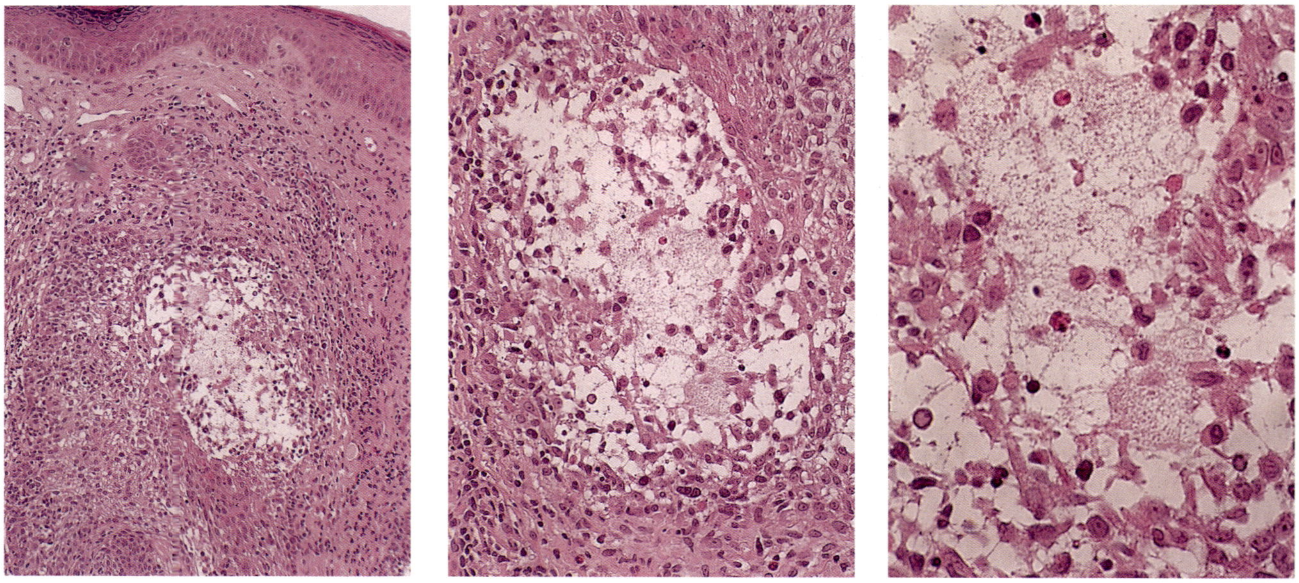

A B C

Figures 27–2A, 27–2B, 27–2C. Follicular mucinosis. Infundibular epithelial mucin with a mixed-cell infiltrate. There are large deposits of gray, granular mucin, separated keratinocytes, lymphocytes, neutrophils, and eosinophils within the infundibulum. A similar inflammatory cell infiltrate is present in the dermis.

TELOGEN EFFLUVIUM

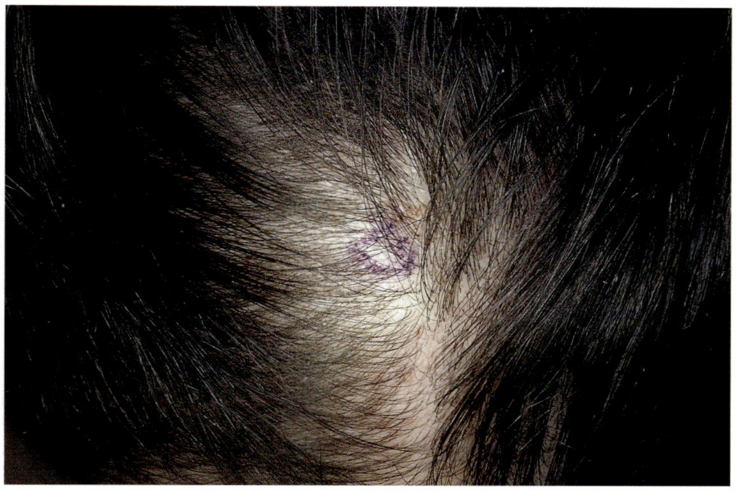

Figure 27–3. Telogen effluvium. Thinning of scalp hair in a woman. Gentian violet marks the site of biopsy.

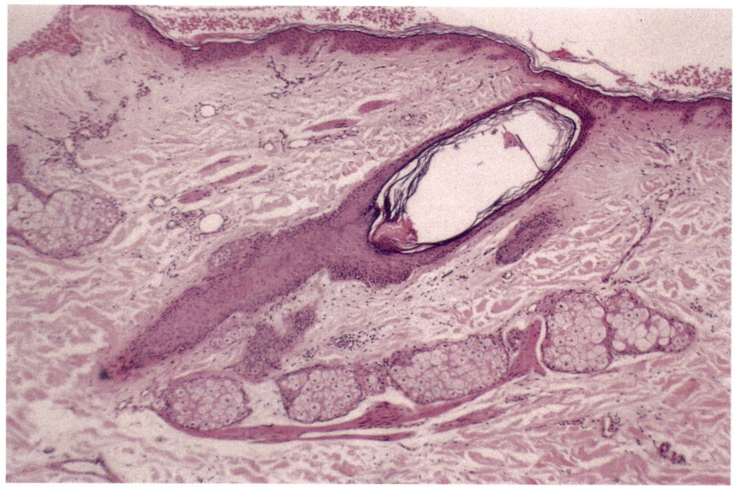

Figure 27–4. Telogen effluvium. Terminal hair follicle in telogen phase. This terminal follicle ends at the isthmus, where the sebaceous duct appears to enter.

PSEUDOPALADE

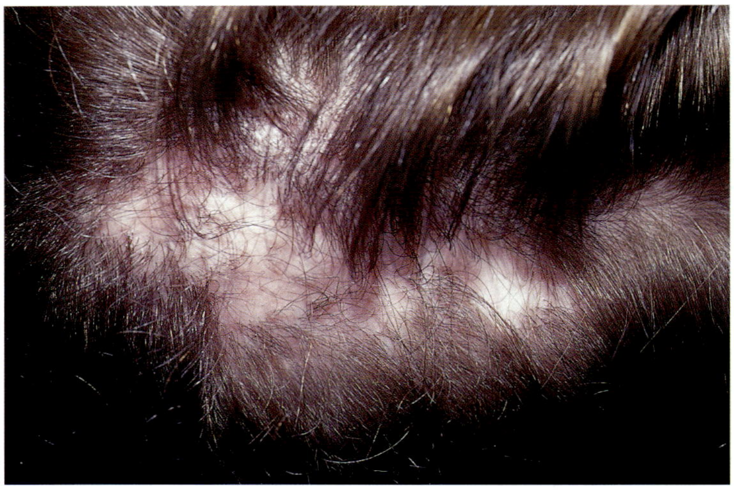

Figure 27–5. Pseudopalade. Scarring alopecia with smooth, hairless, white patches in the scalp. This clinical appearance has been referred to as "footprints in the snow." This pattern is considered nonspecific because it may be seen in the end stages of lichen planopilaris and discoid lupus erythematosus.

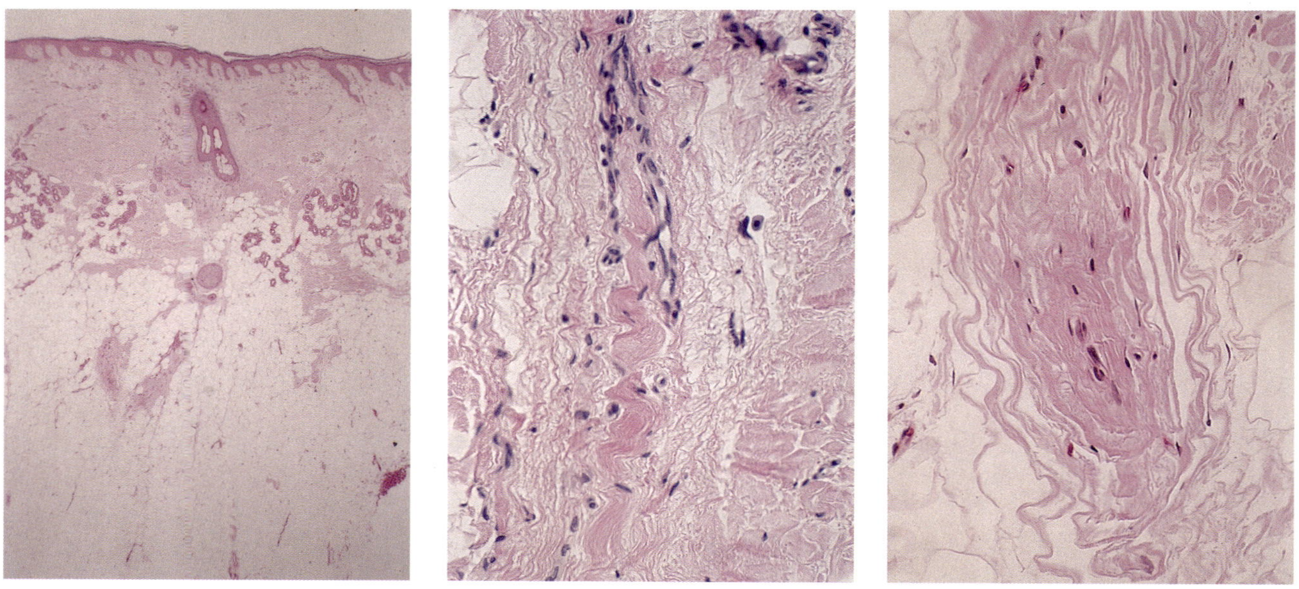

A B C

Figures 27–6A, 27–6B, 27–6C. Pseudopalade. Fibroplasia and absence of terminal hair follicles rooted in the subcutaneous fat. Vertically oriented fibrous bands replace former sites of the inferior segments of terminal scalp folliculosebaceous units. At the site of the original hair bulb, there remains a small nubbin of fibrous tissue.

LICHEN PLANOPILARIS

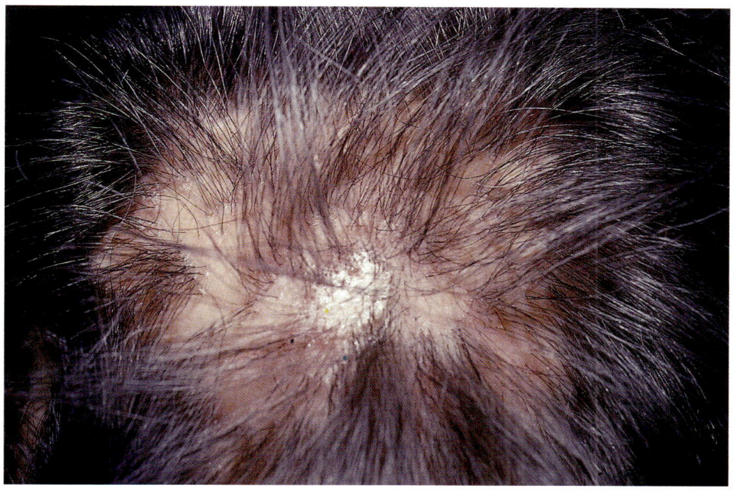

Figure 27–7. Lichen planopilaris. Scarring alopecia with keratotic follicular papules with patulous ostia and pale scars.

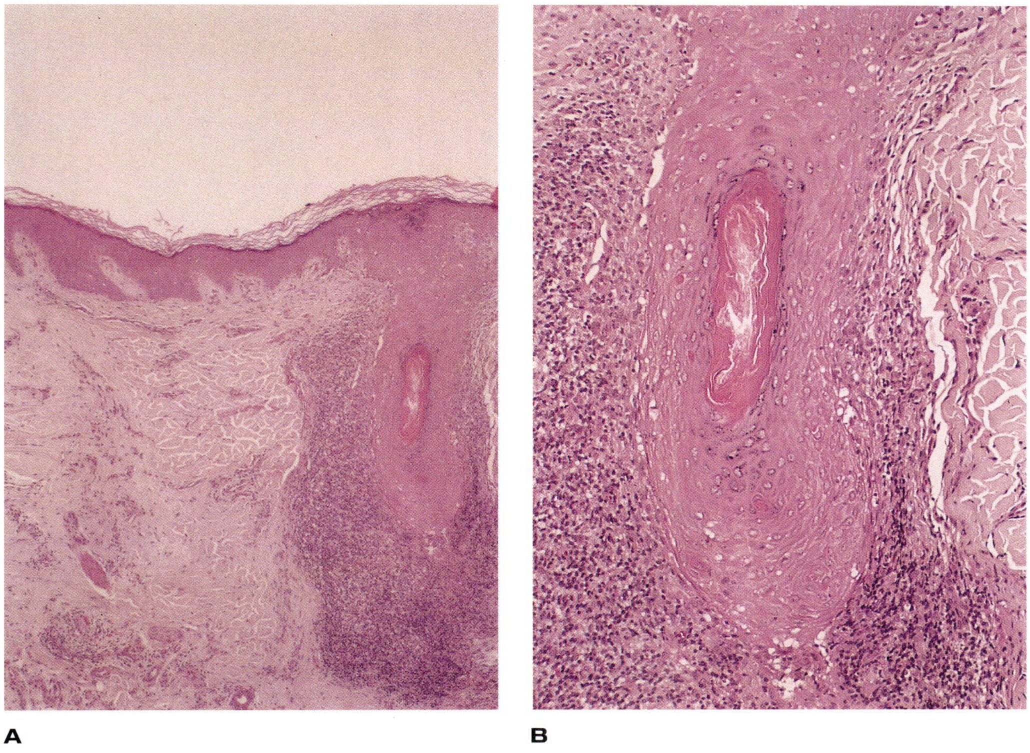

Figures 27–8A, 27–8B. Lichen planopilaris. Dense lichenoid perifollicular infiltrate. There is infundibular hyperkeratosis, wedge-shaped hypergranulosis, and perifollicular clefting surrounded by a dense lichenoid lymphocytic infiltrate and fibroplasia.

ALOPECIA AREATA

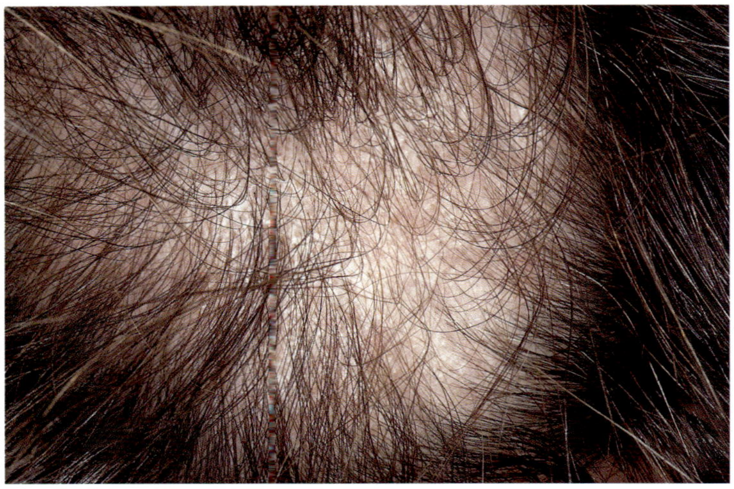

Figure 27–9. Alopecia areata, early. Diffuse, patchy loss of scalp hair.

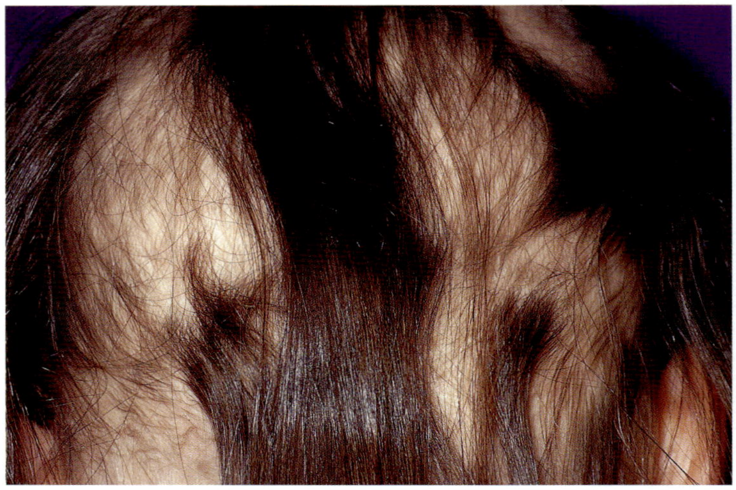

Figure 27–10. Alopecia areata, late. Patchy, bald spots and partial hair loss.

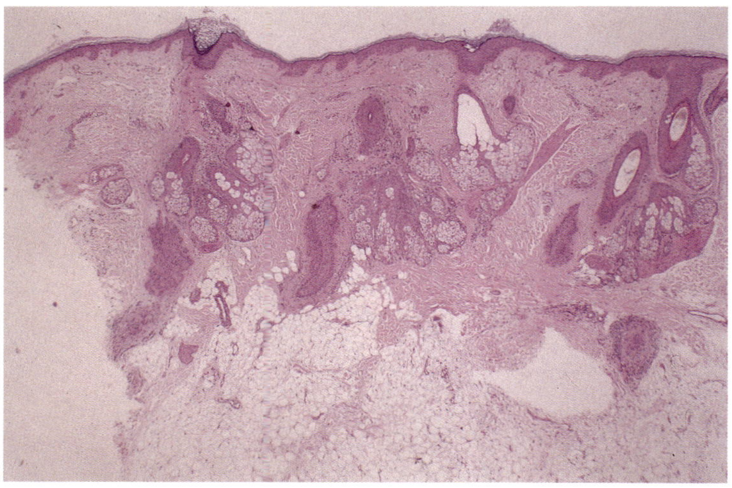

A

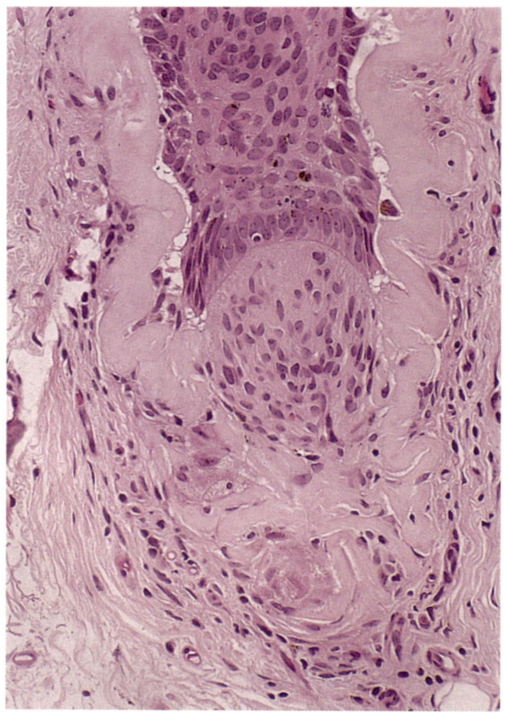

B

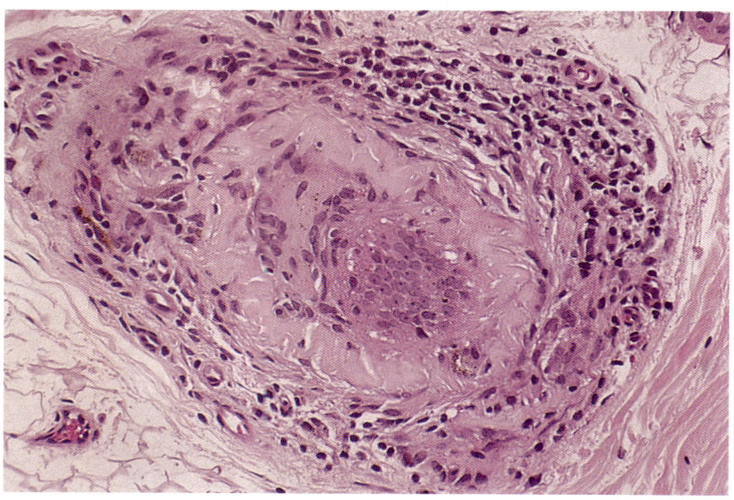

C

Figures 27–11A, 27–11B, 27–11C. Alopecia areata. Three terminal hair follicles in the same catagen stage with thickened, eosinophilic, corrugated basement membrane and patchy, lymphocytic infiltrates around the inferior segments. These changes are typical for alopecia areata.

TRICHOTILLOMANIA

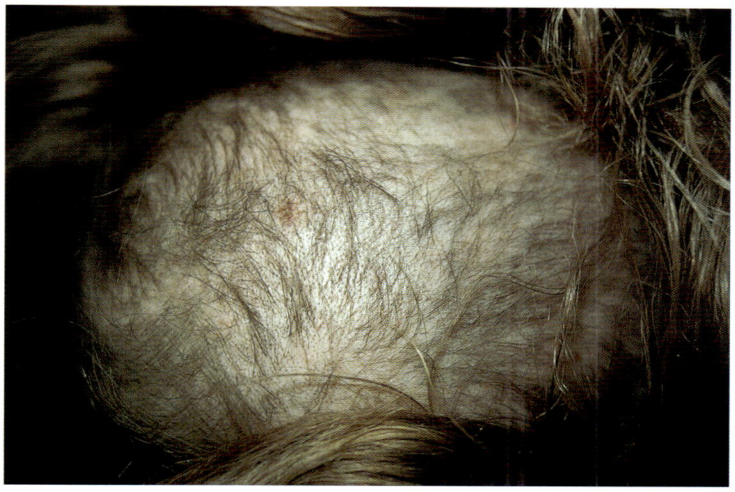

Figure 27–12. Trichotillomania. Alopecia with broken hairs of unequal lengths.

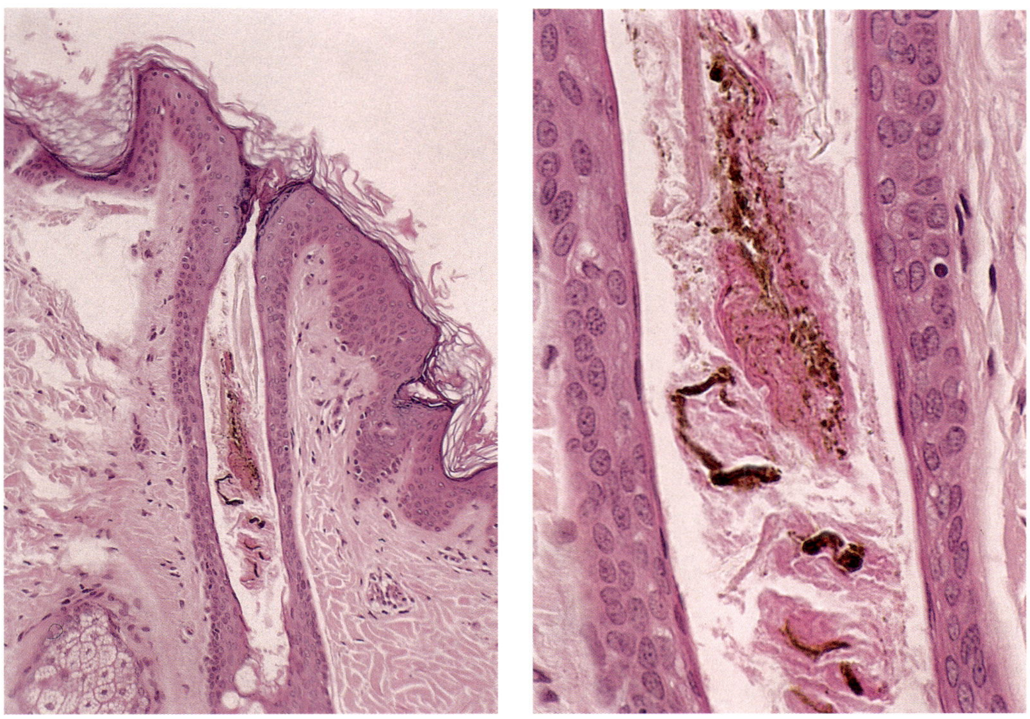

A B

Figures 27–13A, 27–13B. Trichotillomania. Frayed hair shaft with variable-sized clumps of melanin. This finding is referred to as trichomalacia and is characteristic for this condition.

DISCOID LUPUS ERYTHEMATOUS

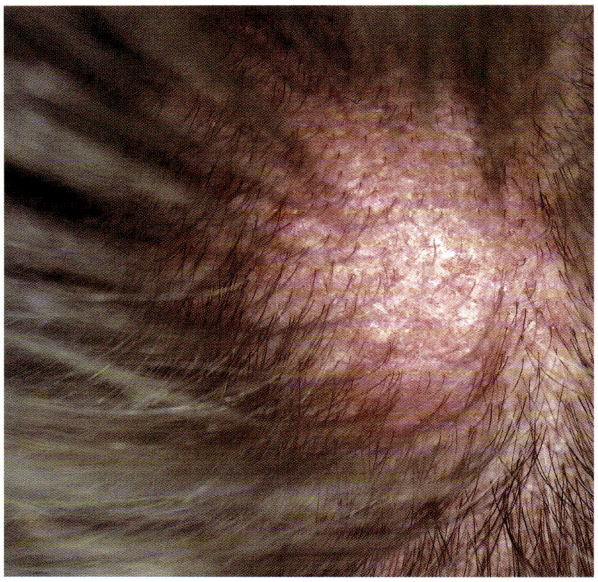

Figure 27–14. Discoid lupus erythematosus. Erythematous plaque with patulous follicular ostia in the scalp of a woman with systemic lupus erythematosus.

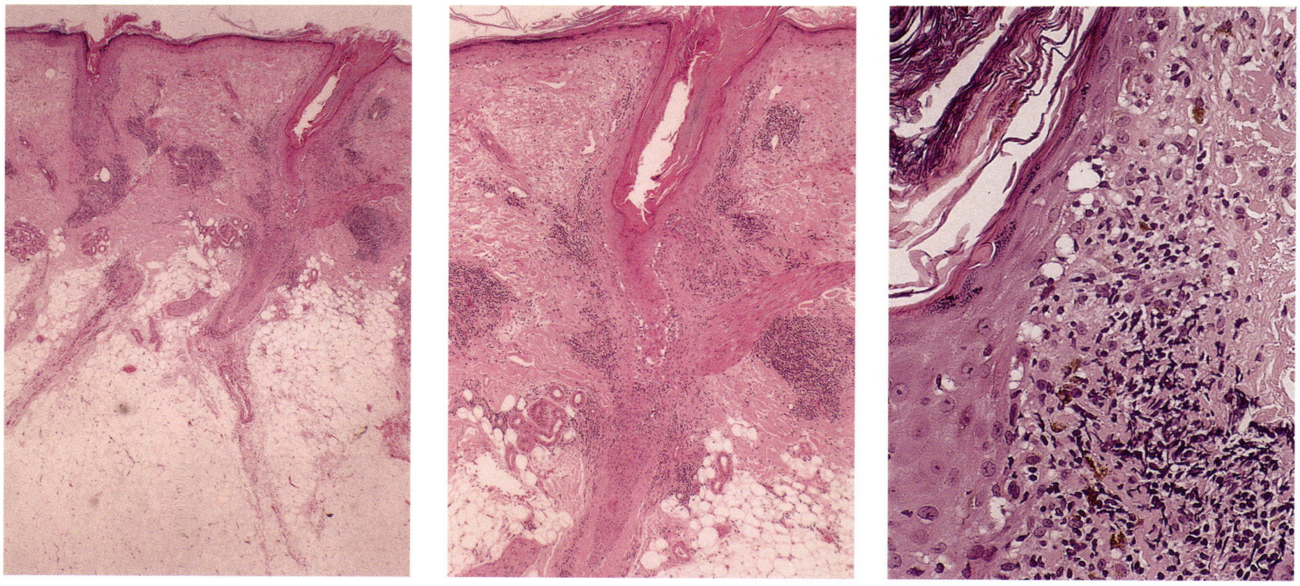

A B C

Figures 27–15A, 27–15B, 27–15C. Discoid lupus erythematosus. Patchy, lichenoid perifollicular and perivascular lymphocytic infiltrate with infundibular and epidermal vacuolar alteration. The epidermis is thinned, and there is dermal mucin deposition and fibroplasia.

28

Inflammatory reactions of the sweat gland unit

- Fox-Fordyce disease
- Pressure necrosis
- Neutrophilic eccrine hidradenitis

FOX-FORDYCE DISEASE

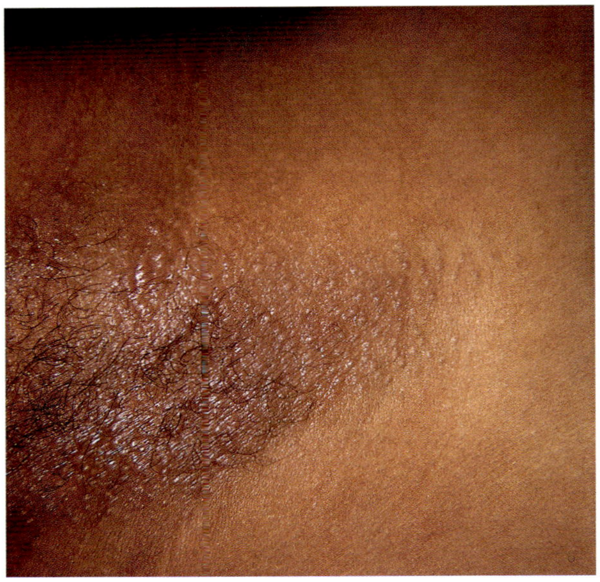

Figure 28–1. Fox-Fordyce disease. Pruritic, agminated, skin-colored papules in the axilla.

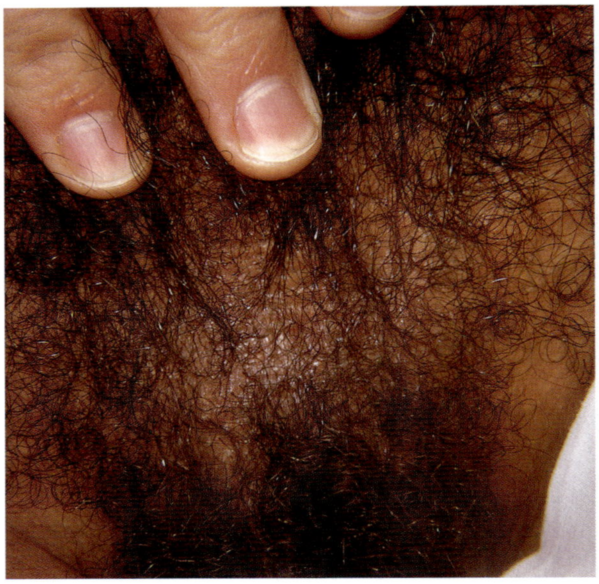

Figure 28–2. Fox-Fordyce disease. Pruritic papules on the pubis in the patient seen in Figure 28–1.

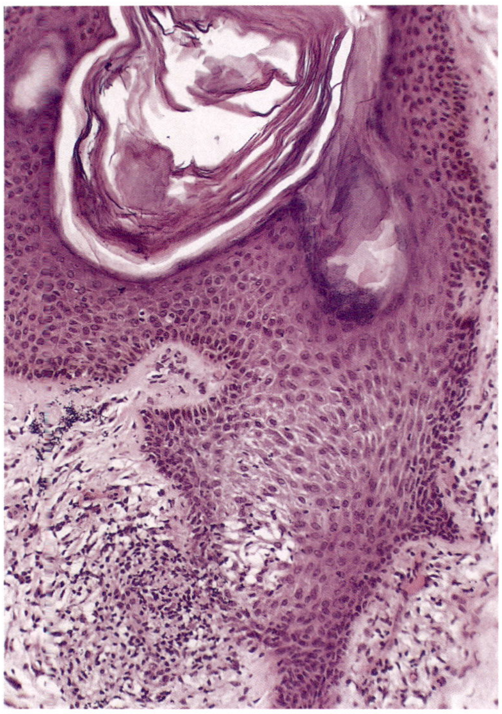

A

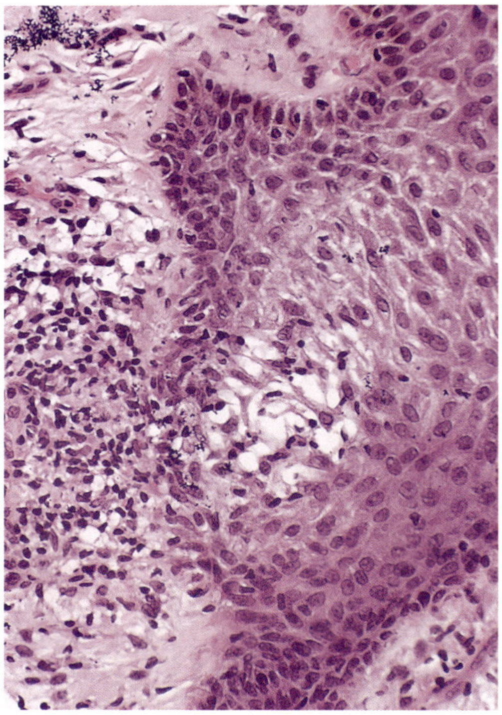

B

Figures 28–3A, 28–3B. Fox-Fordyce disease. Spongiosis of the apocrine duct as it enters the infundibulum. The infundibulum is dilated and hyperkeratotic. The duct is surrounded by a predominantly mononuclear cell infiltrate.

PRESSURE NECROSIS

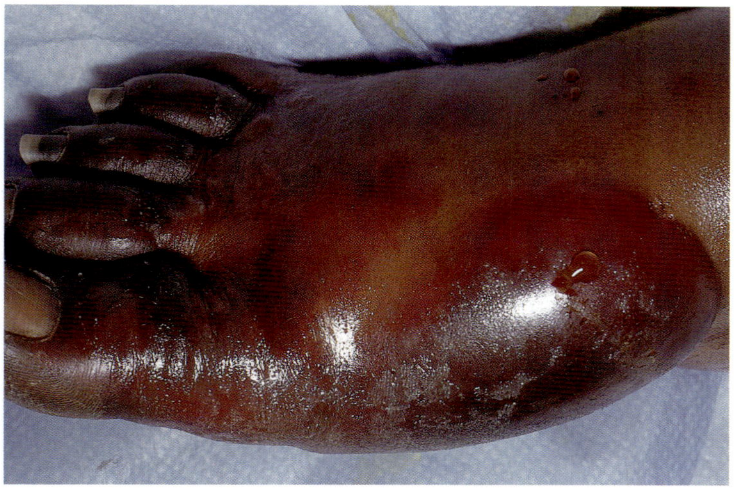

Figure 28–4. Pressure necrosis. Bullae on the foot and toes of a comatose patient.

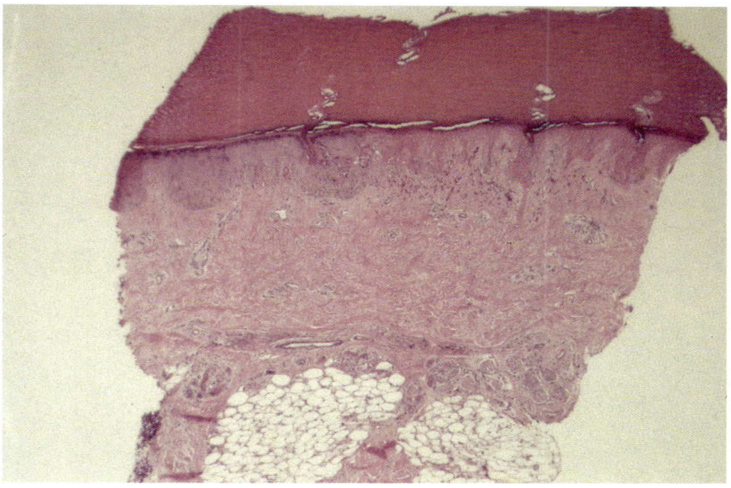

Figure 28–5. Pressure necrosis. Acral skin with necrosis of the epidermis and a patchy, lymphocytic eccrine gland infiltrate.

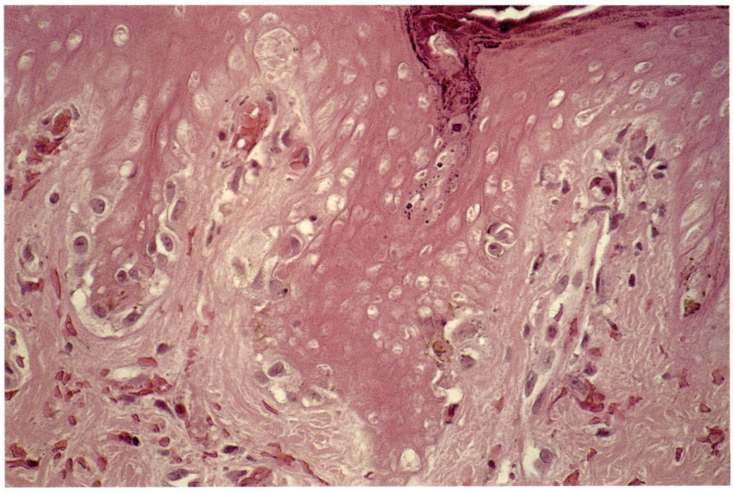

Figure 28–6. Pressure necrosis. Confluent epidermal necrosis with necrosis of the acrosyringium, dermal blood vessel ectasia, and numerous extravasated red blood cells.

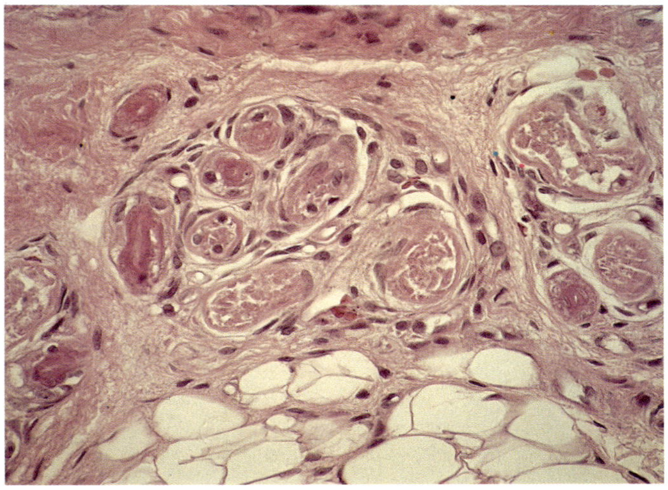

Figure 28–7. Pressure necrosis. Eccrine gland necrosis. Eosinophilic, amorphous material replaces the normal epithelium of the eccrine glands.

NEUTROPHILIC ECCRINE HIDRADENITIS

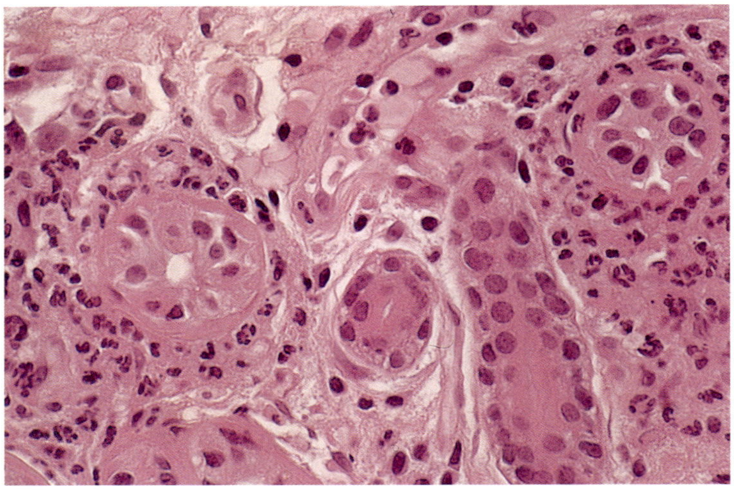

Figure 28–8. Neutrophilic eccrine hidradenitis. Necrotic eccrine epithelial cells surrounded by a neutrophilic infiltrate.

29

Mucous membrane disorders

- Morsicatio buccorum, (cheek and lip biting, and chewing)
- Amalgam tattoo
- Geographic tongue (migratory stomatitis)
- Oral hairy leukoplakia
- Verruciform xanthoma
- Aphthous ulcer
- Balanitis circumscripta plasmacellularis (Zoon's balanitis)
- White sponge nevus
- Verrucous carcinoma

MORSICATIO BUCCORUM (CHEEK AND LIP BITING AND CHEWING)

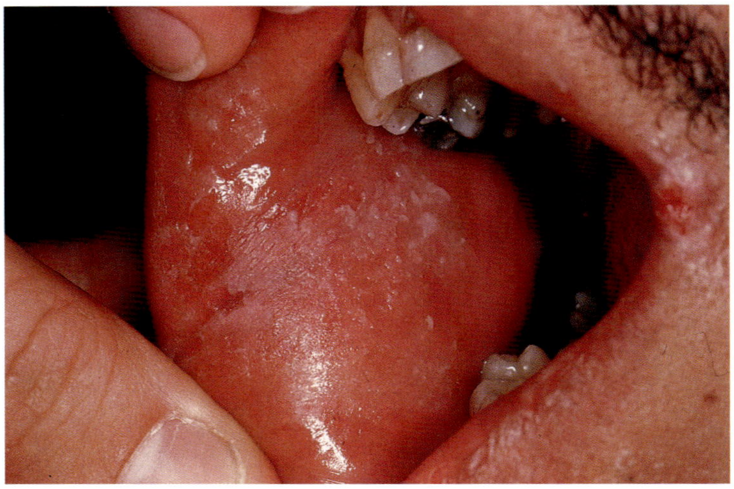

Figure 29–1. Morsicatio buccorum. White, ragged irregular patches on the buccal mucosa of a man who has a history of chewing on his cheek.

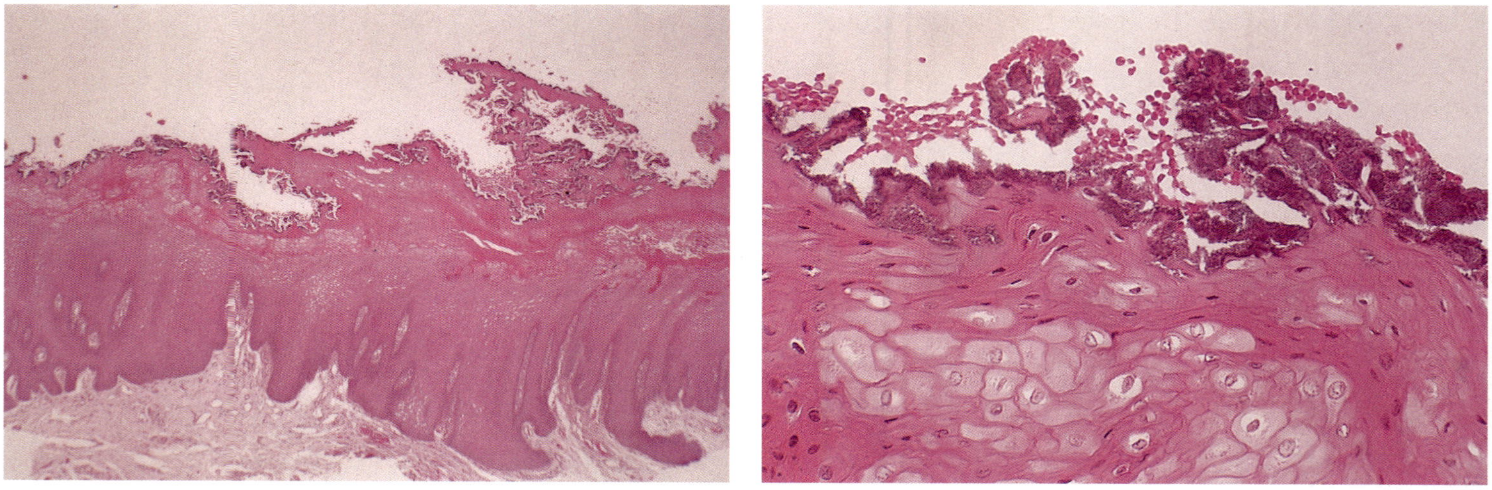

A

B

Figures 29–2A, 29–2B. Morsicatio buccorum. Serrated epithelial surface with epithelial hyperplasia. There are clumps of bacteria along with jagged epithelial surface, a zone of parakeratotic cells, and a subjacent zone of plump cells with abundant pale-staining cytoplasm.

AMALGAM TATTOO

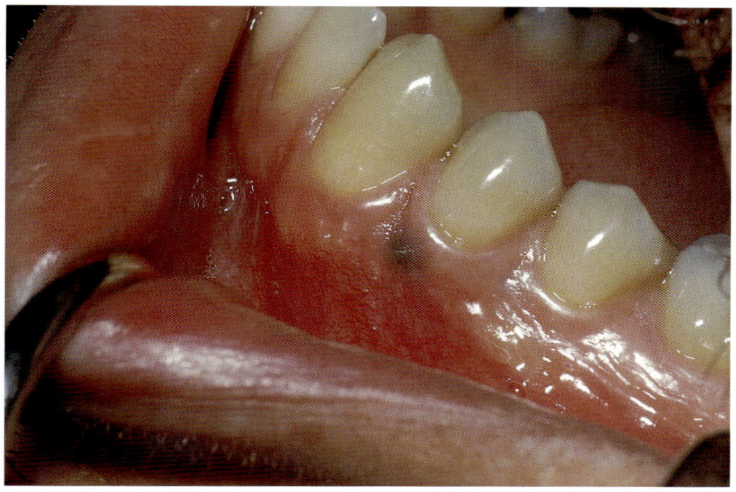

Figure 29–3. Amalgam tattoo. Blue macule on the alveolar ridge.

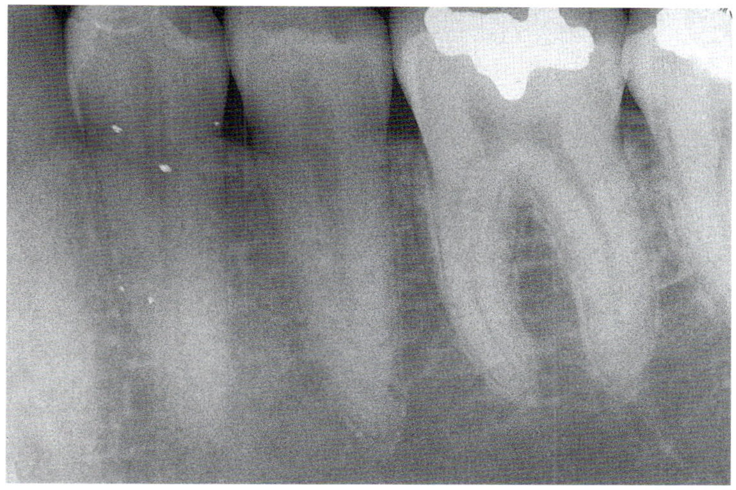

Figure 29–4. Amalgam tattoo. Radiograph shows metallic particles in the alveolar tissue as white speckles.

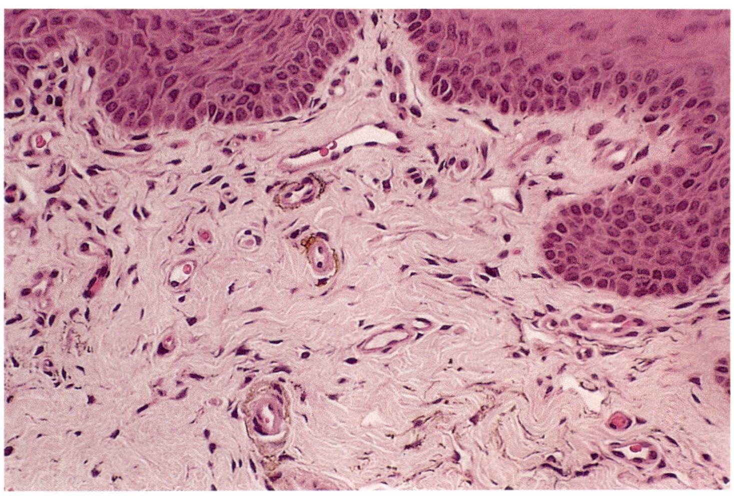

A

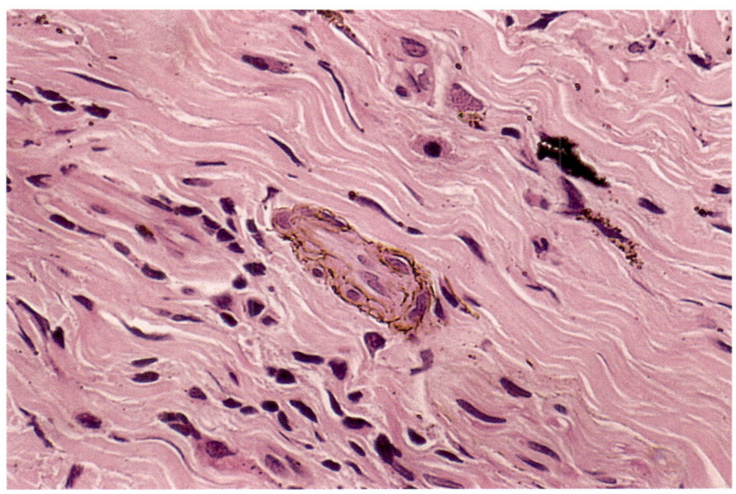

B

Figures 29–5A, 29–5B. Amalgam tattoo. Alloy particles deposited around and within blood vessel walls, on collagen bundles and within macrophages.

GEOGRAPHIC TONGUE (MIGRATORY STOMATITIS)

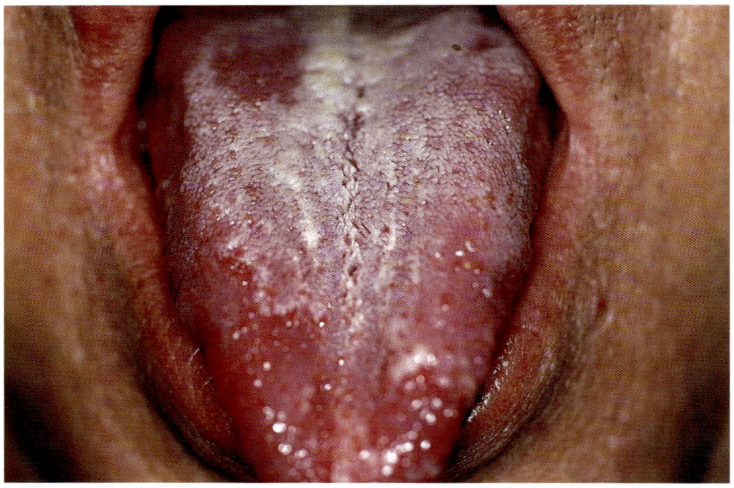

Figure 29–6. Geographic tongue. Multiple irregular circinate, erythematous patches on the dorsum and sides of the tongue.

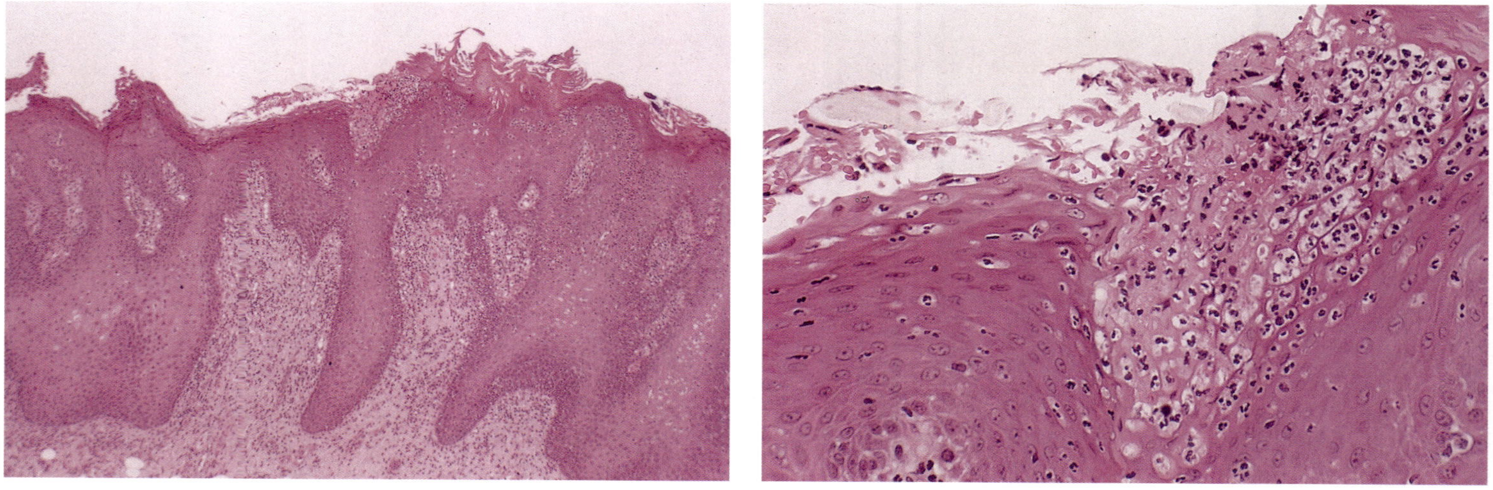

A B

Figures 29–7A, 29–7B. Geographic tongue. Psoriasiform epithelial hyperplasia with a neutrophilic infiltrate. Surface epithelium shows ragged hyperkeratosis, individual neutrophils, and aggregates of neut ophils forming spongiform pustules. In the stroma there are dilated blood vessels and neutrophilic inflammatory infiltrate.

ORAL HAIRY LEUKOPLAKIA

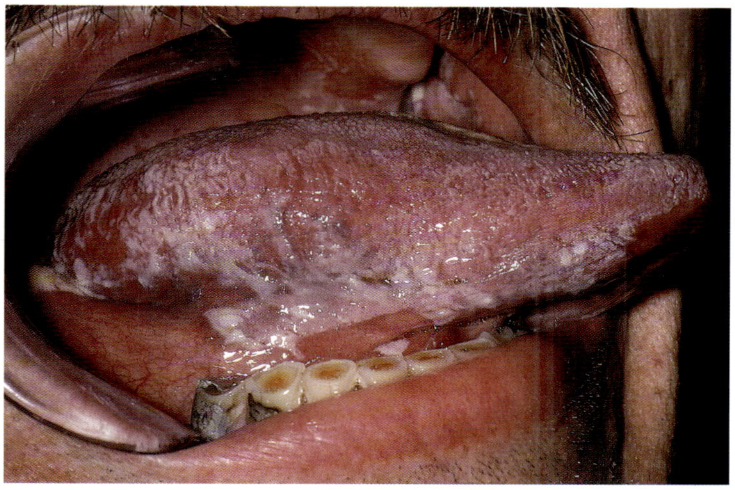

Figure 29–8. Oral hairy leukoplakia. White ruggated lesions on the side of the tongue in an HIV-positive man. There is also evidence of extensive mucosal candidiasis on the tongue and palate.

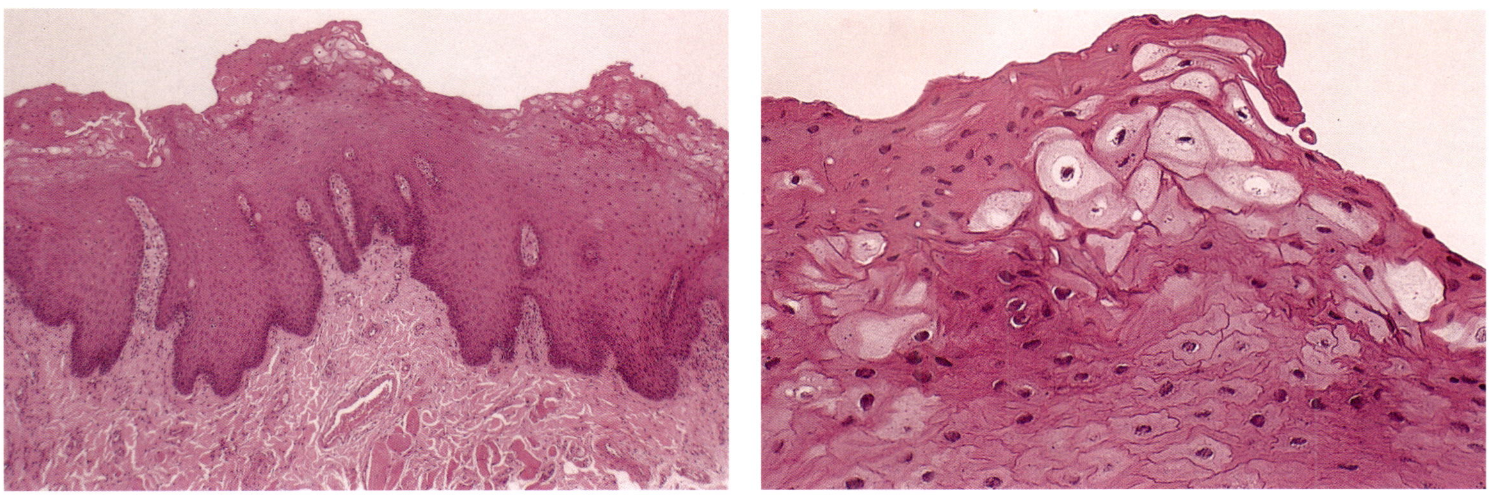

A **B**

Figures 29–9A, 29–B. Oral hairy leukoplakia. Epithelial hyperplasia, hyperkeratosis, and large epithelial cells with perinuclear halo and abundant pale-staining cytoplasm. Candidal hyphal elements are also present, which is not an uncommon finding.

VERRUCIFORM XANTHOMA

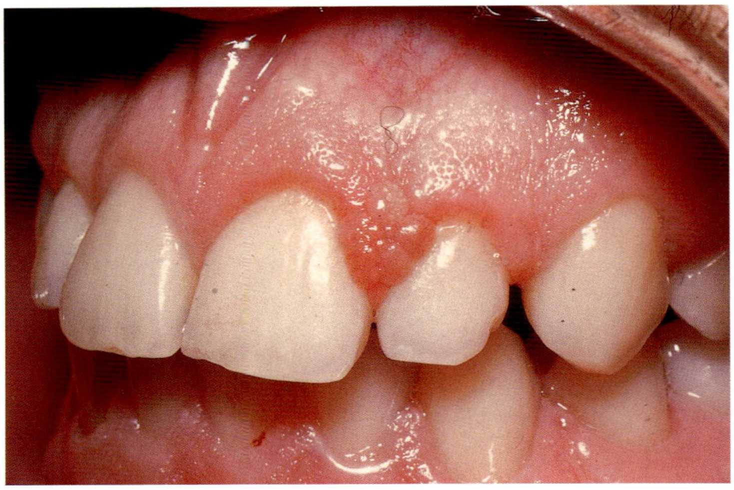

Figure 29–10. Verruciform xanthoma. Erythematous papillated lesion on the gingiva papilla.

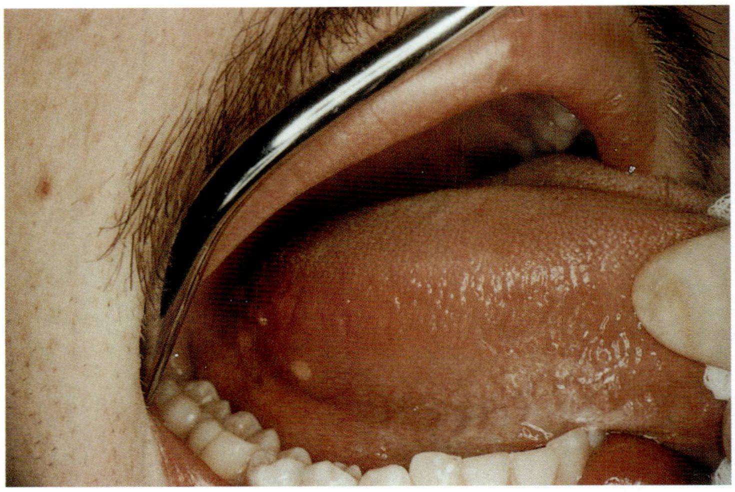

Figure 29–11. Verruciform xanthoma. Raised white papule on the posterior lateral tongue.

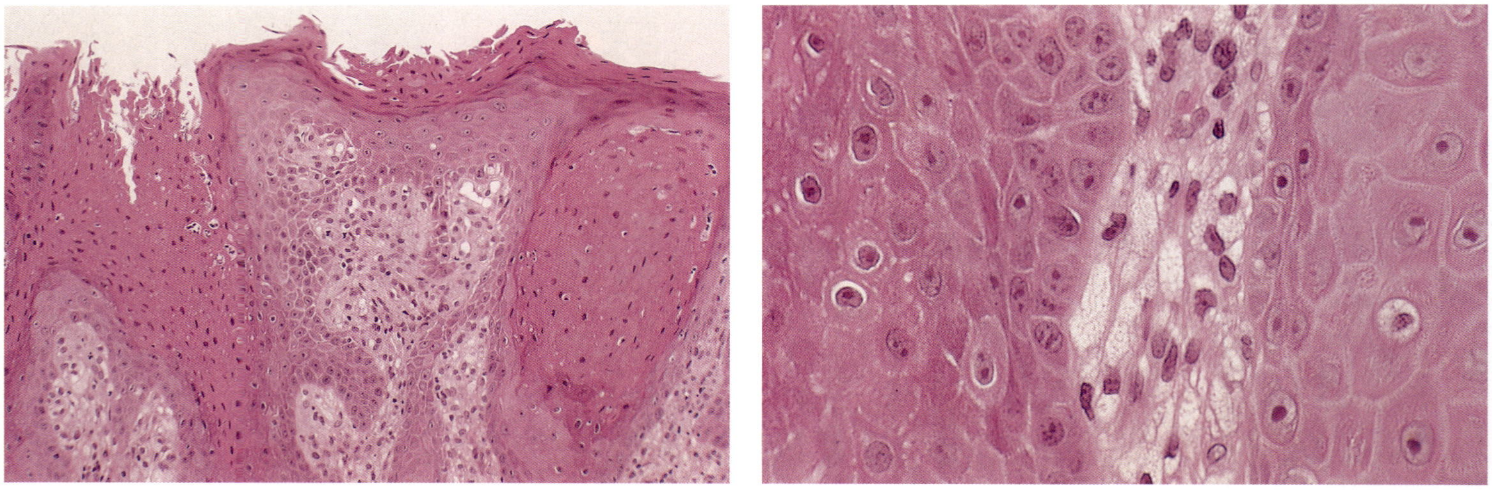

A

B

Figures 29–12A, 29–12B. Verruciform xanthoma. Epithelial hyperplasia, parakeratosis, and foam cells within the widened stromal papilla. Vacuolated histiocytic cells fill the papilla between hyperplastic epithelial ridges.

APHTHOUS ULCER

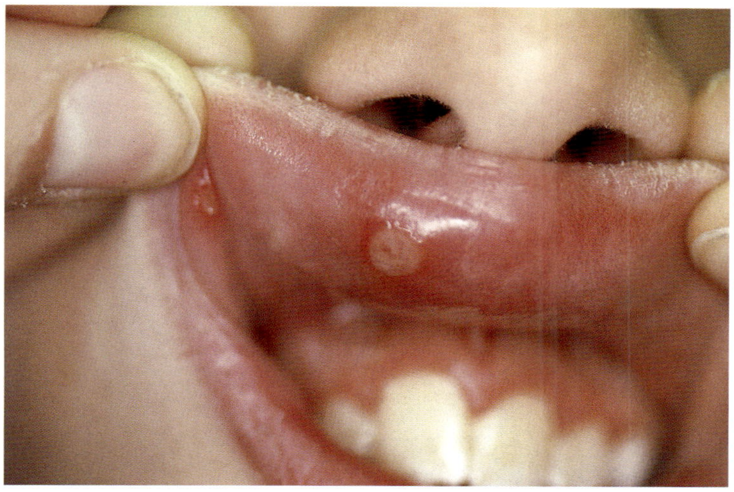

Figure 29–13. Aphthous ulcer. Recurrent gray-white ulcers with slightly raised margins and peripheral erythema on the mucosal surface of the upper lip of a child.

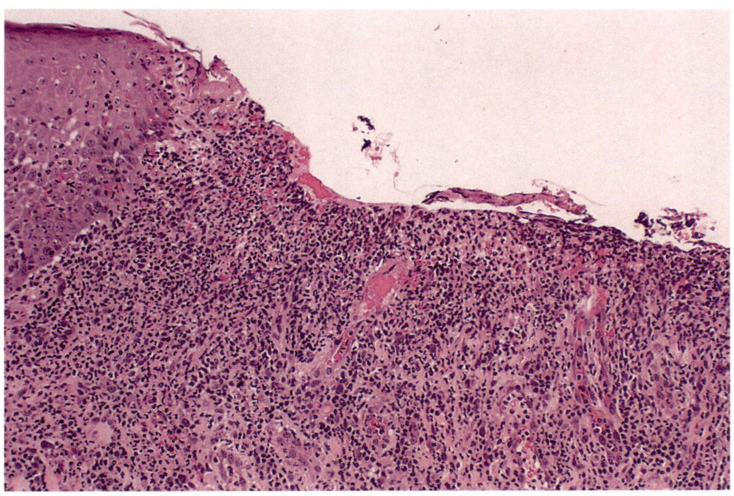

A

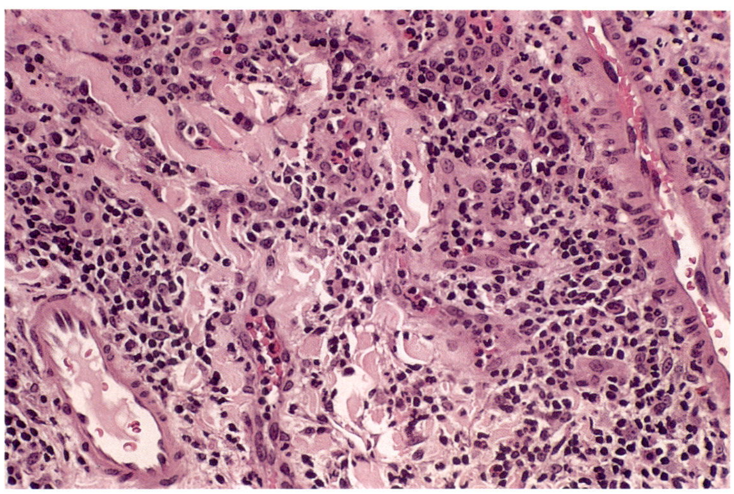

B

Figures 29–14A, 29–14B. Aphthous ulcer. Epithelial ulceration with a dense mixed-cell infiltrate in the lamina propria. There is a prominent perivascular lymphocytic infiltrate, many neutrophils with occasional nuclear fragments, a few eosinophils, and altered congested blood vessels.

BALANITIS CIRCUMSCRIPTA PLASMACELLULARIS (ZOON'S BALANITIS)

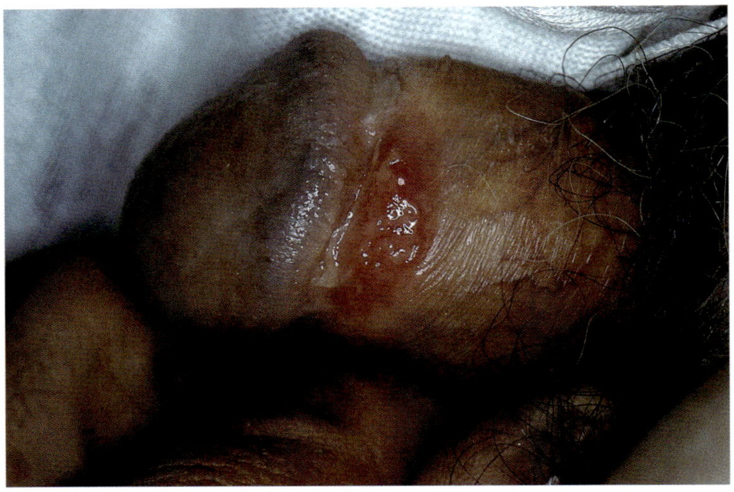

Figure 29–15. Balanitis circumscripta plasmacellularis. Sharply circumscribed ulcer in the sulcus on the penis.

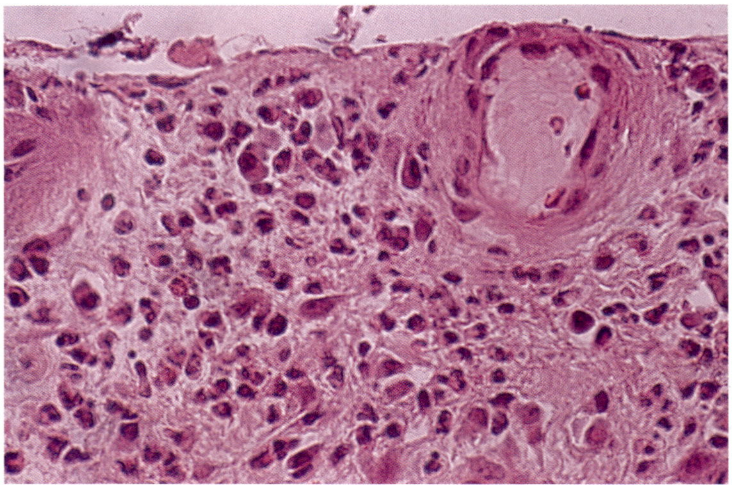

Figure 29–16. Balanitis circumscripta plasmacellularis. Denuded epithelium and a dense mixed-cell infiltrate with numerous plasma cells.

WHITE SPONGE NEVUS

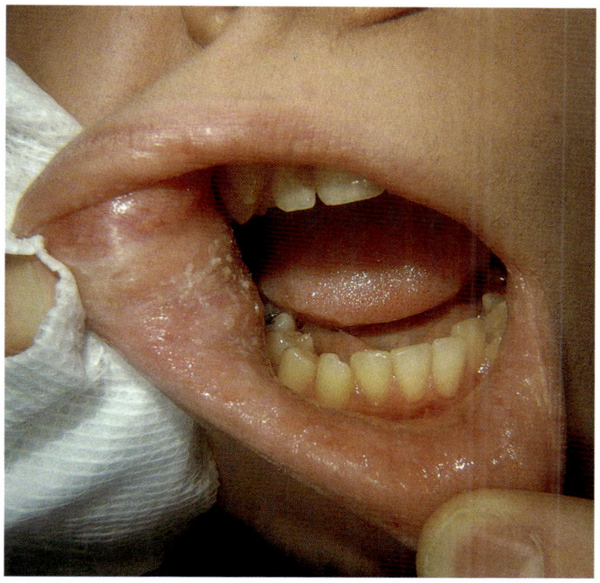

Figure 29–17. White sponge nevus. Asymptomatic white shaggy keratotic lesion on the buccal mucosa of a young boy.

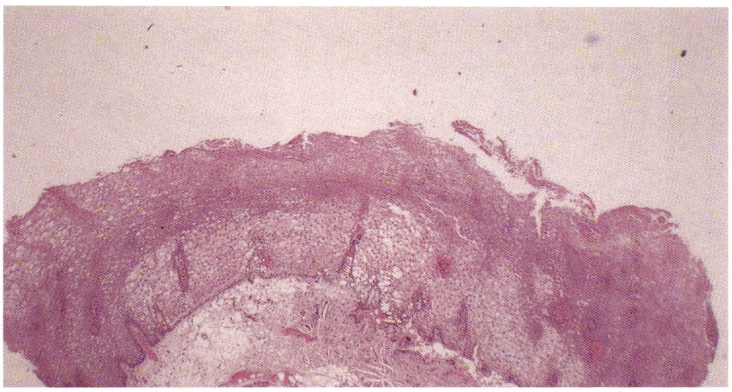

A

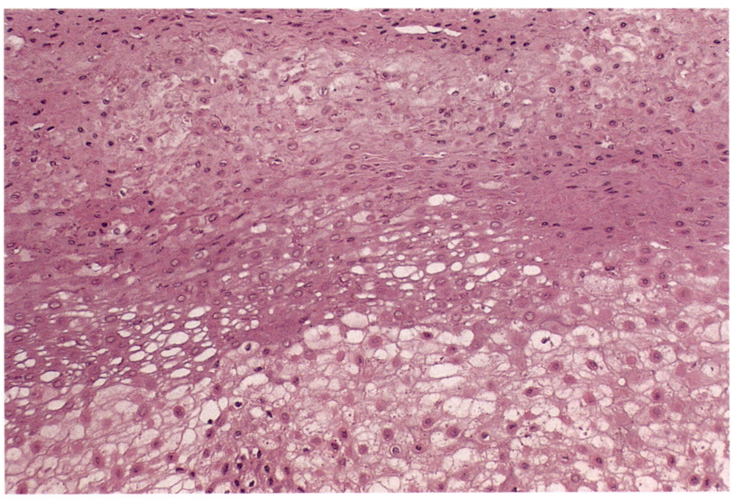

B

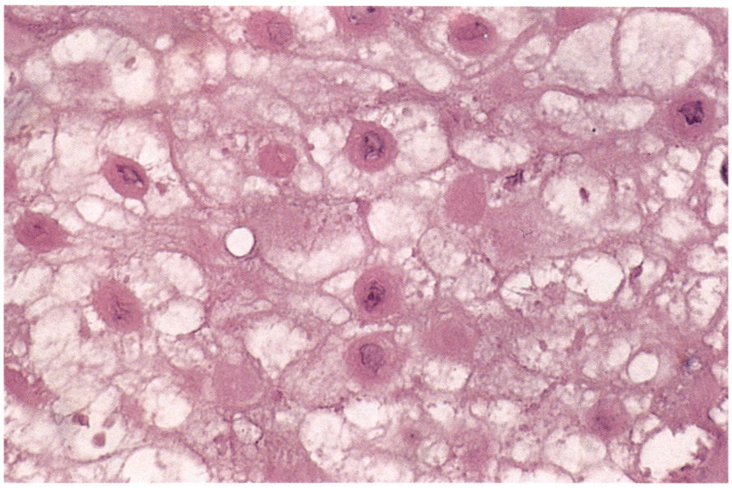

C

Figures 29–18A, 29–18B, 29–18C. White sponge nevus. Hyperkeratosis, parakeratosis, and epithelial hyperplasia with numerous pale and vacuolated mucosal cells. Eosinophilic, paranuclear cytoplasmic condensations are characteristic changes within many of the vacuolated mucosal cells.

VERRUCOUS CARCINOMA

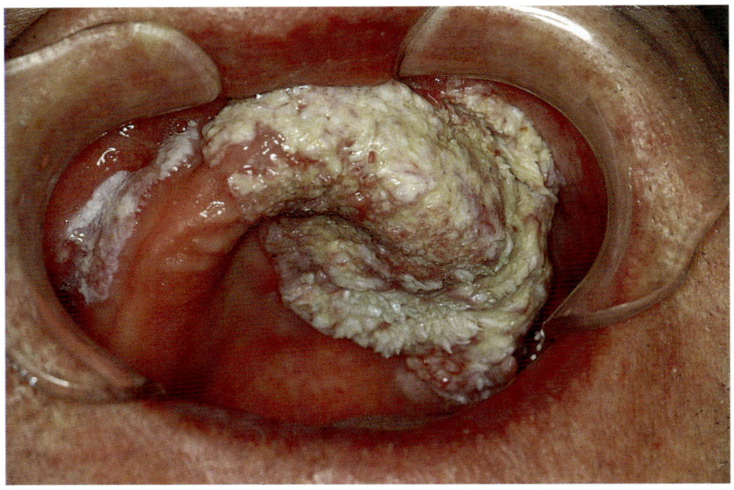

Figure 29–19. Verrucous carcinoma. Extensive verrucous lesion involving palatal and alveolar mucosa.

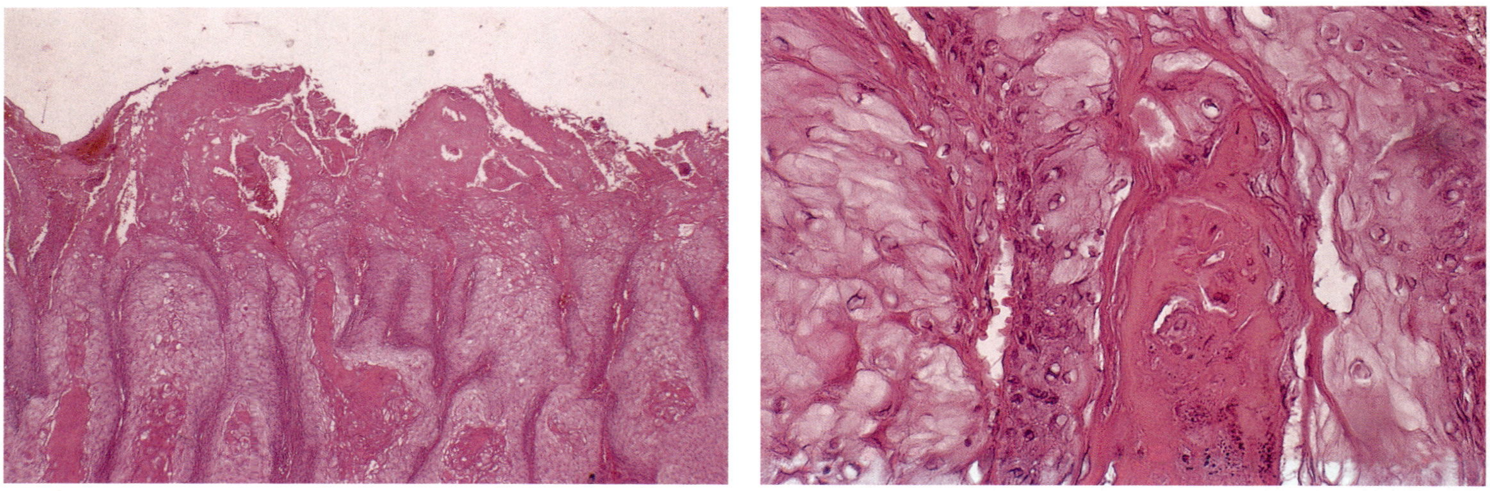

A **B**

Figures 29–20A, 29–20B. Verrucous carcinoma. Hyperkeratosis, papillomatosis, and a proliferation of well-differentiated, deceptively benign-appearing epithelial cells. There are parakeratotic plugs within the nvaginations.

30

Benign epidermal neoplasms

- Epidermal nevus
  - *A) Verrucous epidermal nevus*
  - *B) Inflammatory linear verrucous epidermal nevus (ILVEN)*
  - *C) Epidermolytic hyperkeratosis (ichthyosis hystrix)*
  - *D) Psoriasiform epidermal nevus*
- Seborrheic keratosis
- Solar lentigo
- Lichenoid keratosis
- Pale-cell acanthoma

EPIDERMAL NEVUS

A) Verrucous epidermal nevus

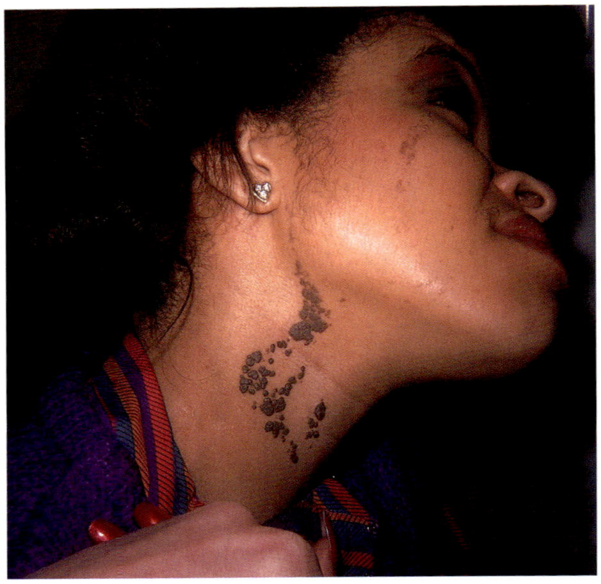

A

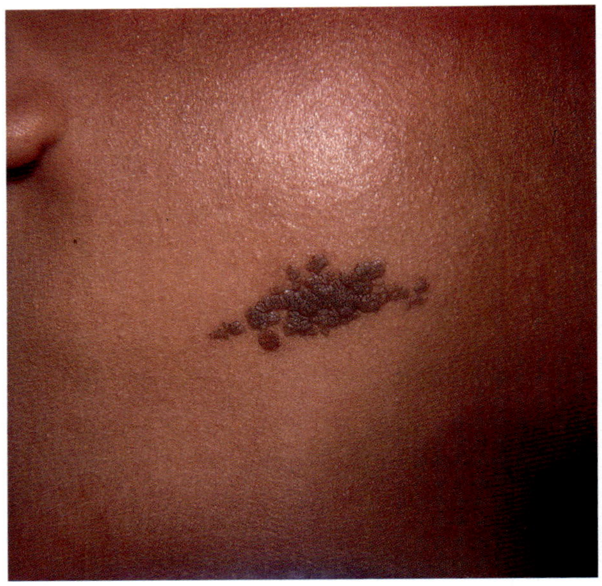

B

Figures 30–1A, 30–1B. Verrucous epidermal nevus. Linear, hyperpigmented confluent papules on the neck.

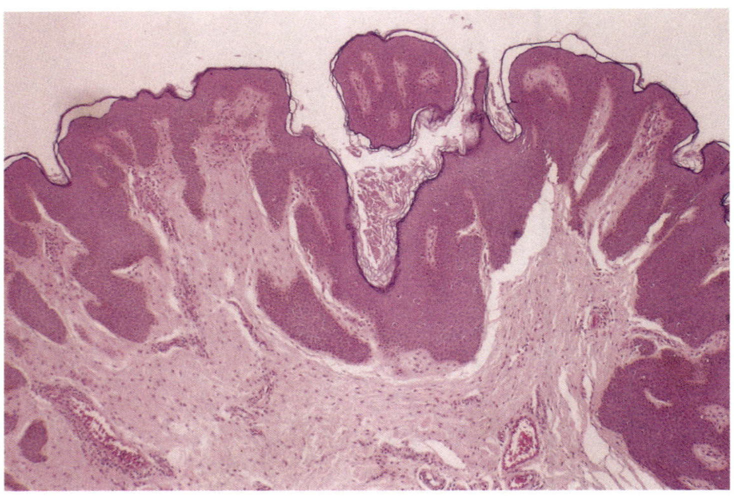

Figure 30–2. Verrucous epidermal nevus. Papillomatosis with epidermal and infundibular hyperplasia. There is a patchy dermal lymphocytic infiltrate and coarse collagen bundles.

EPIDERMAL NEVUS

B) Inflammatory linear verrucous epidermal nevus (ILVEN)

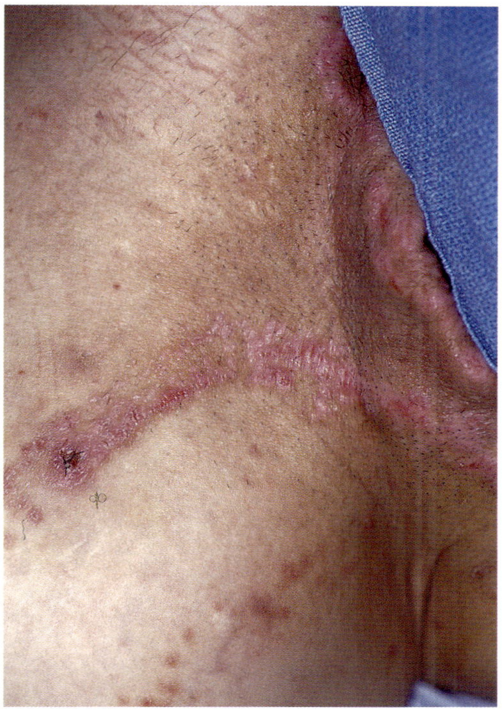

Figure 30–3. Inflammatory linear verrucous epidermal nevus. Erythematous, linear, contiguous keratotic papules involving the labia, groin, inner thigh, and leg.

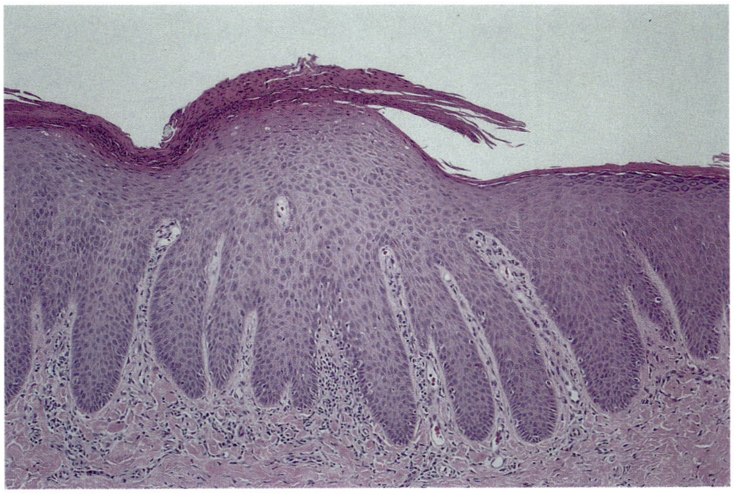

Figure 30–4. Inflammatory linear verrucous epidermal nevus. Psoriasiform epidermal hyperplasia with focal parakeratosis and scale-crust. Coarse collagen bundles, dilated blood vessels, and a mononuclear inflammatory-cell infiltrate is present in the dermis.

EPIDERMAL NEVUS

C) Epidermolytic hyperkeratosis (ichthyosis hystrix)

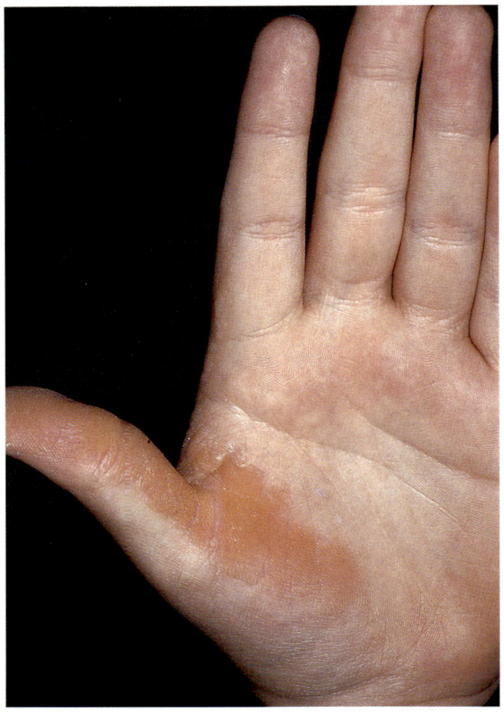

Figure 30–5. Epidermolytic hyperkeratosis. Linear, bronze keratotic plaques involving the palm and thumb.

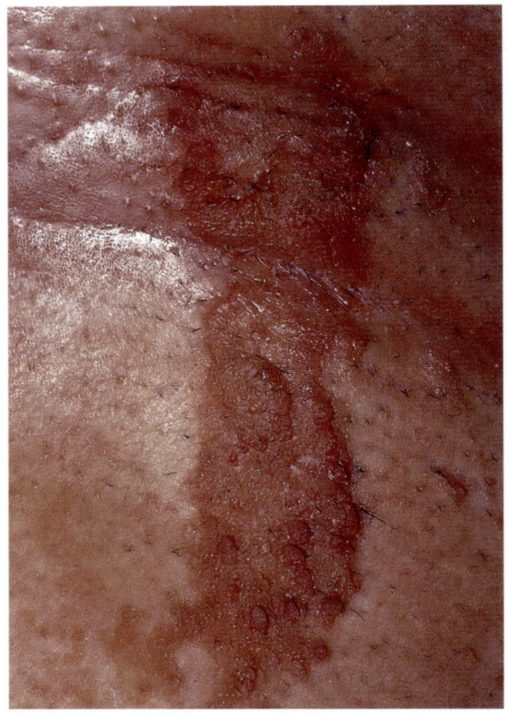

Figure 30–6. Epidermolytic hyperkeratosis. Linear, reddish, verrucous, moist linear plaque.

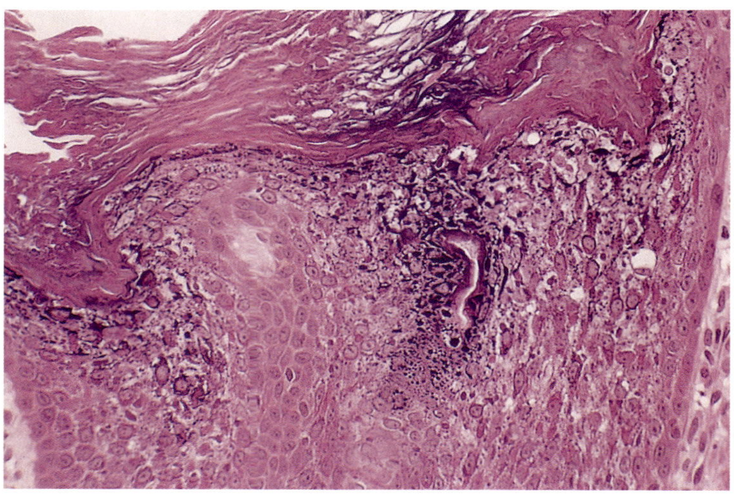

A

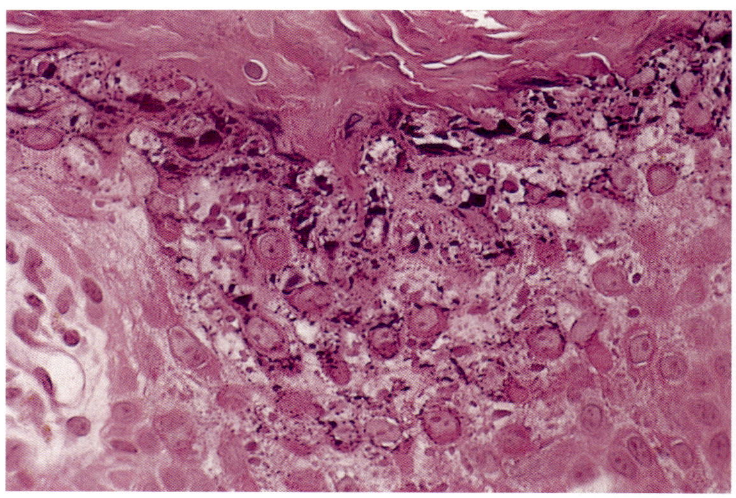

B

Figures 30–7A, 30–7B. Epidermolytic hyperkeratosis. Epidermal hyperplasia, hyperkeratosis, hypergranulosis, and epidermolysis. There are large and irregular shaped keratohyaline granules and pale-staining, dislodged keratinocytes.

EPIDERMAL NEVUS

D) Psoriasiform epidermal nevus

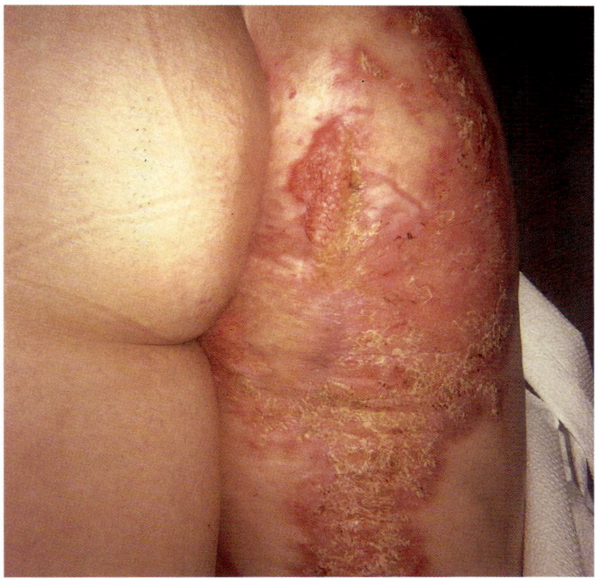

A

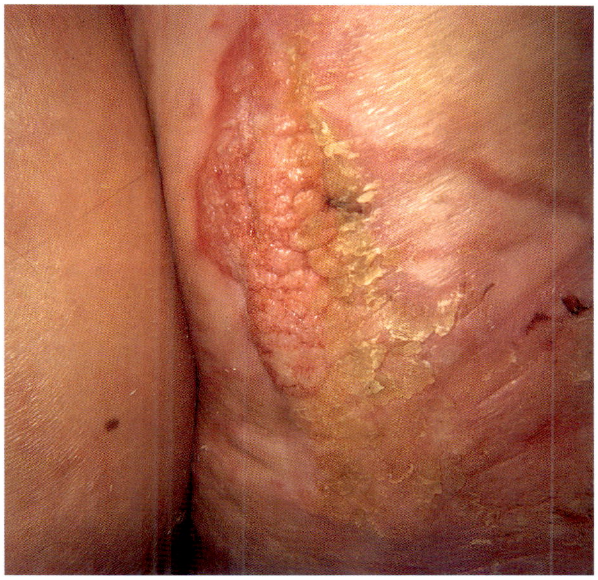

B

Figures 30–8A, 30–8B. Psoriasiform epidermal nevus. Linear, verrucous, crusted, scaly erythematous plaques involving the buttocks, groin, thigh, and leg. Involvement of the distal extremity ultimately resulted in bony destruction and loss of digits.

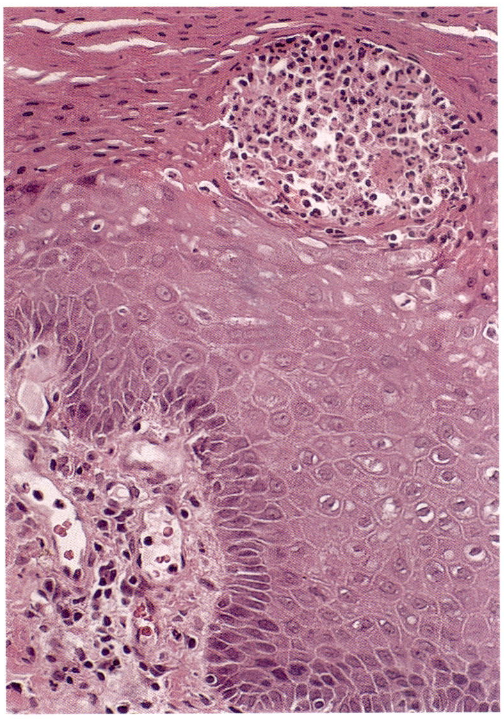

Figure 30–9. Psoriasiform epidermal nevus. Psoriasiform epidermal hyperplasia and parakeratosis, with a large intracorneal collection of neutrophils.

SEBORRHEIC KERATOSIS

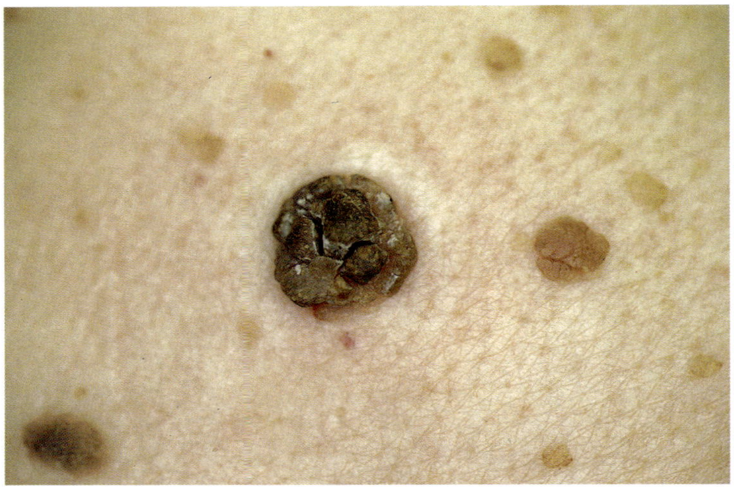

Figure 30–10. Seborrheic keratosis. Hyperkeratotic and hyperpigmented papules and nodules on the back.

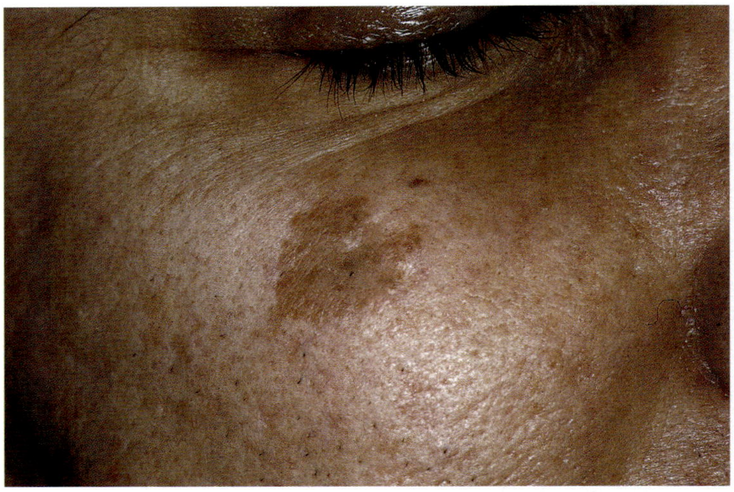

Figure 30–11. Seborrheic keratosis. Irregular, hyperpigmented keratotic plaque contiguous with a hyperpigmented macular lesion on the cheek of a woman. This lesion illustrates the evolution of a solar lentigo into a seborrheic keratosis.

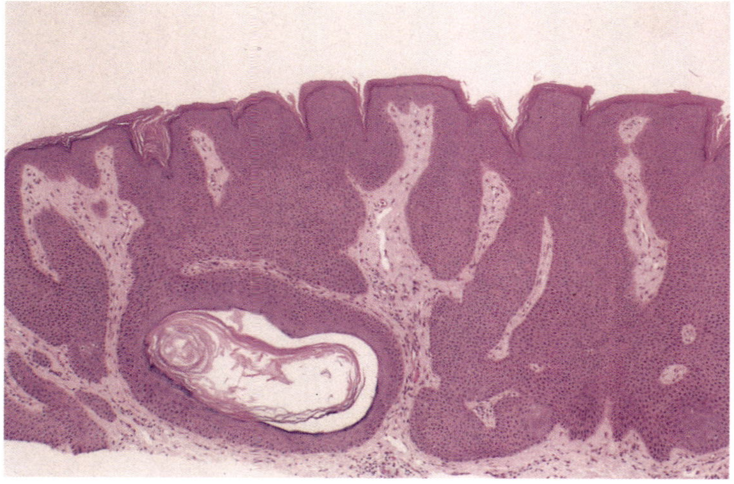

A

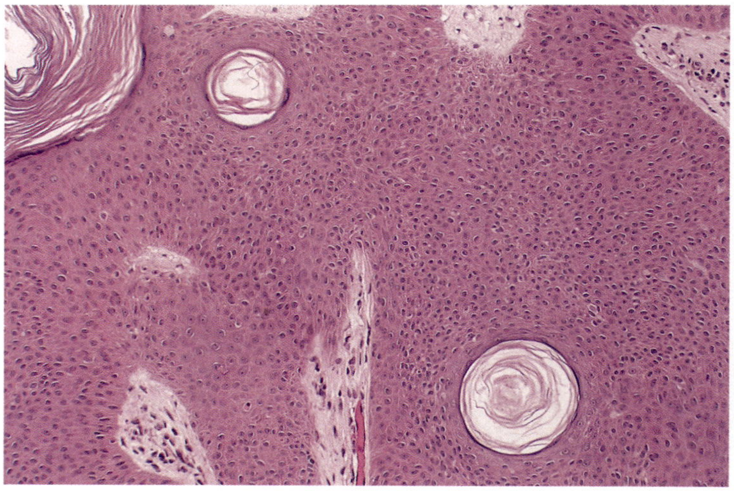

B

Figures 30–12A, 30–12B. Seborrheic keratosis. Proliferation of basiloid cells with dilated, hyperkeratotic infundibula

SEBORRHEIC KERATOSIS

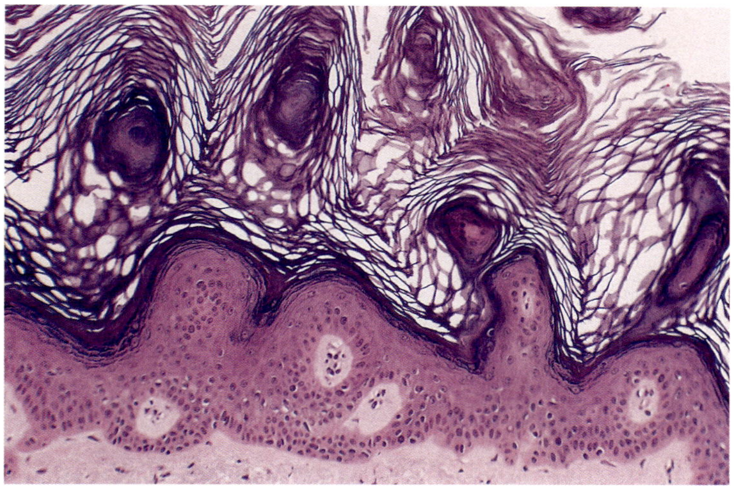

Figure 30–13. Seborrheic keratosis. Digitate epidermal hyperplasia and hyperkeratosis.

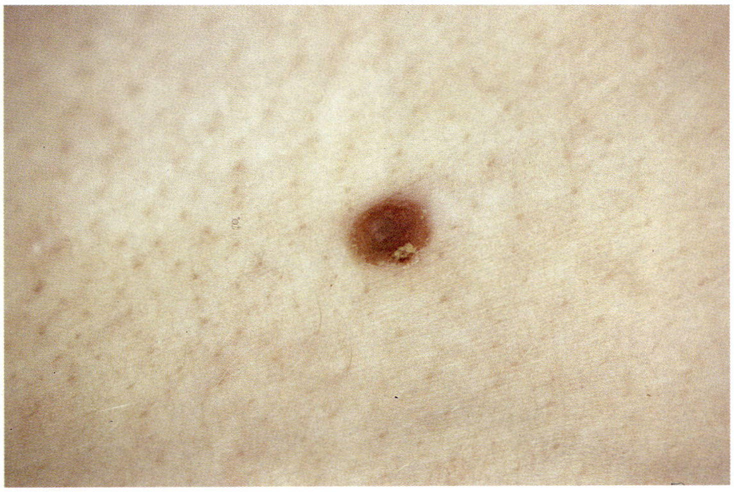

Figure 30–14. Seborrheic keratosis, inflamed. Scaly and crusted, hyperpigmented, keratotic papule in the axilla of a woman.

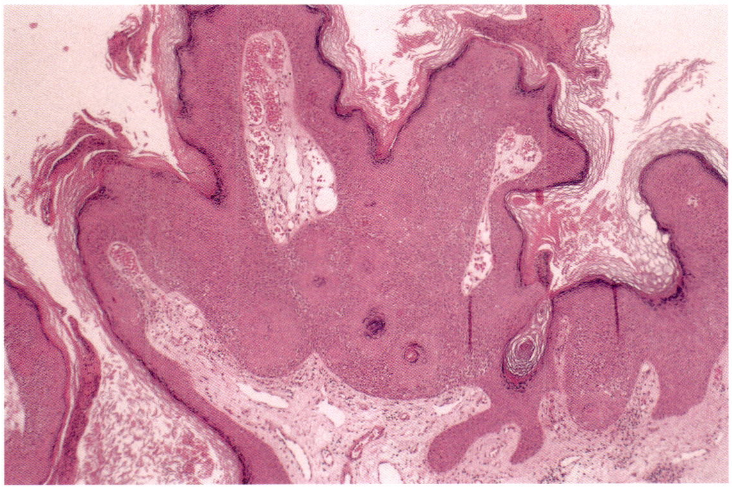

Figure 30–15. Seborrheic keratosis, inflamed. Whorls of eosinophilic-staining epithelial cells (squamous eddies) often with hypergranulosis within hyperplastic infundibula. There is hyperkeratosis, scale-crust, spongiosis, and disarray of adjacent follicular keratinocytes.

SOLAR LENTIGO

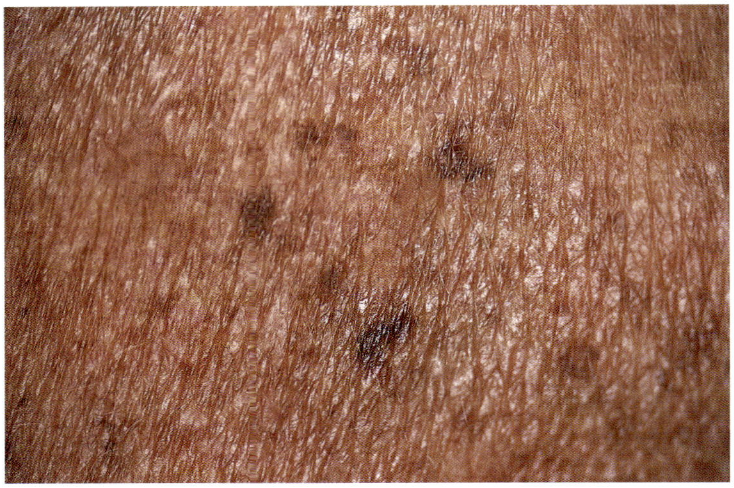

Figure 30–16. Solar lentigo. Irregular, hyperpigmented macules on severely sun-damaged skin.

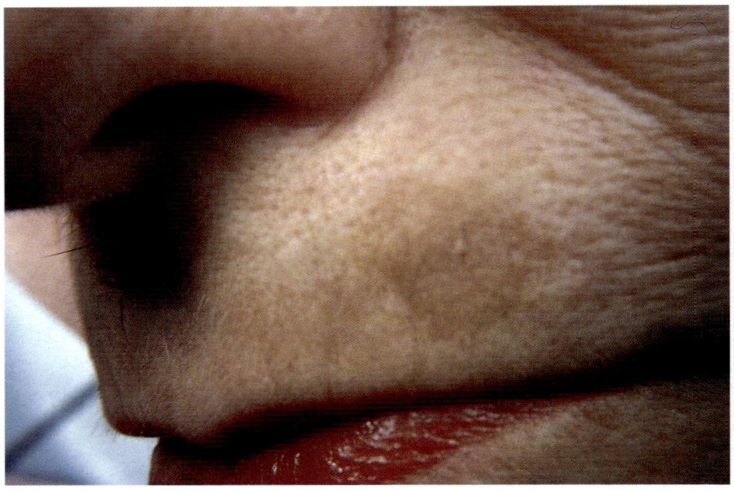

Figure 30–17. Solar lentigo. Uniform tan patch on the lip of a woman.

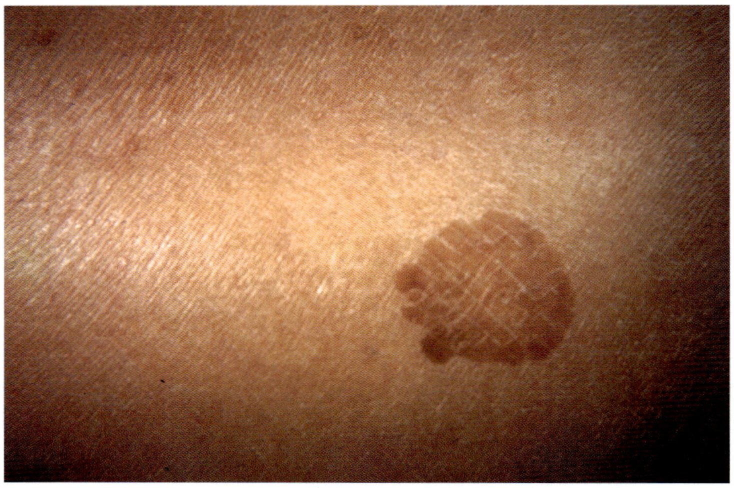

Figure 30–18. Solar lentigo with evolving seborrheic keratosis. Mottled brown, irregular, slightly raised plaque with accentuated skin markings.

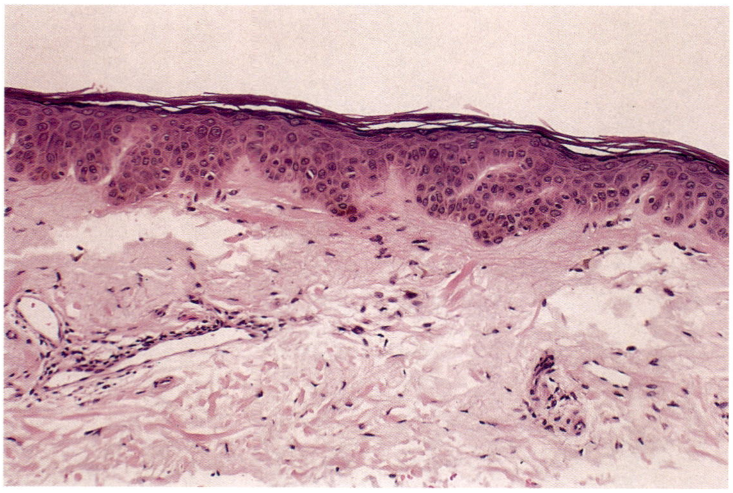

A

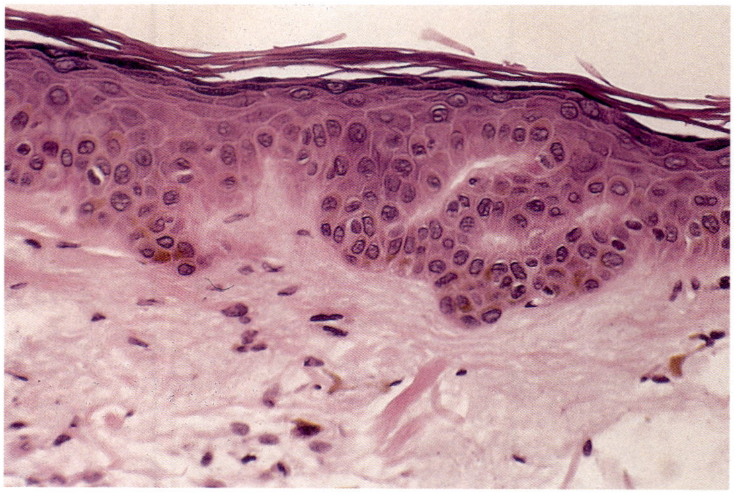

B

Figures 30–19A, 30–19B. Solar lentigo. Hyperplastic and hyperpigmented keratinocytes within elongated rete ridges. There is dermal solar elastosis and dilated blood vessels.

LICHENOID KERATOSIS

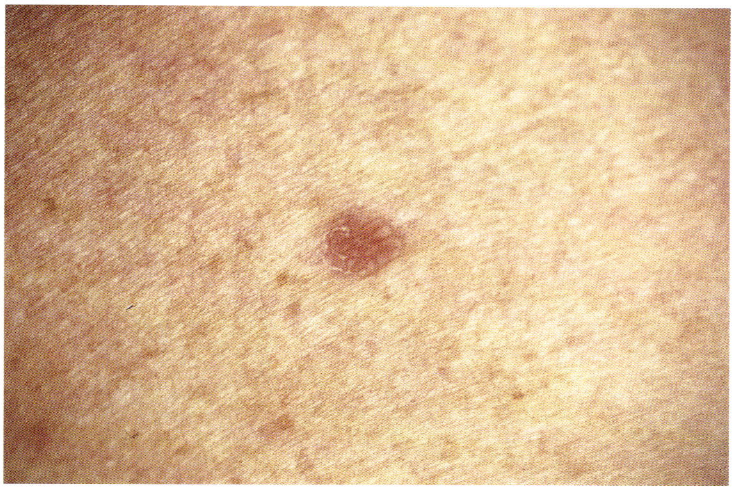

Figure 30–20. Lichenoid keratosis. Slightly raised pink, scaly lesion on the chest, which had changed in size and color.

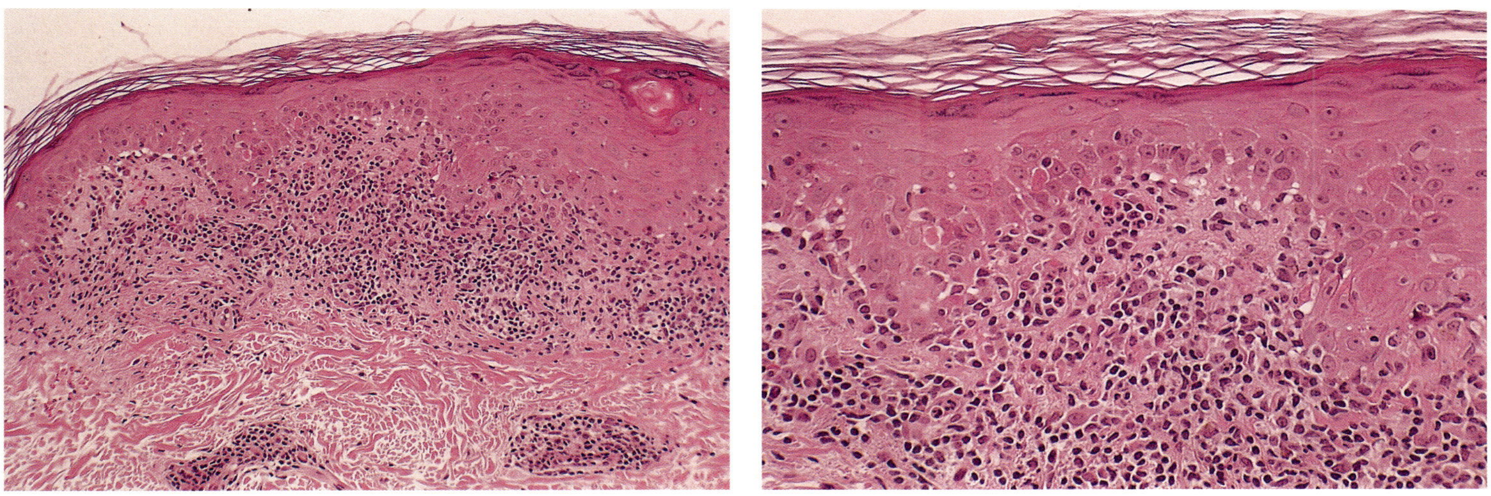

A B

Figures 30–21A, 30–21B. Lichenoid keratosis. Irregular epidermal hyperplasia, vacuolar alteration, numerous necrotic keratinocytes and a dense lichenoid mixed-cell infiltrate filling the thickened papillary dermis.

LICHENOID KERATOSIS

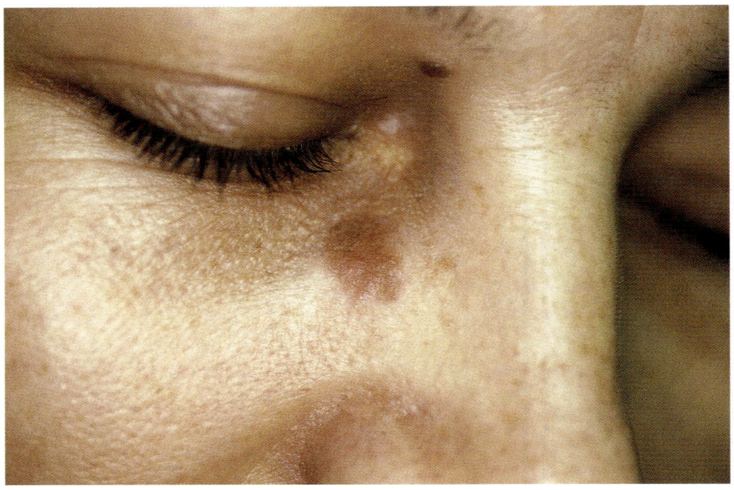

Figure 30–22. **Lichenoid keratosis, pigmented.** Long-standing infraorbital pigmented patch that has recently become elevated.

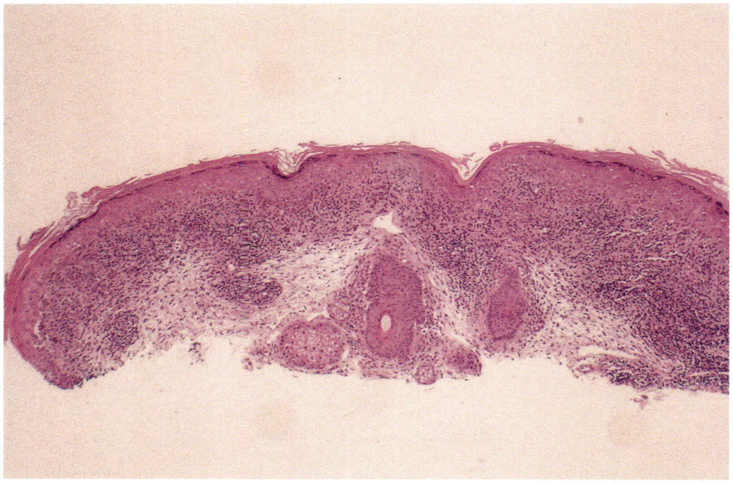

A

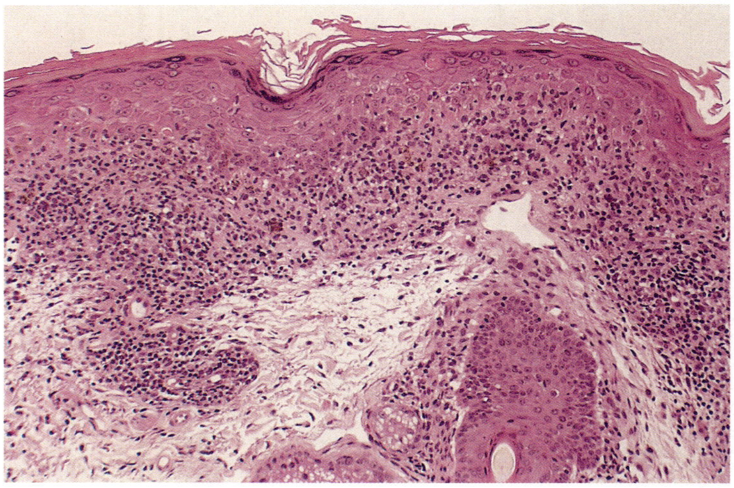

B

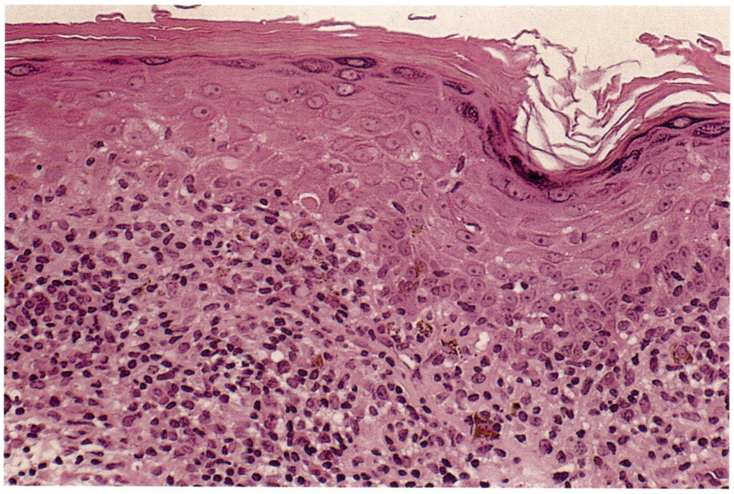

C

Figures 30–23A, 30–23B, 30–23C. Lichenoid keratosis, pigmented. Dense, lichenoid infiltrate with irregular epidermal hyperplasia. There is compact hyperkeratosis, necrotic keratinocytes, melanophages, and a mixed inflammatory cell infiltrate.

PALE-CELL ACANTHOMA

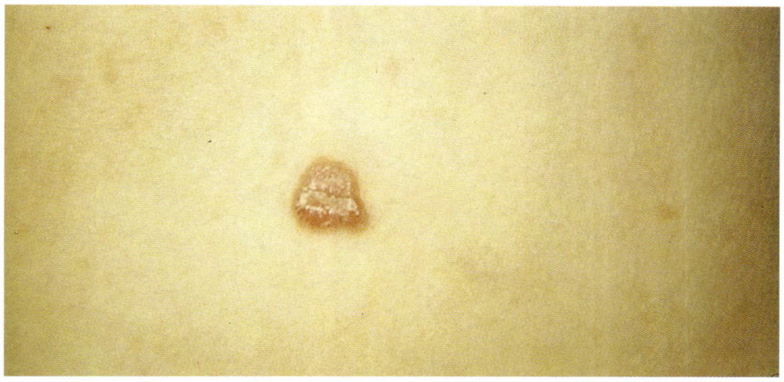

Figure 30–24. Pale-cell acanthoma. Raised, erythematous, crusted plaque on the abdomen of a woman.

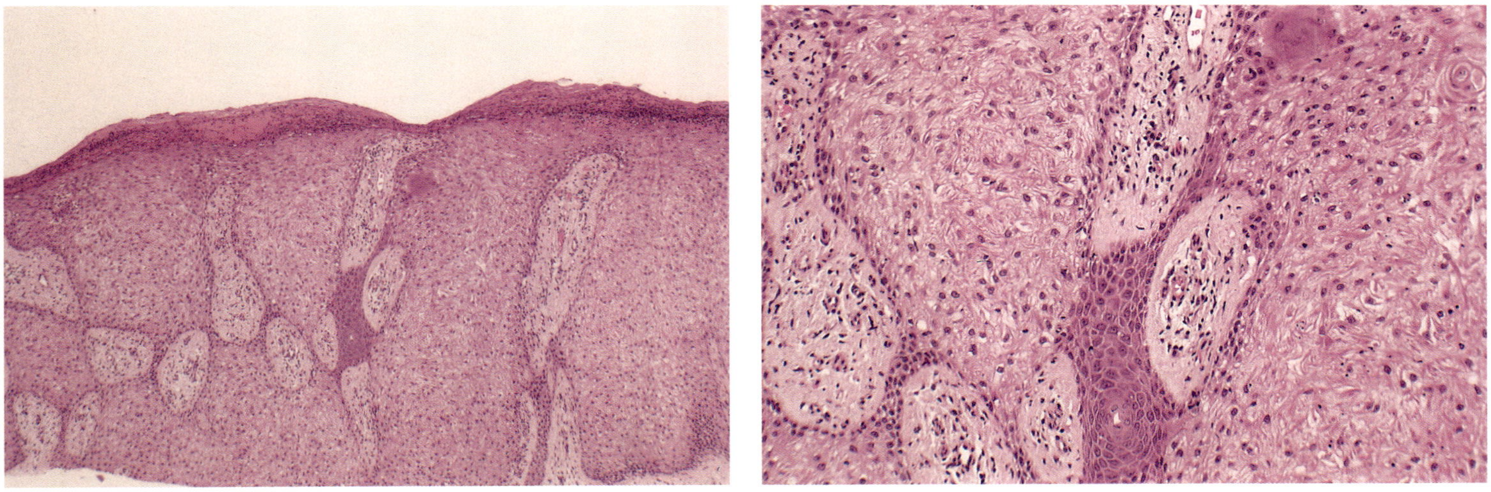

A B

Figures 30–25A, 30–25B. Pale-cell acanthoma. Pale keratinocytes and epidermal hyperplasia. The conspicuous pale keratinocytes spare adnexal structures, and neutrophils are scattered throughout the epidermis and within the overlying scale-crust.

31

PRECANCEROUS AND MALIGNANT NEOPLASMS OF THE EPIDERMIS

- Atypical keratinocytic neoplasms
  - *A) Solar keratosis (actinic keratosis, senile keratosis, squamous-cell carcinoma in situ, evolving squamous-cell carcinoma)*
  - *B) Arsenical keratosis (squamous-cell carcinoma in situ)*
  - *C) Bowen's disease/erythroplasia of Queyrat (squamous-cell carcinoma in situ)*
  - *D) Keratoacanthoma (squamous-cell carcinoma, keratoacanthomatous type)*
- Squamous-cell carcinoma
- Basal-cell carcinoma
- Extramammary Paget's disease

ATYPICAL KERATINOCYTIC NEOPLASMS

A) Solar Keratosis (actinic keratosis, senile keratosis, squamous-cell carcinoma in situ, evolving squamous-cell carcinoma)

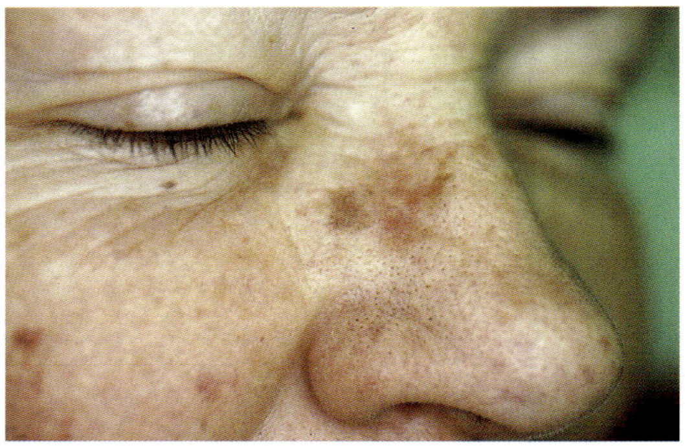

Figure 31–1. Solar keratosis. Pink and brown, rough, keratotic patch on the nose of an older woman.

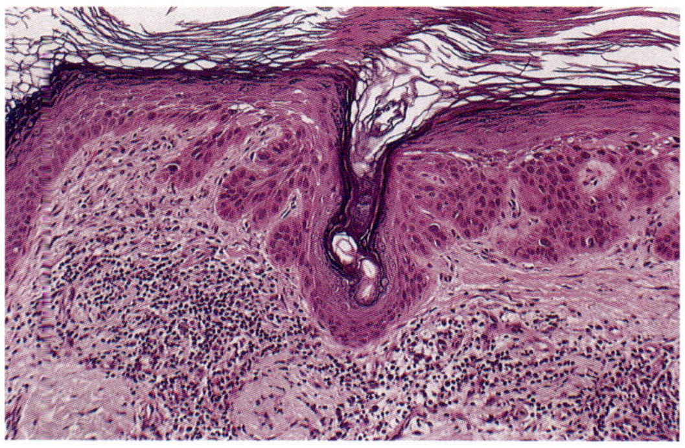

A

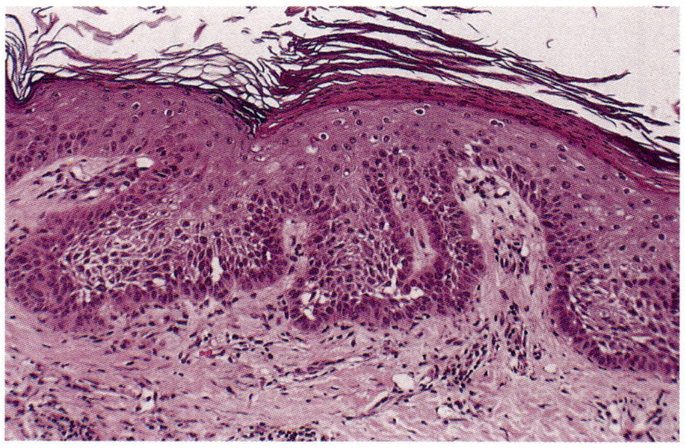

B

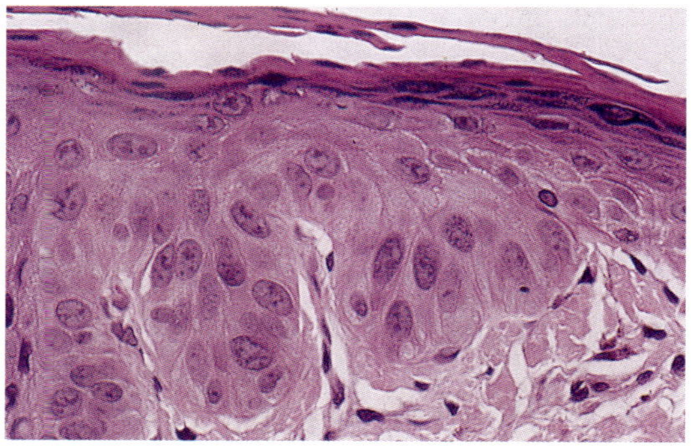

C

Figures 31–2A, 31–2B, 31–2C. Solar keratosis. Atypical, large, pleomorphic keratinocytes extend into the papillary dermis. There is alternating orthokeratosis and parakeratosis, foci of epidermal suprabasilar clefting, and dermal solar elastosis with an accompanying patchy lymphohistiocytic infiltrate.

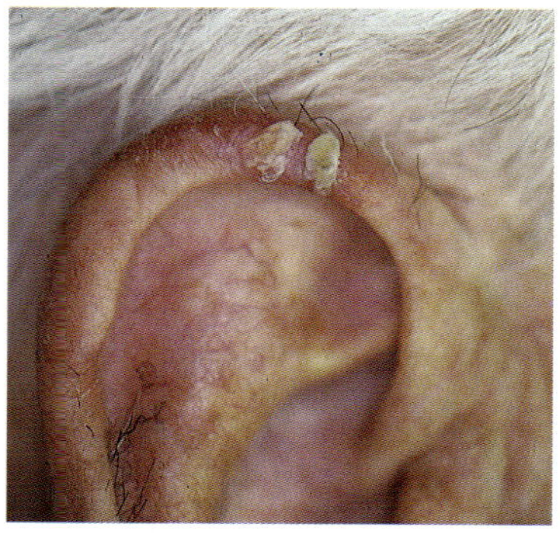

Figure 31–3. Solar keratosis, digitate type. Raised, keratotic horns within a scaly, erythematous patch on the rim of the ear.

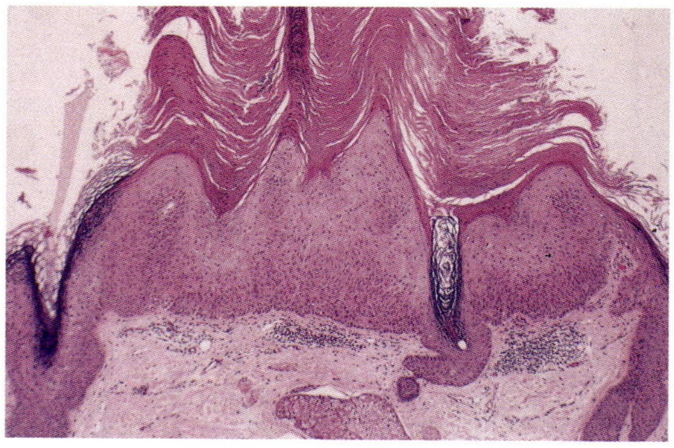

Figure 31–4. Solar keratosis, digitate type. Tiers of parakeratosis, hyperkeratosis, and atypical epidermal keratinocytes. Atypical keratinocytes involve all levels of the epidermis, and there are dilated blood vessels, solar elastosis, and a patchy lymphohystiocytic infiltrate in the dermis.

ATYPICAL KERATINOCYTIC NEOPLASMS

B) Arsenical keratosis (squamous-cell carcinoma in situ)

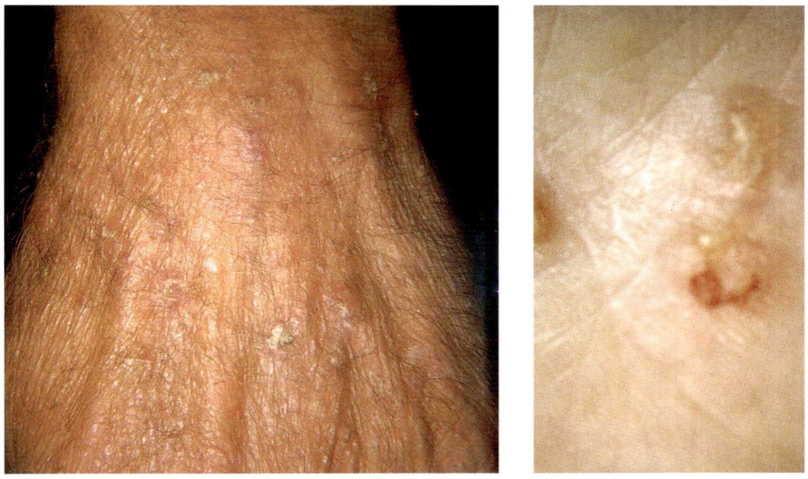

A B

Figures 31–5A, 31–5B. Arsenical keratoses. Keratotic macules and papules on the dorsum and palm of the hand of a patient with arsenical keratoses. Arsenical keratoses on the dorsum of the hand may be mistaken for solar keratoses.

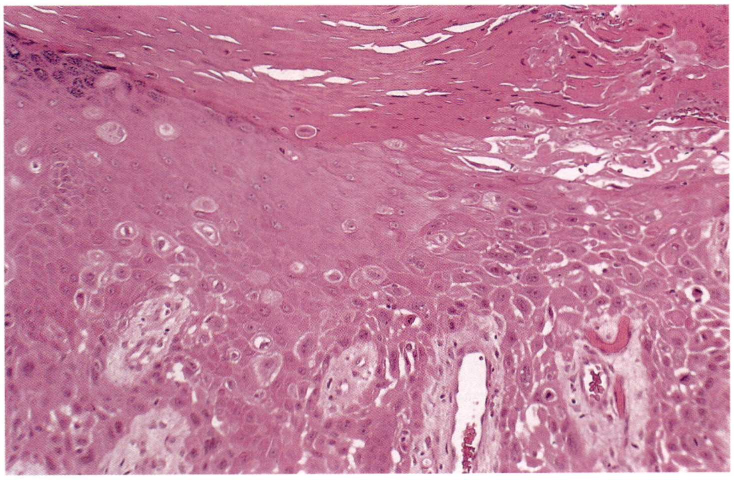

Figure 31–6. Arsenical keratosis. Atypical and pleomorphic keratinocytes involve all levels of the epidermis. There is compact hyperkeratosis, necrotic keratinocytes, and numerous mitotic figures.

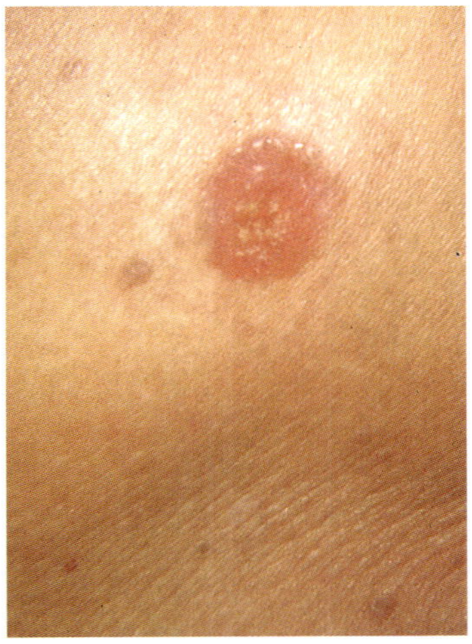

Figure 31–7. Arsenical (squamous-cell) carcinoma. Erythematous plaque on the back of a man with numerous arsenical keratoses. This is an example of the progression of an arsenical keratosis. This lesion came from the same patient shown in Figures 31–5A and 31–5B.

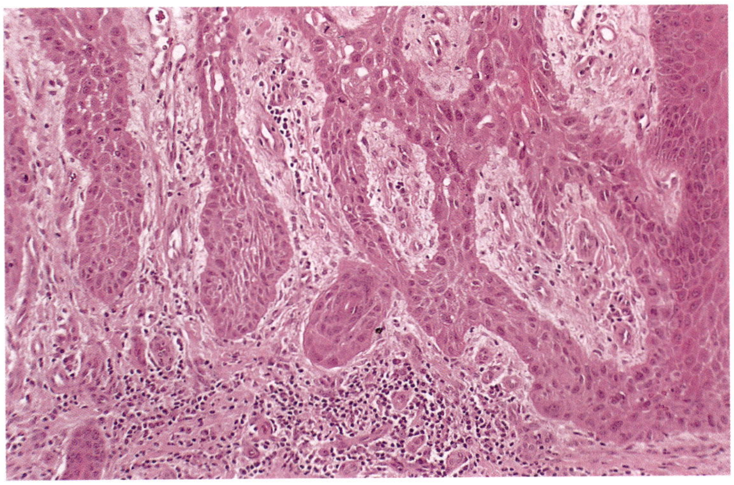

Figure 31–8. Arsenical (squamous-cell) carcinoma. Atypical and pleomorphic keratinocytes extend into the dermis.

ATYPICAL KERATINOCYTIC NEOPLASMS

C) Bowen's disease/erythroplasia of Queyrat (squamous-cell carcinoma in situ)

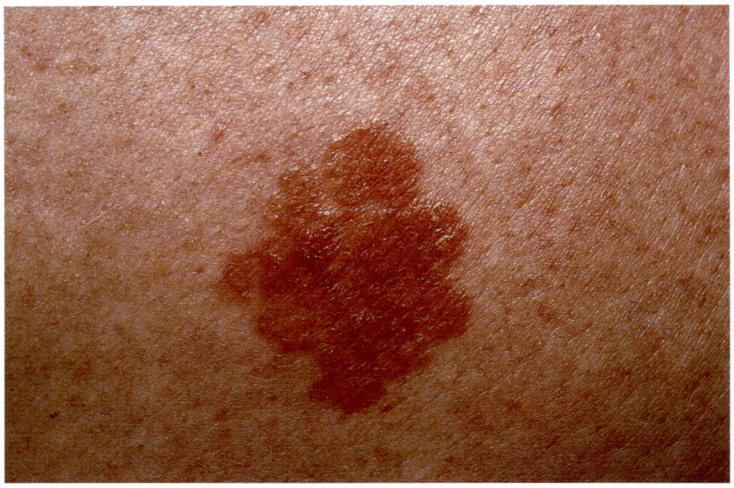

Figure 31–9. Bowen's disease. Irregular erythematous plaque.

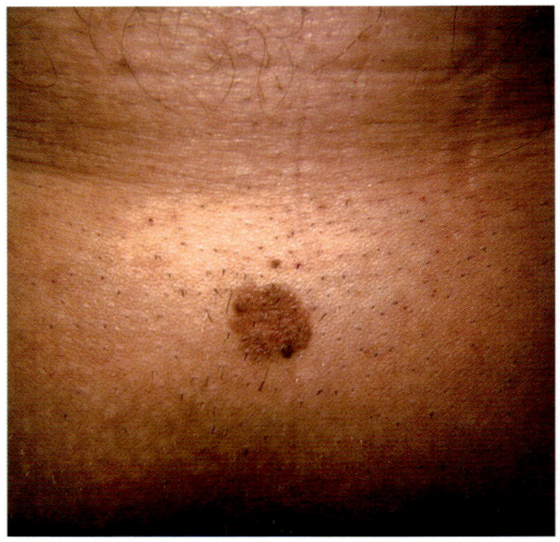

Figure 31–10. Bowen's disease. Irregular pigmented plaque on the pubis.

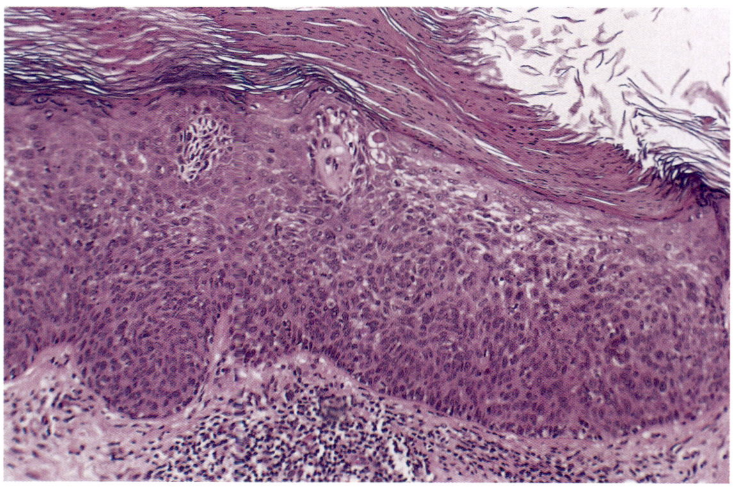

A

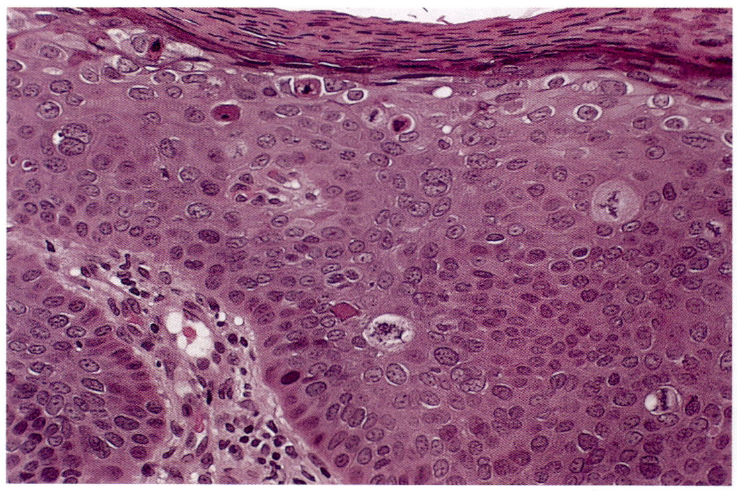

B

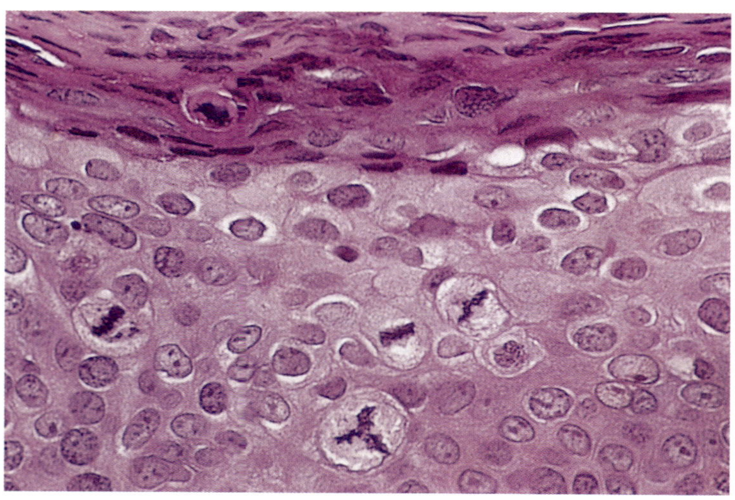

C

Figures 31–11A, 31–11B, 31–11C. Bowen's disease/erythroplasia of Queyrat. Atypical and pleomorphic keratinocytes at all levels of the hyperplastic epidermis. Bizarre, large individual and multinucleate keratinocytes. Necrotic keratinocytes and cells with typical and atypical mitotic figures are also present.

ATYPICAL KERATINOCYTIC NEOPLASMS

D) Keratoacanthoma (squamous-cell carcinoma, keratoacanthomatous type)

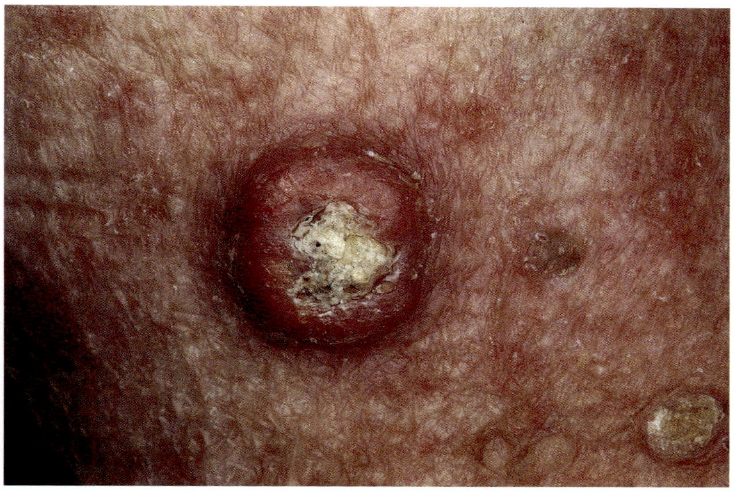

Figure 31–12. Keratoacanthoma. Erythematous nodule with a large, central keratotic crater on severely sun-damaged skin.

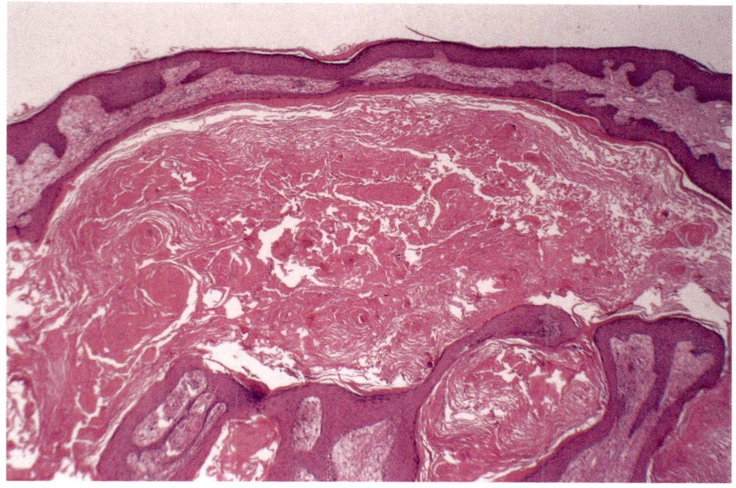

Figure 31–13. Keratoacanthoma. Liplike, epithelial extensions over the keratin-filled crater.

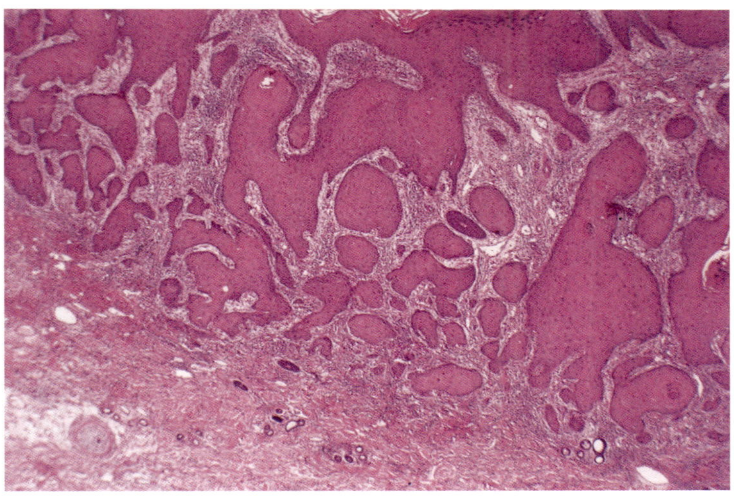

Figure 31–14. Keratoacanthoma. Columns of epithelial cells extend into the dermis where there is fibroplasia and a mixed-cell infiltrate.

ATYPICAL KERATINOCYTIC NEOPLASMS

D) Keratoacanthoma (squamous-cell carcinoma, keratoacanthomatous type) *(con't)*

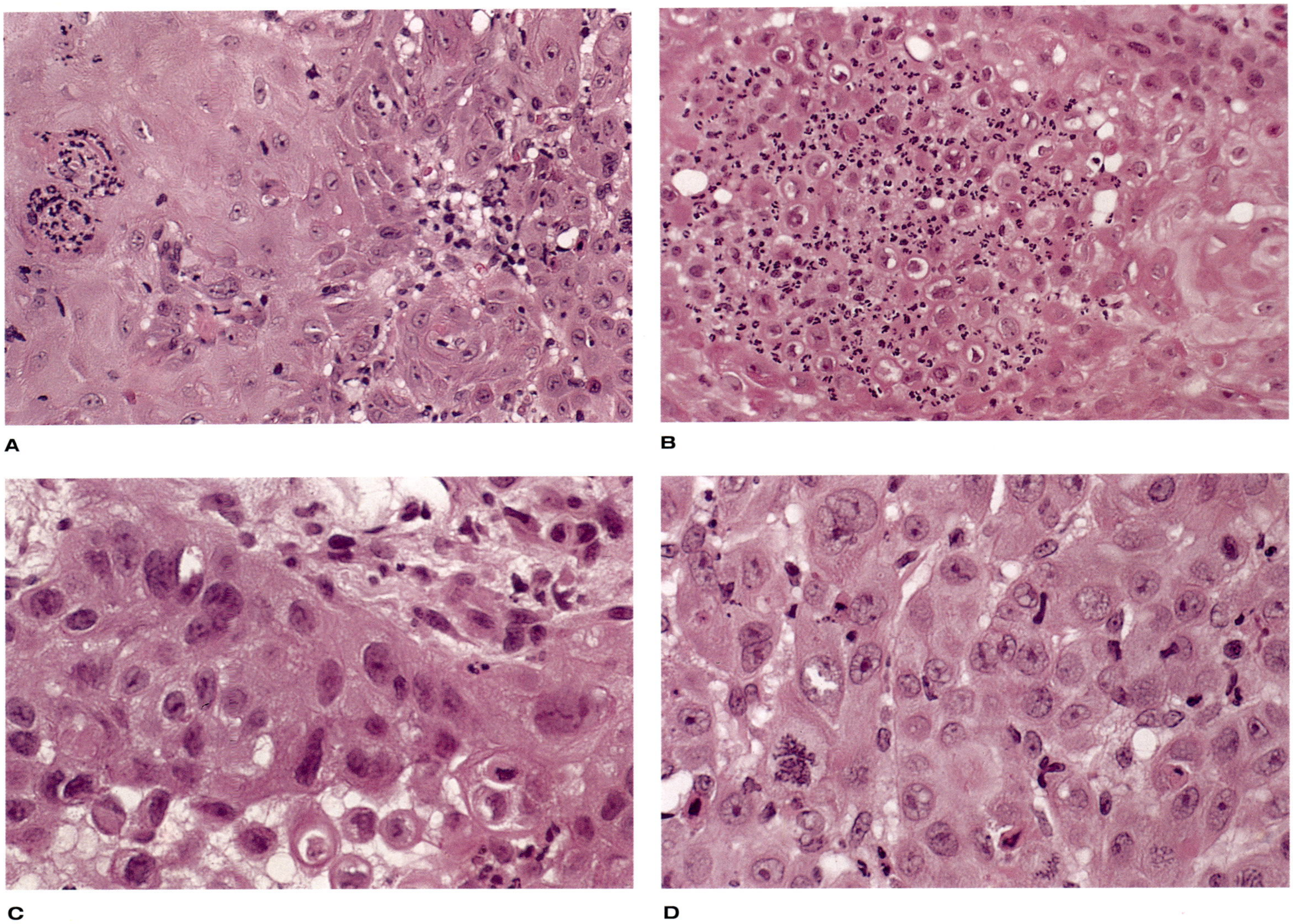

Figures 31–15A, 31–15B, 31–15C, 31–15D. Keratoacanthoma. Large, pale-staining keratinocytes surround neutrophilic abscesses. There are atypical necrotic and acantholytic keratinocytes. Variable numbers of mitotic figures may be seen.

SQUAMOUS-CELL CARCINOMA

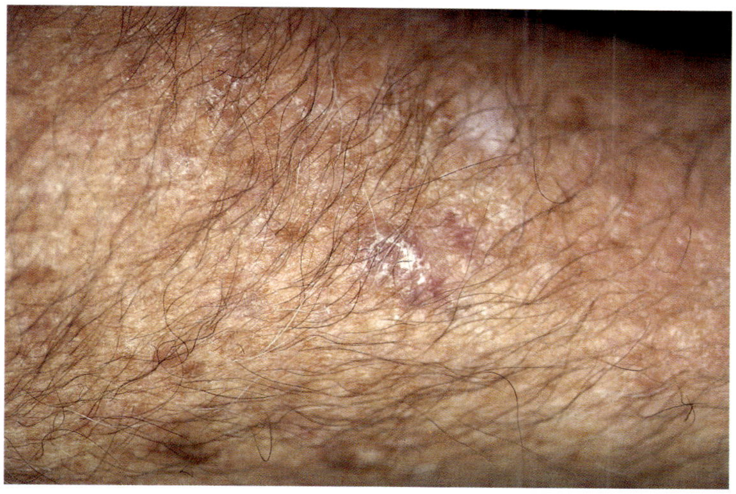

Figure 31–16. Squamous-cell carcinoma, superficial type. Erythematous, scaly, keratotic plaque on the arm of a man with severely sun-damaged skin.

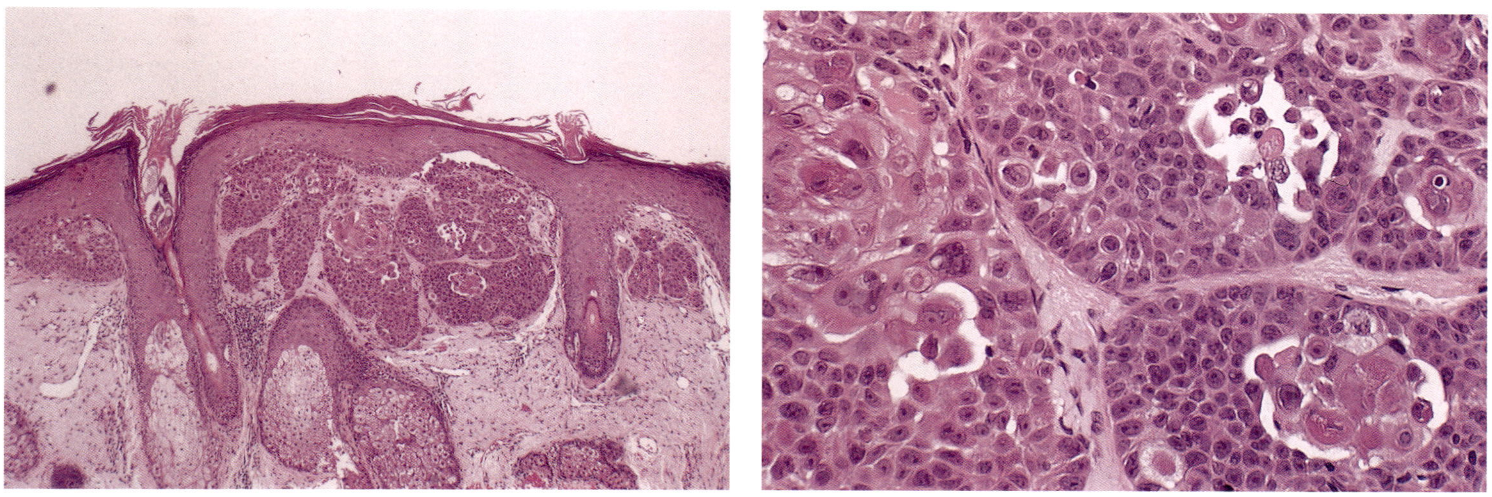

A B

Figures 31–17A, 31–17B. Squamous-cell carcinoma, superficial type. Nests and columns of atypical keratinocytes extend from the epidermis into the superficial dermis where there is severe solar elastosis, dilated blood vessels, and a patchy mononuclear cell infiltrate. There are pleomorphic, dyskeratotic, acantholytic keratinocytes, with occasional mitotic figures. On the left, **(31–17A)**, there is an adjacent, solitary nest of atypical keratinocytes at the dermoepidermal junction, which strongly suggests that this lesion evolved from a solar keratosis.

SQUAMOUS-CELL CARCINOMA

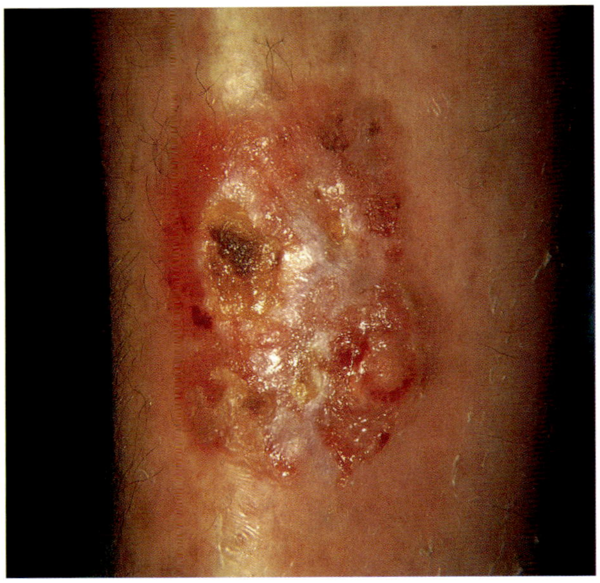

Figure 31–18. Squamous-cell carcinoma. Crusted and ulcerated erythematous plaque on the lower leg of a man.

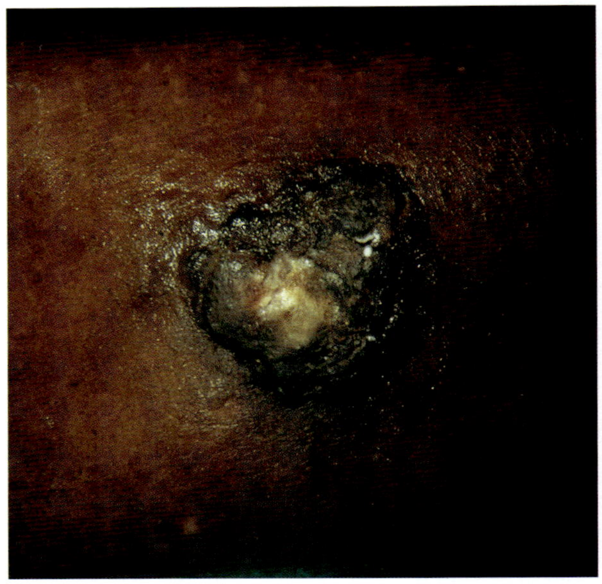

Figure 31–19. Squamous-cell carcinoma. Hyperpigmented, ulcerated, and crusted nodule on the lower leg of an African-American man.

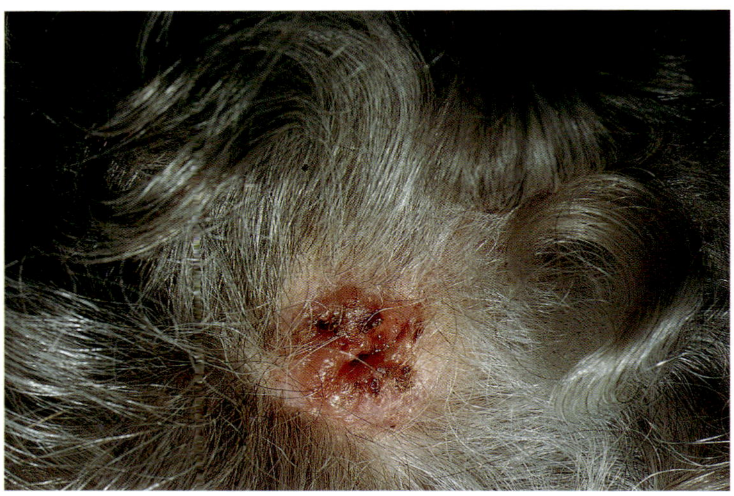

Figure 31–20. Squamous-cell carcinoma. Crusted and ulcerated plaque in the scalp of an older woman.

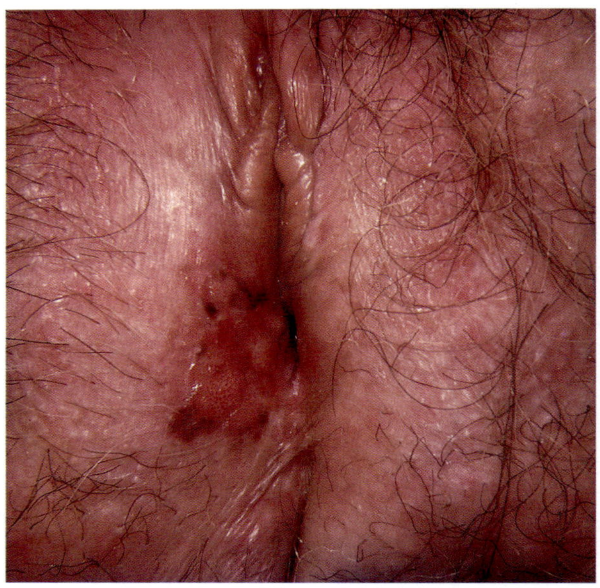

Figure 31–21. Squamous-cell carcinoma. Irregularly pigmented, ulcerated, verrucous plaque on the labia of an older woman.

SQUAMOUS-CELL CARCINOMA

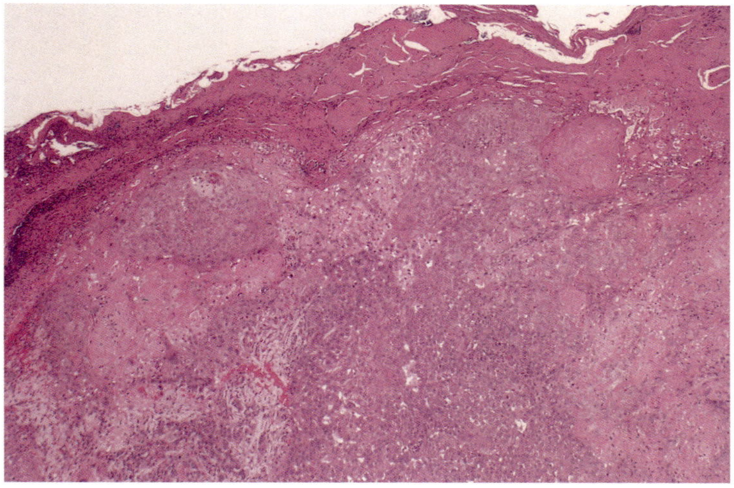

A

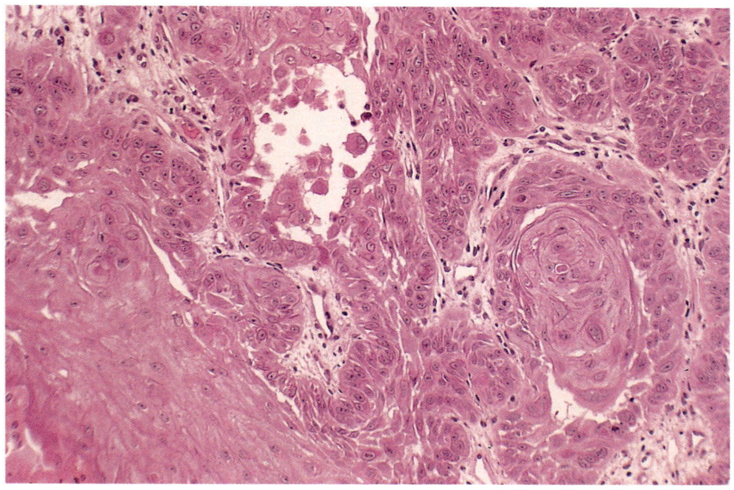

B

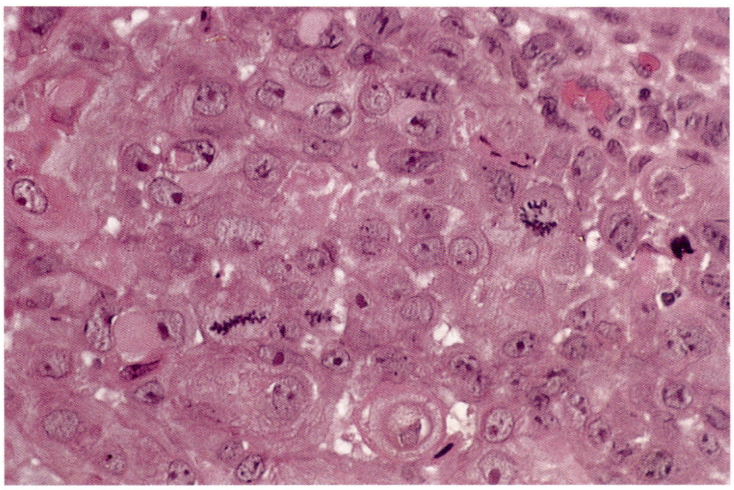

C

Figures 31–22A, 31–22B, 31–22C. Squamous-cell carcinoma. Epidermal scale-crust with sheets of pale-staining, pleomorphic, atypical keratinocytes that extend deep into the reticular dermis. There are ribbons of acantholytic, atypical keratinocytes, and there are many typical and atypical mitotic figures and necrotic cells.

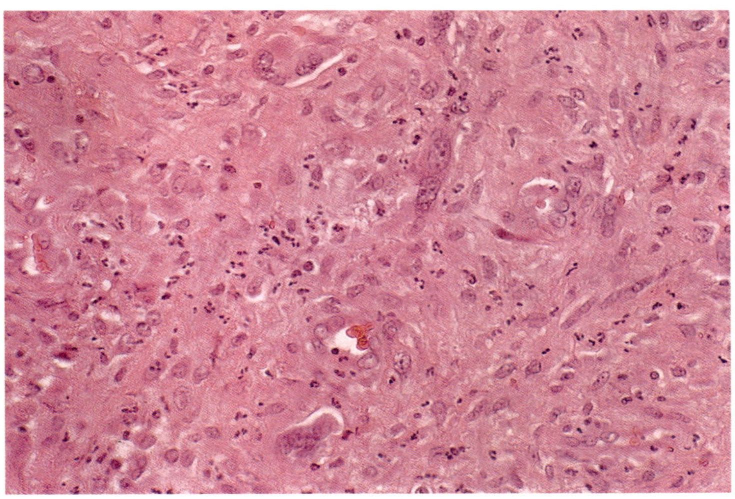

Figure 31–23. Squamous-cell carcinoma, spindle-cell type. Atypical oval and spindle-shaped keratinocytes in the dermis intermingled with many neutrophils.

BASAL-CELL CARCINOMA

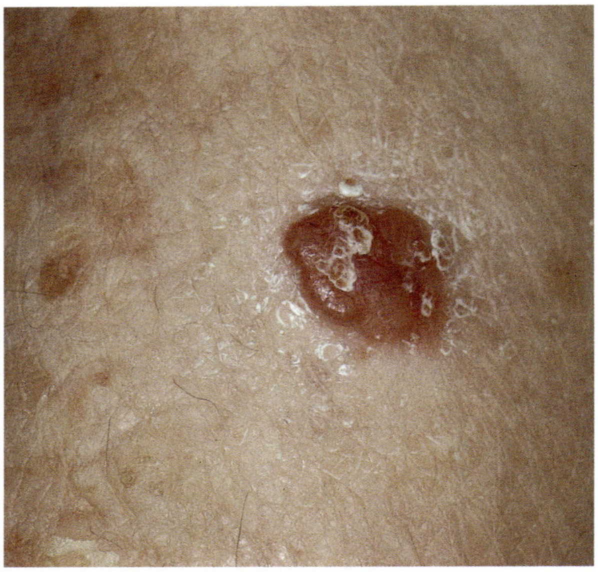

Figure 31–24. Basal-cell carcinoma, nodular type. Erythematous, fleshy, telangiectatic nodule.

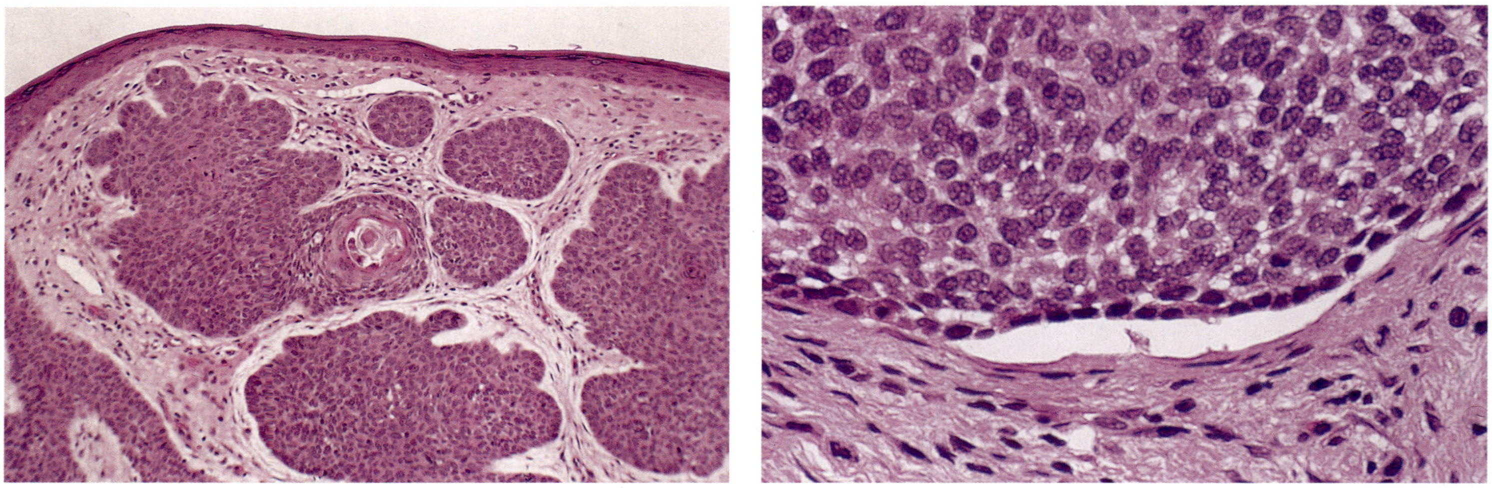

A **B**

Figures 31–25A, 31–25B. Basal-cell carcinoma, nodular type. Small and large irregularly shaped nodules of neoplastic basaloid cells. There are necrotic basaloid cells, and there are clefts separating the tumor nodules from the surrounding stroma.

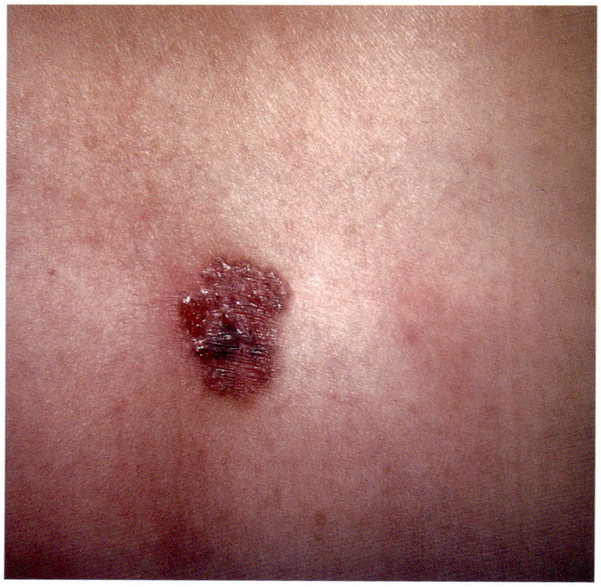

Figure 31–26. Basal-cell carcinoma, pigmented type. Irregularly shaped reddish-brown plaque with stippled blue-gray pigmentation. This clinical appearance may be mistaken for a malignant melanoma.

BASAL-CELL CARCINOMA

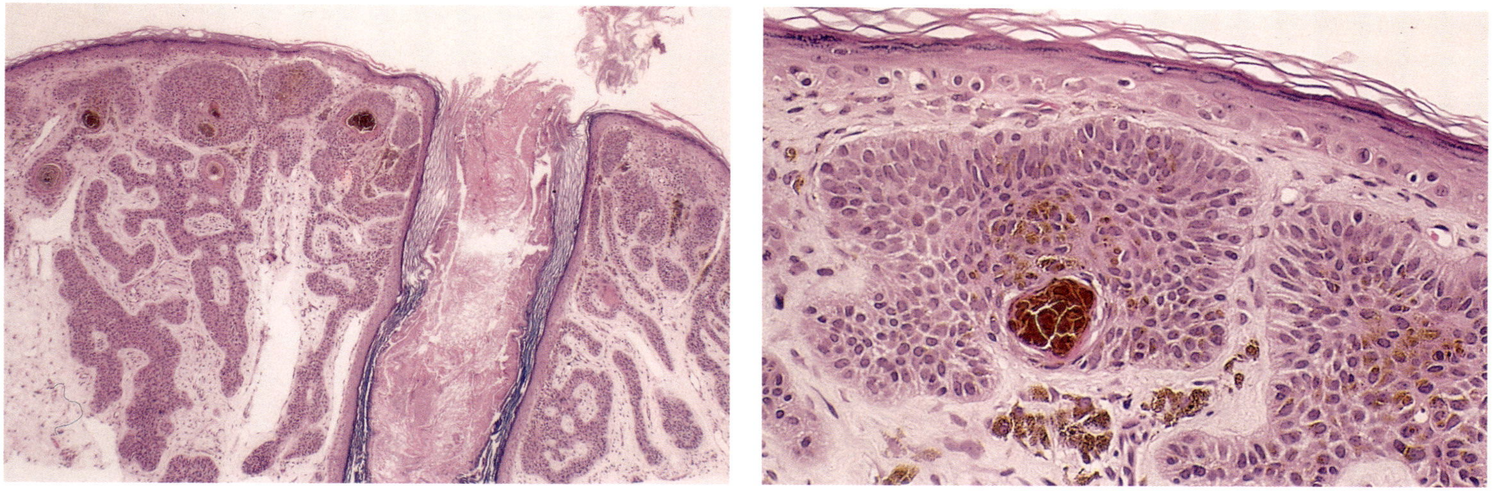

A B

Figures 31–27A, 31–27B. **Basal-cell carcinoma, pigmented type.** Variably shaped intradermal nodules and columns of neoplastic basaloid cells. Melanin is deposited within the cytoplasm of neoplastic cells and within dermal melanophages.

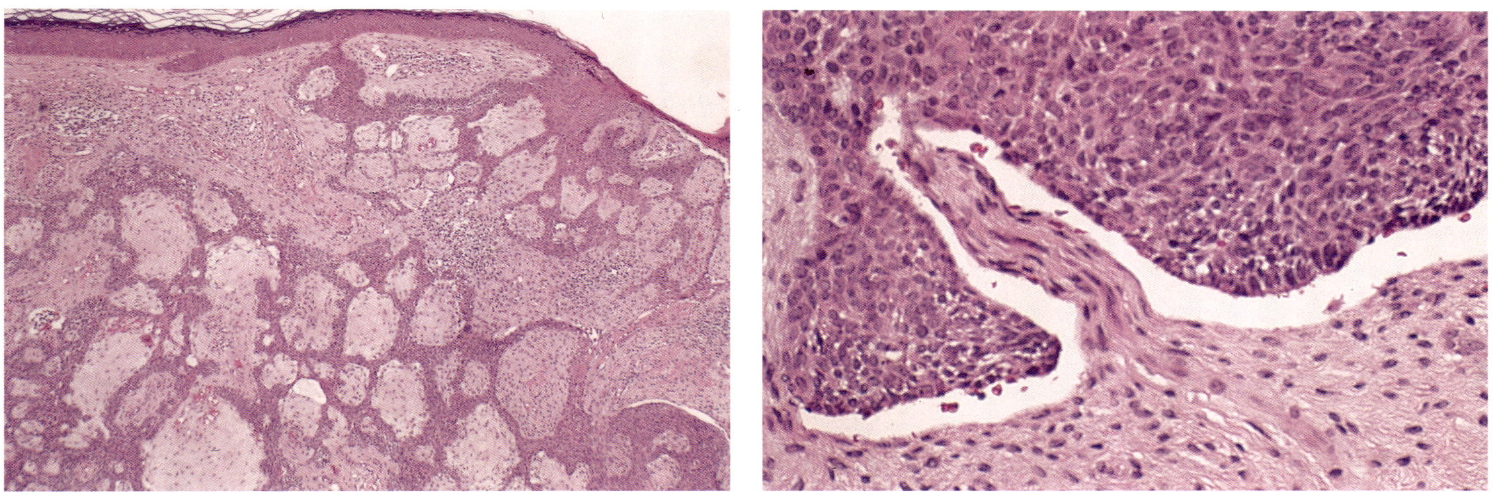

A B

Figures 31–28A, 31–28B. **Basal-cell carcinoma, fibroepithelial type.** Cords and columns of neoplastic basaloid cells in a fenestrated pattern within the dermis. Large nodules are separated by clefts from the surrounding fibrillary dermal collagen.

BASAL-CELL CARCINOMA

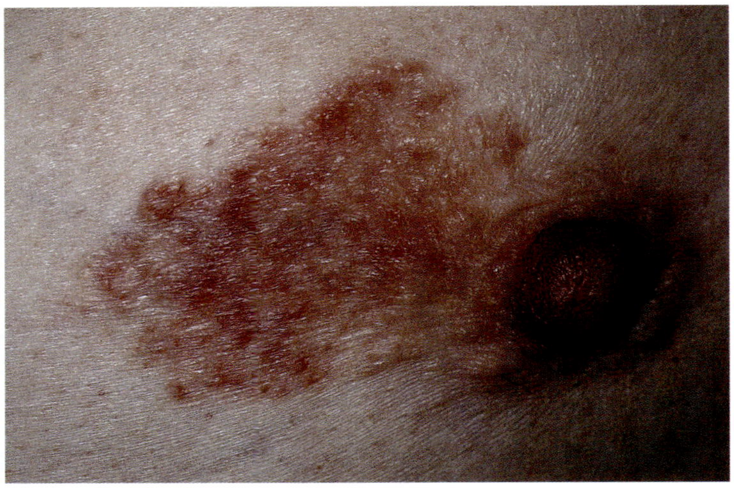

Figure 31–29. Basal-cell carcinoma, superficial type. Erythematous, poorly marginated plaque on the breast present for several years.

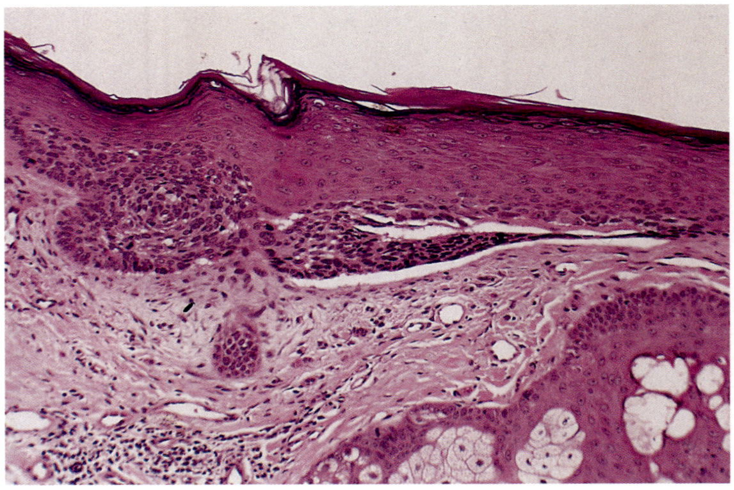

Figure 31–30. Basal-cell carcinoma, superficial type. Nests of neoplastic basaloid cells with a horizontal cleft separating it from the papillary dermis.

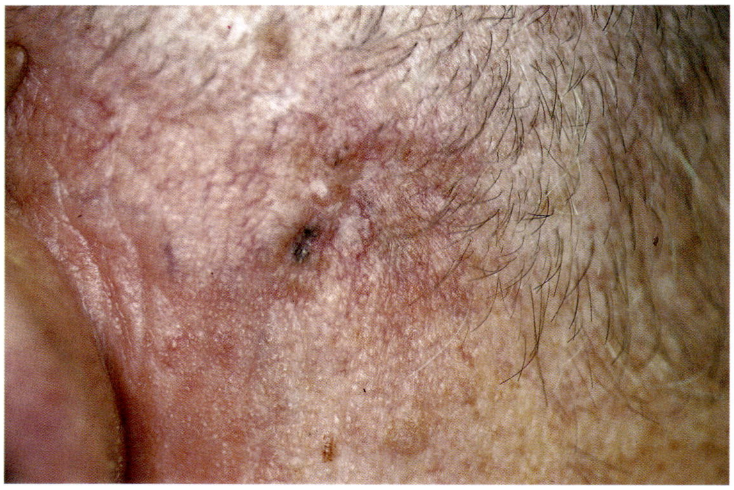

Figure 31–31. Basal-cell carcinoma, morpheaform type. Firm, pale, telangiectatic, poorly circumscribed plaque in the posterior scalp of a man.

BASAL-CELL CARCINOMA

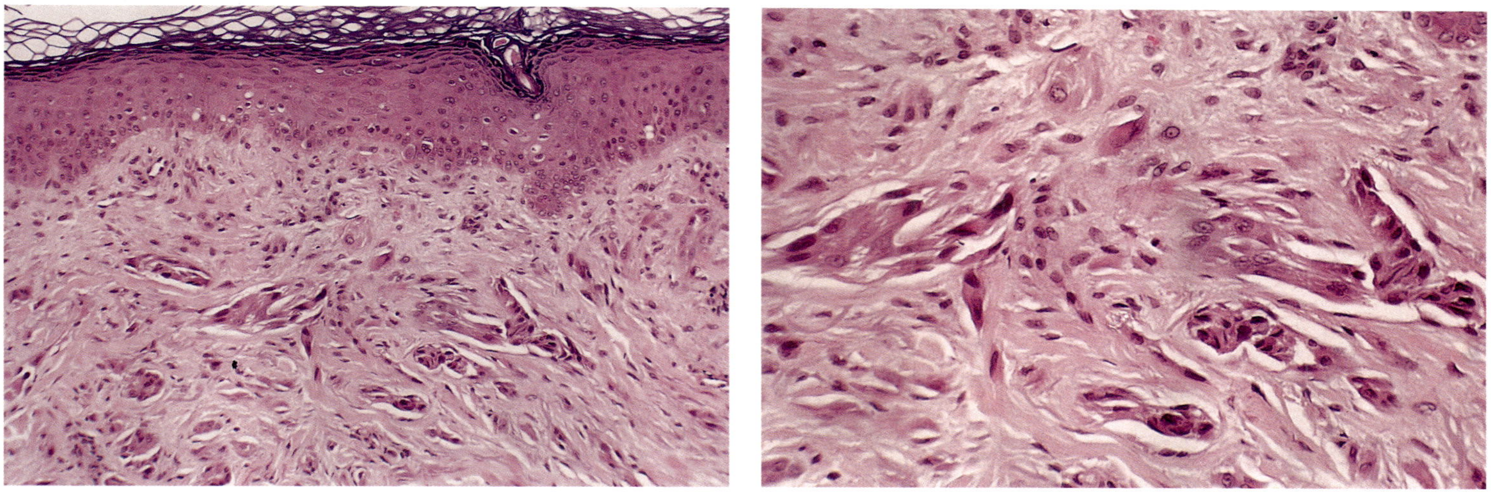

A B

Figures 31–32A, 31–32B. Basal-cell carcinoma, morpheaform type. Strands, cords, and columns and nests of oval and spindle-shaped neoplastic basaloid cells interdigitated between thickened bundles of collagen. There are clefts separating some basaloid cells from the surrounding dermal collagen.

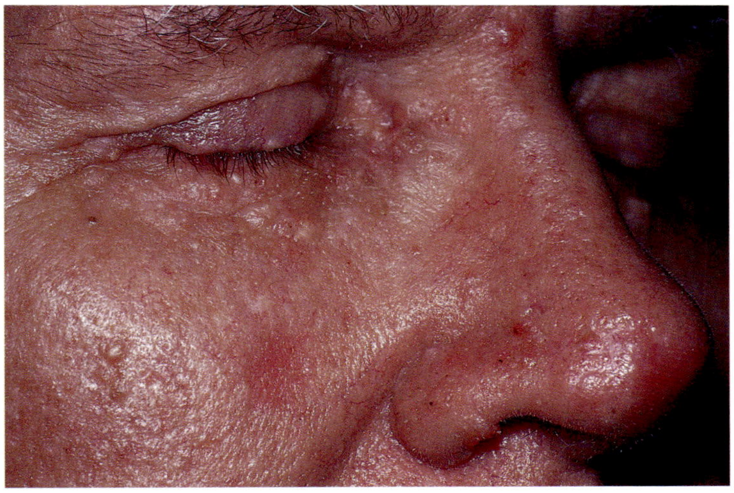

Figure 31–33. Basal-cell carcinoma, infundibulocystic type. Multiple 2 to 3 mm erythematous and skin-colored papules on the cheek, eyelids, and nose of a man.

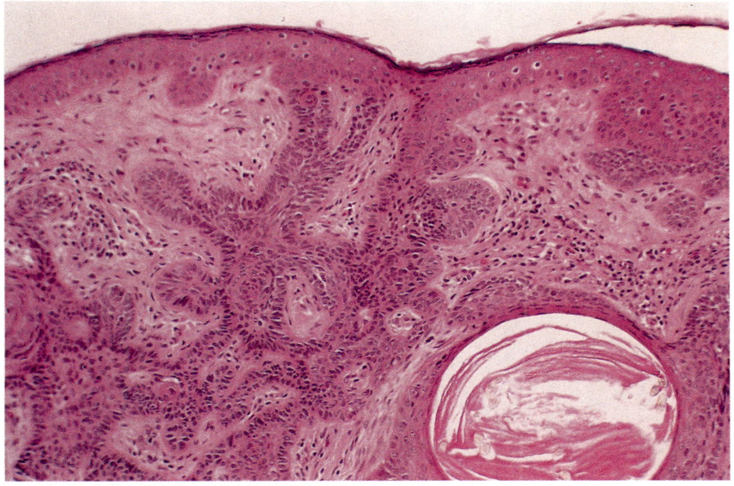

Figure 31–34. Basal-cell carcinoma, infundibulocystic type. Anastomosing columns of pink neoplastic cells continuous with several infundibula, and an infundibulocystic structure.

EXTRAMAMMARY PAGET'S DISEASE

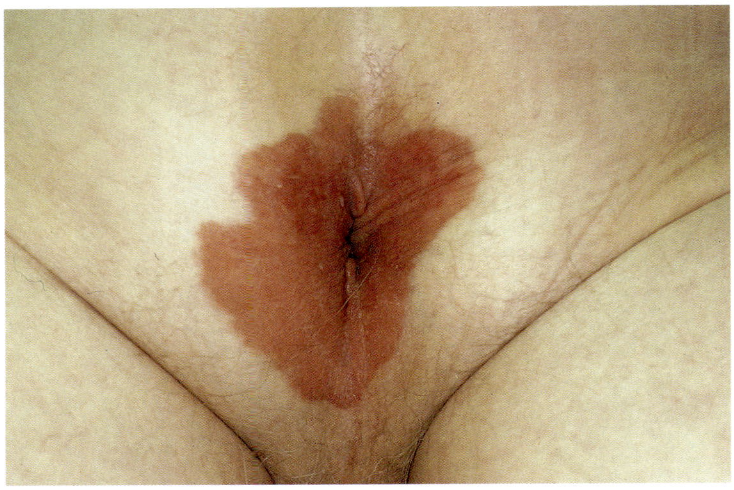

Figure 31–35. Extramammary Paget's disease. Pruritic perianal erythematous patch.

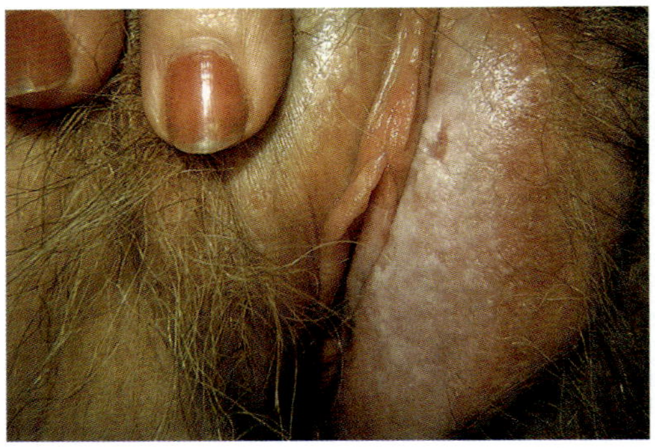

Figure 31–36. Extramammary Paget's disease. White, keratotic, ragged plaque on the labia.

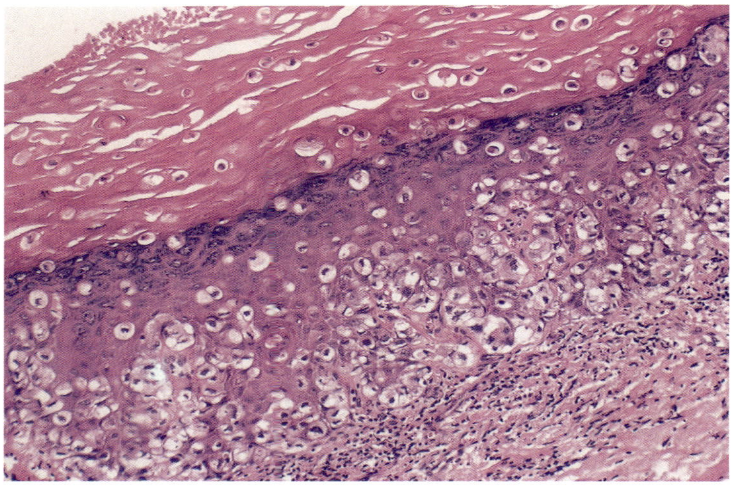

Figure 31–37. Extramammary Paget's disease. Hyperplastic epidermis with diffusely scattered atypical neoplastic cells. Tumor cells are present as solitary units and in nests at all levels of the epidermis, including the basal layer and the stratum corneum. Necrotic cells and mitotic figures are present. There is fibroplasia with a patchy lymphocytic infiltrate in the dermis.

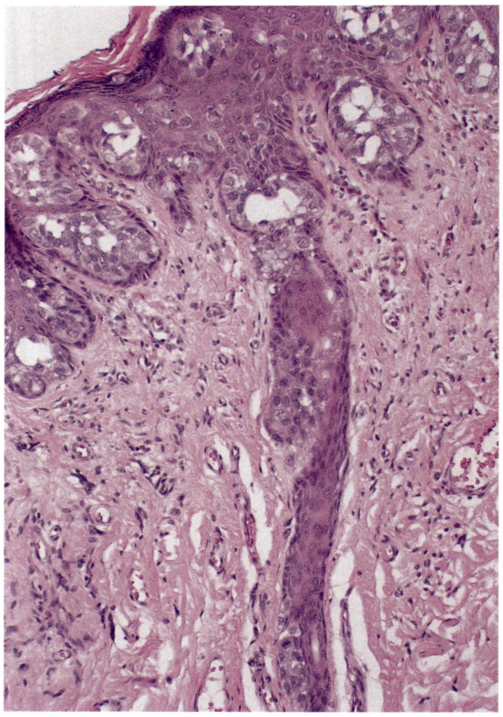

Figure 31–38. Extramammary Paget's disease. Solitary units and tubular structures composed of mucin-containing neoplastic cells are present within an adnexal duct.

EXTRAMAMMARY PAGET'S DISEASE

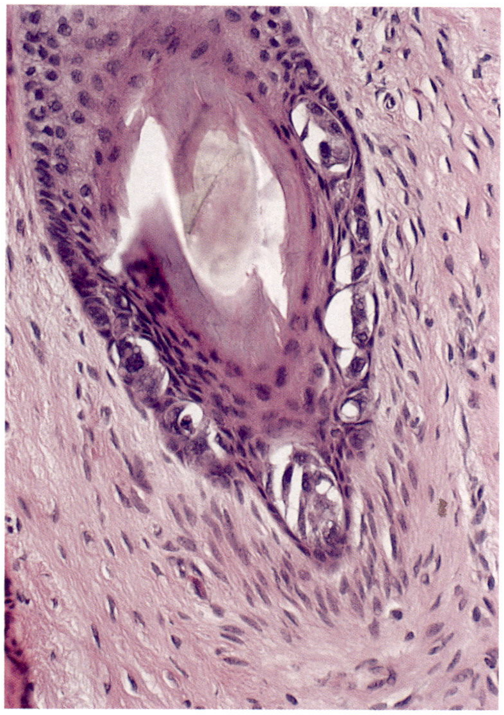

Figure 31–39. Extramammary Paget's disease. Small nests of tumor cells with ductal differentiation involve the infundibulum.

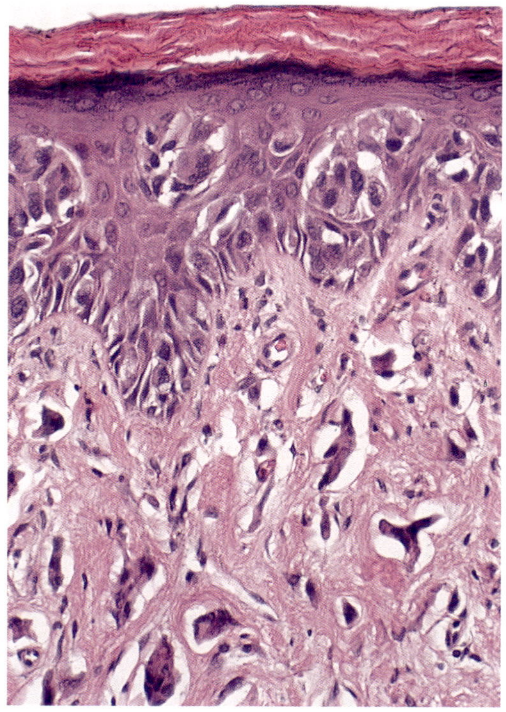

Figure 31–40. Extramammary Paget's disease with dermal involvement. Tumor cells in solitary units and nests fill the epidermis and extend into the dermis.

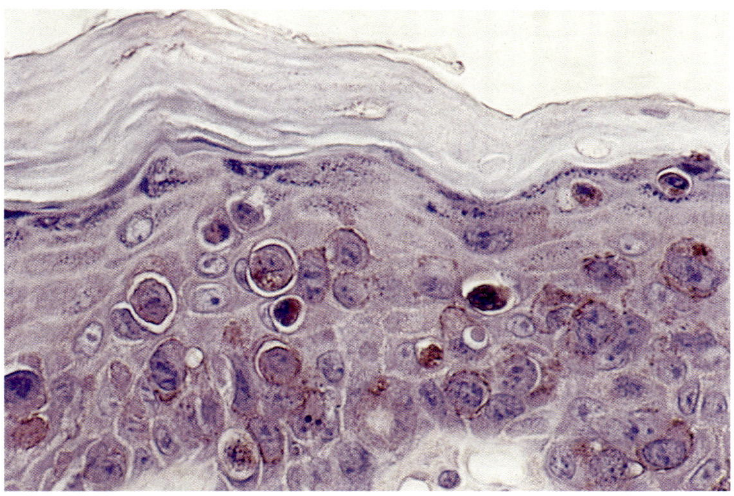

Figure 31–41. Extramammary Paget's disease. Immunoperoxidase staining with carcinoembryonic antigen (CEA) shows positive brown deposits within the neoplastic cells.

32

FOLLICULAR DISORDERS

- Nevus comedonicus
- Fibrous papule
- Trichofolliculoma
- Trichodiscoma/fibrofolliculoma
- Trichoblastoma
- Trichoepithelioma
- Desmoplastic trichoepithelioma
- Tumor of follicular infundibulum
- Pilar sheath acanthoma
- Pilomatrixoma
- Pilar tumor (proliferating follicular cystic neoplasm)
- Tricholemmoma
- Inverted follicular keratosis

NEVUS COMEDONICUS

Figure 32–1. Nevus comedonicus. Cluster of keratotic follicular papules.

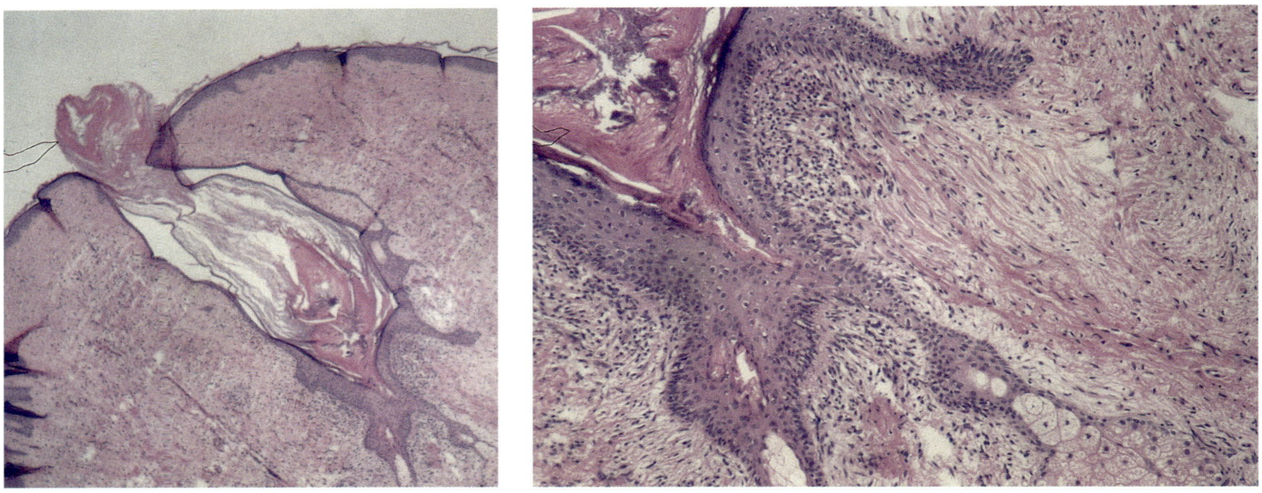

A B

Figures 32–2A, 32–2B. Nevus comedonicus. Distended, hyperkeratotic infundibulum. There is perifollicular, fibrillary fibroplasia and a patchy lymphohistiocytic infiltrate.

FIBROUS PAPULE

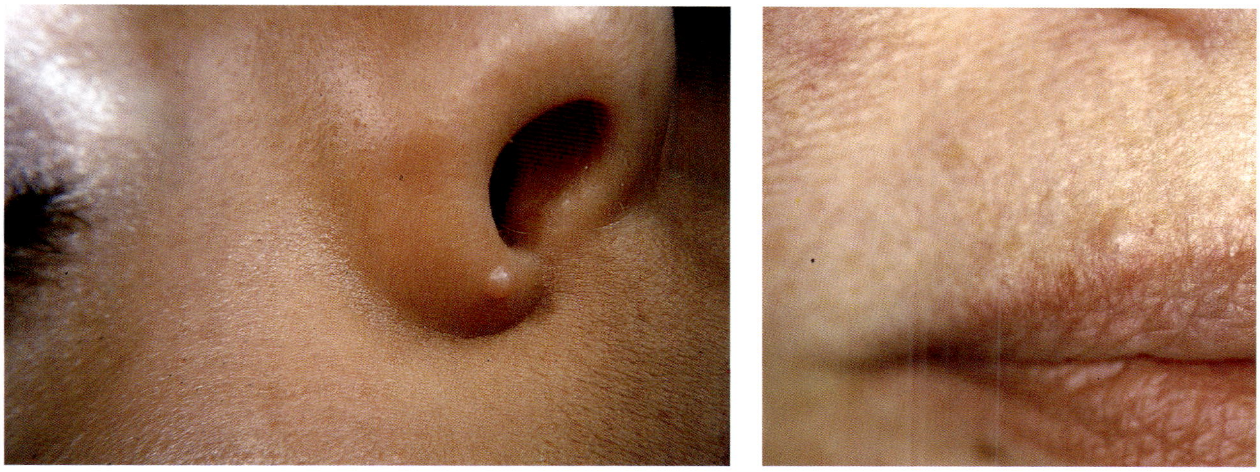

A B

Figures 32–3A, 32–3B. Fibrous papule. Skin-colored papule on the ala nasi of the nose and the upper lip.

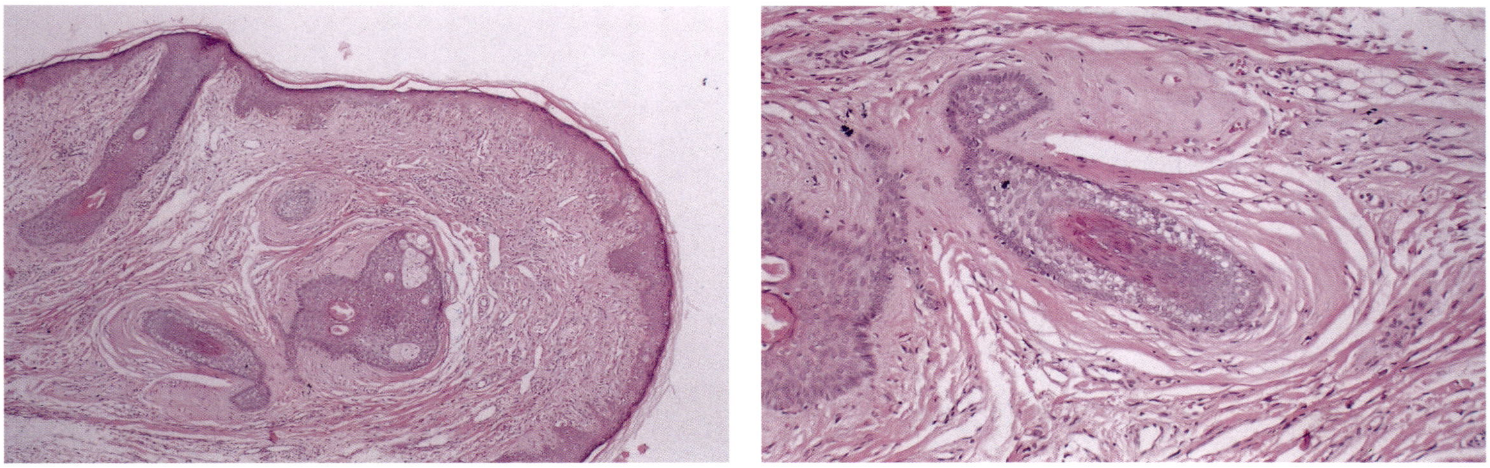

A B

Figures 32–4A, 32–4B. Fibrous papule. Folliculosebaceous units in disarray. There is fibrillary fibroplasia, which is accentuated around adnexal structures and blood vessels. Plump and stellate fibrocytes are common.

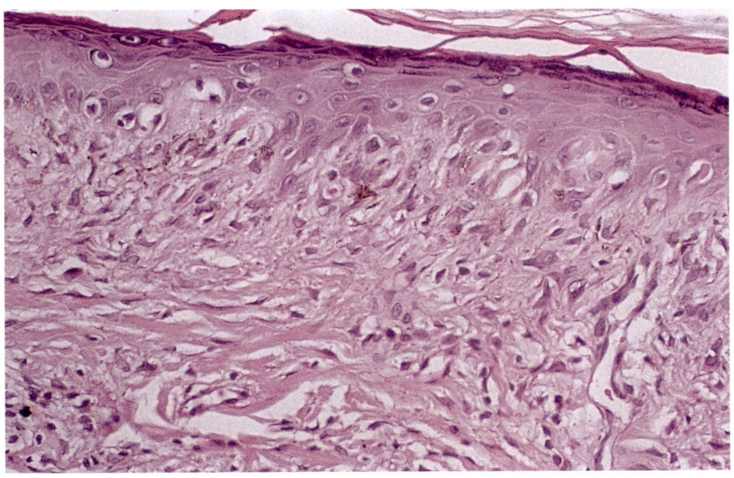

Figure 32–5. Fibrous papule. Melanocytic hyperplasia at the dermoepidermal junction.

TRICHOFOLLICULOMA

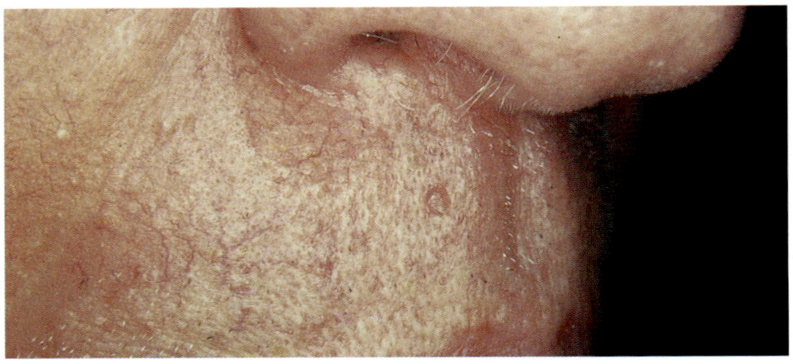

Figure 32–6. Trichofolliculoma. Pink papule with white, wispy hair shafts.

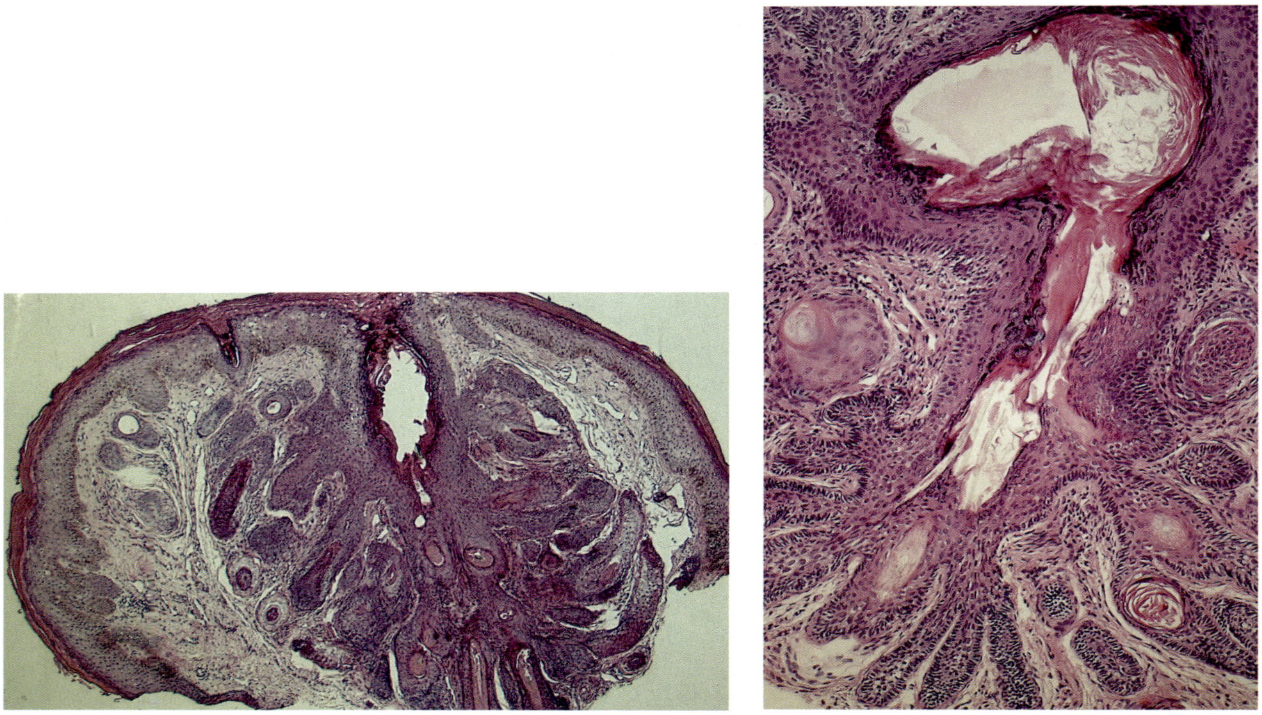

A B

Figures 32–7A. 32–7B. Trichofolliculoma. Numerous folliculosebaceous units radiate from a solitary infundibulum. Follicular germs, papillae, and inner root sheaths are apparent.

TRICHODISCOMA/FIBROFOLLICULOMA

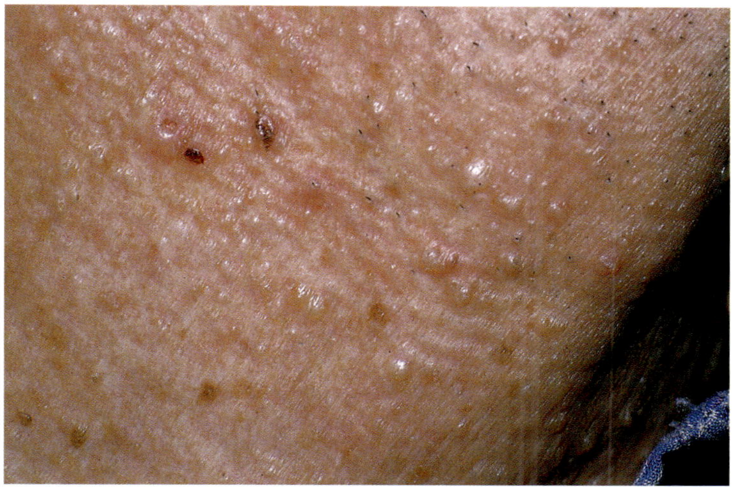

Figure 32–8. **Trichodiscoma/fibrofolliculoma.** Many skin-colored and pink follicular papules on the neck of a man.

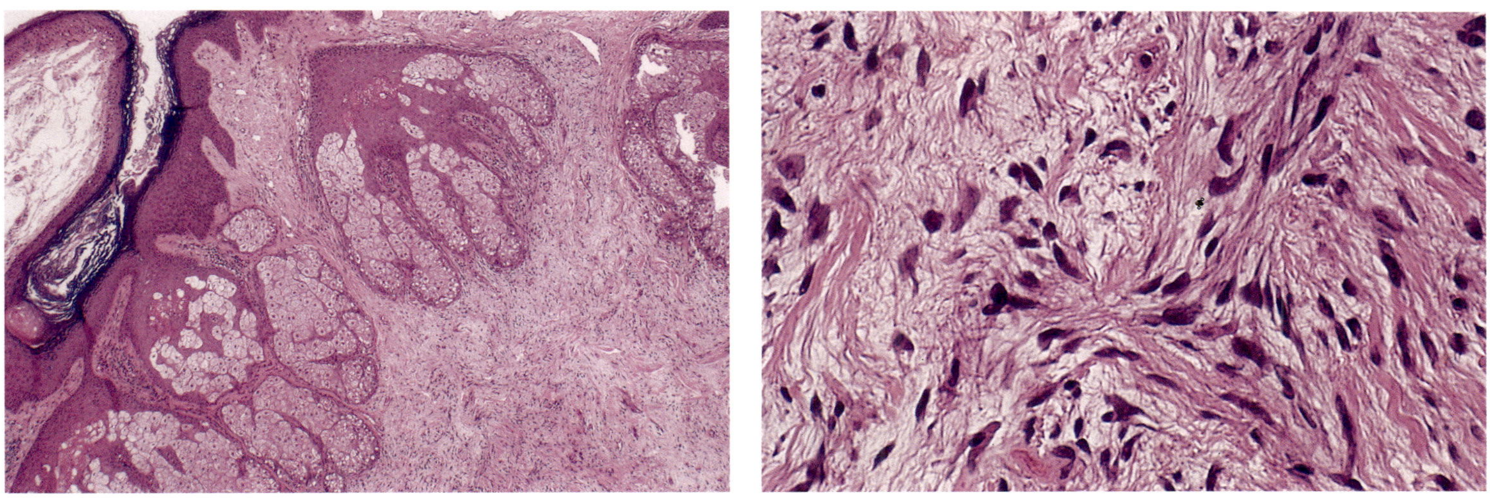

A B

Figures 32–9A, 32–9B. **Trichodiscoma/fibrofolliculoma.** Proliferation of sebaceous lobules contiguous with an infundibulum in association with dermal fibroplasia. There are many plump and stellate-shaped fibrocytes, fibrillary collagen, and mucin in the dermis.

TRICHOBLASTOMA

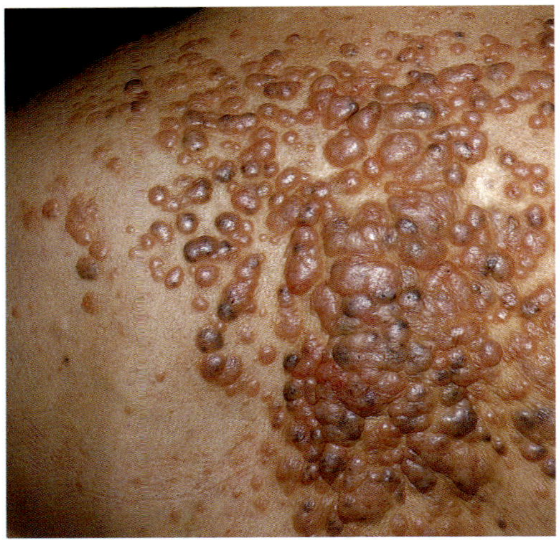

Figure 32–10. Trichoblastoma. A patient with multiple follicular tumors histologically shows various proliferative patterns.

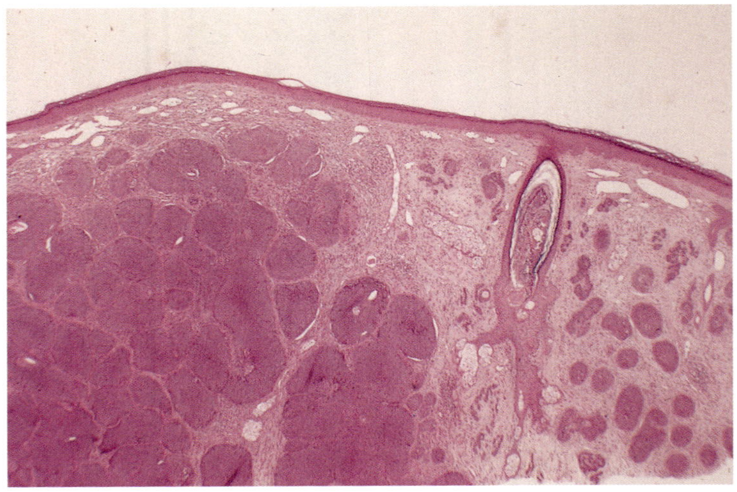

Figure 32–11. Trichoblastoma. Large nodules, small nodules, and columns of uniform basaloid cells in a fibrillary stroma.

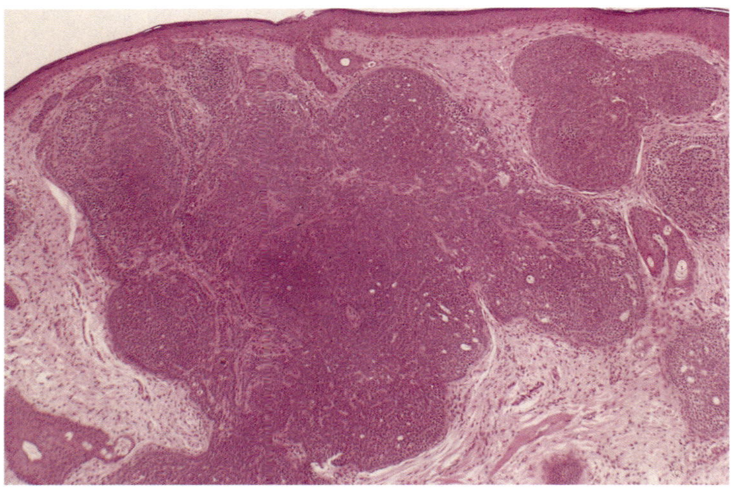

A

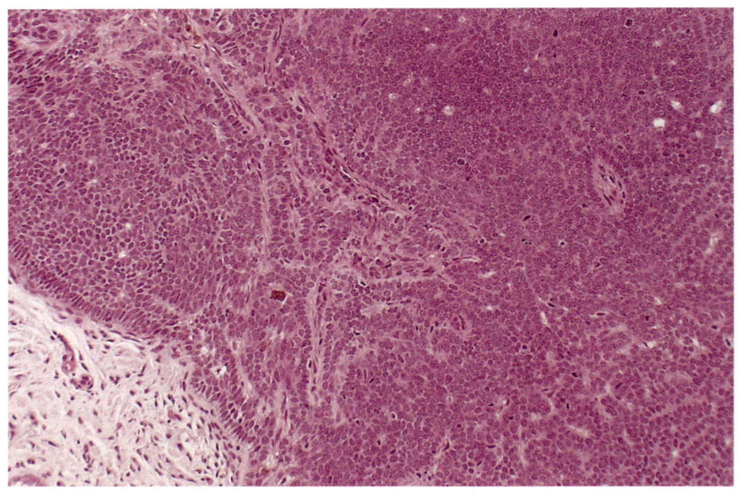

B

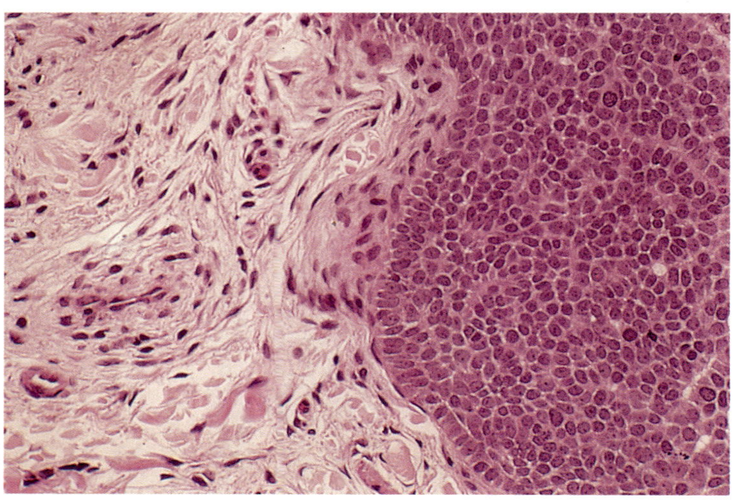

C

Figures 32–12A, 32–12B, 32–12C. Trichoblastoma. Cribriform pattern of basaloid cells. Follicular germ and papilla are identified at the edge of a nodule within fibrocytic stroma.

TRICHOEPITHELIOMA

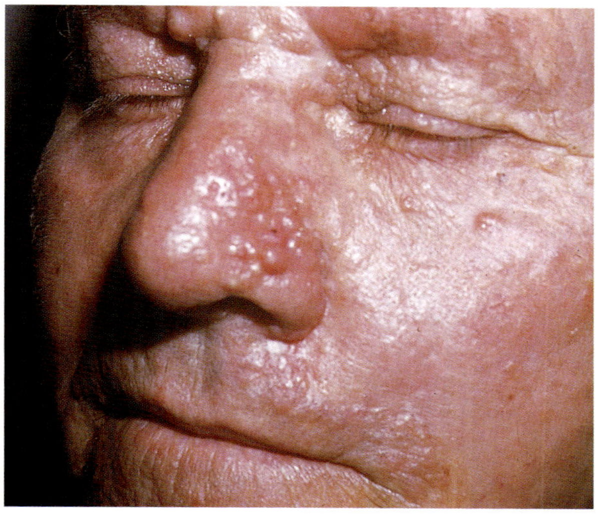

Figure 32–13. **Trichoepithelioma.** Dome-shaped papules on the face of a man.

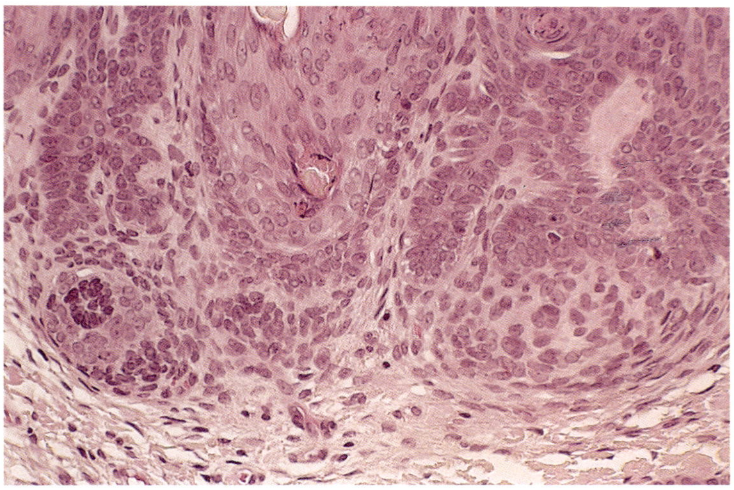

A

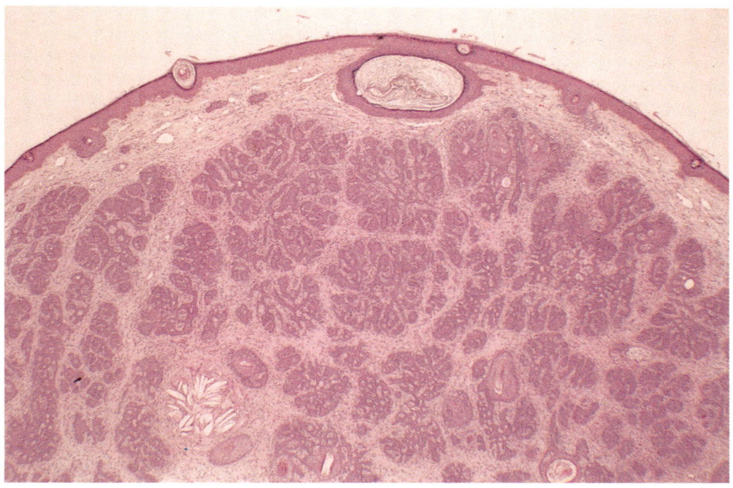

B

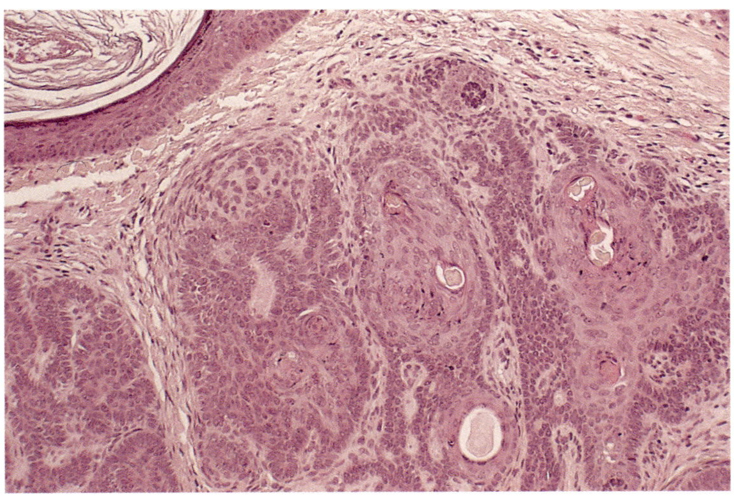

C

Figures 32–14A, 32–14B, 32–14C. **Trichoepithelioma.** Cribriform nodules of uniform basaloid cells in a distinctive fibrocytic stroma. Many follicular germs and papillae are contiguous with the nodules.

DESMOPLASTIC TRICHOEPITHELIOMA

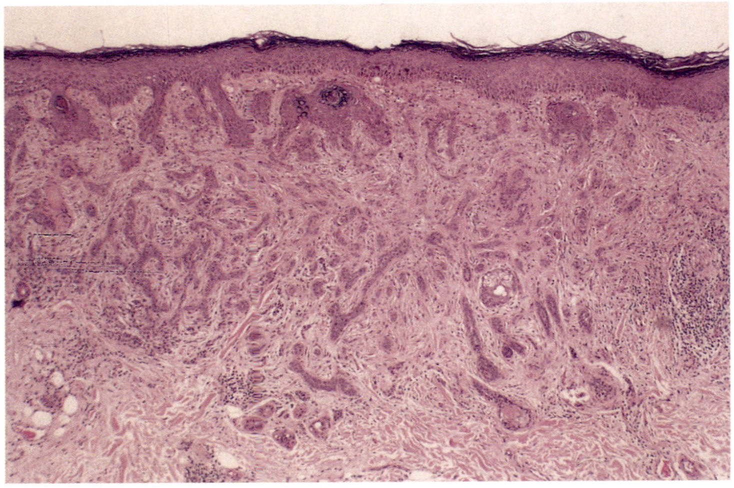

A

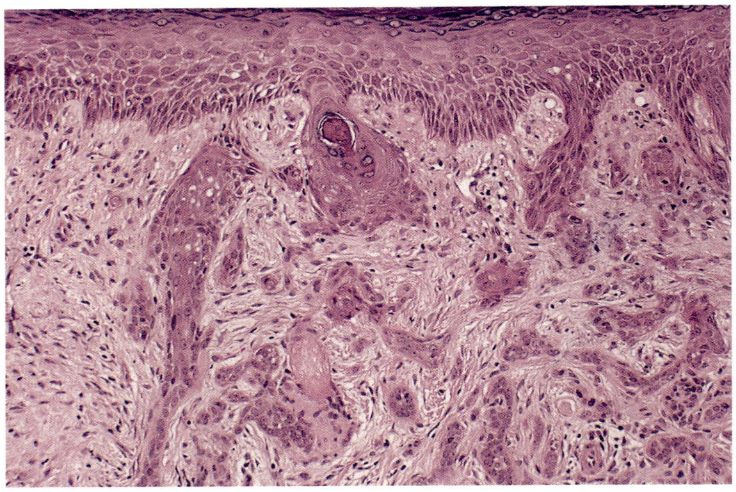

B

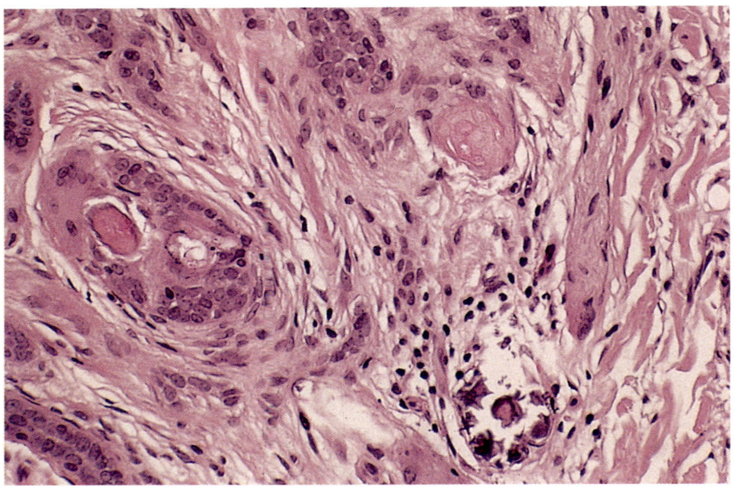

C

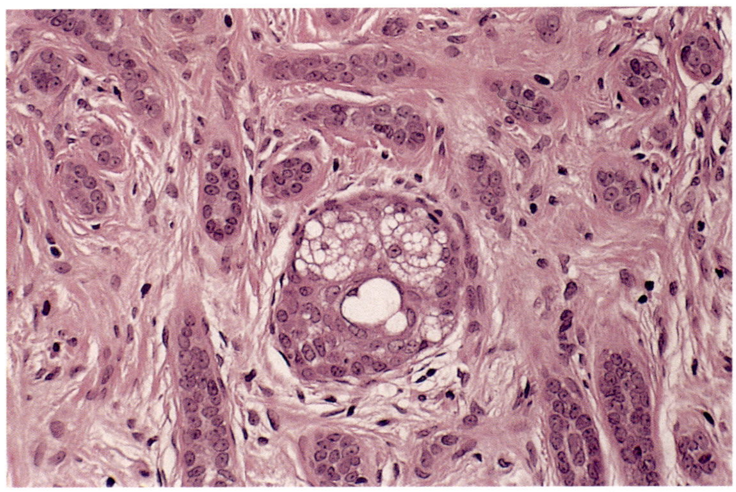

D

Figures 32–15A, 32–15B, 32–15C, 32–15D. Desmoplastic trichoepithelioma. Small cords and columns of uniform, branching basaloid cells in a fibrocytic stroma with a patchy lymphohistiocytic infiltrate. There are cystic structures containing anucleate cells (shadow/ghost cells), sebocytes associated with basaloid cells, and a focus of dermal calcification.

TUMOR OF FOLLICULAR INFUNDIBULUM

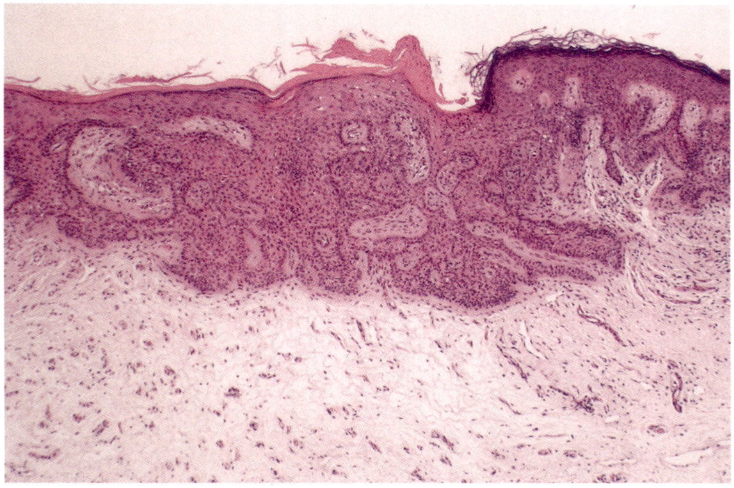

A

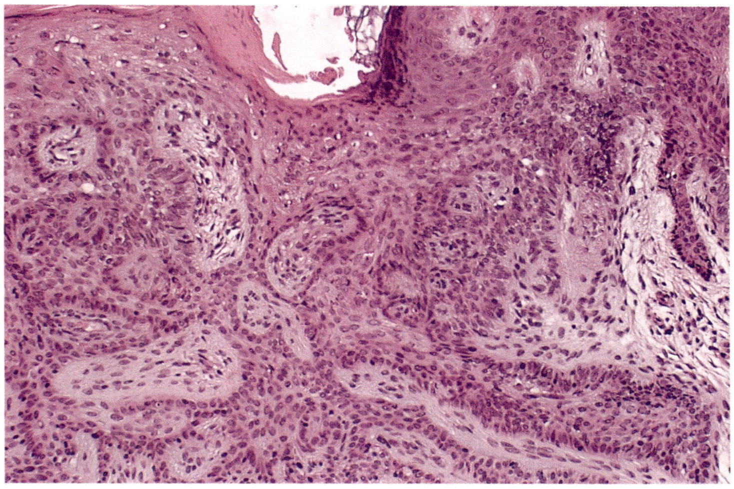

B

Figures 32–16A, 32–16B. Tumor of follicular infundibulum. Proliferation of pink-staining follicular, isthmic epithelium that parallels the epidermis. There is dermal fibroplasia and a lymphohistiocytic infiltrate.

PILAR SHEATH ACANTHOMA

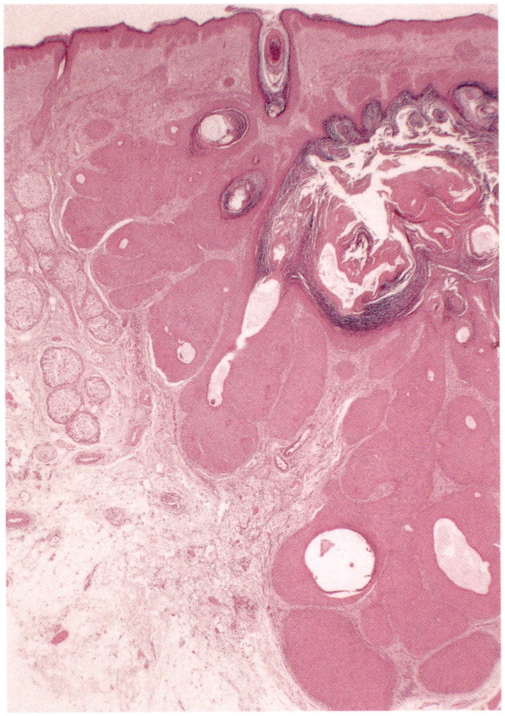

A

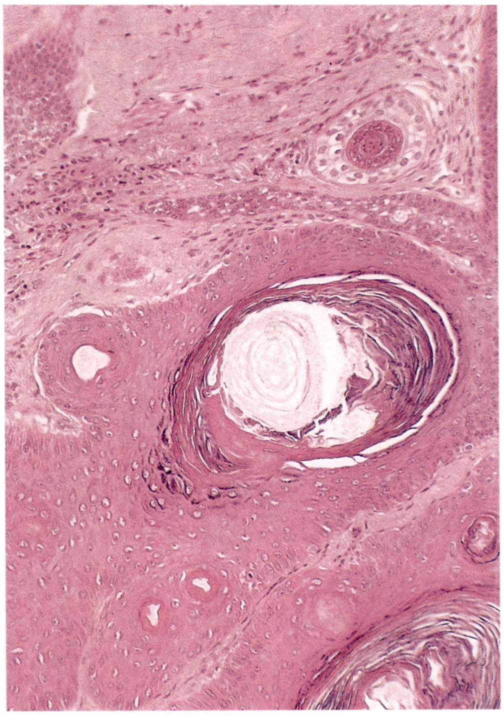

B

Figures 32–17A, 32–17B. Pilar sheath acanthoma. Dilated and hyperkeratotic infundibulum with bulbous pink isthmic epithelial proliferations. Sebaceous ducts are typically seen within the proliferative epithelium.

PILOMATRIXOMA

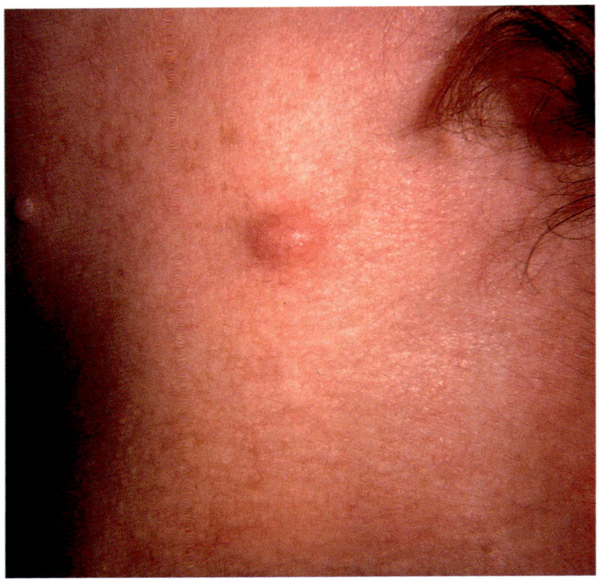

Figure 32–18. Pilomatrixoma. Dome-shaped erythematous nodules on the neck of a girl.

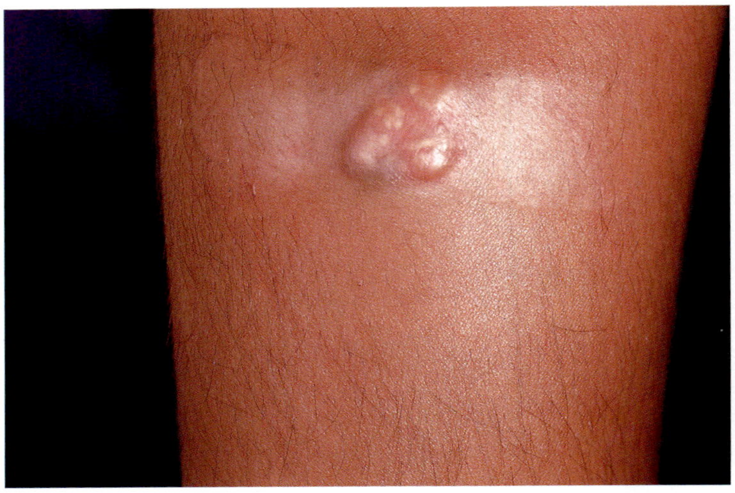

Figure 32–19. Pilomatrixoma. Multinodular lesion on the arm of a boy.

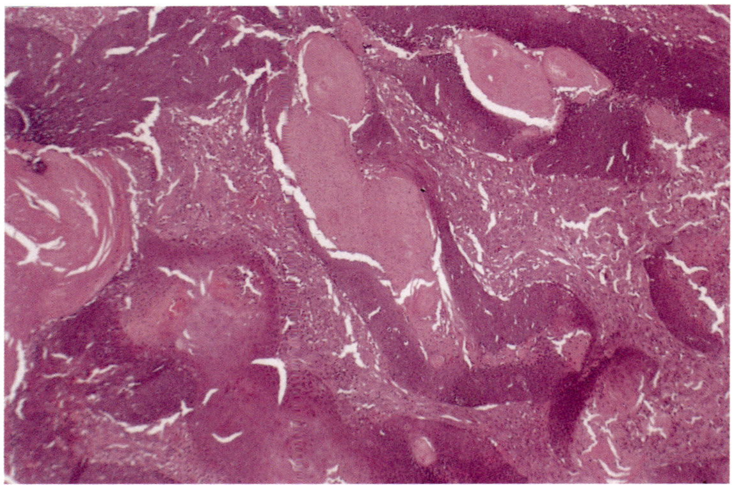

A

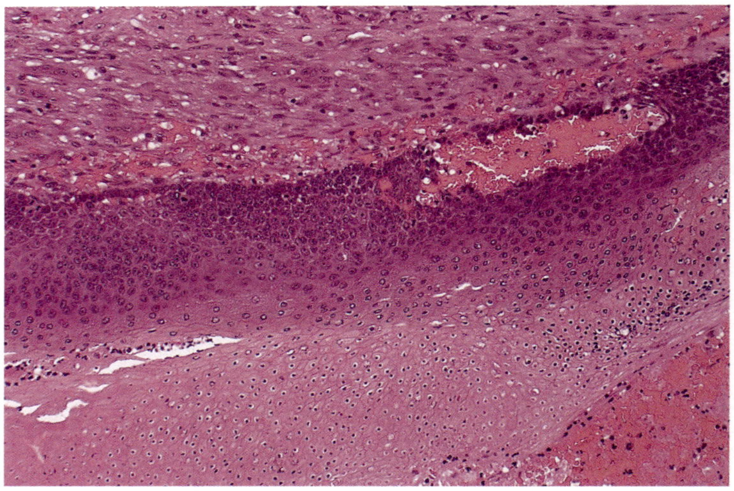

B

Figures 32–20A, 32–20B. Pilomatrixoma. Islands of follicular basophilic, keratinizing matrix cells. Shadow cells (anucleate matrix cells) are prominent, and there is an accompanying fibrosing-granulomatous dermal infiltrate.

PILAR TUMOR (PROLIFERATING FOLLICULAR CYSTIC NEOPLASM)

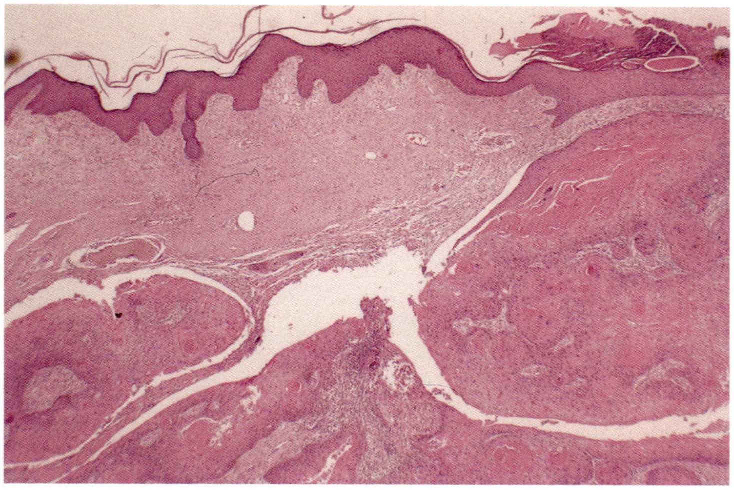

A

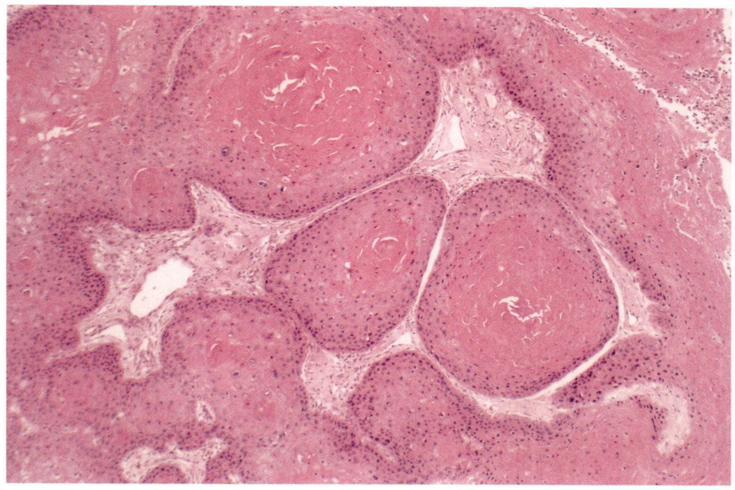

B

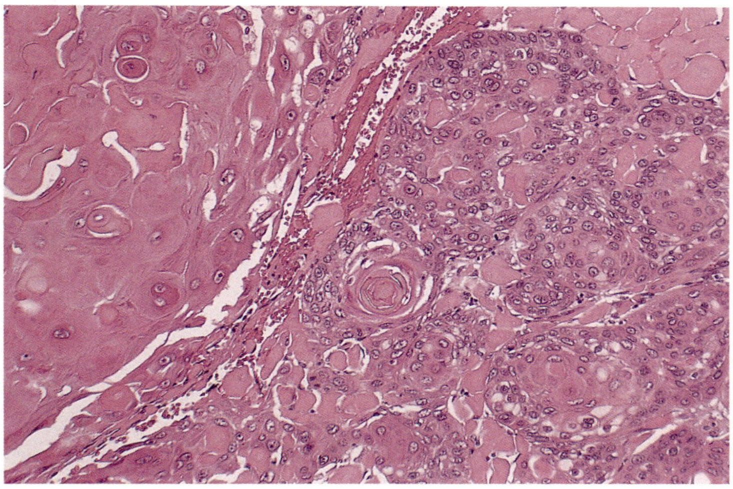

C

Figures 32–21A, 32–21B, 32–21C. Pilar tumor. Smooth, rounded aggregates of keratinizing follicular keratinocytes. The islands of keratinized cells are often separated by clefts from the normal dermis. Individual keratinocytes may appear large and atypical.

TRICHOLEMMOMA

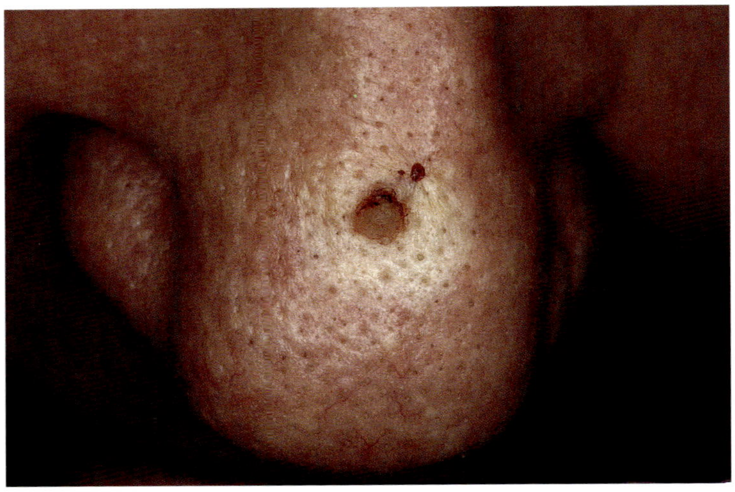

Figure 32–22. Tricholemmoma. Verrucous papule on the nose of an older man.

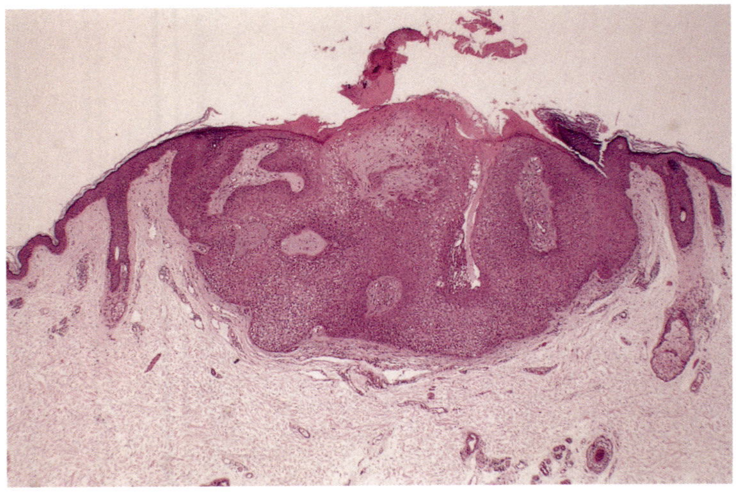

Figure 32–23. Tricholemmoma. Endophytic follicular epithelial proliferation with many clear cells.

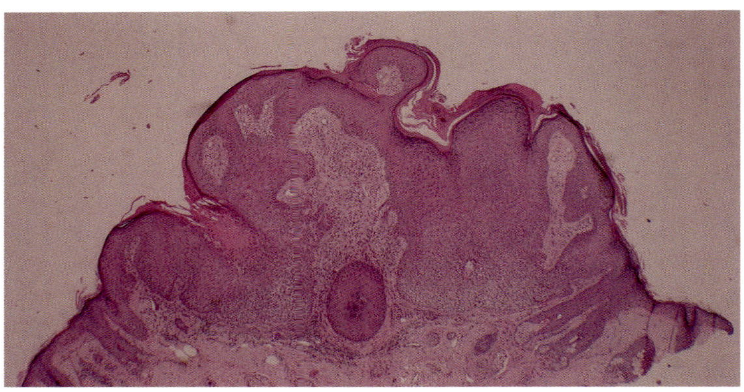

A

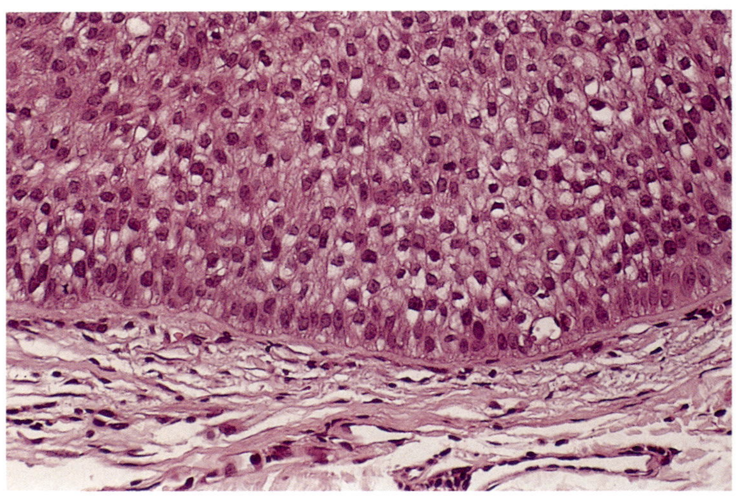

B

Figures 32–24A, 32–24B. Tricholemmoma. Exophytic follicular epithelial proliferation with many clear cells. Clear cells appear similar to the clear cells of the outer root sheath.

INVERTED FOLLICULAR KERATOSIS

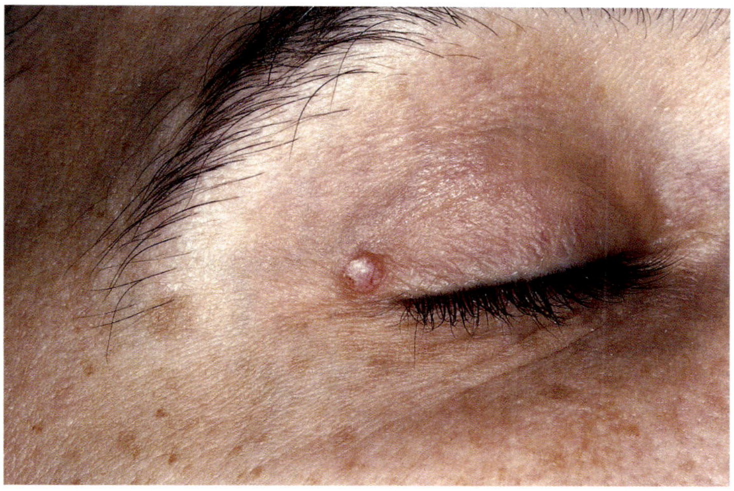

Figure 32–25. Inverted follicular keratosis. Pink keratotic papule on the upper eyelid.

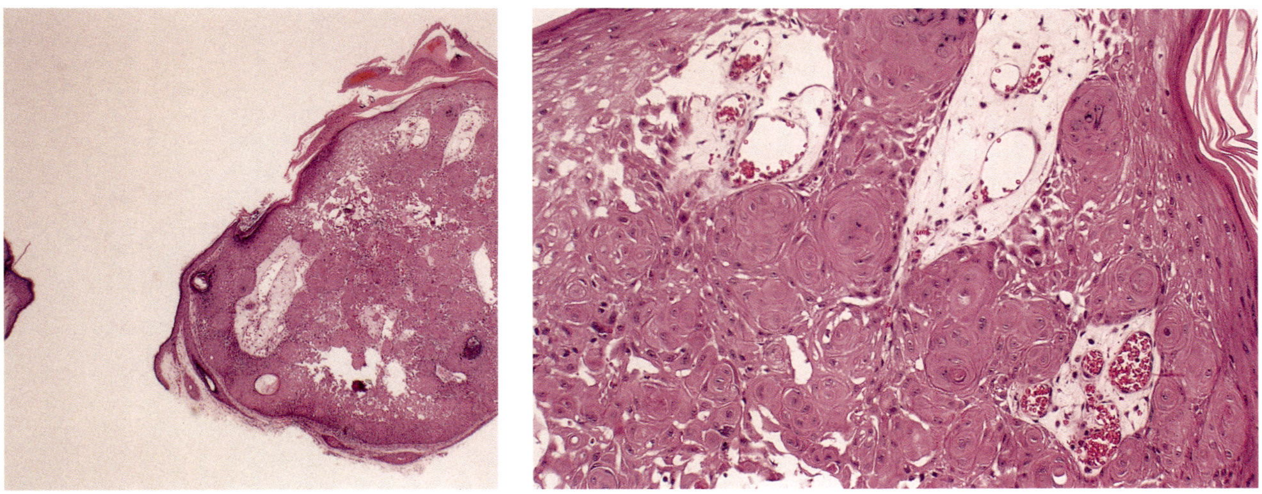

A B

Figures 32–26A, 32–26B. Inverted follicular keratosis. Proliferation of follicular keratinocytes forming numerous squamous eddies. There are atypical and necrotic keratinocytes; vascular ectasia is prominent.

33

SEBACEOUS PROLIFERATIVE DISORDERS

- Steatocystoma
- Nevus sebaceous
- Sebaceous hyperplasia
- Sebaceous adenoma
- Sebaceoma (undifferentiated sebaceous adenoma)
- Sebaceous carcinoma

STEATOCYSTOMA

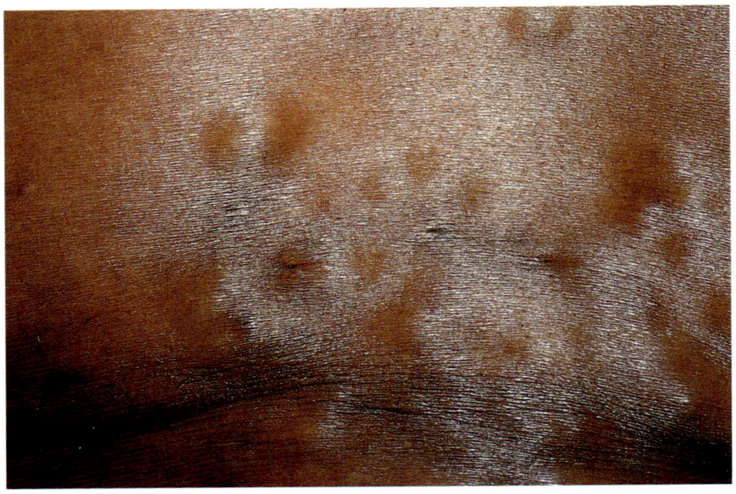

Figure 33–1. **Steatocystoma.** Papules on the chest of a man.

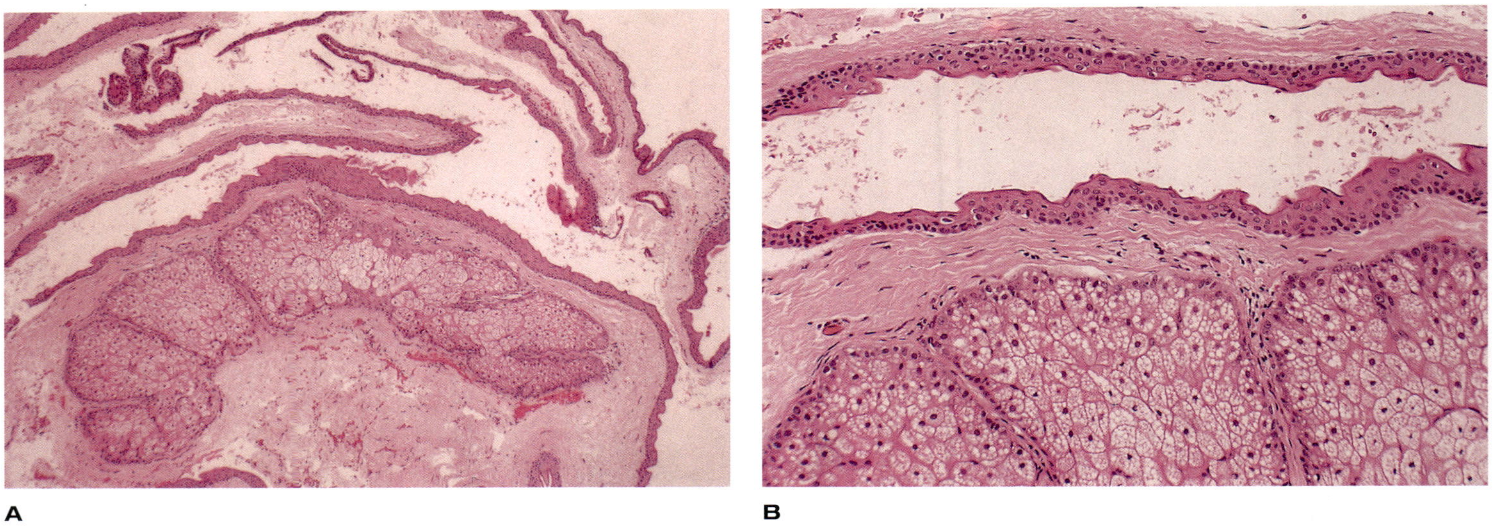

Figures 33–2A, 33–2B. **Steatocystoma.** Anastomosing tubular structures with sebaceous lobules within the wall. There is an eosinophilic, crenulated cuticle lining the tubular structure.

NEVUS SEBACEOUS

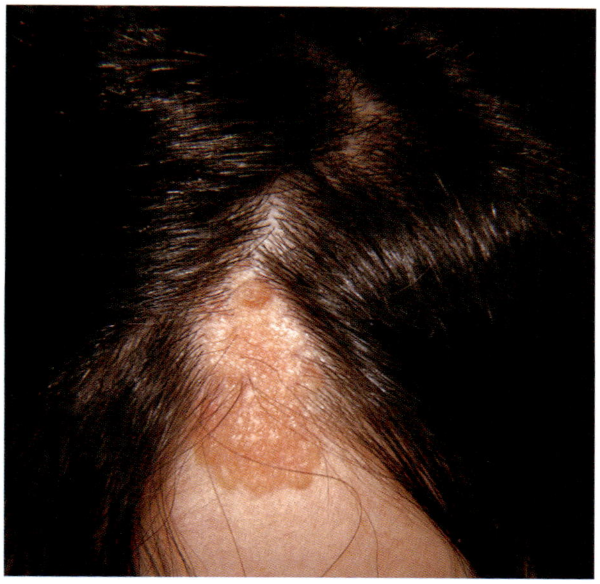

Figure 33–3. Nevus sebaceous. Yellow, cobblestone-surfaced, hairless nodule on the forehead and scalp of a woman.

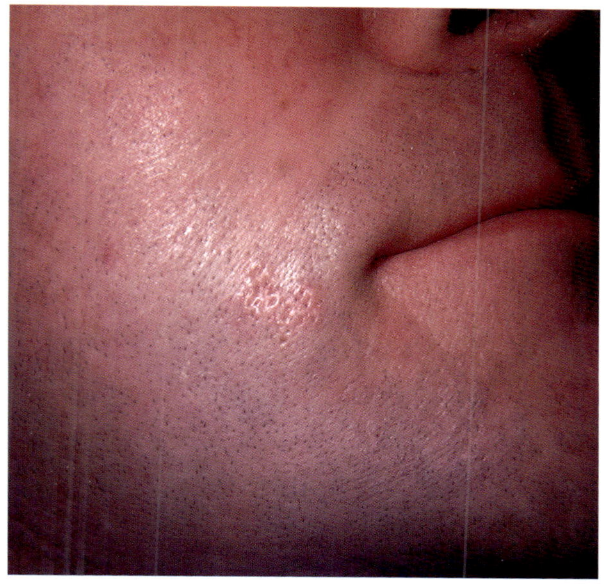

Figure 33–4. Nevus sebaceous. Small, yellowish plaque on the cheek.

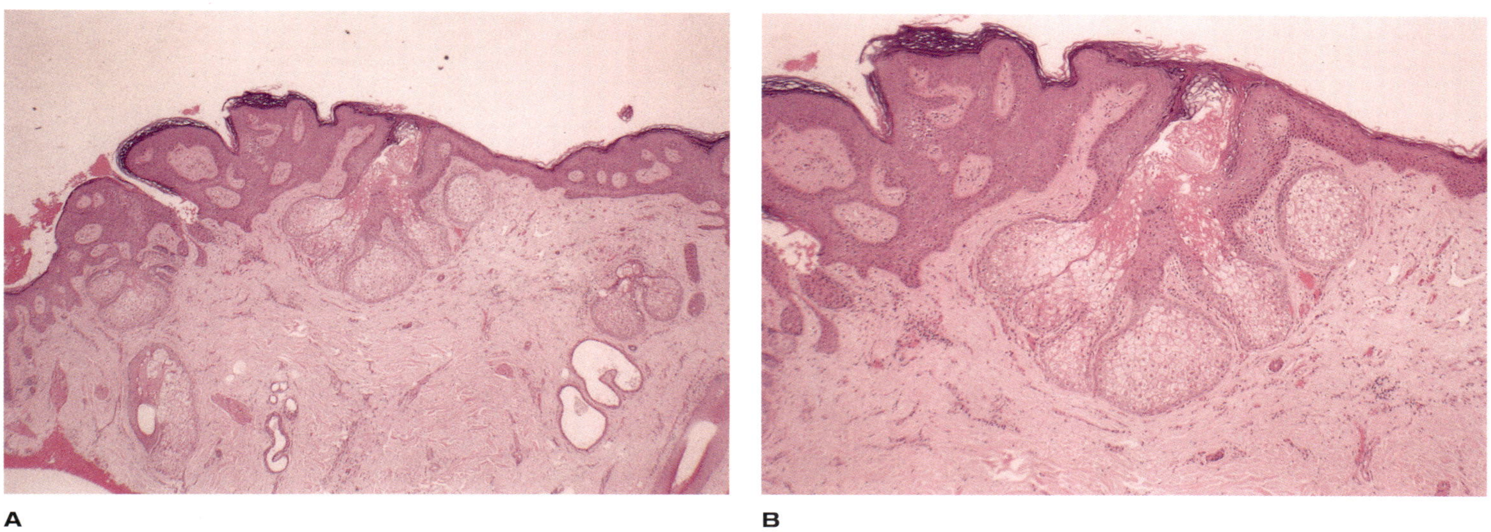

Figures 33–5A, 33–5B. Nevus sebaceous. Sebaceous lobules, hyperkeratosis, and papillomatosis. Sebaceous ducts connect directly with the epidermis. There are apocrine tubular structures and dilated blood vessels in the fibrocytic dermis.

SEBACEOUS HYPERPLASIA

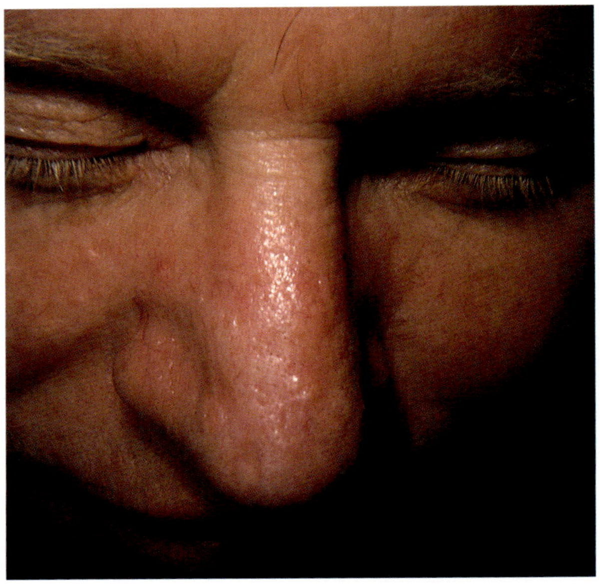

Figure 33–6. Sebaceous hyperplasia. Yellowish, telangiectatic papules on the cheeks and nose of a man.

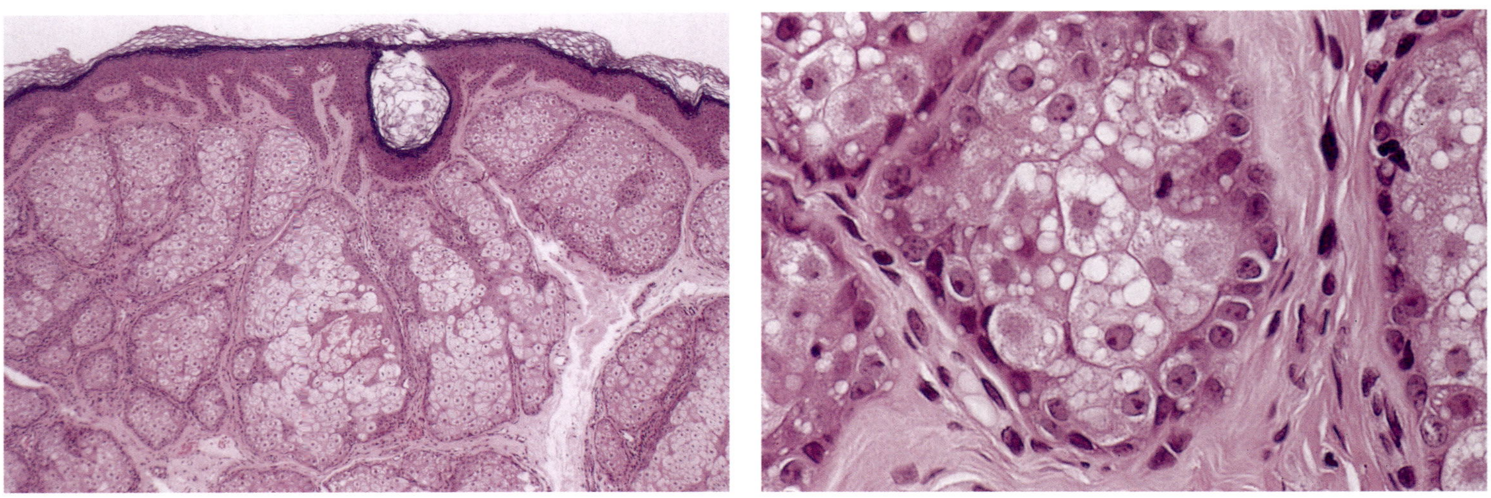

A B

Figures 33–7A, 33–7B. Sebaceous hyperplasia. Numerous normal-appearing sebaceous lobules in the dermis surrounding a dilated infundibulum. Mature sebocytes have a crenulated nucleus and vacuolated cytoplasm.

SEBACEOUS ADENOMA

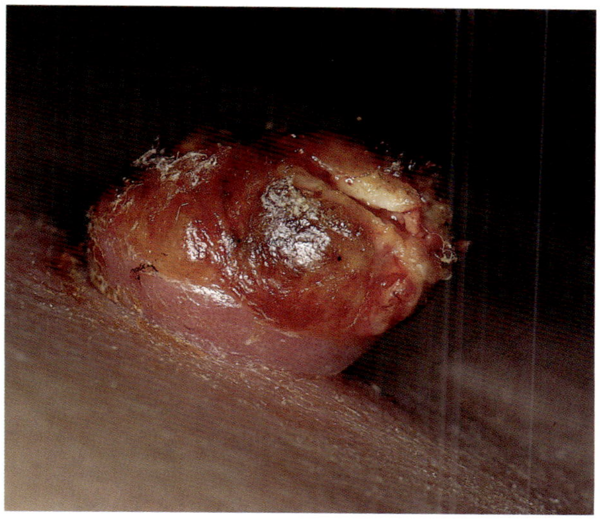

Figure 33–8. Sebaceous adenoma. Sessile, ulcerated and crusted nodule on the shoulder.

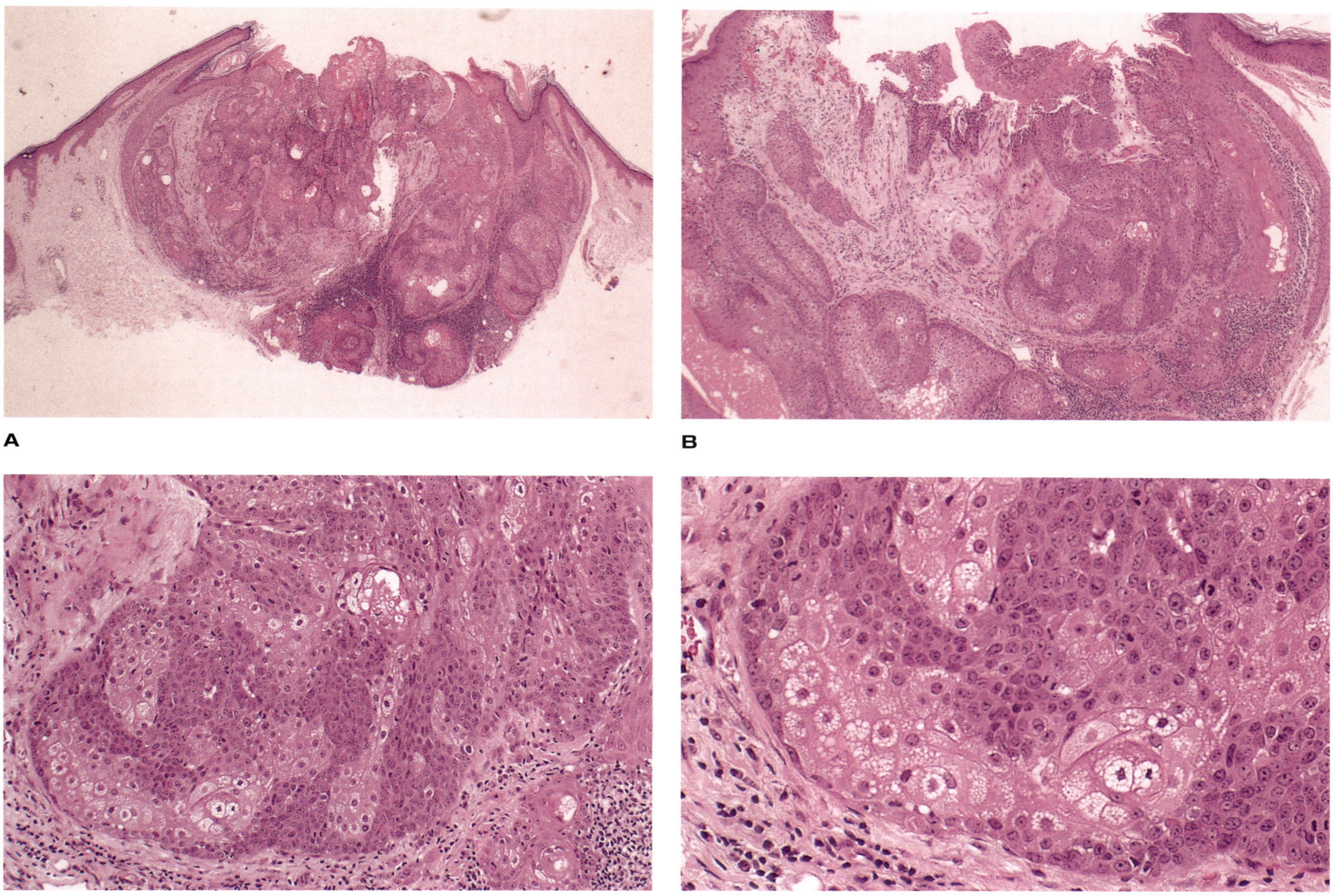

A B C D

Figures 33–9A, 33–9B, 33–9C, 33–9D. Sebaceous adenoma. Proliferation of sebaceous lobules with many immature and mature sebocytes and dilated sebaceous ductal structures. The epidermis is ulcerated, and the dermis is fibrocytic with dilated blood vessels and a mixed-cell infiltrate.

SEBACEOMA (UNDIFFERENTIATED SEBACEOUS ADENOMA)

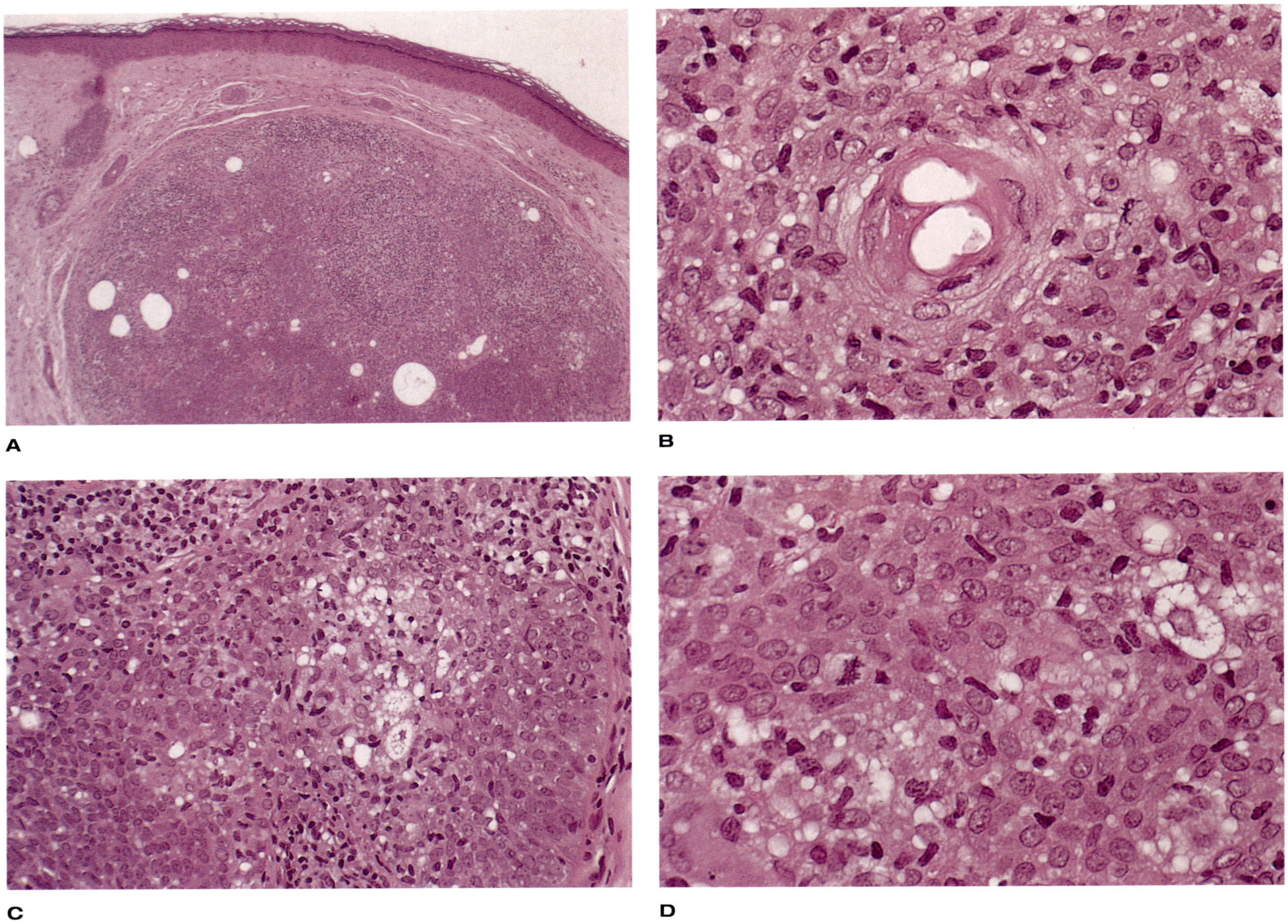

Figures 33–10A, 33–10B, 33–10C, 33–10D. Sebaceoma. Sharply circumscribed dermal nodule with dilated sebaceous ductal structures. There is maturation of round to oval immature sebocytes to mature sebocytes with crenulated nuclei and vacuolated cytoplasms. There are foci of atypical, pleomorphic sebocytes with mitotic figures. Dermal fibroplasia with clefting between collagen bundles is common.

SEBACEOUS CARCINOMA

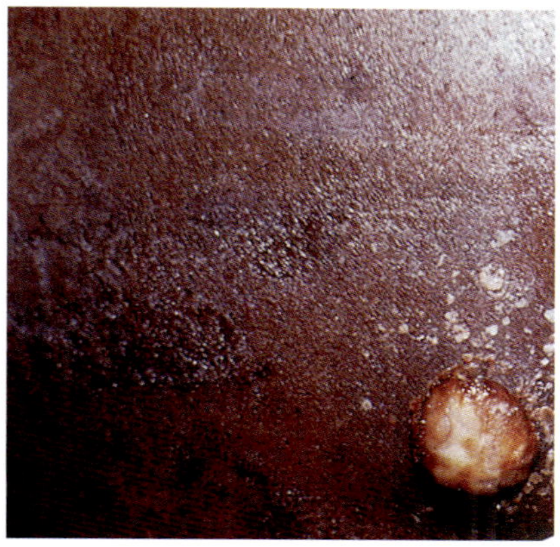

Figure 33–11. Sebaceous carcinoma. Ulcerated yellowish nodule on the back of a man.

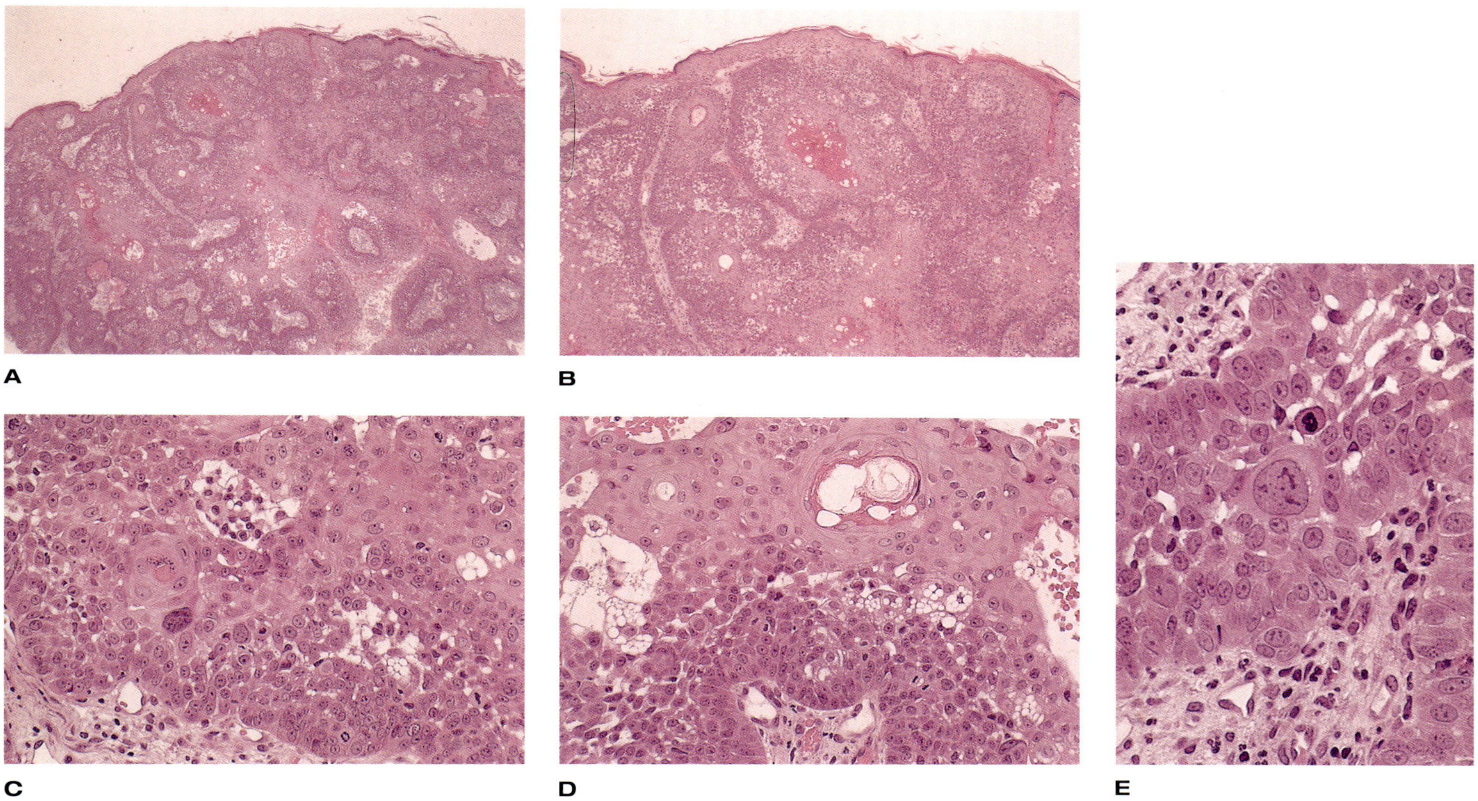

Figures 33–12A, 33–12B, 33–12C, 33–12D, 33–12E. Sebaceous carcinoma. Columns of atypical and pleomorphic undifferentiated sebocytes with and without cytoplasmic vacuoles extend from the epidermis deep into the reticular dermis. There are sebaceous ductal structures, strikingly large and pleomorphic sebocytes, and numerous mitotic figures.

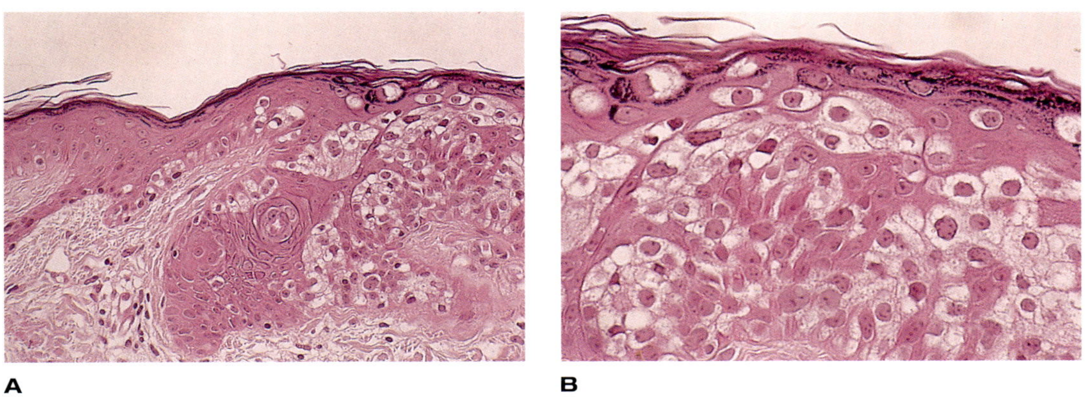

Figures 33–13A, 33–13B. Sebaceous carcinoma of the eyelid. Numerous solitary and nested atypical cells with large round nuclei and abundant pale-staining cytoplasm (pagetoid cells) are scattered at all levels of the epidermis in a pagetoid pattern. Sebaceous carcinoma on the eyelid may have a similar architectural pattern to extramammary Paget's disease, malignant melanoma, and Bowen's disease.

34

Sweat gland proliferative disorders

- Hidrocystoma
- Syringocystadenoma papilliferum
- Syringoma
- Clear-cell hidradenoma
- Cylindroma
- Mixed tumor
- Spiradenoma
- Poromas (hidroacanthoma simplex, dermal duct tumor, hidradenoma)
- Microcystic adnexal carcinoma
- Syringomatous carcinoma
- Mucinous carcinoma

HIDROCYSTOMA

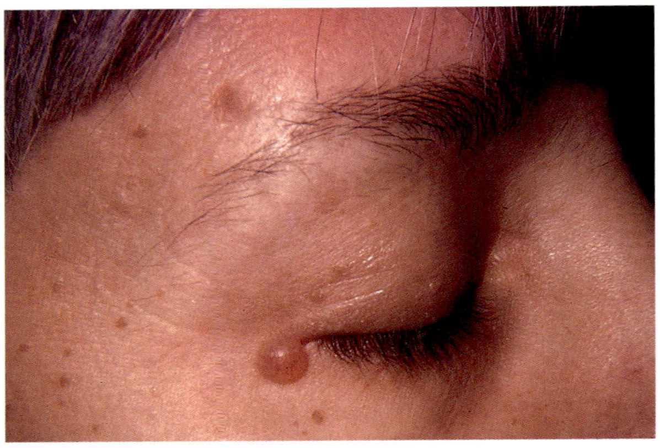

Figure 34–1. Hidrocystoma. Pedunculated, skin-colored, smooth lesion on the eyelid.

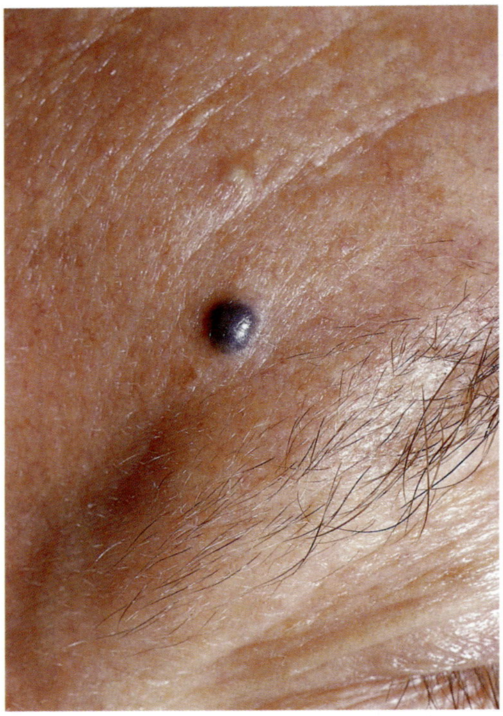

Figure 34–2. Hidrocystoma. Dark-blue, smooth dome-shaped papule on the forehead adjacent to the eyebrow.

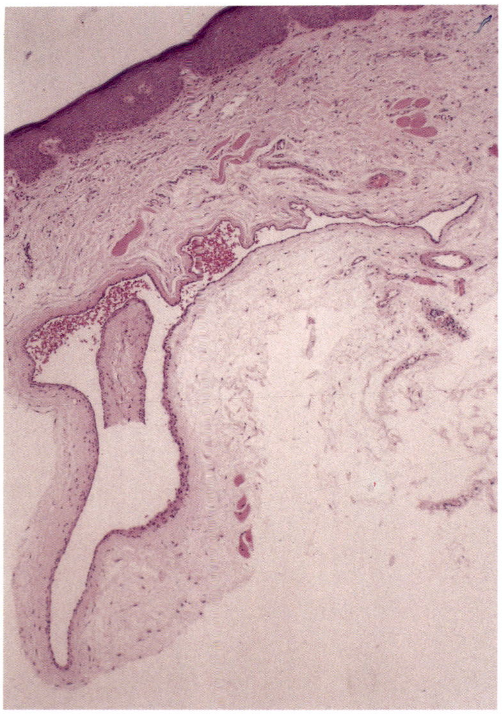

A

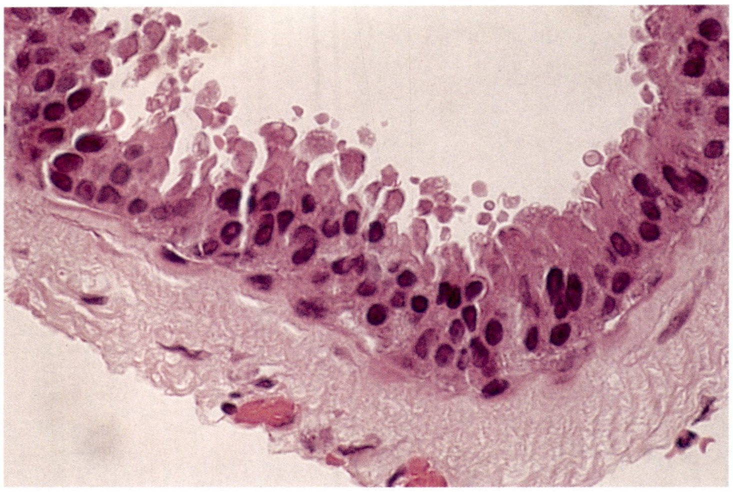

B

Figures 34–3A, 34–3B. Hidrocystoma. Tortuous, elongated tubular structures. There are cuboidal epithelial cells lining the tubule with characteristic decapitation secretion, which is characteristic of apocrine secretion.

SYRINGOCYSTADENOMA PAPILLIFERUM

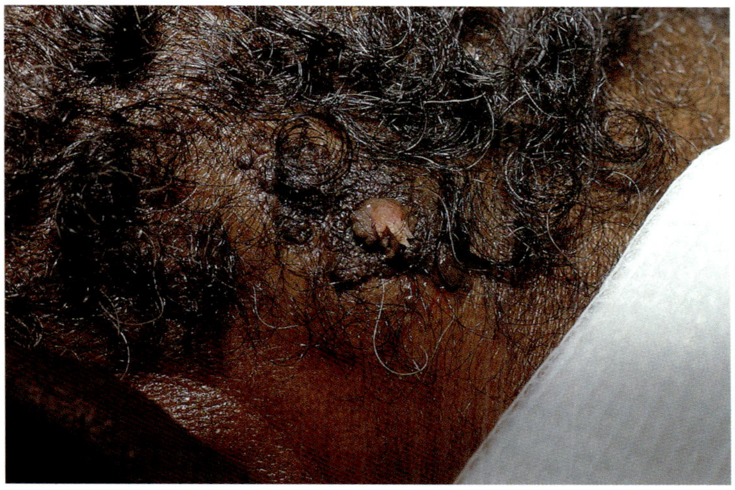

Figure 34–4. Syringocystadenoma papilliferum. Fleshy, protuberant papule within a verrucous nevus sebaceous.

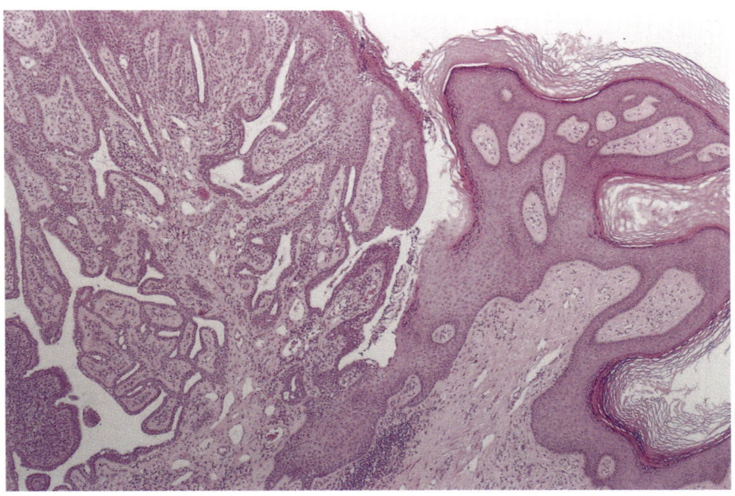

A

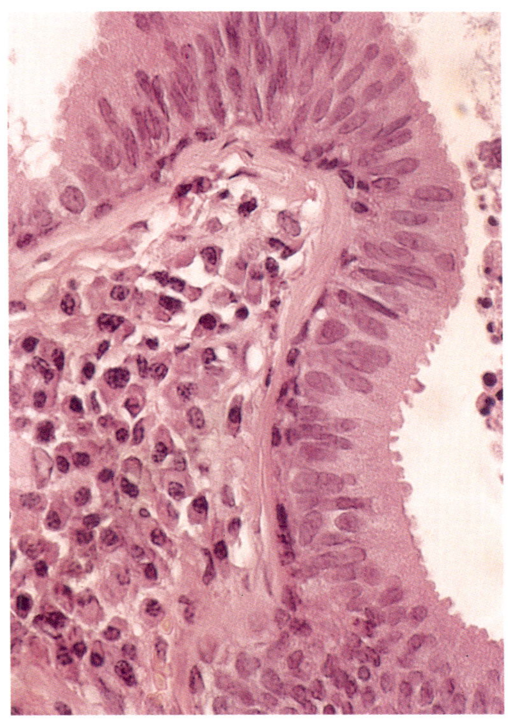

B

Figures 34–5A, 34–5B. Syringocystadenoma papilliferum. Papillated tubular structures contiguous with a dilated infundibulum. Columnar epithelial cells with decapitation secretion line the tubules. Plasma cells are scattered throughout the stroma.

SYRINGOMA

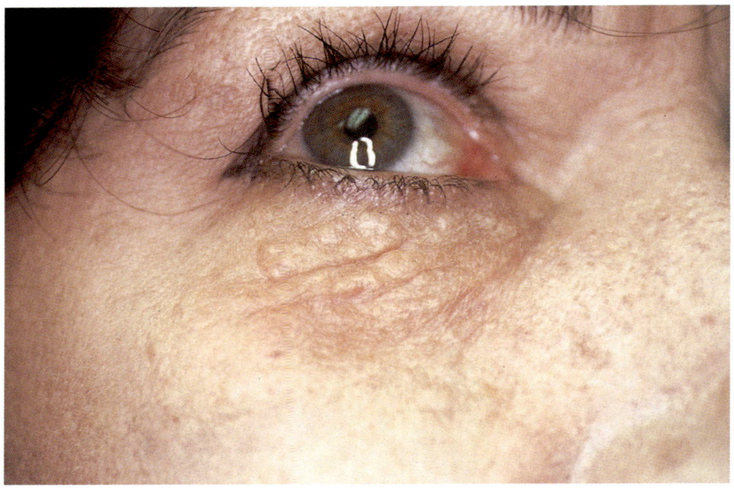

Figure 34–6. Syringoma. Grouped skin-colored papules on the lower eyelid.

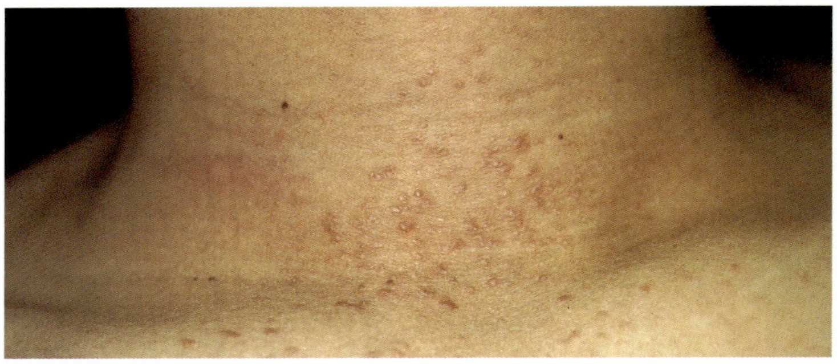

Figure 34–7. Syringoma. Dome-shaped, tan papules on the neck and chest of a woman.

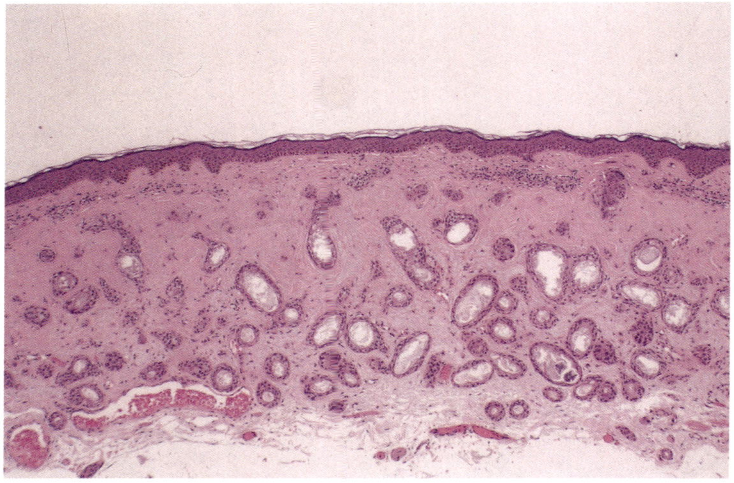

A

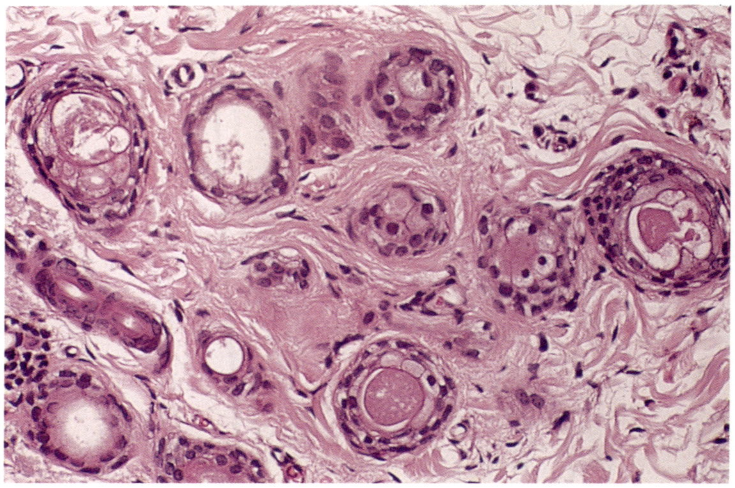

B

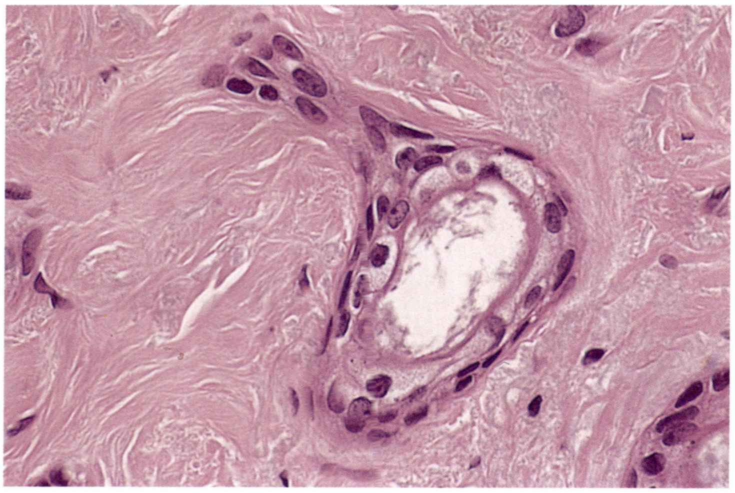

C

Figures 34–8A, 34–8B, 34–8C. Syringoma. Round and oval tubular structures within a fibrocytic dermis. There is eosinophilic, homogeneous material within the lumen of the tubules, which are lined by dark and clear cells.

CLEAR-CELL HIDRADENOMA

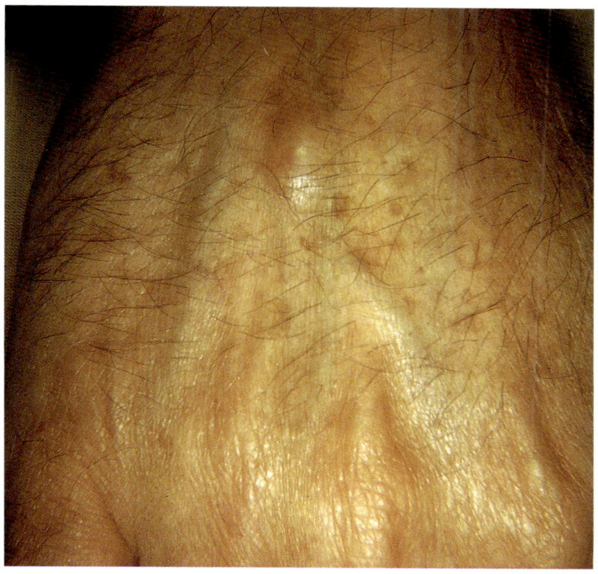

Figure 34–9. Clear-cell hidradenoma. Skin-colored nodule on the dorsum of the hand.

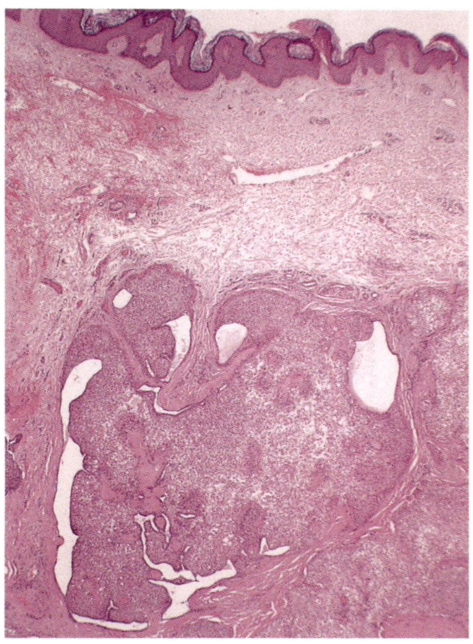

A

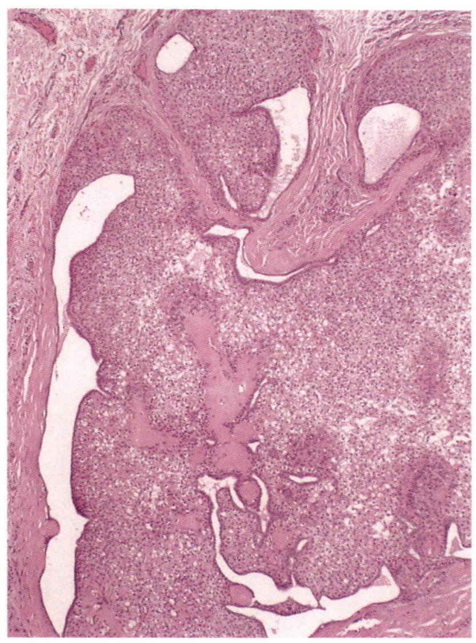

B

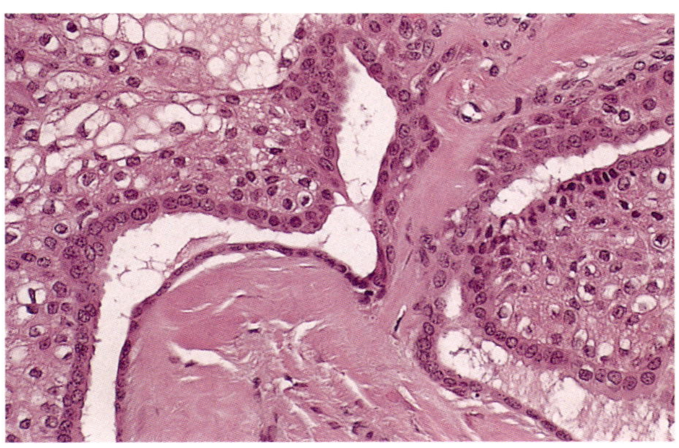

C

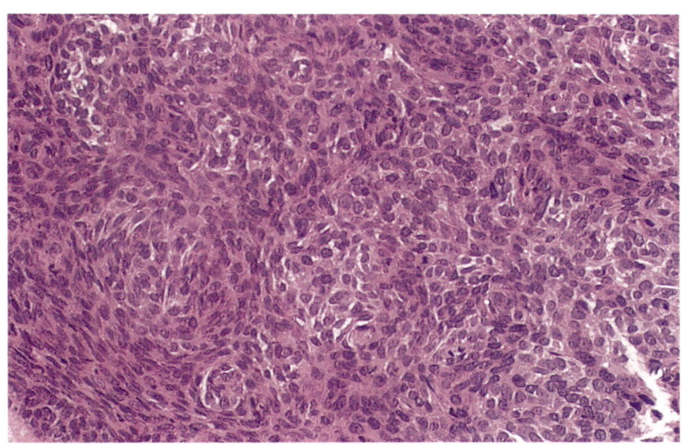

D

Figures 34–10A, 34–10B, 34–10C, 34–10D. Clear-cell hidradenoma. Elongated, tortuous tubular structures with decapitation secretion. There are sheets of pale, clear, mucinous and spindle-shaped cells within a fibrocytic dermis.

CYLINDROMA

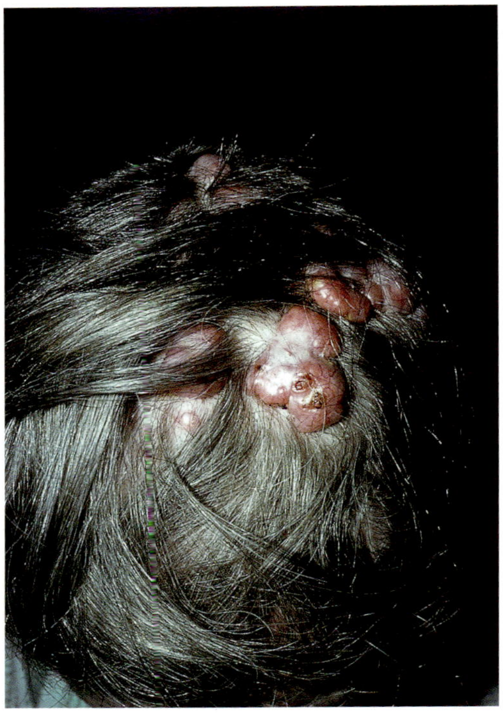

Figure 34–11. Cylindroma. Multiple large polypoid, erythematous, telangiectatic, crusted nodules on the scalp.

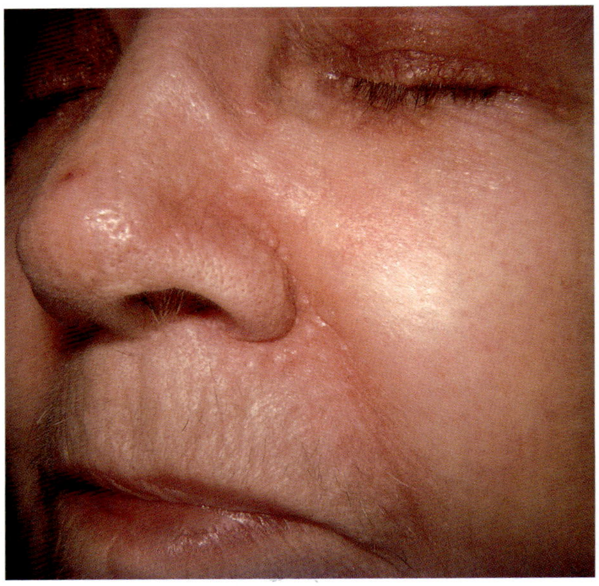

Figure 34–12. Cylindroma. Multiple small erythematous papules on the nose, cheek, lip, and eyelid of a woman.

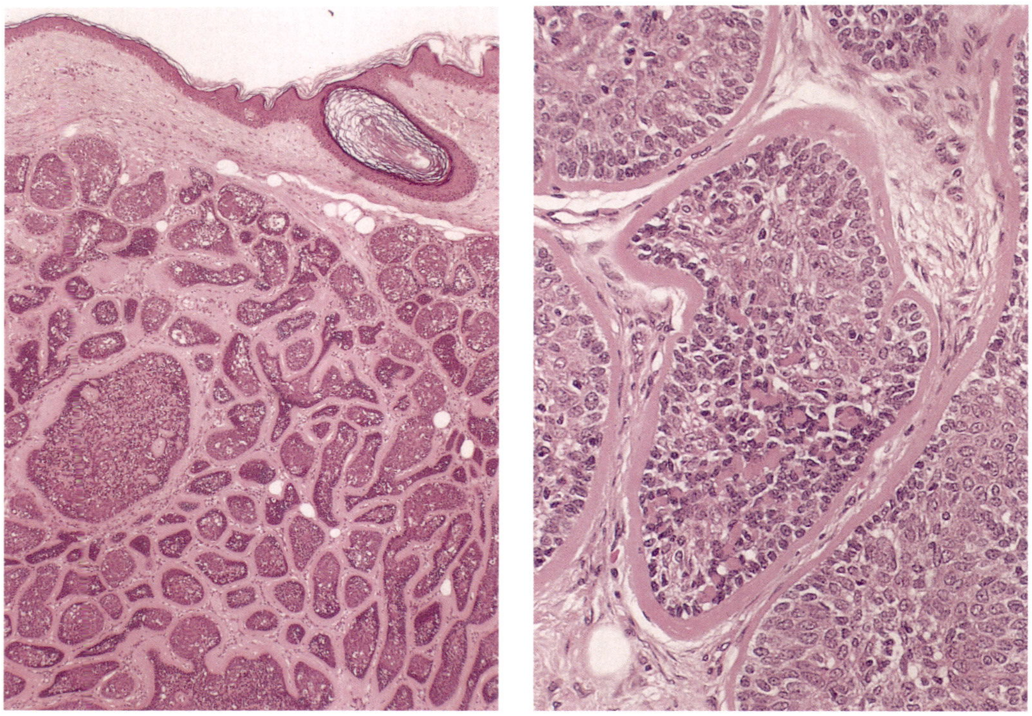

A B

Figures 34–13A, 34–13B. Cylindroma. Irregularly shaped nodules composed of clear and dark cells. Homogeneous eosinophilic material is deposited in round globules within the nodules and as a thick band around each aggregate in the fibrocytic dermis.

MIXED TUMOR

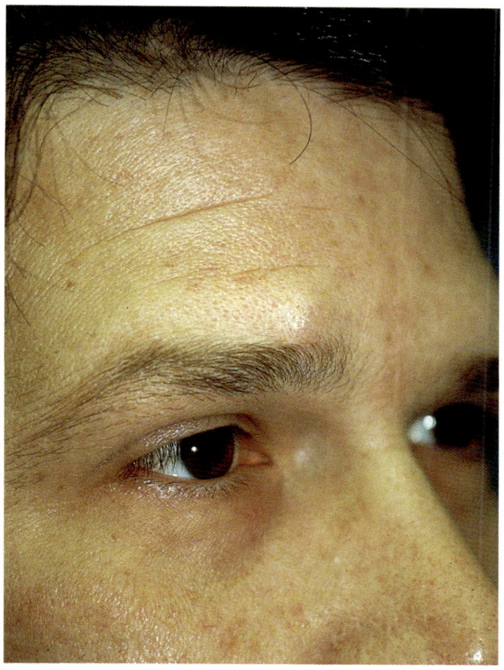

Figure 34–14. Apocrine mixed tumor. Skin-colored nodule on the forehead just above the eyebrow.

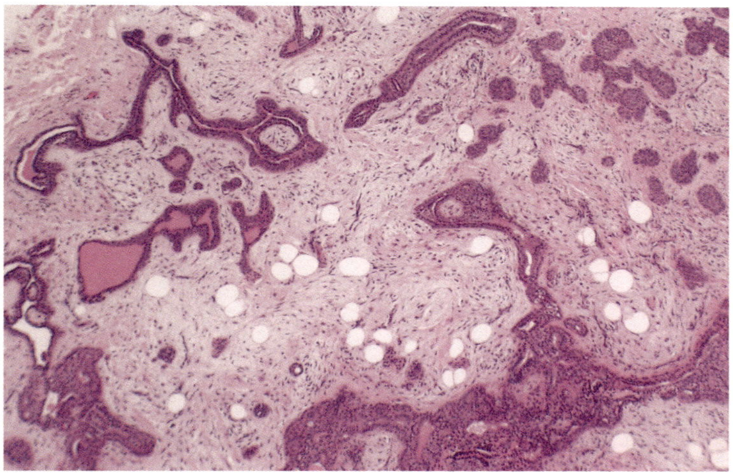

A

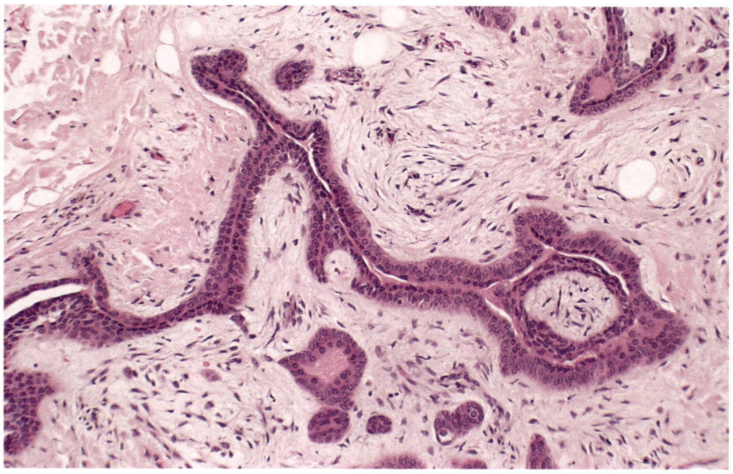

B

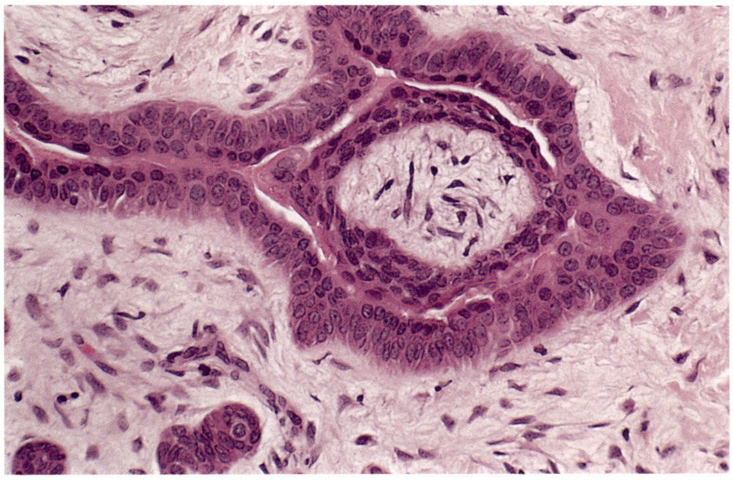

C

Figures 34–15A, 34–15B, 34–15C. Apocrine mixed tumor. Interconnecting, elongated tubular structures lined by a double row of epithelial cells, embedded in a pale, mucinous, chondroidal, and fibrocytic stroma. There are deposits of homogeneous eosinophilic material within the lumen of the tubular structures as well as evidence of decapitation secretion.

MIXED TUMOR

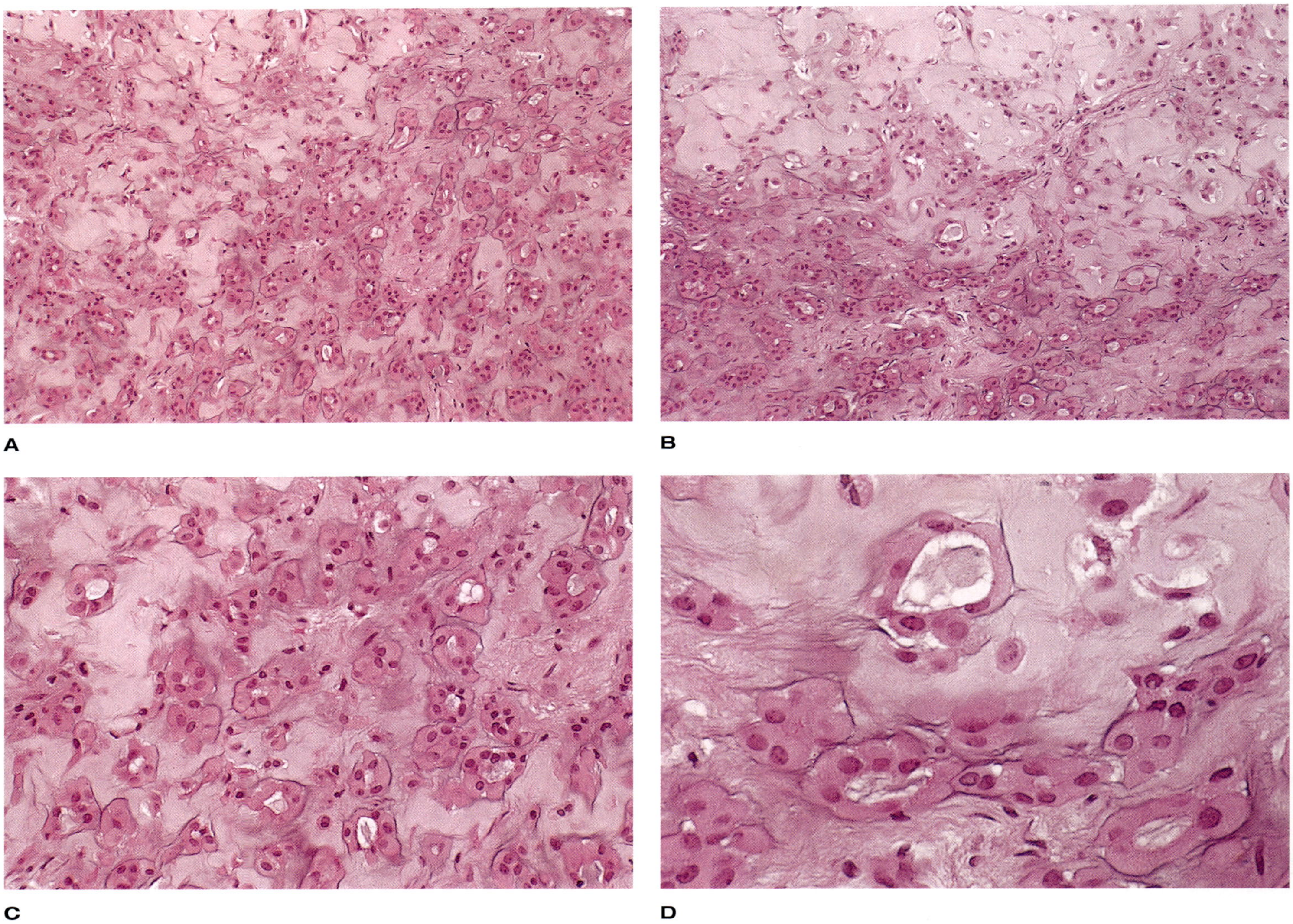

Figures 34–16A, 34–16B, 34–16C, 34–16D. Eccrine mixed tumor. Round tubules lined by a single row of cuboidal epithelial cells. The tubules are found within a gray mucinous and chondroidal stroma.

SPIRADENOMA

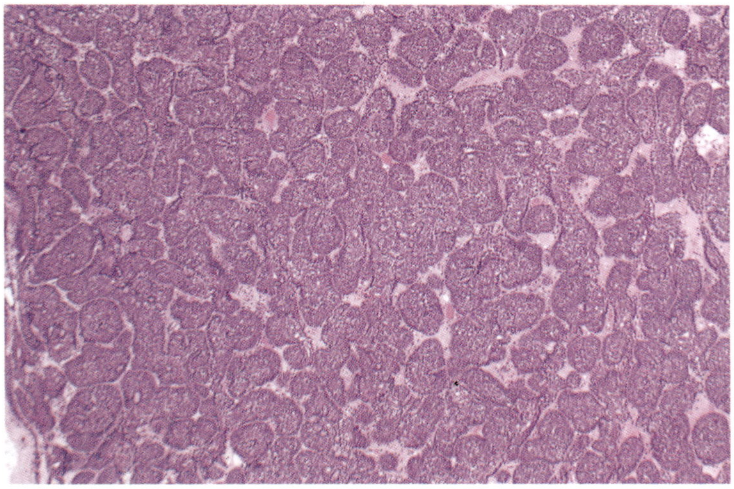

A

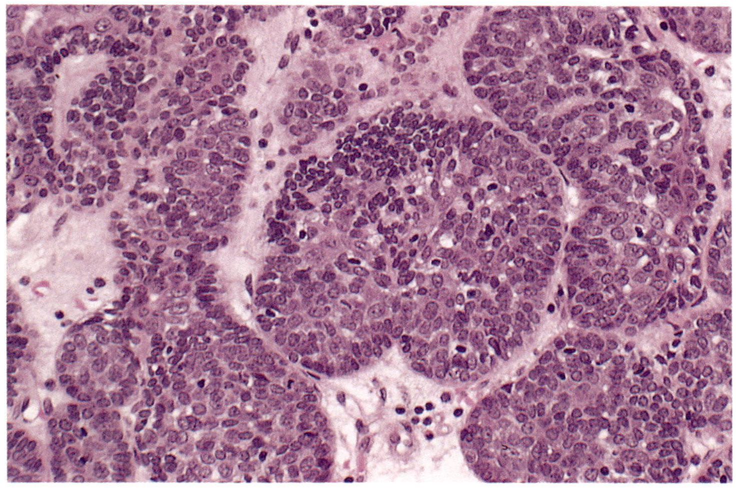

B

Figures 34–17A, 34–17B. Spiradenoma. Closely aligned aggregates of small dark and large pale-staining epithelial cells. There are lymphocytes scattered within the nodules.

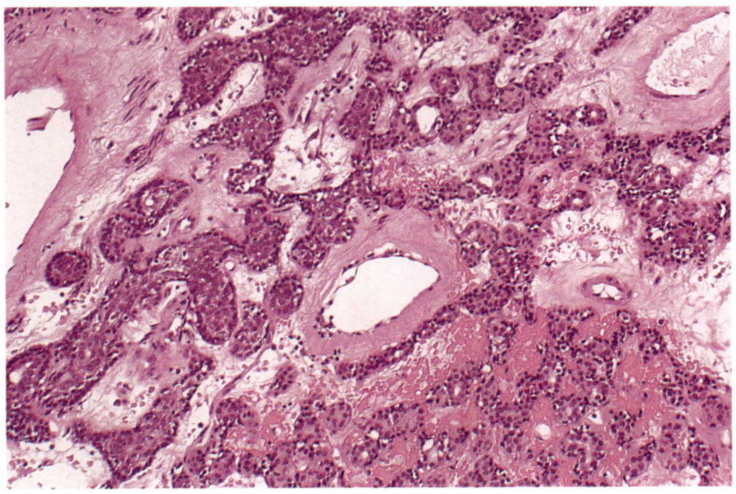

Figure 34–18. Spiradenoma, ancient type. Aggregates of dark and pale-staining epithelial cells. Sclerotic, eosinophilic bands around blood vessels and mucin deposits in the dermis are the distinguishing features.

POROMAS (HIDROACANTHOMA SIMPLEX, DERMAL DUCT TUMOR, HIDRADENOMA)

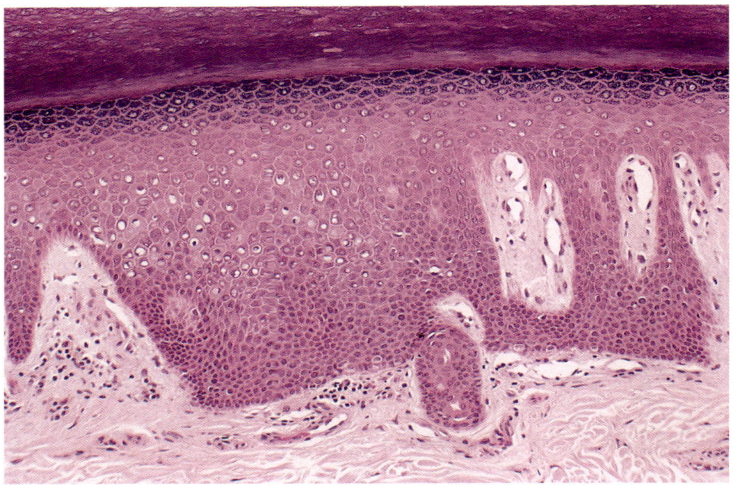

A

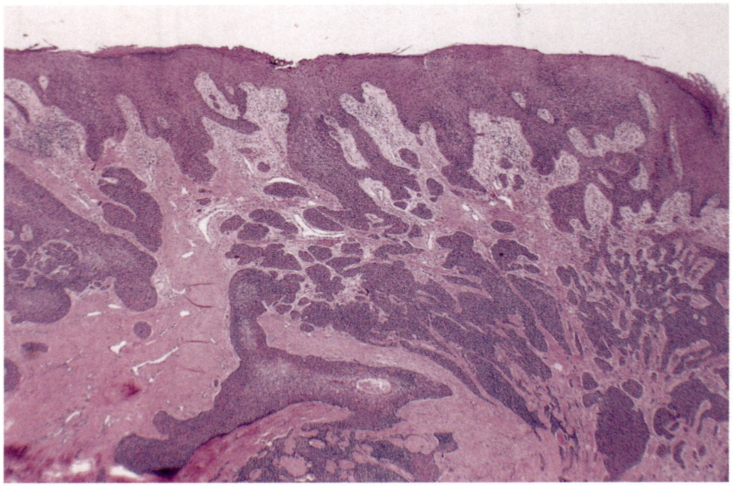

B

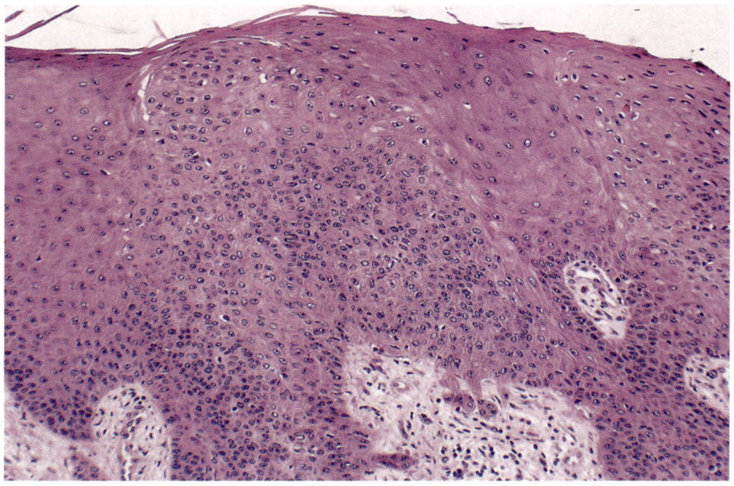

C

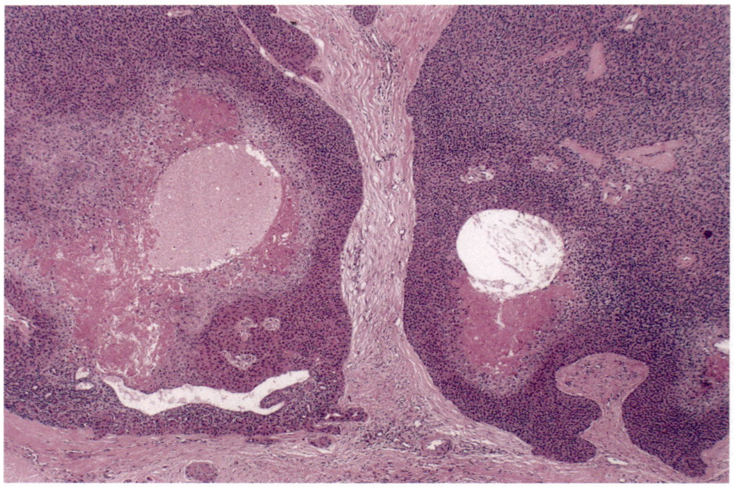

D

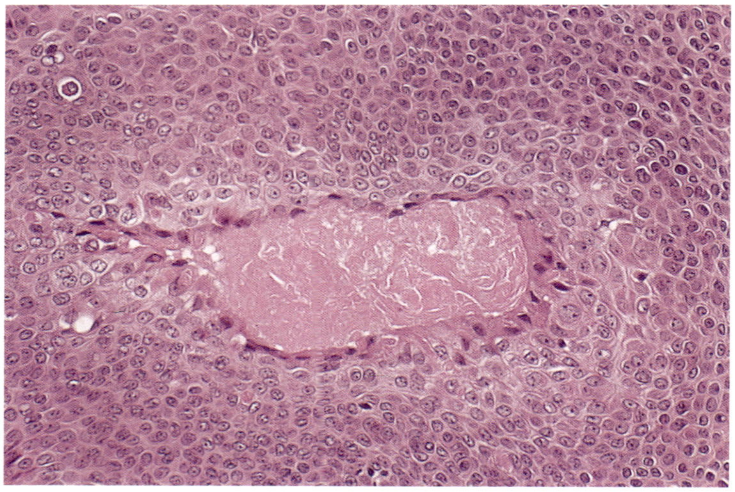

E

Figures 34–19A, 34–19B, 34–19C, 34–19D, 34–19E. Poromas. Aggregates of small, dark, round epithelial cells (poroid cells) and large, pale, eosinophilic, polygonal epithelial cells (cuticular cells) are located either within the epidermis (hidroacanthoma simplex), or within the epidermis and dermis (dermal duct tumor), or within the dermis as large, solid, cystic nodules (hidradenoma). Closely crowded poroid cells have scant cytoplasm, whereas the cuticular cells have abundant cytoplasm and are associated with ductal structures. Individual cell necrosis or large areas of necrosis may be common.

MICROCYSTIC ADNEXAL CARCINOMA

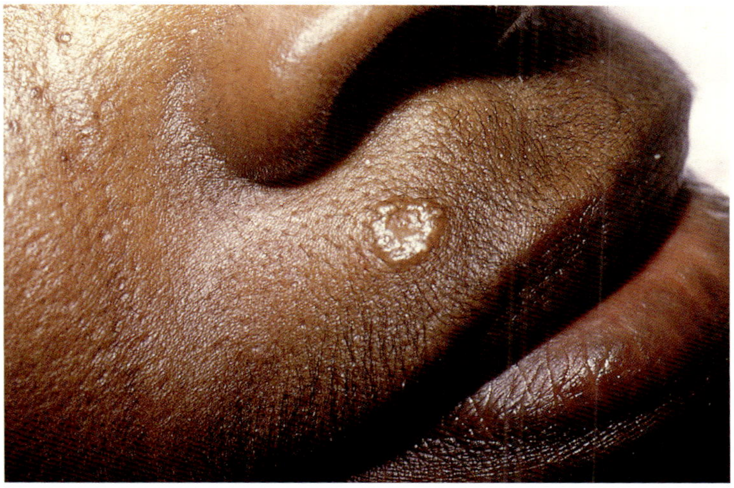

Figure 34–20. Microcystic adnexal carcinoma. Firm, umbilicated plaque on the lip of a woman.

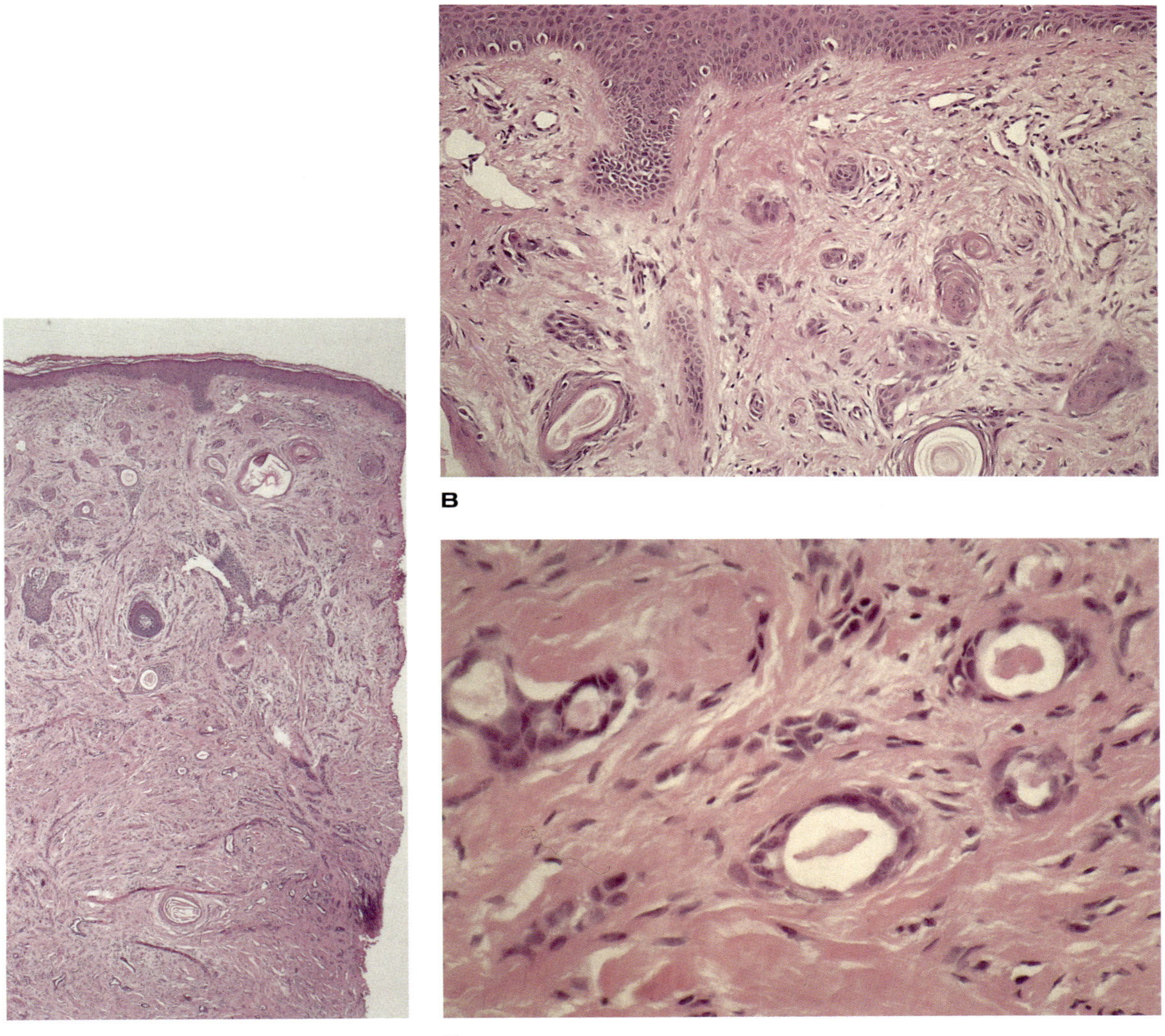

B

A

C

Figures 34–21A, 34–21B, 34–21C. Microcystic adnexal carcinoma. Monomorphous, small epithelial cells in strands, cords, columns, and nests, in addition to infundibulocystic structures, involve the upper and lower reticular dermis. The dermis is fibrocytic and has a lymphohistiocytic infiltrate. Ductal structures with deposits of eosinophilic material are seen.

MICROCYSTIC ADNEXAL CARCINOMA

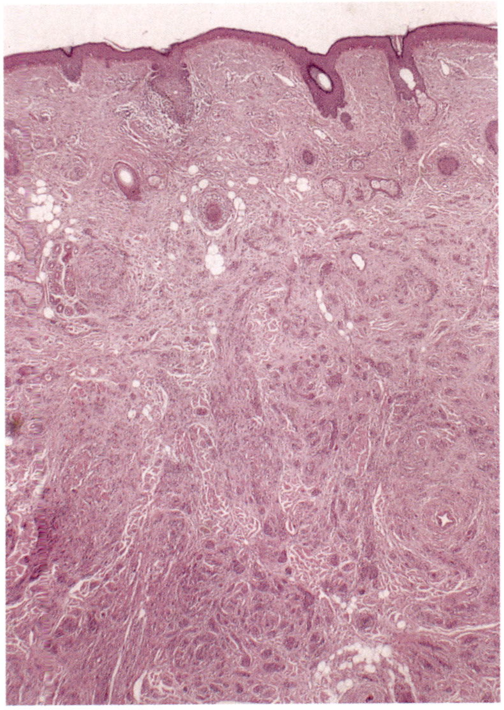

A

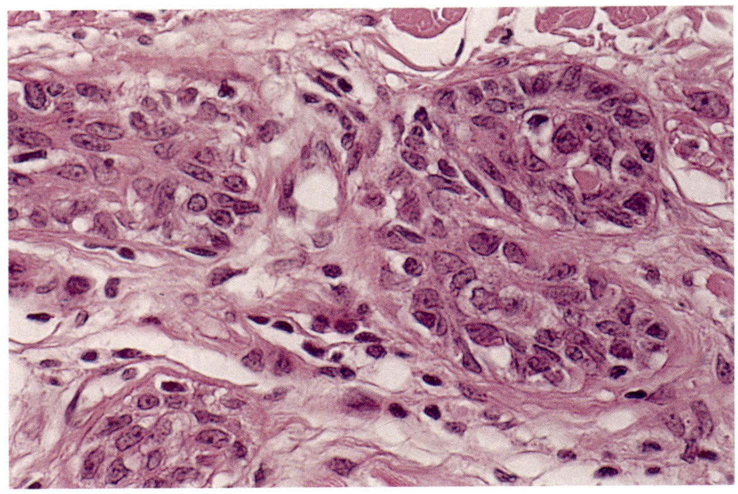

B

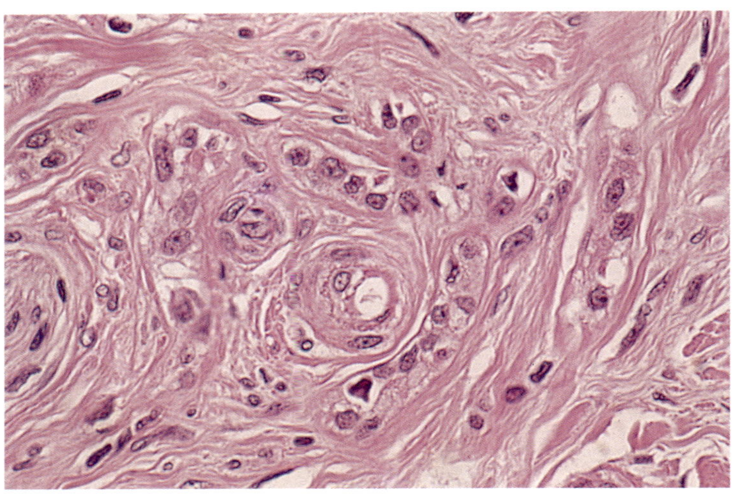

C

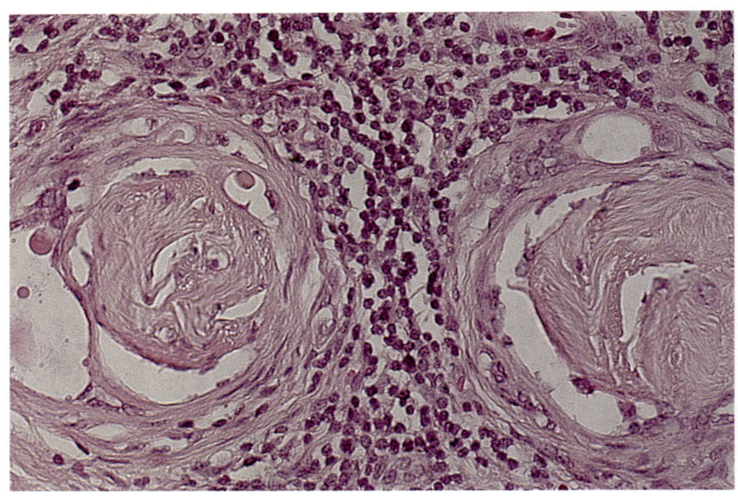

D

Figures 34–22A, 34–22B, 34–22C, 34–22D. Microcystic adnexal carcinoma. Superficial and deep dermal infiltrate of monomorphous, adnexal, epithelial cells as strands, columns, and nests, but with an absence of infundibulocystic structures. Neoplastic cells form small ductal structures and involve nerve fascicles.

SYRINGOMATOUS CARCINOMA

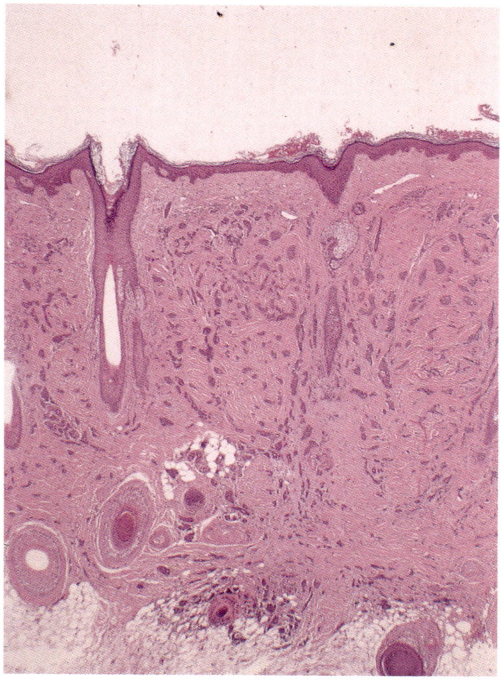

A

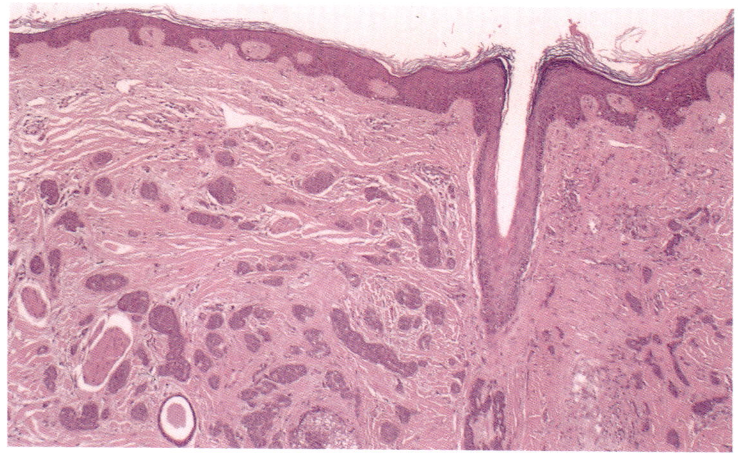

B

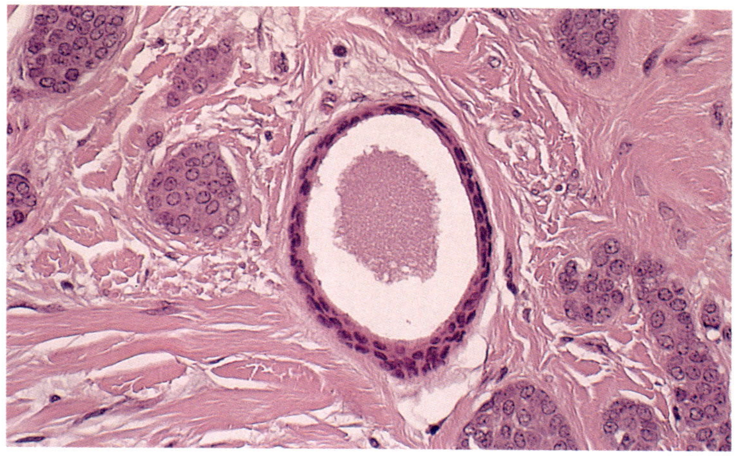

D

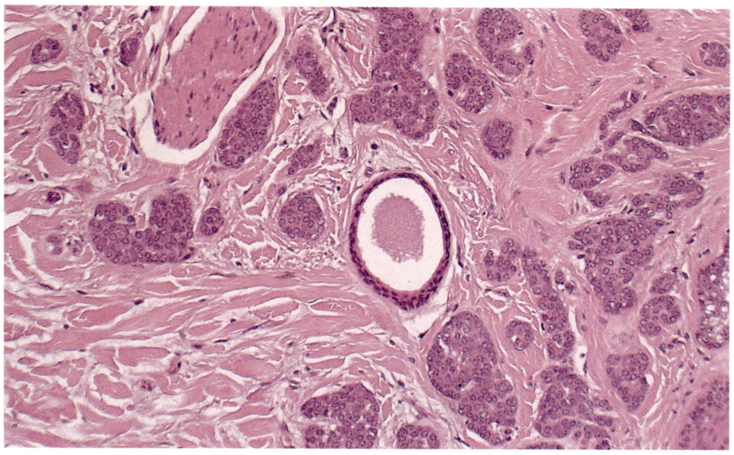

C

Figures 34–23A, 34–23B, 34–23C, 34–23D. Syringomatous carcinoma. Irregularly shaped tubular and nested aggregates of atypical eosinophilic epithelial cells. The aggregates extend deep into the reticular dermis and subcutaneous tissue. The dilated tubular structures contain eosinophilic amorphous material.

MUCINOUS CARCINOMA

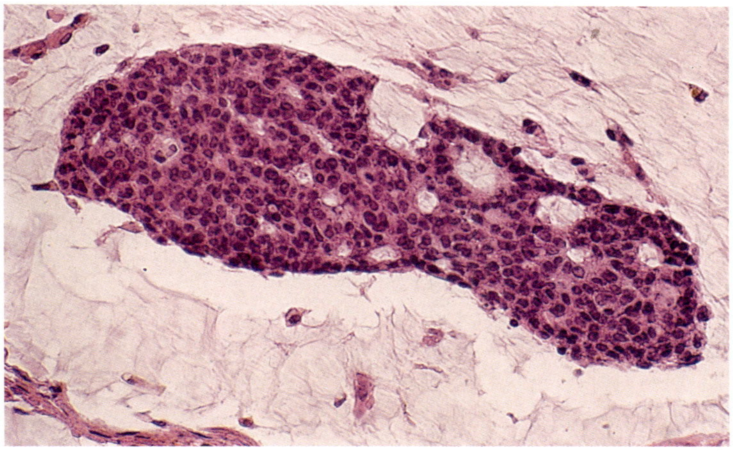

Figure 34–24. Mucinous carcinoma. Aggregate of eosinophilic, atypical epithelial cells, forming tubular structures and surrounded by copious deposits of stromal mucin.

35

Benign melanocytic neoplasms

- Simple lentigo
- Junctional melanocytic nevus
- Compound melanocytic nevus
- Intradermal melanocytic nevus
- Clark's (dysplastic) melanocytic nevus
- Halo melanocytic nevus
- Congenital melanocytic nevus
  - *A) Superficial congenital melanocytic nevus*
  - *B) Deep congenital melanocytic nevus*
- Recurrent (persistent) melanocytic nevus
- Spitz's melanocytic nevus
- Genital melanocytic nevus
- Acral melanocytic nevus
- Keratotic melanocytic nevus
- Ancient melanocytic nevus
- Blue melanocytic nevus
- Melanocytic nevus of Ota/Ito

SIMPLE LENTIGO

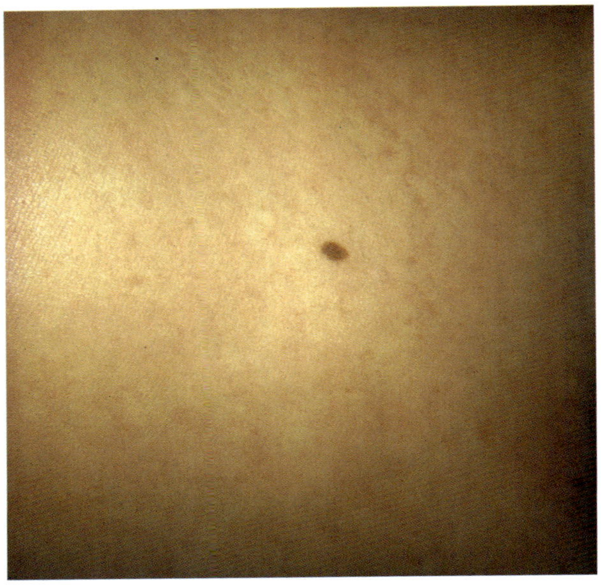

Figure 35–1. Simple lentigo. Small, brown, irregular macule on the calf.

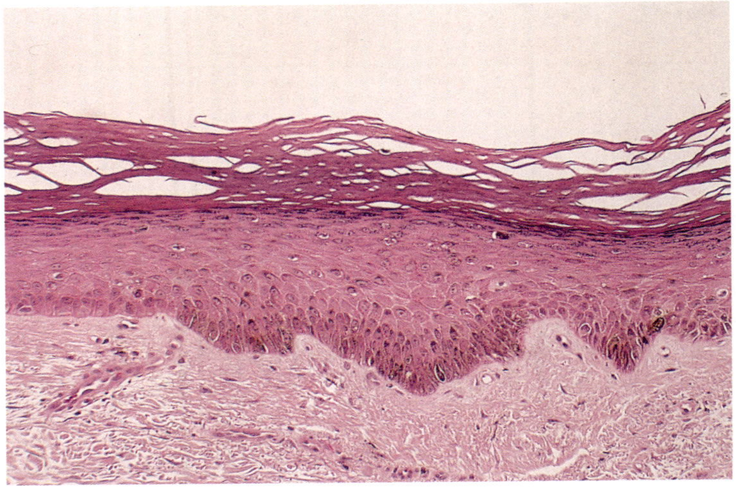

Figure 35–2. Simple lentigo. Increased number of melanocytes in the basal layer. There are melanin granules in the stratum corneum, and in melanophages in the dermis.

JUNCTIONAL MELANOCYTIC NEVUS

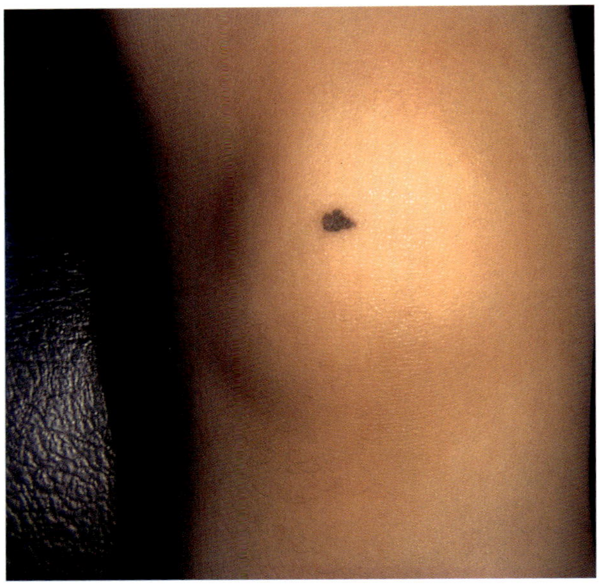

Figure 35–3. Junctional melanocytic nevus. Dark-brown irregular macule on the knee of a girl.

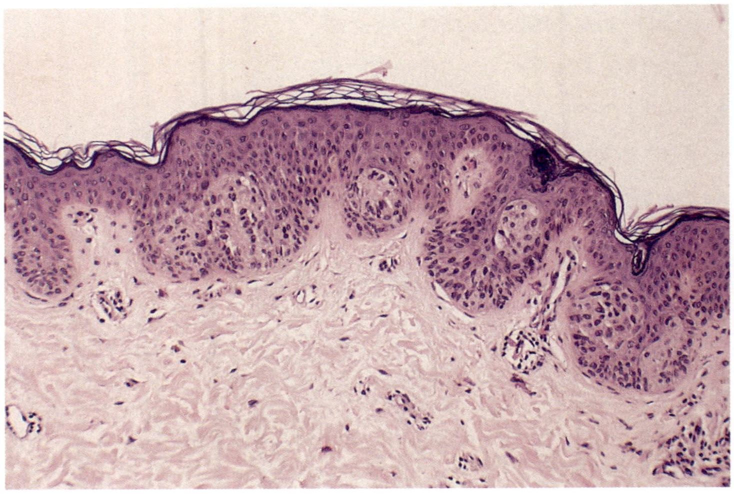

Figure 35–4. Junctional melanocytic nevus. Uniform-sized and -shaped nests of small, oval, monomorphous melanocytes at the dermoepidermal junction.

COMPOUND MELANOCYTIC NEVUS

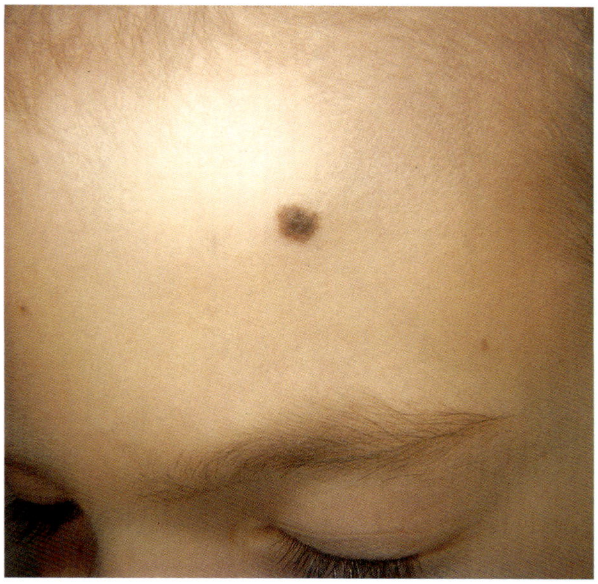

Figure 35–5. Compound melanocytic nevus. Dark-brown, slightly raised papule on the forehead of a boy.

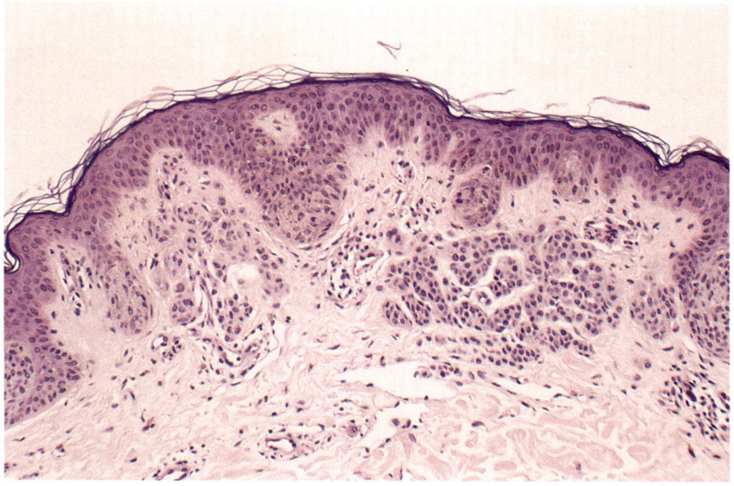

Figure 35–6. Compound melanocytic nevus. Uniform-sized and -shaped nests of small, oval, monomorphous melanocytes at the dermoepidermal junction and within the dermis.

INTRADERMAL MELANOCYTIC NEVUS

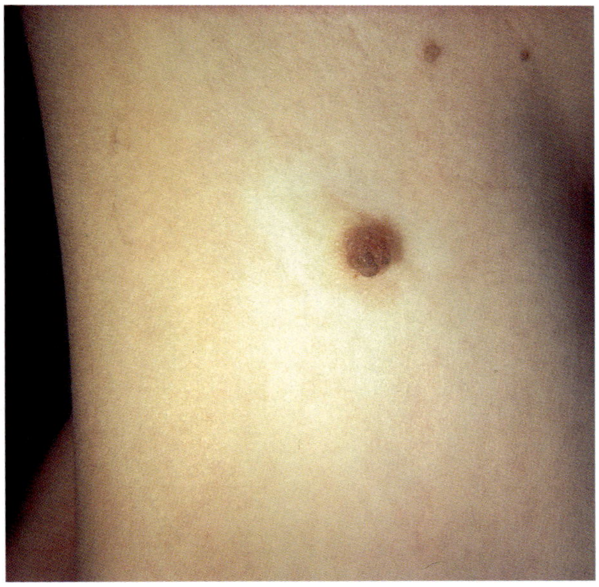

Figure 35–7. Intradermal melanocytic nevus. Soft, pedunculated brown papule on the leg of a girl.

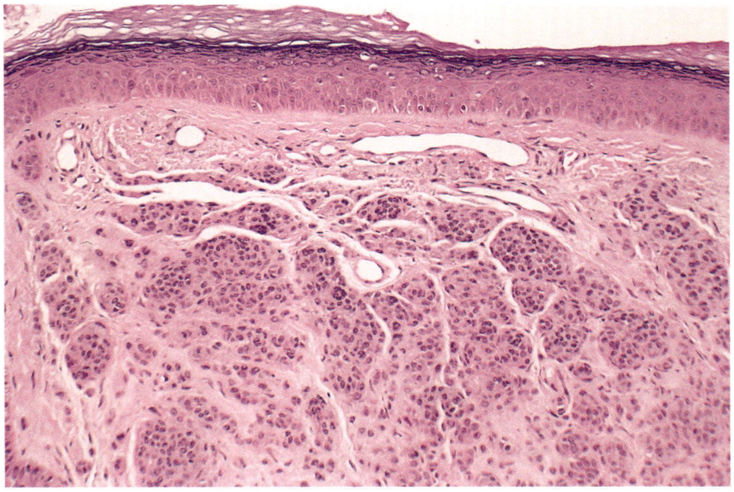

Figure 35–8. Intradermal melanocytic nevus. Round and oval nests of small round and oval monomorphous melanocytes within the dermis.

CLARK'S (DYSPLASTIC) MELANOCYTIC NEVUS

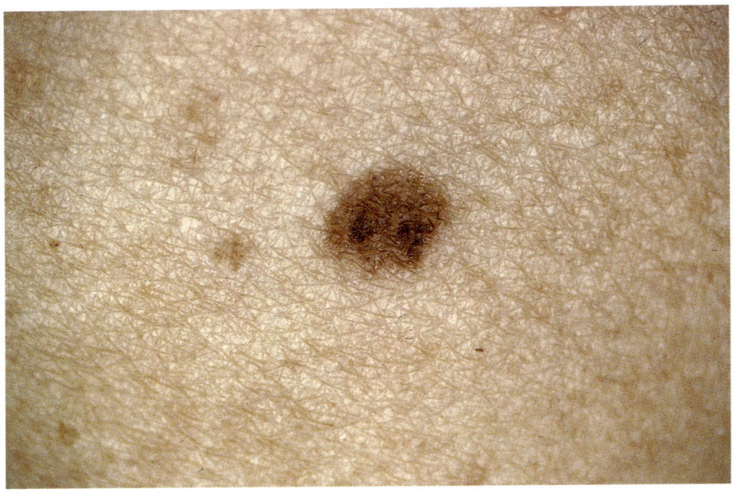

Figure 35–9. Clark's melanocytic nevus, junctional type. Tan macule with central dark-brown pigmentation and an irregular border.

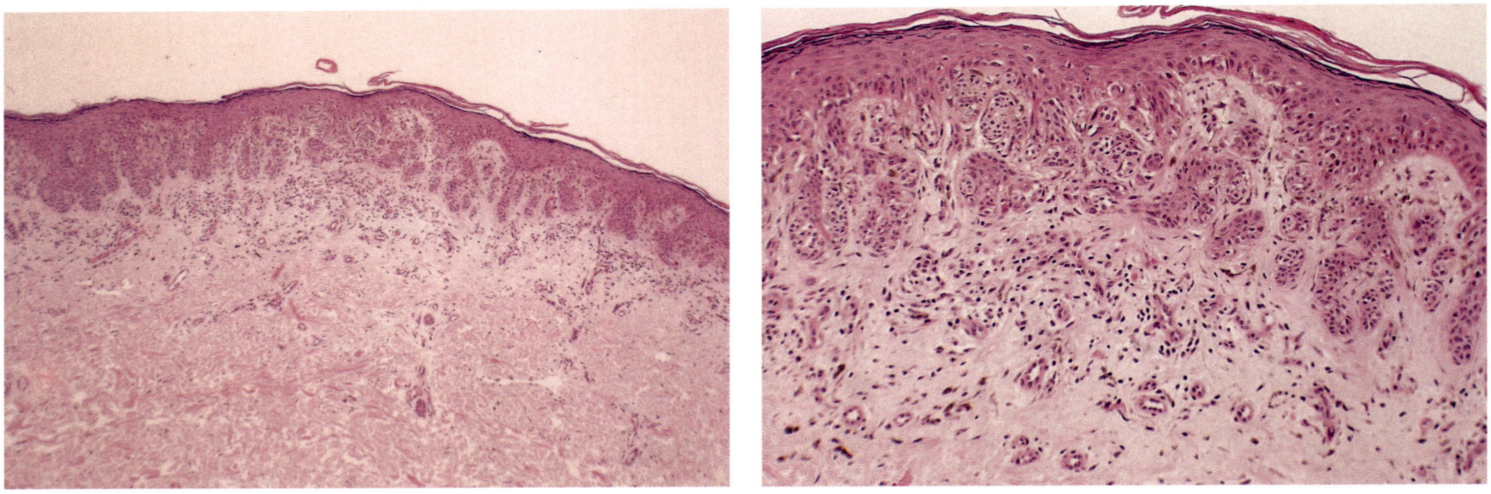

A

B

Figures 35–10A, 35–10B. Clark's melanocytic nevus, junctional type. Small oval melanocytes singly and in nests at the dermoepidermal junction. Atypical melanocytes may be present. There are elongated rete ridges, dilated blood vessels, melanophages, and a patchy superficial dermal lymphohistiocytic infiltrate.

CLARK'S (DYSPLASTIC) MELANOCYTIC NEVUS

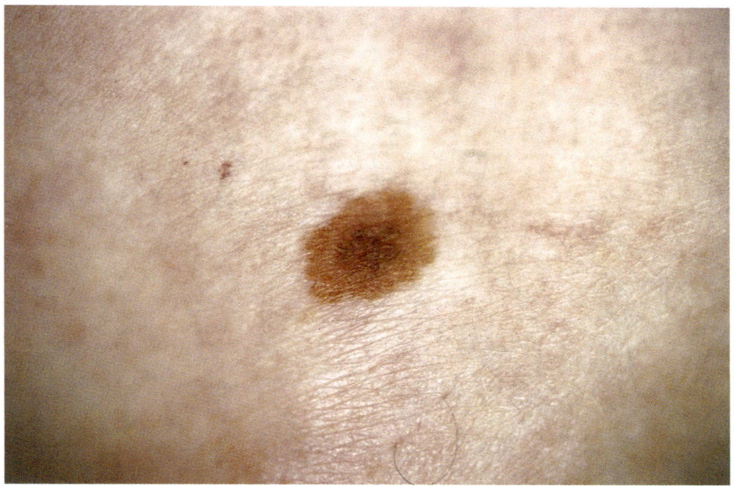

Figure 35–11. Clark's melanocytic nevus, compound type. Two-toned, slightly elevated, irregularly shaped plaque on the breast.

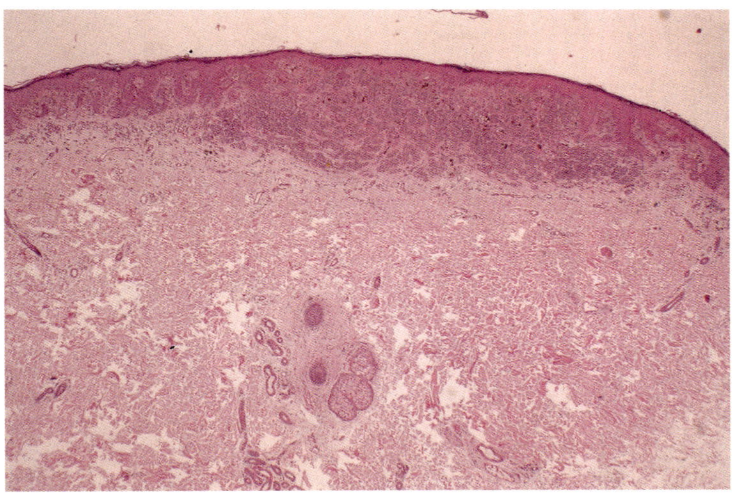

A

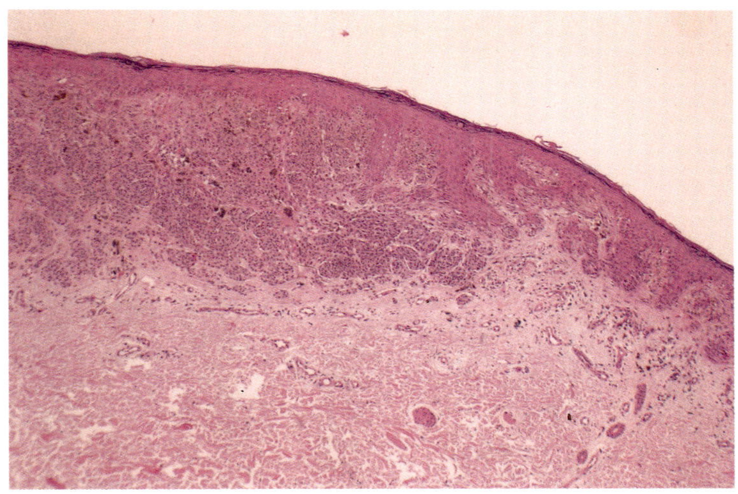

B

Figures 35–12A, 35–12B. Clark's melanocytic nevus, compound type. Symmetrical melanocytic nevus. The dermal component is confined to the thickened papillary dermis, and the junctional component extends laterally beyond the central portion of the lesion.

CLARK'S (DYSPLASTIC) MELANOCYTIC NEVUS

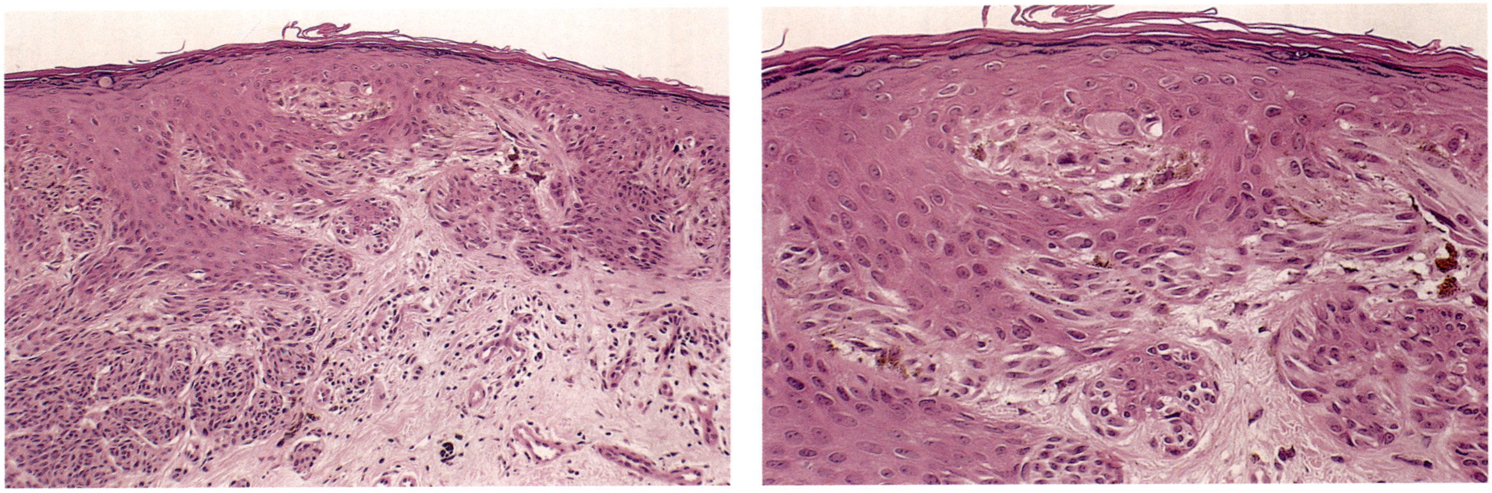

A B

Figures 35–13A, 35–13B. Clark's melanocytic nevus, compound type. Uniform nests of round and oval melanocytes at the dermoepidermal junction and within the thickened papillary dermis. Atypical melanocytes may occur at the dermoepidermal junction or within the papillary dermis. There are elongated rete ridges, fibroplasia, dilated blood vessels, melanophages, and a patchy lymphohistiocytic infiltrate.

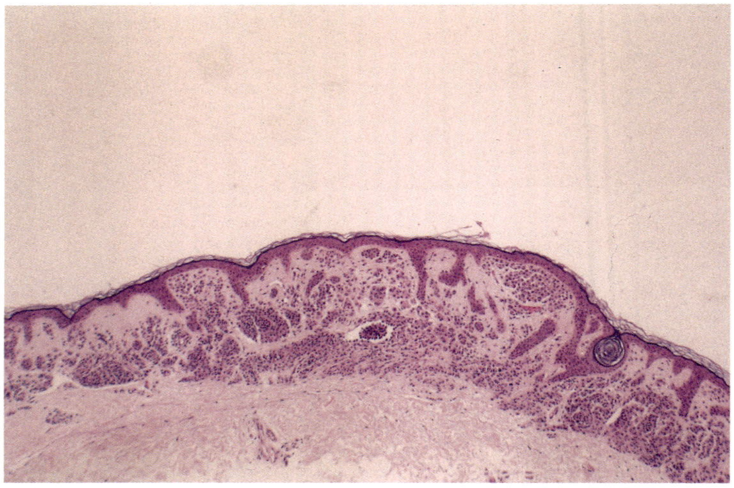

Figure 35–14. Clark's melanocytic nevus, intradermal type. Uniform nests of small oval melanocytes confined to and filling the thickened, flat-bottomed papillary dermis. There are elongated rete ridges and dilated blood vessels.

HALO MELANOCYTIC NEVUS

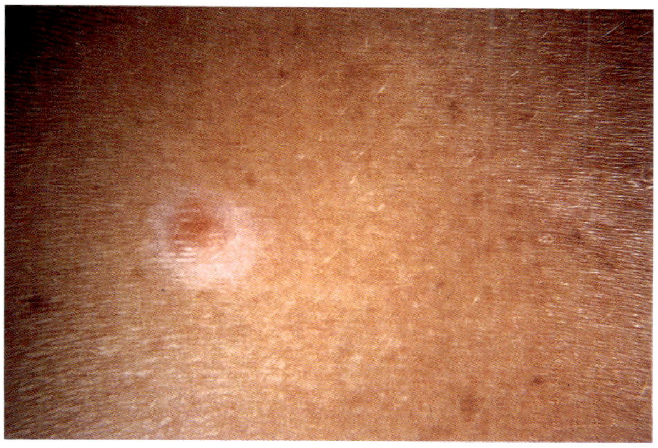

Figure 35–15. Halo melanocytic nevus. Central raised pink papule with surrounding hypopigmentation on the back.

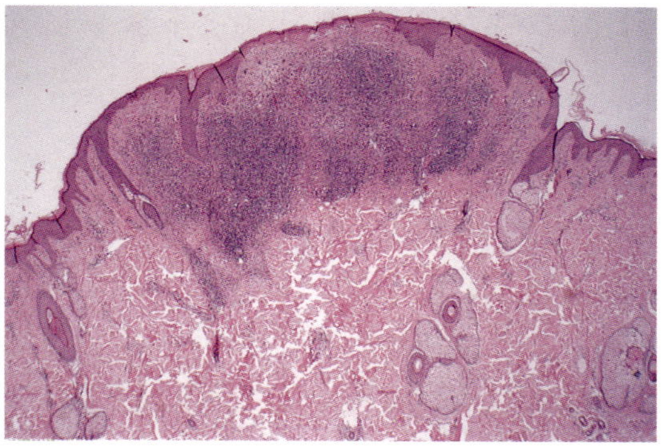

A

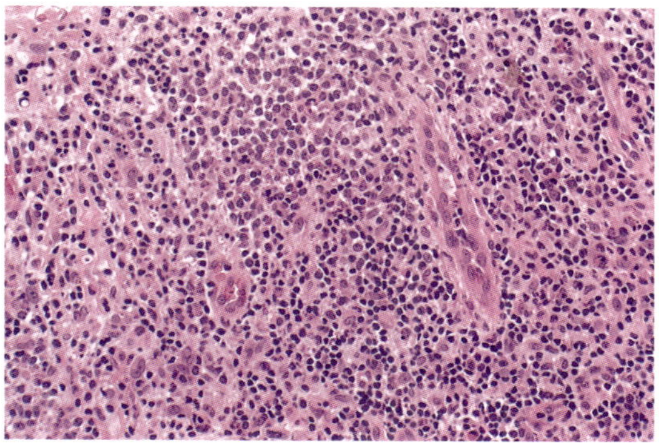

B

Figures 35–16A, 35–16B. Halo melanocytic nevus. Dome-shaped lesion with a dense lymphocytic infiltrate that obscures and destroys the melanocytes. There are dilated blood vessels and melanophages in the dermis.

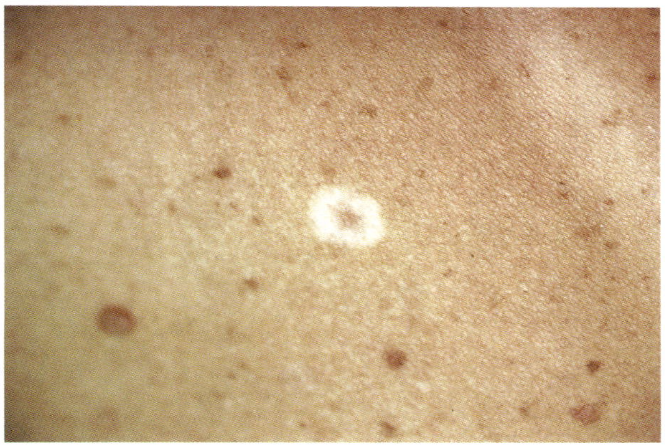

Figure 35–17. Halo melanocytic nevus, regressed. Pale, slightly raised papule with a surrounding area of hypopigmentation.

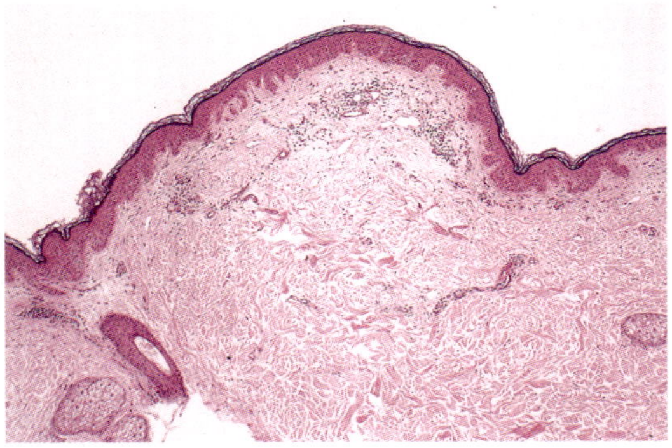

A

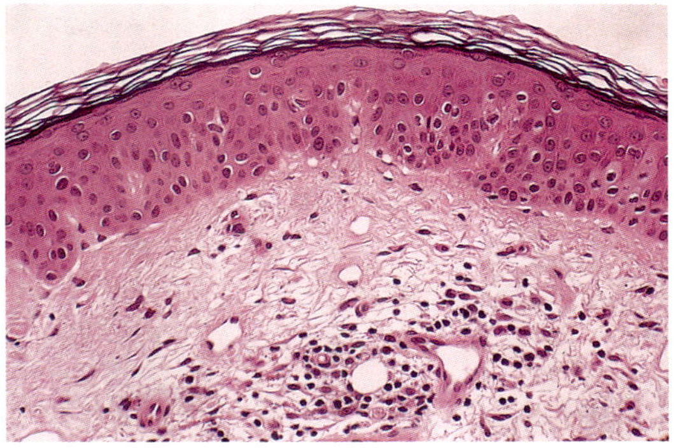

B

Figures 35–18A, 35–18B. Halo melanocytic nevus, regressed. Dome-shaped lesion with fibroplasia, dilated blood vessels, melanophages, and a patchy lymphocytic infiltrate. No melanocytes remain.

CONGENITAL MELANOCYTIC NEVUS

A) Superficial congenital melanocytic nevus

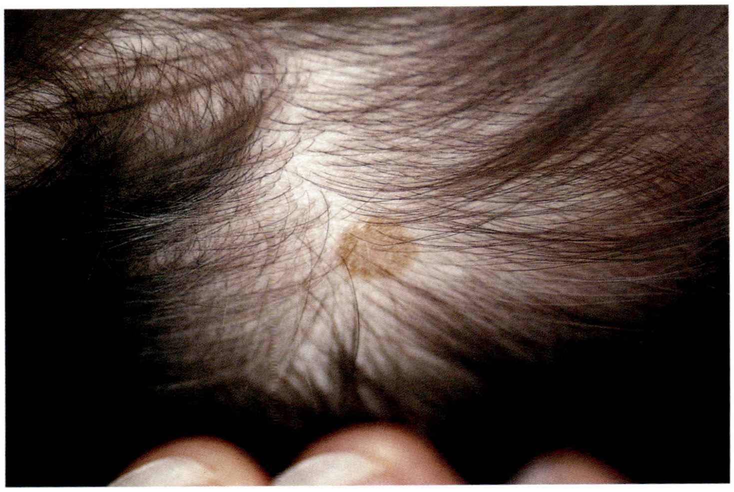

Figure 35–19. Superficial congenital melanocytic nevus. Darkening tan patch on the scalp of a four-year-old girl that has been present since birth.

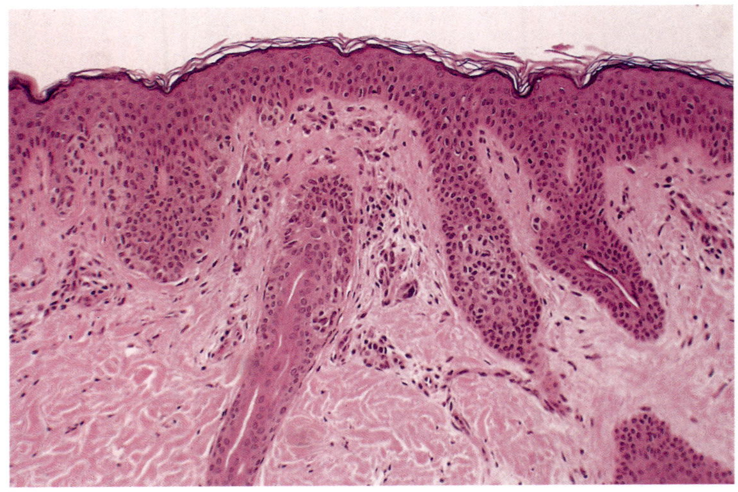

Figure 35–20. Superficial congenital melanocytic nevus, junctional type. Biopsy is from the patient shown in Figure 35–19. There are nests of melanocytes confined to the epidermis and structures of adnexa.

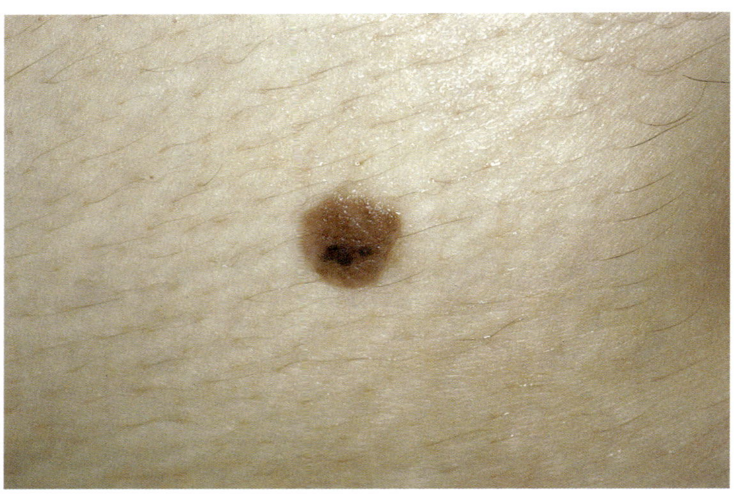

Figure 35–21. Superficial congenital melanocytic nevus. Irregularly pigmented light- and dark-brown nodule with an irregular border on the abdomen of a woman. The nevus had been present all her life.

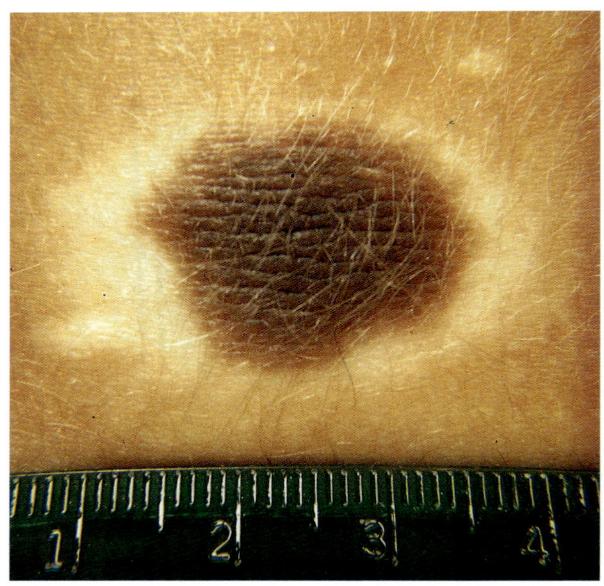

Figure 35–22. Superficial congenital melanocytic nevus. Brown nodule with numerous terminal hair shafts was present since birth. Surrounding hypopigmentation (halo) is of recent onset.

CONGENITAL MELANOCYTIC NEVUS

A) Superficial congenital melanocytic nevus

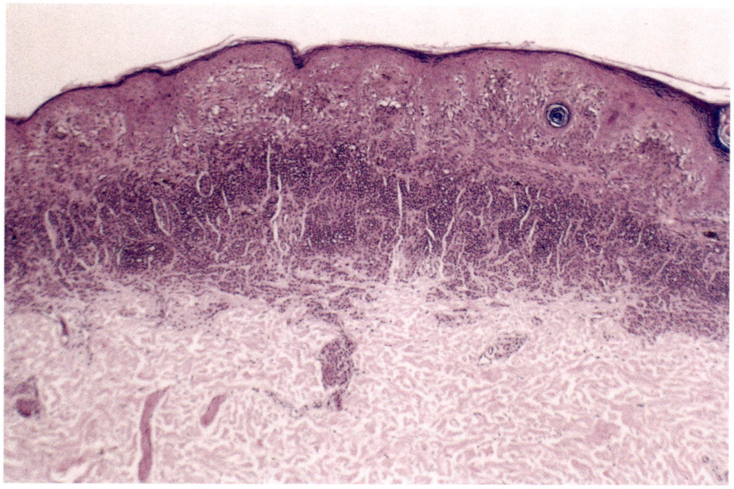

Figure 35–23. Superficial congenital melanocytic nevus, compound type. Nests of uniform melanocytes at the dermoepidermal junction, in the papillary and reticular dermis. There is adnexocentricity, angiocentricity, and solitary melanocytes between collagen bundles.

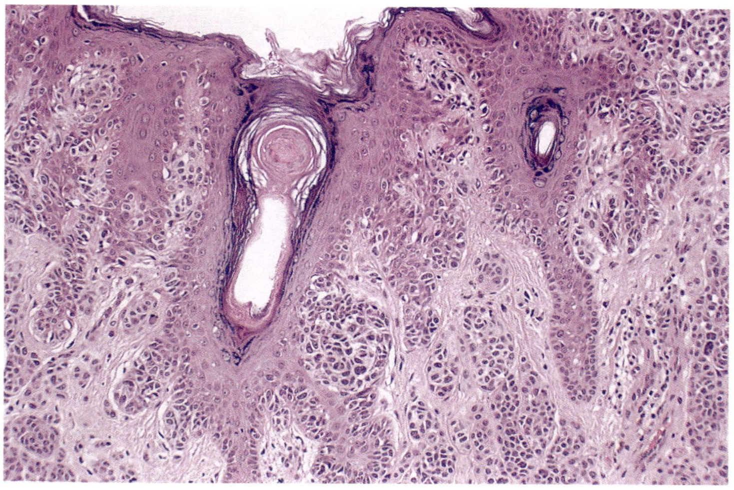

Figure 35–24. Superficial congenital melanocytic nevus, compound type. Solitary melanocytes and nests of melanocytes involve folliculosebaceous units. Nests of small round and oval melanocytes are present in the dermis.

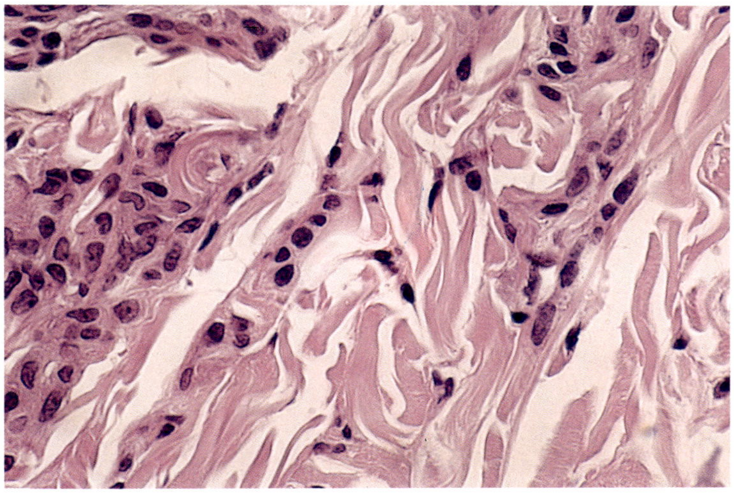

Figure 35–25. Superficial congenital melanocytic nevus. Uniform round and oval melanocytes between collagen bundles.

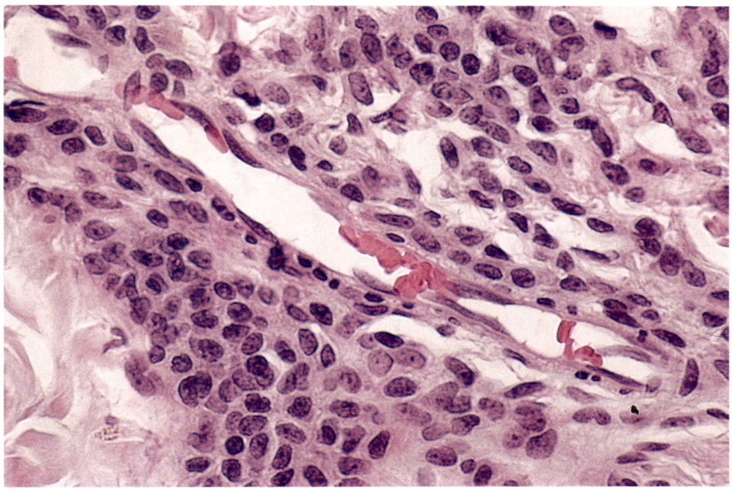

Figure 35–26. Superficial congenital melanocytic nevus. Monomorphous melanocytes within and around blood-vessel wall.

CONGENITAL MELANOCYTIC NEVUS

A) Superficial congenital melanocytic nevus

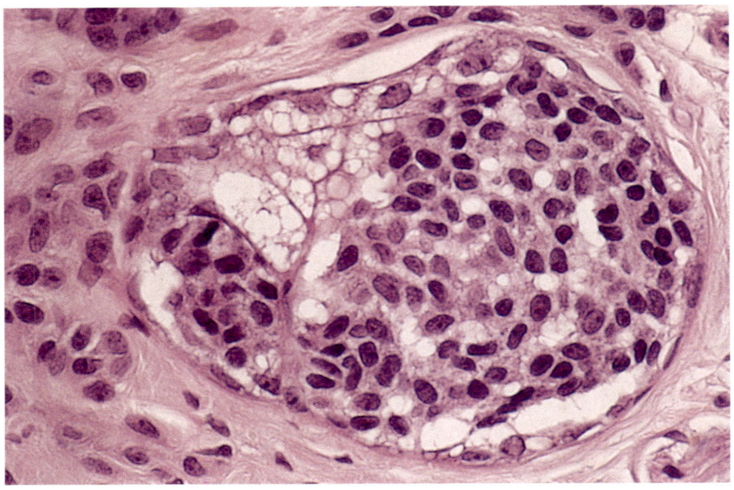

Figure 35–27. Superficial congenital melanocytic nevus. Nest of uniform oval melanocytes within a sebaceous lobule. Sebocytes have vacuolated cytoplasm.

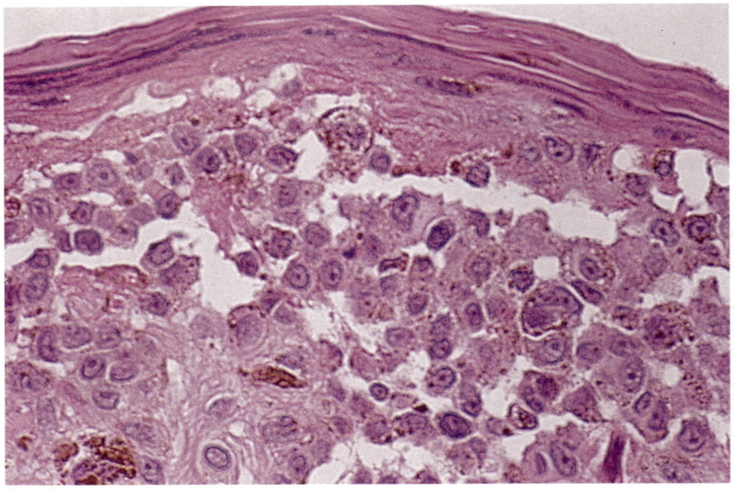

Figure 35–28. Superficial congenital melanocytic nevus, compound type. Round and plump-oval melanocytes as solitary units, in disheveled nests, and with loss of cohesion within the upper levels of the epidermis. These changes in a superficial congenital compound melanocytic nevus occur sporadically and may simulate a malignant melanoma.

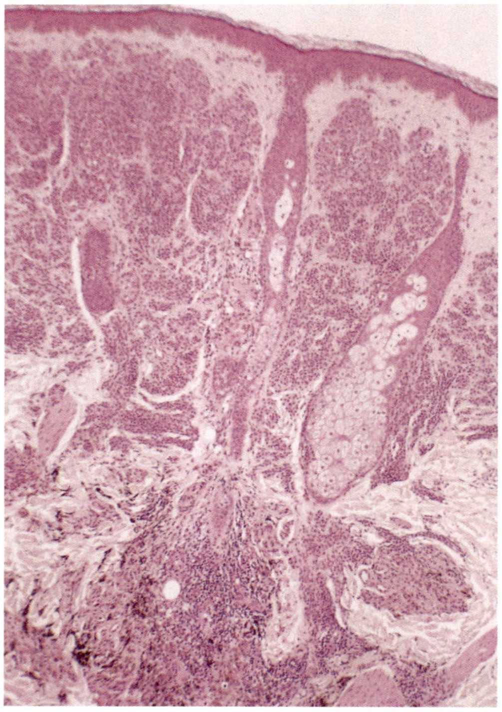

A

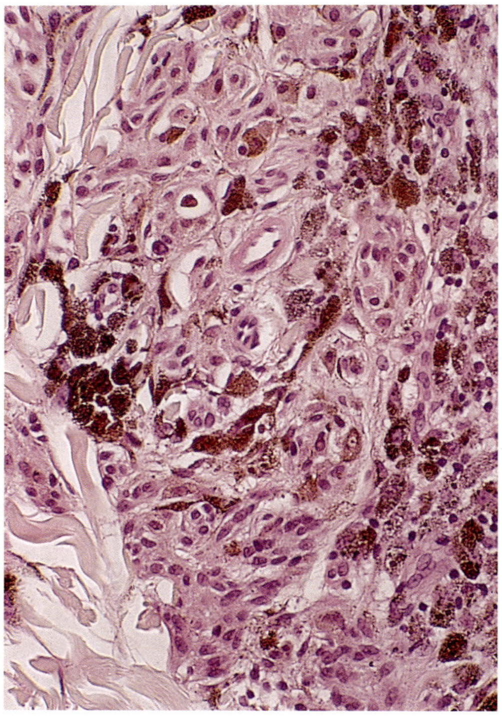

B

Figures 35–29A, 35–29B. Superficial congenital melanocytic nevus, combined/deep penetrating type. Vertically oriented nests of melanocytes within the reticular dermis with adnexocentricity. There are round, oval, spindle-shaped pigmented dendritic melanocytes and small typical pagetoid melanocytes (large cell with abundant pale-staining cytoplasm and small round nucleus). Prominent intra- and extracellular melanin deposition is present.

CONGENITAL MELANOCYTIC NEVUS

B) Deep congenital melanocytic nevus

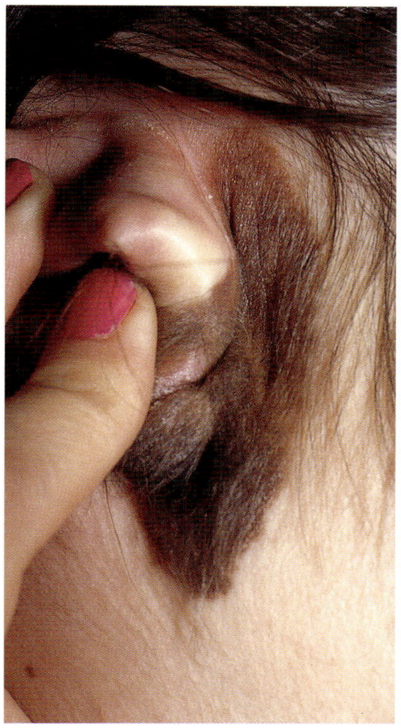

Figure 35–30. Deep congenital melanocytic nevus. Large, irregular hyperpigmented plaque with an abundance of terminal hairs located on the ear and postauricular area.

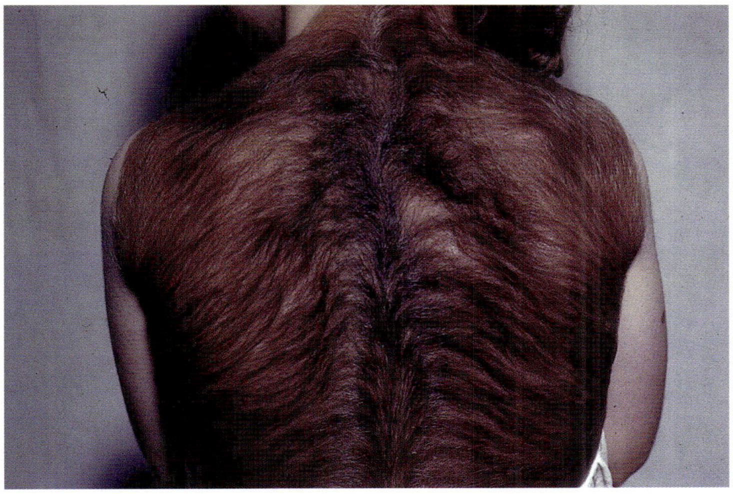

Figure 35–31. Deep congenital melanocytic nevus. Large, dark-brown confluent lesion with increased hair involving the back and neck of a young girl.

CONGENITAL MELANOCYTIC NEVUS

B) Deep congenital melanocytic nevus

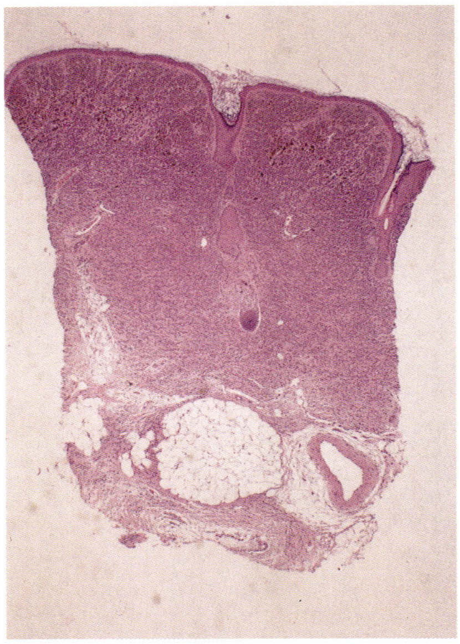

A

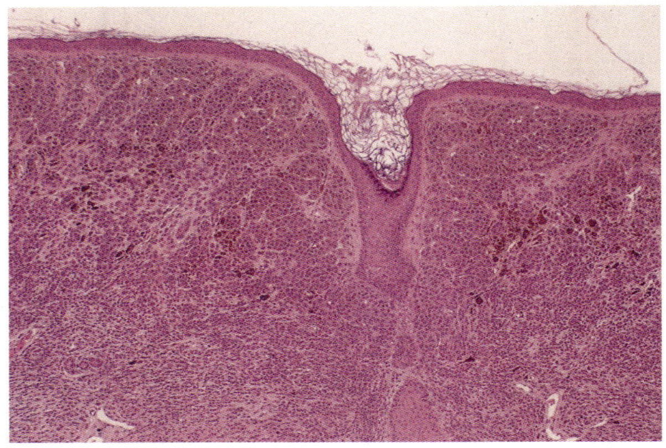

B

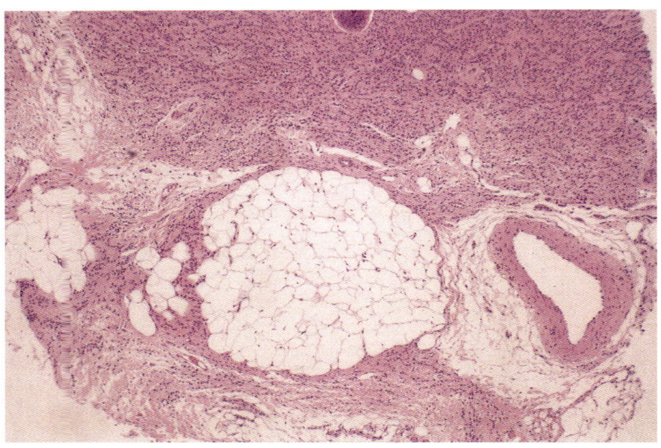

C

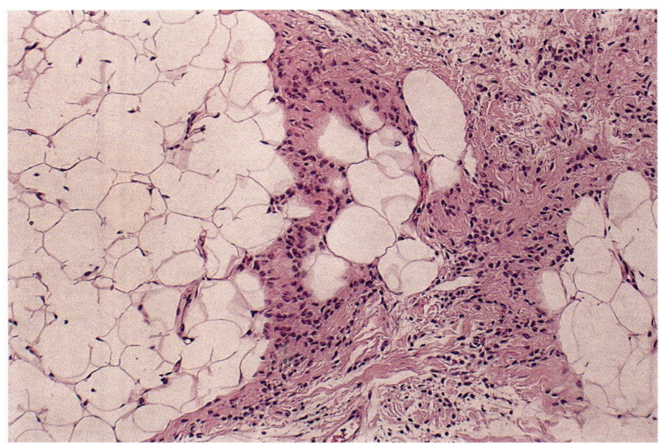

D

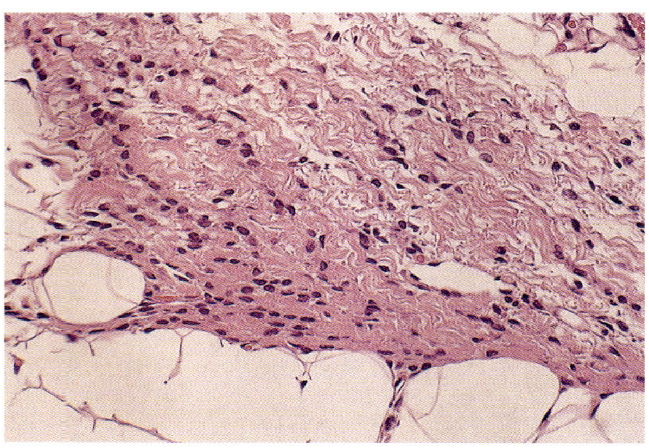

E

Figures 35–32A, 35–32B, 35–32C, 35–32D, 35–32E. **Deep congenital melanocytic nevus.** Nests and sheets of small oval and round melanocytes involve the full thickness of the reticular dermis and extend into the subcutaneous tissue.

RECURRENT (PERSISTENT) MELANOCYTIC NEVUS

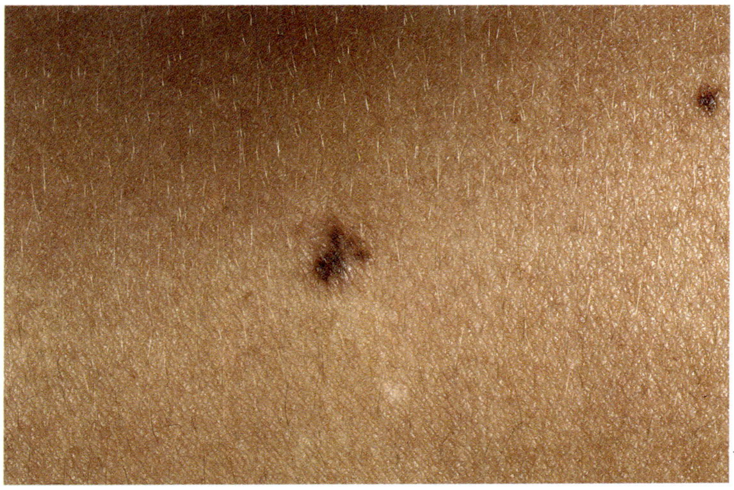

Figure 35–33. Recurrent melanocytic nevus. Irregularly pigmented brown lesion on the back of a woman. A benign melanocytic nevus was partially removed from the site four months earlier.

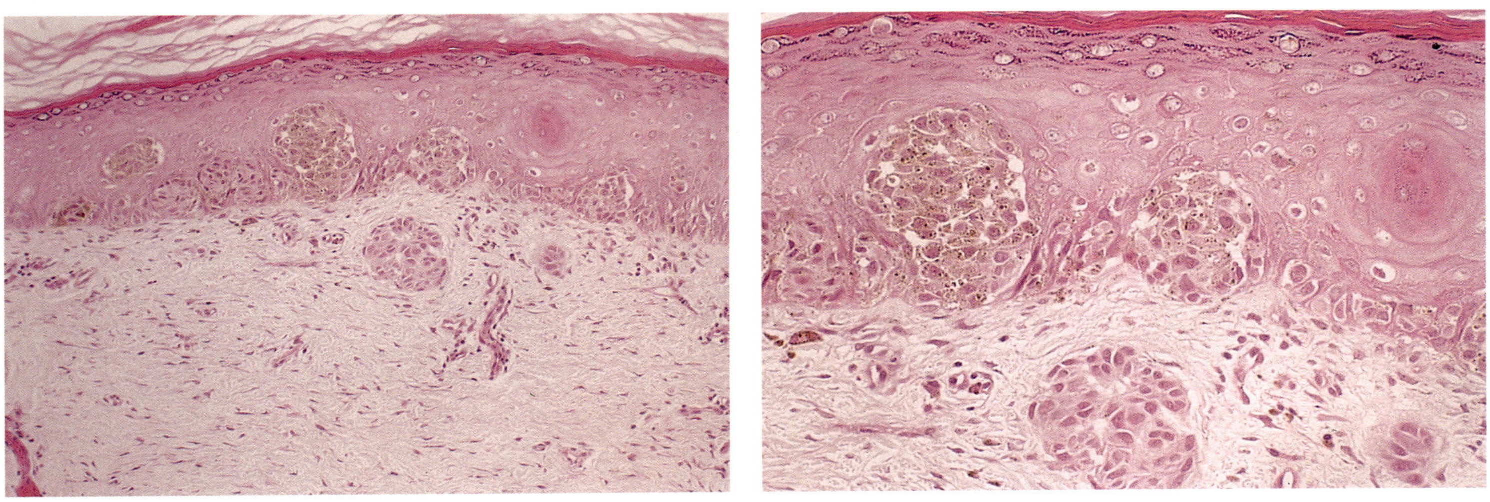

A B

Figures 35–34A, 35–34B. Recurrent melanocytic nevus. Solitary and irregular nested melanocytes within the lower and mid-epidermis and dermis. There is horizontal dermal fibroplasia and vertically oriented blood vessels in the dermis, which are the dermal changes of a scar. These changes simulate malignant melanoma. Histologic examination of the original nevus is judicious.

SPITZ'S MELANOCYTIC NEVUS

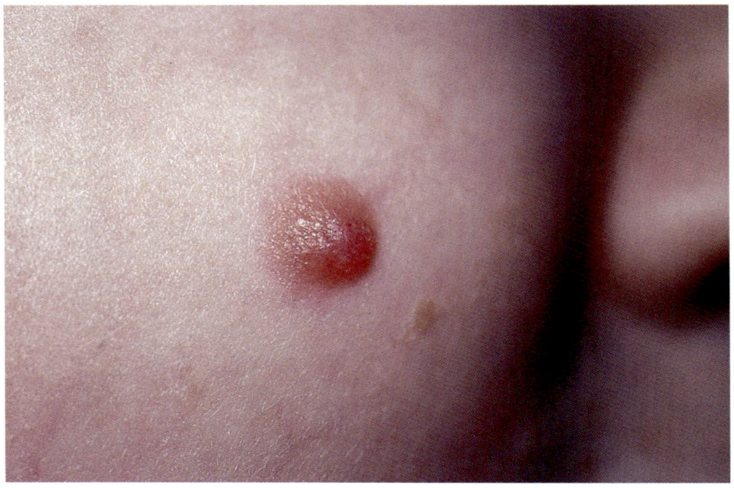

Figure 35–35. Spitz's melanocytic nevus. Red, dome-shaped nodule on the cheek of a child. The nodule had grown rapidly in the previous four months.

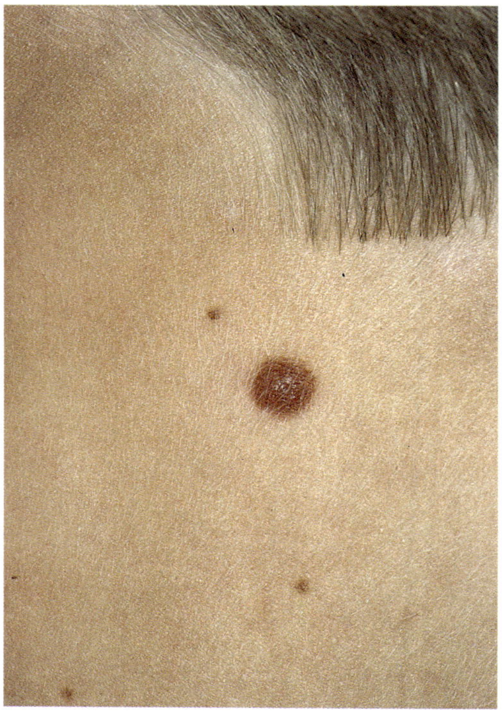

Figure 35–36. Spitz's melanocytic nevus. Brown, dome-shaped nodule, which had recently enlarged in a young boy.

SPITZ'S MELANOCYTIC NEVUS

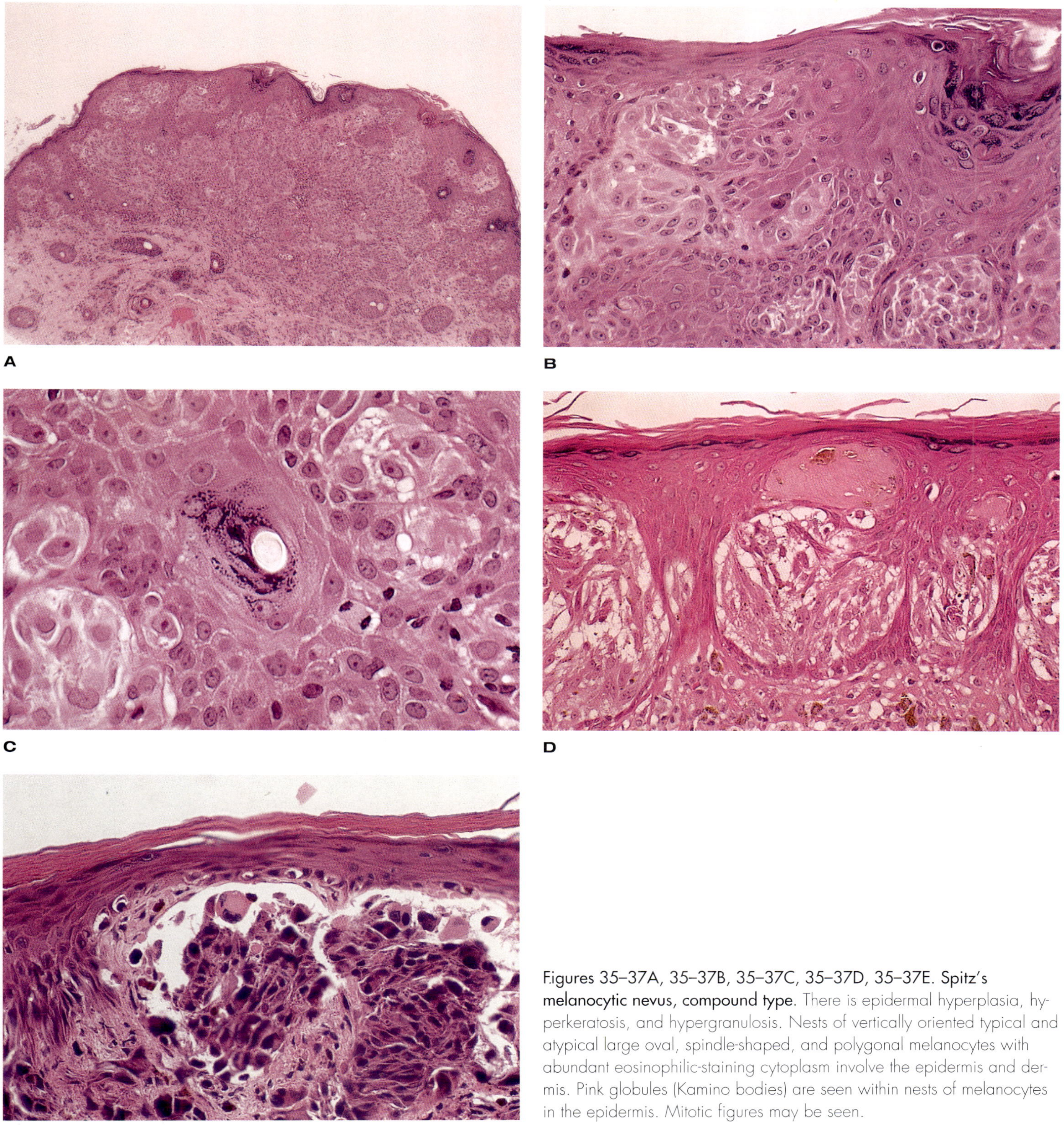

A B C D E

Figures 35–37A, 35–37B, 35–37C, 35–37D, 35–37E. **Spitz's melanocytic nevus, compound type.** There is epidermal hyperplasia, hyperkeratosis, and hypergranulosis. Nests of vertically oriented typical and atypical large oval, spindle-shaped, and polygonal melanocytes with abundant eosinophilic-staining cytoplasm involve the epidermis and dermis. Pink globules (Kamino bodies) are seen within nests of melanocytes in the epidermis. Mitotic figures may be seen.

SPITZ'S MELANOCYTIC NEVUS

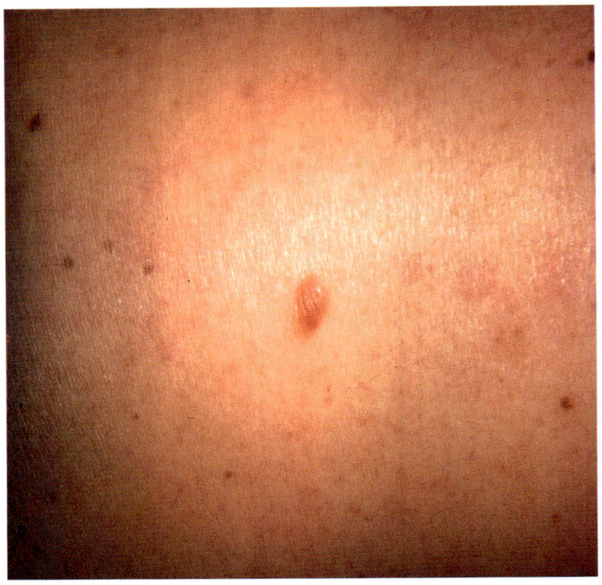

Figure 35–38. Spitz's melanocytic nevus, intradermal type. Pink, firm nodule on the back of a young man.

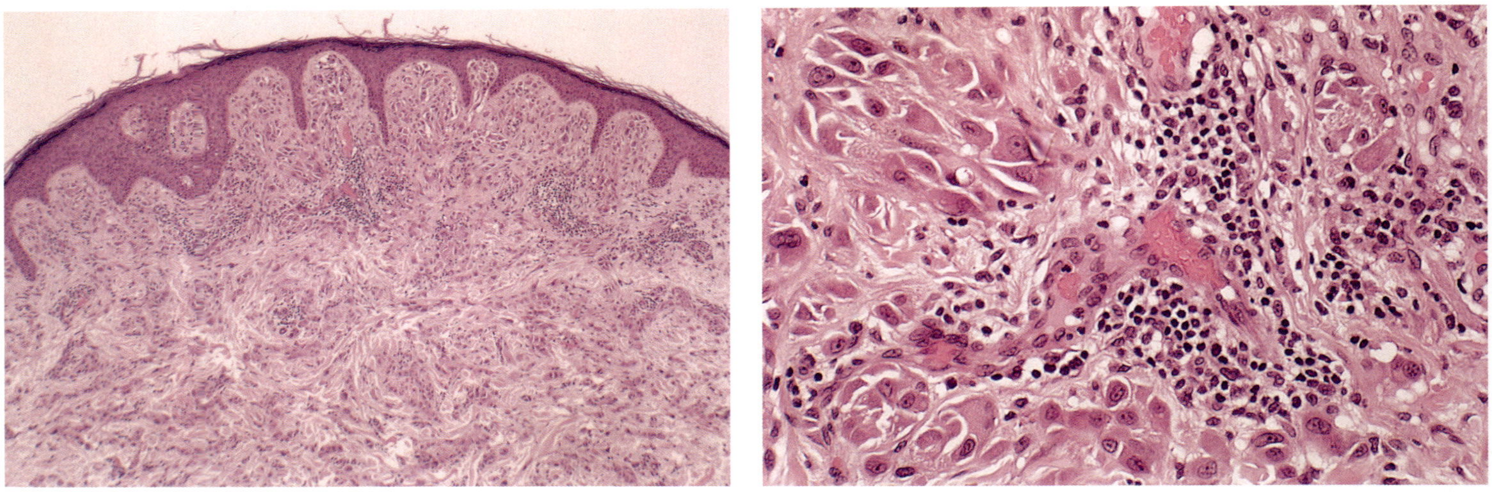

A B

Figures 35–39A, 35–39B. Spitz's melanocytic nevus, intradermal type. Dome-shaped nodule with large single and many multinucleated polygonal and oval melanocytes with abundant eosinophilic-staining cytoplasm confined to the dermis. The dermis is fibrocytic, and there is a patchy perivascular lymphocytic infiltrate.

SPITZ'S MELANOCYTIC NEVUS

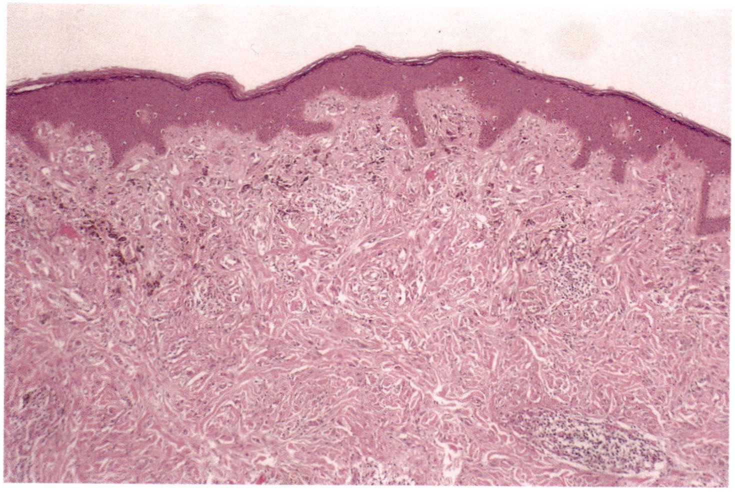

A

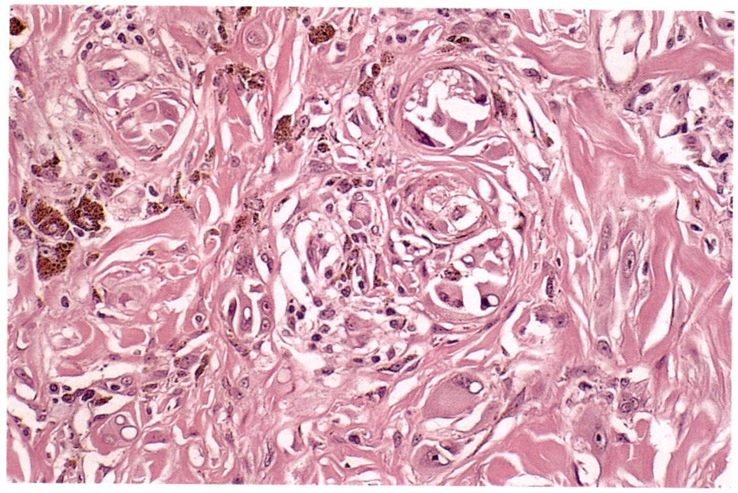

B

Figures 35–40A, 35–40B. Spitz's melanocytic nevus, desmoplastic type. Extensive desmoplasia with thick collagen bundles, many fibrocytes, and numerous large polygonal and oval single and multinucleated melanocytes with abundant eosinophilic-staining cytoplasm.

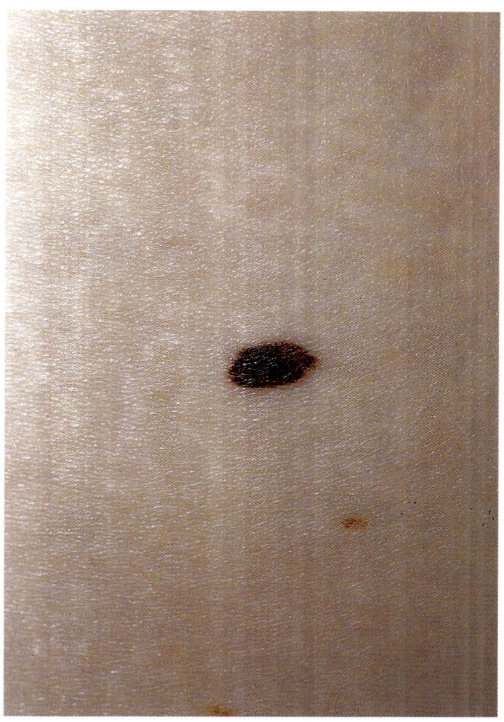

Figure 35–41. Spitz's nevus, pigmented spindle-cell variant. Dark-brown pigmented plaque on the buttocks of a young woman.

SPITZ'S MELANOCYTIC NEVUS

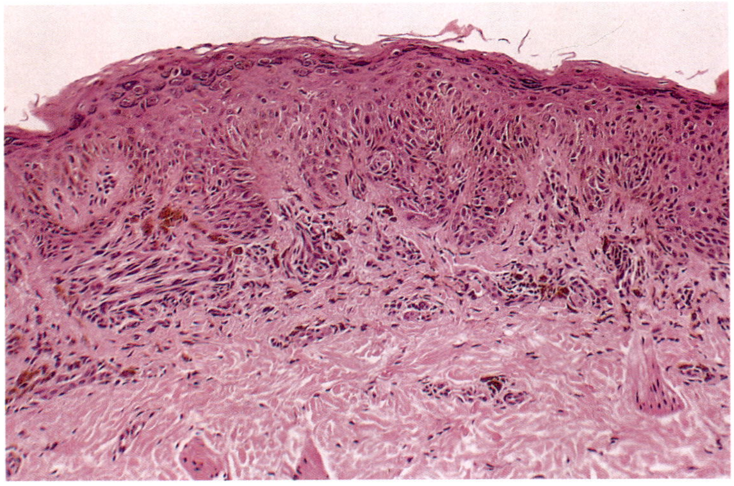

A

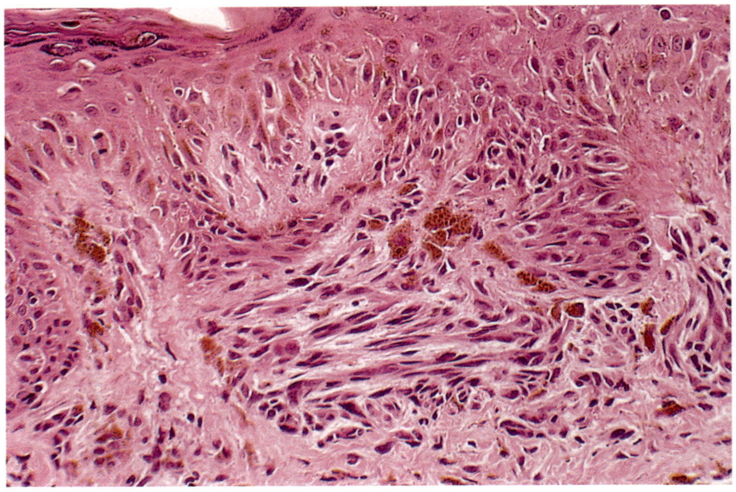

B

Figures 35–42A, 35–42B. Spitz's nevus, pigmented spindle-cell variant. Nests of large, spindle-shaped melanocytes within the lower epidermis and thickened papillary dermis. These cells have abundant eosinophilic-staining cytoplasm and melanin. There is hyperkeratosis, hypergranulosis and epidermal hyperplasia.

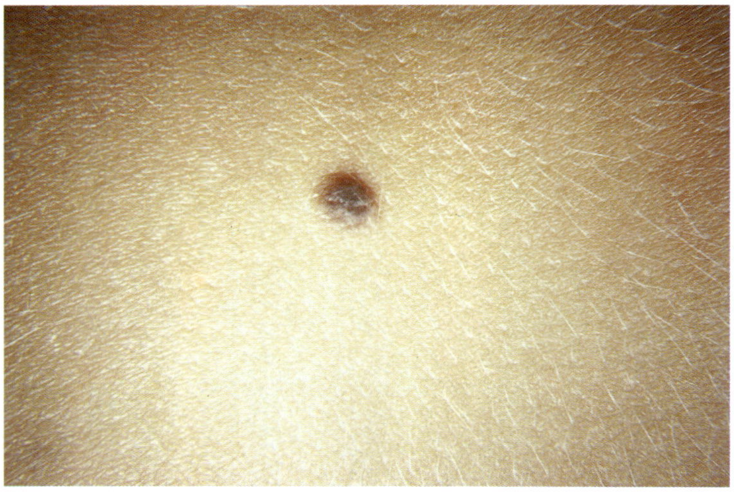

Figure 35–43. Spitz's nevus, combined type. Irregular blue-gray pigmented papule on the back of a nine-year-old boy.

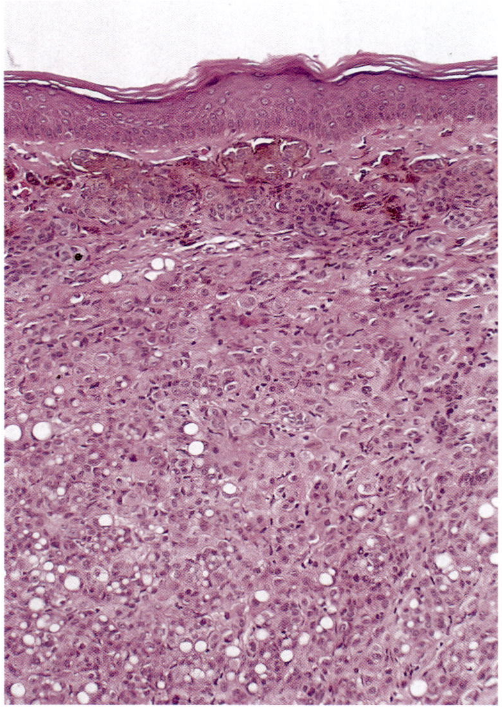

Figure 35–44. Spitz's nevus, combined type. Nests of monomorphous small, round and oval pigmented melanocytes overlying sheets of large, polygonal single and multinucleated melanocytes with abundant eosinophilic-staining cytoplasm. There are necrotic cells, mitotic figures, and atypical melanocytes.

GENITAL MELANOCYTIC NEVUS

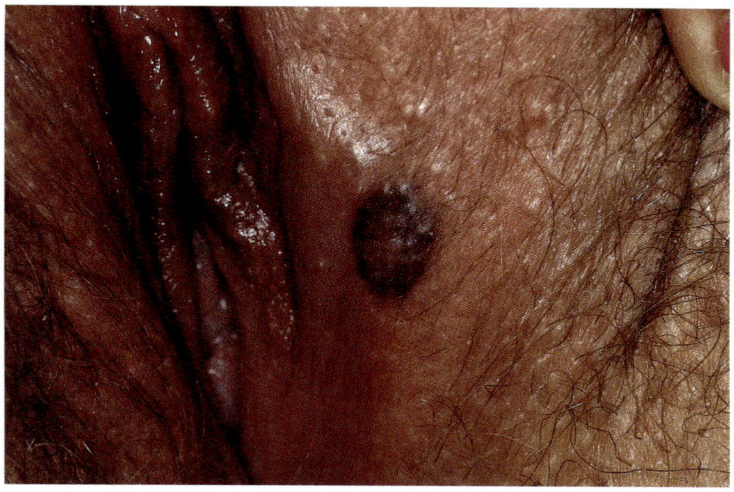

Figure 35–45. Genital melanocytic nevus. Long-standing hyperpigmented plaque on the labia of a woman. This melanocytic nevus may be a superficial congenital melanocytic nevus.

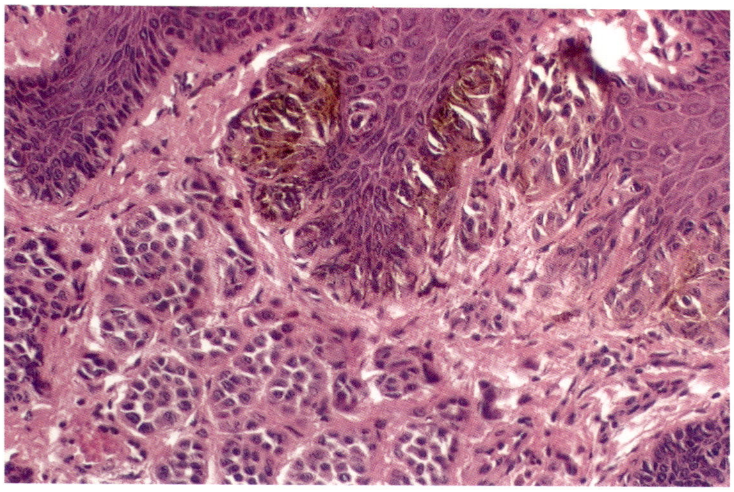

Figure 35–46. Genital melanocytic nevus. Single and nested pigmented spindle-shaped and oval melanocytes within the lower layers of the epidermis. The nuclei become smaller with progressive descent into the papillary dermis. Atypical and necrotic melanocytes with occasional mitotic figures may be present.

ACRAL MELANOCYTIC NEVUS

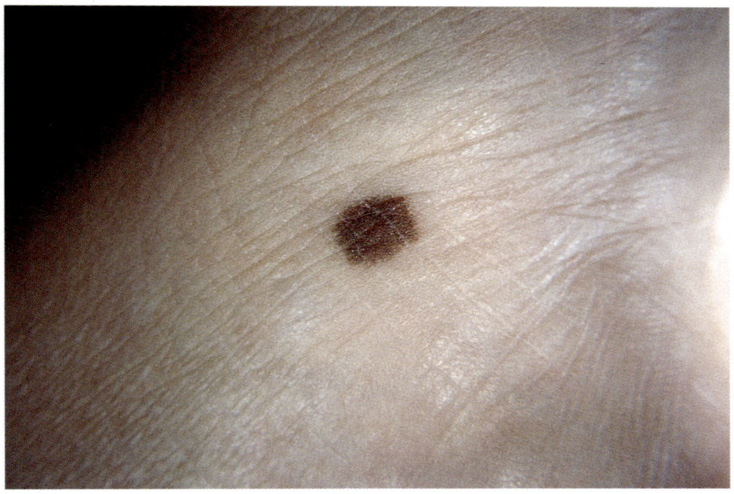

Figure 35–47. Acral melanocytic nevus. Hyperpigmented raised plaque on the foot. Surface of the lesion retains normal skin markings.

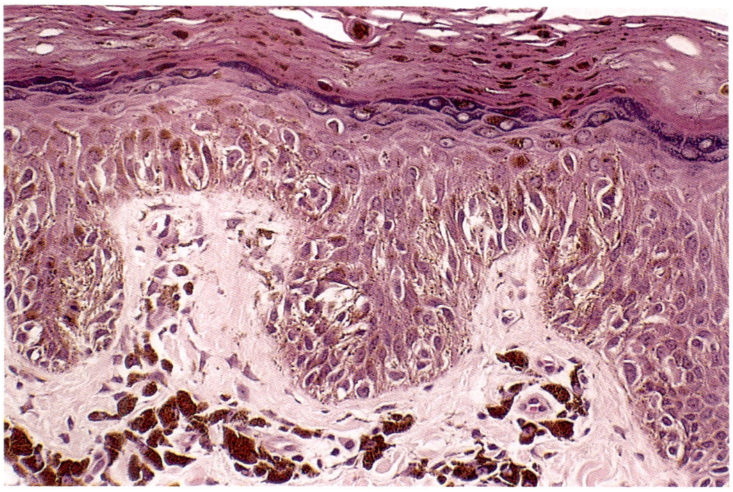

Figure 35–48. Acral melanocytic nevus. Single and nested spindle-shaped and oval melanocytes are present at all levels of the epidermis, where there are necrotic and mitotic melanocytes. Clefted, pigmented melanocytes are present within the stratum corneum along with copious deposits of melanin. Within the dermis, there are numerous melanophages and fibrocytes.

KERATOTIC MELANOCYTIC NEVUS

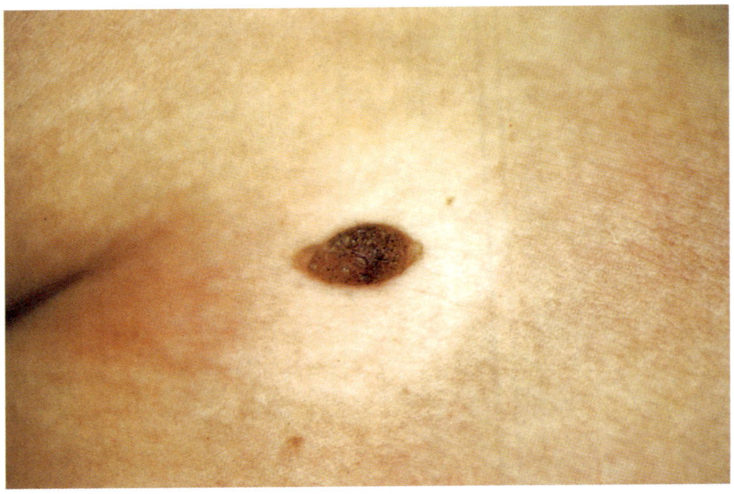

Figure 35–49. Keratotic melanocytic nevus. Raised brown corrugated papule with prominent follicular ostia. This lesion is commonly mistaken clinically for a seborrheic keratosis.

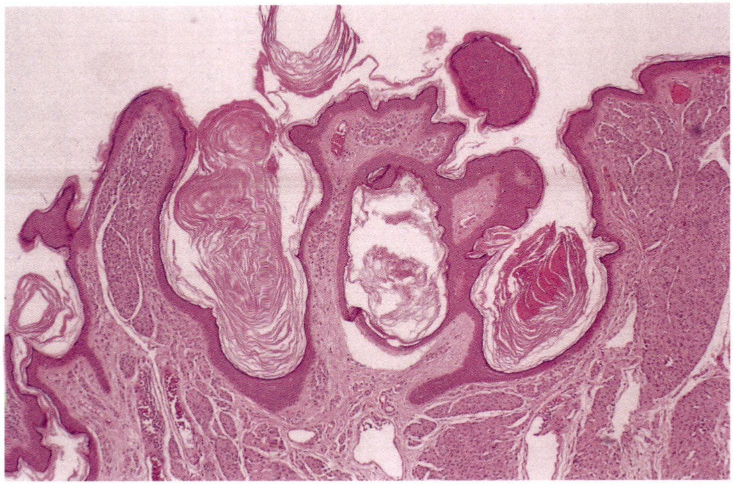

A

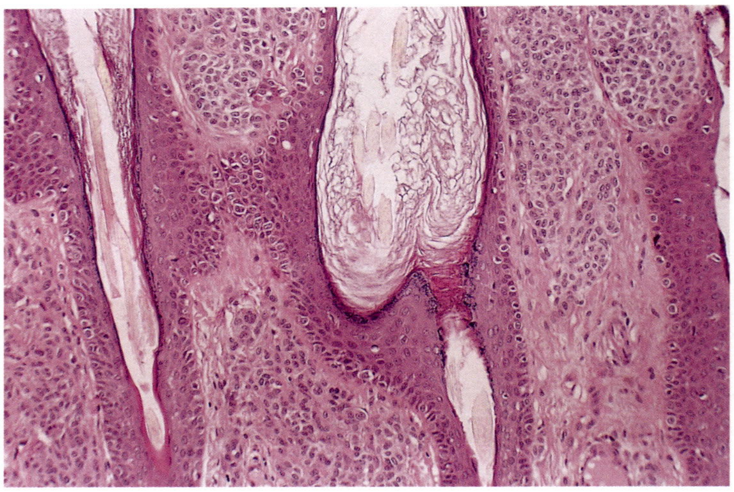

B

Figures 35–50A, 35–50B. Keratotic melanocytic nevus. Hyperkeratotic and distended infundibula encircled by normal-appearing, mostly nested small oval and round melanocytes in the dermis. The hyperkeratotic infundibula often contain hair shaft fragments. The melanocytes may be present in either the dermis or the epidermis or both.

ANCIENT MELANOCYTIC NEVUS

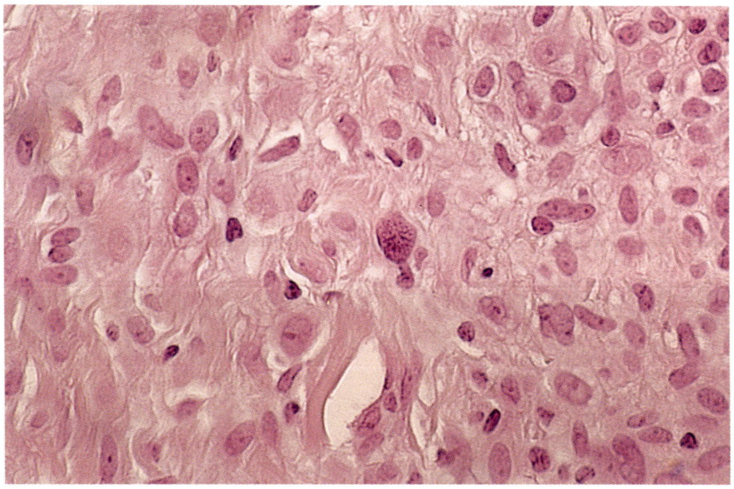

A

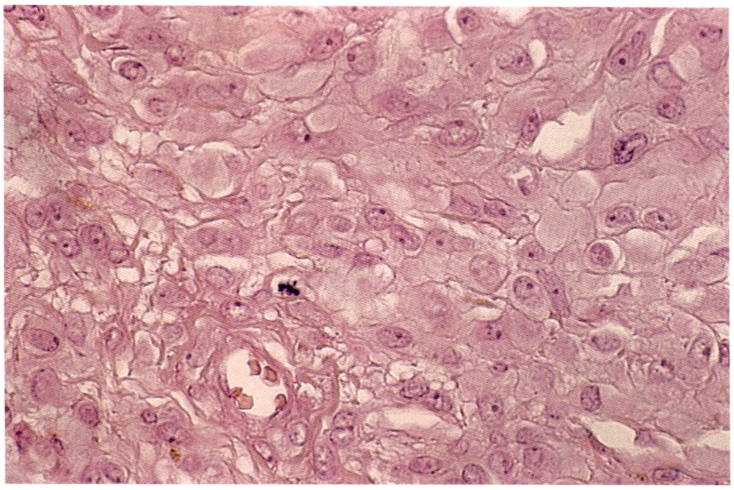

B

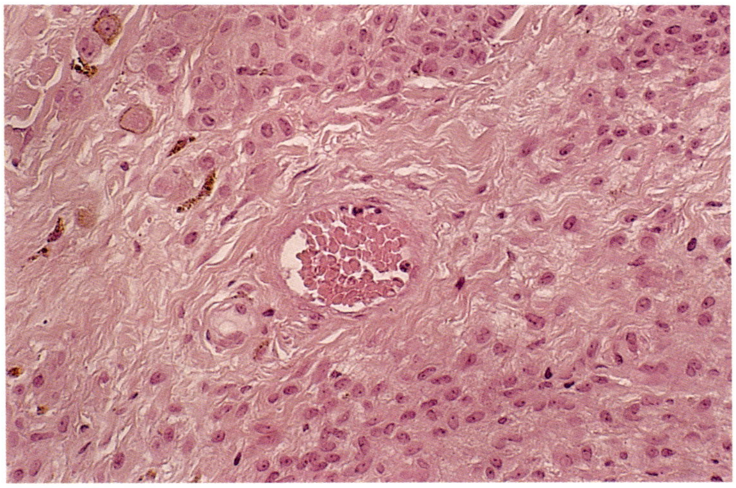

C

Figures 35–51A, 35–51B, 35–51C. Ancient melanocytic nevus. Scattered pleomorphic dermal melanocytes with an occasional mitotic figure admixed with normal-appearing dermal melanocytes. There are areas with predominantly perivascular sclerosis, dilated venules, and dermal mucin deposition.

BLUE MELANOCYTIC NEVUS

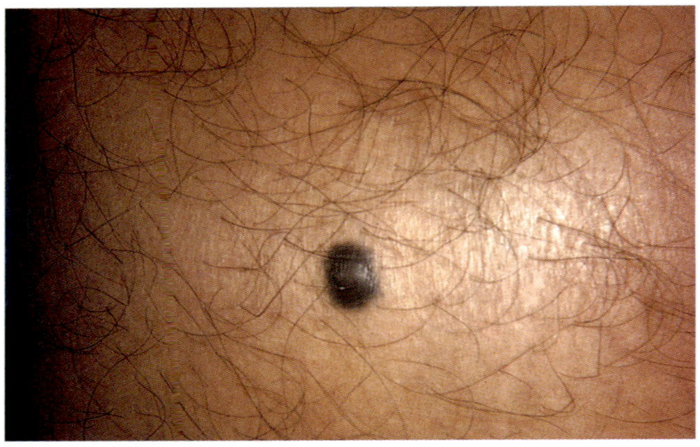

Figure 35–52. Blue melanocytic nevus. Blue-gray dome-shaped papule on the calf of a man.

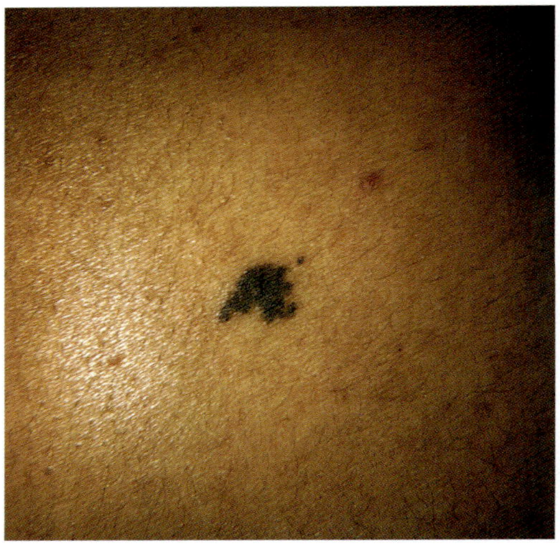

Figure 35–53. Blue melanocytic nevus. Strikingly irregular, blue papillated plaque with notched margins. Blue melanocytic nevi may represent a type of congenital melanocytic nevus.

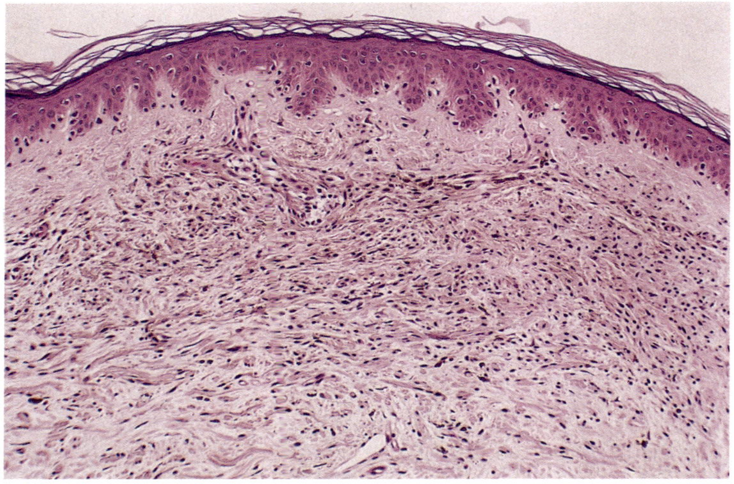

A

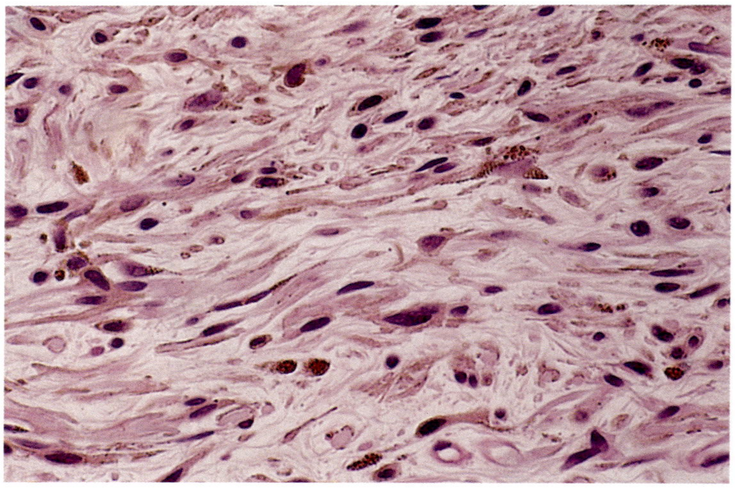

B

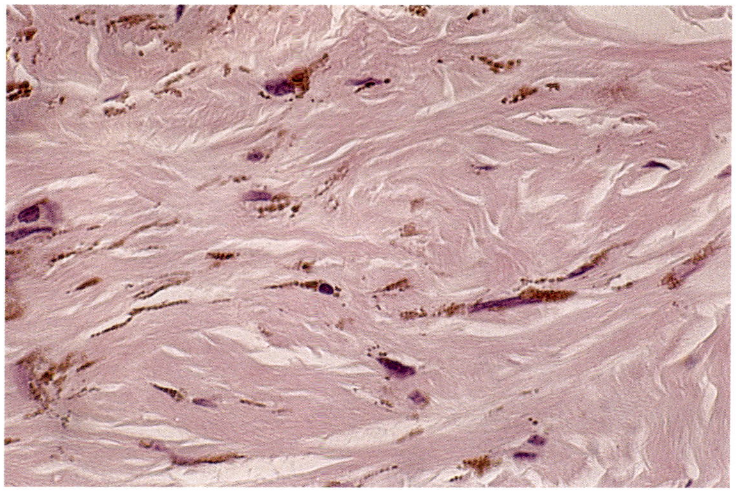

C

Figures 35–54A, 35–54B, 35–54C. Blue melanocytic nevus. Dome-shaped lesion with prominent dermal fibroplasia intermixed with spindle-shaped, and pigmented dendritic melanocytes. Melanin granules are present in the bipolar dendritic processes and extend between thickened collagen bundles.

MELANOCYTIC NEVUS OF OTA/ITO

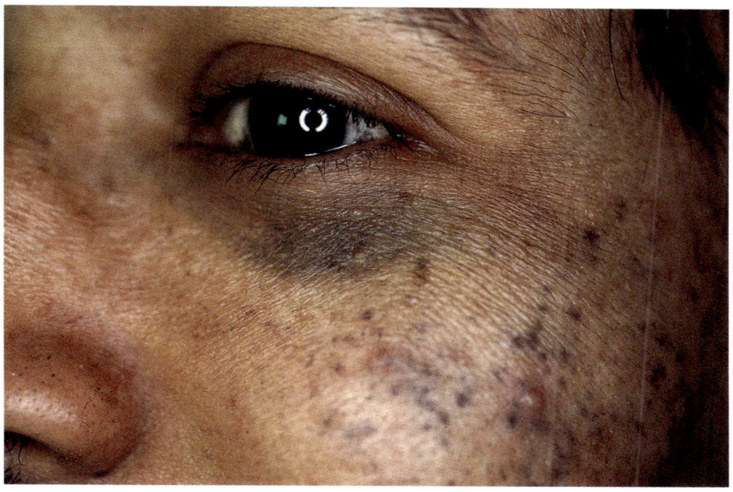

Figure 35–55. **Melanocytic nevus of Ota.** Blue pigmentation of the sclera, eyelid, and cheek.

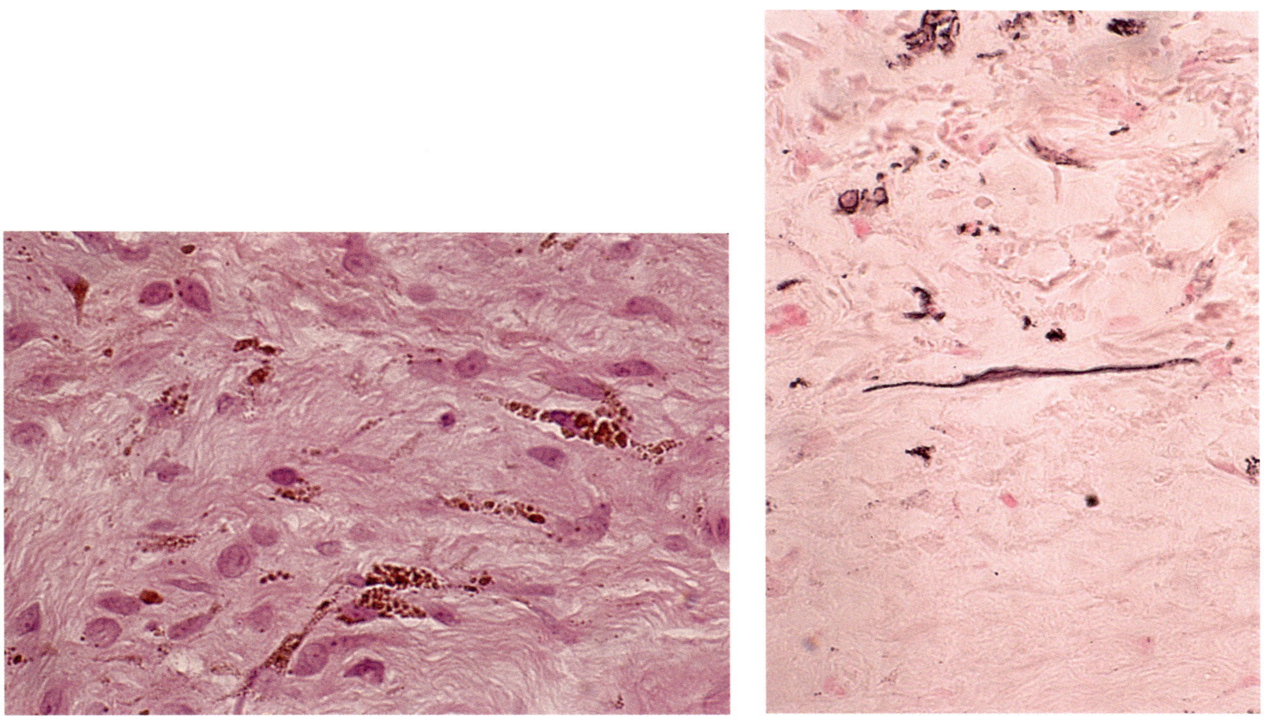

A B

Figures 35–56A, 35–56B. **Melanocytic nevus of Ota/Ito.** Bipolar dendritic melanocytes containing melanin granules in the reticular dermis.

36

MALIGNANT MELANOCYTIC NEOPLASMS

- Malignant melanoma in situ
- Malignant melanoma
- Malignant melanoma arising in a superficial congenital melanocytic nevus

MALIGNANT MELANOMA IN SITU

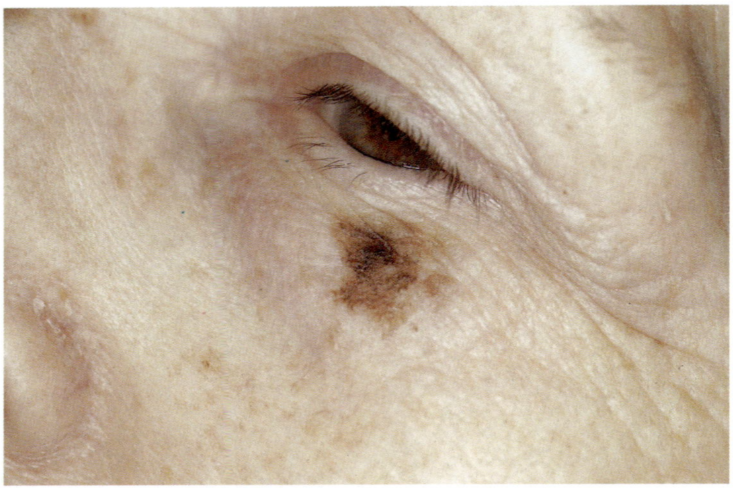

Figure 36–1. Malignant melanoma in situ. Mottled tan and dark-brown pigmented patch with irregular margins on the eyelid of a woman.

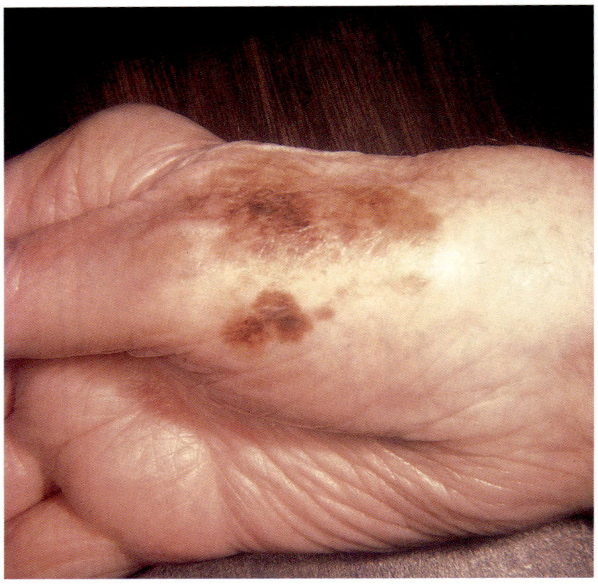

Figure 36–2. Malignant melanoma in situ. Irregular-sized and -shaped, multicolored brown patches on the hand of an elderly woman.

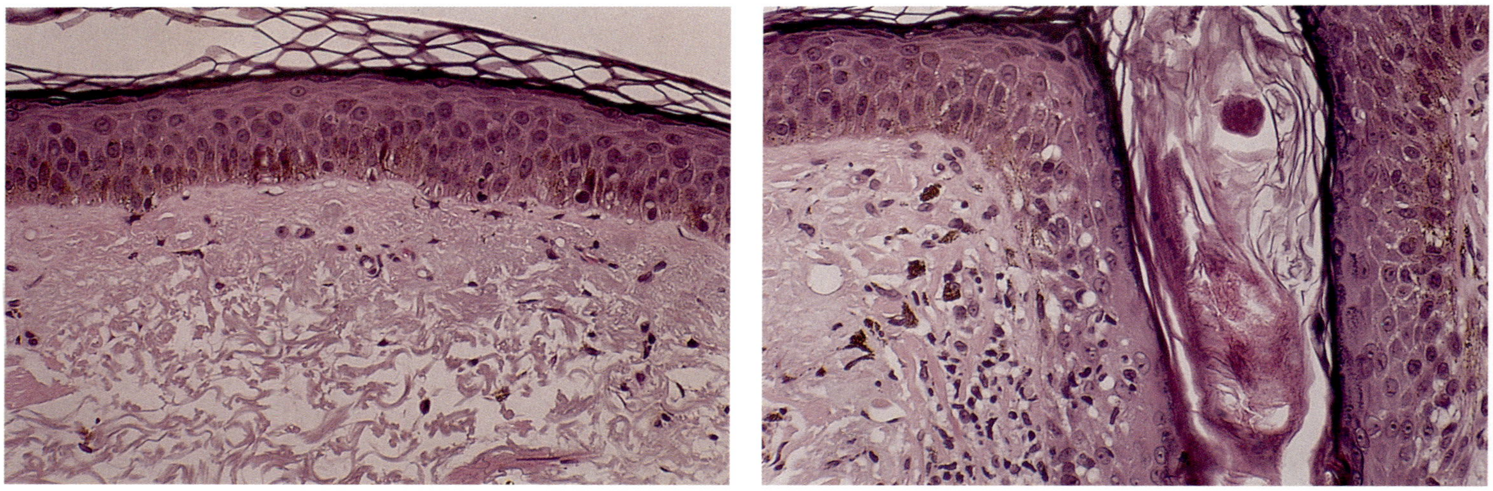

A

B

Figures 36–3A, 36–3B. Malignant melanoma in situ, evolving lesion without nests of atypical melanocytes. Solitary, atypical melanocytes are present within the lower layer of the epidermis and infundibulum. There is extensive dermal solar elastosis, dilated blood vessels, and a patchy lymphocytic infiltrate.

MALIGNANT MELANOMA IN SITU

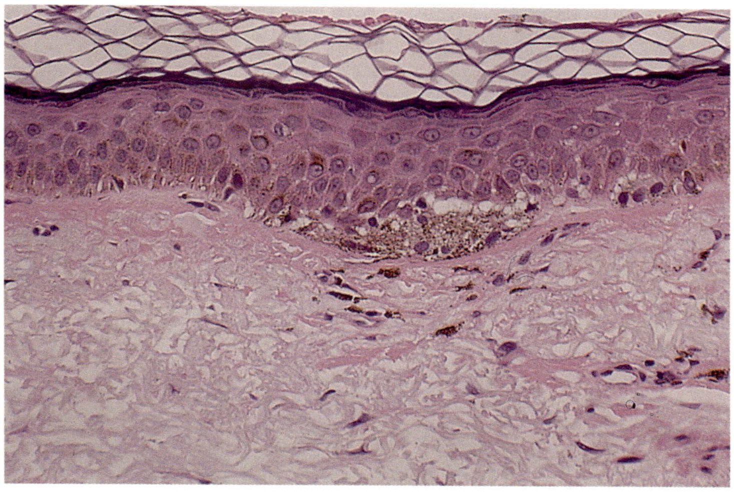

A

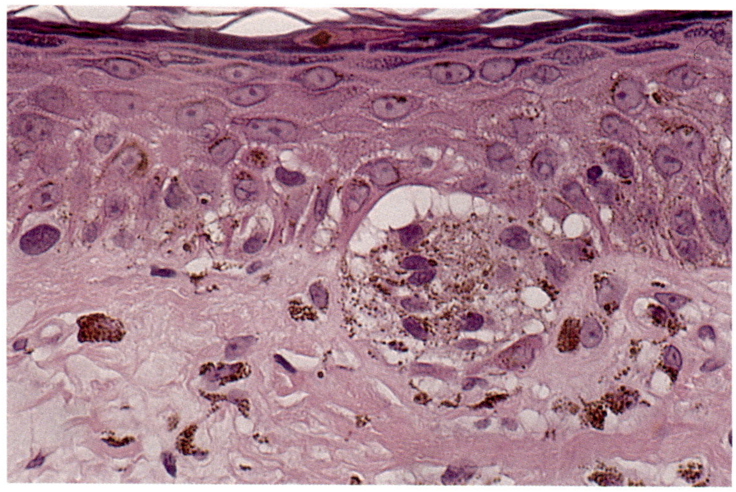

B

Figures 36–4A, 36–4B. Malignant melanoma in situ, early, with nests of atypical melanocytes. Nests of atypical melanocytes at the dermoepidermal junction are adjacent to solitary atypical melanocytes in the lower layer of the epidermis.

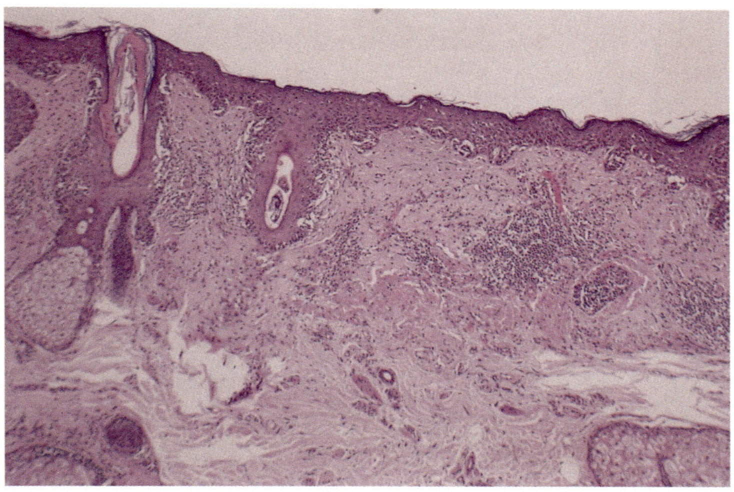

A

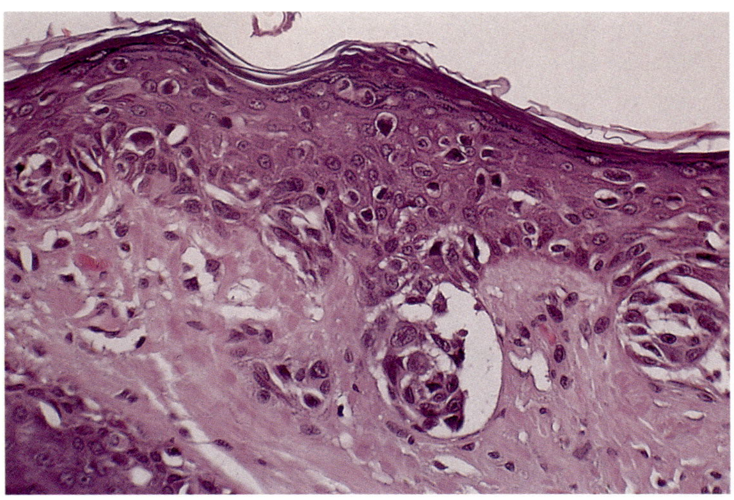

B

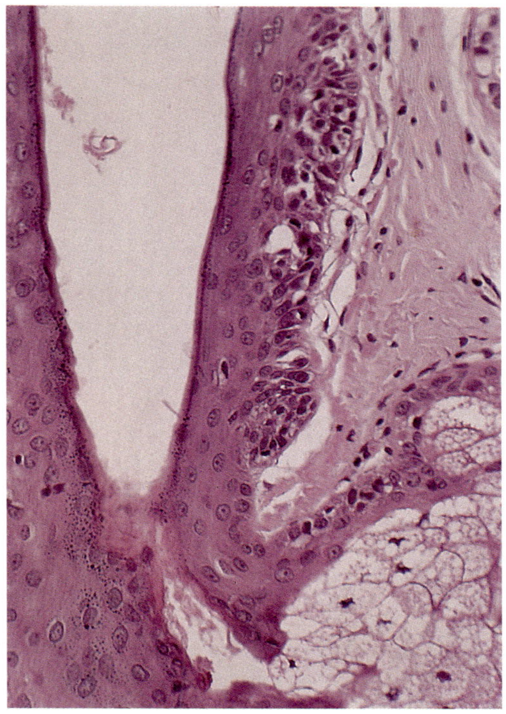

C

Figures 36–5A, 36–5B, 36–5C. Malignant melanoma in situ, mature lesion. Atypical melanocytes as solitary units and in nests at all levels of the epidermis and adnexal epithelium. Cells extend into the cornified layer. Nests of atypical melanocytes vary in size and shape, are not equidistant from one another, and are often confluent. There is severe dermal solar elastosis, melanophages, dilated blood vessels, and a patchy lymphocytic infiltrate.

MALIGNANT MELANOMA

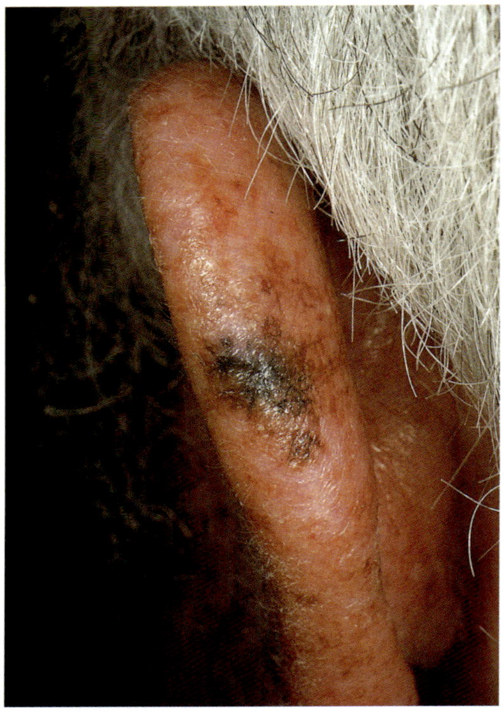

Figure 36–6. Malignant melanoma. Reticulated, irregular, dark- and light-brown pigmented patch on sun-damaged skin of a man's ear.

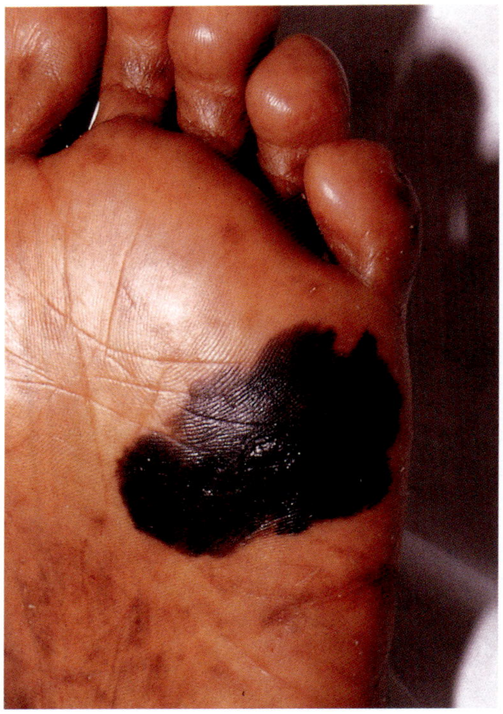

Figure 36–7. Malignant melanoma. Black pigmented irregular plaque on the foot.

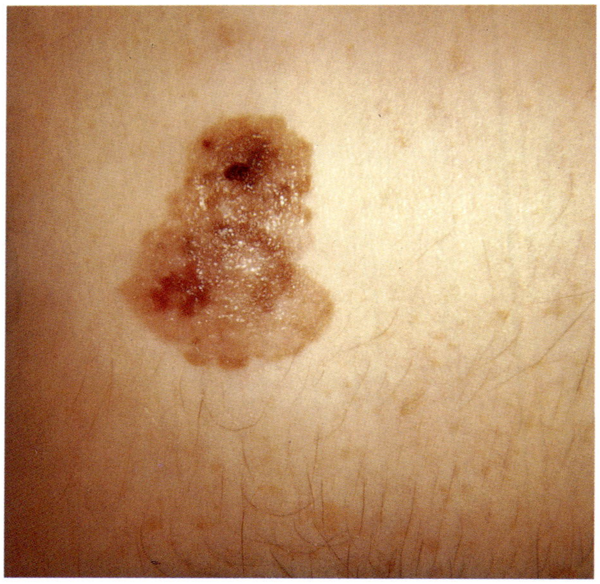

Figure 36–8. Malignant melanoma. Multicolored tan, red, and dark-brown irregular plaque on the abdomen.

MALIGNANT MELANOMA

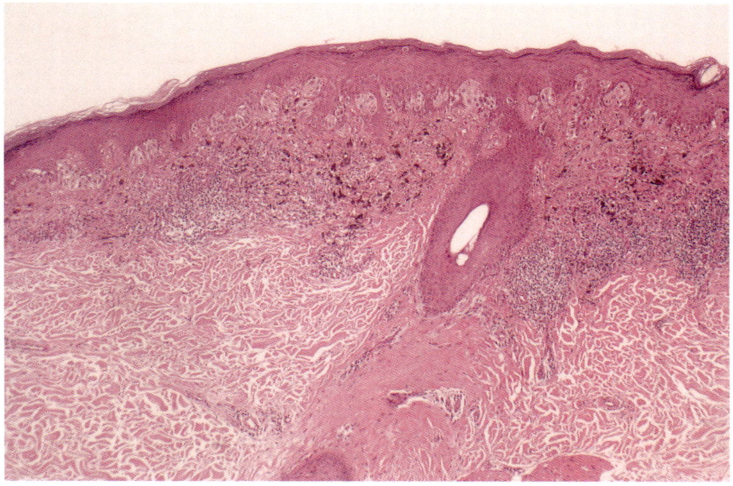
A

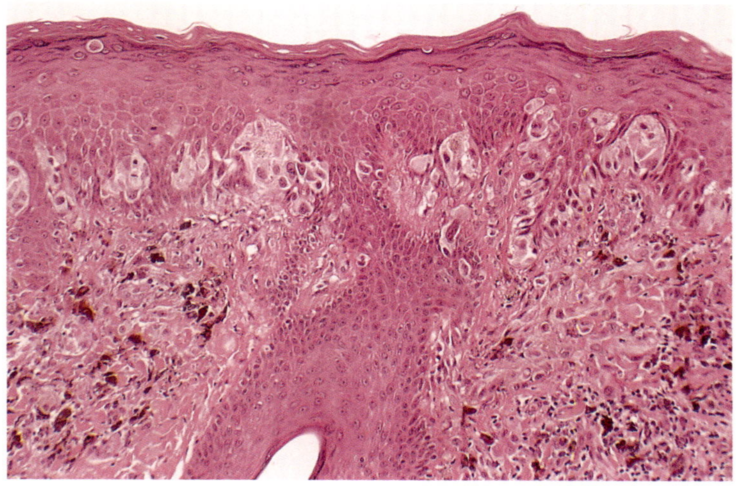
B

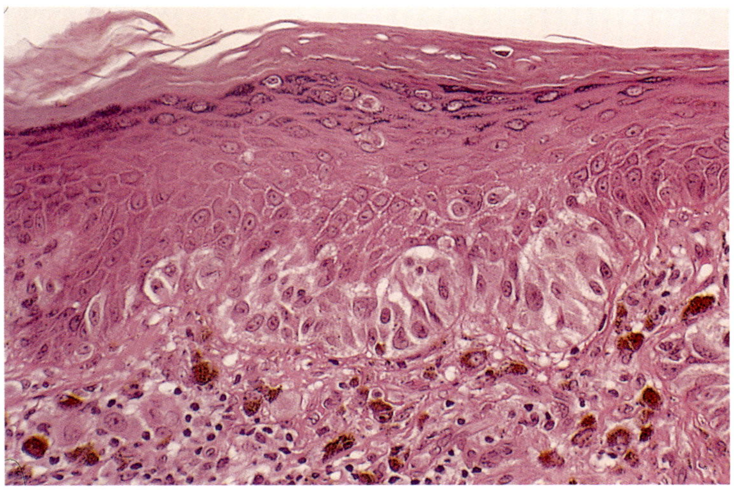
C

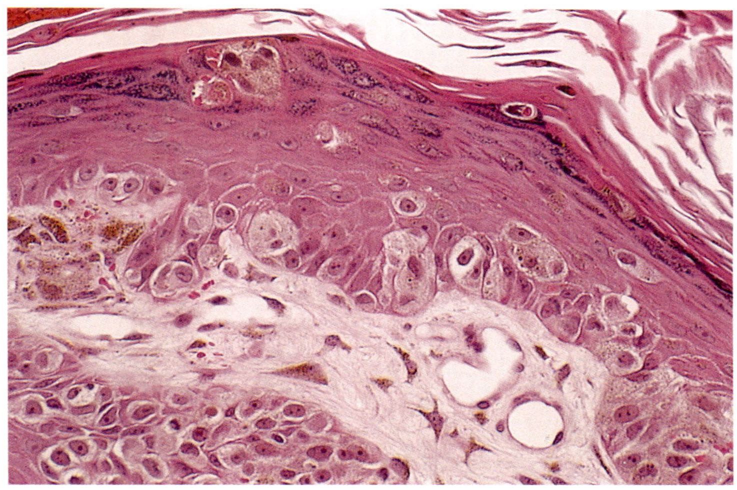
D

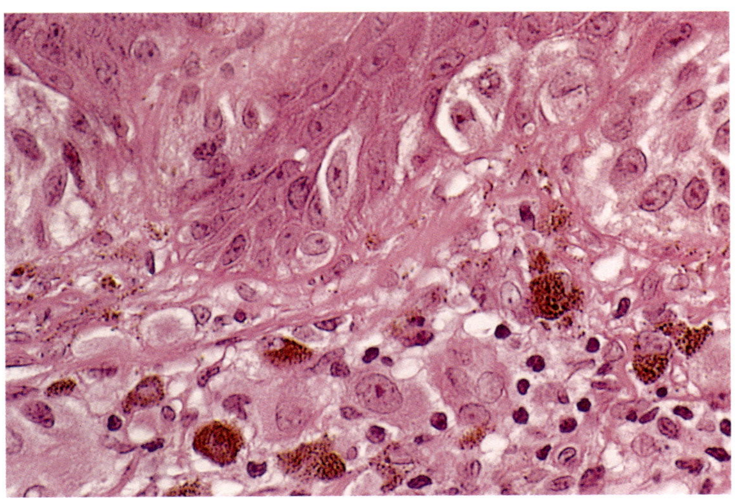
E

Figures 36–9A, 36–9B, 36–9C, 36–9D, 36–9E. Malignant melanoma. Atypical melanocytes, with many atypical pagetoid melanocytes, as solitary units and in nests asymmetrically located in the epidermis and dermis. The atypical melanocytes are present at all levels of the epidermis. Nests of atypical melanocytes are not equidistant, vary in size and shape, and are often confluent without signs of maturation with progression into the dermis. There are melanophages, dilated blood vessels, and a patchy lymphocytic infiltrate.

MALIGNANT MELANOMA

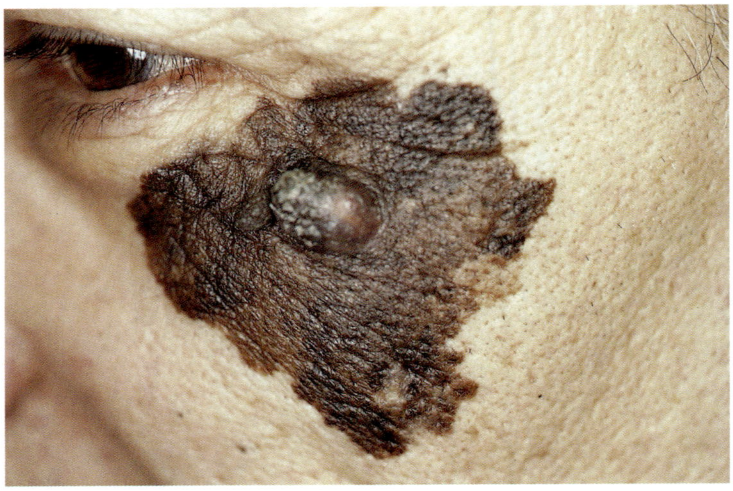

Figure 36–10. Malignant melanoma. Multiple crusted nodules within a markedly hyperpigmented dark-brown and black plaque on the face.

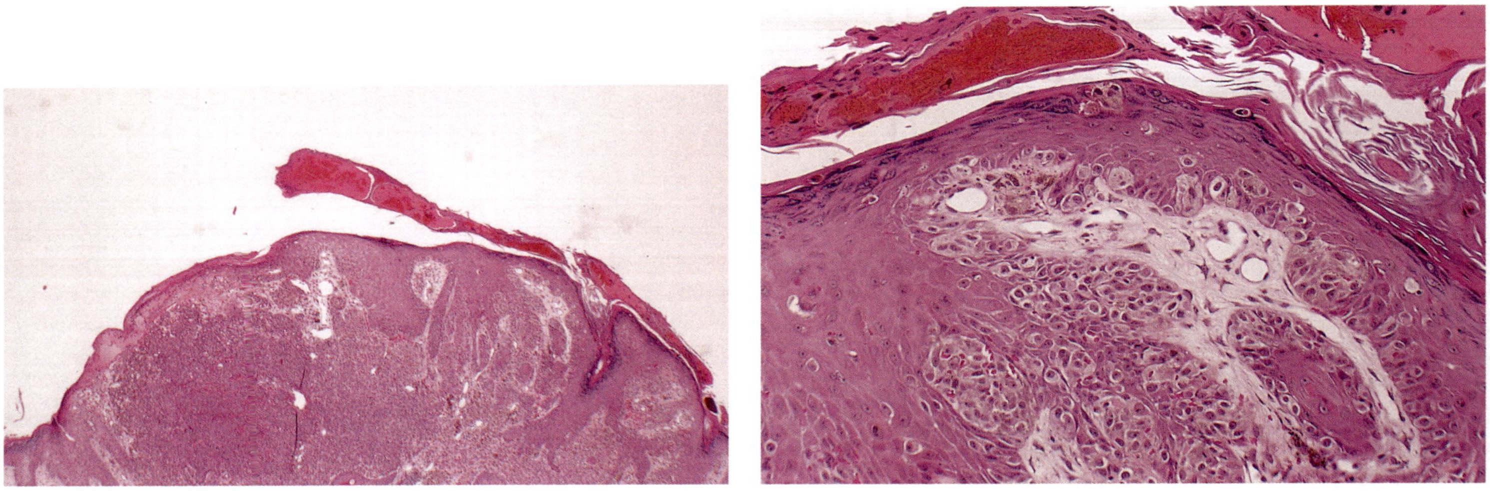

A B

Figures 36–11A, 36–11B. Malignant melanoma. Dome-shaped nodule of atypical melanocytes. There are atypical melanocytes at all levels of the epidermis and extending into the dermis.

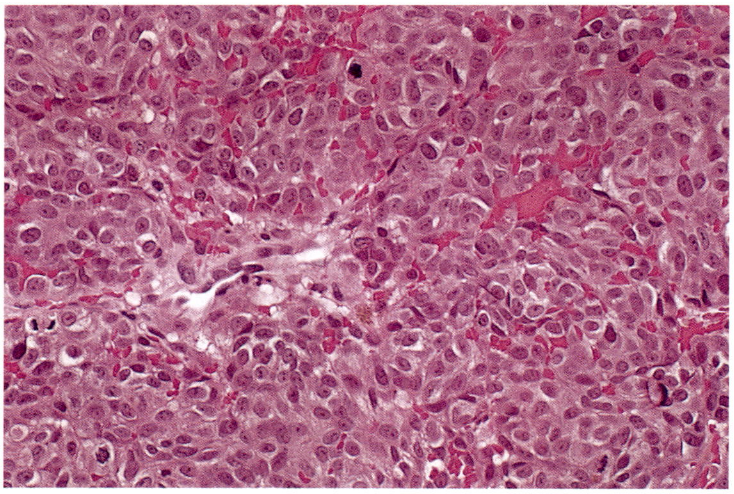

Figure 36–12. Malignant melanoma. Sheets of atypical oval, round, and polygonal melanocytes in the dermis. There are necrotic and mitotic melanocytes, melanin deposition, and congested blood vessels.

MALIGNANT MELANOMA

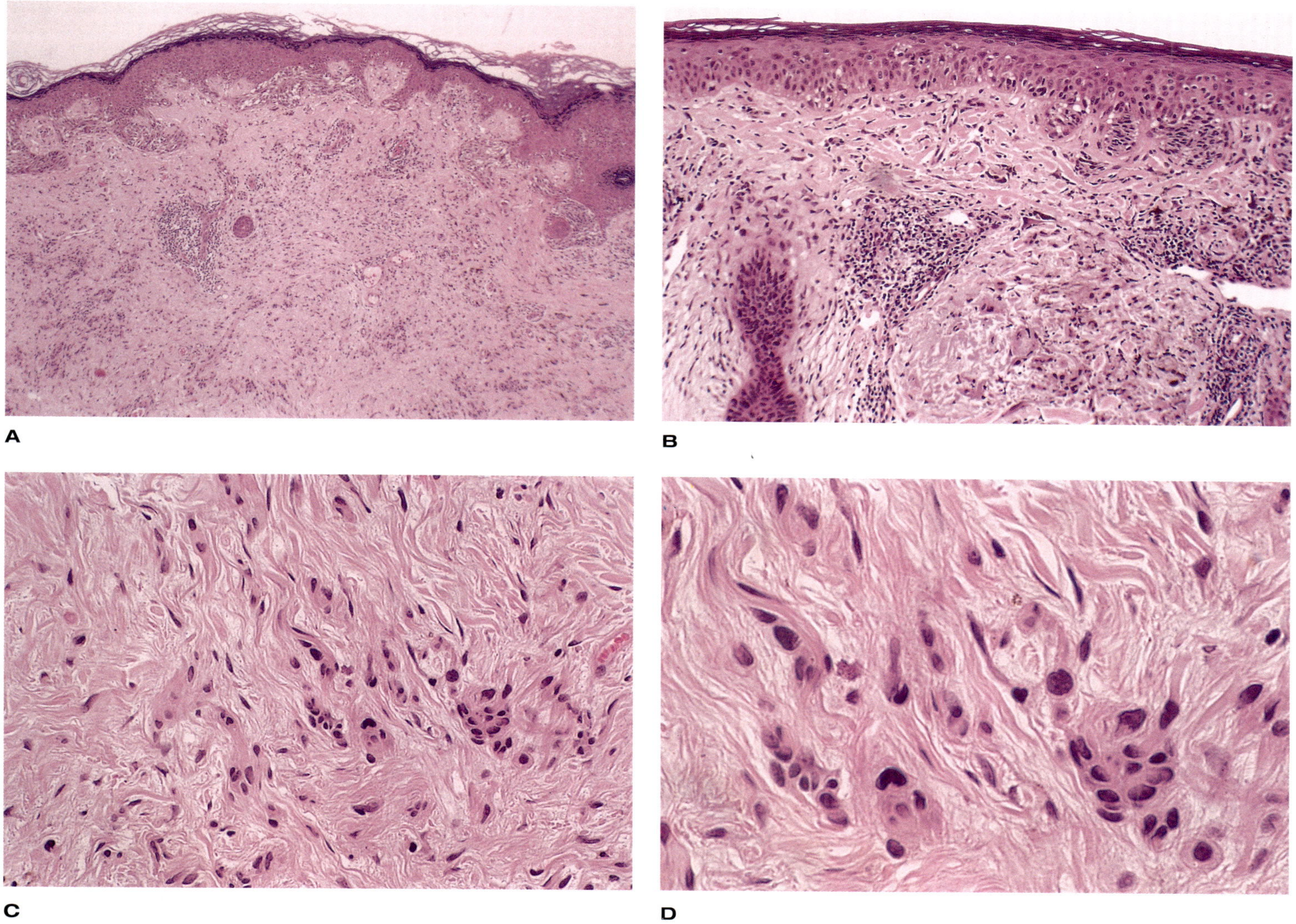

Figures 36–13A, 36–13B, 36–13C, 36–13D. Malignant melanoma, desmoplastic type. Atypical melanocytes within the epidermis as solitary units and in nests. Strands of oval and spindle-shaped atypical melanocytes are intermingled in the fibrocytic dermis with coarse collagen bundles, fibrocytes, and a patchy lymphocytic infiltrate.

MALIGNANT MELANOMA

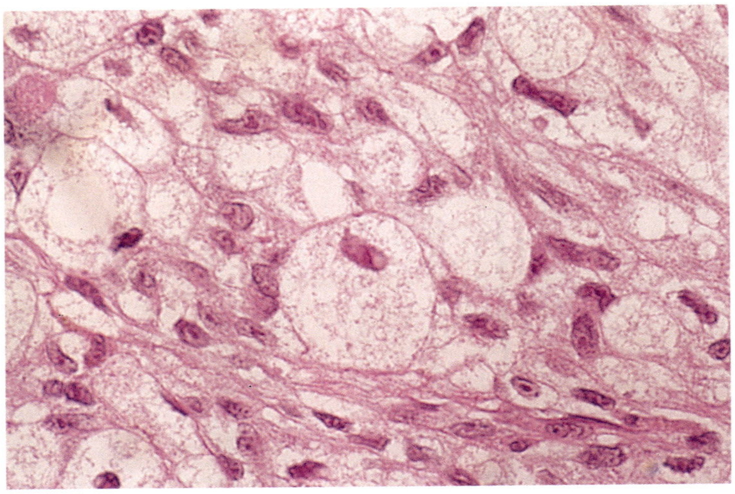

Figure 36–14. Malignant melanoma, balloon-cell type. There are atypical and pleomorphic melanocytes with voluminous amounts of cytoplasm.

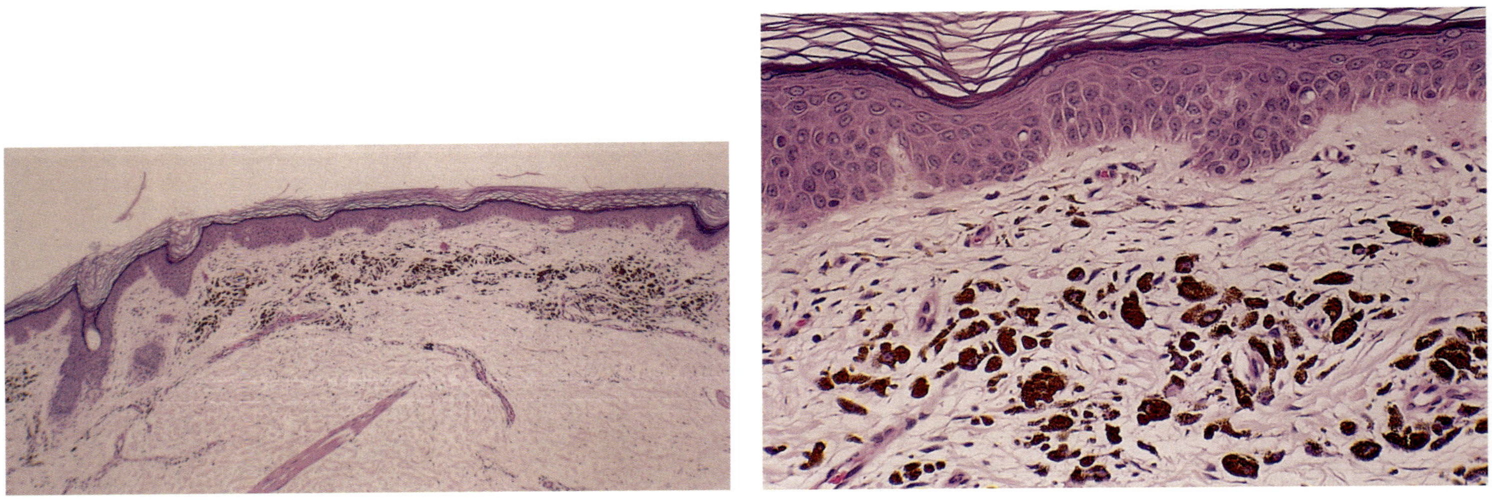

A B

Figures 36–15A, 36–15B. Malignant melanoma, complete regression, melanosis type. Dense band of melanophages fill the thickened papillary dermis, where there is fibroplasia, dilated blood vessels, and lymphocytes.

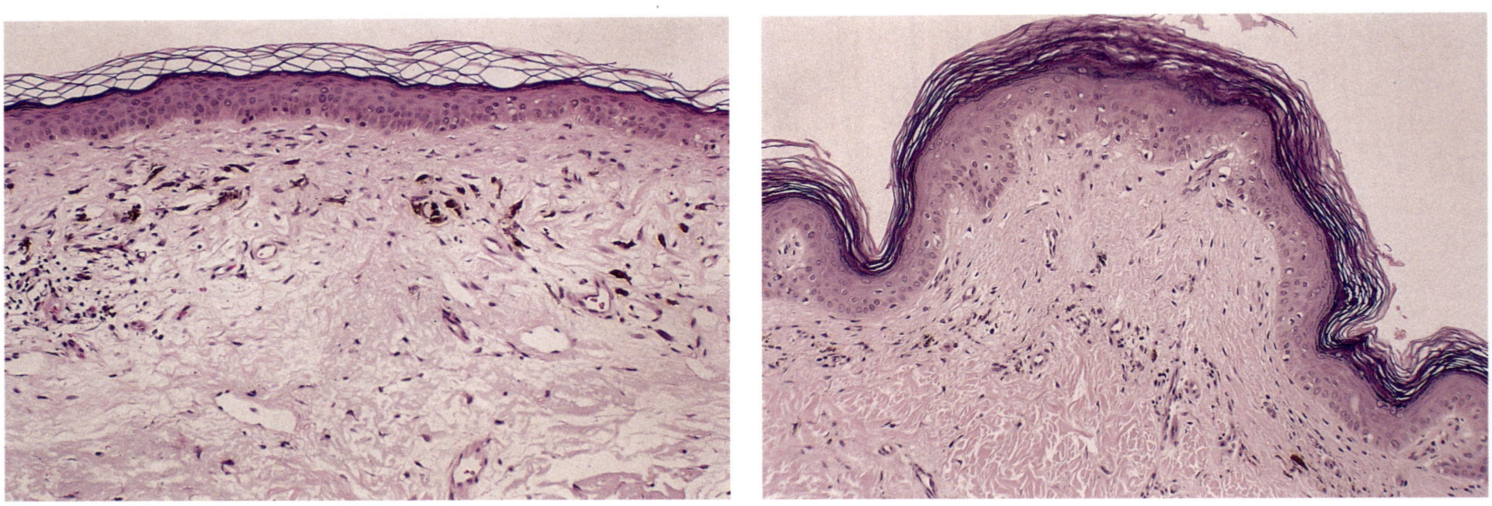

A B

Figures 36–16A, 36–16B. Malignant melanoma, complete regression, fibrocytic type. Fibroplasia, solar elastosis, dilated blood vessels, lymphocytes, and scattered melanophages fill the thickened papillary dermis.

MALIGNANT MELANOMA ARISING IN A SUPERFICIAL CONGENITAL MELANOCYTIC NEVUS

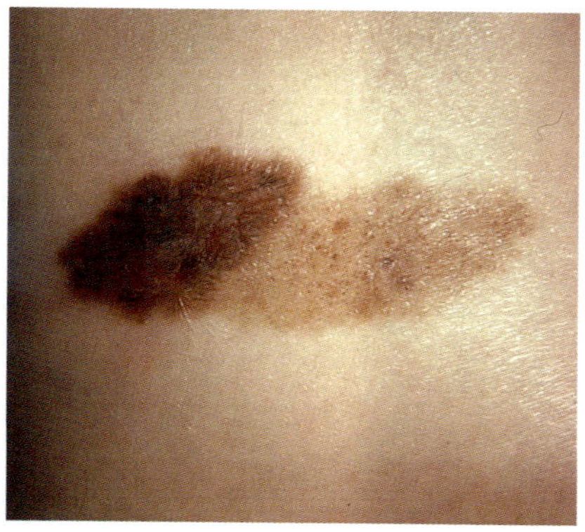

Figure 36–17. Malignant melanoma arising in a superficial congenital melanocytic nevus. The area on the right is a light-brown pigmented plaque present since birth. Contiguous with it, on the left, there is a more recently developed irregular, multicolored, dark-brown pigmented plaque with raised dark-brown papules and notched borders.

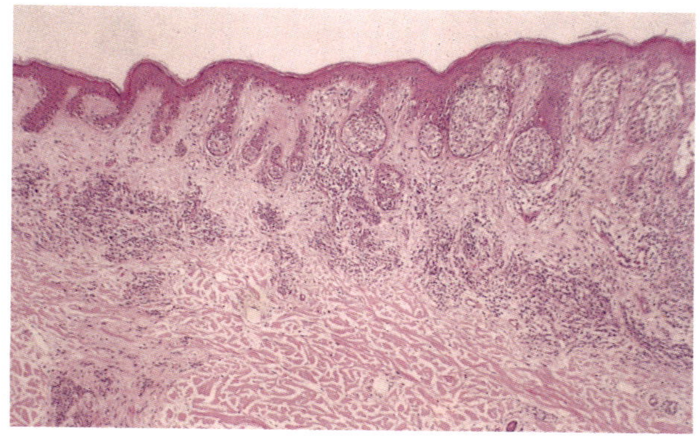

Figure 36–18. Malignant melanoma arising in a superficial congenital melanocytic nevus. Intradermal superficial congenital melanocytic nevus on the left. Small, round and oval uniform melanocytes with adnexocentricity, angiocentricity, and interdigited among collagen bundles in the reticular dermis. Atypical melanocytes are present in the overlying epidermis and in the dermis to the right of the congenital melanocytic nevus.

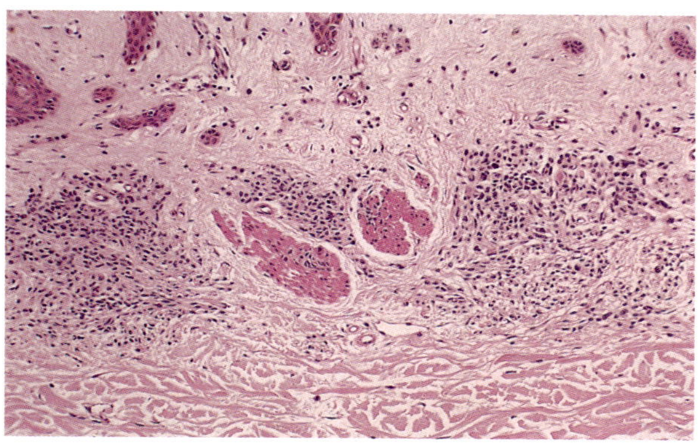

Figure 36–19. Intradermal superficial congenital melanocytic nevus. Adnexocentricity, angiocentricity, and solitary melanocytes among collagen bundles.

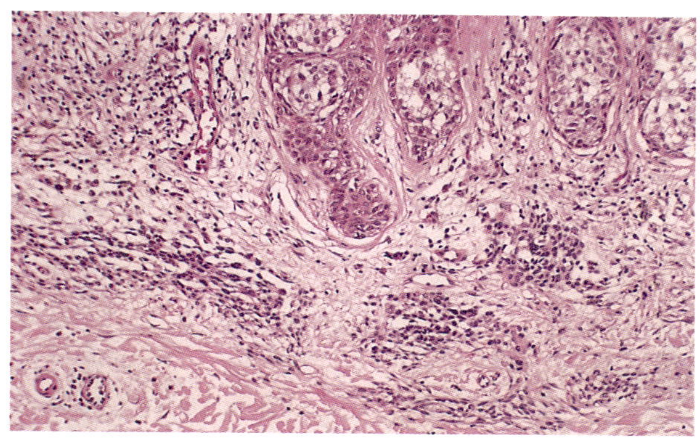

Figure 36–20. Malignant melanoma in situ and intradermal superficial congenital melanocytic nevus. Nests of atypical melanocytes in the epidermis and typical melanocytes in the dermis.

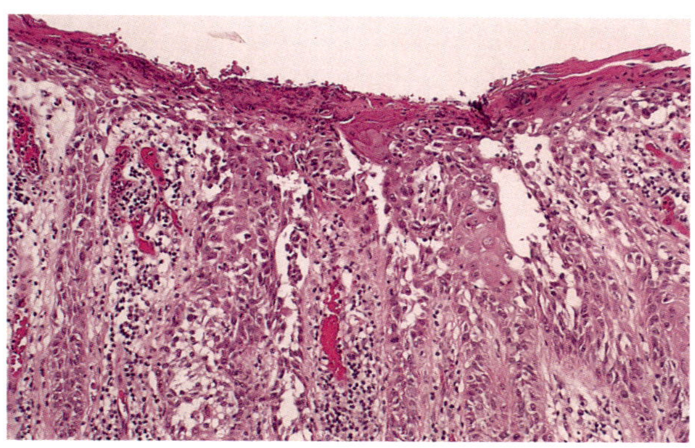

Figure 36–21. Malignant melanoma arising in a superficial congenital melanocytic nevus. Malignant melanoma with atypical melanocytes as solitary units and in nests in the epidermis and dermis. There is epidermal ulceration with scale crust.

37

Neural and Neuroendocrine Neoplasms

- Neurofibroma
- Schwannoma
- Granular cell tumor
- Nerve sheath myxoma
- Palisaded encapsulated neuroma
- Amputation neuroma
- Merkel cell carcinoma

NEUROFIBROMA

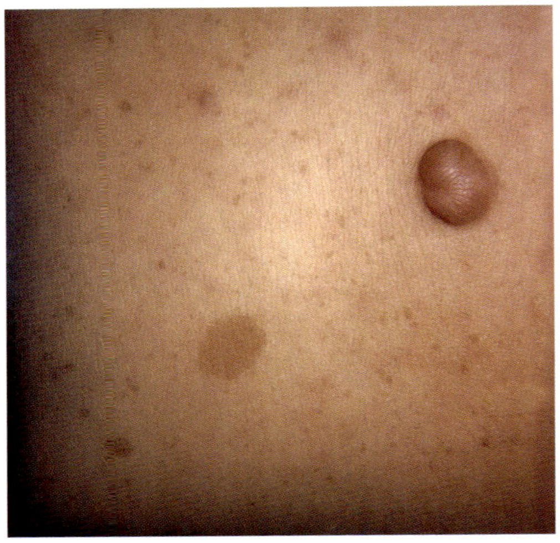

Figure 37–1. Neurofibroma. Sessile, tan, soft nodule on the abdomen of a woman with neurofibromatosis. Café-au-lait macules are present.

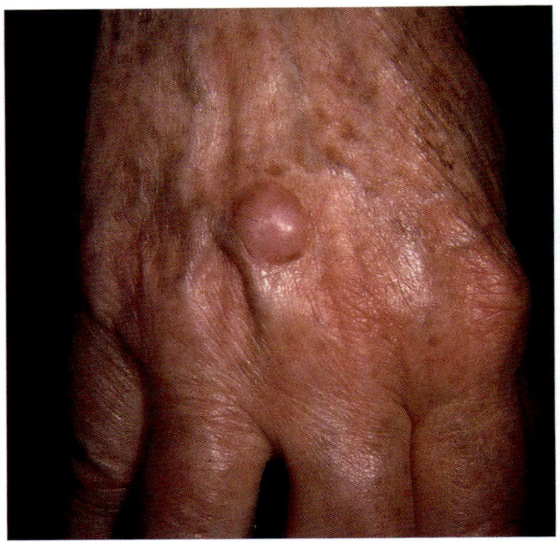

Figure 37–2. Neurofibroma. Smooth skin-colored nodule on the dorsum of the hand.

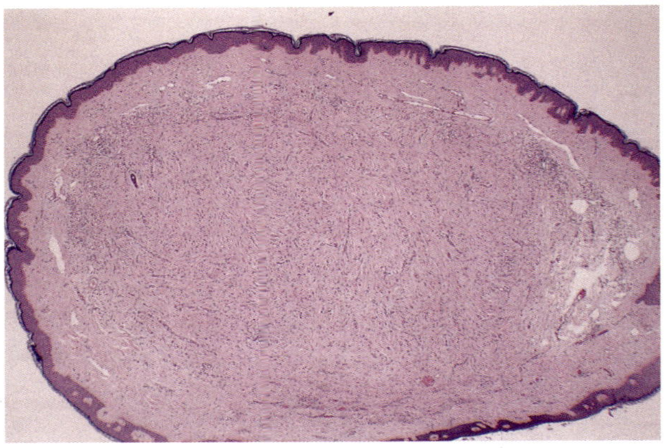

A

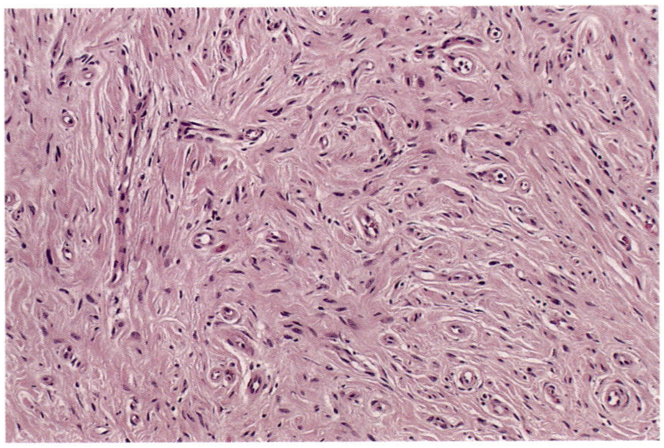

B

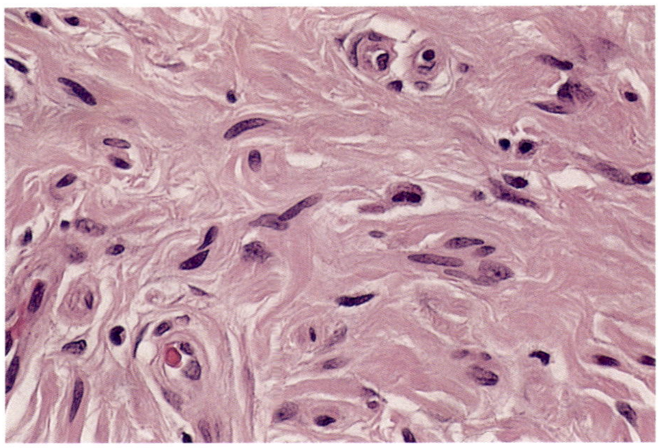

C

Figures 37–3A, 37–3B, 37–3C. Neurofibroma. Circumscribed, cellular dermal nodule with oval and wavy nuclei. There is fibrillary collagen, numerous blood vessels, mucin, mast cells, and clefting among the collagen bundles.

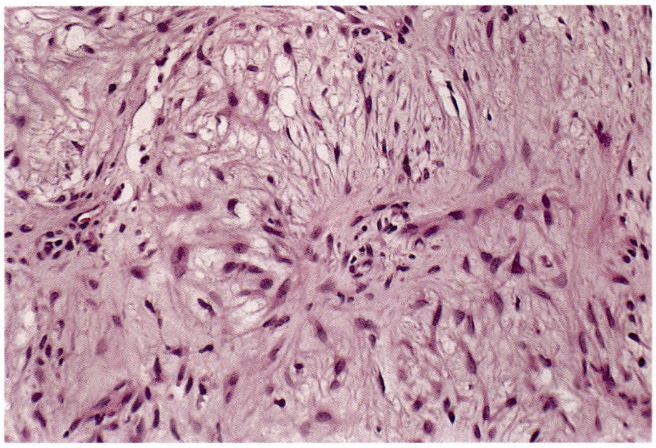

Figure 37–4. Neurofibroma. Neurofibroma, myxoid type. Extensive deposits of mucin among fibrillary collagen bundles and wavy oval nuclei.

SCHWANNOMA

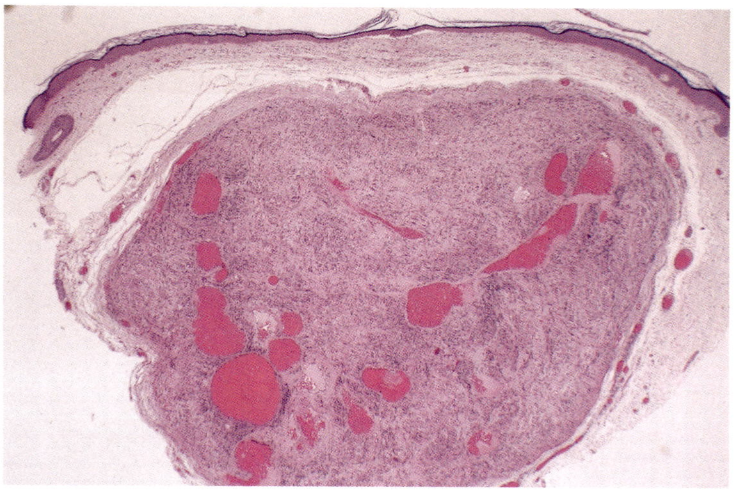

A

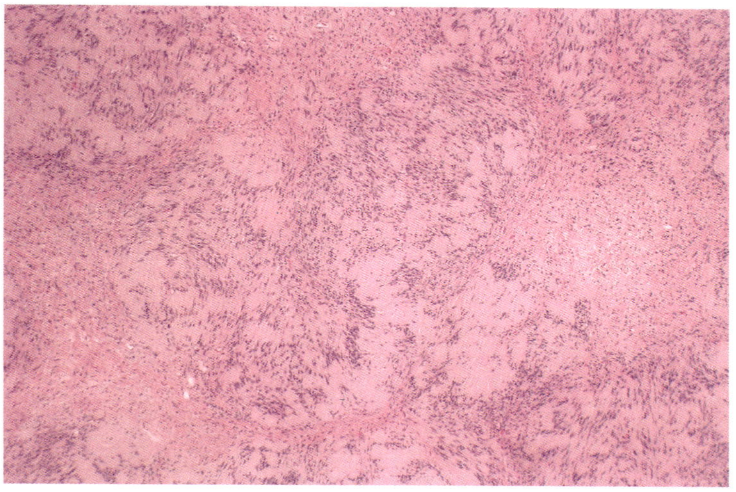

B

Figures 37–5A, 37–5B. Schwannoma. Sharply demarcated, clefted dermal nodule with oval and spindle-shaped Schwann cells forming Verocay bodies. There are zones with nuclei of Schwann cells in palisade (Antoni A) adjacent to areas with Schwann cells in loose disarray (Antoni B), with dilated and congested blood vessels.

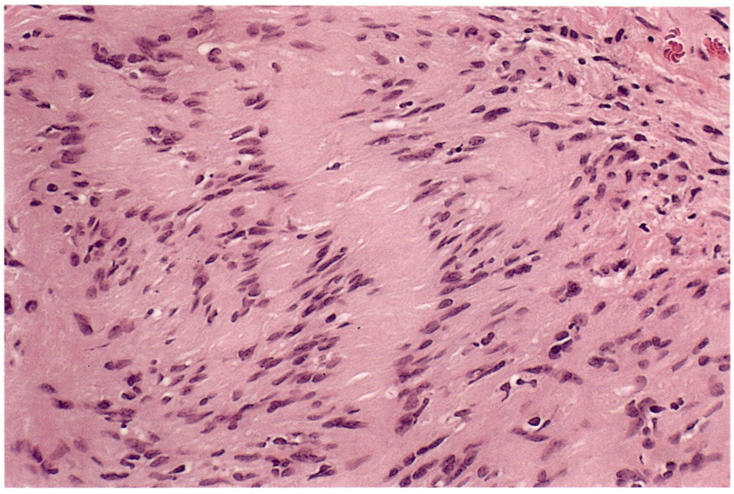

Figure 37–6. Schwannoma, Antoni A. Verocay body with palisaded nuclei of Schwann cells encircles their eosinophilic, fibrillary cytoplasmic processes.

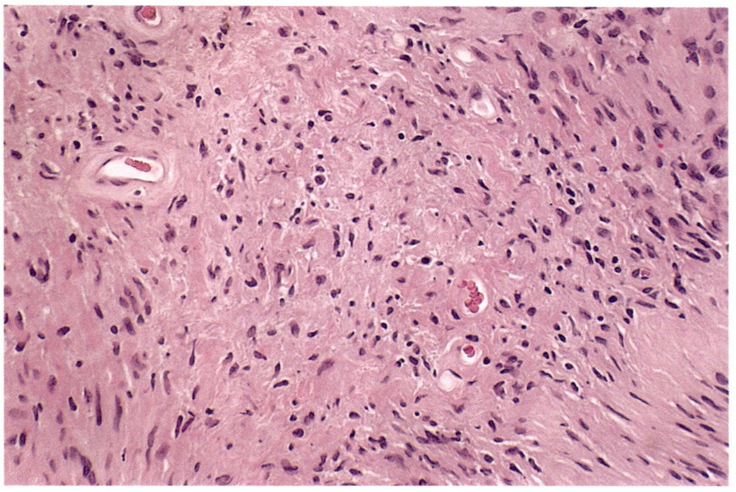

Figure 37–7. Schwannoma, Antoni B. Wavy and oval Schwann cells in disarray within loose connective tissue, where there is mucin deposition and dilated blood vessels.

GRANULAR CELL TUMOR

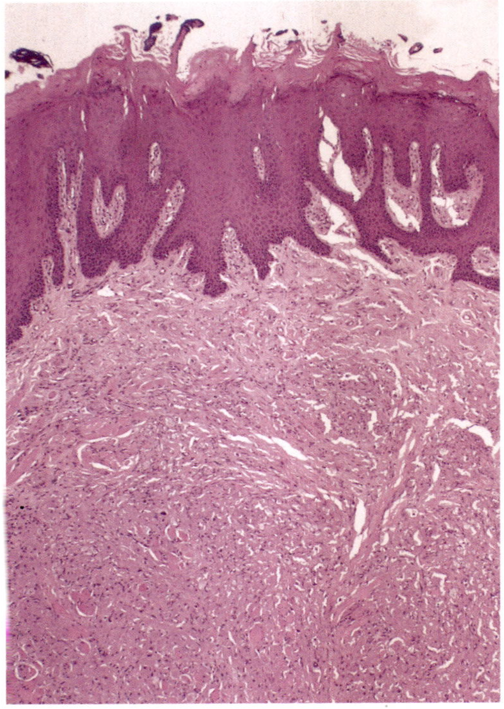

A

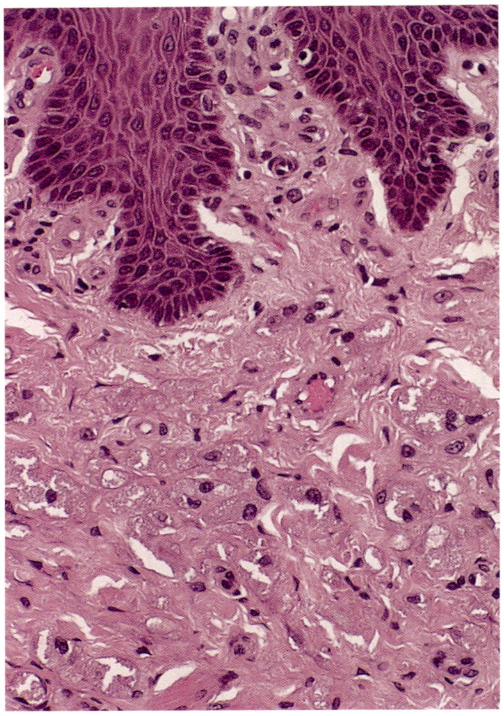

B

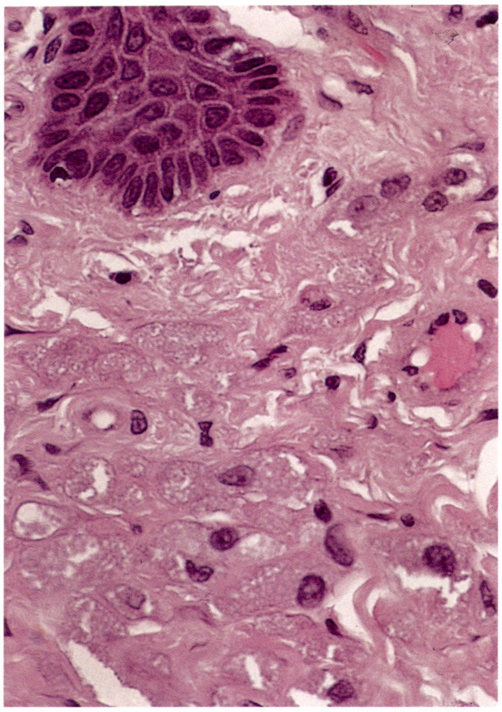

C

Figures 37–8A, 37–8B, 37–8C. Granular cell tumor, tongue. Epithelial hyperplasia, sheets of polygonal cells packed with amphophilic-staining cytoplastic granules. The nuclei of the polygonal cells are mostly uniform, round, and oval.

NERVE SHEATH MYXOMA

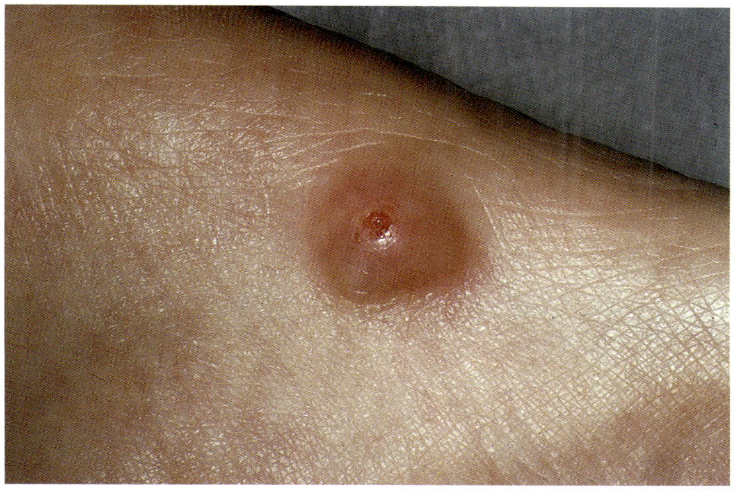

Figure 37–9. Nerve sheath myxoma. Dome-shaped, erythematous nodule with central ulceration on the foot.

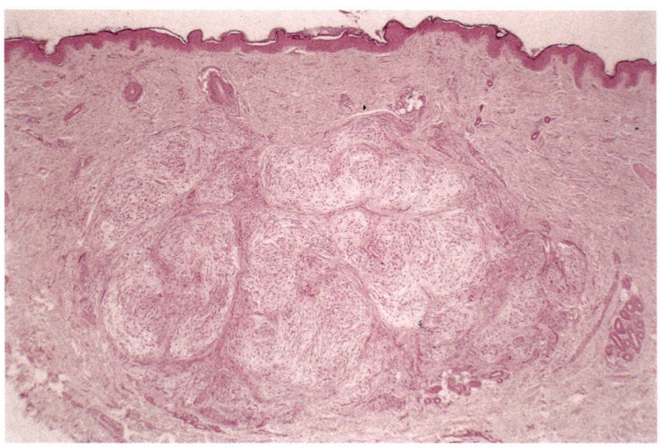

A

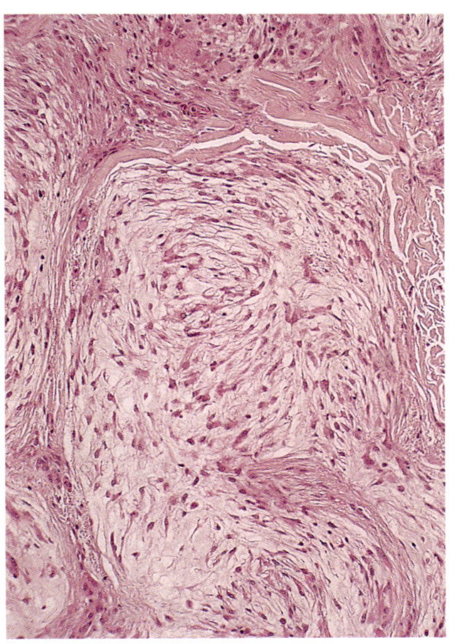

B

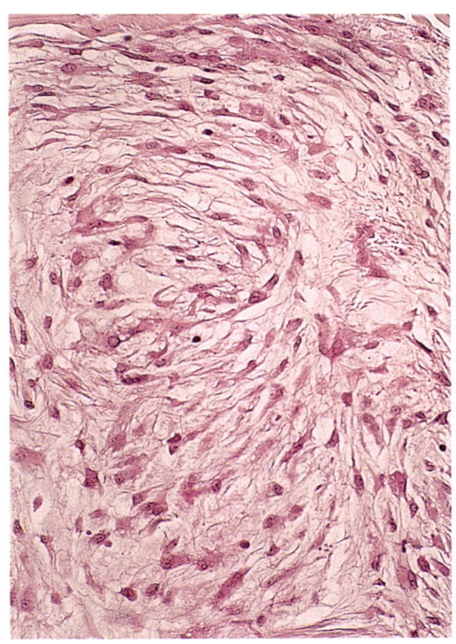

C

Figures 37–10A, 37–10B, 37–10C. Nerve sheath myxoma. Multilobulated dermal nodule. The aggregates are composed of oval and spindle-shaped cells within a pale-staining myxomatous stroma.

Young people
♀ : ♂ 2 : 1
head & neck

cellular variant (neuro thekeoma)
S100 ⊖
EMA ⊖

Reticular dermis

encapsulated
++ mucin ++
↓
(myxoma)

PALISADED ENCAPSULATED NEUROMA

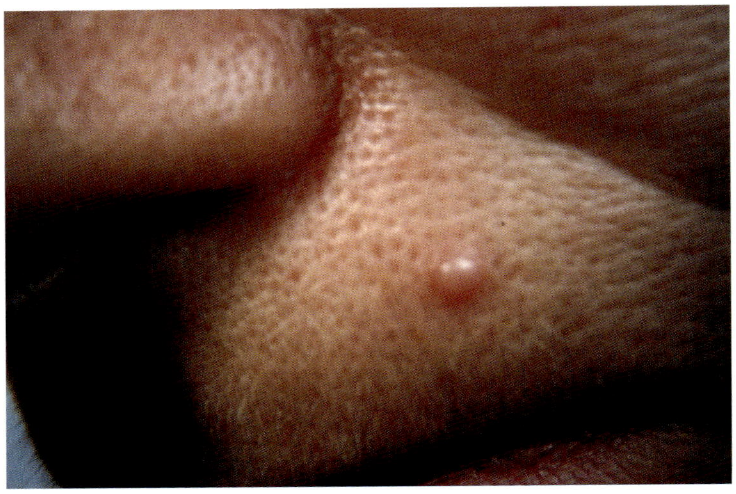

Figure 37–11. Palisaded encapsulated neuroma. Pink, dome-shaped papule on the lip of a woman.

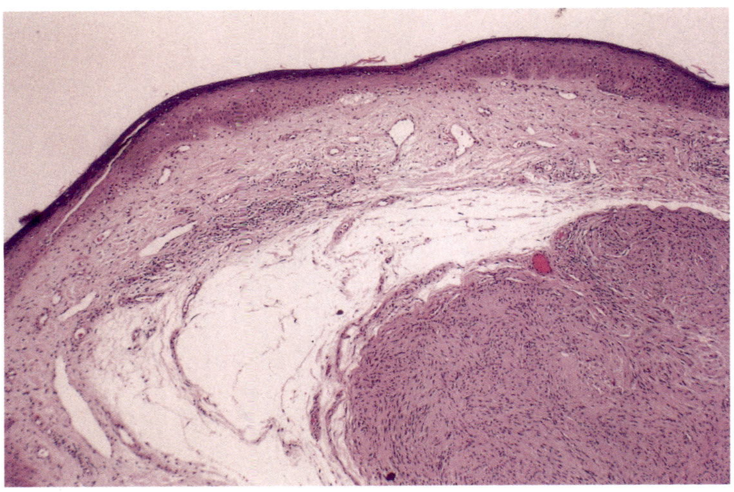

A

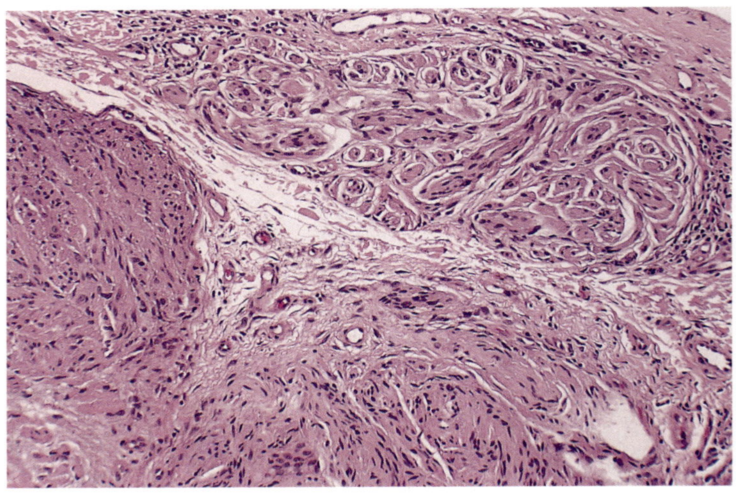

B

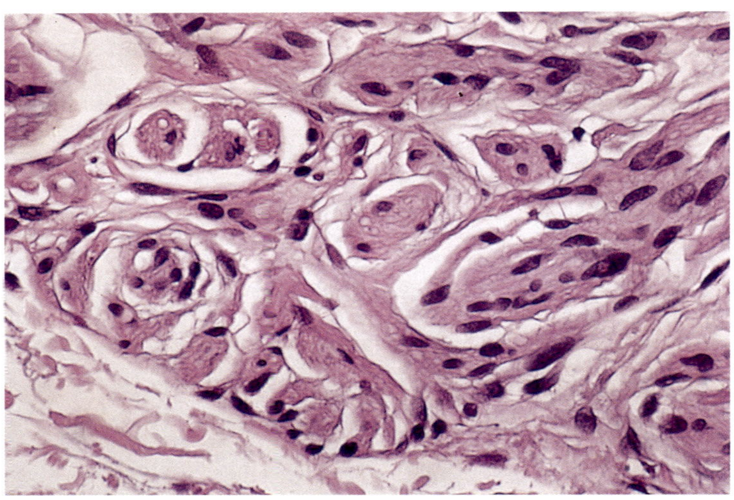

C

Figures 37–12A, 37–12B, 37–12C. Palisaded encapsulated neuroma. Clefts around and within elongated fascicles of neural structures. There are oval and wavy nuclei.

38

Vascular proliferative disorders

- Pyogenic granuloma
- Hemangioma
- Glomus tumor
- Capillary malformation
- Lymphangioma
- Nevus araneus
- Intravascular papillary endothelial hyperplasia
- Venous lake
- Arteriovenous malformation
- Angiolymphoid hyperplasia with eosinophilia
- Angiokeratoma
- Kaposi's sarcoma
- Angiosarcoma

PYOGENIC GRANULOMA

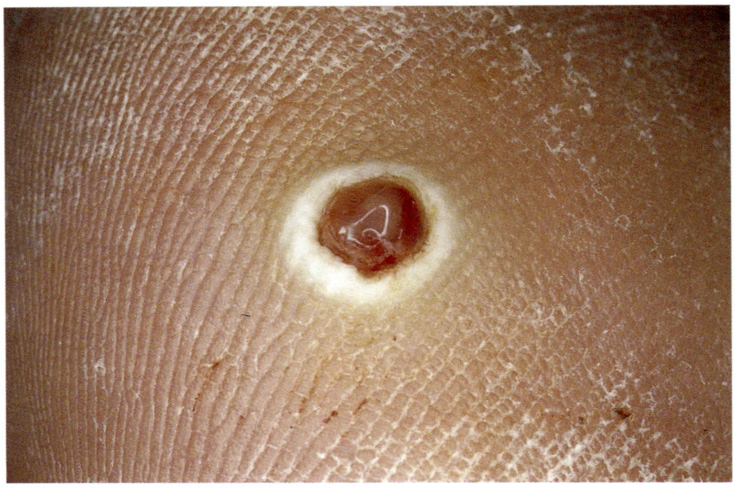

Figure 38–1. Pyogenic granuloma. Soft, erythematous, oozing nodule on the heel of a man.

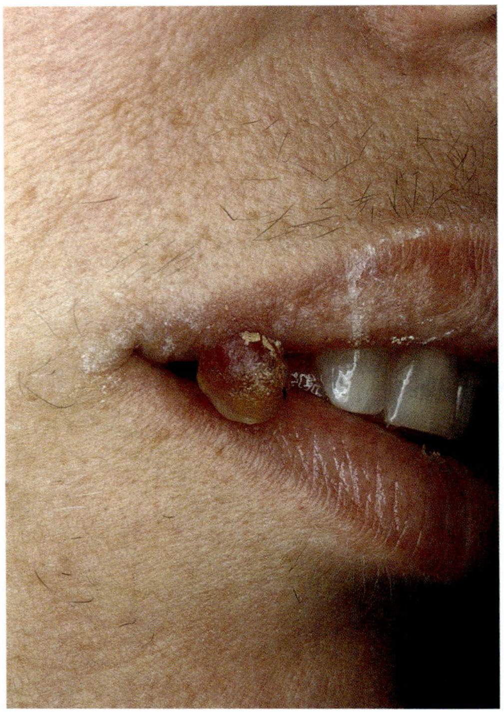

Figure 38–2. Pyogenic granuloma. Sessile, erythematous, crusted nodule on the upper lip of a woman in her last trimester of pregnancy. This lesion grew rapidly, and in this clinical setting it has been referred to as a pregnancy tumor.

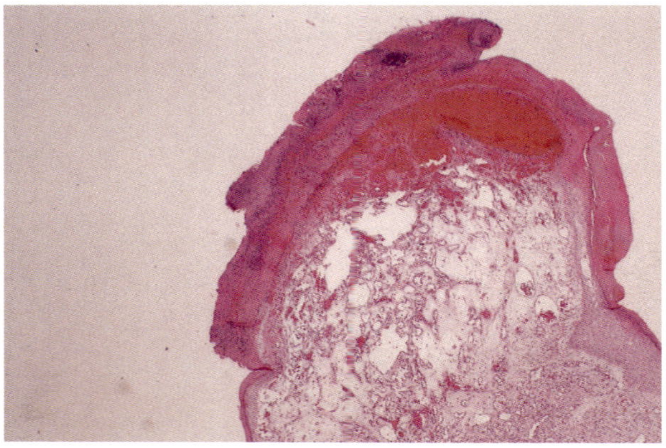

A

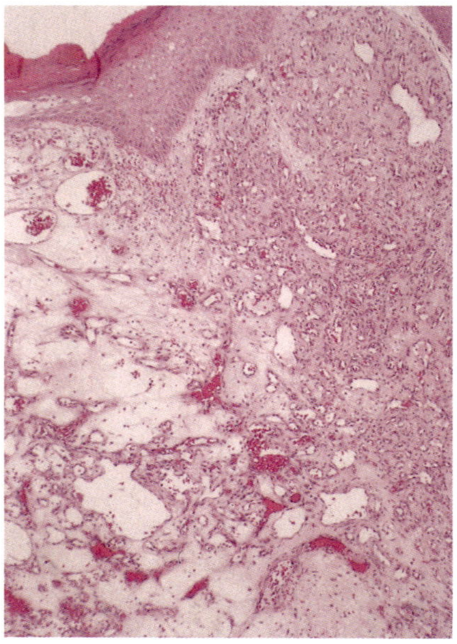

B

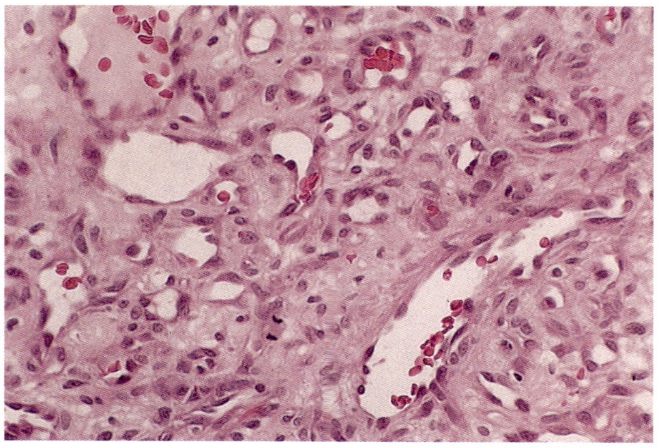

C

Figures 38–3A, 38–3B, 38–3C. Pyogenic granuloma. Pedunculated, ulcerated, and crusted nodule with numerous dilated vascular channels. There is a proliferation of capillaries, fibroplasia, and an edematous stroma.

HEMANGIOMA

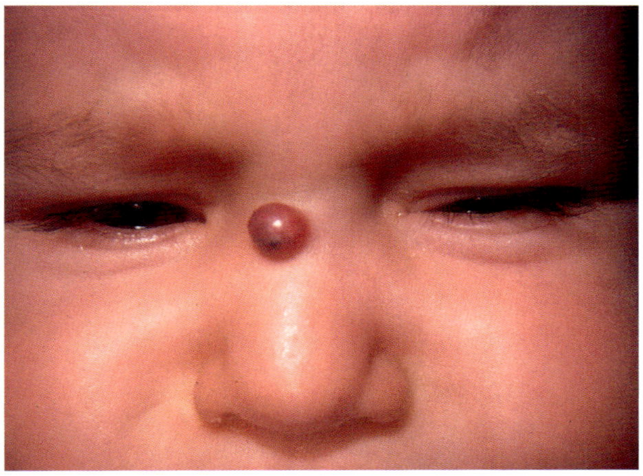

Figure 38–4. **Hemangioma.** Smooth, dome-shaped, erythematous nodule on the dorsum of the nose of an infant.

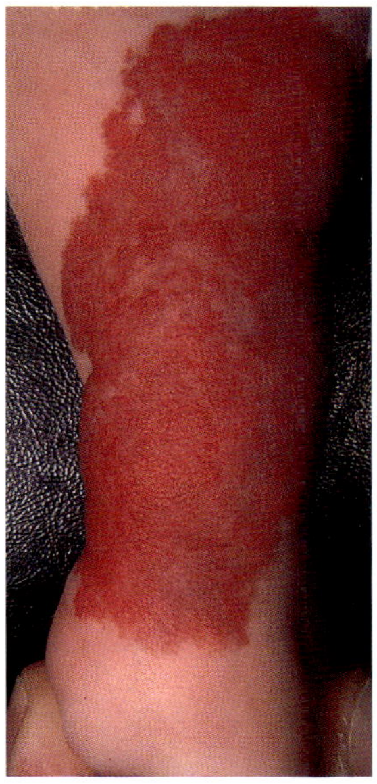

Figure 38–5. **Hemangioma.** Large, papillated, erythematous plaque on the arm of a four-week-old girl.

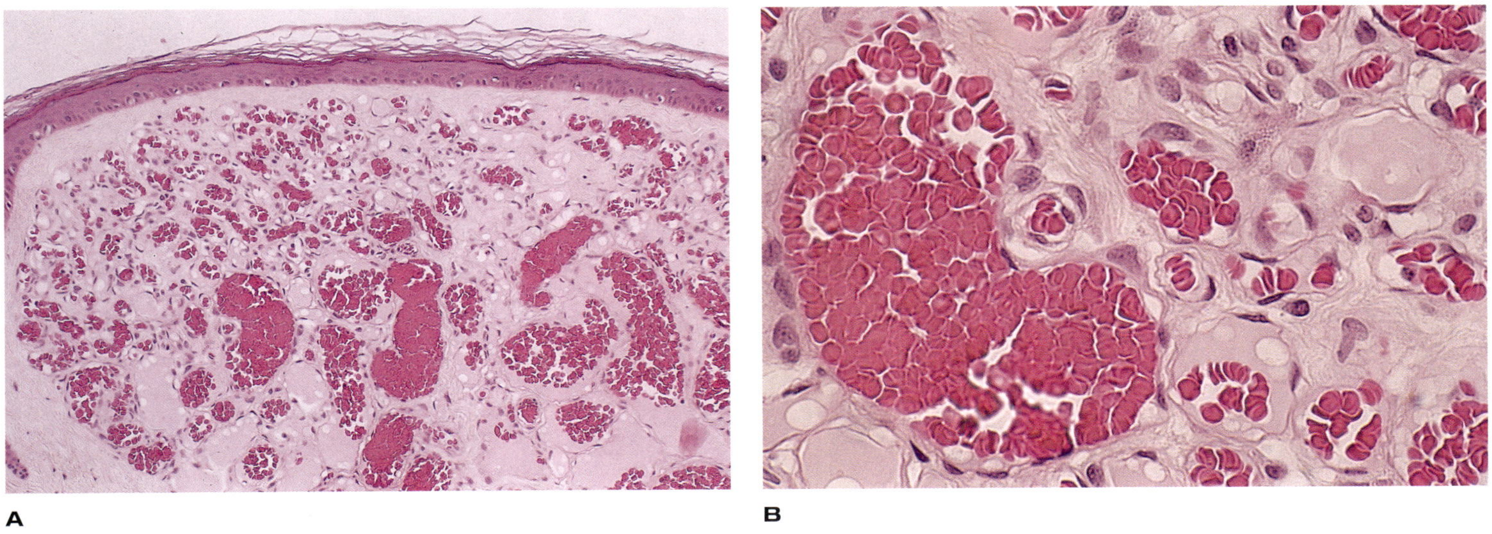

Figures 38–6A, 38–6B. **Hemangioma.** Dilated and congested capillaries that vary in size and shape.

GLOMUS TUMOR

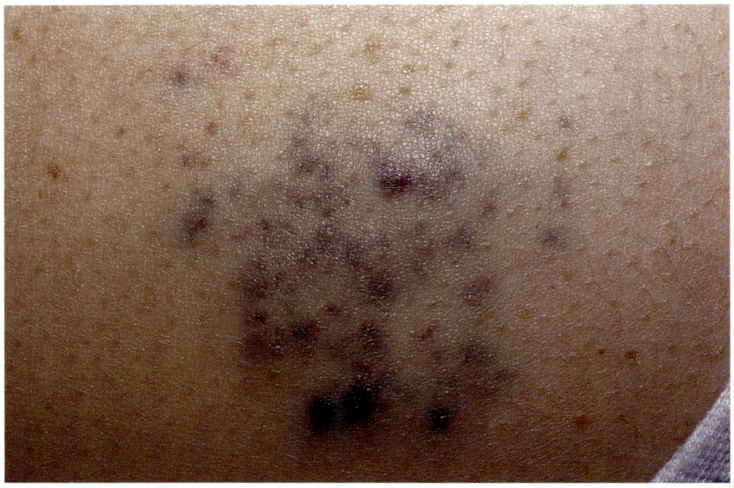

Figure 38–7. Glomus tumor. Agminated blue papules on the back of a woman.

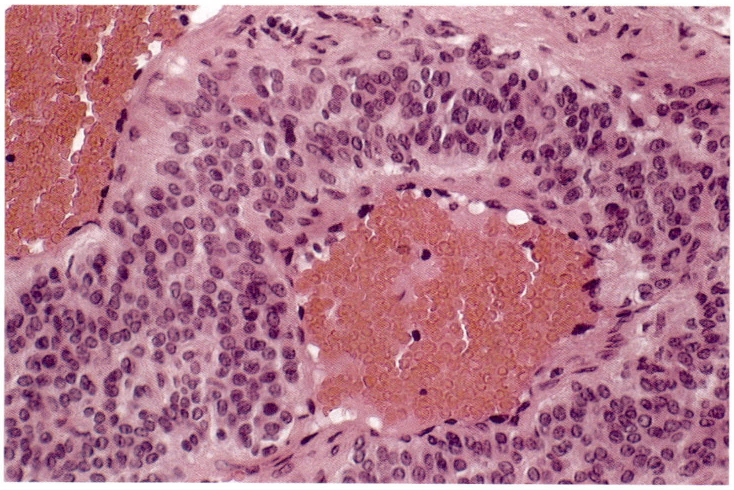

Figure 38–8. Glomus tumor. Sheets of monomorphous, round glomus cells surround a dilated and congested blood vessel.

CAPILLARY MALFORMATION

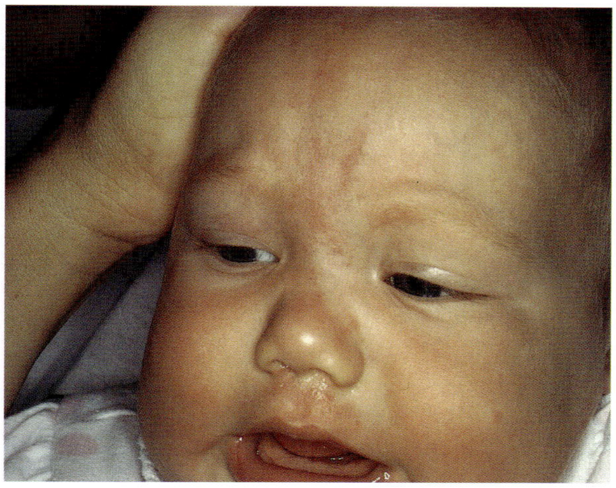

Figure 38–9. Capillary malformation, nevus flammeus type. Pink macules and patches on the lip, nose, glabella, and forehead in an infant since birth.

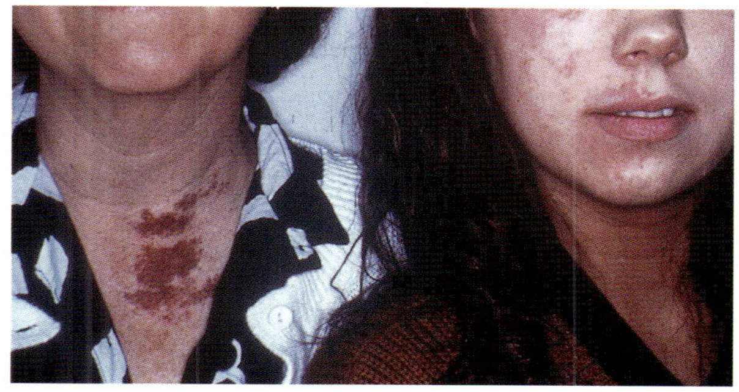

Figure 38–10. Capillary malformation, port wine type. Irregular purple patches and plaques on the neck and chest of the mother, and pink patches on the cheek, lip, chin, neck, and chest of her daughter. Both lesions were present at birth.

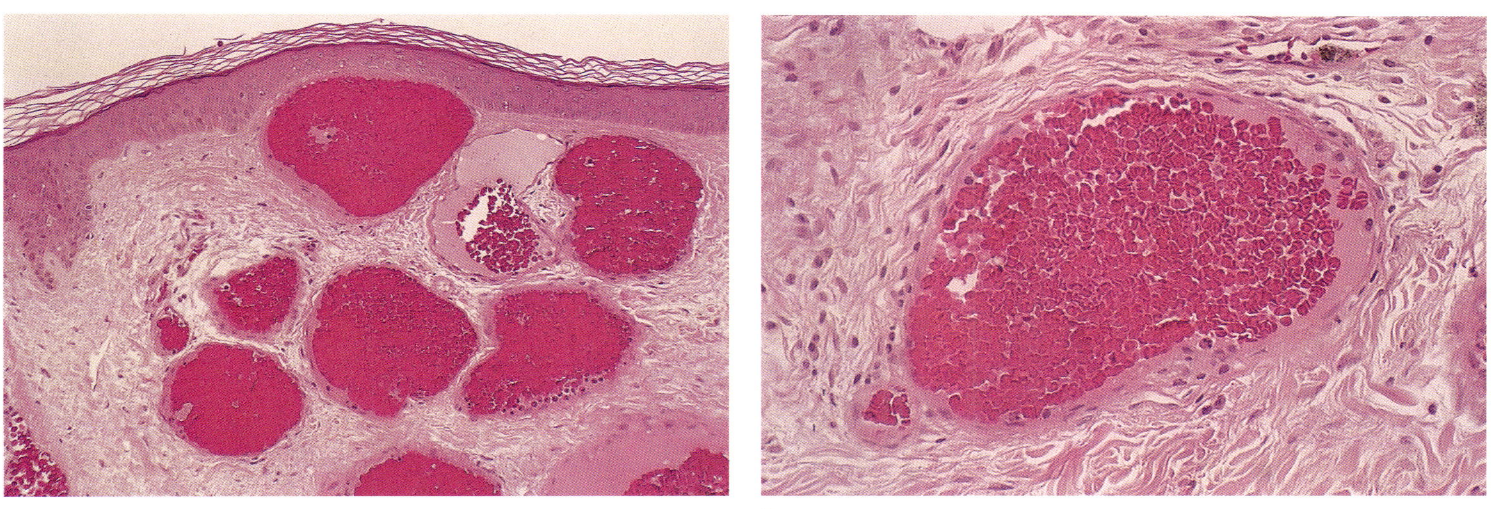

Figures 38–11A, 38–11B. Capillary malformation. Numerous markedly ectatic and congested blood vessels in the dermis.

LYMPHANGIOMA

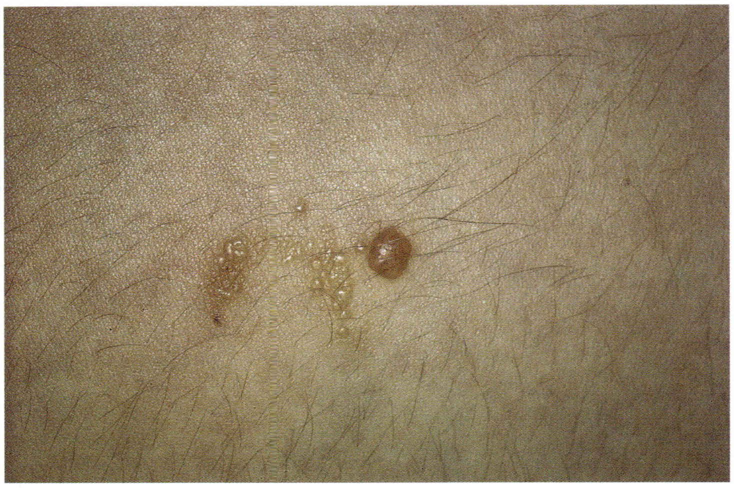

Figure 38–12. Lymphangioma. Aggregate of skin-colored papules on the thigh of a young girl.

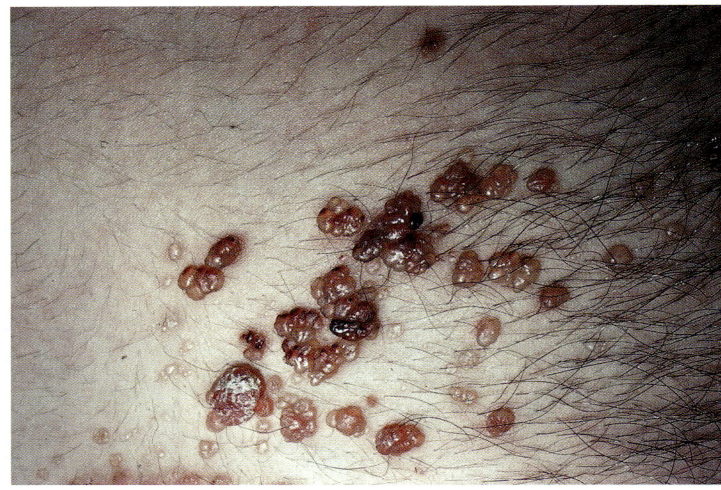

Figure 38–13. Lymphangioma. Agminated, hemorrhagic and skin-colored, smooth and crusted papules on the lower abdomen of a man.

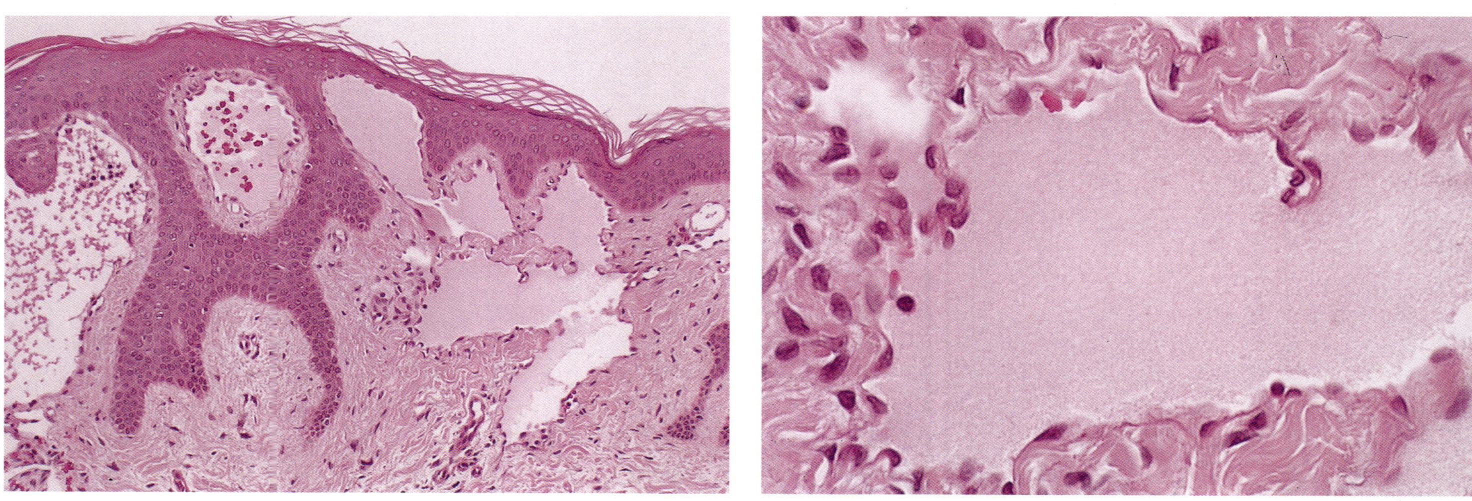

A B

Figures 38–14A, 38–14B. Lymphangioma. Dilated and irregular-shaped lymph channels filled with a pale eosinophilic granular material, and a sprinkling of red and white blood cells.

NEVUS ARANEUS

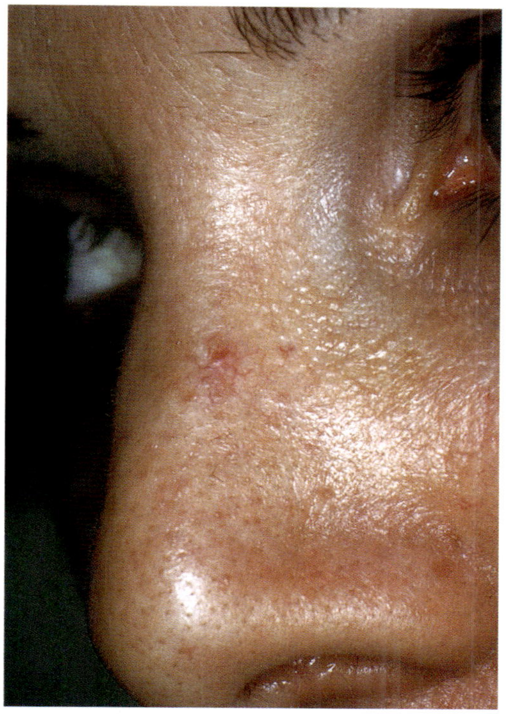

Figure 38–15. Nevus araneus. Central raised red papule with radiating branches. This lesion is commonly referred to as a spider nevus.

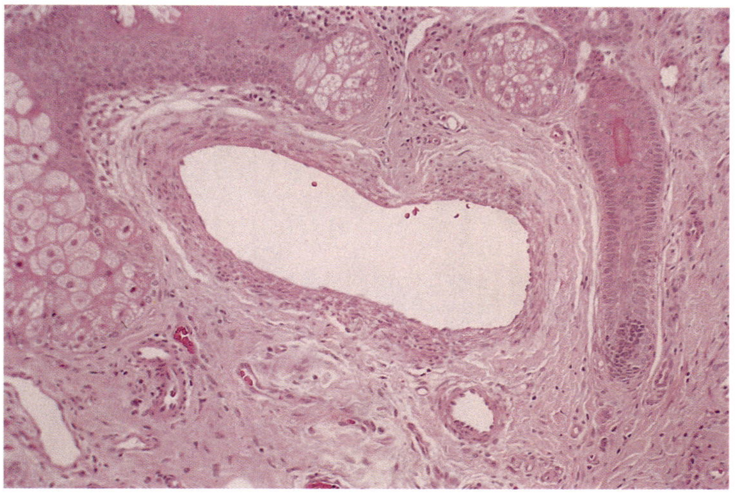

Figure 38–16. Nevus araneus. Dilated dermal arteriole and its adjacent tributaries.

INTRAVASCULAR PAPILLARY ENDOTHELIAL HYPERPLASIA

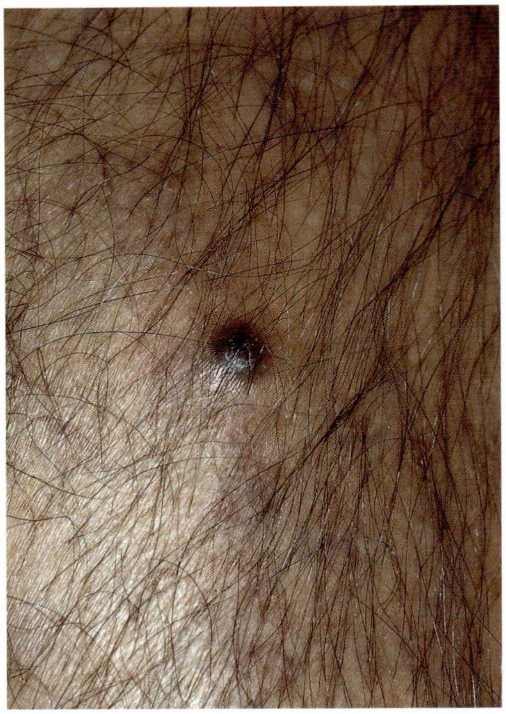

Figure 38–17. Intravascular papillary endothelial hyperplasia. Dark blue-gray dome-shaped papule on the arm of a man.

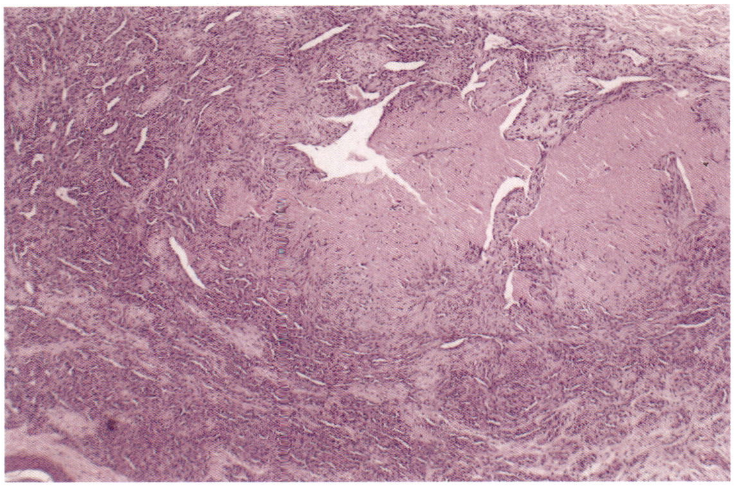

A

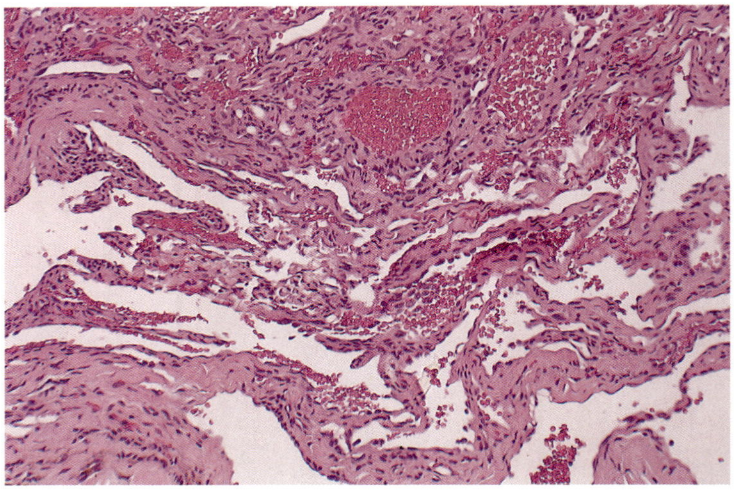

B

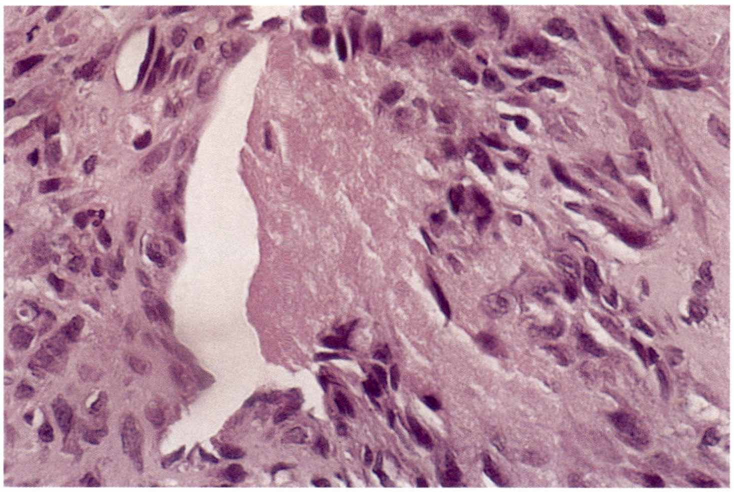

C

Figures 38–18A, 38–18B, 38–18C. Intravascular papillary endothelial hyperplasia. Proliferation of vascular channels containing coarse collagen bundles, plump endothelial cells, and fibrin. These changes are usually associated with a preexisting vascular lesion such as hemangioma.

VENOUS LAKE

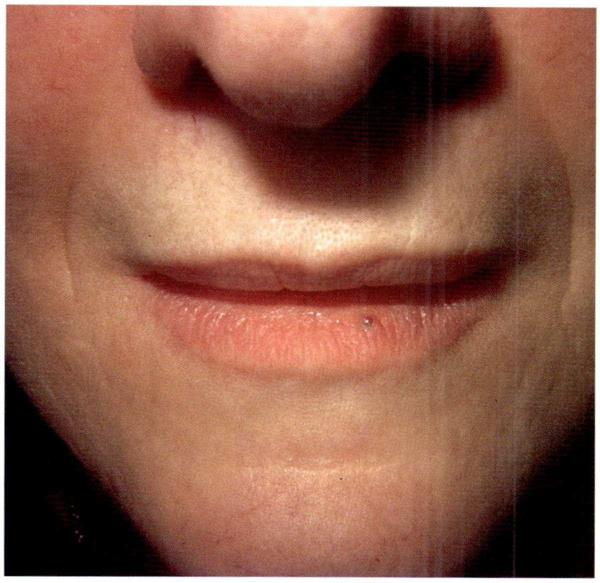

Figure 38–19. Venous lake. Purple papule on the lip of a woman.

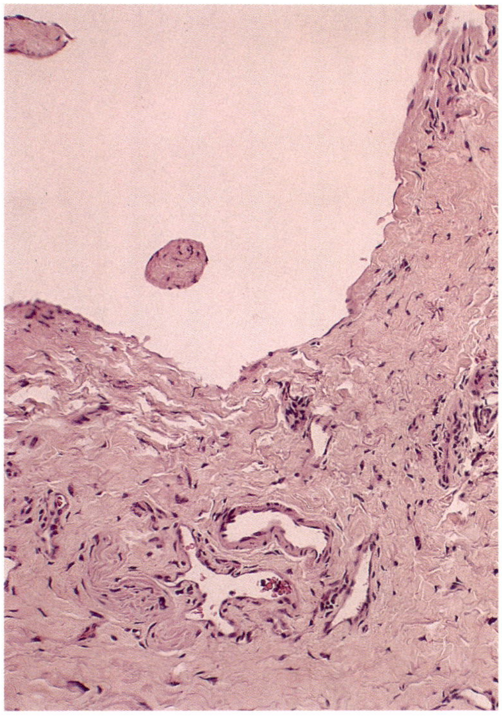

Figure 38–20. Venous lake. Widely dilated and ectatic dermal venules.

ARTERIOVENOUS MALFORMATION

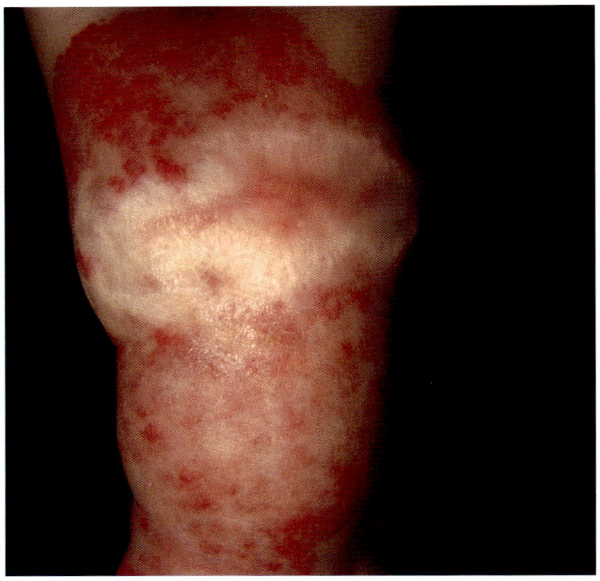

Figure 38–21. Arteriovenous malformation. Markedly enlarged and distorted arm of a six-month-old boy with confluent erythematous papules and nodules.

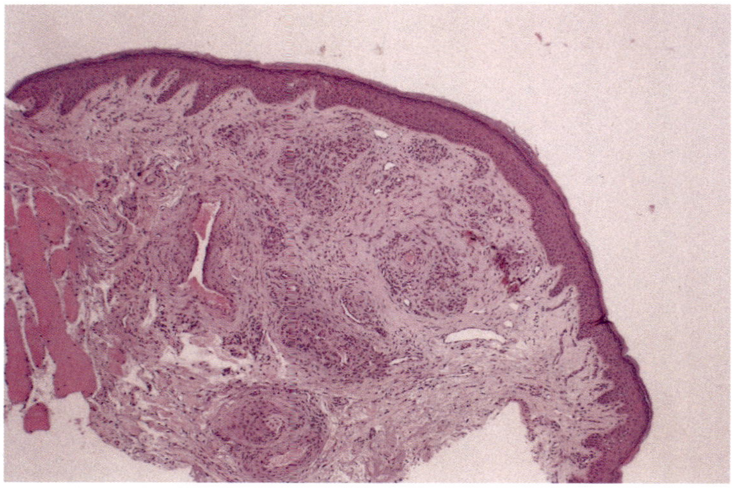

A

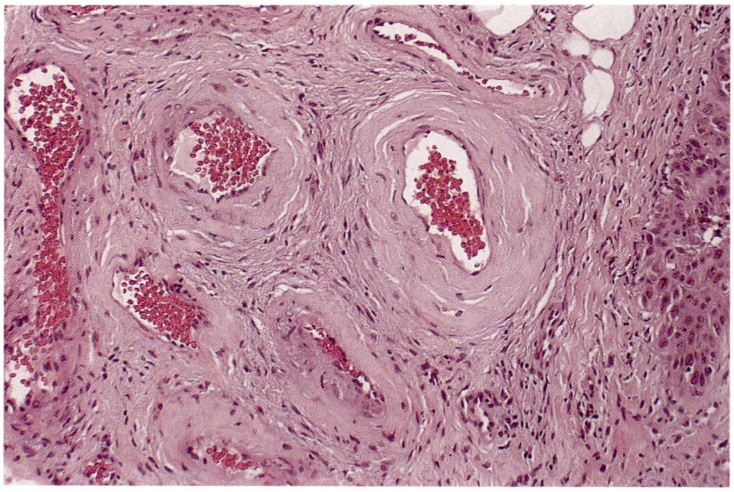

B

Figures 38–22A, 38–22B. Arteriovenous malformation. Anastomosing, thick-walled dermal blood vessels.

ANGIOLYMPHOID HYPERPLASIA WITH EOSINOPHILIA

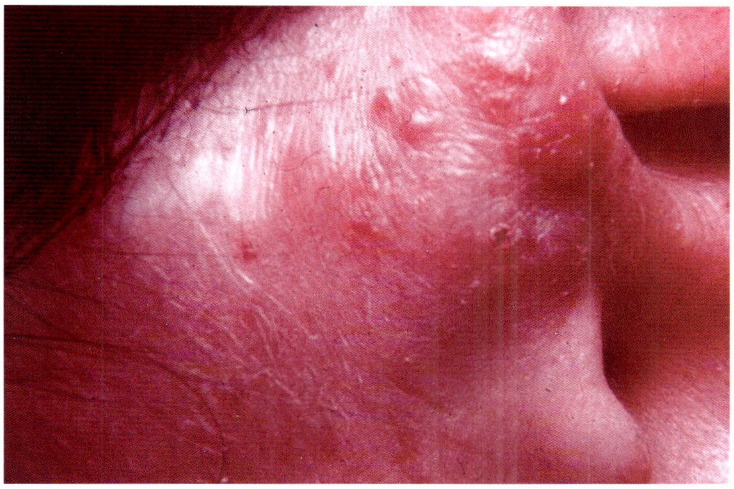

Figure 38–23. Angiolymphoid hyperplasia with eosinophilia. Preauricular, erythematous, asymptomatic nodules in a 34-year-old woman.

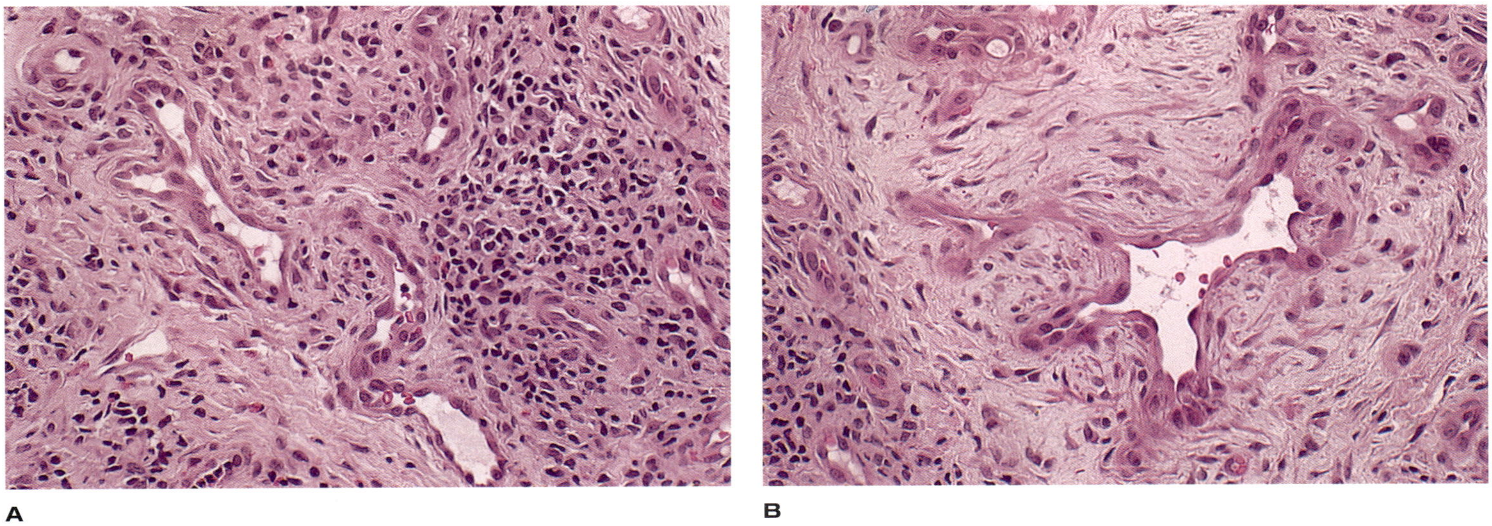

Figures 38–24A, 38–24B. Angiolymphoid hyperplasia with eosinophilia. Bizarre-shaped blood vessels in a fibrocytic dermis surrounded by a dense mononuclear cell infiltrate containing eosinophils. The thickened blood vessel walls contain mucin deposits and are lined with plump endothelial cells.

ANGIOKERATOMA

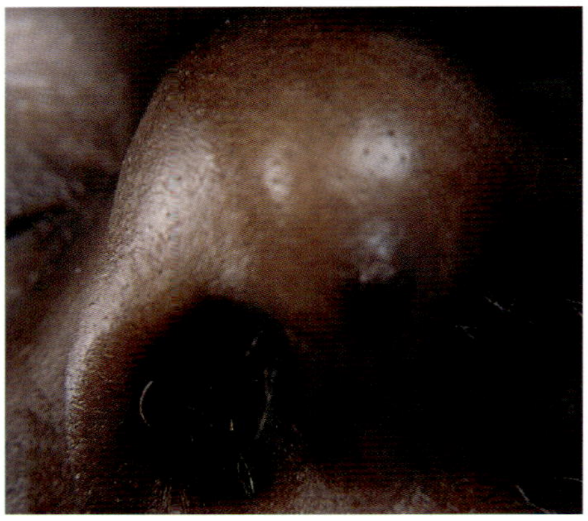

Figure 38–25. Angiokeratoma, solitary type. Hyperkeratotic, dome-shaped papule on the tip of the nose.

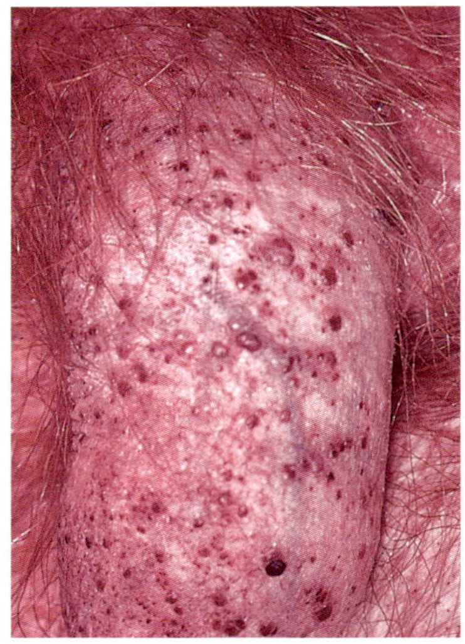

Figure 38–26. Angiokeratomas, multiple type. Variably sized and shaped red and dark-blue papules on the penis and scrotum. This man has Fabry's disease, but similar lesions may be seen in individuals without Fabry's disease.

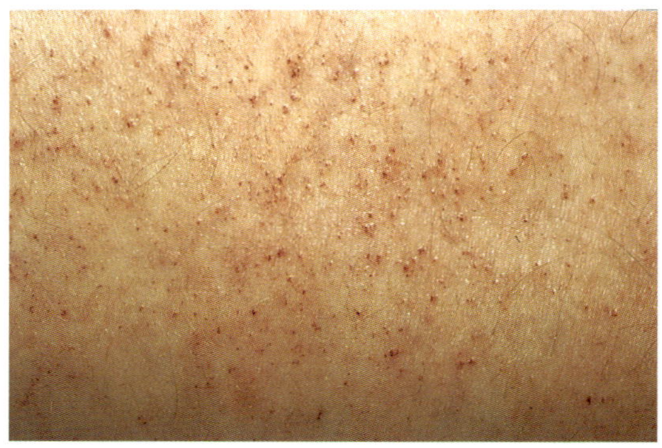

Figure 38–27. Angiokeratomas, multiple type. Small, erythematous keratotic papules on the abdomen of a man with Fabry's disease.

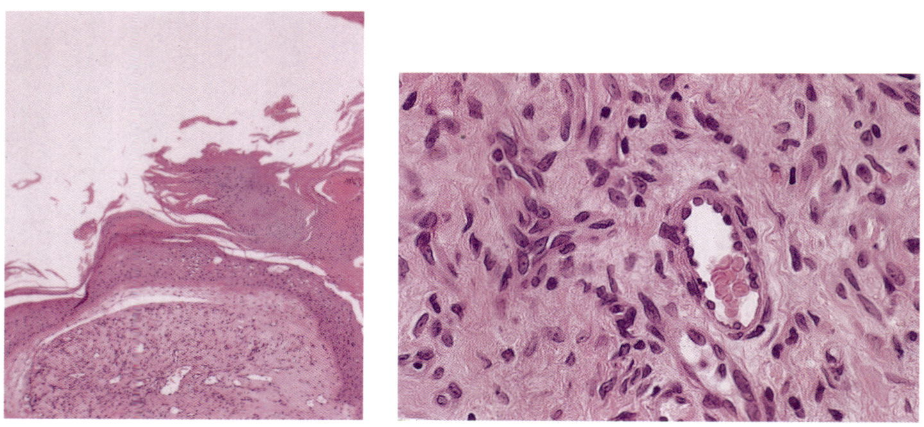

A **B**

Figures 38–28A, 38–28B. Angiokeratoma. Epidermal hyperplasia, hyperkeratosis, and papillomatosis with scale-crust. There is a proliferation of blood vessels filling the thickened and fibrocytic papillary dermis.

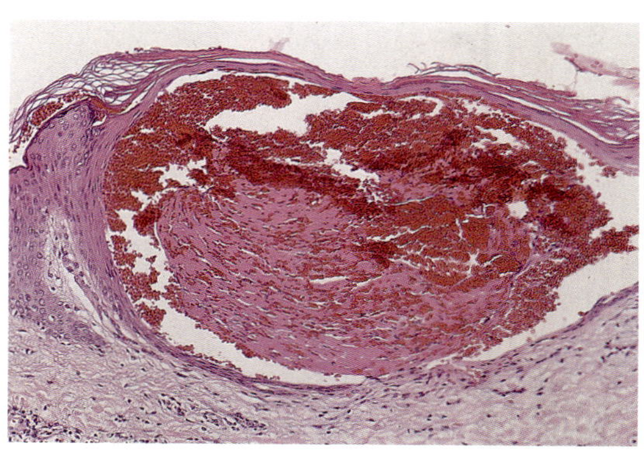

Figure 38–29. Angiokeratoma. Epidermal collarette surrounds a dilated dermal blood vessel filled with erythrocytes and fibrin.

KAPOSI'S SARCOMA

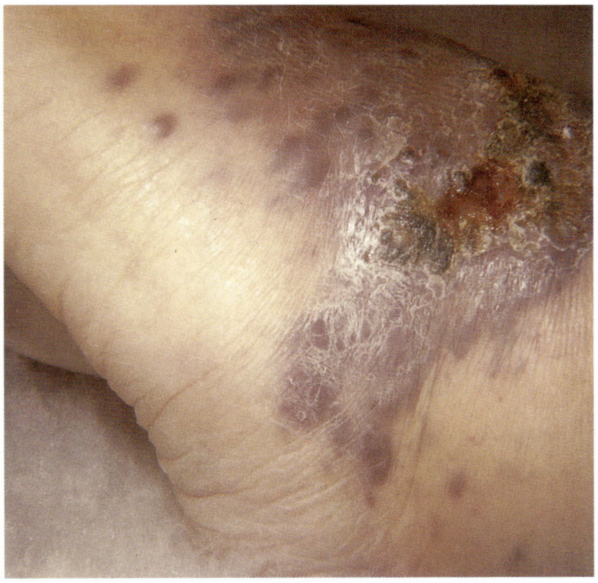

Figure 38–30. Kaposi's sarcoma. Crusted, violaceous papules and nodules on the lower leg and foot of an elderly woman with the classic type of Kaposi's sarcoma. At autopsy, she had multiple internal organs involved.

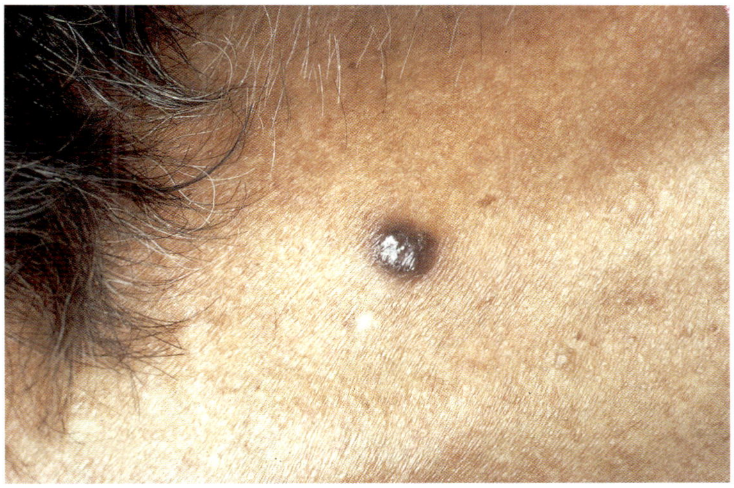

Figure 38–31. Kaposi's sarcoma. Blue-gray nodule on the neck of a young man who is HIV-positive.

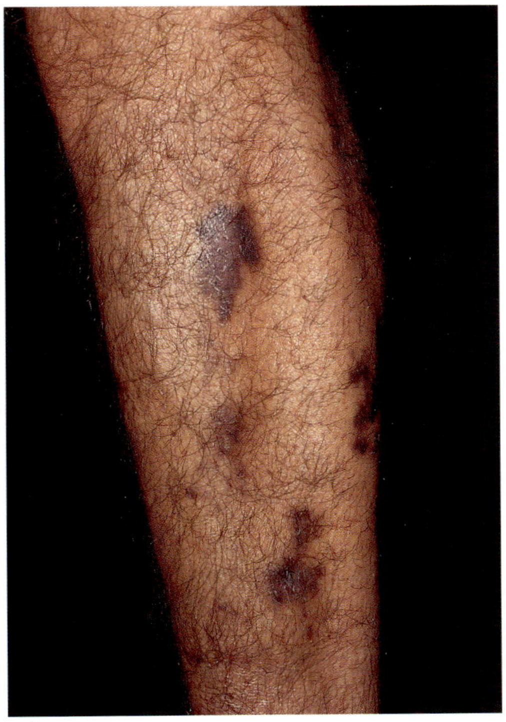

Figure 38–32. Kaposi's sarcoma. Multiple blue-gray plaques on the lower leg of an HIV-positive man.

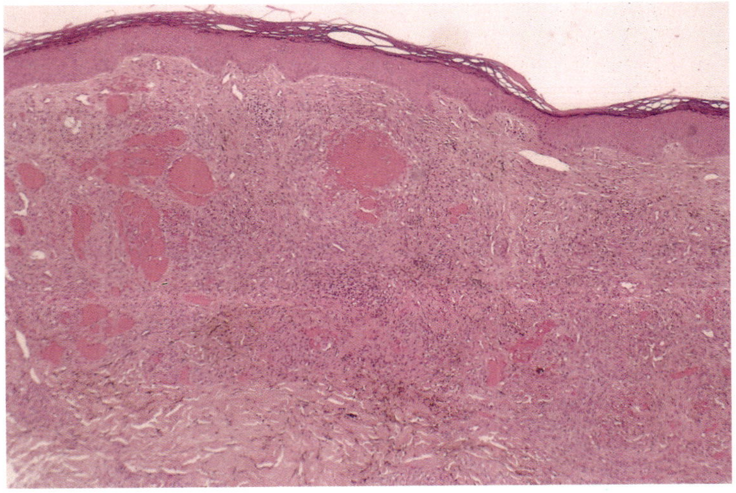

Figure 38–33. Kaposi's sarcoma. Dilated, congested, and irregularly shaped blood vessels within a dense, cellular stroma.

KAPOSI'S SARCOMA

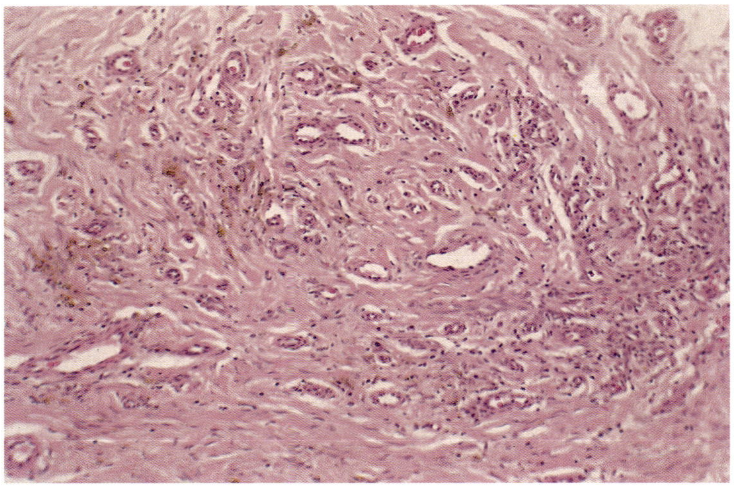

Figure 38–34. Kaposi's sarcoma. Blood vessels appear within irregularly shaped clear vascular channels lined by endothelial cells. This is referred to as the promontory sign.

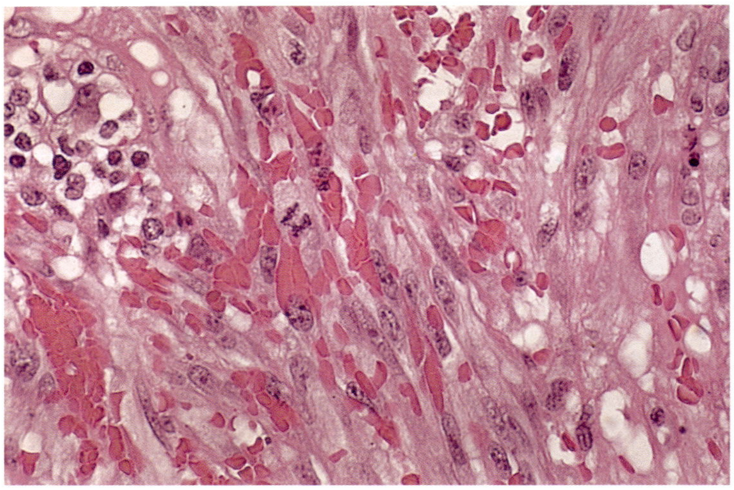

Figure 38–35. Kaposi's sarcoma. Erythrocytes in single file between atypical and mitotic endothelial cells.

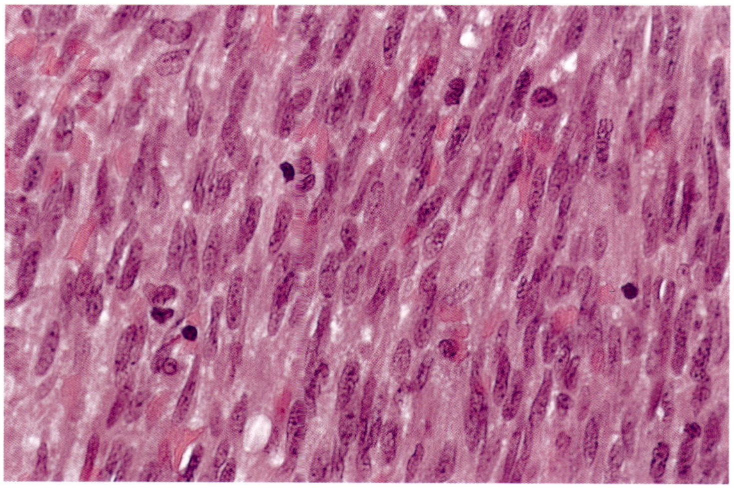

Figure 38–36. Kaposi's sarcoma. Solitary erythrocytes among fascicles and sheets of atypical endothelial cells.

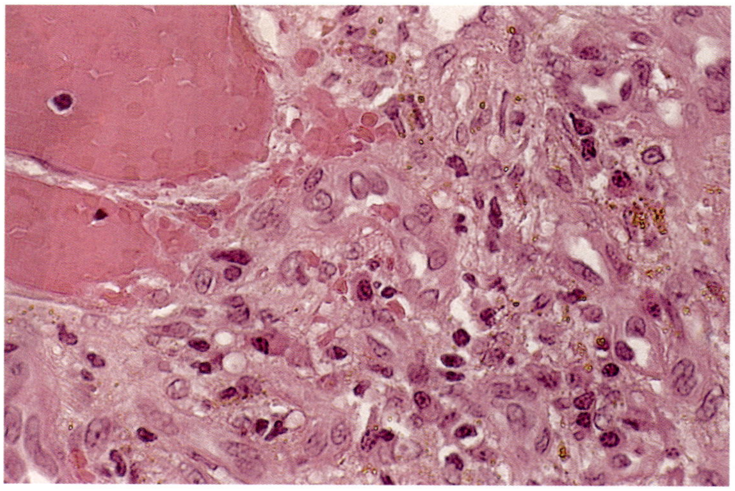

Figure 38–37. Kaposi's sarcoma. Plasma cells and siderophages surround severely congested vascular channels.

KAPOSI'S SARCOMA

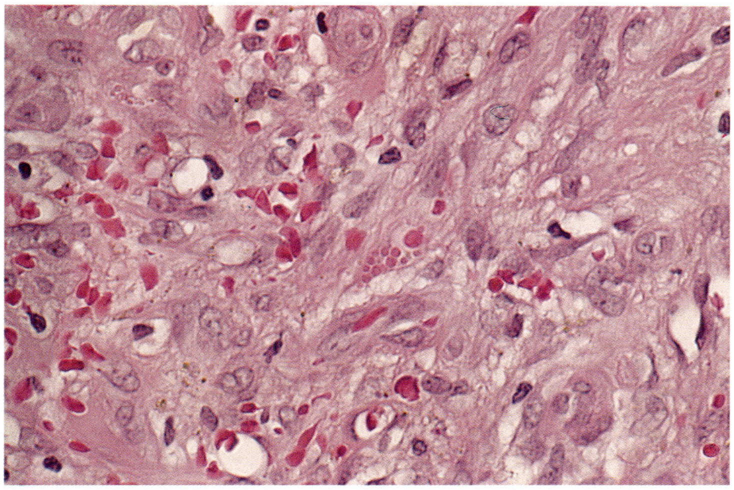

Figure 38–38. Kaposi's sarcoma. Pink globules (phagocytosed and degenerated erythrocytes) within the cytoplasm of an atypical endothelial cell.

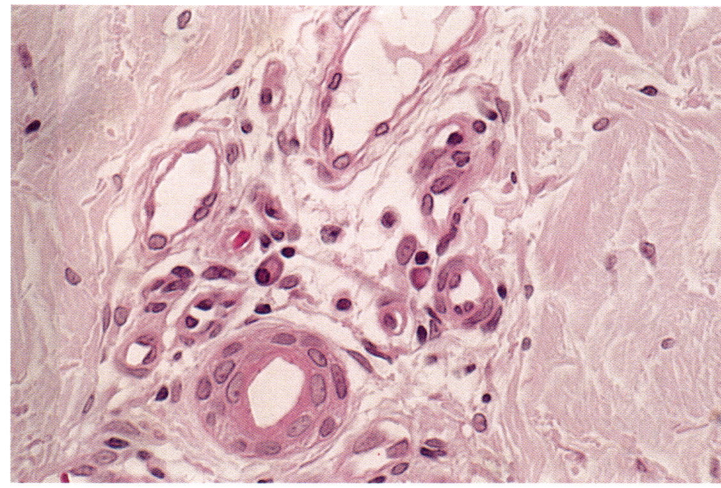

Figure 38–39. Kaposi's sarcoma. Bizarre-shaped, endothelial-lined vascular channels encircle an adnexal structure and blood vessels. There are lymphocytes and plasma cells.

ANGIOSARCOMA

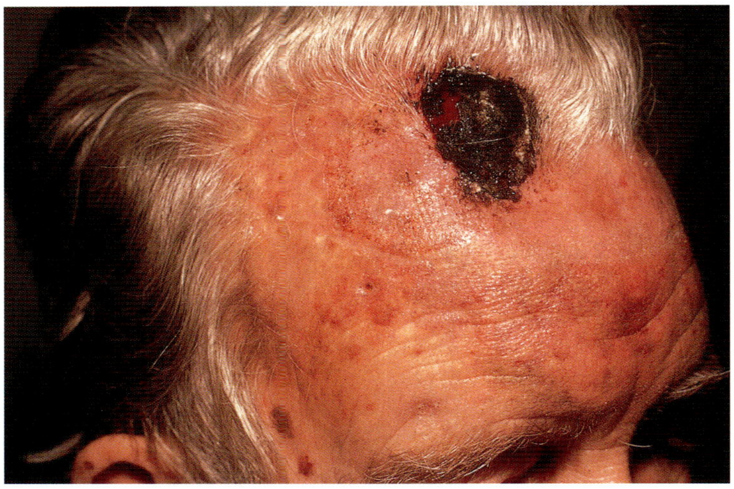

Figure 38–40. **Angiosarcoma.** Ulcerated and crusted plaque on the frontal scalp of an elderly man.

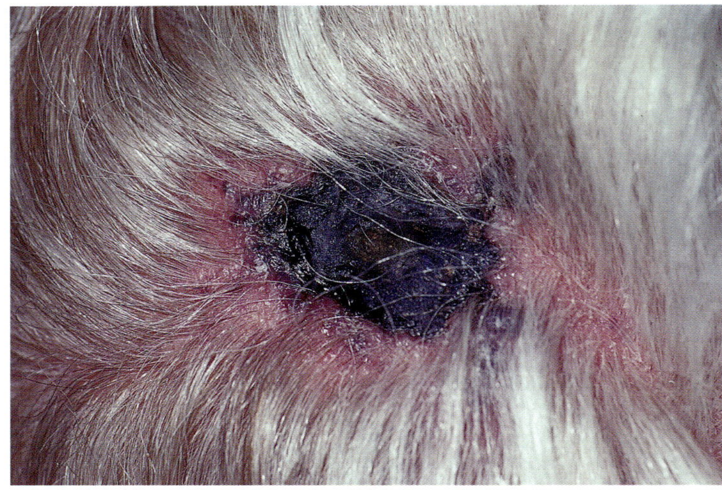

Figure 38–41. **Angiosarcoma.** Erythematous, ulcerated, and crusted plaque in the scalp of a woman.

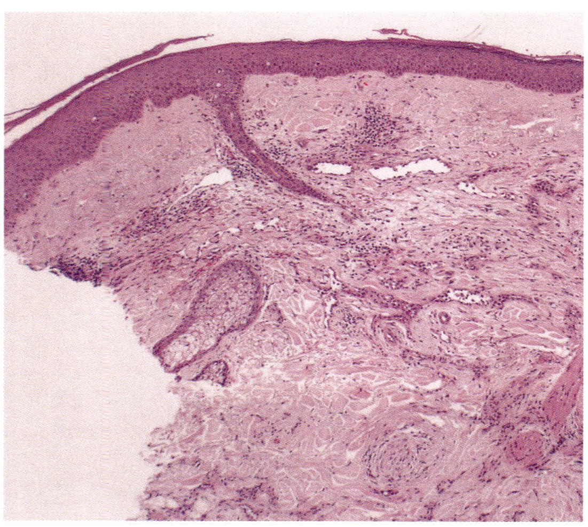

A

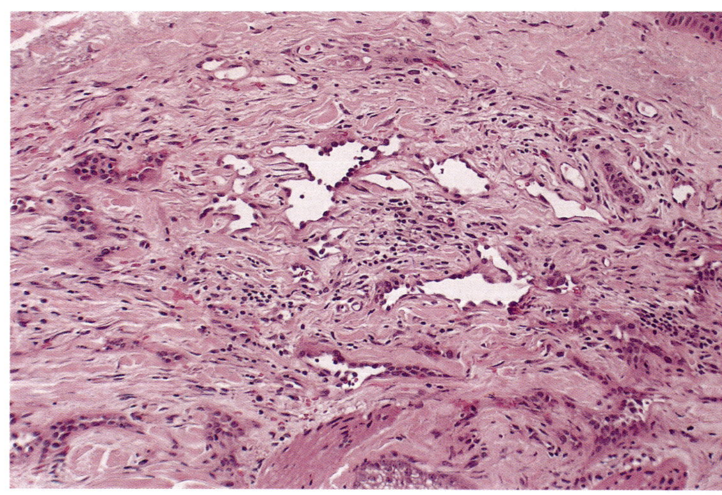

B

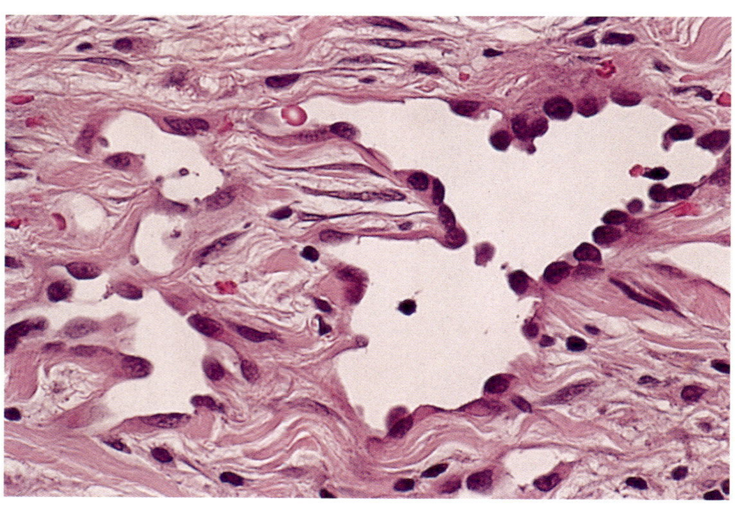

C

Figures 38–42A, 38–42B, 38–42C. **Angiosarcoma.** Bizarre-shaped blood vessels in a fibrocytic dermis. Large, atypical, crowded, and protruding endothelial cells line the vascular channels. A few tumor cells appear to be floating within the lumen (pseudoacantholytic), while others are present between collagen bundles.

39

Smooth muscle and adipose proliferative disorders

- Piloleiomyoma
- Smooth-muscle hamartoma
- Angioleiomyoma
- Leiomyosarcoma
- Lipoma
- Angiolipoma
- Spindle-cell lipoma
- Myxoid lipoma
- Pleomorphic lipoma
- Hibernoma
- Lipoblastoma
- Liposarcoma

PILOLEIOMYOMA

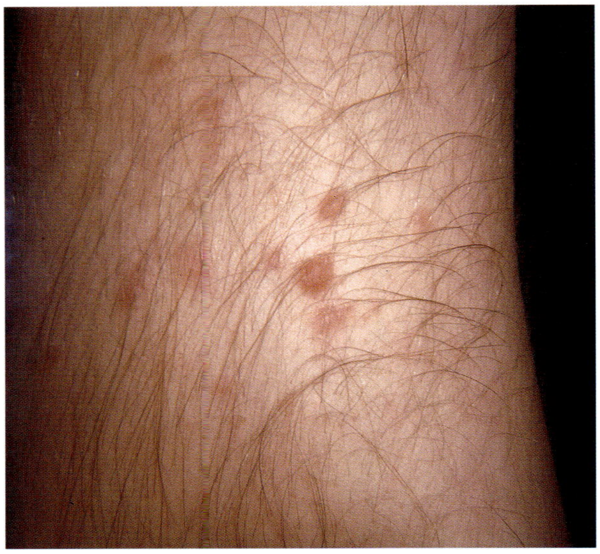

Figure 39–1. Piloleiomyoma. Tender pink papules on the arm of a man.

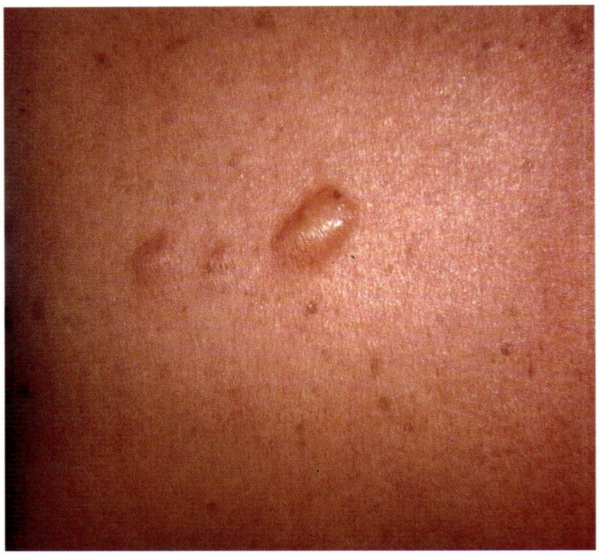

Figure 39–2. Piloleiomyoma. Smooth, tender pink papules and nodule on the back.

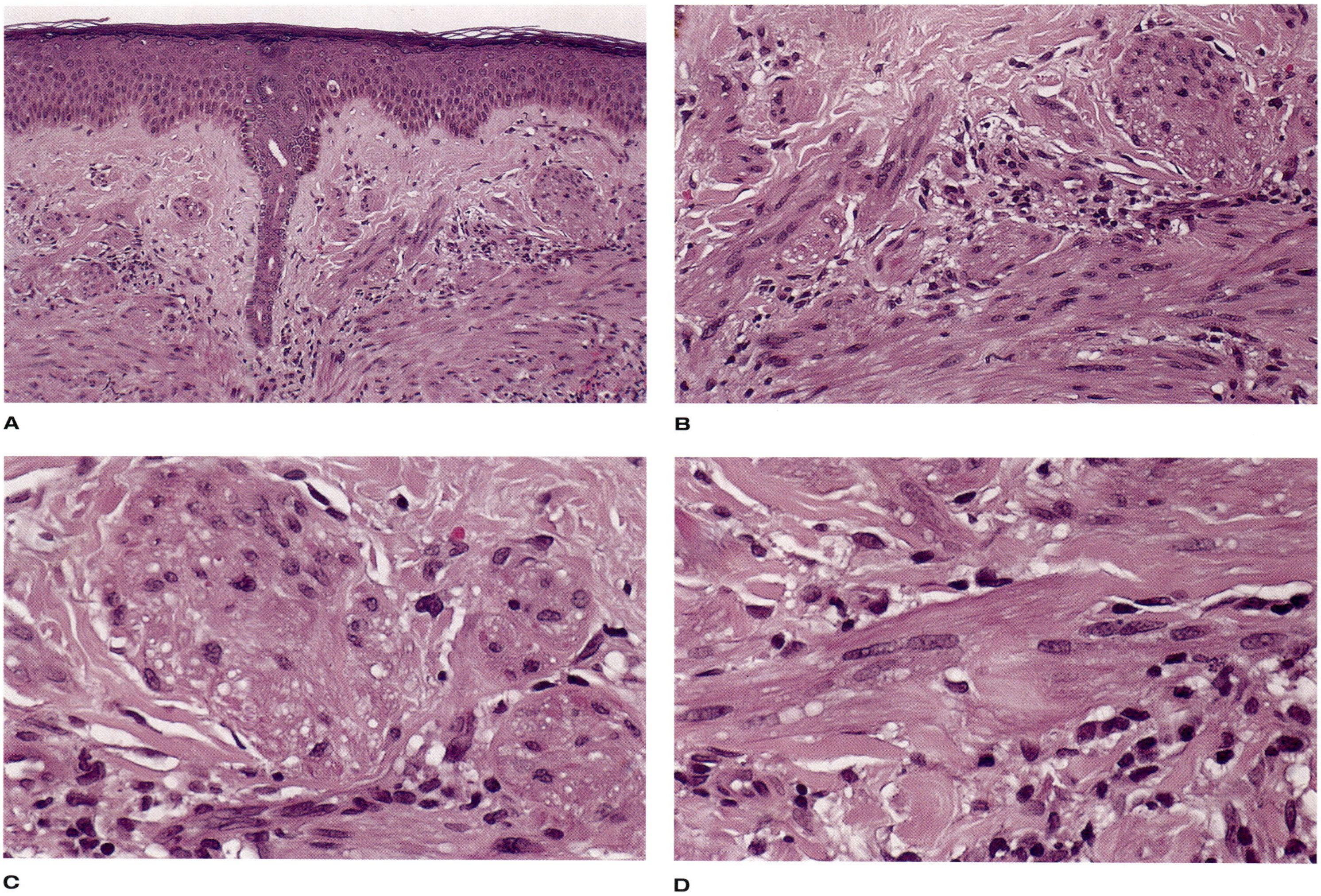

Figures 39–3A, 39–3B, 39–3C, 39–3D. Piloleiomyoma. Discrete, interlacing fascicles of smooth-muscle bundles contiguous with, but separated from, collagen bundles. The muscle bundles are more eosinophilic than the surrounding collagen, and their nuclei are elongated and blunt-tipped. Perinuclear vacuoles are noted in fascicles cut on cross-section.

SMOOTH-MUSCLE HAMARTOMA

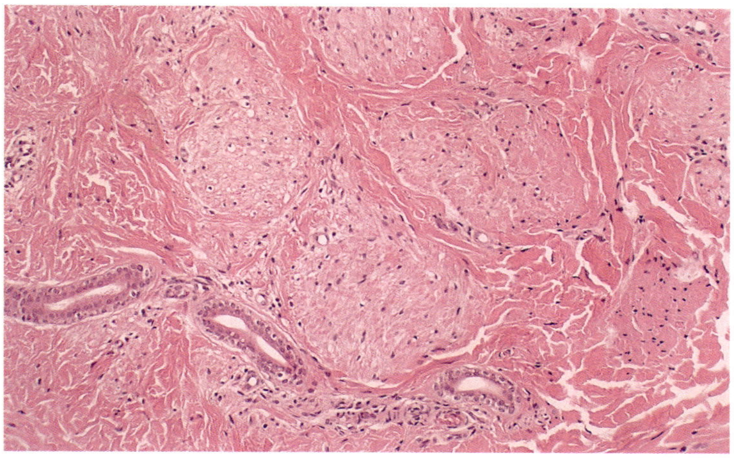

Figure 39–4. Smooth-muscle hamartoma. Fascicles of smooth-muscle bundles. There are elongated blunt-ended oval nuclei and perinuclear halos.

ANGIOLEIOMYOMA

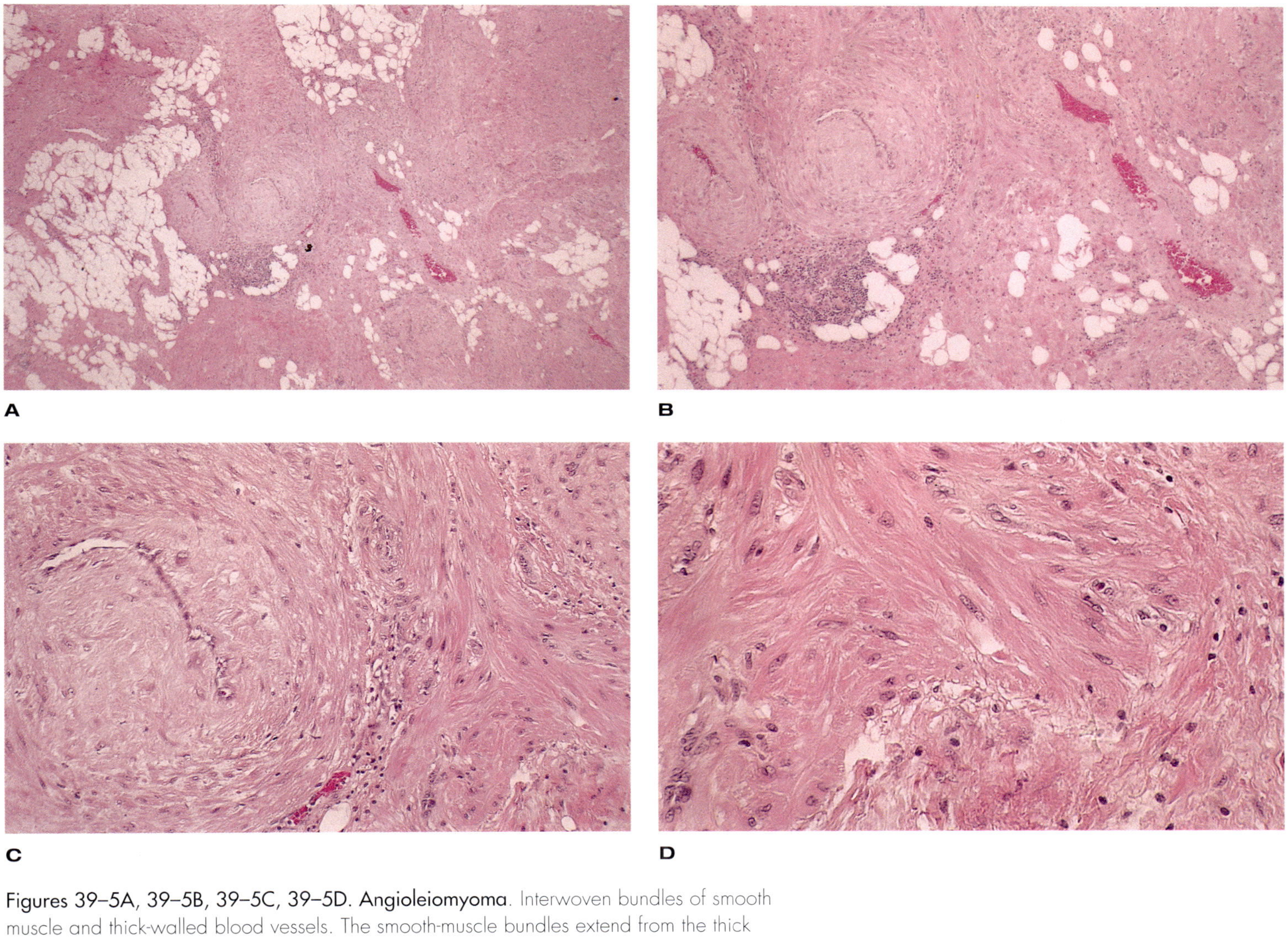

A B C D

Figures 39–5A, 39–5B, 39–5C, 39–5D. Angioleiomyoma. Interwoven bundles of smooth muscle and thick-walled blood vessels. The smooth-muscle bundles extend from the thick blood vessel walls.

LEIOMYOSARCOMA

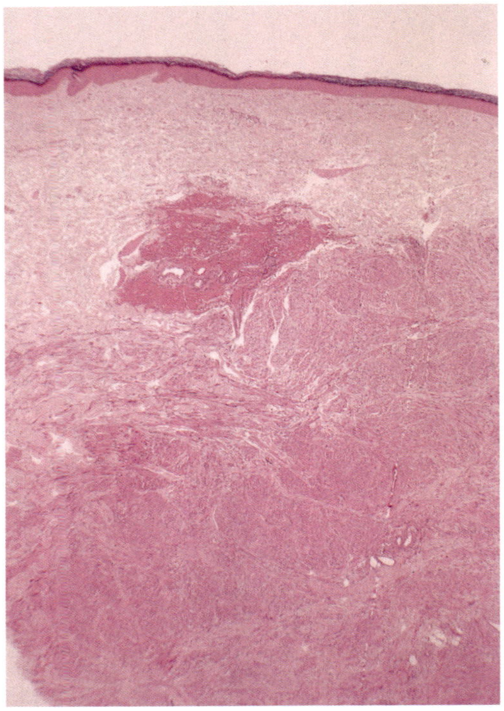

A

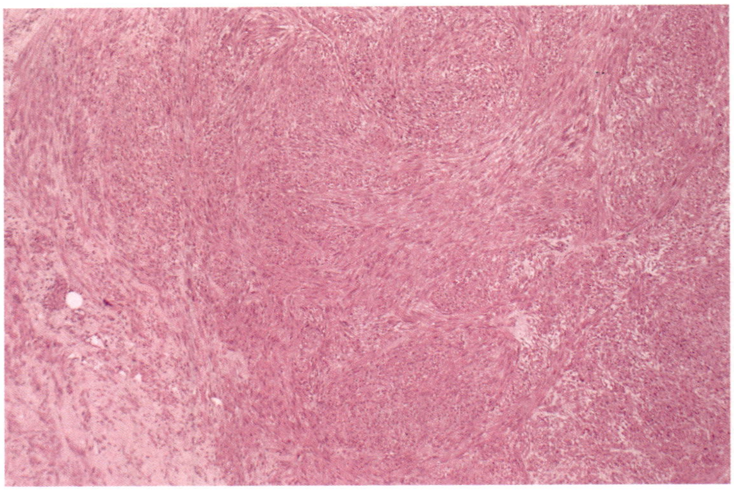

B

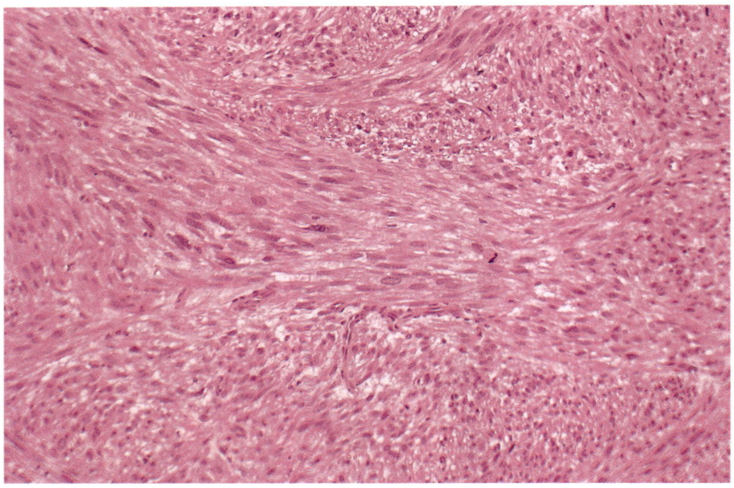

C

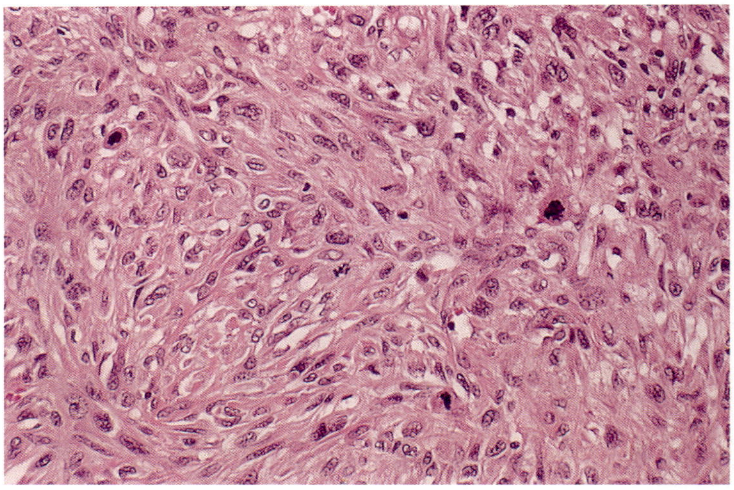

D

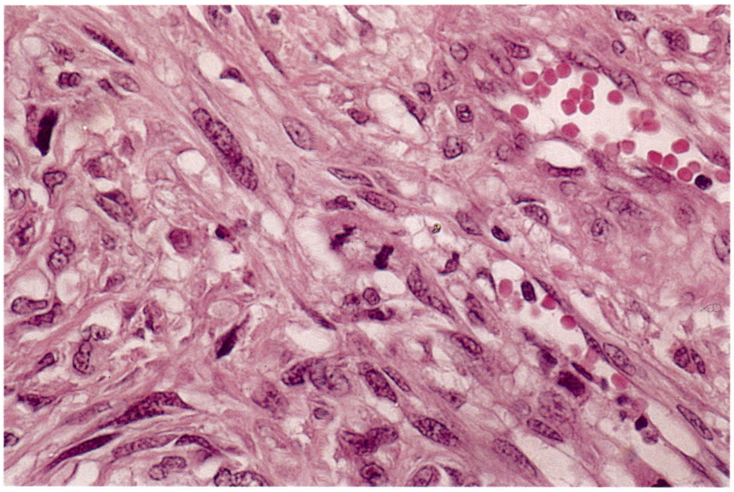

E

Figures 39–6A, 39–6B, 39–6C, 39–6D, 39–6E. Leiomyosarcoma. Poorly circumscribed, highly cellular, interlacing fascicles of atypical and pleomorphic oval and spindle-shaped cells. There are zones where mitotic figures and necrotic cells predominate, while in other areas they are sparse.

LIPOMA

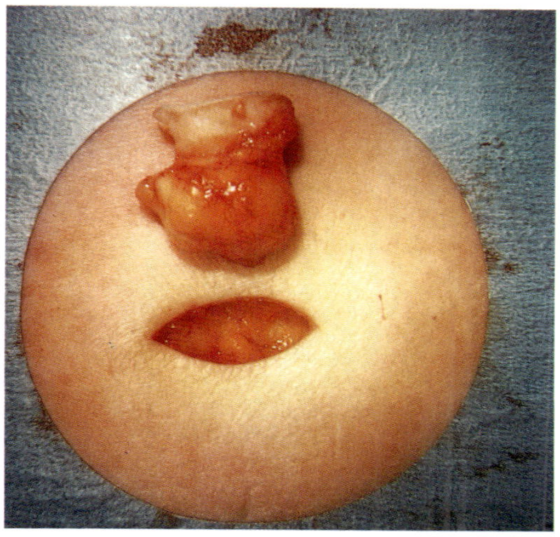

Figure 39–7. Lipoma. Flesh-colored, circumscribed, lobulated, and firm subcutaneous mass subjacent and attached to an elliptical piece of skin.

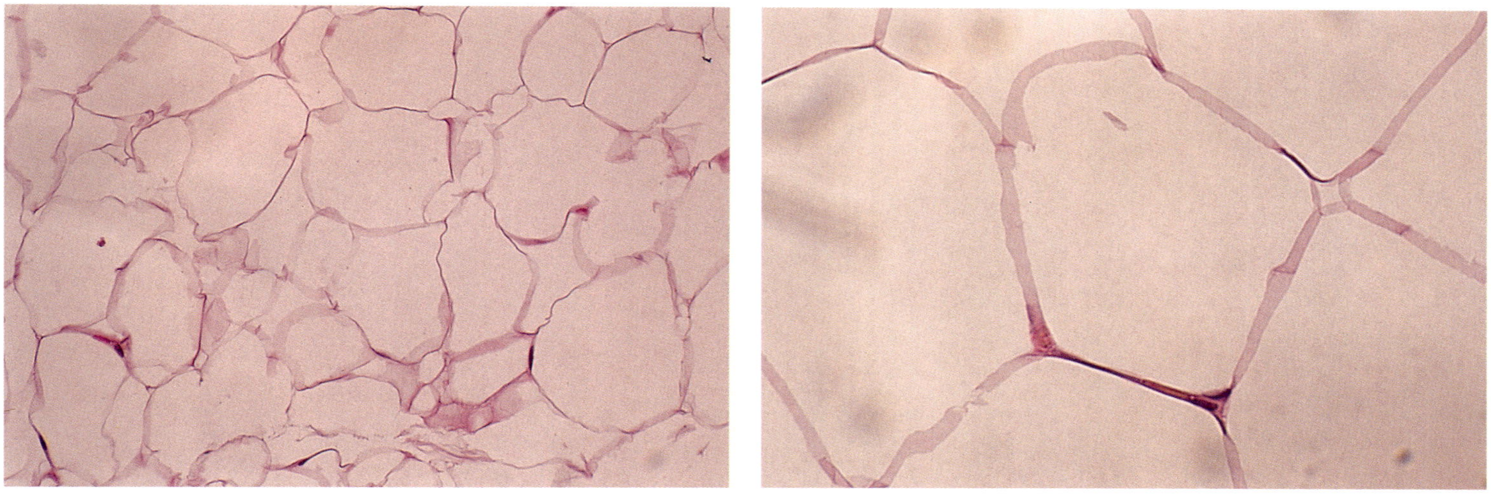

A **B**

Figures 39–8A, 39–8B. Lipoma. Lipocytes in lobular pattern. Polygonal lipocytes with a single large, central vacuole with a flattened nucleus to one side.

ANGIOLIPOMA

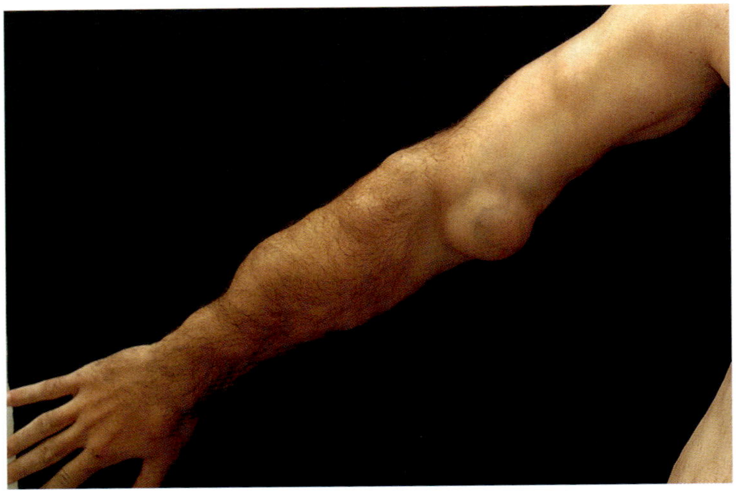

Figure 39–9. Angiolipoma. Multiple skin-colored nodules on the arm of a man.

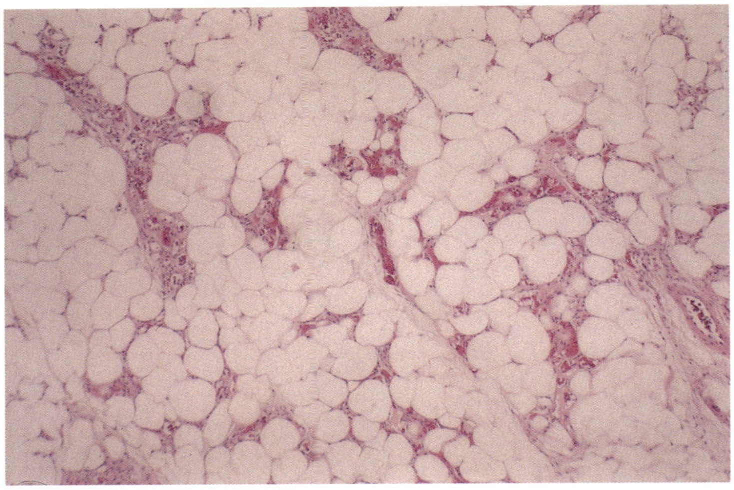

A

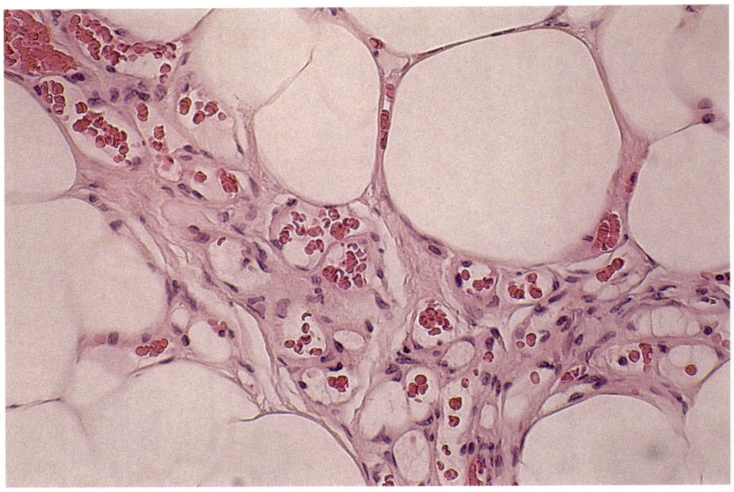

B

Figures 39–10A, 39–10B. Angiolipoma. Numerous blood vessels separating lobules of uniform lipocytes.

SPINDLE-CELL LIPOMA

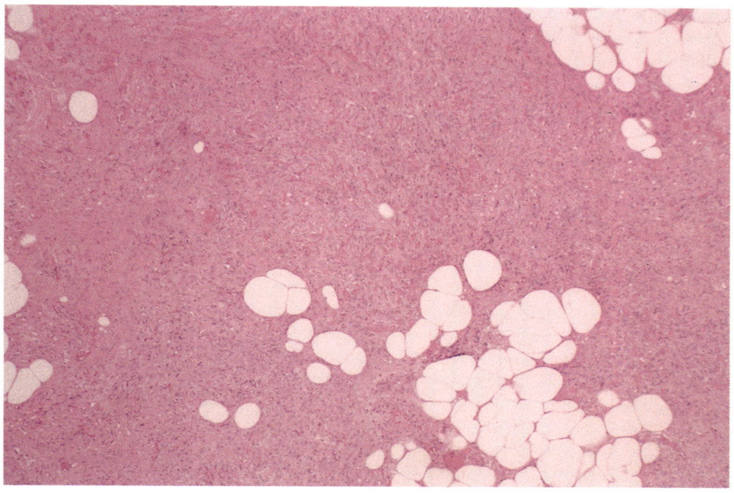

A

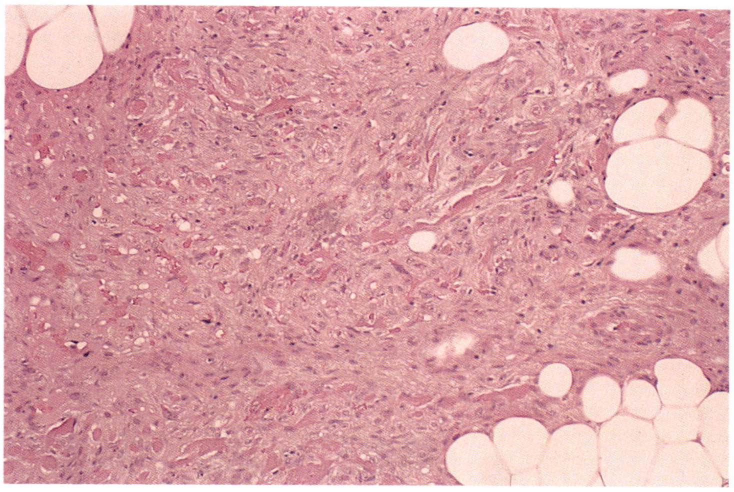

B

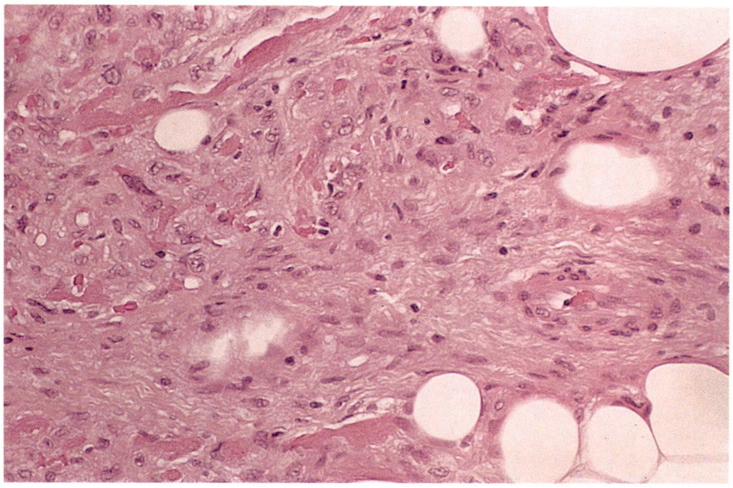

C

Figures 39–11A, 39–11B, 39–11C. Spindle-cell lipoma. Mature fat lobules intersected by thick fascicles of oval and spindle-shaped cells separated by collagen bundles and dilated blood vessels.

MYXOID LIPOMA

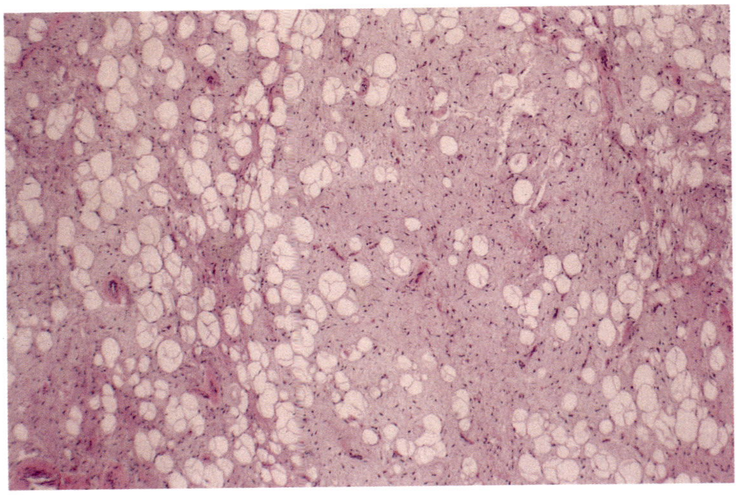

A

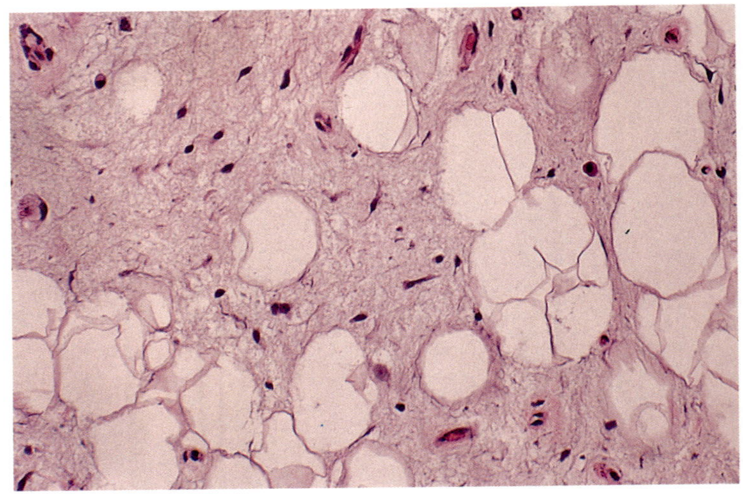

B

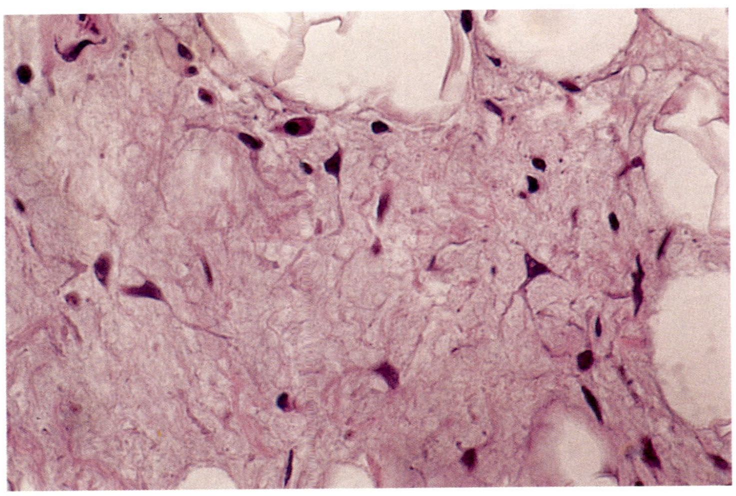

C

Figures 39–12A, 39–12B, 39–12C. Myxoid lipoma. Abundant mucin and mature lipocytes. There are spindle- and stellate-shaped cells, mast cells, gray-staining mucin, and dilated blood vessels.

PLEOMORPHIC LIPOMA

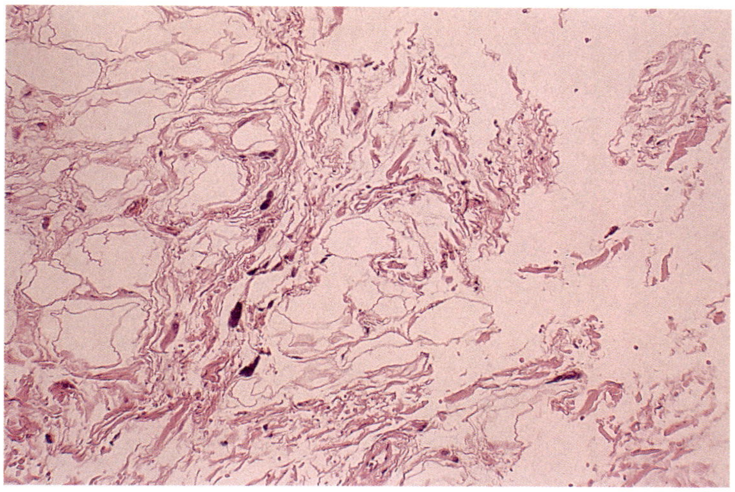

A

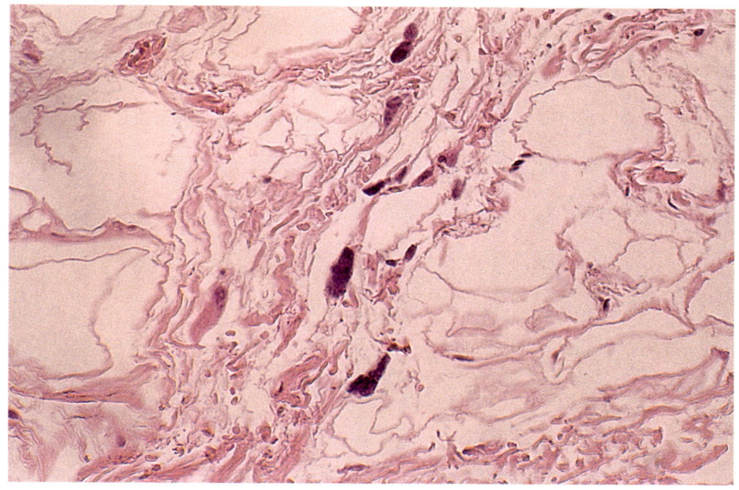

B

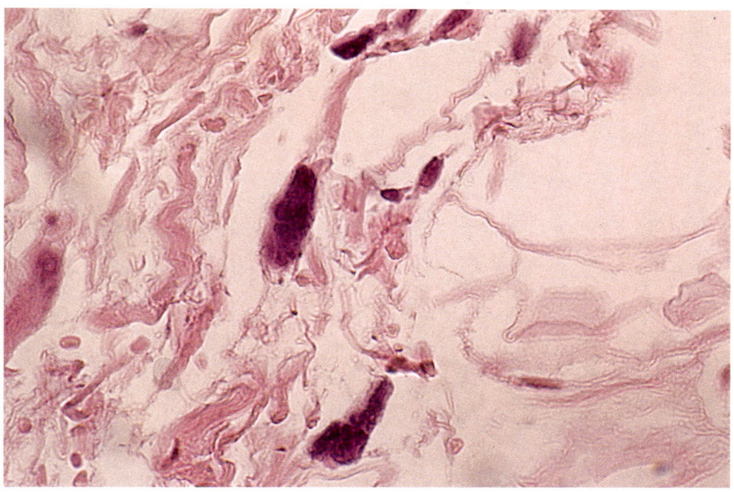

C

Figures 39–13A, 39–13B, 39–13C. Pleomorphic lipoma. Mature lipocytes and multinucleate giant cells with hyperchromatic and overlapping nuclei.

(Floret giant cells)

HIBERNOMA

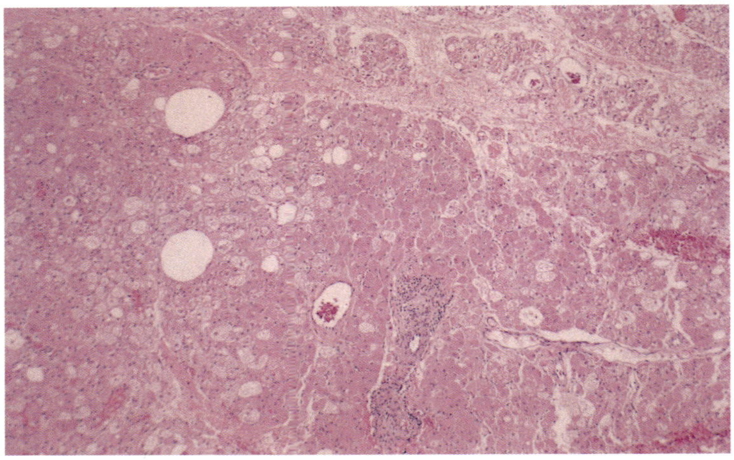

A

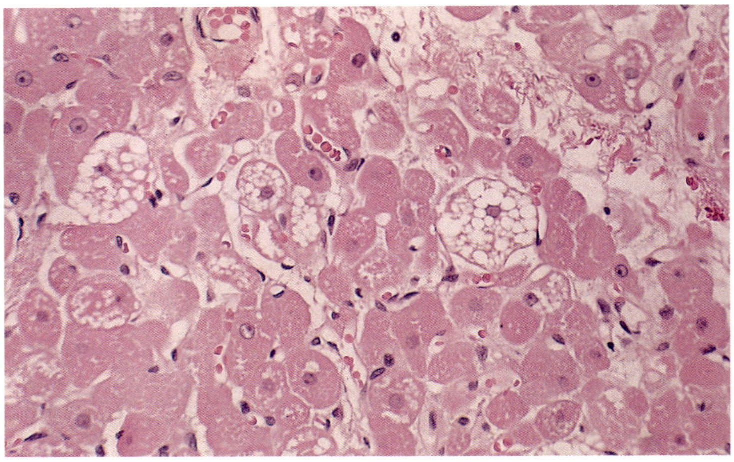

B

Figures 39–14A, 39–14B. H bernoma. Lobules of eosinophilic, vacuolated lipocytes within a fibrovascular stroma. There are a variety of lipocytes with central nuclei that have either prominent granular, eosinophilic cytoplasm with few vacuoles; or an extensive number of vacuoles with no granular, eosinophilic cytoplasm. The latter cell is referred to as a mulberry cell.

mulberry cells

LIPOBLASTOMA

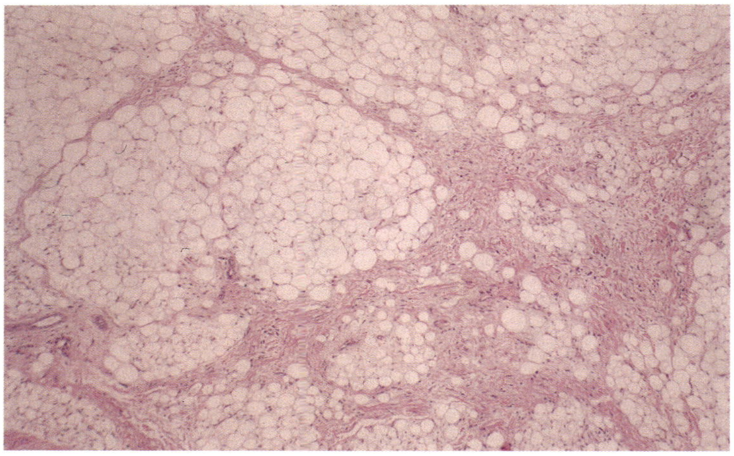

A

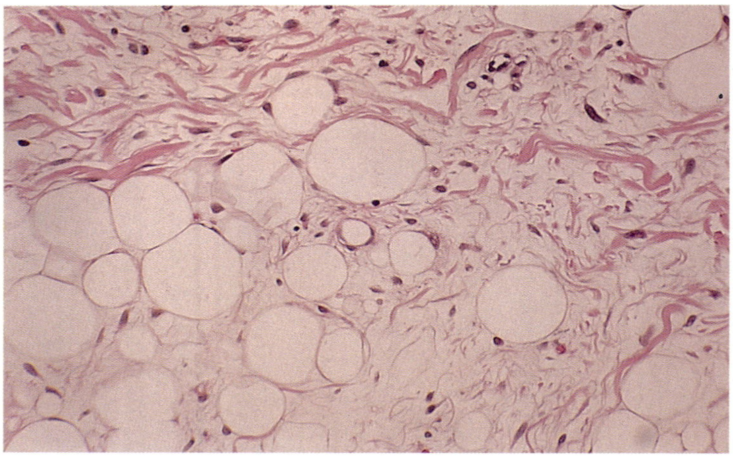

B

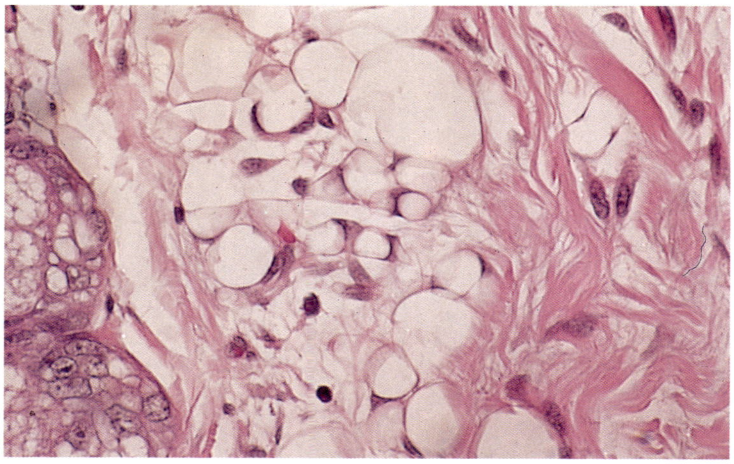

C

like a liposarc but it's in a kid?

Figures 39–15A, 39–15B, 39–15C. Lipoblastoma. Multiple irregular fat lobules within a fibrovascular stroma. There are mature lipocytes with thin nuclei as well as immature, vacuolated lipocytes with plump nuclei having a "signet ring" appearance.

LIPOSARCOMA

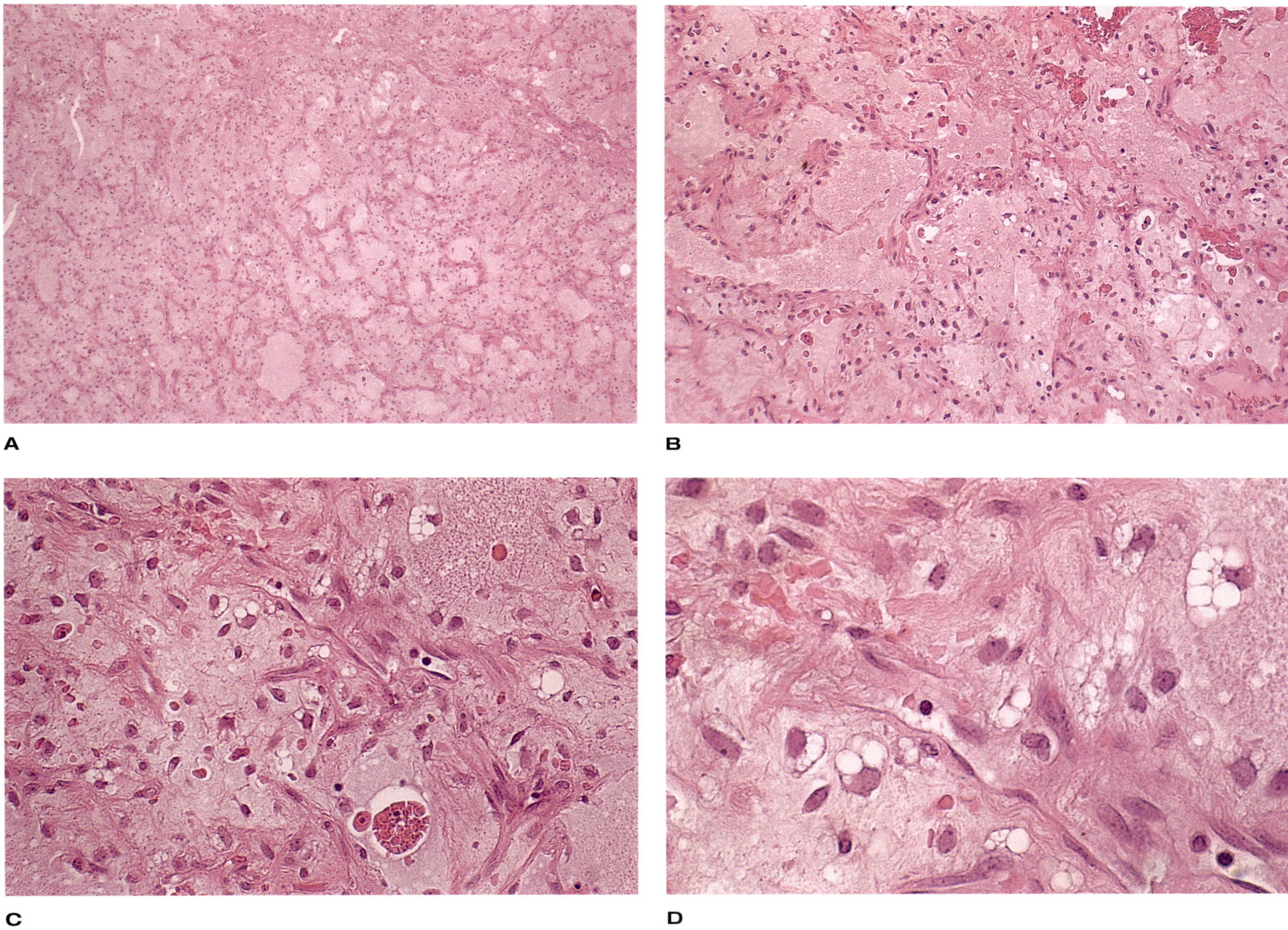

Figures 39–16A, 39–16B, 39–16C, 39–16D. **Liposarcoma, myxoid type.** Abundant mucin deposition, extensive blood vessel proliferation, and numerous characteristic multivacuolated lipoblasts.

40

Metastatic neoplasms

- Metastatic malignant melanoma
- Metastatic adenocarcinoma
- Metastatic renal-cell carcinoma
- Metastatic breast carcinoma

METASTATIC MALIGNANT MELANOMA

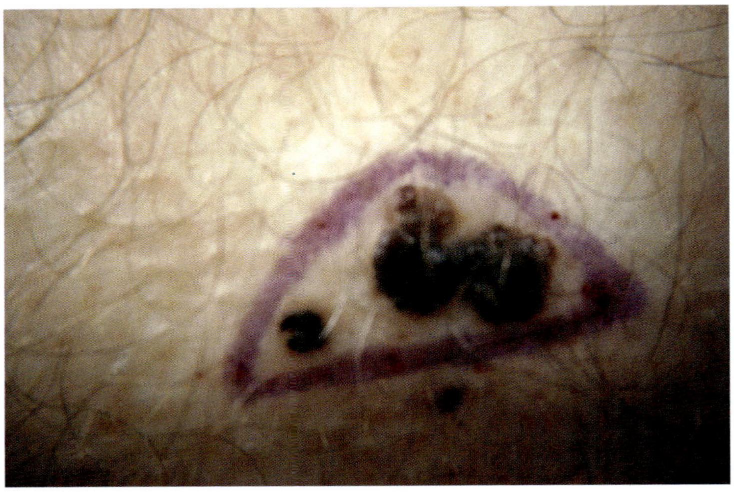

Figure 40–1. Primary and metastatic malignant melanoma. Darkly pigmented brown nodules (right) denote primary malignant melanoma. Smaller peripheral lesions are satellite metastases. The histology of these lesions is shown in Figures 40–2, 40–3A, and 40–3B.

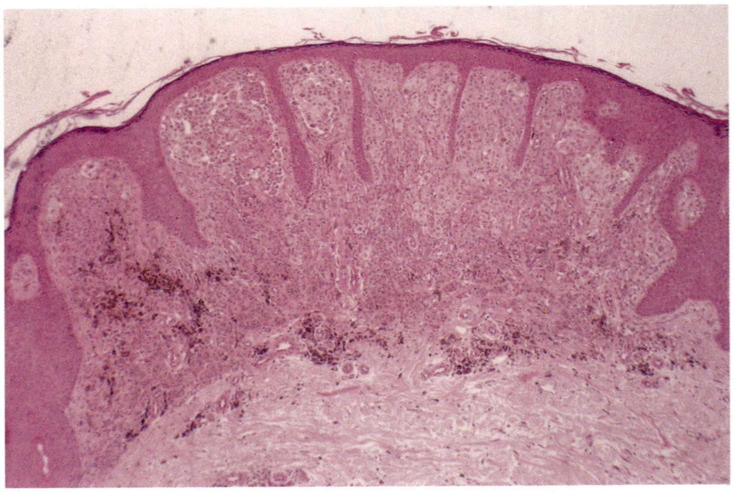

Figure 40–2. Primary malignant melanoma. Sheets of atypical melanocytes extend into the reticular dermis where melanophages are scattered in an asymmetrical distribution.

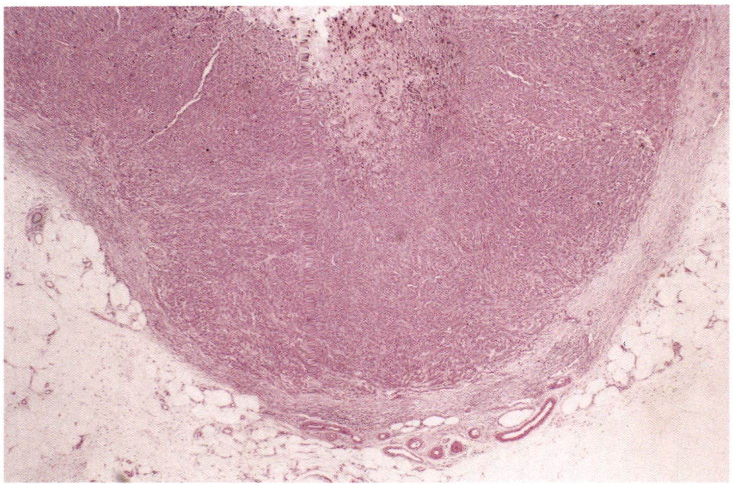

A

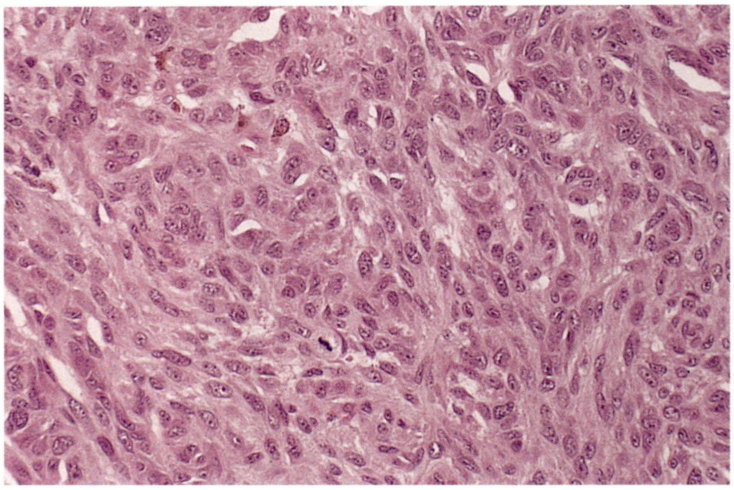

B

Figures 40–3A, 40–3B. Metastatic malignant melanoma. Circumscribed nodule of atypical melanocytes with central necrosis. There are sheets of atypical plump, oval melanocytes, melanin granules, and a mitotic figure.

METASTATIC MALIGNANT MELANOMA

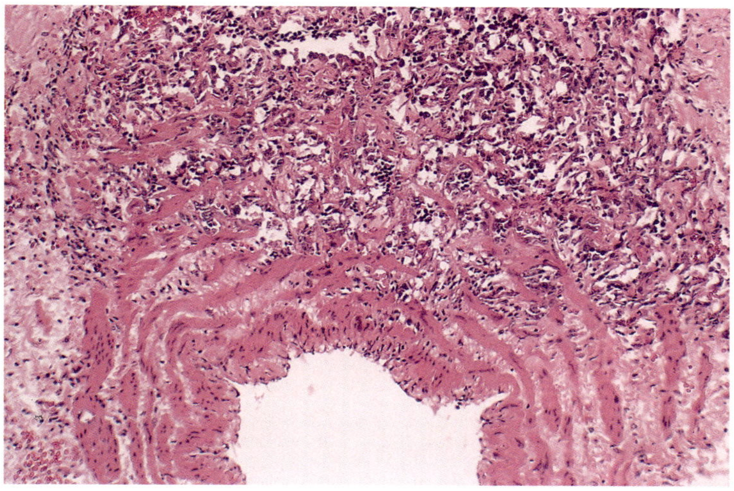

Figure 40–4. Metastatic malignant melanoma. Solitary and nested atypical melanocytes involve the muscular wall of a blood vessel.

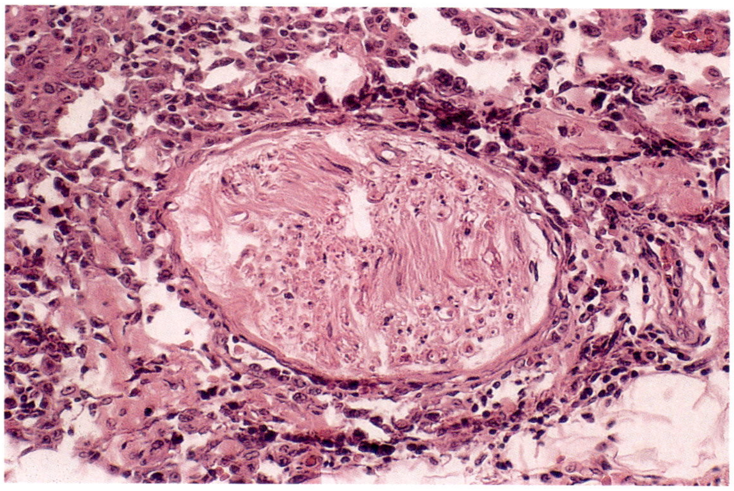

Figure 40–5. Metastatic malignant melanoma. Atypical melanocytes involve the perineural sheath of a large nerve bundle.

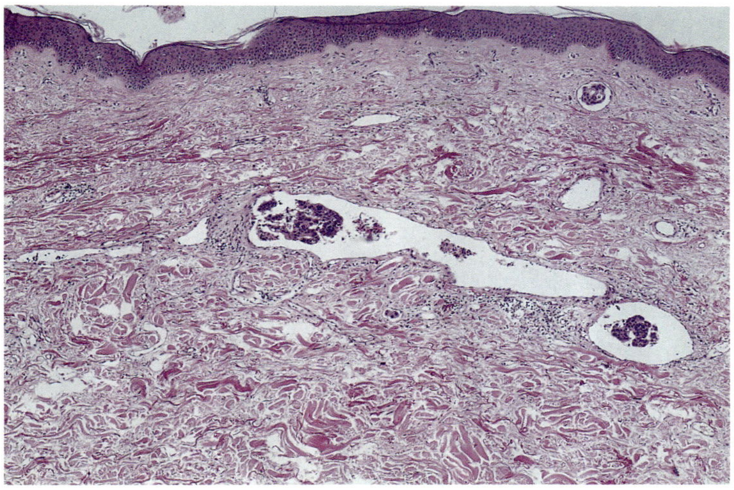

Figure 40–6. Metastatic malignant melanoma. Intralymphatic clusters of melanoma cells.

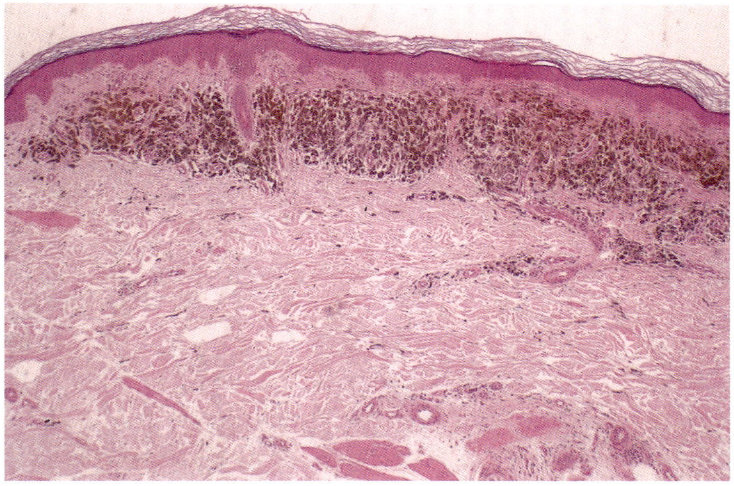

Figure 40–7. Metastatic malignant melanoma with complete regression, melanosis type. Dense bandlike infiltrate of melanophages fills the papillary dermis and involves the adventitial dermis around adnexal and vascular structures in the reticular dermis.

METASTATIC ADENOCARCINOMA

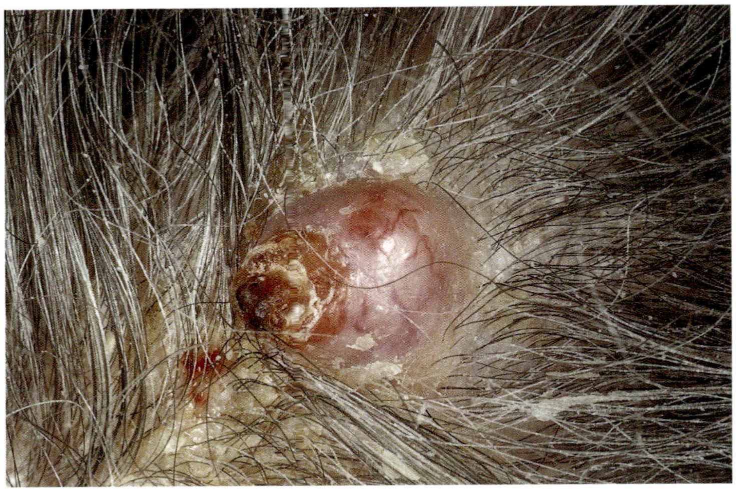

Figure 40–8. Metastatic adenocarcinoma. Protuberant dome-shaped, crusted, telangiectatic, skin-colored nodule on the scalp of an older woman.

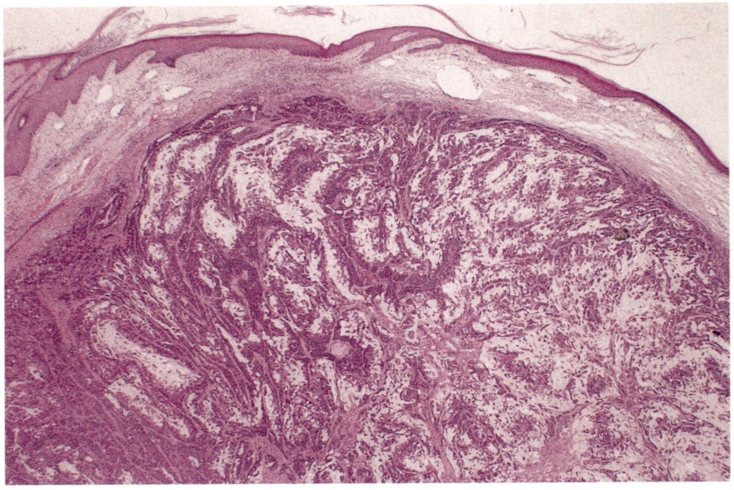

Figure 40–9. Metastatic adenocarcinoma. Sheets of tubular structures composed of eosinophilic, atypical polygonal epithelial cells separated by copious amounts of dermal mucin.

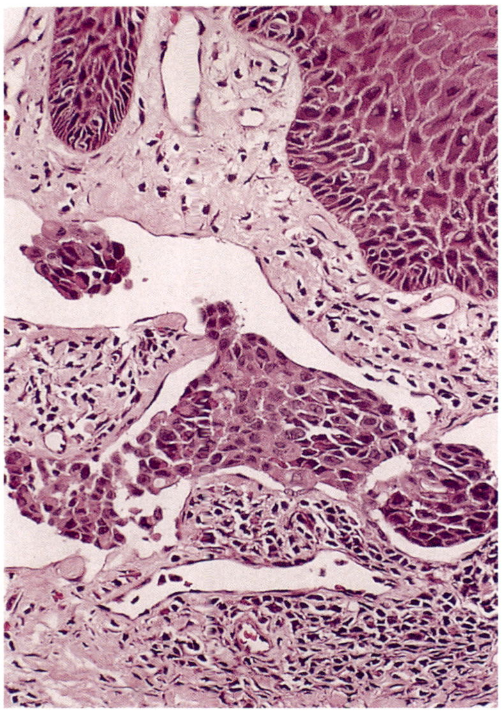

Figure 40–10. Metastatic adenocarcinoma. Atypical polygonal epithelial cells within widely dilated lymphatic channels beneath the epidermis.

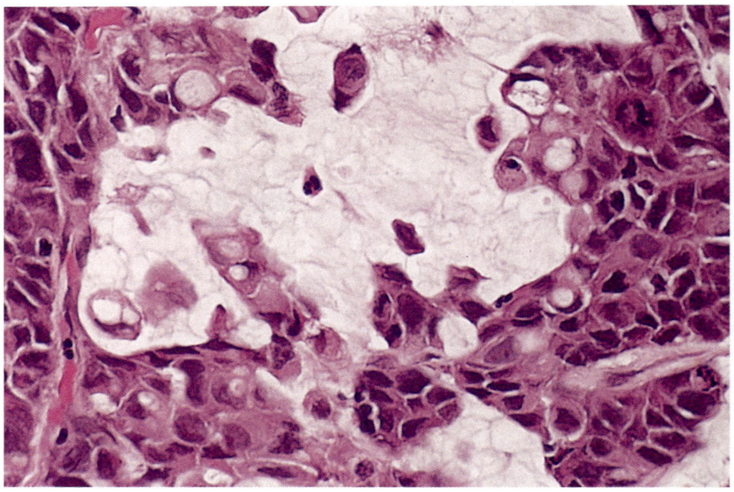

Figure 40–11. Metastatic adenocarcinoma. Pleomorphic, atypical neoplastic cells with hyperchromatic nuclei and eosinophilic cytoplasm. The cells lie within a sea of mucin. There are signet-ring cells, mitotic figures, and tumor cells with abundant cytoplasmic mucin.

METASTATIC RENAL-CELL CARCINOMA

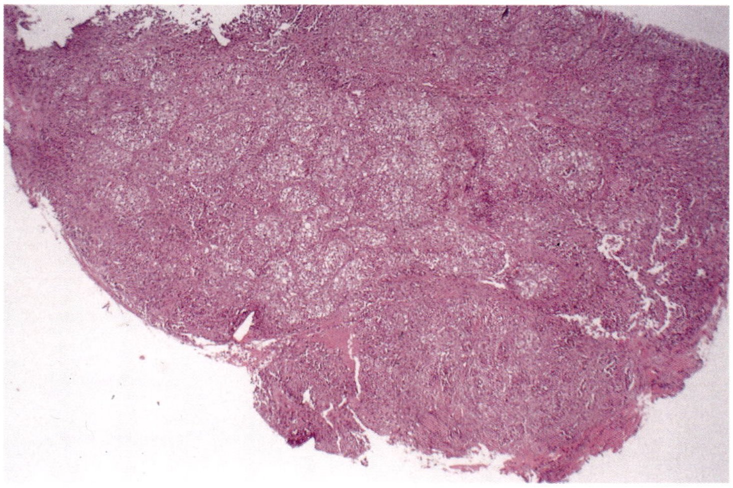

Figure 40–12. **Metastatic renal-cell carcinoma.** Lobular pattern of clear cells intermixed with an intertwining network of vascular channels.

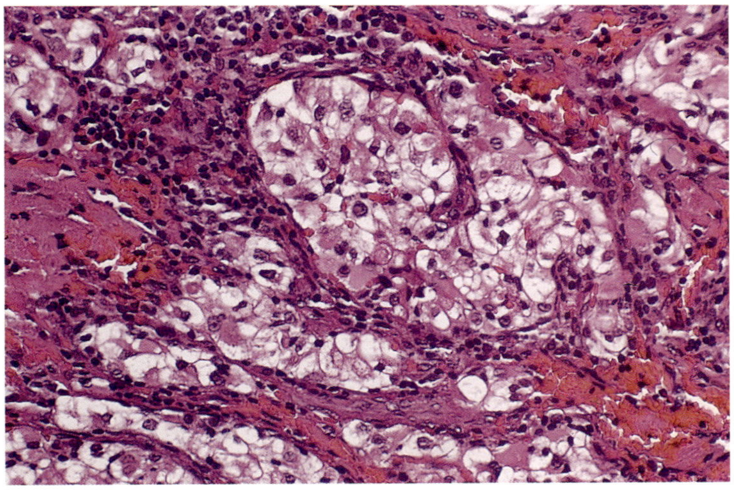

A

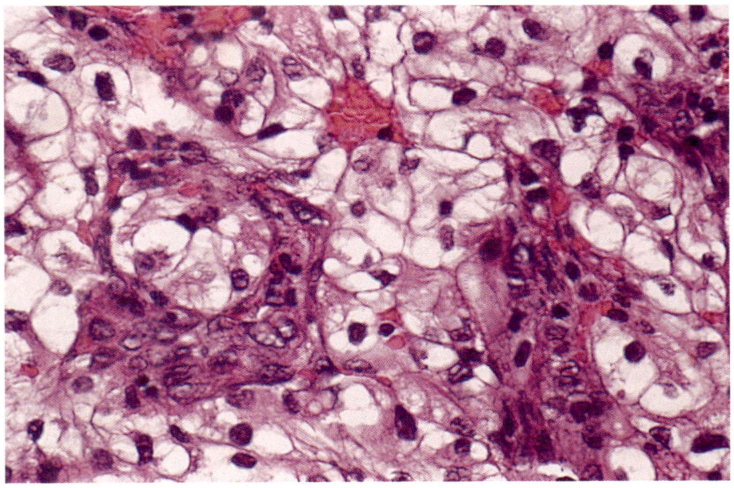

B

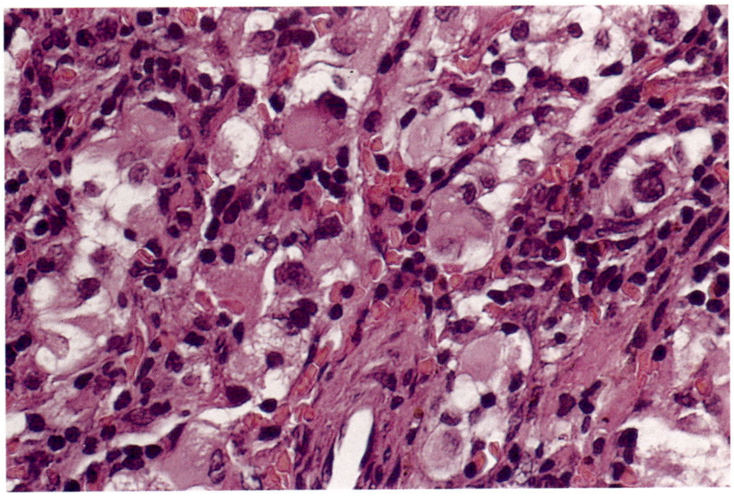

C

Figures 40–13A, 40–13B, 40–13C. **Metastatic renal-cell carcinoma.** Atypical and pleomorphic neoplastic cells with hyperchromatic nuclei and clear or eosinophilic cytoplasm. Polygonal epithelial cells are surrounded by dilated and congested blood vessels.

METASTATIC BREAST CARCINOMA

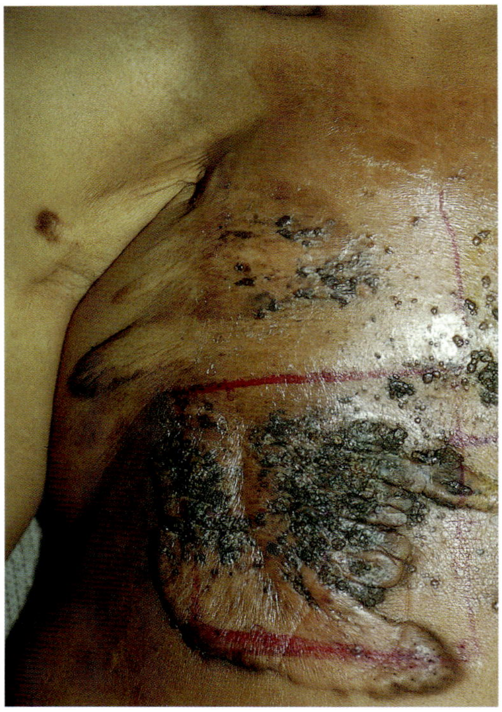

Figure 40–14. Metastatic breast carcinoma. Numerous solitary and confluent crusted papules and nodules on the chest of a woman previously treated for breast carcinoma.

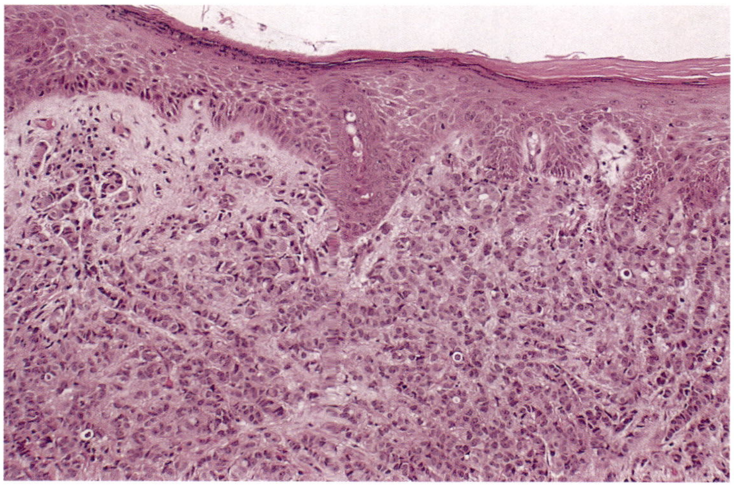

A

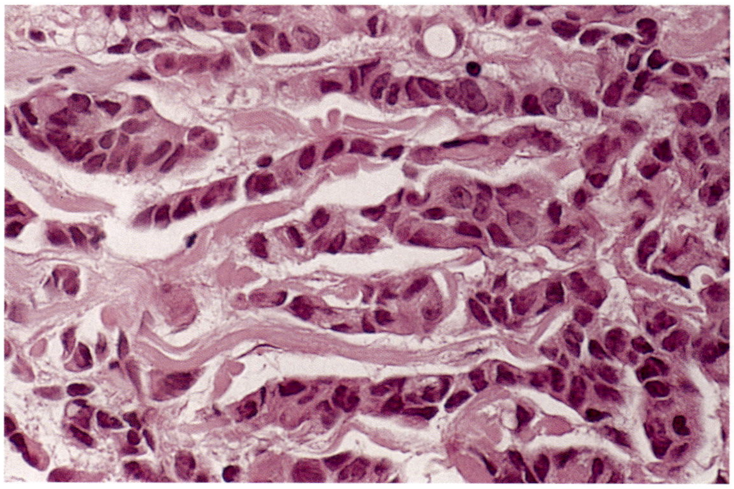

B

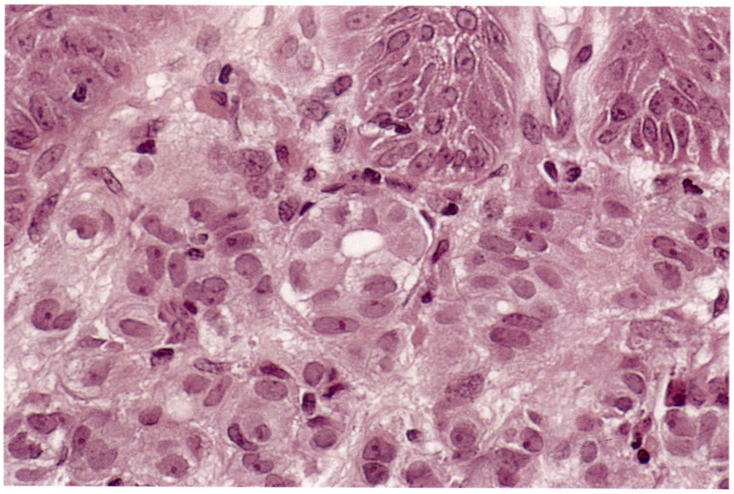

C

Figures 40–15A, 40–15B, 40–15C. Metastatic breast carcinoma. Atypical dermal neoplastic cells in strands, cords, and columns. Tubular forms are also seen among thickened collagen bundles. There are necrotic and mitotic epithelial cells.

41

LYMPHOMAS

- Lymphomatoid papulosis
- Mycosis fungoides
- Cutaneous Hodgkin's disease
- Extramedullary hematopoiesis
- B-cell lymphoma
- Angiotrophic T-cell lymphoma
- Leukemia cutis

LYMPHOMATOID PAPULOSIS

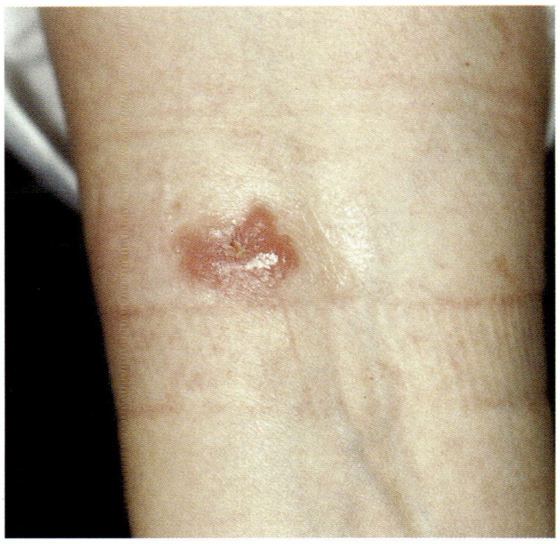

A

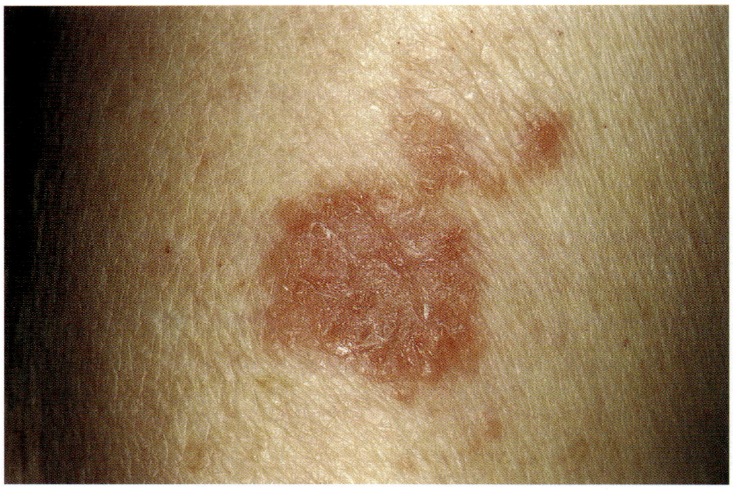

B

Figures 41–1A, 41–1B. Lymphomatoid papulosis. Evolving (left) and regressing (right) lesions on the arm of an elderly woman.

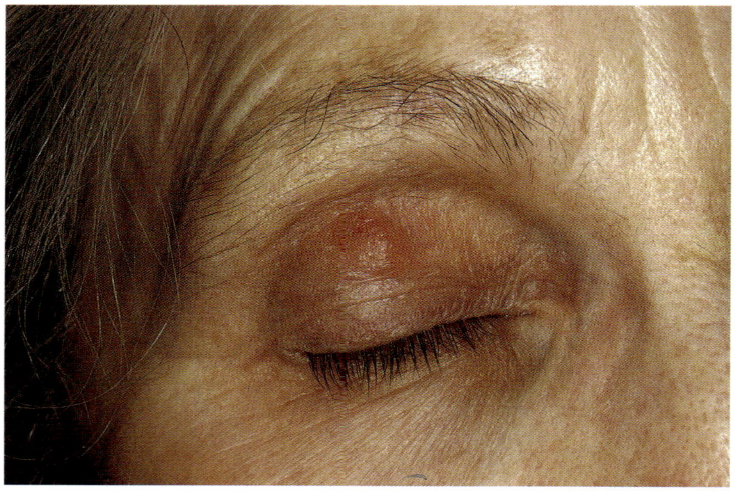

Figure 41–2. Lymphomatoid papulosis. Erythematous nodule on the upper eyelid.

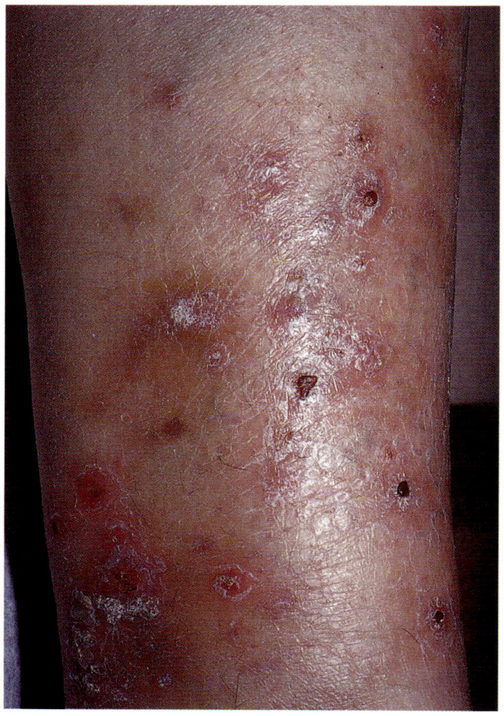

Figure 41–3. Lymphomatoid papulosis. Crusted erythematous papules on the leg.

LYMPHOMATOID PAPULOSIS

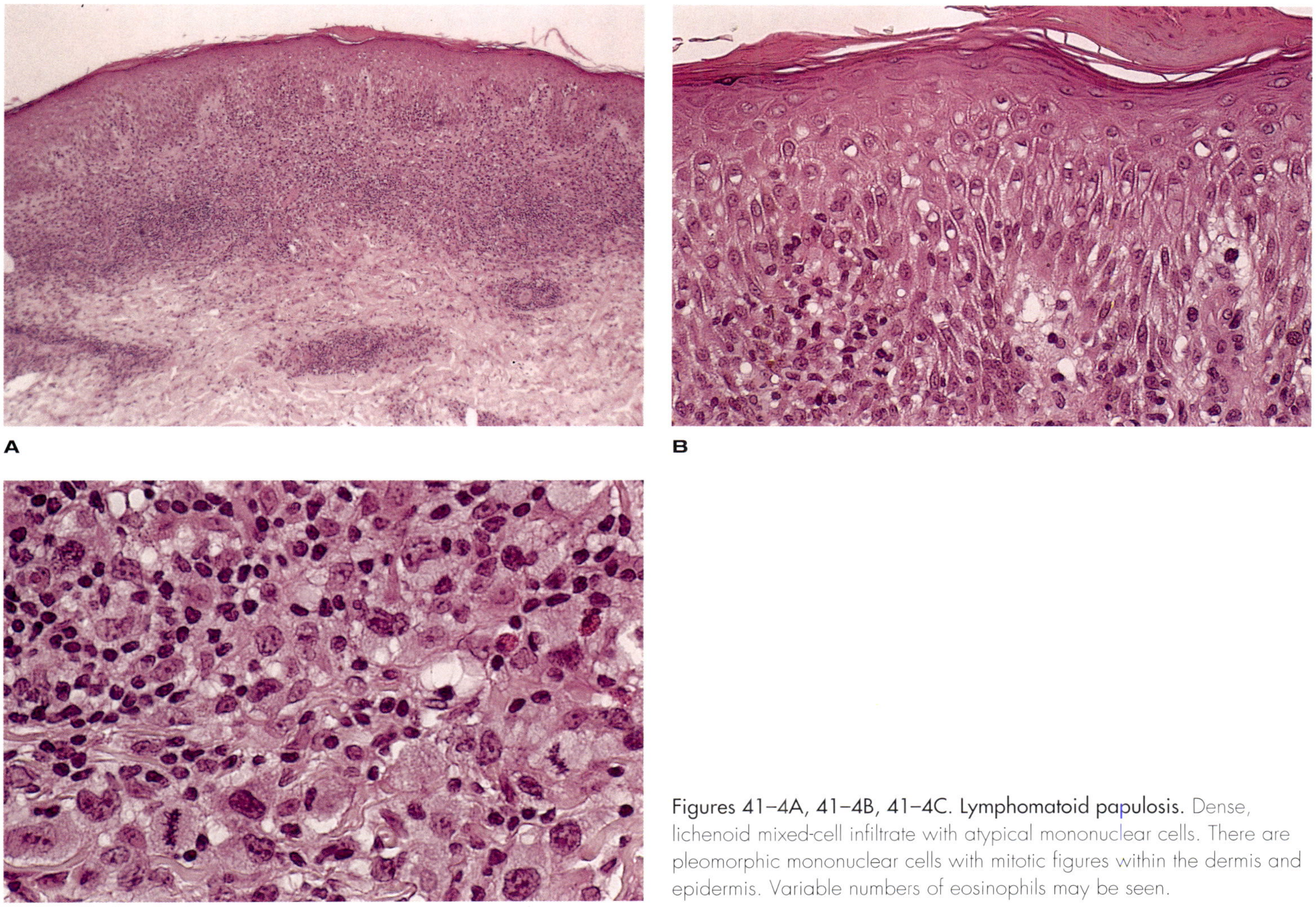

A B C

Figures 41–4A, 41–4B, 41–4C. **Lymphomatoid papulosis.** Dense, lichenoid mixed-cell infiltrate with atypical mononuclear cells. There are pleomorphic mononuclear cells with mitotic figures within the dermis and epidermis. Variable numbers of eosinophils may be seen.

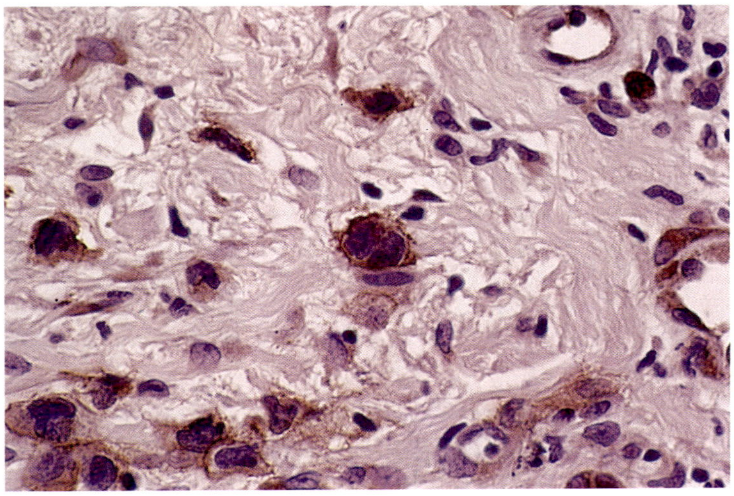

Figure 41–5. **Lymphomatoid papulosis.** CD 30 (Ki-1) antibody stains the atypical mononuclear cells brown.

MYCOSIS FUNGOIDES

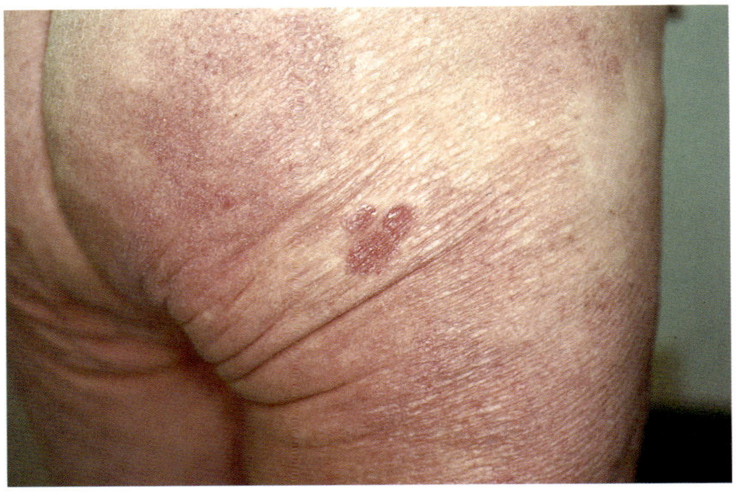

Figure 41–6. Mycosis fungoides. Pruritic scaly erythematous patches and an irregular plaque on the buttocks of a woman.

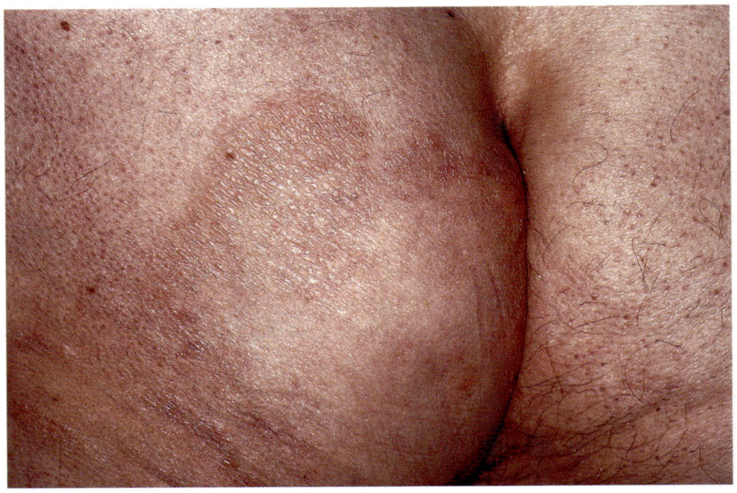

Figure 41–7. Mycosis fungoides. Annular, scaly, erythematous patches on the hip and buttocks.

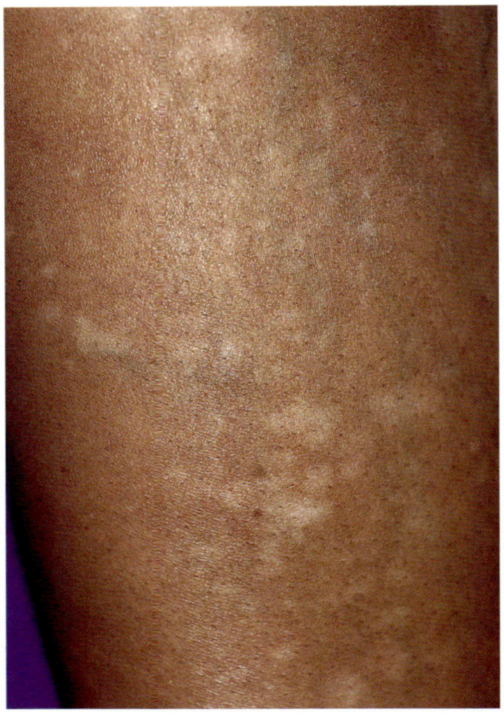

Figure 41–8. Mycosis fungoides. Hypopigmented macules and patches on the thigh.

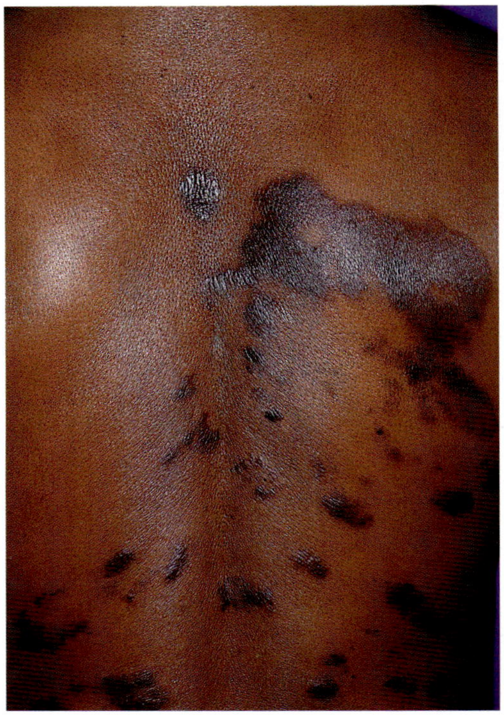

Figure 41–9. Mycosis fungoides. Widespread hyperpigmented patches and plaques on the back of a man.

MYCOSIS FUNGOIDES

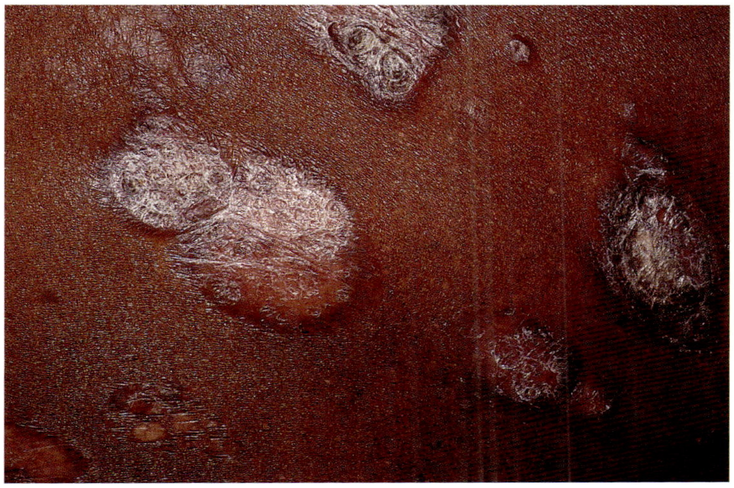

Figure 41–10. **Mycosis fungoides.** Numerous keratotic papules and nodules on the back of a woman with mycosis fungoides for many years.

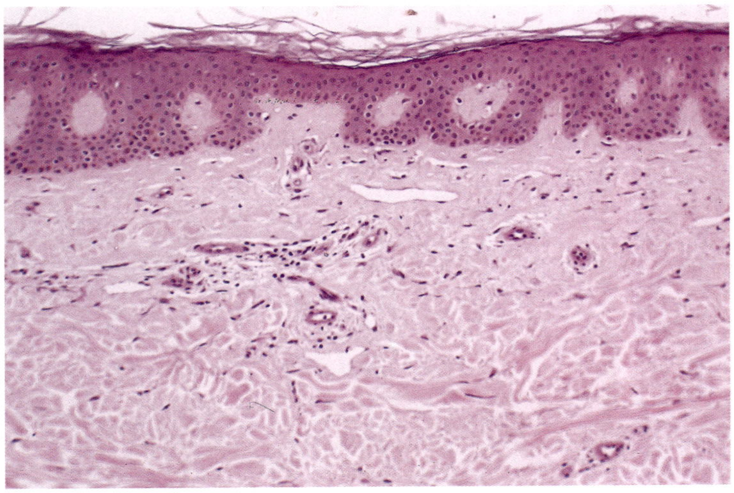

A

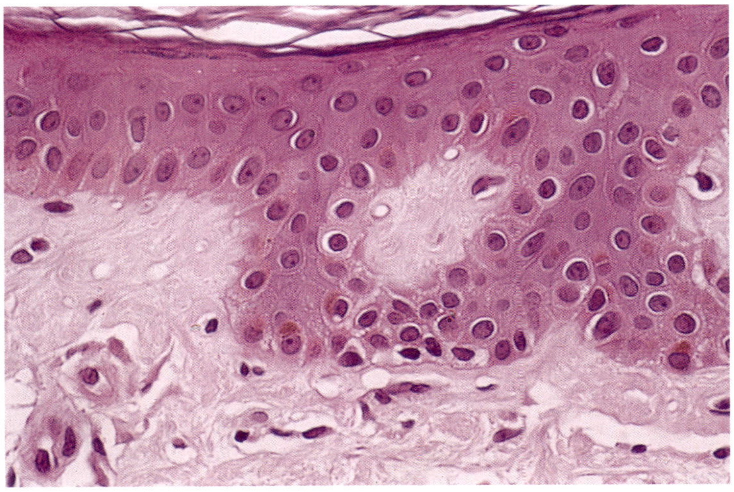

B

Figures 41–11A, 41–11B. **Mycosis fungoides.** Very early changes of mycosis fungoides. There are an increased number of solitary lymphocytes aligned in the basal cell layer. There is very mild fibroplasia of the papillary dermis.

MYCOSIS FUNGOIDES

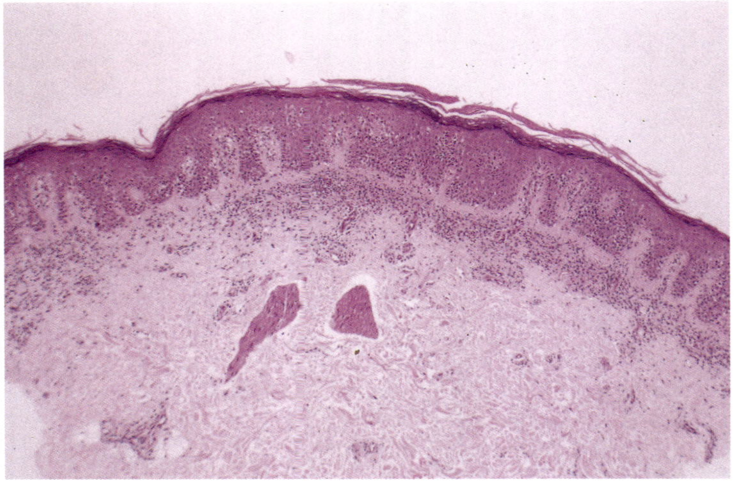

Figure 41–12. Mycosis fungoides. Psoriasiform lichenoid dermatitis. One of the patterns of plaque-stage mycosis fungoides.

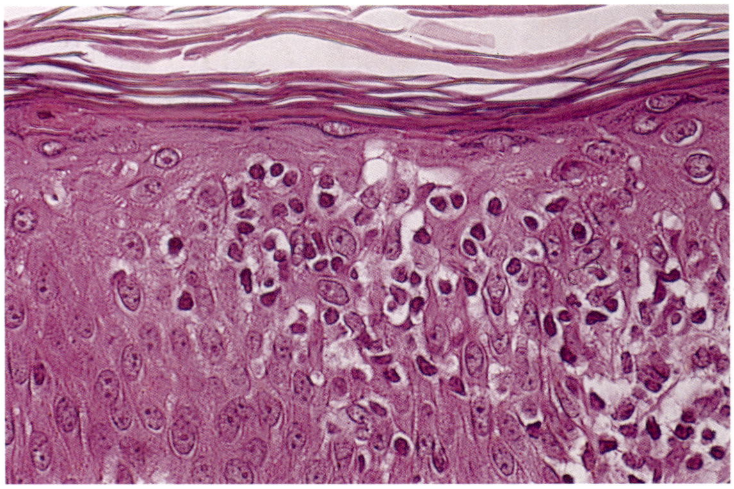

Figure 41–13. Mycosis fungoides. Increased numbers of solitary lymphocytes at all levels of the epidermis with minimal spongiosis.

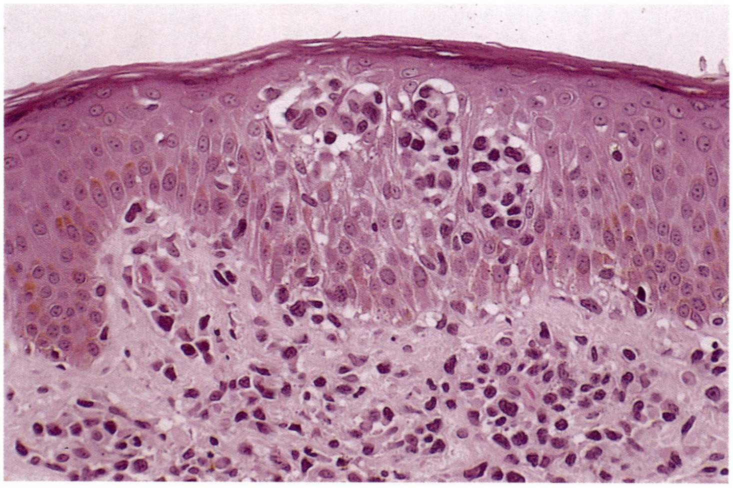

Figure 41–14. Mycosis fungoides. Collections of atypical mononuclear cells (Pautrier's microabscess) within the epidermis. Similarly atypical mononuclear cells are present in the papillary dermis.

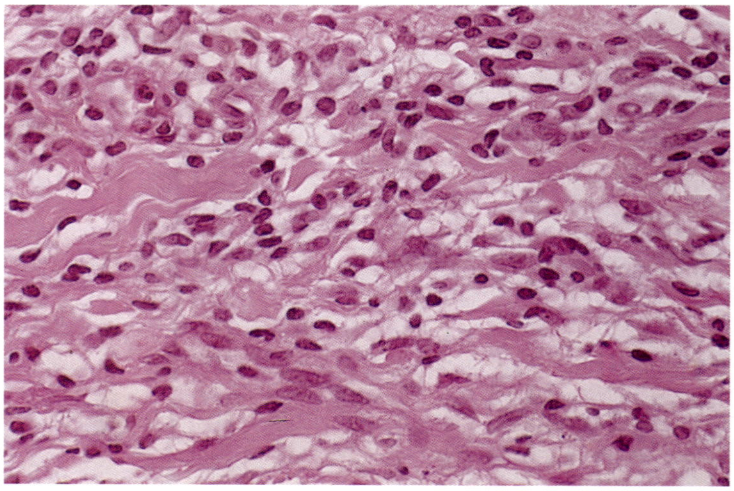

Figure 41–15. Mycosis fungoides. Coarse collagen bundles in disarray, intermixed with mononuclear cells in a thickened papillary dermis. This is a characteristic finding in mycosis fungoides.

MYCOSIS FUNGOIDES

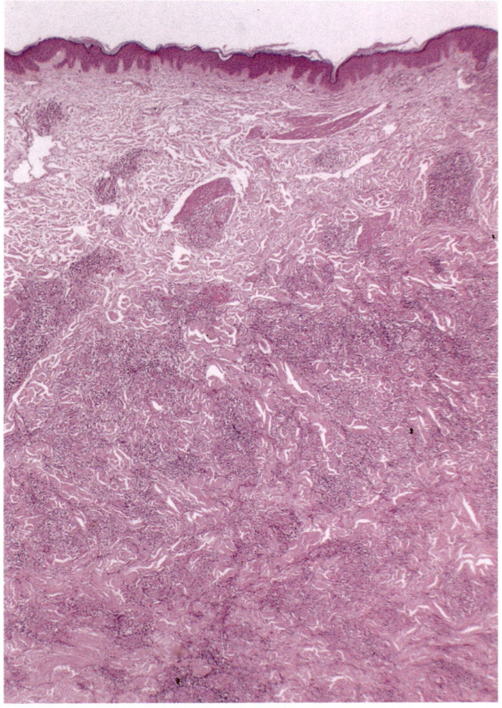

A

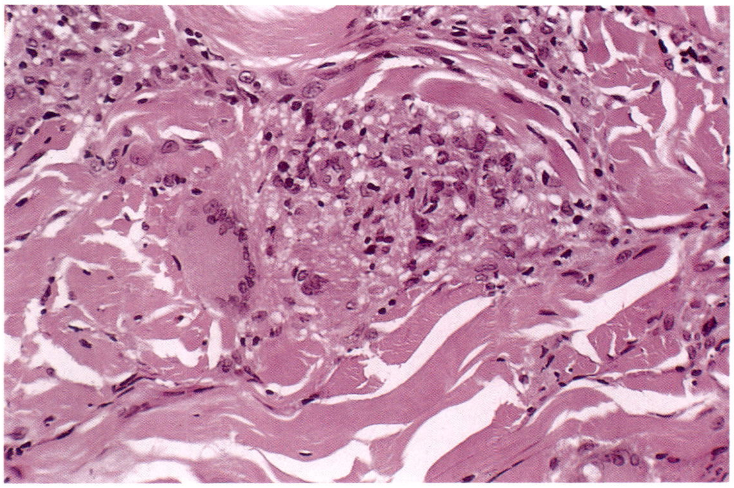

B

Figures 41–16A, 41–16B. **Mycosis fungoides.** Granulomatous dermal infiltrate with multinucleated histiocytic giant cells and atypical mononuclear cells.

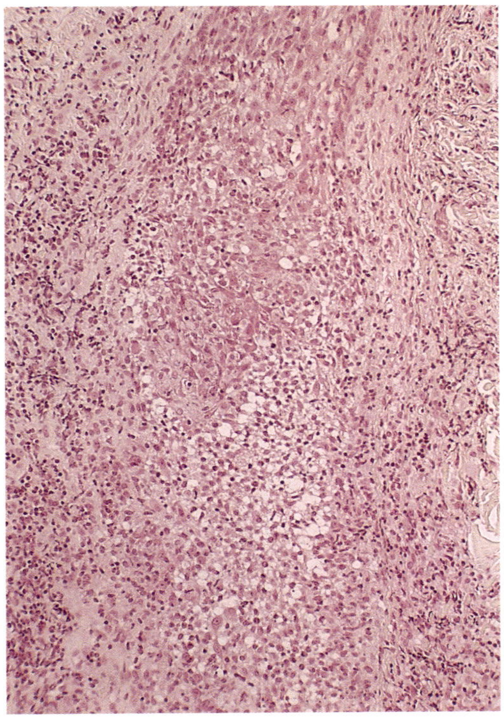

A

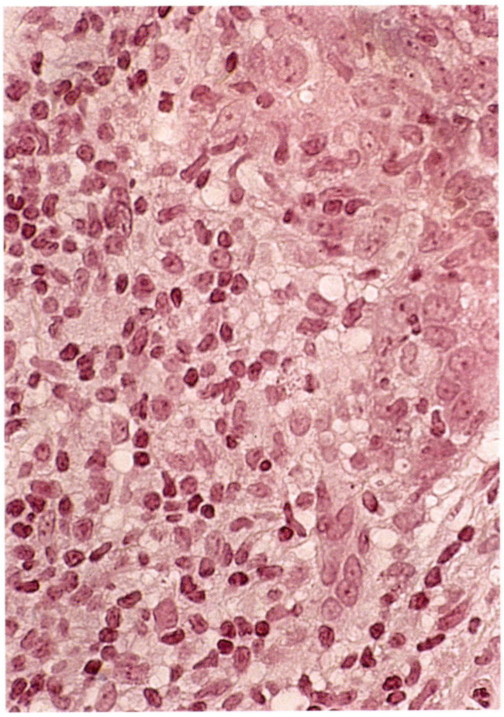

B

Figures 41–17A, 41–17B. **Mycosis fungoides.** Atypical mononuclear cells and epithelial mucin (follicular mucinosis) fill a distorted infundibulum.

CUTANEOUS HODGKIN'S DISEASE

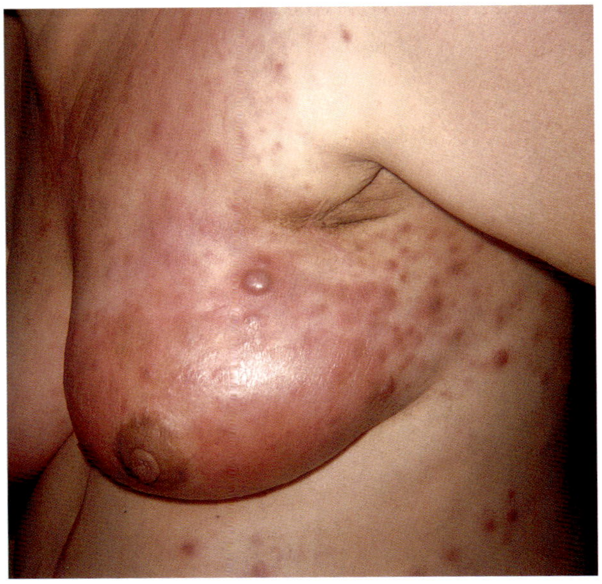

Figure 41–18. Cutaneous Hodgkin's disease. Erythematous plaques and nodules on the breast of a woman with Hodgkin's disease.

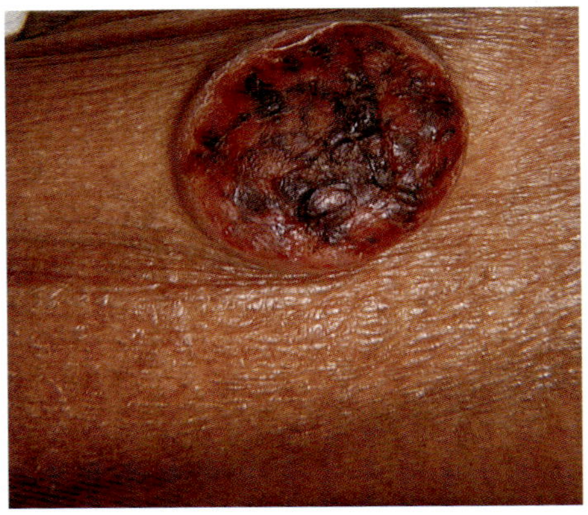

Figure 41–19. Cutaneous Hodgkin's disease. Crusted nodule on the arm of a woman with Hodgkin's disease.

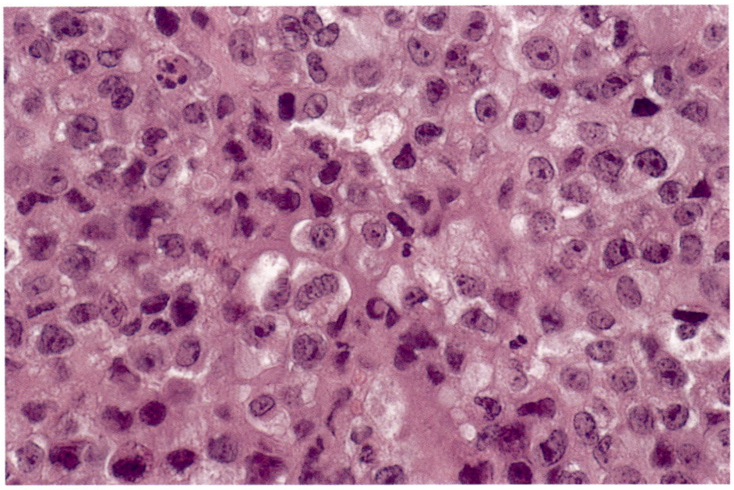

Figure 41–20. Cutaneous Hodgkin's disease. Sheets of large, atypical, pleomorphic mononuclear and bilobed cells with vesicular nuclei with prominent nucleoli.

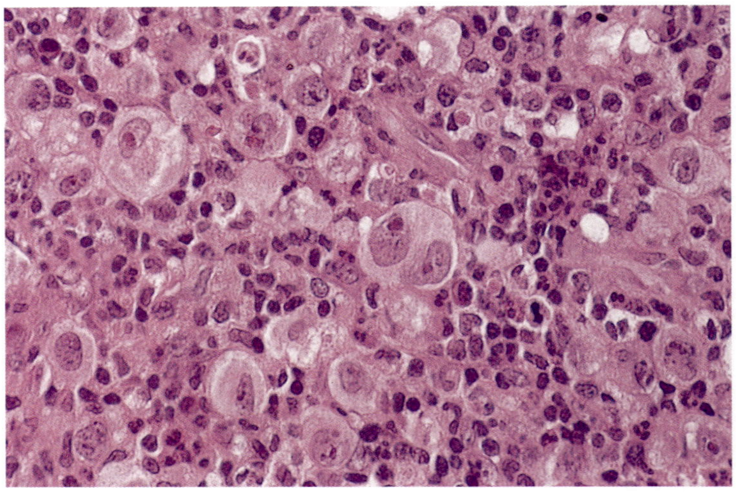

Figure 41–21. Cutaneous Hodgkin's disease. Lymph node from woman with cutaneous Hodgkin's disease seen in Figure 41–18, with characteristic Reed–Sternberg cells.

EXTRAMEDULLARY HEMATOPOIESIS

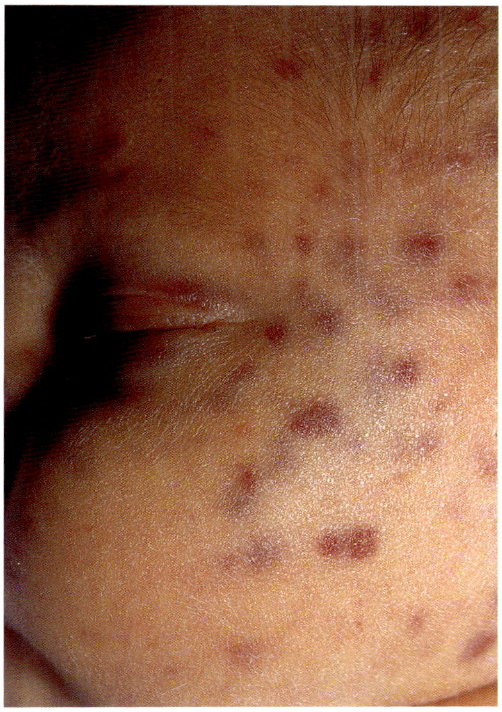

Figure 41–22. Extramedullary hematopoiesis. Bluish-red macules and papules on the face and scalp of an infant.

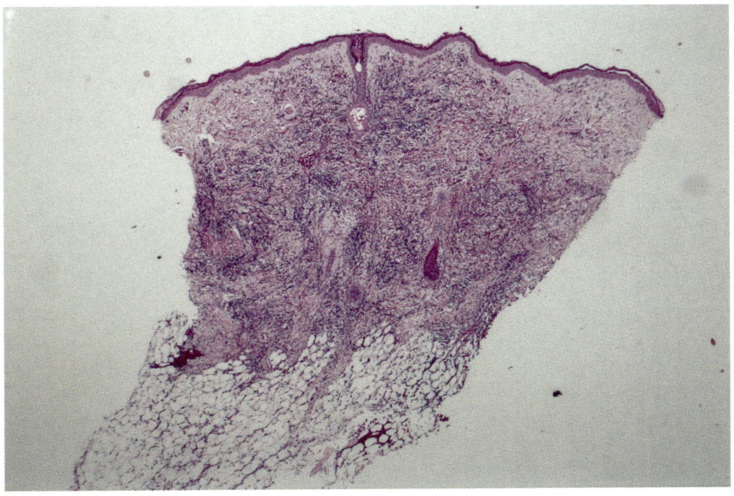

A

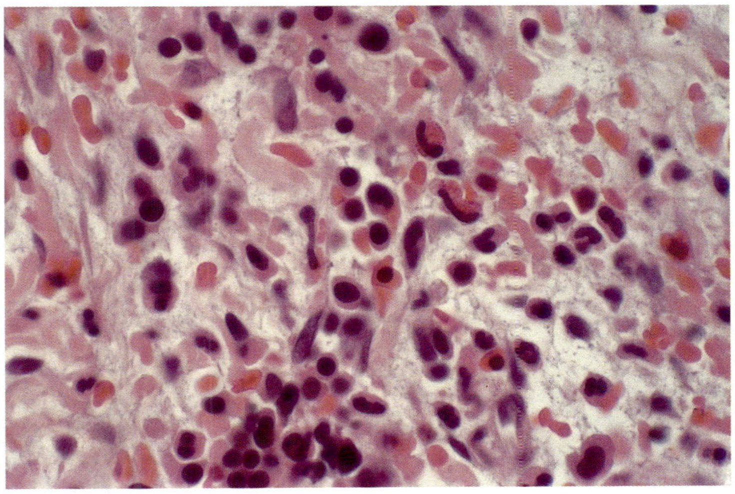

B

Figures 41–23A, 41–23B. Extramedullary hematopoiesis. Diffuse bone marrow-like infiltrate in the dermis and subcutaneous fat. There are mature and immature erythrocytes, with nucleated red blood cells.

B-CELL LYMPHOMA

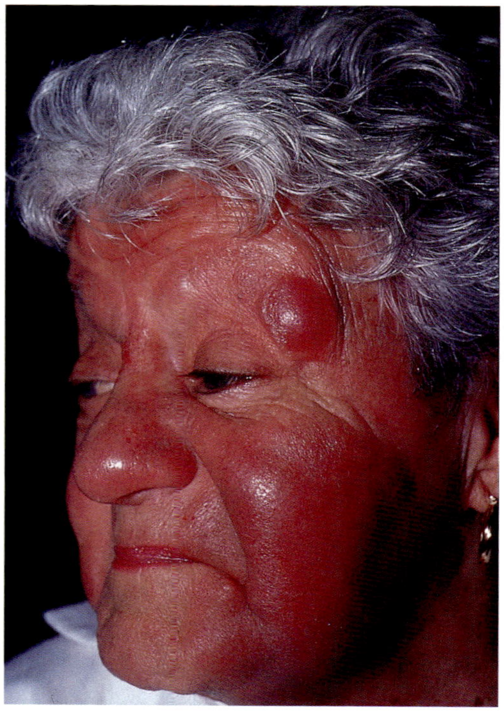

Figure 41–24. B-cell lymphoma. Large, erythematous, smooth nocules on the face.

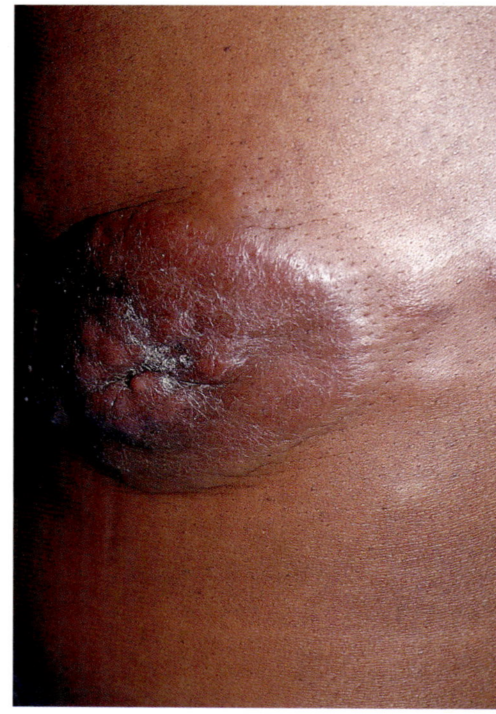

Figure 41–25. B-cell lymphoma. Multinodular crusted plaque.

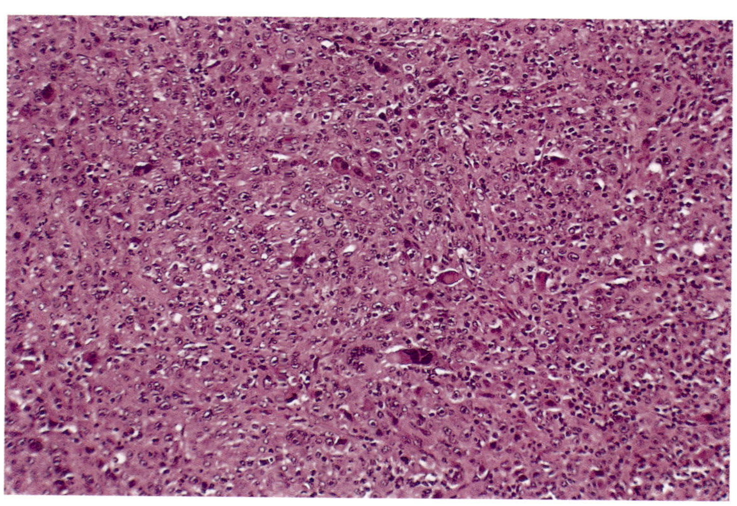

A

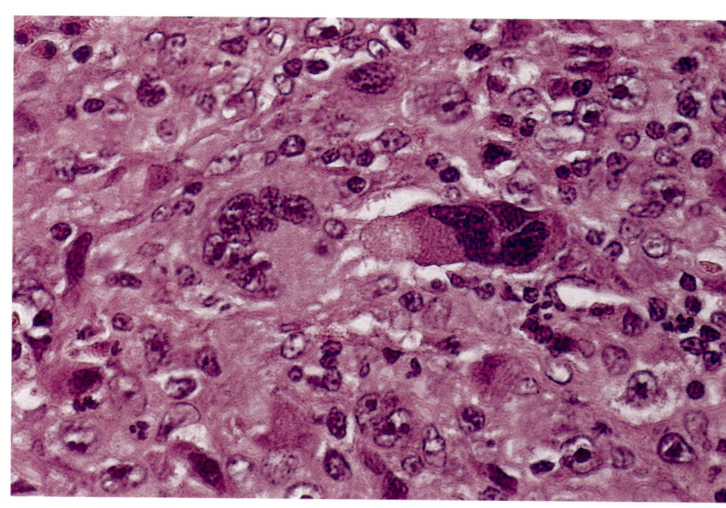

B

Figures 41–26A, 41–26B. 3-cell lymphoma. Sheets of atypical and pleomorphic mononuclear and multinucleated giant cells with hyperchromatic and bizarre-shaped nuclei. There are mitotic figures and necrotic cells.

ANGIOTROPHIC T-CELL LYMPHOMA

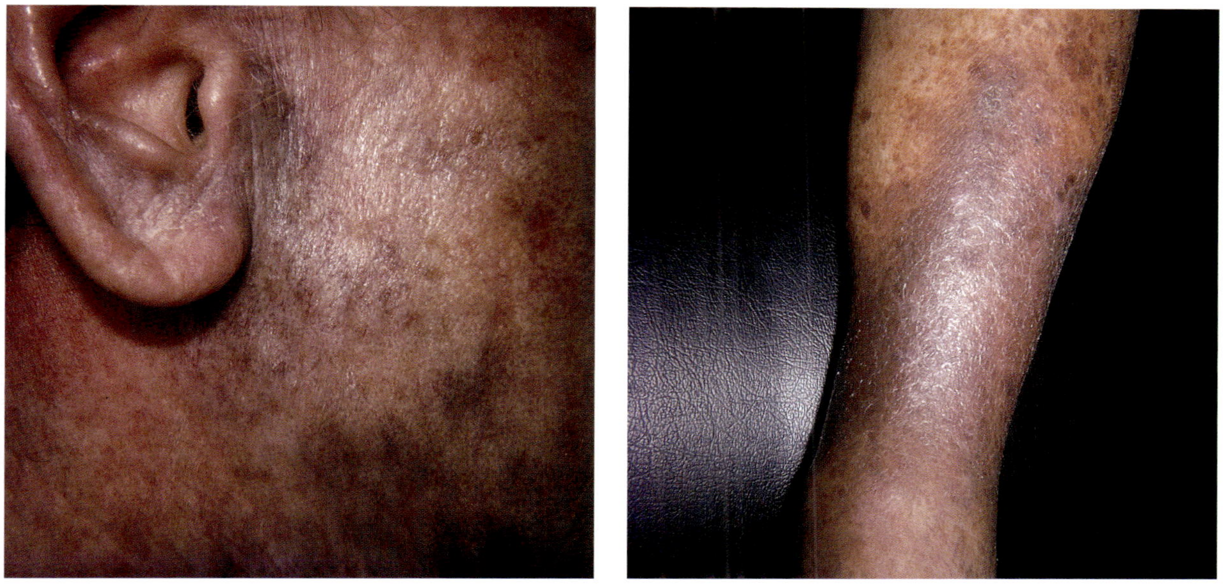

A B

Figures 41–27A, 41–27B. Angiotrophic T-cell lymphoma. Gray patches and plaques on the preauricular cheek (left) and lower leg (right) of a man.

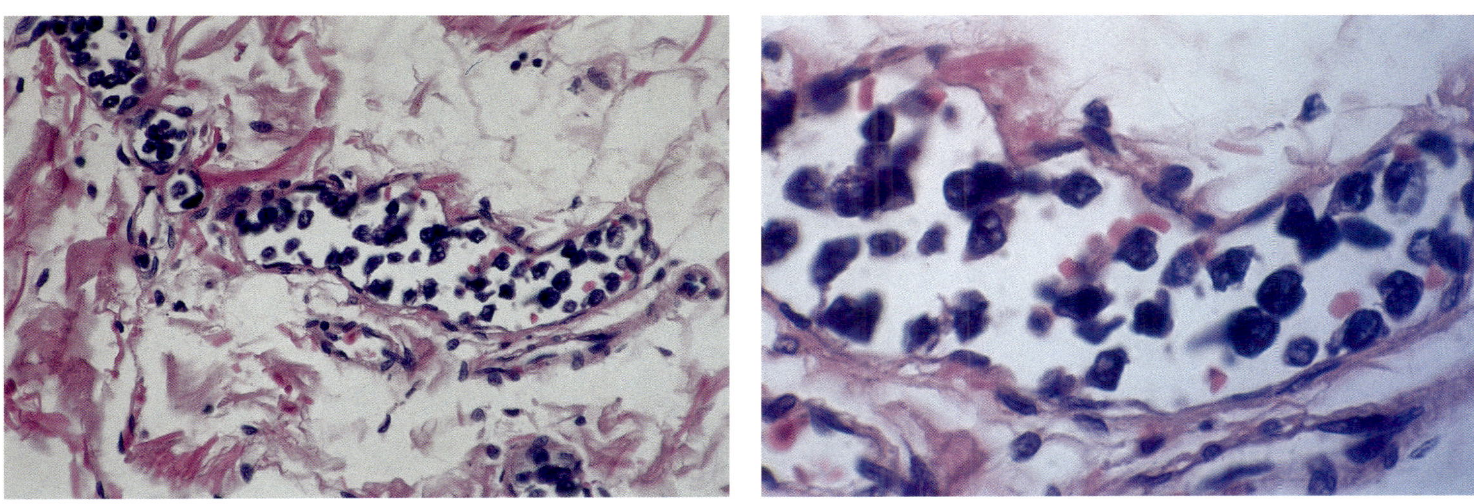

A B

Figures 41–28A, 41–28B. Angiotrophic T-cell lymphoma. Intravascular atypical mononuclear cells.

LEUKEMIA CUTIS

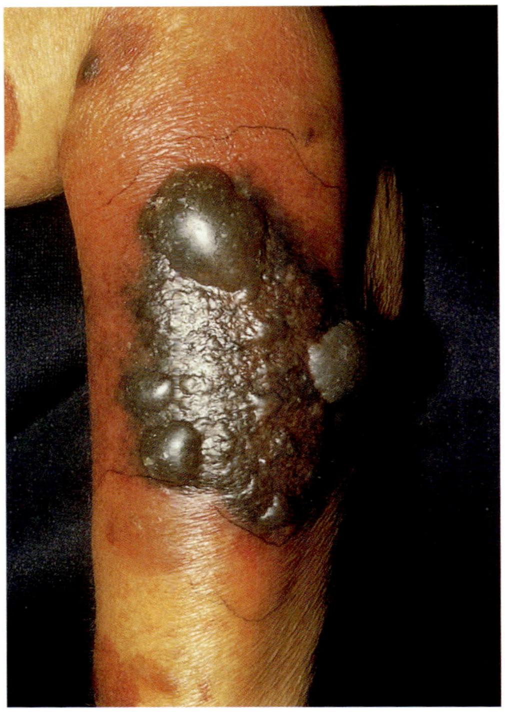

Figure 41–29. Leukemia cutis. Dark-gray bullae on top of an erythematous plaque on the arm.

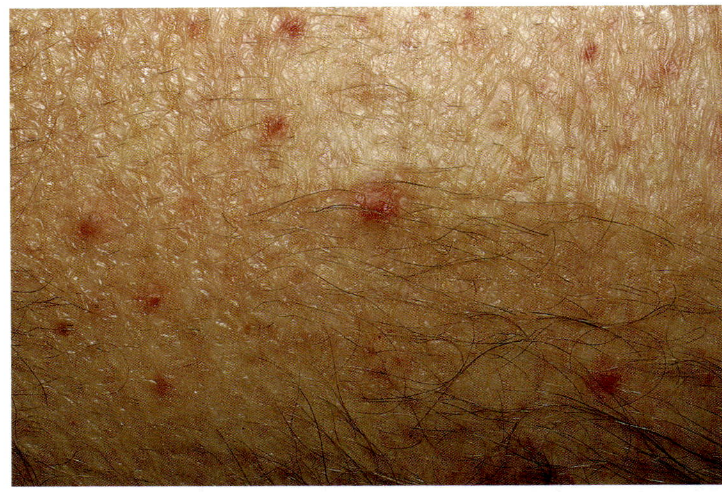

Figure 41–30. Leukemia cutis. Erythematous papules.

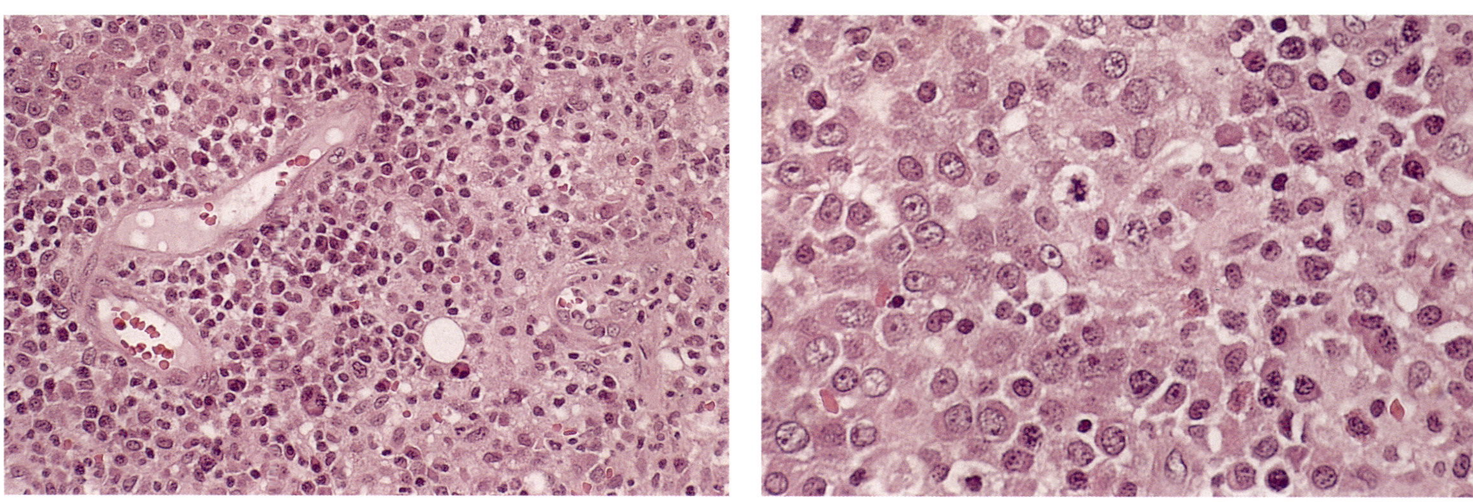

A B

Figures 41–31A, 41–31B. Leukemia cutis. Sheets of atypical cells with frequent mitotic figures in a patient with myelocytic leukemia.

42

Cysts

- Follicular cyst, infundibular (epidermoid)
- Eruptive vellus hair cyst
- Follicular cyst, isthmic (pilar, tricholemmal)
- Dermoid cyst
- Hybrid cyst
- Median raphe cyst
- Bronchogenic cyst
- Branchial cleft cyst
- Thyroglossal duct cyst
- Ciliated cyst

FOLLICULAR CYST, INFUNDIBULAR (EPIDERMOID)

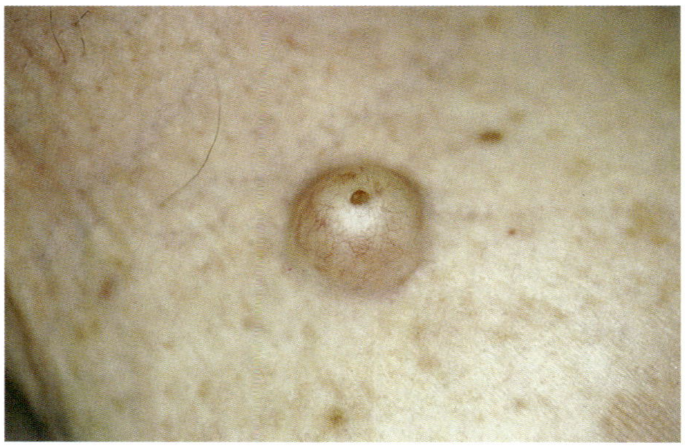

Figure 42–1. Follicular cyst, infundibular. Dome-shaped, skin-colored nodule with central dilated, keratotic infundibular plug.

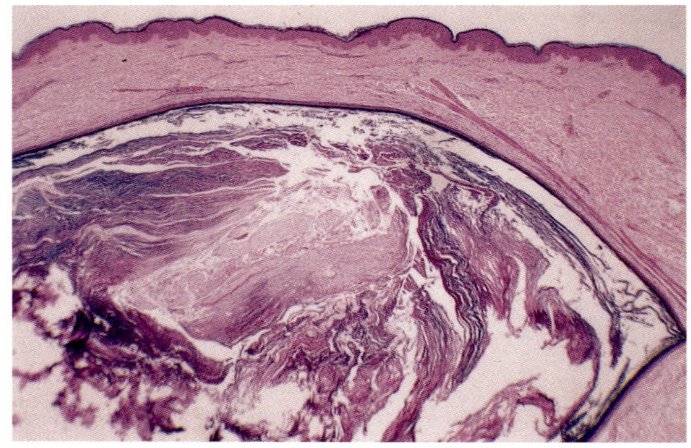

Figure 42–2. Follicular cyst, infundibular. Distended infundibulum with keratinous debris.

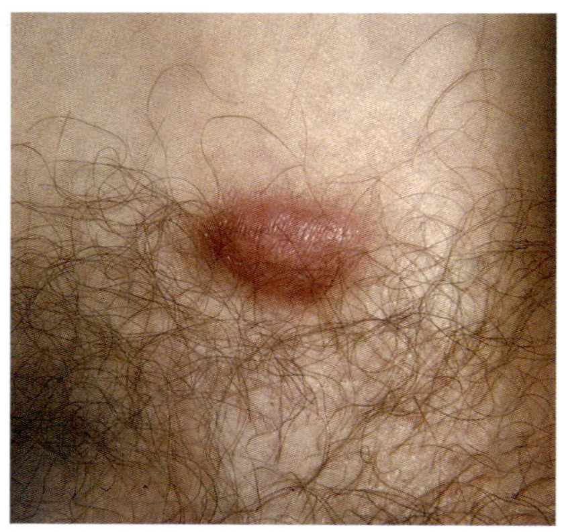

Figure 42–3. Follicular cyst, infundibular, ruptured. Erythematous, tender nodule on the chest of a man.

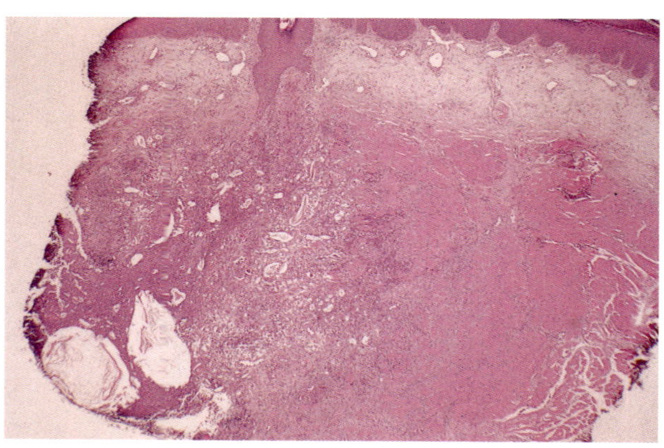

A

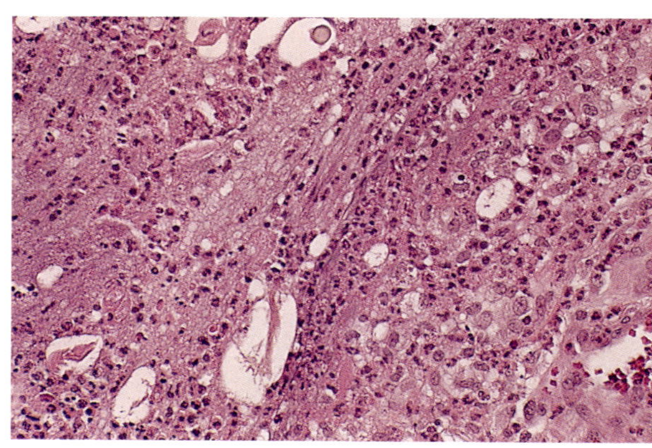

B

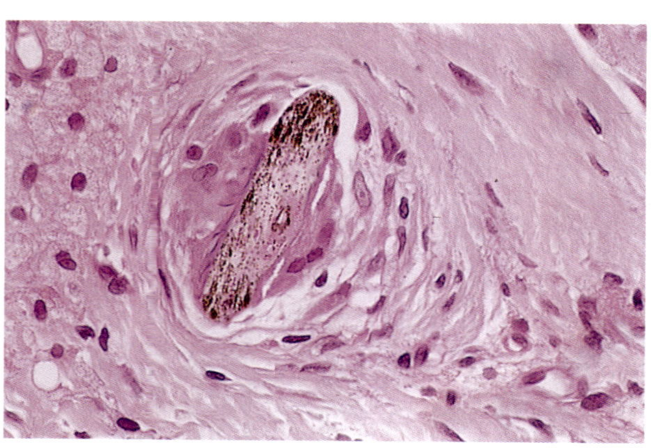

C

Figures 42–4A, 42–4B, 42–4C. Follicular cyst, infundibular, ruptured. Suppurative-granulomatous dermal infiltrate. There are squames (parakeratotic cells) lying free within the dermis and within multinucleated histiocytic giant cells, remnants of the infundibular wall, and engulfed hair-shaft fragments.

ERUPTIVE VELLUS HAIR CYST

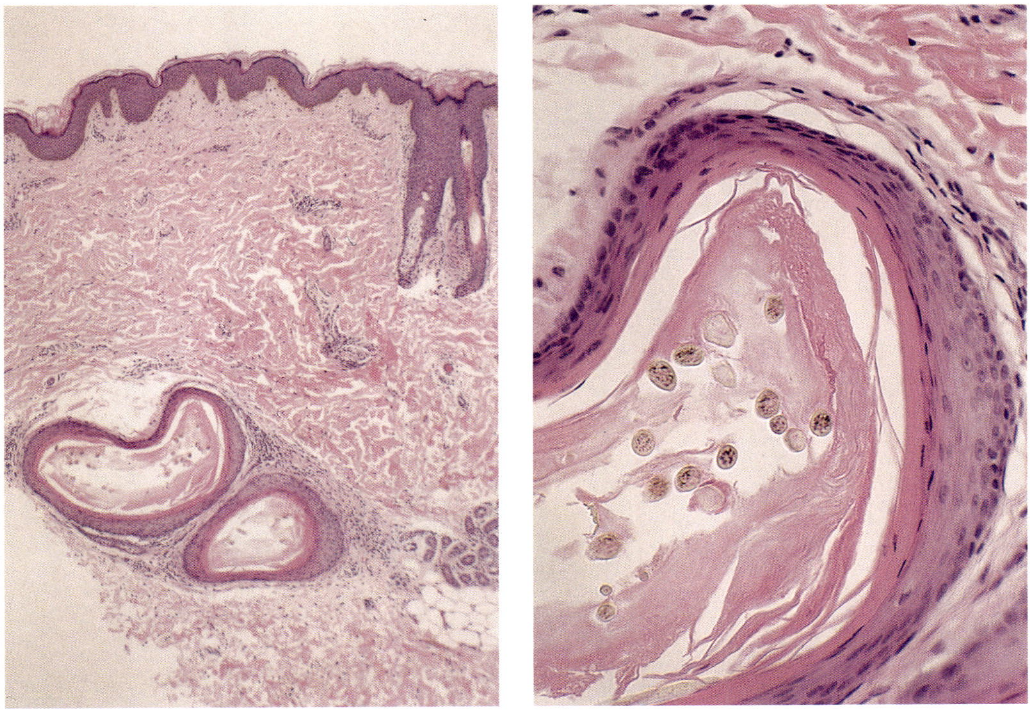

A B

Figures 42–5A, 42–5B. Eruptive vellus hair cyst. Epithelial-lined cystic structures contain numerous vellus hair shafts.

FOLLICULAR CYST, ISTHMIC (PILAR, TRICHOLEMMAL)

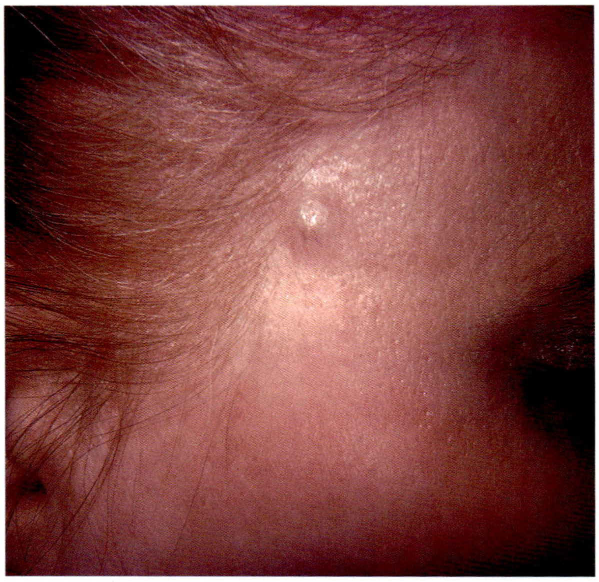

Figure 42–6. Follicular cyst, isthmic. Firm, skin-colored nodule on the temple of a young girl.

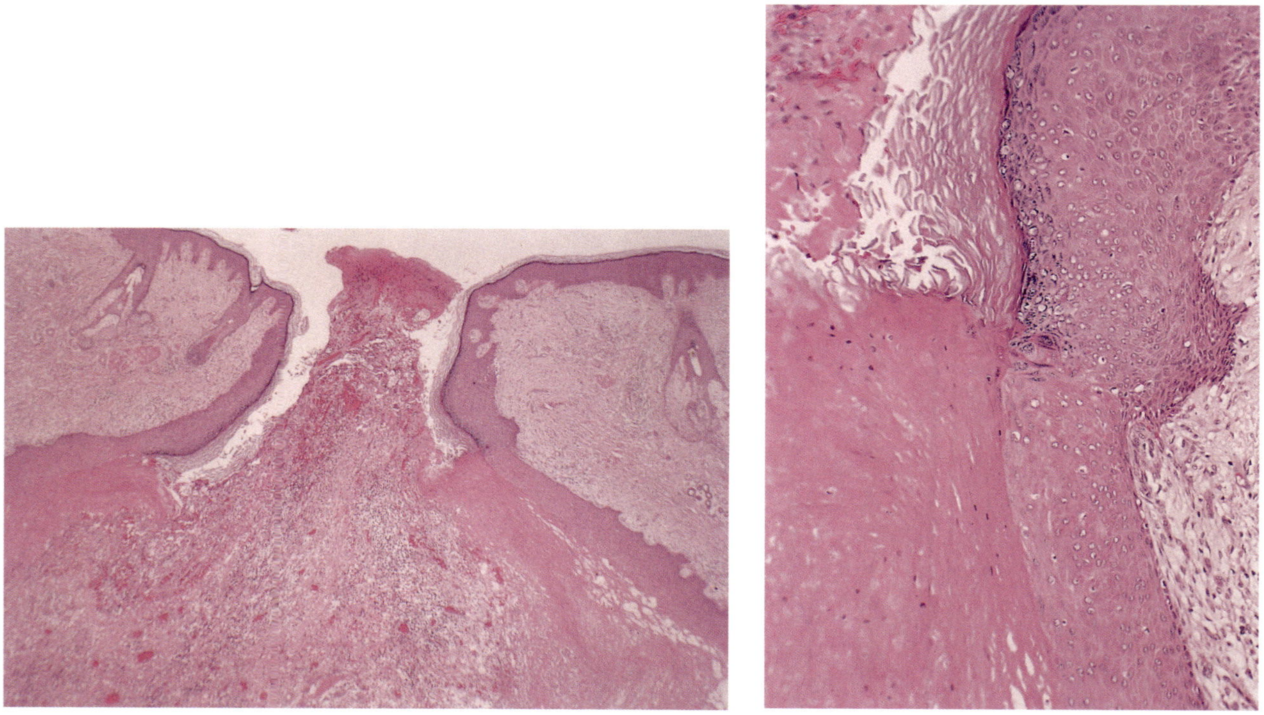

A B

Figures 42–7A, 42–7B. Follicular cyst, isthmic. Eosinophilic, keratinous debris within a distended folliculosebaceous unit. This photomicrograph shows two types of epithelium and two types of keratinization. The infundibulum shows basket-weave hyperkeratosis and a granular layer; the isthmus shows compact hyperkeratosis without a granular cell layer.

DERMOID CYST

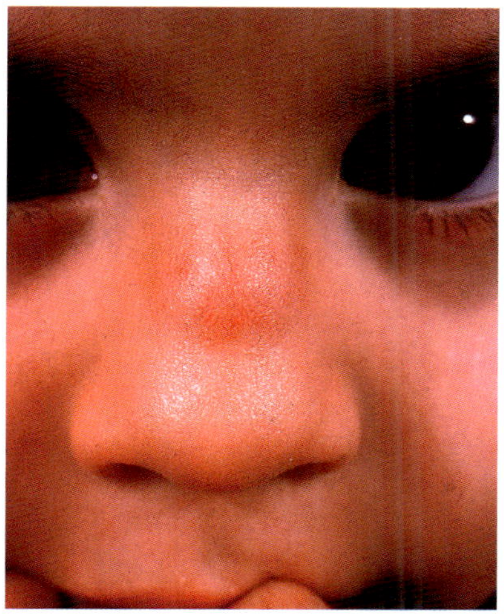

Figure 42–8. Dermoid cyst. Midline, dome-shaped erythematous nodule on the nose of a child.

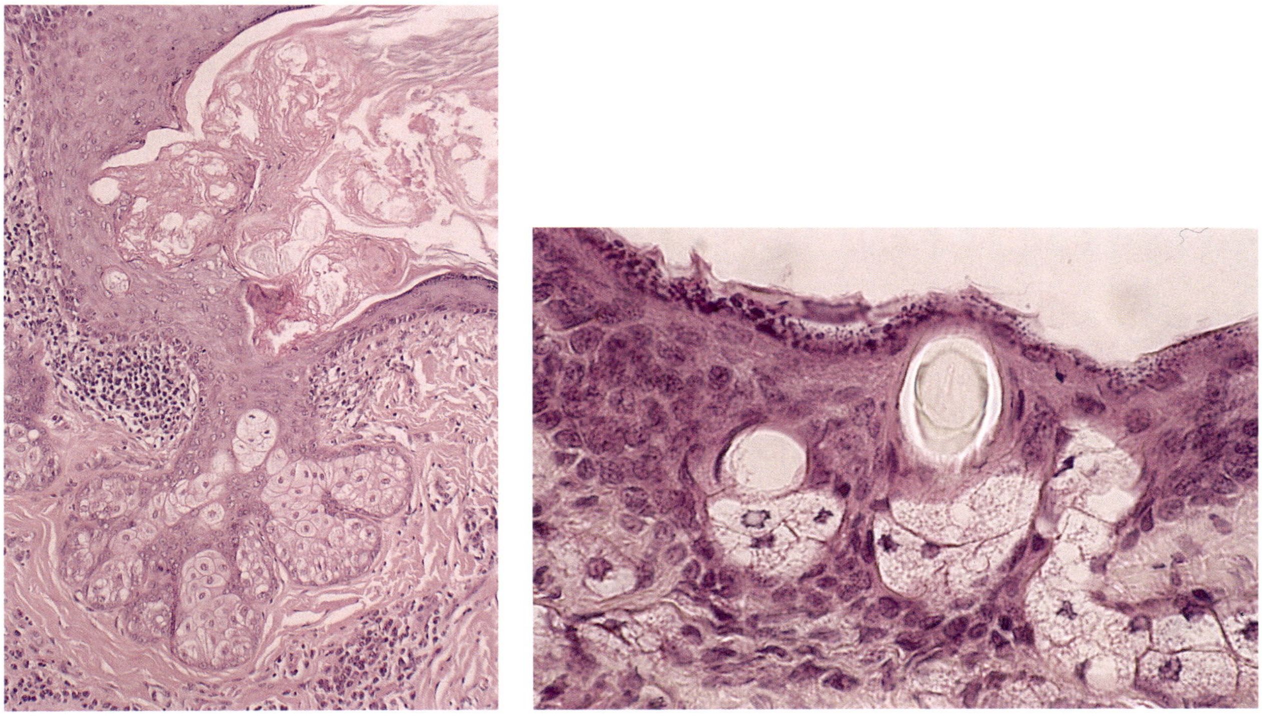

A B

Figures 42–9A, 42–9B. Dermoid cyst. Folliculosebaceous structure and hair-shaft fragment within the wall of a keratinous cyst, which is lined by stratified squamous epithelium with a prominent granular cell layer.

HYBRID CYST

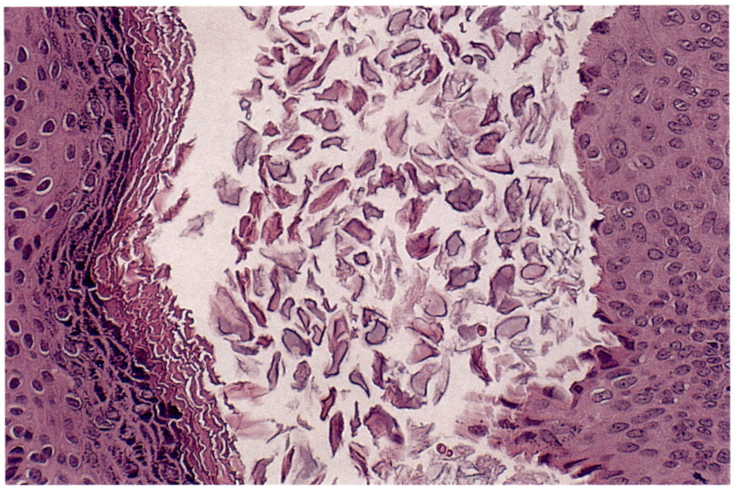

Figure 42–10. Hybrid cyst. Cystic lesion with two forms of keratinization. On the left, the cyst wall resembles the stratified squamous epithelium and prominent granular layer of the infundibulum, while on the right the epithelium resembles that of the isthmus, without a granular layer.

MEDIAN RAPHE CYST

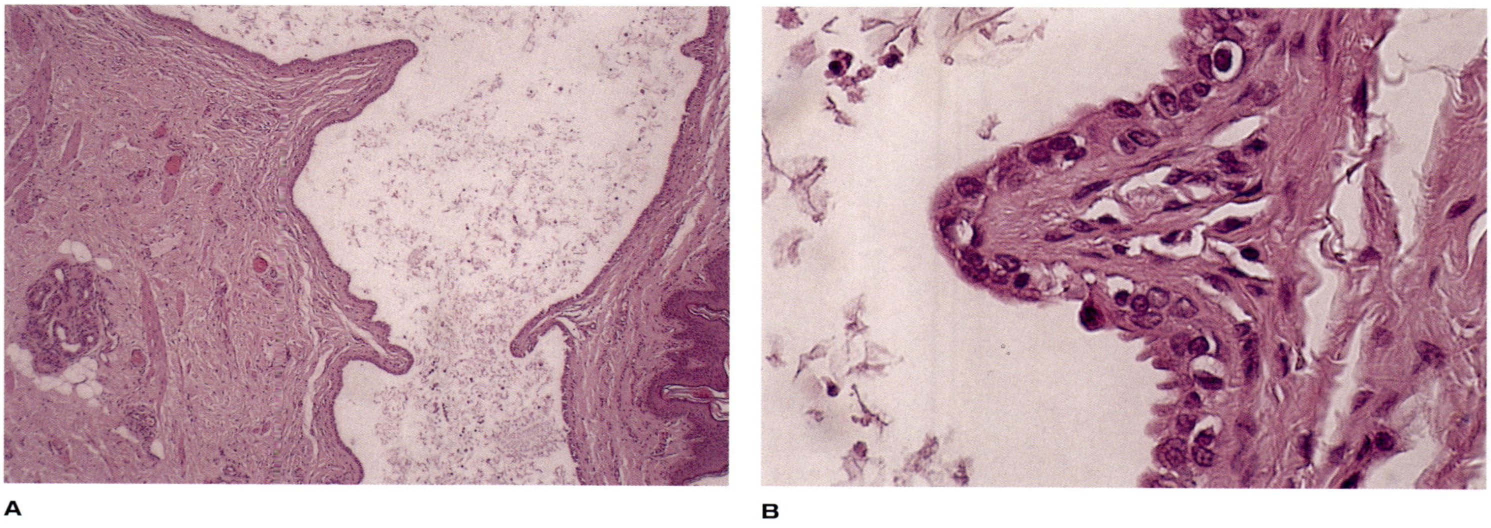

Figures 42–11A, 42–11B. Median raphe cyst. Irregularly shaped cystic structure lined with columnar, vacuolated epithelium, which may be a single cell layer or pseudostratified. There is no connection to the skin surface epithelium.

BRONCHOGENIC CYST

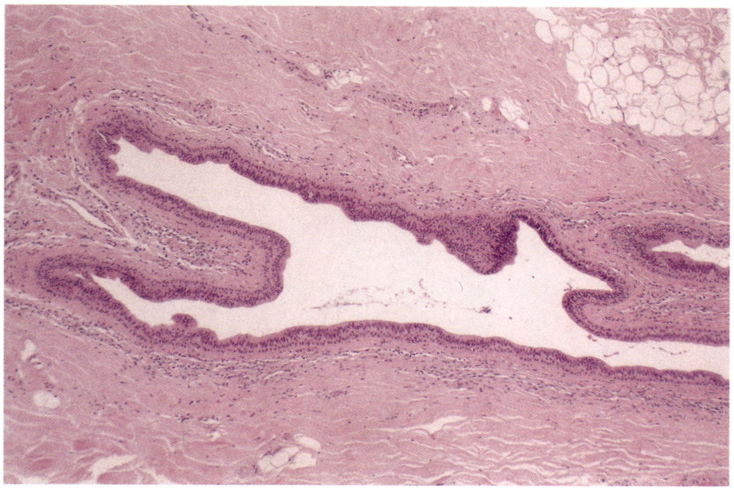

A

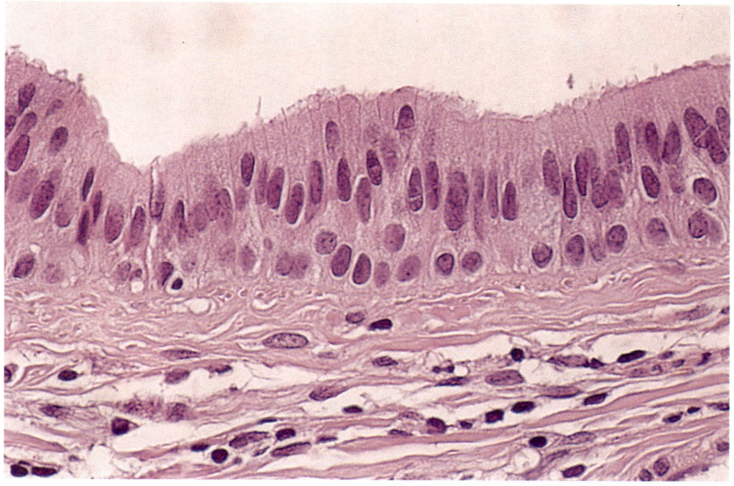

B

Figures 42–12A, 42–12B. Bronchogenic cyst. Pseudostratified, ciliated columnar epithelium.

BRANCHIAL CLEFT CYST

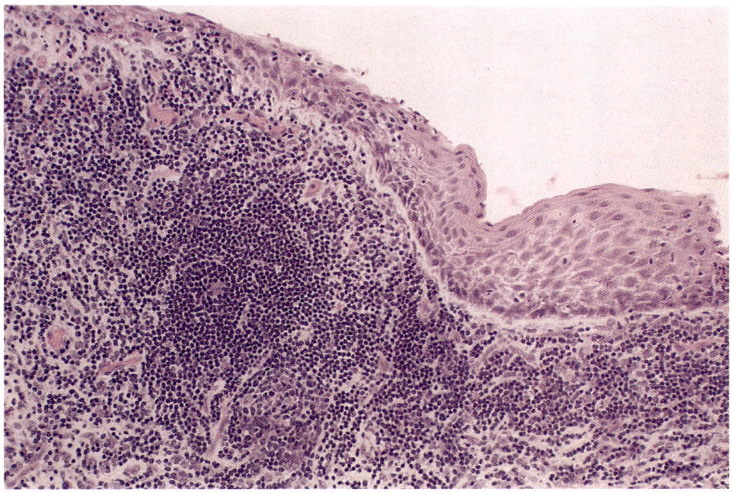

A

Figures 42–13A, 42–13B. Branchial cleft cyst. Dense zone of lymphoid cells surround the wall of the cyst. There is pseudostratified squamous epithelium lining the cyst, a result of squamous metaplasia that replaces the usual columnar epithelium.

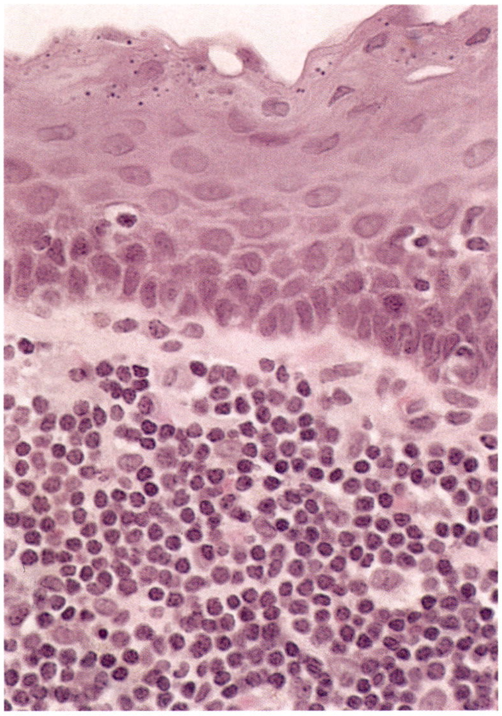

B

THYROGLOSSAL DUCT CYST

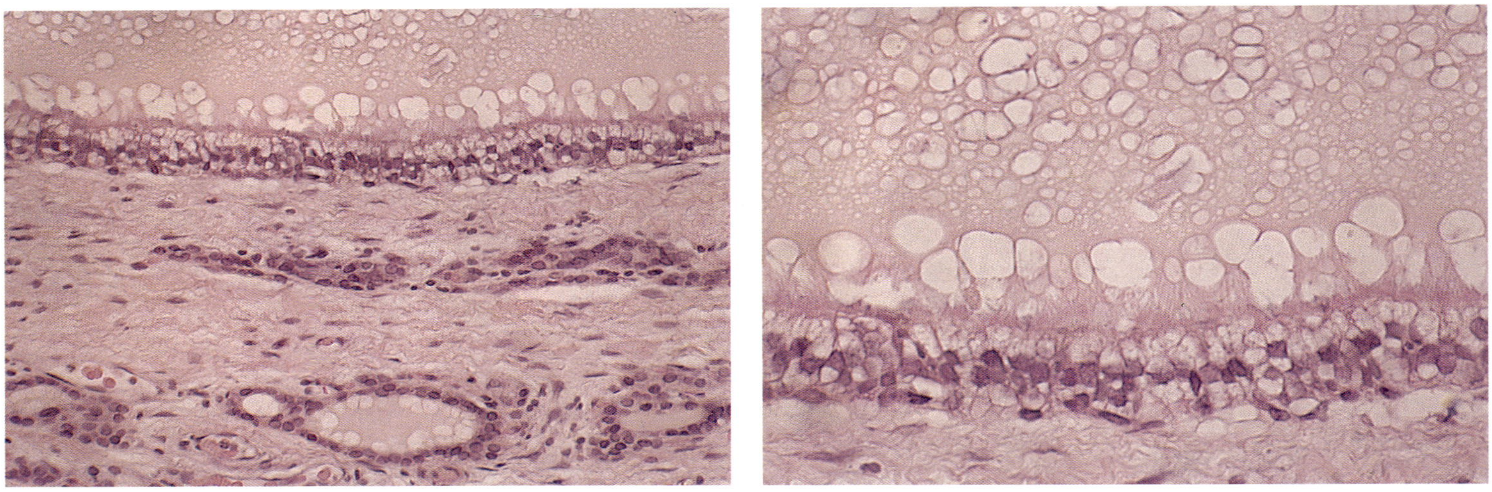

A B

Figures 42–14A, 42–14B. Thy-oglossal duct cyst. Ciliated respiratory epithelium. There are numerous vacuolated cuboidal cells.

CILIATED CYST

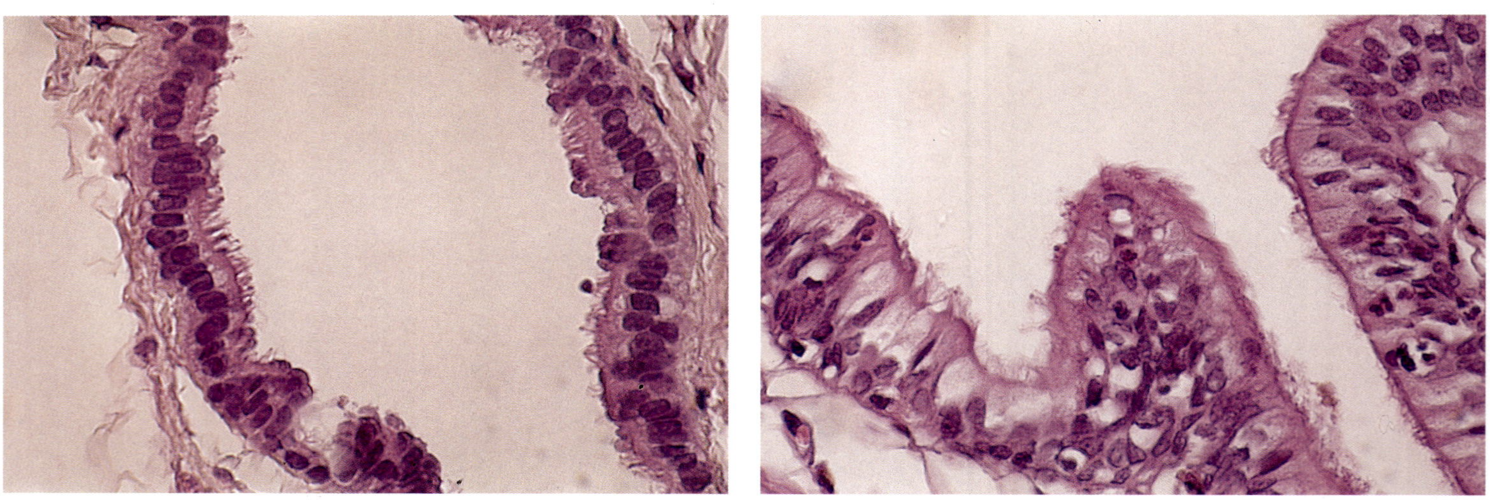

A B

Figures 42–15A, 42–15B. Cilicted cyst. Pseudostratified, columnar ciliated epithelium lines the cyst.

43

CUTANEOUS DRUG REACTIONS

- Perivascular and interstitial dermatitis
- Interface dermatitis
  - *A) Macular-papular*
  - *B) Photodermatitis*
  - *C) Bleomycin*
  - *D) Fixed drug*
  - *E) Dermatomyositis-like*
  - *F) Lichenoid*
- Spongiotic dermatitis
  - *A) Vancomyin*
  - *B) Mycosis fungoides-like*
- Vesiculobullous dermatitis
  - *A) Pemphigus-like*
  - *B) Linear IgA-like (dermatitis herpetiformis-like)*
  - *C) Erythema multiforme/toxic epidermal necrolysis/Stevens-Johnson syndrome*
  - *D) Allergic urticarial vesiculobullous*
  - *E) Pseudoporphyria*
  - *F) Pemphigoid-like*
- Pustular dermatitis
  - *A) Lithium*
  - *B) Trimethoprim-sulfamethoxazole*
  - *C) Phenytoin*
- Adnexal alteration
  - *A) Iododerma*
  - *B) Neutrophilic eccrine hidradenitis*
- Vasculopathy
  - *A) Coumadin necrosis*
  - *B) Leukocytoclastic vasculitis*
  - *C) Tissue plasminogen activator (tPA)*
- Pigmentary alteration
  - *A) Clofazimine hyperpigmentation*
  - *B) Minocycline hyperpigmentation*
  - *C) Chloroquine*
  - *D) Argyria*

PERIVASCULAR AND INTERSTITIAL DERMATITIS

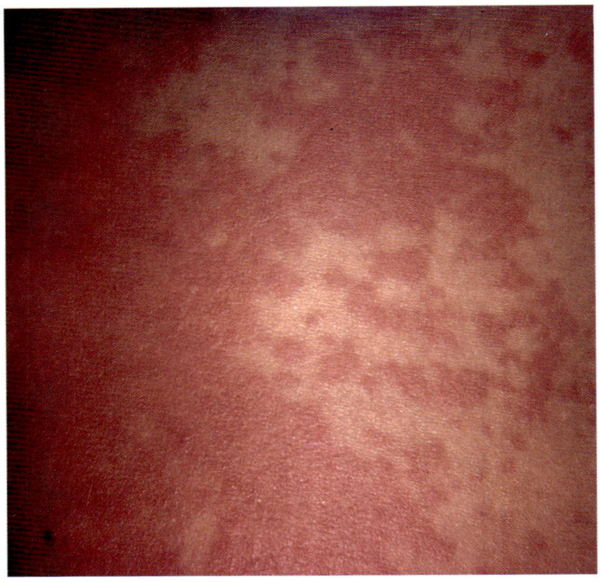

Figure 43–1. Macular-papular eruption. Solitary and confluent erythematous macules and papules.

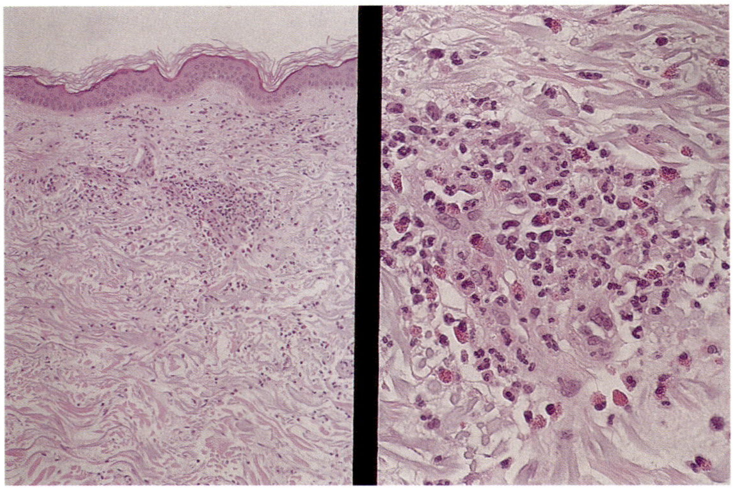

Figure 43–2. Macular-papular eruption. Perivascular and interstitial mixed-cell infiltrate with lymphocytes, neutrophils, and eosinophils.

INTERFACE DERMATITIS

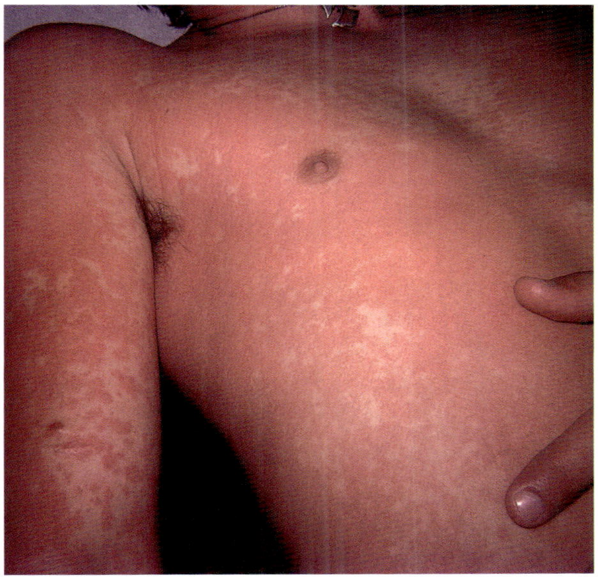

Figure 43–3. Macular-papular erythema, ibuprofen induced. Diffuse erythematous patches and papules on the trunk and extremities.

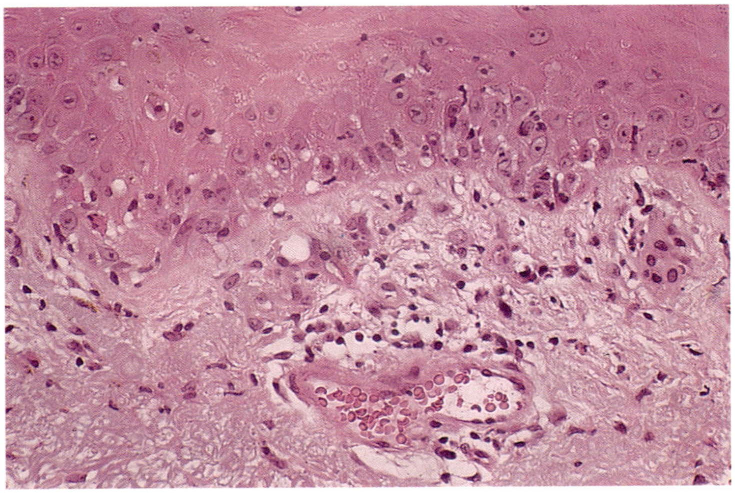

Figure 43–4. Macular-papular erythema. Vacuolar alteration, necrotic keratinocytes, papillary edema, dilated blood vessels, and a dermal mixed-cell infiltrate.

INTERFACE DERMATITIS

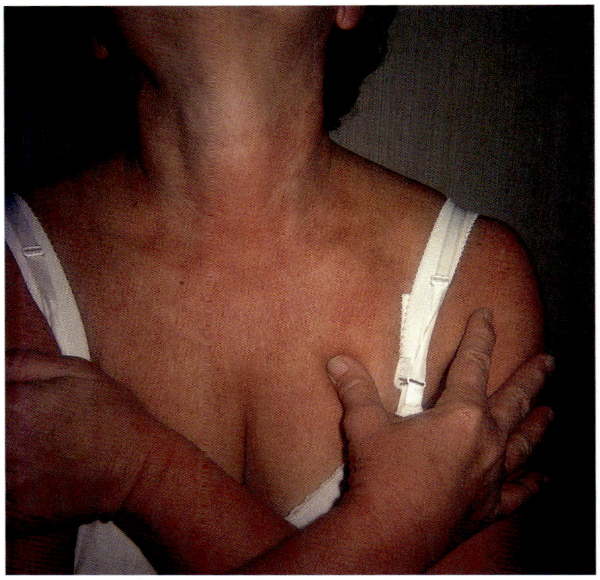

A

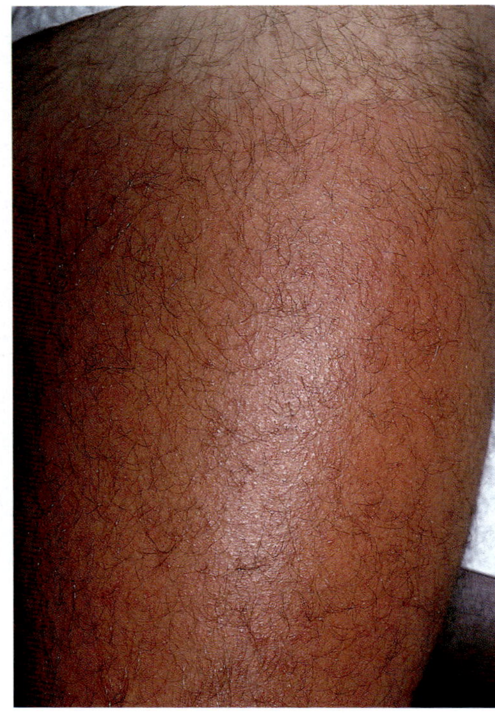

B

Figures 43–5A, 43–5B. Photodermatitis, Diazide induced (left), piroxicam incuced (right). Macular erythema on sun-exposed sites of the skin. (There is submental sparing in areas covered by cothing.)

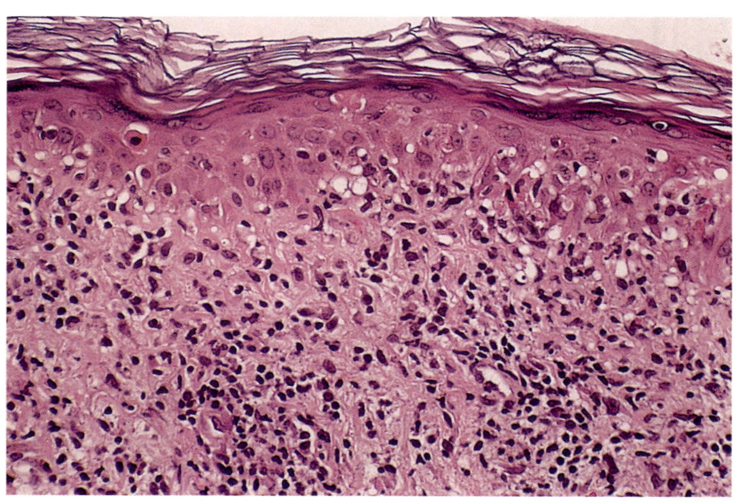

Figure 43–6. Photodermatitis. Vacuolar alteration, necrotic keratinocytes, basket-weave orthokeratosis, papillary edema, and a dermal lichenoid mixed-cell infiltrate.

INTERFACE DERMATITIS

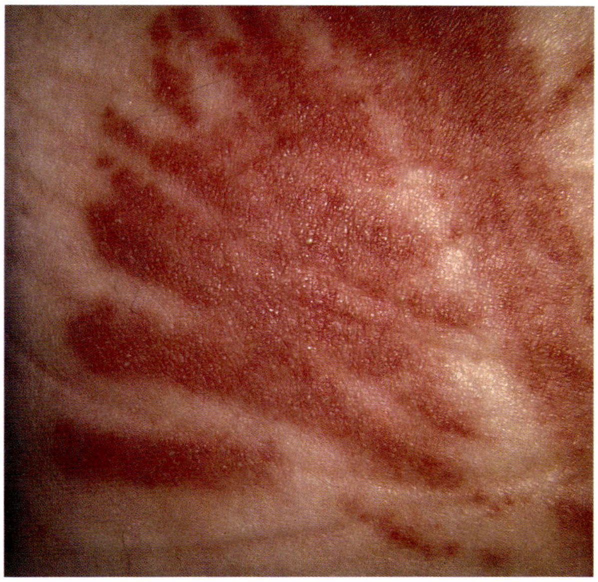

Figure 43–7. Bleomycin. Bizarre-shaped erythematous linear plaques.

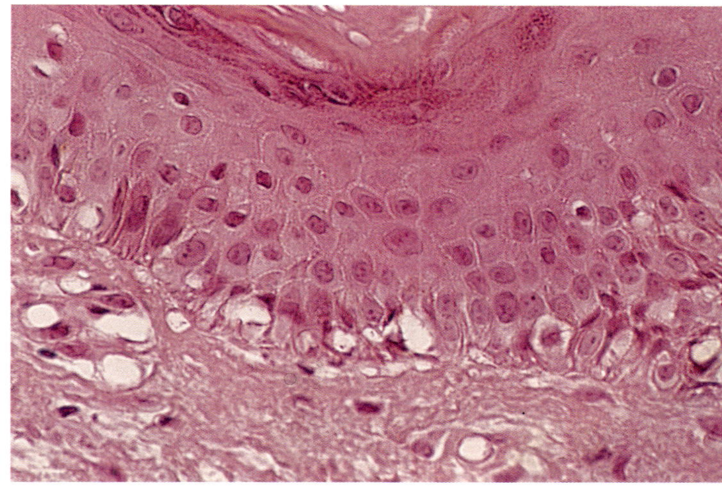

Figure 43–8. Bleomycin. Vacuolar alteration and necrotic keratinocytes.

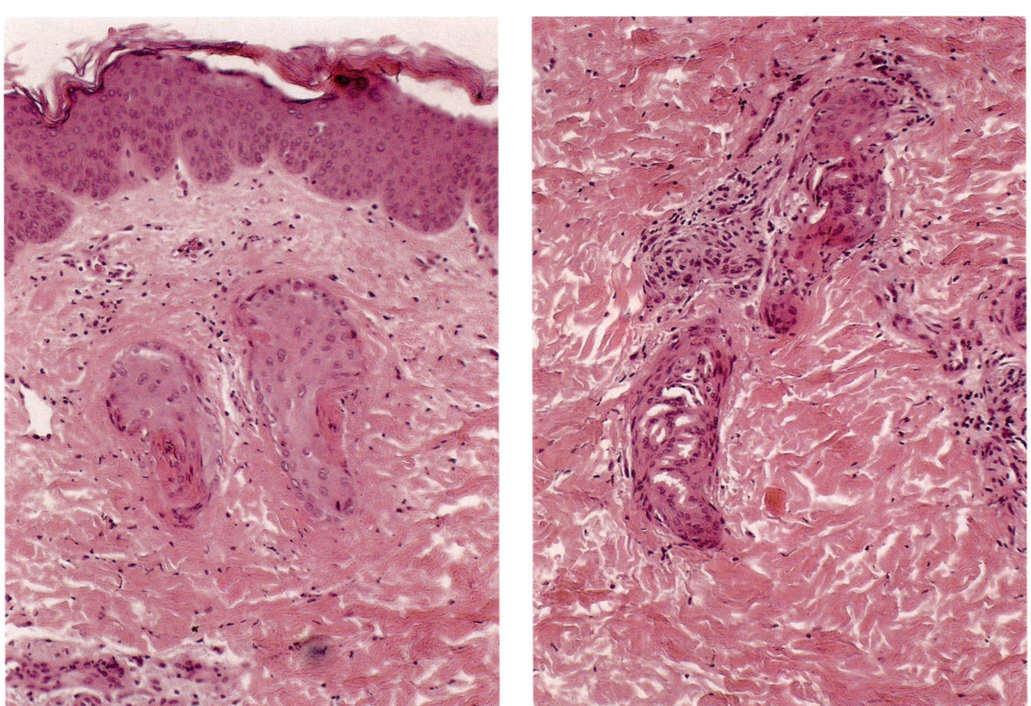

A B

Figures 43–9A, 43–9B. Bleomycin. Follicular and syringomatous metaplasia.

INTERFACE DERMATITIS

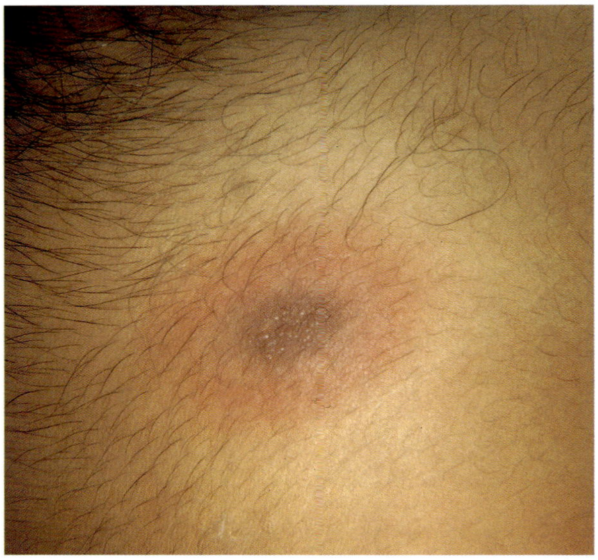

Figure 43–10. Fixed drug eruption, tetracycline induced, evolving lesion. Gray patch with central vesicles and surrounding erythema.

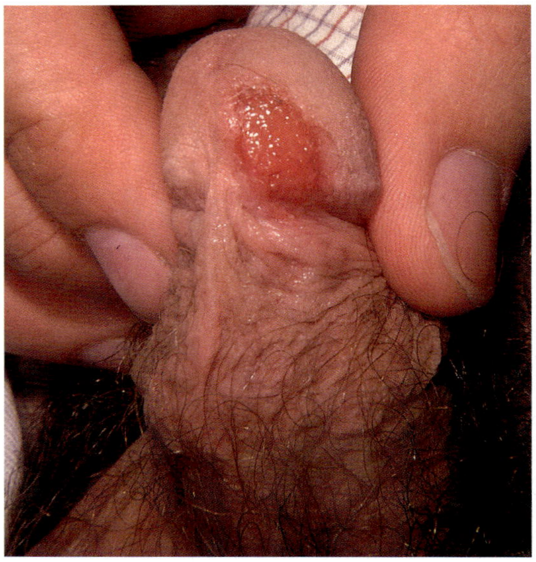

Figure 43–11. Fixed drug eruption, mature lesion. Ruptured bulla on the glans penis.

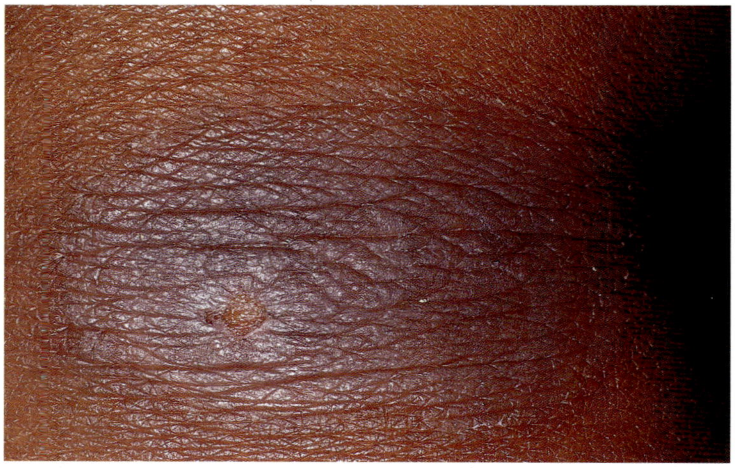

Figure 43–12. Fixed drug eruption, resolving lesion. Erythematous and hyperpigmented patch with ulceration.

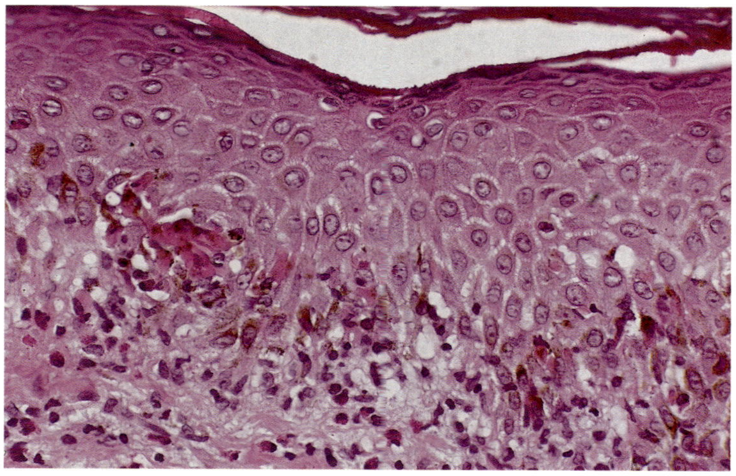

A

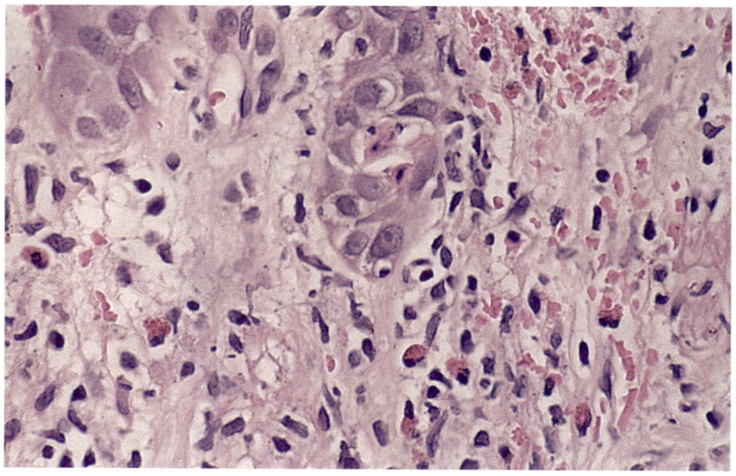

B

Figures 43–13A, 43–13B. Fixed drug eruption. Vacuolar alteration, spongiosis, and necrotic keratinocytes. There is a dermal, lichenoid mixed-cell infiltrate containing lymphocytes, neutrophils, many eosinophils, and melanophages. Papillary edema may be prominent.

INTERFACE DERMATITIS

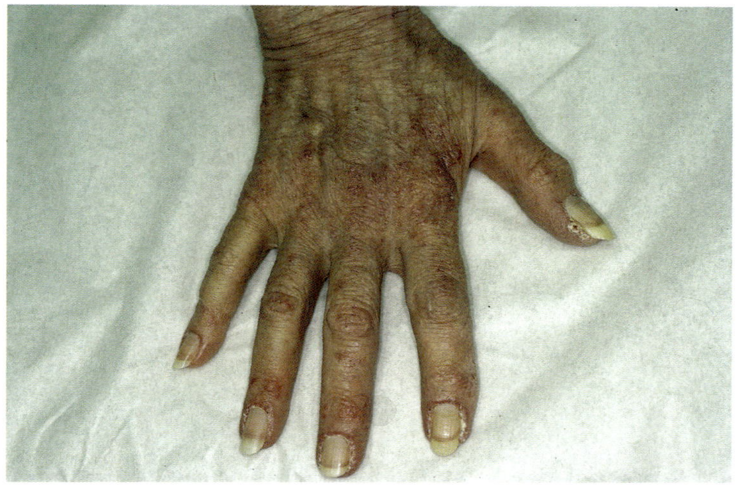

Figure 43–14. Dermatomyositis-like, paclitaxel induced. Flat-topped erythematous papules on the dorsum of the hand and fingers with accompanying periungual erythema and telangiectases.

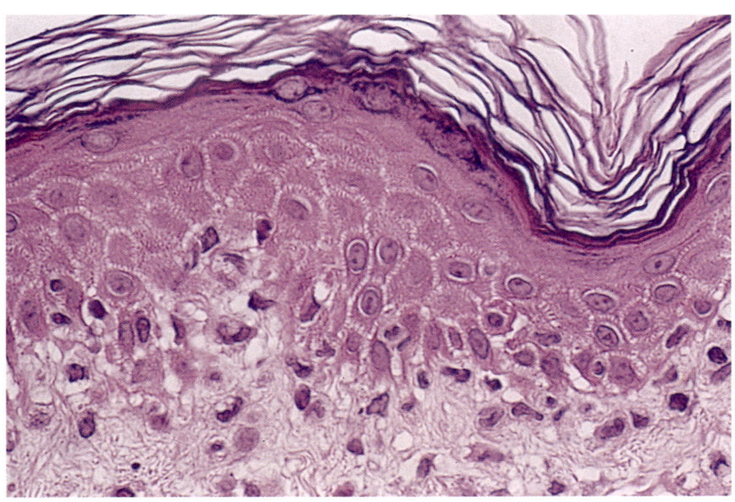

Figure 43–15. Dermatomyositis-like. Vacuolar alteration, spongiosis, and basket-weave orthokeratosis.

INTERFACE DERMATITIS

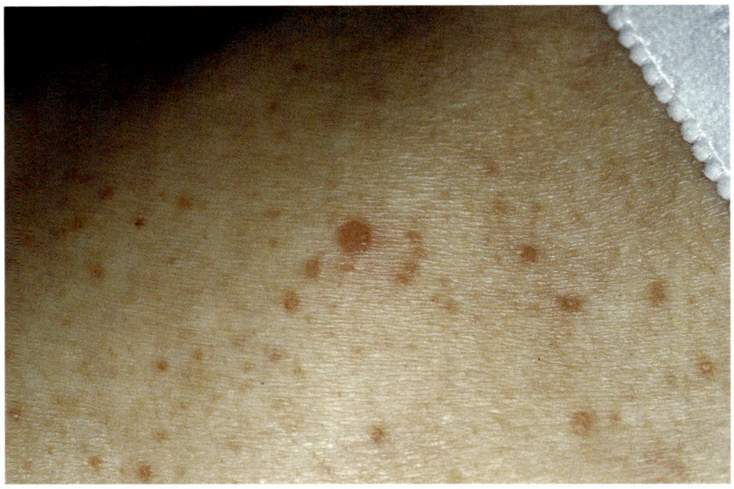

Figure 43–16. **Lichenoid drug eruption.** Erythematous flat-topped papules on the thigh of a woman.

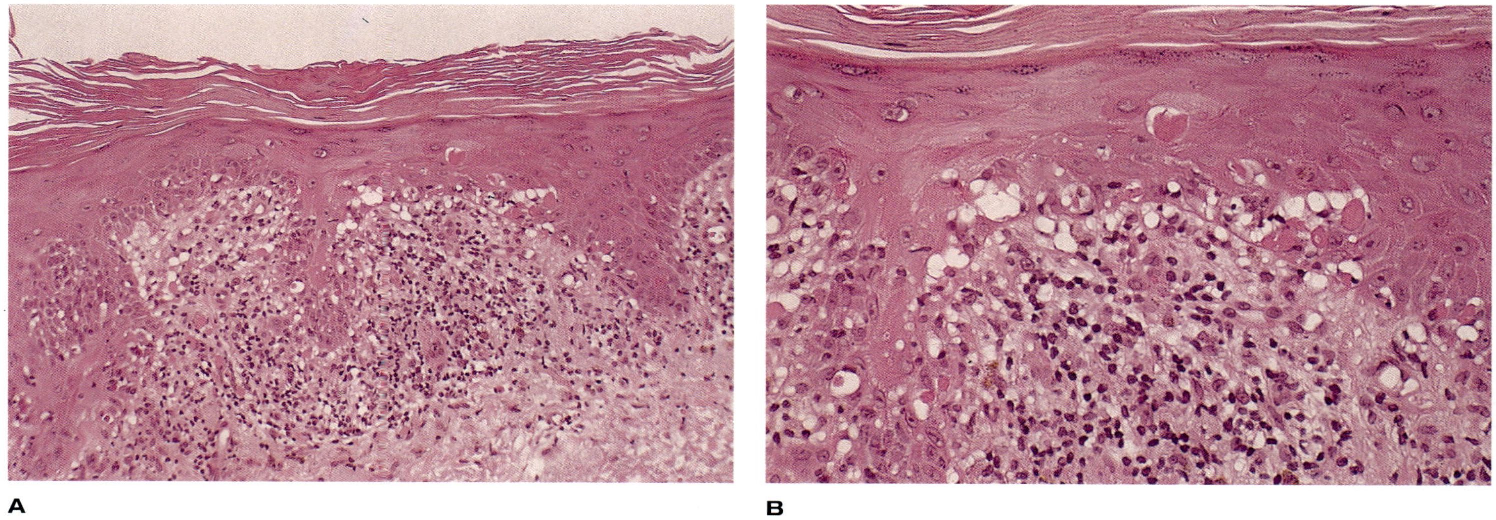

Figures 43–17A, 43–17B. **Lichenoid drug eruption.** Irregular epidermal hyperplasia, vacuolar alteration, and necrotic keratinocytes. There is marked papillary edema and a dermal lichenoid mononuclear cell infiltrate.

SPONGIOTIC DERMATITIS

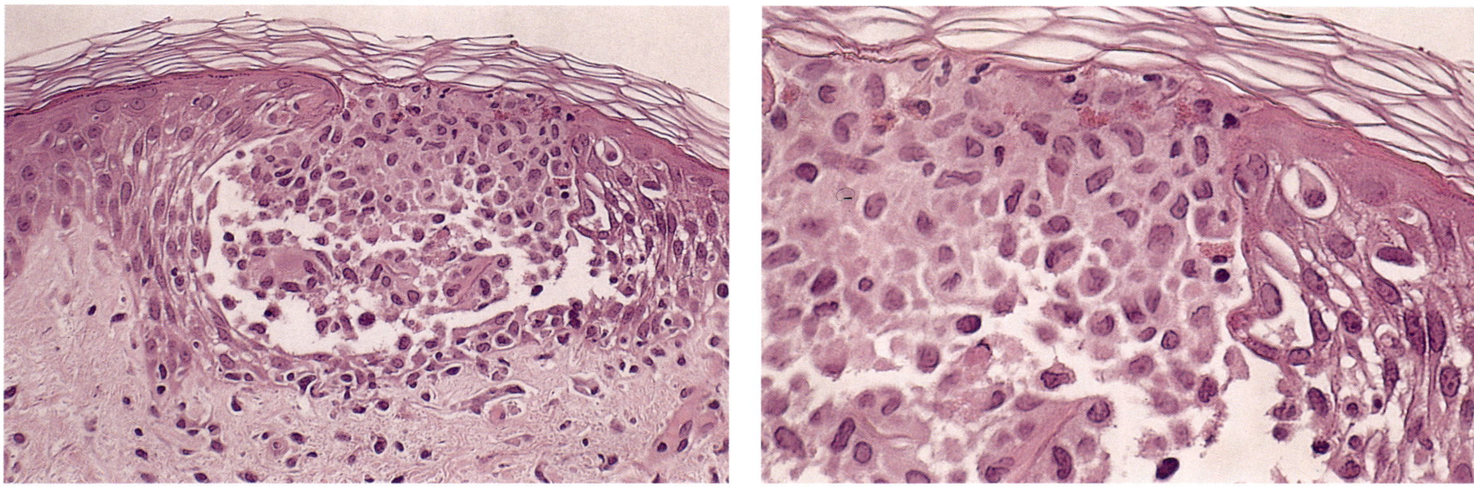

A B

Figures 43–18A, 43–18B. Spongiotic dermatitis, vancomycin induced. Intraepidermal spongiosis with microvesiculation. There are lymphocytes and eosinophils within the epidermis and dermis.

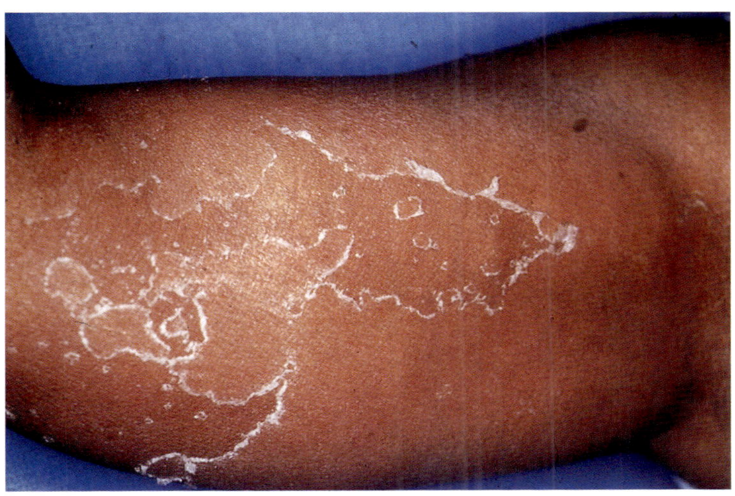

Figure 43–19. Mycosis fungoides-like, phenytoin induced. Patchy erythema and desquamation on the arm.

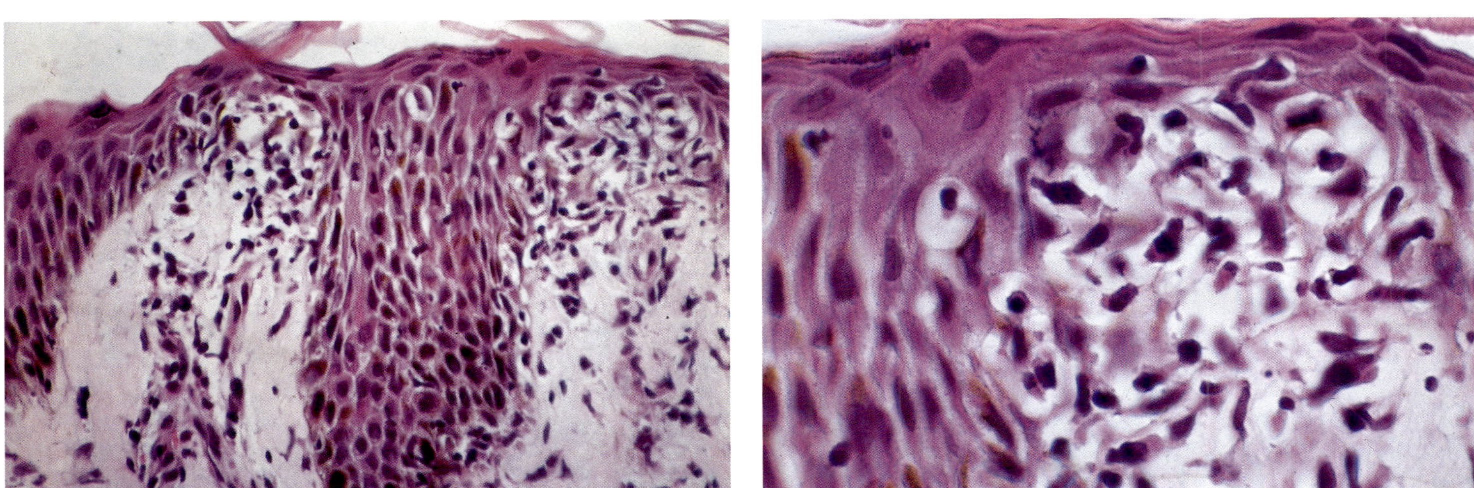

A B

Figures 43–20A, 43–20B. Mycosis fungoides-like, phenytoin induced. Increased number of large lymphocytes in the epidermis and dermis. Keratinocytes with tails of eosinophilic cytoplasm lie within the spongiotic epidermis. Marked papillary dermal edema is present.

VESICULOBULLOUS DERMATITIS

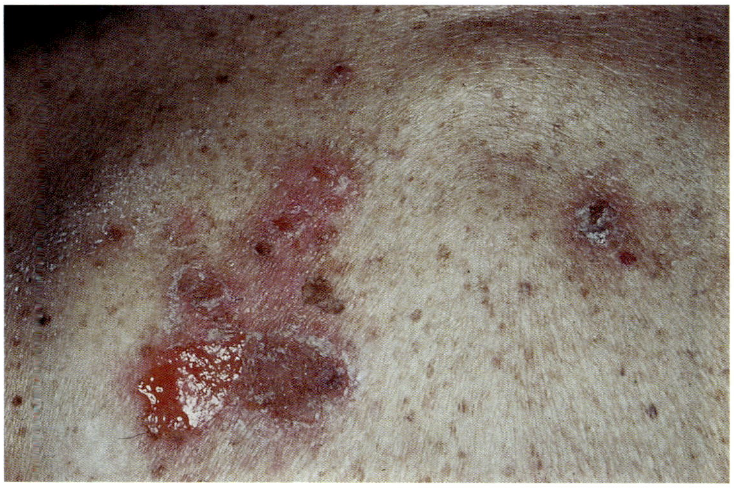

Figure 43–21. **Pemphigus vulgaris–like, Captopril induced.** Erythematous erosive patches on the chest.

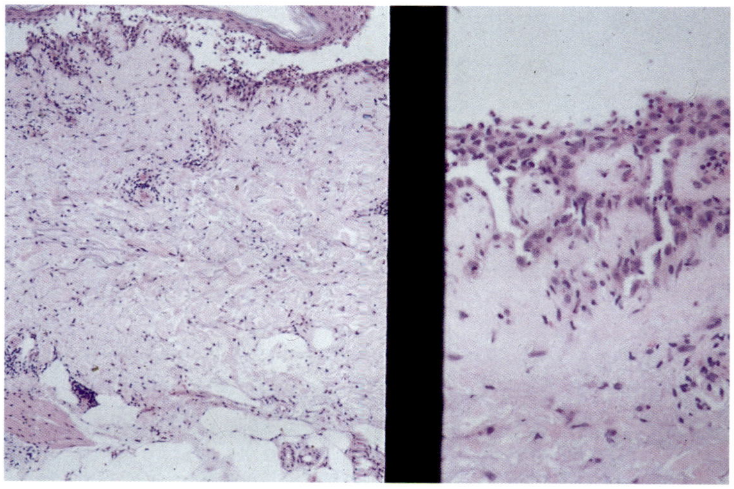

A

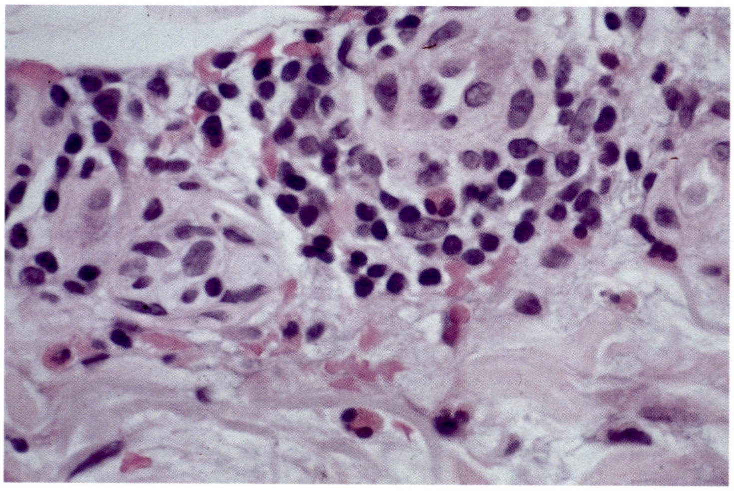

B

Figures 43–22A, 43–22B. **Pemphigus vulgaris–like, Captopril induced.** Suprabasilar and intraepidermal acantholysis. There is an infiltrate of lymphocytes and eosinophils in the epidermis and dermis.

VESICULOBULLOUS DERMATITIS

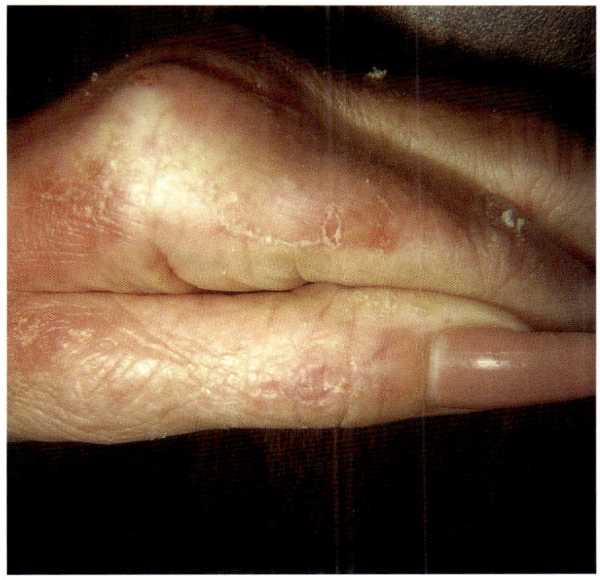

Figure 43–23. Pemphigus vulgaris–like, penicillamine induced. Erythema, desquamation, and clusters of vesicles on the hand and fingers.

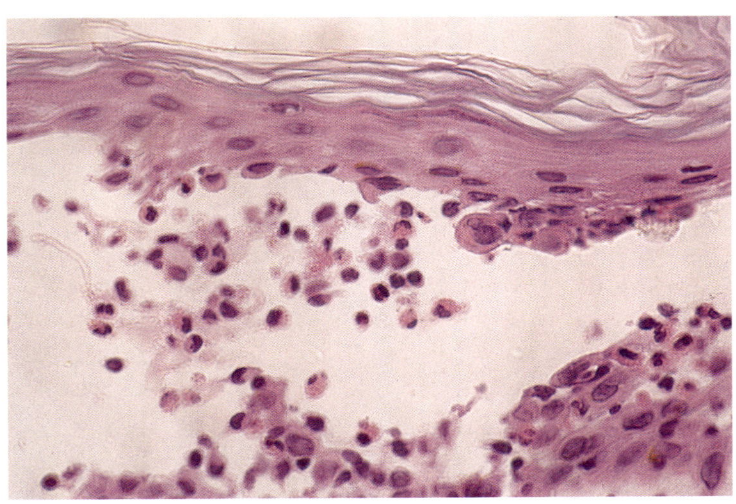

Figure 43–24. Pemphigus vulgaris–like, penicillamine induced. Intraepidermal acantholysis and spongiosis with neutrophils and eosinophils in the bulla cavity.

VESICULOBULLOUS DERMATITIS

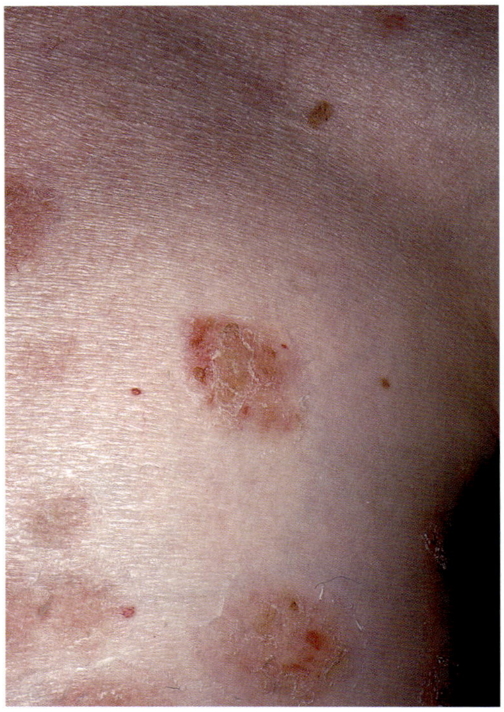

Figure 43–25. Pemphigus foliaceus–like, penicillamine induced. Superficial crusted patches on the back.

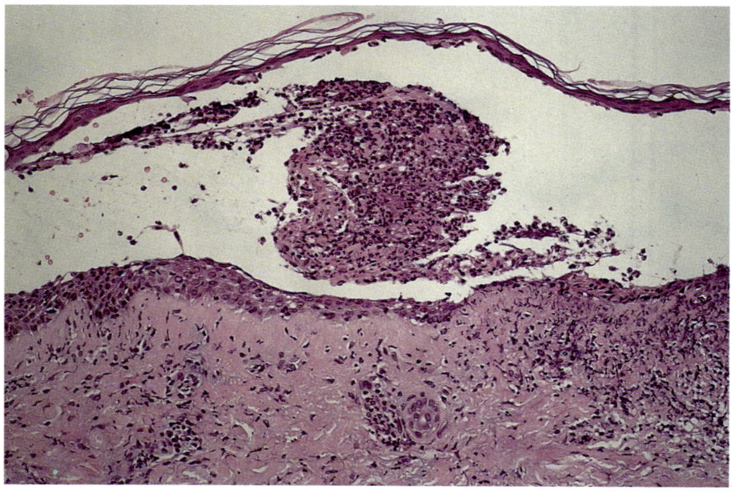

Figure 43–26. Pemphigus foliaceus–like, penicillamine induced. Subcorneal, intragranular, and upper spinous layer vesiculation. There are acantholytic keratinocytes dispersed amid numerous neutrophils within the vesicle.

VESICULOBULLOUS DERMATITIS

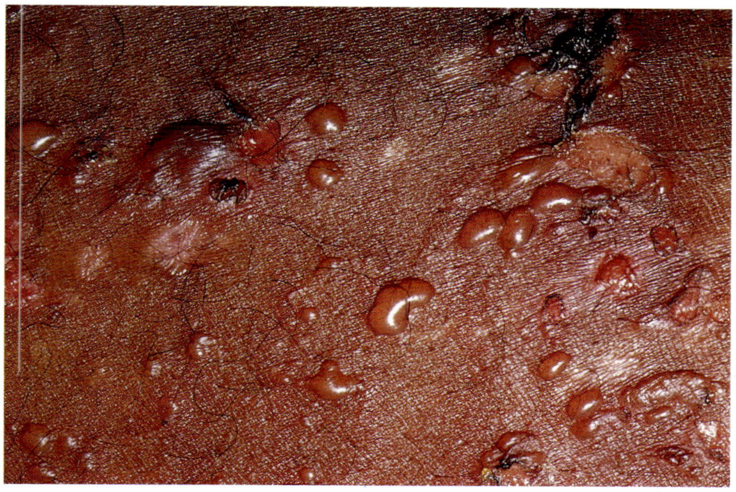

Figure 43–27. Linear IgA--like (dermatitis herpetiformis–like), vancomycin induced. Vesicles, bullae, and crusts.

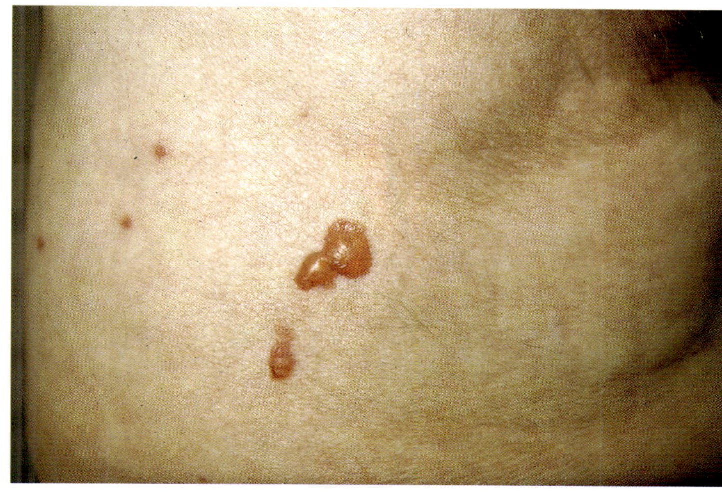

Figure 43–28. Linear IgA–like (dermatitis herpetiformis–like). Vesicles and bulla on the side of a man.

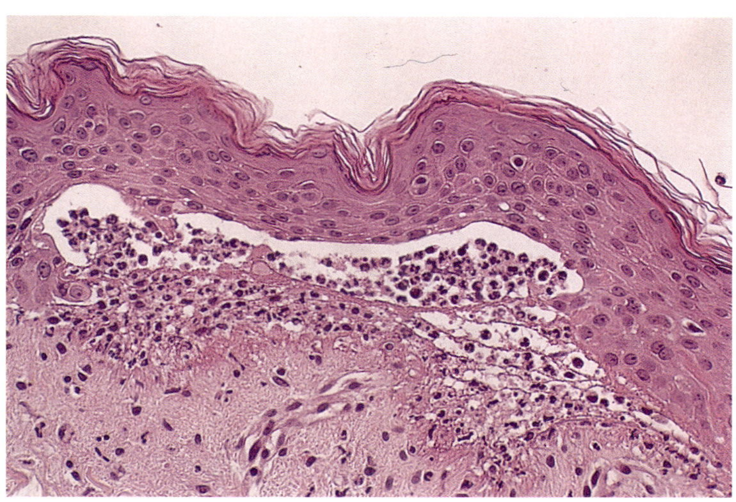

Figure 43–29. Linear IgA–like (dermatitis herpetiformis–like). Subepidermal vesicle. There are numerous neutrophils, nuclear fragments, and fibrin within the papillary dermis.

VESICULOBULLOUS DERMATITIS

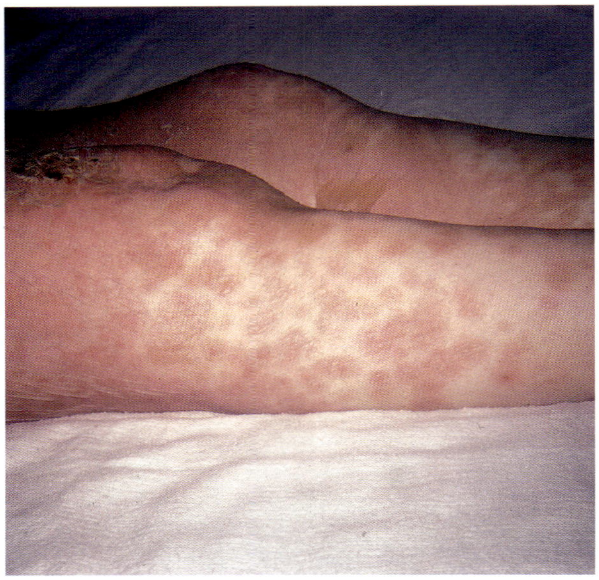

A

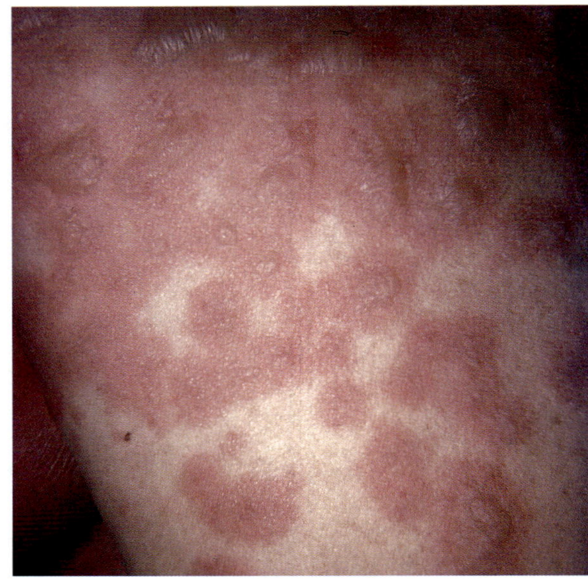

B

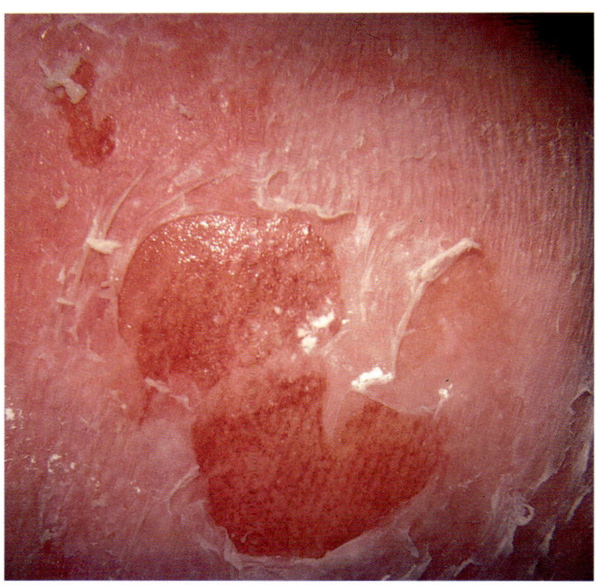

C

Figures 43–30A, 43–30B, 43–30C. Erythema multiforme/toxic epidermal necrolysis/Stevens-Johnson syndrome, Captopril induced. Erythematous macules, papules, vesicles, bullae, and erosions.

VESICULOBULLOUS DERMATITIS

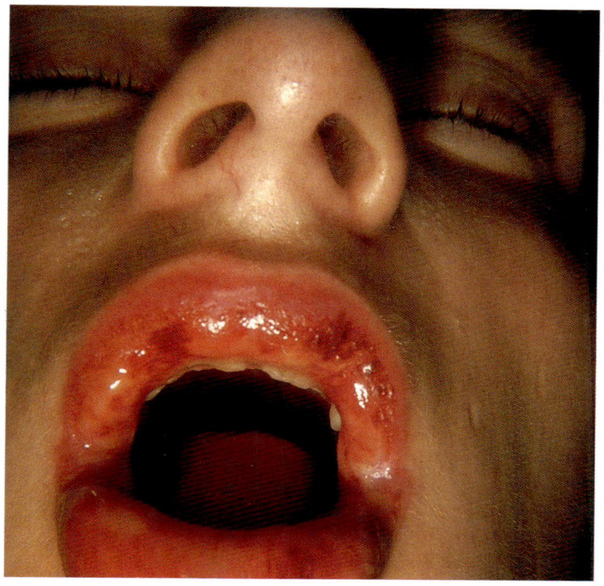

A

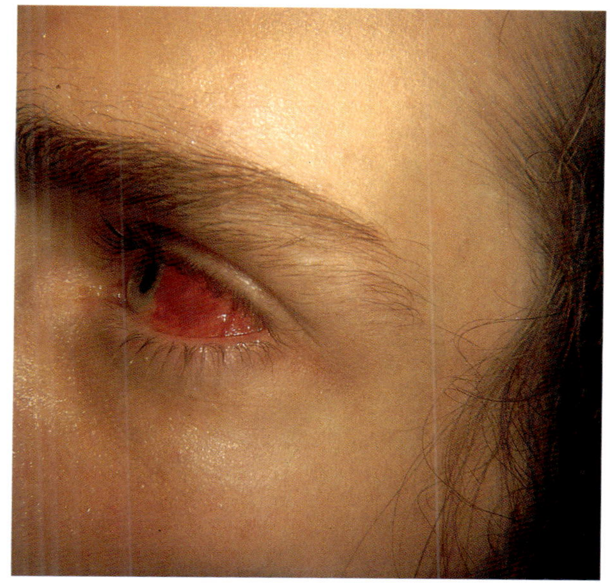

B

Figures 43–31A, 43–31B. Erythema multiforme/toxic epidermal necrolysis/Stevens-Johnson syndrome. Exudative, erosive, erythematous lesions involving the oral mucous membranes. There is also conjunctival hemorrhage.

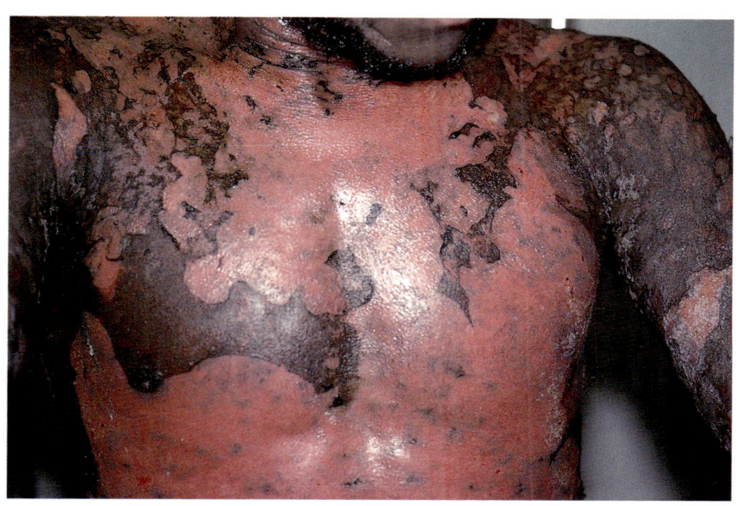

Figure 43–32. Erythema multiforme/toxic epidermal necrolysis/Stevens-Johnson syndrome. Islands of regenerated skin after total body denudation.

VESICULOBULLOUS DERMATITIS

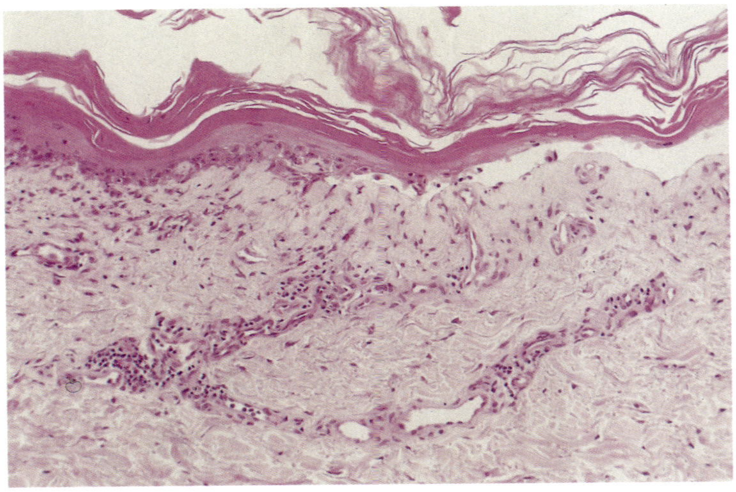

A

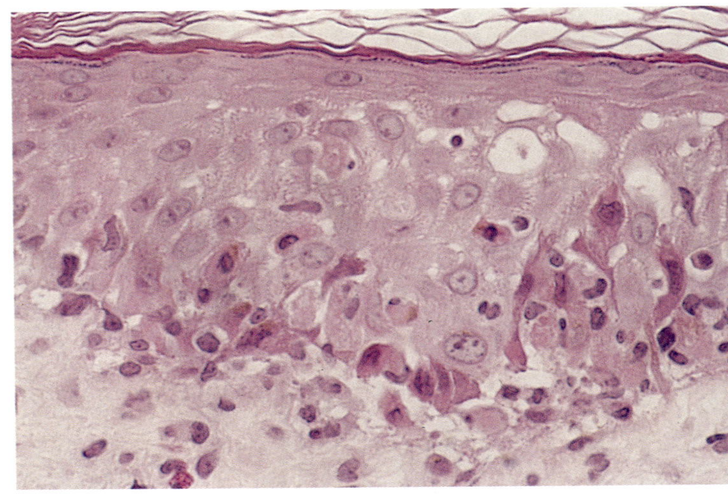

B

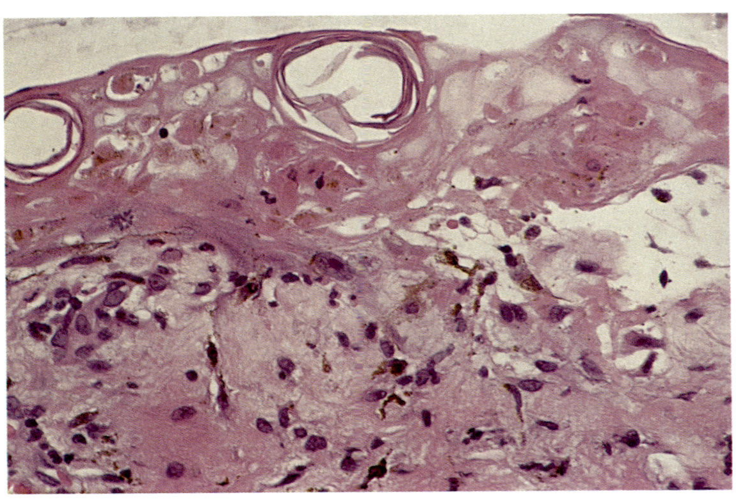

C

Figures 43–33A, 43–33B, 43–33C. Erythema multiforme/toxic epidermal necrolysis/Stevens-Johnson syndrome. Subepidermal vesiculation, solitary and confluent necrotic keratinocytes, with ballooning and spongiosis. There is marked papillary edema, predominantly mononuclear cell infiltrate with sporadic eosinophils, dilated blood vessels, and melanophages.

VESICULOBULLOUS DERMATITIS

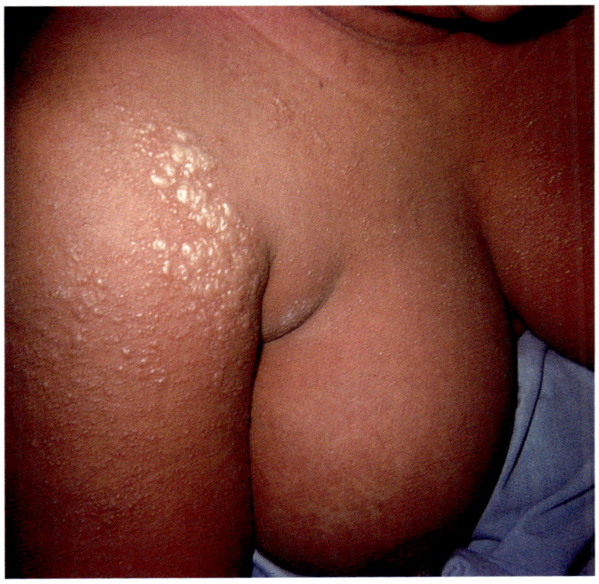
A

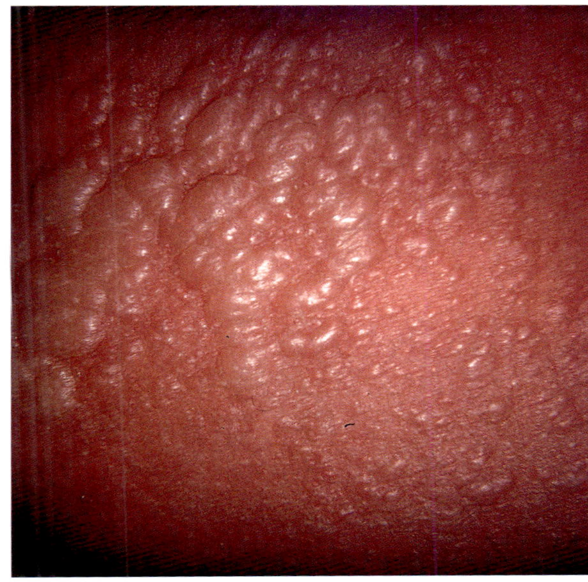
B

Figures 43–34A, 43–34B. Allergic urticarial vesiculobullous reaction. Diffuse erythema with solitary and confluent tense, clear vesicles and bullae on the trunk, breast, and extremities.

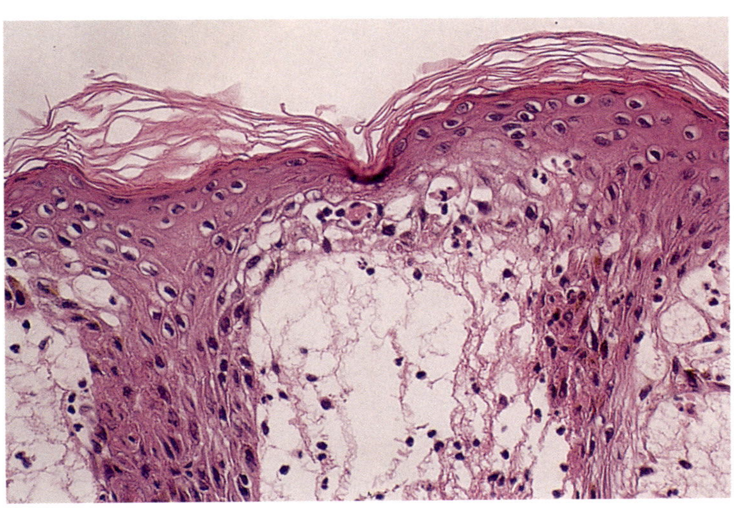
A

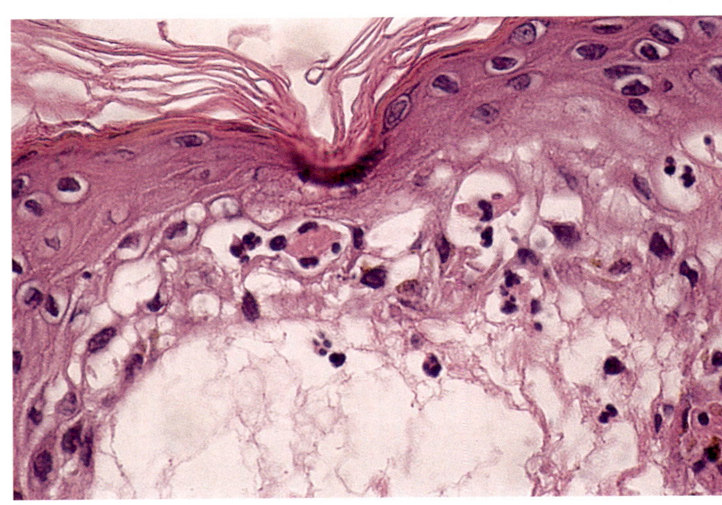
B

Figures 43–35A, 43–35B. Allergic urticarial vesiculobullous reaction. Severe papillary edema with gossamer collagen fibers and subepidermal vesiculation with basket-weave orthokeratosis, ballooned and necrotic keratinocytes, and spongiosis. There is reticular alteration of the papillary dermis and a mixed-cell infiltrate with neutrophils and eosinophils.

VESICULOBULLOUS DERMATITIS

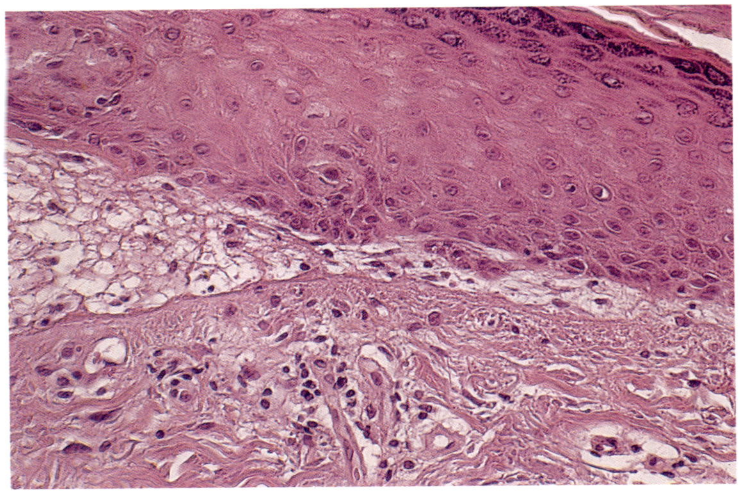

Figure 43–36. Pseudoporphyria. Subepidermal vesiculation with thick-walled papillary dermal blood vessels.

VESICULOBULLOUS DERMATITIS

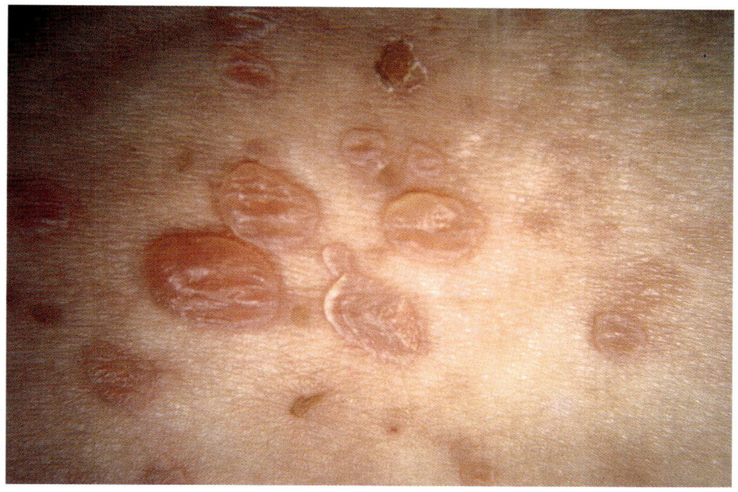

Figure 43–37. Pemphigoid-like. Flaccid bullae on the abdomen of a woman.

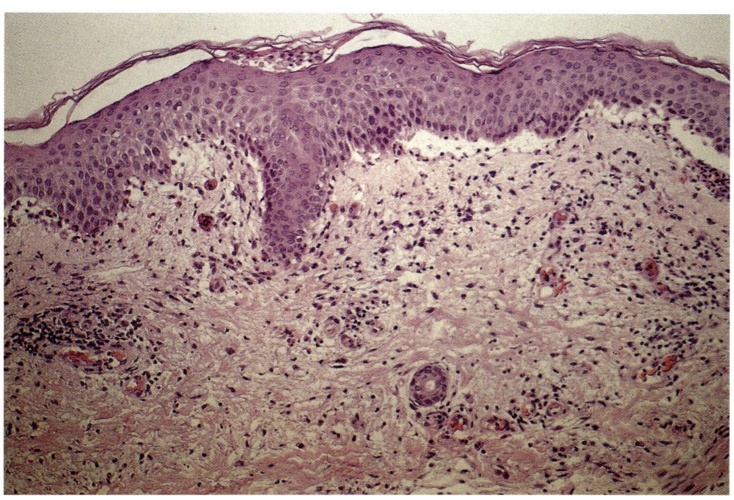

A

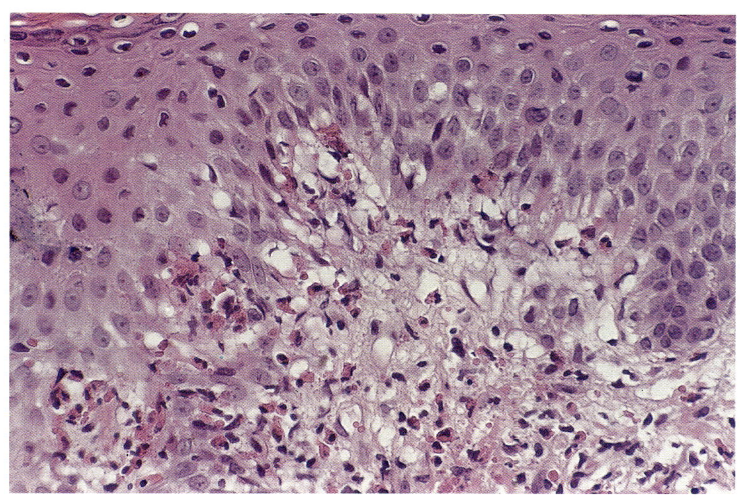

B

Figures 43–38A, 43–38B. Pemphigoid-like. Subepidermal vesiculation with an inflammatory infiltrate containing numerous eosinophils. There is marked papillary edema and spongiosis.

PUSTULAR DERMATITIS

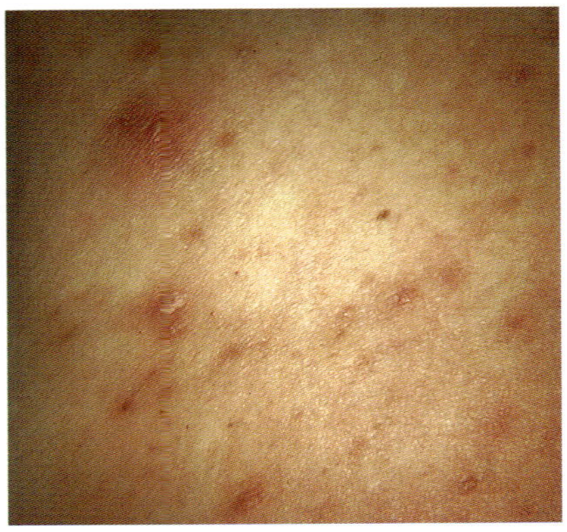

Figure 43–39. Pustular dermatitis, lithium induced. Scattered pustules surrounded by erythema.

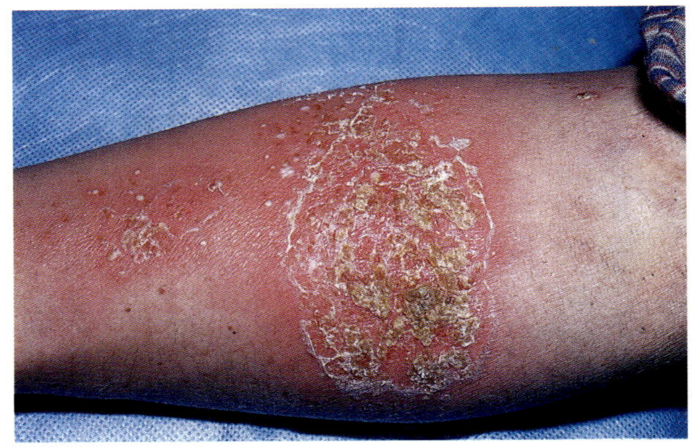

Figure 43–40. Pustular dermatitis. Pustules scattered within an area of erythema and edema on the arm.

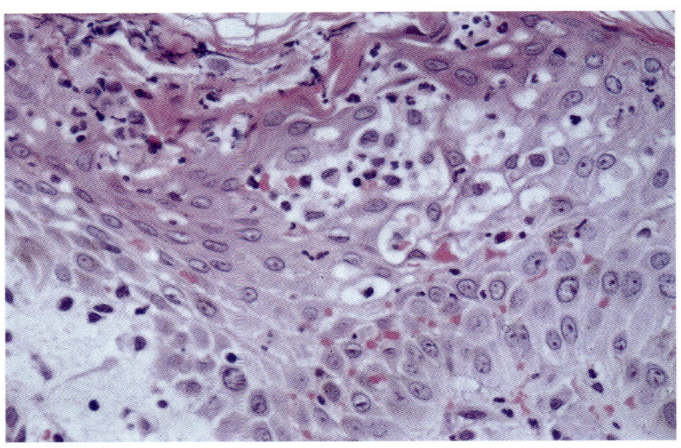

Figure 43–41. Pustular dermatitis. Subcorneal and intraspinous spongiosis with many neutrophils.

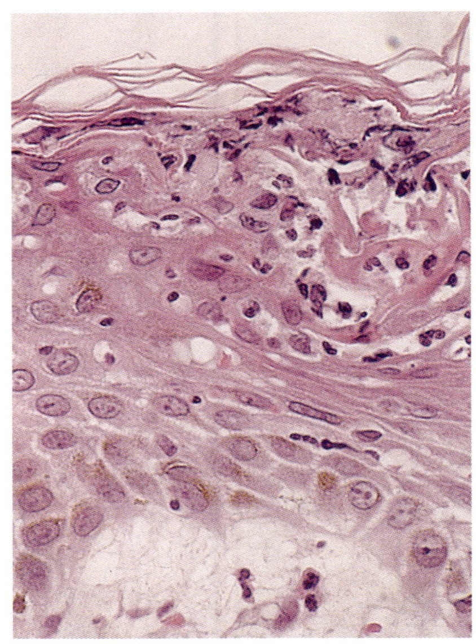

Figure 43–42. Pustular dermatitis, trimethoprim-sulfamethoxazole induced. Subcorneal aggregate of neutrophils. There is marked papillary edema.

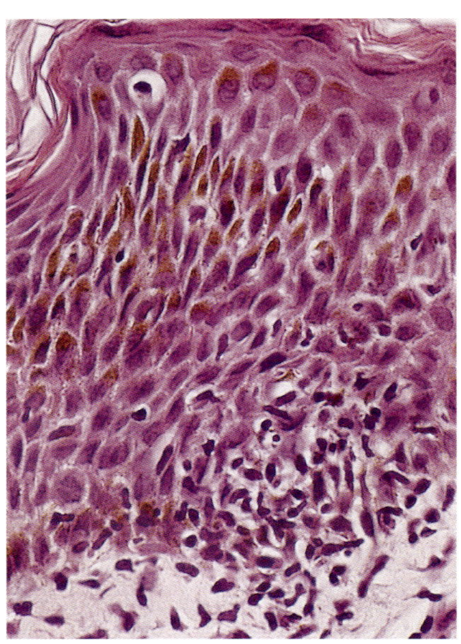

A

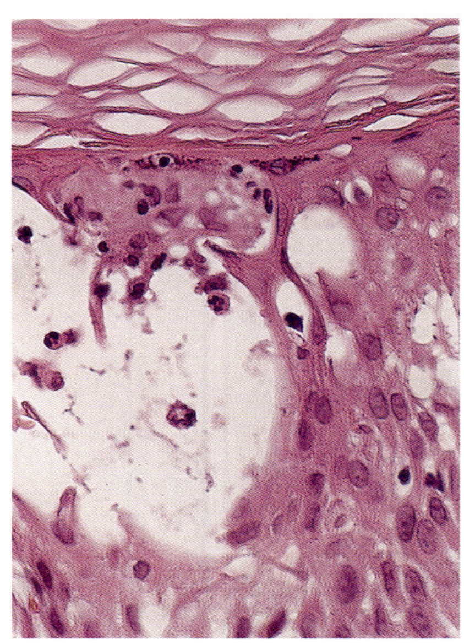

B

Figures 43–43A, 43–43B. Pustular dermatitis, phemytoin induced. There is intraepidermal spongiosis and microvesiculation with many neutrophils.

ADNEXAL ALTERATION

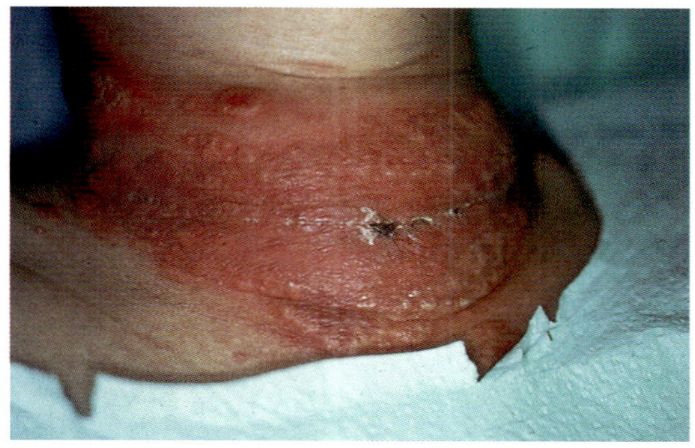

Figure 43–44. Iododerma. Confluent erythematous nodules and plaques on the neck and chest.

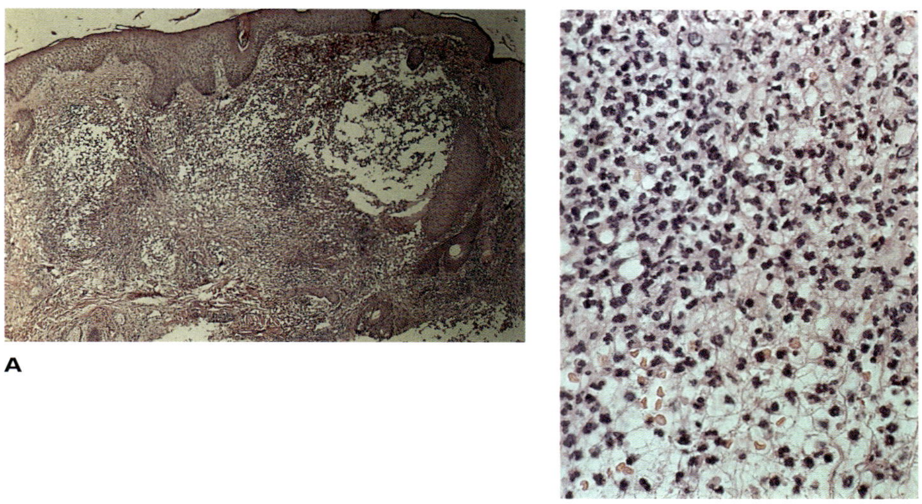

A

B

Figures 43–45A, 43–45B. Iododerma. Expansive infundibular hyperplasia with extensive neutrophilic infiltration with abscess formation.

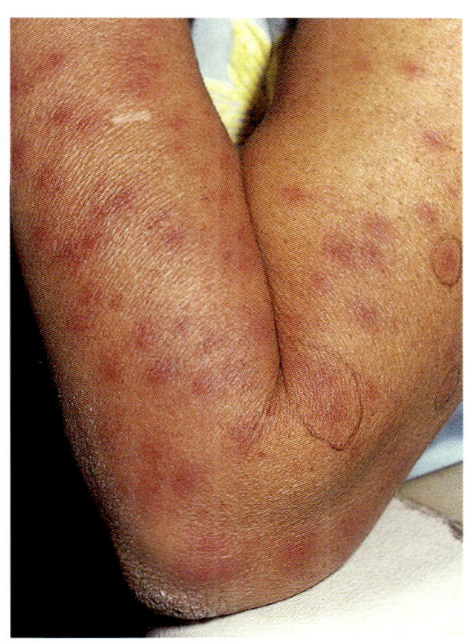

Figure 43–46. Neutrophilic eccrine hidradenitis. Scattered erythematous macules and papules on the leg.

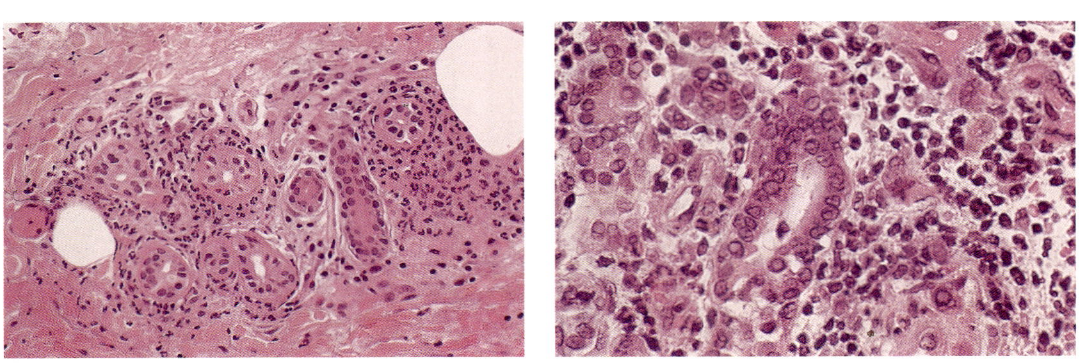

A

B

Figures 43–47A, 43–47B. Neutrophilic eccrine hidradenitis. Neutrophils within and around eccrine ducts and glands. There are mitotic figures and necrotic tubular epithelial cells.

VASCULOPATHY

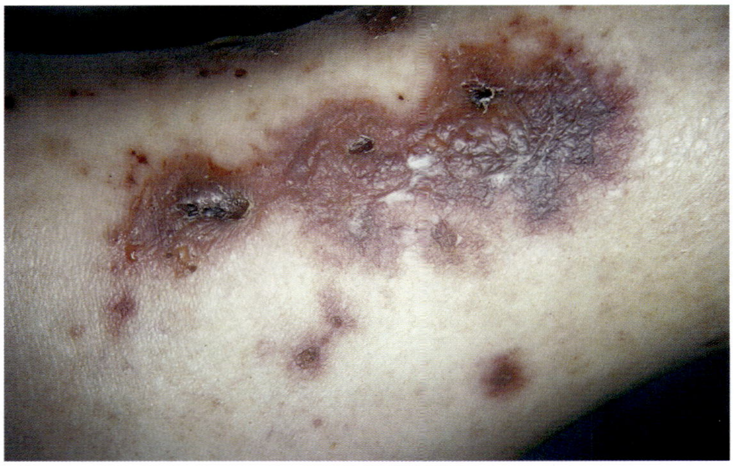

Figure 43–48. **Coumadin necrosis.** Reddish-gray vesicular and crusted lesions on the leg.

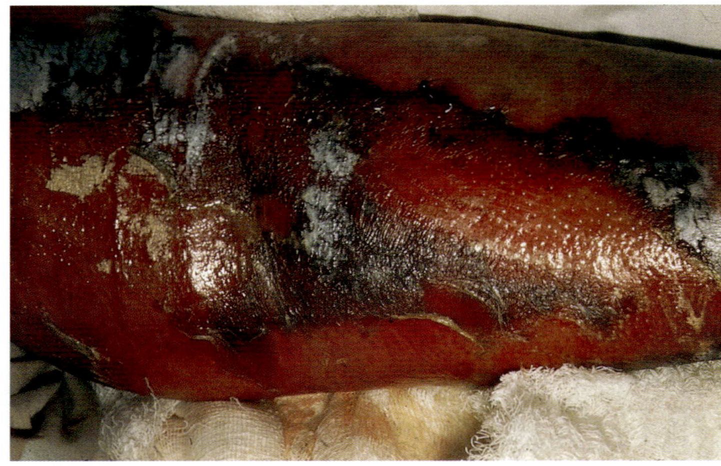

Figure 43–49. **Coumadin necrosis.** Crusted gray bullae on an erythematous and edematous leg.

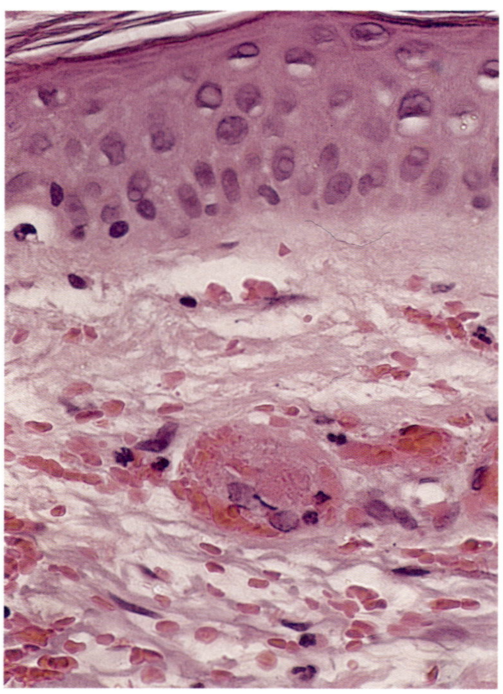

A

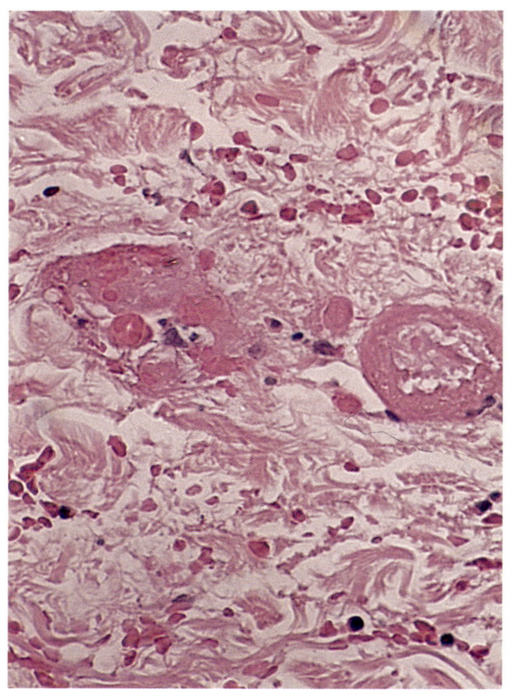

B

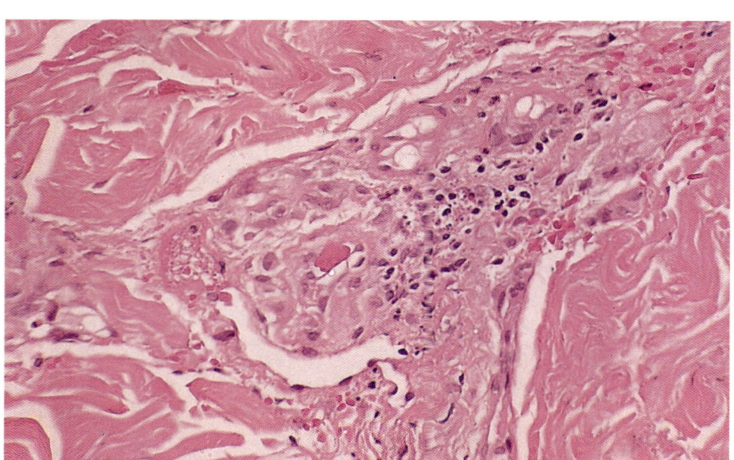

C

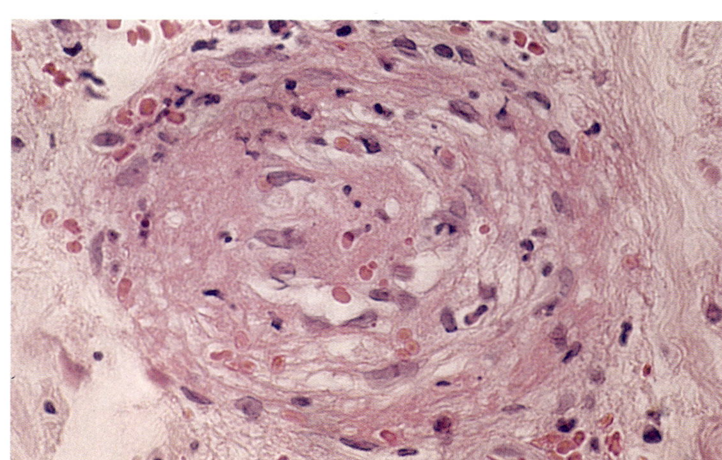

D

Figures 43–50A, 43–50B, 43–50C, 43–50D. **Coumadin necrosis.** Fibrin thrombi within dermal blood vessels with little inflammatory cell infiltrate. On occasion, there are mild changes of a leukocytoclastic vasculitis, but these changes are more commonly seen with heparin necrosis.

VASCULOPATHY

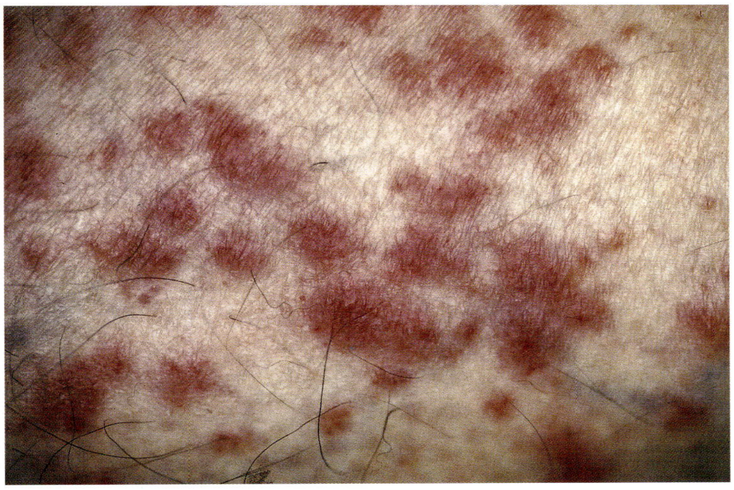

Figure 43–51. Leukocytoclastic vasculitis. Erythematous macules and papules with central hemorrhage.

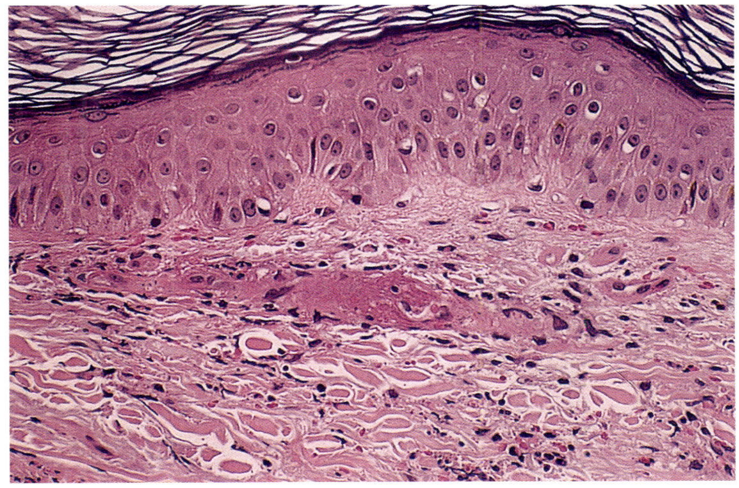

Figure 43–52. Leukocytoclastic vasculitis. Fibrin within blood-vessel wall and lumen. There are neutrophils, nuclear dust, extravasated erythrocytes, and dermal edema, which are the characteristic changes.

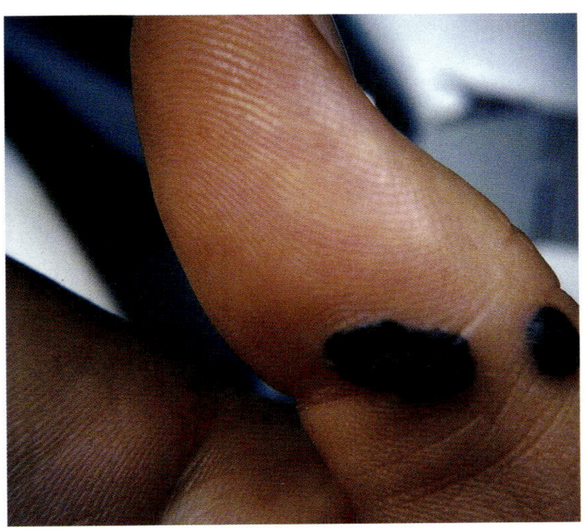

Figure 43–53. Tissue plasminogen activator (tPA). Painful hemorrhagic blisters on the thumb of a man 24 hours after intravenous tPA treatment for an acute myocardial infarction. The lesions occurred in areas of prior trauma.

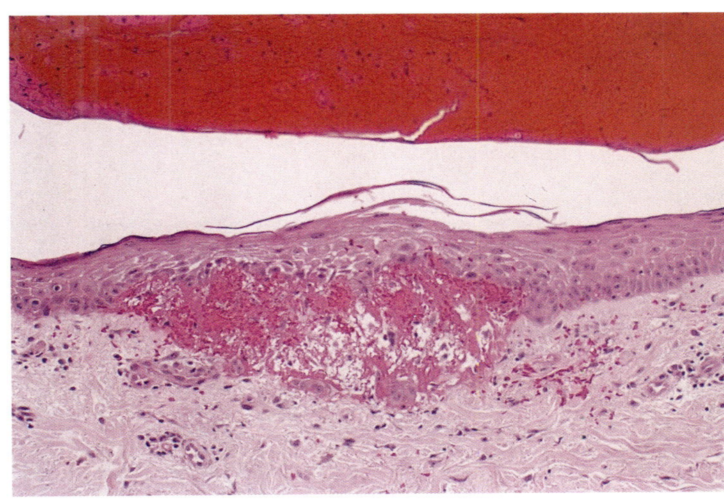

Figure 43–54. Tissue plasminogen activator (tPA). Hemorrhagic crust. There is fibrin and hemorrhage in the epidermis and papillary dermis, and a mild dermal perivascular mixed-cell infiltrate.

PIGMENTARY ALTERATION

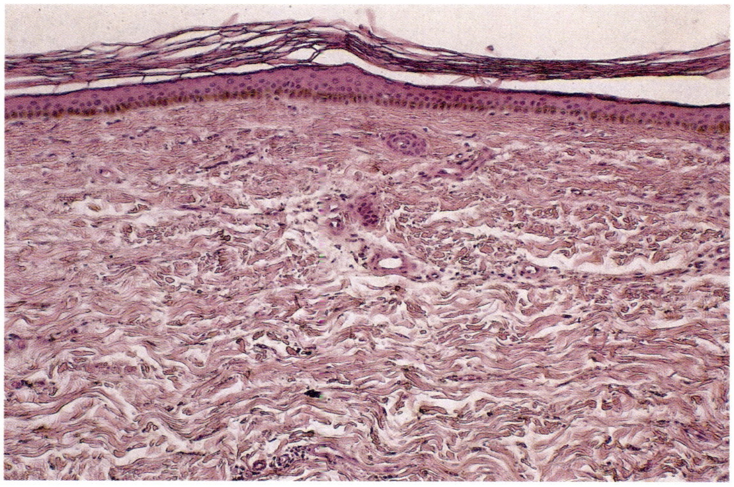

A

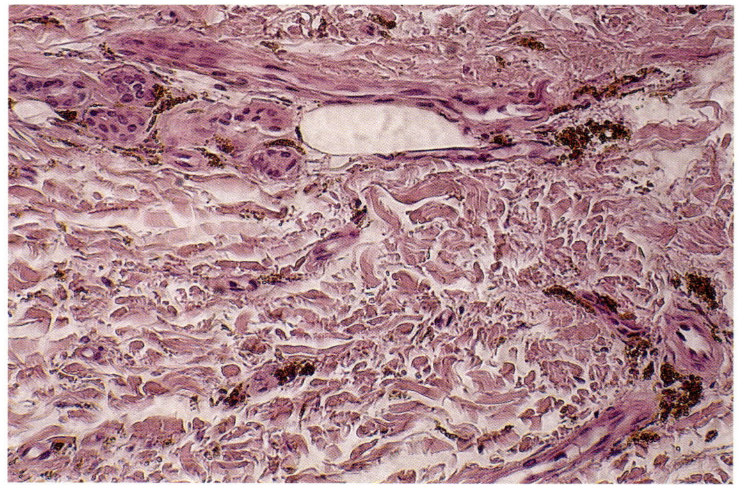

B

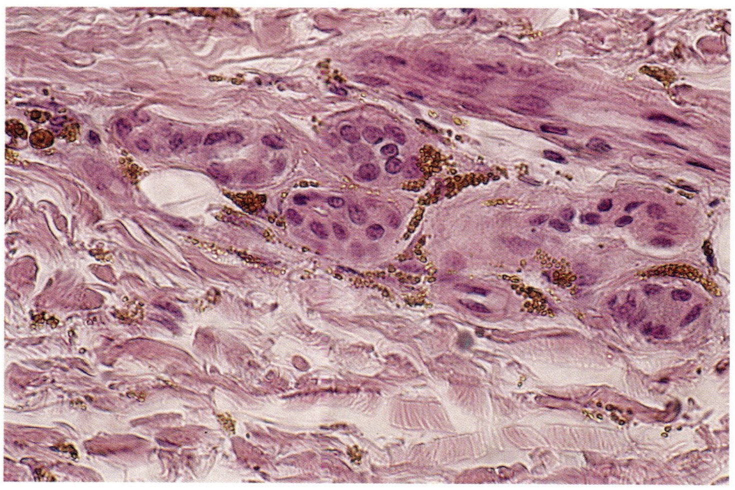

C

Figures 43–55A, 43–55B, 43–55C. Clofazimine hyperpigmentation. Golden-brown granular deposits among collagen bundles and adnexal structures.

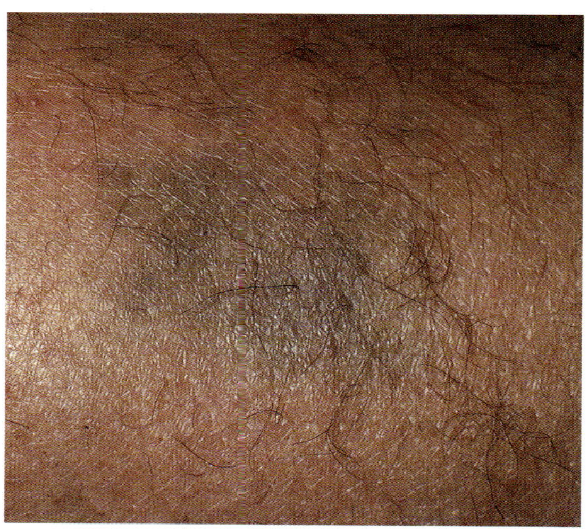

Figure 43–56. Minocycline hyperpigmentation. Irregular gray-pigmented patch.

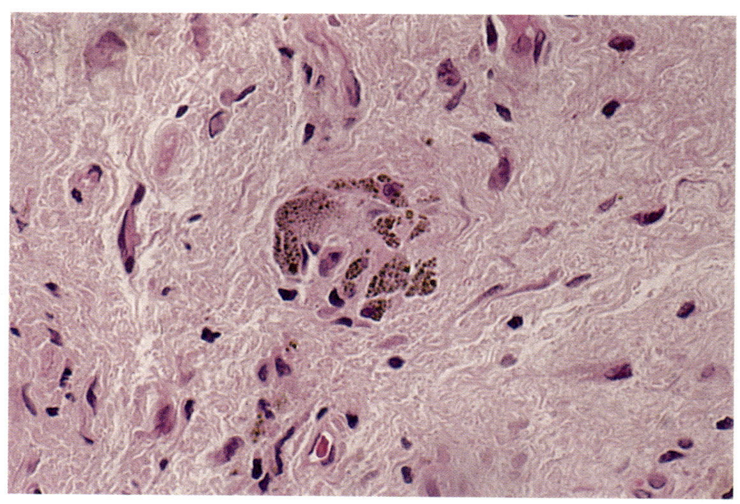

Figure 43–57. Minocycline hyperpigmentation. Brownish-black irregular granules lying free and within histiocytic cells in the dermis. Silver and iron methods stain the granules positively.

PIGMENTARY ALTERATION

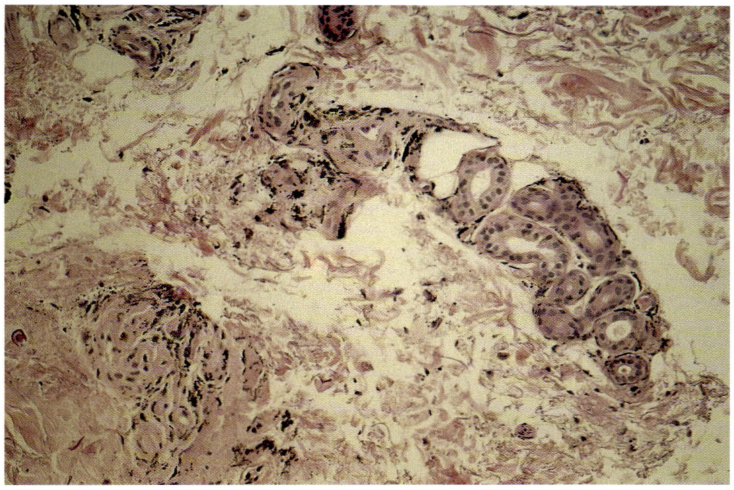

A

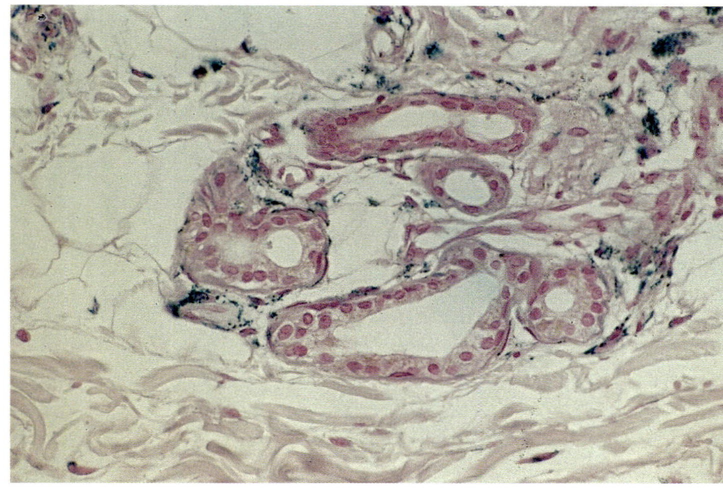

B

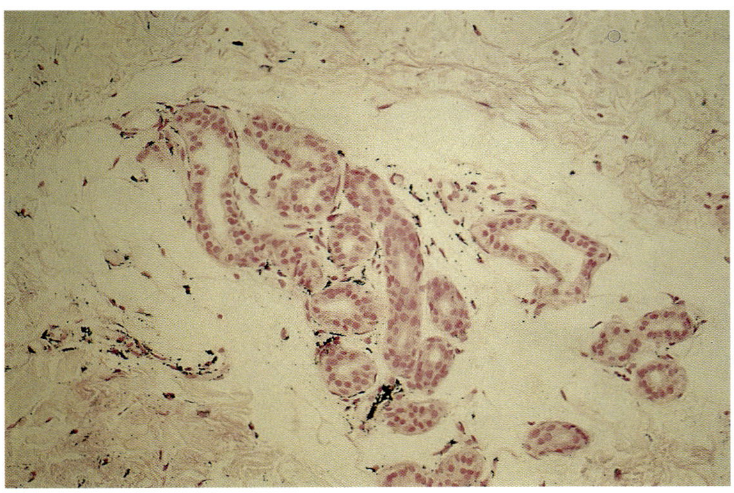

C

Figures 43–58A, 43–58B, 43–58C. Chloroquine hyperpigmentation. Black granules around adnexal structures. The granules stain blue with iron stains and black with melanin stains.

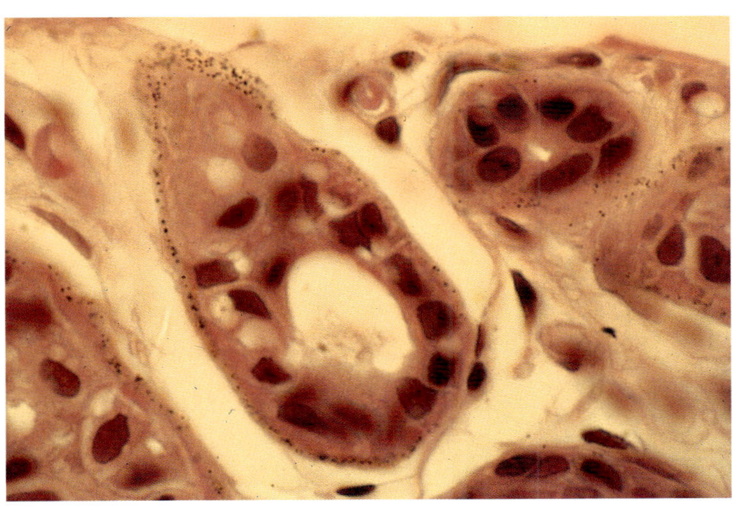

Figure 43–59. Argyria. Black silver particles within the wall of adnexal tubular structures.

INDEX

A

B

C

D

E

F

L

M

Q

R

S

T

U

V

W

X

Z